GYNECOLOGY

*A Study by Age Groups of the Developmental,
Functional and Pathological Aspects of the
Female Reproductive System and Its Disorders*

(From Fluhmann: The Cervix Uteri and Its Diseases. Color photographs courtesy of Wilson Footer, M.D. and L. A. Emge, M.D.)

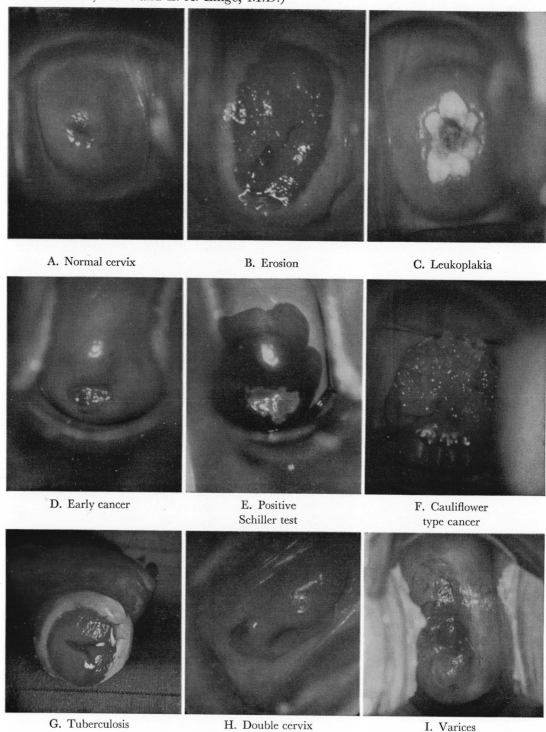

A. Normal cervix   B. Erosion   C. Leukoplakia

D. Early cancer   E. Positive Schiller test   F. Cauliflower type cancer

G. Tuberculosis   H. Double cervix   I. Varices

FACING PAGE: Large tissue section of cancer of the cervix.

GYNECOLOGY

By LANGDON PARSONS, M.D.

Professor of Obstetrics and Gynecology, Boston University School of Medicine
Chief of Gynecology, Massachusetts Memorial Hospitals

And SHELDON C. SOMMERS, M.D.

Pathologist, Scripps Memorial Hospital,
La Jolla, California
Clinical Professor of Pathology,
University of Southern California
School of Medicine

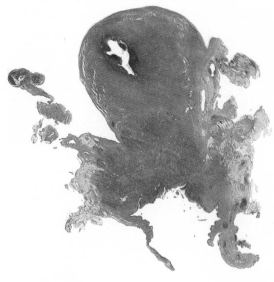

W. B. SAUNDERS COMPANY

Philadelphia and London

TO OUR WIVES

Foreword

Every once in a while a new idea in writing a book on an old subject is born. This book, written by a clinician and by a pathologist, is definitely unique. In the first place, many gynecologic textbooks have been written by clinicians well versed in gynecologic pathology, but to my knowledge this is the first written in collaboration with an excellent general pathologist. In the Boston hospitals a strictly gynecologic pathologist is a great rarity, and yet the amount of material coming to our laboratories is large and diversified. The great scientific gynecologic reports of such pathologists as Hertig, Warren, Castleman, Hicks and Scully, to name a few, demonstrate the expertness of our group. There can be no doubt of the excellence and ability of Dr. Sommers.

Dr. Parsons has contributed really a new organization of the field of gynecology. The division of the subject into age groups is new and should be of the greatest value to the student of gynecology. Rarely has such a comprehensive text been presented, ranging from infant problems to those of old age. Dr. Parsons has wisely refrained from technical descriptions of gynecologic operations, since surgical procedures and techniques represent a separate area of teaching. One look at the outline of this text will startle the average gynecologist because of the diversity of topics. Dr. Parsons himself is one of the few physicians I know who could write this book, for he has had a great deal of experience in surgical as well as gynecologic problems, and because of this training has the advantage of a very broad exposure to medicine, surgery and gynecology. Incidentally, and this is meant only to further my idea of his capacity, he is a great student, was a most satisfactory assistant to those of us whom he helped in his early days, and is one of the most able writers on medical subjects that I have been privileged to know.

As a gynecologist and as one interested in the problems he and Dr. Sommers have elucidated, I can recommend this book highly and can advise any one who is a doctor of medicine to read and to use it, for it is one of the great books of recent years.

Joe V. Meigs, M.D.

Foreword

DURING THE PAST 150 years there have been numerous books, monographs and reference works written upon the various aspects of gynecology. Such writings have tended to cover the general, the medical, the pediatric, the endocrinologic, the dermatologic, the anatomic, the pathologic or the operative aspects of this multifaceted special branch of medicine. Therefore these books have been written primarily for the medical student, the general practitioner, the pathologist or the gynecologic specialist, but usually not for all these groups. Such treatises might be described as having been horizontally integrated, focusing their attention on one of the many special aspects of gynecology. Age groups are mentioned in such writing only as an incidental aspect of the particular problem under discussion.

The present text is by Drs. Langdon Parsons and Sheldon C. Sommers, the former a gynecologic clinician, the latter a general pathologist interested in reproductive pathology. These two authors became associated, quite by chance, in their respective capacities as gynecologist and pathologist at the Massachusetts Memorial Hospitals, the teaching center of Boston University's School of Medicine. Both men are outstandingly competent in their own fields and have collaborated synergistically and even symbiotically in a figurative manner. They have written a unique book on gynecologic problems as oriented and integrated vertically by biologically significant age groups. They have perhaps subconsciously been swayed by Sir William Osler's concept that it is more important to know what kind of person had a disease than to know what specific disease a person had. Trousseau said it somewhat differently when he indicated that there are no diseases, only sick persons.

Parsons and Sommers unwittingly, or perhaps deliberately, borrowed Shakespeare's concept of the seven ages of man in describing beautifully and completely the gynecologic problems encountered during the seven ages of woman. The neat division of the book into seven parts allows each subdivision to correspond precisely or generally with the seven decades in the life of the female. That this grouping is not only temporally accurate but also biologically sound is due to the natural predominance of specific problems during well defined periods of growth, development, maturation, maturity, senescence and senility.

The practicing gynecologic clinician will ultimately learn to correlate, almost reflexly, the main problems with the age group in which such problems occur. This text will enable him to arrive at this state of clinical maturity earlier and more easily. Since the integrated approach is necessary to the teaching as well as the learning process, this book will make it easier and more pleasant for the medical student as well as the general practitioner to see the whole field of gynecology from birth to old age. Such readers will learn more quickly, understand more clearly and remember longer the essential problems in this broad and important field of medicine.

Both authors are experienced writers who produce lucid and flowing prose that is pleasant to read. The problems are so well presented from a comprehensive patho-physiologic point of view that it is difficult for this reviewer, who has known both authors as friends and colleagues for years, to determine just what part was written by whom.

This book is a monument to an extensive experience and reading in the broad fields of gynecology and its pathology. As such it is a superb synthesis of the many facets which pathology presents to the student, the practitioner and the gynecologic specialist.

ARTHUR T. HERTIG, M.D.
Shattuck Professor of Pathological Anatomy and
Chairman of the Department of Pathology
Harvard Medical School

Winchester, Mass.

Preface

WHEN THE ORIGINAL suggestion was made that a clinician and a pathologist should collaborate to report their combined experience in gynecology, we were reluctant to undertake the task because there seemed to be too many good textbooks already available.

The chief point of difference between this book and others, we believe, is that we have tried to relate gynecologic symptoms, which are actually few, to various disease processes and derangements in function as they manifest themselves in different age groups. To explain the symptoms and physical findings there is a wide spectrum of possibilities, both local and systemic. No longer can the gynecologist focus on the pelvis alone. We realize more and more that the generative organs, their anatomic and functional derangements, can be dealt with intelligently only if we consider women as a whole.

An attempt has been made to discuss each particular problem in the age group in which it is frequently found and in which there is the greatest chance of confusion in both diagnosis and treatment. Since we elected to discuss gynecologic problems in all age groups, it was essential that we include sections on gynecology in the infant as well as in the geriatric patient. Until recently gynecologists have been interested in women chiefly after they reached the years of reproductivity and have tended to lose interest afterward. Many problems that may appear in the reproductive years and later actually have their beginnings during infancy and childhood.

We have not included any formal section on anatomy or embryology, nor have we attempted to outline the details of operative procedures. Medicine has become a multidisciplined art and science, and we have felt that the student and the practitioner of today already have had the basic exposure to female anatomy. Their primary concern should be the recognition and proper interpretation of departures from the normal. We have chosen, instead of a synopsis or outline form, to try to paint word pictures of gynecologic problems, in the hope that though they may take longer to read, some point of the discussion will be retained.

No combination of authors has equal facility in all fields. The observations in this book represent a compilation of our own ideas and those of others. Gratitude is therefore owed to all who have contributed by articles in books and periodicals, and by word of mouth, to a discussion of the expanding scope of gynecologic problems. We wish to pay particular tribute to Dr. J. V. Meigs and Dr. Arthur T. Hertig, who have tutored and sponsored us through the years. We have attempted some recognition of the vast gynecologic literature by including references in the bibliography, which has been subdivided into the various aspects of the subjects discussed.

It is impossible to write a textbook without acquiring a deep sense of humility, which undoubtedly was not present at the outset, or one would never have contemplated such a project. With it goes a profound feeling of gratitude to all concerned with the various phases of its production. Our associates have been most kind, considerate and cooperative in complying with our whims. To them we will be eternally thankful and solemnly promise never to do this sort of thing again. This promise is made particularly to our wives. The loss of contact with the world and friends may be small sacrifice for the authors, but offers a considerable problem for the wives.

Specifically we wish to thank our devoted secretaries. Miss Signe Windhol labored to interpret the original handwritten manuscript without losing either her disposition or her sanity. Mrs. Maureen Drummy, Miss Elizabeth Foley, Mrs. Ann Preece, Mrs. Marcia Saitow and Miss Judith Merrill provided invaluable service. Mrs. Marian Adam and Mrs. Merry Ann Lewis assisted with references and proof.

Mr. Jerome Hartzberg prepared the new photographs, and Mr. Lawrence Turner assisted in photography. Mr. Bill Osburn made a number of original drawings and diagrams and supervised the art work. We wish to thank them. Several friendly physicians provided illustrations which are acknowledged in the legends. We are particularly indebted to Dr. F. Ronchese for many fine photographs of dermatologic lesions.

We are indebted to Dr. Sydney S. Gellis, Dr. Thomas H. Green, Jr., and Dr. Francis M. Ingersoll for helpful criticism and suggestions on the sections devoted respectively to pediatric gynecology, problems of the 40- to 50-year age group and the chapters on fertility.

Finally, the courtesy and patience of the publishers, particularly Mr. John Dusseau and Mr. Robert Rowan, were almost beyond belief.

LANGDON PARSONS

SHELDON C. SOMMERS

Contents

Part III.   GYNECOLOGIC PROBLEMS OF THE YOUNG WOMAN (AGE 20 TO 30)

Part VI. GYNECOLOGIC PROBLEMS IN THE POSTMENOPAUSAL ERA (AGE 50 TO 65)

Part VII. GYNECOLOGIC PROBLEMS IN OLD AGE

PART I

Gynecologic Problems
of Infancy and Childhood

Chapter 1

General Survey

ONLY in recent years has the gynecologist become interested in the infant and the growing child. This has been particularly true of the adolescent age group, since the pediatrician has felt that the female child has passed beyond his province, but the internist and the gynecologist have been slow to assume the burden of her care. Gradually we have become aware of the fact that many of the problems seen in adult life stem from physiologic or organic abnormalities which began at or about or even preceding puberty. Actually, the physicians most likely to come in contact with the problems of the young child from birth on are the family doctor and the pediatrician. Only rarely has the gynecologist been called into the picture for consultation. Then all too frequently he is discomfited by his unfamiliarity with the problems of the infant or young child. In order that the physician may successfully cope with the irregularities he must (*a*) be familiar with the normal to recognize the deviation from it; (*b*) be aware of the anatomic differences between child and adult anatomy as well as the growth pattern and stages of functional development of both bony and organic structures; (*c*) be cognizant of the techniques which are basic in a proper examination; (*d*) be alert to the psychologic impact of a complete physical examination on the infant as well as the parent; (*e*) be informed concerning the various laboratory studies which may be helpful in making a diagnosis in the problems of childhood.

The problems are many and change with advancing years, since it is within this age span from birth to puberty that the greatest development occurs both in terms of bony growth and glandular maturation. By the time the menarche appears the young girl has developed all her standard equipment to carry her through life. From then on it is largely a question of how well it functions and how well she uses it. It is a challenge for the medical profession to see that the child receives the best of medical care during this period of development. Since the problems vary with the individual child and are constantly changing as she matures, great skill and judgment will be required from the physician in charge.

What Are the Major Problems in Infancy and Childhood?

The basic problems are not unlike those that occur in adult life with one exception: namely, congenital malformations. In too many instances the basic defects go unrecognized until the patient is about to be married or has been married, but is unable to have a child. The problem is particularly acute when the sex of the infant is in question. The recognition of basic defects should be made in early infancy. One

3

can then select the proper age in which to carry out corrective measures. The adjustments then follow a calculated plan rather than becoming an improvisation based on a pre-existing but an unrecognized state.

In addition to the various forms of congenital malformations in structure and in the normal growth pattern that may appear in infancy and childhood, the remaining problems are those of infection, abnormal bleeding from the genital tract and tumor formation.

DEVIATION FROM THE NORMAL.   If the physician is to decide whether the female child deviates from the normal in skeletal or glandular development, he must have a working knowledge of what is expected in order to determine the significance of the departure. In most instances the family, and frequently the physician, attribute any variation from the normal to endocrine failure, particularly if there is no obvious explanation at hand. This is especially true if the external genitalia do not develop along anticipated lines. The effect may be due to hormonal cause of permanent or temporary origin, but it is also possible that genetic, nutritional or constitutional factors are at work which modify the action of the hormones. The explanation lies in the presence of congenital anomalies and has nothing to do with the endocrine system at all.

It is not always an easy matter to place the responsibility for the deviation in its proper category, for in some instances overlapping may occur. Thus a child whose proper sex is in question may have an unusual sex chromatin pattern and a congenital abnormality in the gonad as well. Furthermore, when there are abnormalities in sex differentiation, it is important to know whether these have come about because of gonadal defect or simply reflect the virilizing influence of the adrenal hormones

What Is the Normal Progression in Skeletal Development?

One of the chief factors which disturb the parent and bring the child to the physician is the apparent failure to follow what the parents feel are normal patterns of growth. To them either the child is too short or too tall for her age, or she is too fat or too thin.

Since no two children are alike and development may occur in spurts rather than slow progression in any given child, it is somewhat difficult to deter mine just what is the average for a child in each of the years from birth to puberty. Forexample, the bone age may not correspond with the chronologic age at one particular phase of development, but with a sudden acceleration in the growth rate the proportions may later become entirely normal. It is important, then, to measure and record growth and development not only at the time, but also at periodic intervals thereafter.

The chief indicators of skeletal growth and development in addition to height and size are (1) the relative proportion of skeletal growth in both upper and lower segments of the body. The various sections of the body develop with different time schedules. For example, the upper portion of the body as measured from the top of the symphysis to the top of the head is approximately twice as long as the measurement from the symphysis to the soles of the feet. From birth on the lower extremities grow much faster under normal conditions than the trunk, so that they become equal in length shortly before puberty. The ratio between the two is of basic importance, since the balance is either undisturbed or shifts in one direction or the other, depending on factors which disturb the normal process of growth (Fig. 1–1). For example, the pituitary dwarf is stunted in growth, but the ratio between the upper and lower

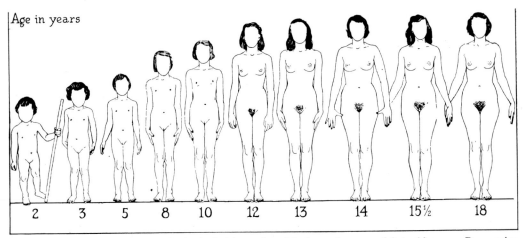

Fig. 1-1. The changes in body habitus of a girl, from the age of 2 to 18 years. Progressive elongation of the extremities is notable. (From photographs in Berkeley Growth Study. Institute of Human Development, University of California.)

portions of the body is in proper proportion. On the other hand, the hypothyroid dwarf, in whom the entire growth process is retarded, continues to have a long trunk and short extremities despite advancing years.

Another important measurement is the span, which is the distance between the finger tips when both arms are fully extended.

It is important to know the standing height in relation to age, but the information will be more meaningful if the physician will compare it with x-ray evidence of ossification in the bony epiphyses as well as the relative proportions in growth between the upper and lower segments of the body. The variation from the mean or average can be plotted on charts (Engelbach) that record such measurements as span, skeletal proportions, and circumference of the head, chest and abdomen in relation to age, height and sex. In this manner it is possible to observe the growth and development of the individual child.

2. The second indicator of skeletal growth is the changing appearance of the bony structure of the head and face. Any physician or mother is aware of the changes that occur in the face of a young infant as she matures. The broad-based, short nose and rounded contour are characteristic of the baby face. Under normal conditions as the infant grows older the jaw elongates as the nose lengthens in relation to its width at the point where it merges with the skull. In some instances, again using the hypothyroid infant as an example, this type of transfiguration does not occur, and the contour retains the broad flat nasal bridge and rounded face.

3. Another important indicator of progress in skeletal growth comprises the changes that appear in the various ossification centers of the bones. The appearance time and union of epiphysial centers in bones of the skeleton follow a definite pattern from birth to puberty under normal conditions. The time schedule is bound to vary to a minor extent, depending on the individual, but the pattern is standard enough so that tables have been devised by which osseous development may be followed through x-ray interpretation (Tables 1, 2).

A variety of pathologic entities, disease processes and disorders of function will influence not only epiphysial development, but the structure of the bone as well

Table 1.   Comparison of Chronologic and Bone Ages

AGE	MEASURE OF OSSEOUS DEVELOPMENT
Birth	Distal epiphysis of femur, astragalus, cuboid, calcaneus
1st year	Wrist—capitate, hamate, distal epiphysis of radius
	Ankle—addition of cuneiform III, distal epiphysis of tibia
2nd year	Capitellum of humerus
	Wrist—no change
	Ankle—addition of epiphysis of fibula
3rd year	Wrist—addition of triangularis
	Ankle—addition of cuneiform I
4th year	Wrist—addition of lunate
	Ankle—addition of cuneiform II, navicular
	Hip—epiphysis of greater trochanter
5th year	Wrist—addition of major multangulum, navicular
	Knee—patella
6th year	Wrist—addition of minor multangulum, epiphysis of ulna
	Shoulder—union of head and tuberosity of humerus
8th year	Ankle—epiphysis of calcaneus
	Union of ischium and pubis
10th year	Wrist—pisiform
12th year	External condyle of humerus
	Union of trochlear and capitellum of humerus
14th year	Union of proximal epiphysis of radius
	Union of olecranon and ulna
16th year	Union of epiphyses of metacarpals and metatarsals
	Appearance of crest of ilium
18th year	Union of distal epiphyses of radius and ulna
	Union of distal epiphyses of tibia and fibula

From Watson and Lowrey.

Table 2.   Average Age of Union of the More Important Epiphyses

AGE	UNION OF EPIPHYSES
6th year	Head and greater tuberosity of humerus
7th year	Ischium and pubis
12th year	Trochlear and capitellum of humerus
13th–14th year	Olecranon and ulna
	Epiphysis of calcaneus
14th–16th year	Proximal epiphysis of radius
	Trochanter and head of femur

Bone length increases 0.25 cm. per month during the first year, and then drops to 0.12 cm. per month in the latter part of the second year.

From Watson and Lowrey.

The stunted structure of the hypothyroid infant is traceable to the impairment of epiphysial growth which is common to this disorder.

4. Another index of skeletal growth is the alteration in the time schedule of the appearance of teeth. Under normal conditions the eruptions and final disappearance of baby teeth follow a fairly standard pattern (Table 3). The same thing may be said of the appearance of tooth buds as seen by x-ray film. This sequence of events

Table 3.   Chronology of Human Dentition

TOOTH	ERUPTION[*]	EXFOLIATION OR SHEDDING[†]
Primary		
Maxilla:		
Central	8–10 months	6–7 years
Lateral	8–10 months	7–8 years
Cuspid	16–20 months	10–12 years
1st molar	12–16 months	9–11 years
2nd molar	20–30 months	10–12 years
Mandible:		
Central	6–8 months	6–7 years
Lateral	10–14 months	7–8 years
Cuspid	16–20 months	9–12 years
1st molar	12–16 months	9–11 years
2nd molar	20–30 months	10–12 years
Permanent		
Maxilla:		
Central	7–8 years	
Lateral	8–9 years	
Cuspid	11–12 years	
1st bicuspid	10–11 years	
2nd bicuspid	10–12 years	
1st molar	6–7 years	
2nd molar	12–14 years	
3rd molar	17–30 years	
Mandible:		
Central	6–7 years	
Lateral	7–8 years	
Cuspid	10–11 years	
1st bicuspid	10–12 years	
2nd bicuspid	11–12 years	
1st molar	6–7 years	
2nd molar	12–13 years	
3rd molar	17–30 years	

* From Holt and McIntosh.
† From Watson and Lowrey.

and the abnormalities seen in the tooth buds may be interrupted by a number of factors that retard growth. Again, hypothyroidism in the young child is such a factor.

5. To the indicators of bony growth mentioned above must be added observations on mental development. For example, hypofunction of the thyroid in infancy and childhood is reflected in the maturation of the central nervous system as well as the bony skeleton. If the problem is congenital, it must be corrected within the first few months following birth if the brain is to develop and function. This is less true when hypothyroidism develops later in childhood, but it is still obvious that the brain is less sensitive and responsive.

6. As the child approaches maturity the physician must be aware of the impact of the hormones and the development of both the sexual organs and the secondary sex characteristics.

What Effects Do the Hormones Have on Skeletal Growth and Development?

In early infancy and childhood we are largely concerned with the problem of somatic growth. In the normal process of growth three hormones are implicated: (*a*) the thyroid, (*b*) the growth hormone of the pituitary, and (*c*) androgen, produced by the adrenal cortex.

There are many factors other than hormones which are responsible for alterations in growth and development. It is unwise, therefore, to assume simply because the child has a growth defect that a faulty production or utilization of the hormones elaborated by the pituitary, adrenal or thyroid is the cause. It is well known, through observations on the growing child as well as by animal experiments, that normal growth and development are dependent on an adequate supply of minerals, vitamins and amino acids. Nutritional deficiencies or debilitating disease which deprive the child of these elements either before or after birth will result in retardation of growth. For example, congenital anomalies noted in the child at birth are occasionally traceable to rubella acquired by the mother in the early weeks of pregnancy.

WHAT EFFECT DOES THE THYROID HAVE ON GROWTH? Proper function of the thyroid appears to be a prime necessity for orderly growth and development, not only of bone, but other organs as well. In earlier discussions we have noted that the thyroid hormone was instrumental in promoting skeletal growth, in molding the facial bones, in stimulating the development of osseous centers in bone, in furthering the process of dental evolution and finally in developing the central nervous system and brain. Any time during childhood when the output of thyroid hormone is diminished or withdrawn the growth process comes to a standstill. Both the thyroid and growth hormone of the pituitary are particularly important in the few years following birth, when the greatest degree of development takes place. Of the two, the thyroid seems to be the more important. Support for this statement is found in the observation that the pituitary dwarf is usually of normal size at birth and continues to grow at a reasonably normal rate for three or four years. It would seem, then, that the growth factor immediately after birth is due either to the action of the thyroid hormone or to a property of growth inherent in the tissues themselves.

WHAT ABOUT THE PITUITARY GROWTH HORMONE? In the early stages of development the pituitary seems to be involved in stimulating skeletal growth rather than in secreting the sex hormones. The exact action of the growth hormone and the life span during which it operates are actually unknown. It is possible that its production and release are regulated by the thyrotropic or adrenotropic hormones, or vice versa. For example, the delay in epiphysial ossification which occurs in pituitary dwarfs may actually be the result of thyroid lack, since the pituitary is not capable of putting out adequate amounts of the thyrotropic hormone. This is not true of all pituitary dwarfs, however, for many never show the clinical signs of thyrotropic or adrenotropic failure, at least in the early stages of development. Later on, when the gonadotropic factor should make its appearance, the lack of genital development may point to the basic pituitary deficiency.

The function of growth hormone is linked to the sex hormones, for it is due to the action of estrin that the epiphyses finally fuse with the long bones and linear growth ceases. This may be the result of direct action of estrin on the epiphysial plate itself, but it is also probable that estrin might suppress the output of growth hormone through its effect upon the pituitary gland.

WHAT ROLE DOES THE ADRENAL PLAY IN SKELETAL GROWTH? The role of the adrenal gland in normal development is not apparent until approximately the time of puberty. During this period a sudden increase in the growth measurement is apparent. Since estrin apparently does not increase the rate of growth when given to girls who are slow in maturing, it is probable that the sudden increase in growth at the time of puberty is due to androgen produced by the adrenal.

When Do Hormones Have the Most Effect on Skeletal Development?

There are two periods in infancy and childhood when the growth factors are abundantly evident. After birth and for the next two or three years a great increase in skeletal development takes place. This gives way to a slower, more orderly development until the gonadotropic hormones begin to exert their effects. At or about the time of puberty another spurt in the growth pattern appears (Fig. 1–2).

Do the Fetal Gonads Have Any Part in Development?

In the normal process of early embryologic development the gonad contains both female and male structures. The final differentiation into ovary or testicle, if inhibiting factors do not appear, will be determined by the sex chromatin pattern of the individual. For the embryo to continue in the male pattern there must appear some component within the medullary portion of the embryonic gonad which is capable of secreting what Wilkins calls the "male organizing substance." It must be present before the male differentiation into ducts and gonads can take place.

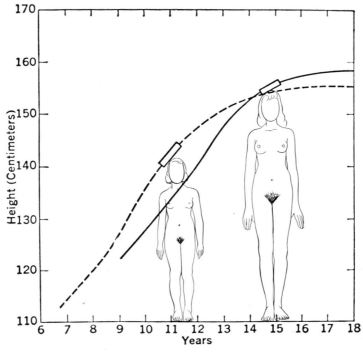

Fig. 1-2. The relation between height in centimeters, age in years, and the onset of the menarche, indicated by the rectangles. The taller girl had a later menarche. (Modified from L. E. Holt, Jr., and R. McIntosh: *Diseases of Infancy and Childhood*. 11th Ed. New York, D. Appleton-Century Company, Inc.)

For the gonad to become a testis the müllerian duct elements must disappear nearly completely and the wolffian components develop to form the vas deferens and the seminal vesicles. Just what the male organizing substance is, is not known. Apparently it is different from testosterone and the sex steroids, for testosterone injected experimentally into the female fetus will produce proliferation of the wolffian duct system, but no suppression of the female müllerian duct structures occurs. The differentiation takes place early in the development of the embryo, probably before the eighth week.

Until recently there was general belief that there was a profound tendency upon the part of the individual to develop as a female unless the male hormones were present. For example, if no gonad is present, as in the syndrome of gonadal aplasia, or if the gonads are removed in the young embryo of experimental animals, the development always takes place along female lines. It would, therefore, seem to be true that the differentiation of the duct systems is dependent upon the male and female hormones secreted by the embryo's own gonad.

These observations may not be entirely correct, however, in view of the recent discovery that in patients who have female external genitalia, but gonadal agenesis, there is a departure from the normal in the chromosomal pattern. Studies of buccal smears in patients with Turner's syndrome (ovarian agenesis) now reveal that these subjects are often chromatin-negative, or, in other words, they lack the nuclear sex pattern of the female. Furthermore, such patients have less than the normal number of forty-six chromosomes. In ovarian agenesis the chromosomal number is now believed to be forty-five. Apparently the male component is absent, and only one half that of the female is present. Such a patient would then be regarded as having the sex chromosomal constitution of XO.

It would therefore seem probable that, although the fetal gonad and its secretion play a role in the normal development of the female, genetic factors are operating in addition.

What Evidence Do We Have of Hormonal Function at Birth?

At birth the infant must have a functioning glandular system to survive in the new, extrauterine environment. Some help may be forthcoming from the maternal hormones, but they cannot be expected to persist for long. That they do exert an effect upon the infant is well documented by the frequent observation of vaginal bleeding, vulvar enlargement, desquamation of the vaginal epithelium and swelling of the breasts complete with secretion from the nipple (witch's milk). There has obviously been endocrine stimulation from some source, probably the placenta or the maternal ovary, which are known to secrete estrin (Fig. 1–3).

The adrenal probably has little effect on sexual maturation early in infancy. The effect of the adrenal hormones will be evident later in childhood. It is true that the adrenal glands at birth are relatively larger than they are at any other time of life and that the quantity of the 17-ketosteroids in both urine and plasma approaches normal adult levels. Within the first two weeks after birth, however, the levels of the urinary 17-ketosteroids have dropped from 1.5 to 2.5 mg. a day to less than 0.5 mg. daily. The adrenal enlargement which had taken place, largely in the inner fetal cortical areas, gradually undergoes involution, which is complete within a span of a few weeks to months.

The thyroid gland often is well developed at the time of birth. Since hyperemia

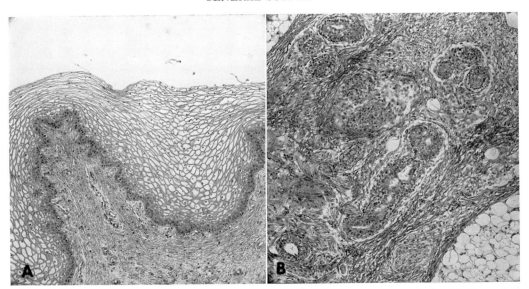

Fig. 1-3.   *A,* There is an adult type of estrogen effect in the uterine cervical epithelium of all newborn girls. *B,* Breast ducts, ductules and intrinsic stroma of both sexes show evidence of endocrine stimulation at birth. From a stillborn girl. × 125. (All photomicrographs were made from slides stained with hematoxylin and eosin, unless otherwise noted.)

and adequate amounts of colloid are noted in the fetal thyroid, it is probable that it is actively functioning before birth occurs. One might expect this, since we noted previously that thyroid function is intimately concerned with the development of both the skeletal and the central nervous systems.

Disorders in Skeletal Growth

Deviations from the normal pattern of growth manifest themselves in a variety of ways throughout childhood. Some may be traced to the genes or abnormal environmental factors which occur in intrauterine life. Many of these cases are recognizable at birth; others are due to faulty endocrine influence. They may be obvious at birth or may not put in an appearance until the time the sex factors become active. The growth disorders can be generalized or restricted to a particular structure. The underlying cause may be traced to (*a*) some inhibiting influence which prevents the child from developing normally, the defect then taking the form of a developmental arrest, or (*b*) some factor which produces overdeve'opment of tissue in a given area. In this case there is no element of deficiency nor is the growth inhibited.

Since the various causative agents operate on different time schedules, it is difficult to assign particular entities to any one period in the child's life. It is, nevertheless, important to detect abnormalities as early as possible, for some of them are amenable to treatment if they are discovered early enough. This can often be done at birth. Normal growth and development then proceed in an uninterrupted fashion. Other growth defects should be recognized so that the family can be informed early in the child's life. The psychologic impact of this discovery is far less at this time than it will be later, if there is no mention of the fact that the child is not normal. It is also important to know the true sex of the child when developmental abnormalities are present to avoid all the problems that may arise if the child is inadvertently brought up in the wrong sex environment. Later in childhood when abnormal patterns of skeletal growth appear we should be able to differentiate between the different types in order to spot those that have an endocrine cause which may be amenable to treatment. Conversely, overenthusiastic attempts to stimulate growth can be curtailed in a child who will develop normally if left alone.

The developmental abnormalities which manifest themselves at birth take precedence in the discussion of pediatric problems. Some of them have genetic cause, but those that are hormonal are frequently amenable to treatment. Later in childhood we are primarily concerned with skeletal growth. In late childhood the sex hormones become active and precipitate a new train of events which may or may not follow a normal pattern.

Before we can discuss the problems of the neonatal period and those of early infancy we must have some idea of the normal anatomy of the child's genital tract and what to look for in the way of deviations.

REFERENCES

General and Skeletal Growth and Development

Bayley, N., and Pinneau, S. R.: Tables for Predicting Adult Height from Skeletal Age: Revised for Use with Greulich-Pyle Hand Standards. *J. Pediat.*, 40: 423, 1952.

Broadbent, B. H.: The Face of the Normal Child. *Angle Orthodontist*, 7: 183, 1937.

Idem: Bolton Standards and Technique in Orthodontic Practice. *Angle Orthodontist*, 7: 209, 1937.

Christie, A.: Prevalence and Distribution of Ossification Centers in the Newborn Infant. *Am. J. Dis. Child.*, 77: 355, 1949.

Crump, E. P., Horton, C. P., Masuoka, J., and Ryan, D.: Relation of Birth Weight in Negro Infants to Sex, Maternal Age, Parity, Prenatal Care, and Socioeconomic Status. *J. Pediat.*, 51: 678, 1957.

Engelbach's Tables of Normal Measurements; in L. Wilkins: *The Diagnosis and Treatment of Endocrine Disorders in Childhood and Adolescence.* 2nd Ed. Springfield, Ill., Charles C Thomas, 1957, pp. 34–7.

Francis, C. C.: Factors Influencing Appearance of Centers of Ossification during Early Childhood. *Am. J. Dis. Child.*, 57: 817, 1939.

Greulich, W. W.: Growth of Children of the Same Race under Different Environmental Conditions. *Science*, 127: 515, 1958.

Greulich, W. W., and Pyle, S. I.: *Radiographic Atlas of Skeletal Development of the Hand and Wrist.* Stanford, Stanford University Press, 1959.

Holt, L. E., Jr., and McIntosh, R.: *Holt Pediatrics.* 12th Ed. New York, Appleton-Century-Crofts, Inc., 1953, pp. 8–44.

House, R. W.: A Summary of Forty-Nine Radiologists' Opinions on Skeletal Age Limits of Apparently Normal Six Year Old Children. *Am. J. Roentgenol.*, 64: 442, 1950.

Krogman, W. M.: The Physical Growth of Children—An Appraisal of Studies 1950–1955. Child Development Publications. Lafayette, Ind., Purdue University, 1956.

Li, C. H., Evans, H. M., and Simpson, M. E.: Isolation and Properties of the Anterior Hypophyseal Growth Hormone. *J. Biol. Chem.*, 159: 353, 1945.

Logan, W. H. G., and Kronfeld, R.: Development of Human Jaws and Surrounding Structures from Birth to Age of Fifteen Years. *J. Am. Dent. A.*, 20: 379, 1933.

Mainland, D.: Evaluation of the Skeletal Age Method of Estimating Children's Development; Variable Errors in Assessment of Roentgenograms. *Pediatrics*, 13: 165, 1954.

Meredith, H. V., and Meredith, E. M.: The Body Size and Form of Present-Day White Elementary School Children Residing in West-Central Oregon. *Child Develop.*, 24: 83, 1953.

Scammon, R. E.: The Measurement of Man; in J. A. Harris, C. M. Jackson, D. C. Patterson and R. E. Scammon: Section on Measurement of Body in Childhood. Minneapolis, University of Minnesota Press, 1930.

Scott, R. B., Ferguson, A. D., Jenkins, M. E., and Cutter, F. F.: Growth and Development of Negro Infants: Neuromuscular Patterns of Behavior during First Year of Life. *Pediatrics*, 16: 24, 1955.

Smith, C. A.: *The Physiology of the Newborn Infant.* 3rd Ed. Springfield, Ill., Charles C Thomas, 1959.

Sontag, L. W., and Lipford, J.: Effect of Illness and Other Factors on Appearance Pattern of Skeletal Epiphyses. *J. Pediat.*, 23: 391, 1943.

Wagner, R.: Nonendocrine Deviations from Normal Pattern of Osseous Development. A.M.A. *Am. J. Dis. Child.*, 82: 519, 1951.

Watson, E. H., and Lowrey, G. H.: *Growth and Development of Children*. 3rd Ed. Chicago, Year Book Publishers, Inc., 1958.

Widdowson, E. M., and Spray, C. M.: Chemical Development in Utero. *Arch. Dis. Childhood*, 26: 205, 1951.

Hormonal Effects on Growth

Bartlett, P. D.: Growth Hormone and Nitrogen Retention; in R. W. Smith, Jr., O. H. Gaebler and C. N. H. Long, Eds.: *The Hypophyseal Growth Hormone, Nature and Actions*. New York, McGraw-Hill Book Company, Inc., 1955, p. 204.

Bergstrand, C. G., and Gemzell, C. A.: Plasma Levels of 17-Hydroxycorticosteroids and Urinary Excretion of 17-Ketosteroids in Normal Children. *Acta paediat.*, 44: 318, 1955.

Dye, J. A., and Maughan, G. H.: Thyroid Gland as Growth-Promoting and Form-Determining Factor in Development of Animal Body. *Am. J. Anat.*, 44: 331, 1929.

Gardner, L. I.: *Adrenal Function in Infants and Children, a Symposium*. New York, Grune & Stratton, Inc., 1956.

Idem: Adrenocortical Metabolism of the Fetus, Infant and Child. *Pediatrics*, 17: 897, 1956.

Jost, A.: The Secretory Activities of Fetal Endocrine Glands and Their Effect upon Target Organs; in C. A. Villee, Ed.: *Gestation*. New York, Josiah Macy, Jr. Foundation, 1957, p. 129.

Kinsell, L. W.: Human Studies with Purified Pituitary Growth Hormone Preparations; in R. W. Smith, O. H. Gaebler and C. N. H. Long: *The Hypophyseal Growth Hormone, Nature and Actions*. New York, McGraw-Hill Book Company, Inc., 1955, p. 507.

Moore, C. R.: The Role of Fetal Endocrine Glands in Development. *J. Clin. Endocrinol.*, 10: 942, 1950.

Ober, W. B., and Bernstein, J.: Observation on the Endometrium and Ovary in the Newborn. *Pediatrics*, 16: 445, 1955.

Patten, B. M.: *Human Embryology*. Philadelphia, Blakiston Company, 1946.

Read, C. H., Venning, E. H., and Ripstein, M. P.: Adrenal Cortical Function in Newly-Born Infants. *J. Clin. Endocrinol.*, 10: 845, 1950.

Van Wyk, J. J.: Hypothyroidism in Childhood. *Pediatrics*, 17: 427, 1956.

Wilkins, L.: Epiphysial Dysgenesis Associated with Hypothyroidism. *Am. J. Dis. Child.*, 61: 13, 1941.

Idem: Disturbances in Growth. *Bull. New York Acad. Med.*, 29: 280, 1953.

Idem: Hormonal Influences on Skeletal Growth. *Ann. New York Acad. Sc.*, 60: 763, 1955.

Chapter 2

Normal Anatomic

Development of the

External Genitalia in the Child

To DETECT deviations from the normal development of the external genitalia it is important that we recognize the normal anatomic architecture in infancy and early childhood. At birth and for a short period thereafter the genital tract is stimulated by the maternal hormones. It is not uncommon to find that (*a*) the child bleeds from the vagina; (*b*) the breasts are engorged; (*c*) the vaginal epithelium is estrogenized; (*d*) the uterus is relatively larger compared to body weight than it will be at any time until puberty; (*e*) the epithelium of the uterine cavity and cervix shows typical estrogenic effects (Figs. 1–3, 2–1). Within the first month the effects of the maternal

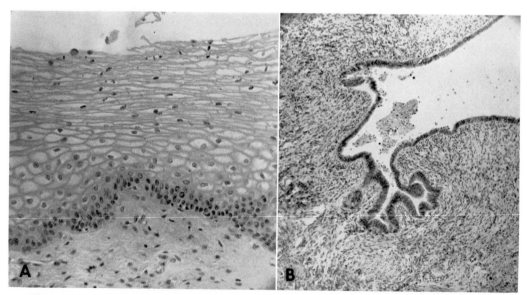

Fig. 2-1.   *A,* The glycogen-rich uterine cervix with watery-appearing epithelial cells indicates estrogenic stimulation in the newborn girl. × 400. *B,* Endometrial glands at birth are slightly hyperplastic, owing to intrauterine maternal estrogenic stimulation. × 125.

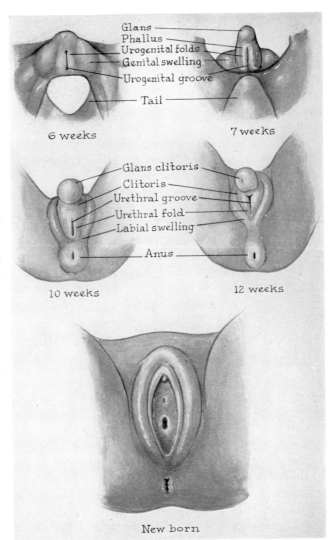

Fig. 2-2. Development of the female external genitalia, shown from the embryo of 6 weeks to birth. (Modified from M. H. Spaulding: *Carnegie Contrib. Embryol.*, 1921, 13, No. 61, 67–88.)

hormones disappear, and the development of the external genitalia remains in a relatively quiescent state until the child begins to produce her own hormones and the secondary sex characteristics appear.

The anatomy of the genital tract in the child differs considerably from that of the adolescent girl. The differences are important and must be taken into consideration before any observations can be made about any possible developmental arrest or departure from the normal (Fig. 2–2).

What Are the Characteristics of the Vulva in the Child?

The normal anatomic development of the vulva in the child has many variables. In general the clitoris, urethra, labia and other components of the external genitalia lie in a more exposed position than in the adult, owing largely to the fact that in early childhood the labia majora are poorly formed and the labia minora attenuated. Some subcutaneous fat is present in and around the vulva, but by and large there is less in proportion to that found in the adult. The amount of subcutaneous fat has a direct relation to the state of nutrition. The more malnutrition, the less fat and the more exposed the position of the clitoris and urethra. Though diminished in size, the child's vulva frequently resembles that of the castrate or menopausal woman. At times, however, it appears to be hypertrophied. There is no particular cause for alarm in this, provided there are no obvious genital defects.

The vulva and the clitoris keep pace with the normal somatic growth pattern. Under normal conditions nothing is seen in the way of secondary sex characteristics until the full impact of the child's hormones is felt about the time of puberty. If the child begins to show evidence of estrogenic stimulation such as engorgement of the vulva or growth of pubic hair, the physician should suspect either precocious puberty, adrenal hyperplasia or the presence of a feminizing tumor of the ovary such as a granulosa cell tumor. Tumors with endocrine effect have been reported as early as eighteen months.

It is also advisable to keep in mind that the child may have swallowed, either inadvertently or by design, some of the estrin tablets her mother has in the medicine closet. A number of such instances have been reported in the literature.

Labial adhesions are occasionally found. They may have a congenital cause, but are far more likely to be due to inflammation of the vulva, which is readily traumatized because of its exposed position.

What Does the Clitoris Look Like in the Child?

At birth the clitoris is rather prominent in relation to the other elements that go to make up the external genitalia (Fig. 2–2). It never grows to any appreciable size under normal conditions, nor does it increase in its dimensions to any great extent as the child approaches puberty. The measurements commonly recorded range from 0.6 to 2 cm. in length with a breadth varying from 0.3 to 0.9 cm. Under the influence of the child's own hormones the external genitalia enlarge appreciably at the time of puberty, but the clitoris takes part in this increase to only a slight degree. In the adult it may be only moderately larger than in childhood. No two children are alike in the size of the clitoris. The arrangement of the foreskin varies widely in the female. Fusion of the prepuce to the glans, for example, is a common finding. It tends to disappear under the influence of the child's own estrogenic hormone.

In most instances obvious clitoral enlargement suggests that either the clitoris has been stimulated by some androgenic source or the child has acquired the habit of masturbation.

What Are the Anatomic Characteristics of the Hymen?

There can be little doubt that much of the protective attitude toward the young female child which prevails in the minds of both parents and practitioners of medicine stems from ancient sex folklore which places the hymen in the untouchable category. The inviolability of the hymen is an extremely serious matter to many races, particularly those of Latin or Mediterranean origin. It is precisely for this reason that many girls reach the age of puberty or even the marital state without ever having been examined. The same mother who will insist upon her young daughter being vaccinated for smallpox or inoculated against poliomyelitis or having her teeth examined regularly will shy away from a pelvic examination for the female child. As a result there is a wide variety of misconceptions about the hymen. It is not uncommon, even in this day of free conversation about sex, to have a girl in her twenties ask on premarital examination whether the hymen has been "broken." The mental picture created is one of an inviolable space sealed by a protective membrane—this despite the fact that the girl menstruates regularly through the vagina!

The hymen is a membranous diaphragm with a central aperture which surrounds the outlet of the vagina from a depressed position within the orifice. At birth it is fairly thick, owing to the influence of the maternal hormones. When the estrinizing influence of the mother's hormones is withdrawn, the hymen becomes thin and flat with a rather delicate edge fanning out from the periphery toward the central opening. This opening is approximately 0.4 cm. in diameter at birth and remains at this size until late childhood, when the vagina and vulva begin to respond to estrin stimulation initiated by the child herself. The increase then is approximately twofold, so that with the onset of the menarche the hymenal opening will normally admit an instrument 1 cm. in diameter.

In the older children the area is extremely sensitive, but at birth and for a few years thereafter the child can be examined vaginally both digitally and with a vaginoscope. The base as well as the leaves of the membranous cuff varies in thickness and hence in distensibility in late childhood. As the child approaches the menarche the hymen becomes thicker and its cufflike appearance more pronounced. It is very vascular and bleeds freely when traumatized. The more fibrous the base, the more resistant and the more likely is it to tear.

The true anatomic nature of the hymen is obvious when the child is placed in the knee-chest position and the buttocks are gently separated. As the vagina fills with air the hymen bulges outward. Rarely is the diaphragm imperforate, although the type of opening follows no constant pattern. Actually, the size of the hymenal orifice is the most variable structural abnormality one sees in the genital tract. The opening may appear as a single, irregularly rounded central aperture, multiple perforations or a longitudinal split. If two openings are seen with a central bridge, the child may have a double vagina. If no opening is seen, an imperforate hymen or congenital absence of the vagina should be suspected.

What Is the Anatomic Arrangement of the Child's Vagina?

In the normal embryologic process following fusion of the two müllerian ducts the epithelium of the urogenital sinus invades the central portion of the genital cord, forming a tube which becomes the vagina. The uterus differentiates from the upper areas of the fused portion of the müllerian ducts, while the tubes and ovaries spring from the parts which do not join (Fig. 2–3). It is obvious that there is a wide variety of anomalies that may develop if growth does not proceed according to the normal pattern. Thus we see on rare occasions congenital absence of the vagina and a variety of vaginal partitions and abnormalities of uterine growth.

When the vagina develops normally, it is a simple elastic tube lined with epithelium which falls into convoluted folds, ridges and crevices running in the long axis of the vagina, but tending to be arranged in circular fashion in the upper part of the vagina. At birth the vaginal canal is approximately 4 cm. in depth. As long as the maternal estrogen stimulates the epithelium lining the tube the vagina has many of the characteristics of the adult vagina. One may then expect to find evidence of cornification in the vaginal smear, a pH in the range of 4.0 to 5.0, abundance of glycogen in the epithelial cells and the vaginal flora of an adolescent girl. As the

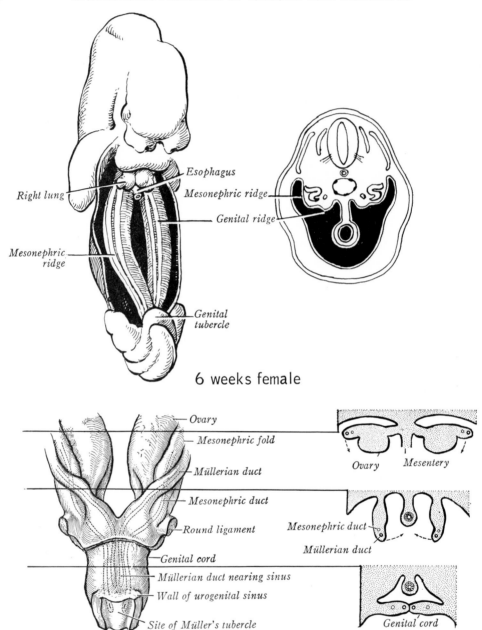

6 weeks female

8 weeks female

Fig. 2-3.   *(Legend on page 19.)*

estrogenic influence recedes the lactobacilli are replaced by other organisms and the acidity shifts toward the alkaline side as lactic acid disappears from the vaginal fluid.

This condition at birth lasts only a few weeks, after which the vaginal epithelium rapidly regresses from the thick succulent type of epithelium containing twenty or more cell layers to the thin atrophic membrane two to eight cells deep of childhood, which we see also following the menopause, when ovarian activity ceases. No longer do we find glycogen or evidence of cornification in the vaginal smears (Fig. 2–4, *A*).

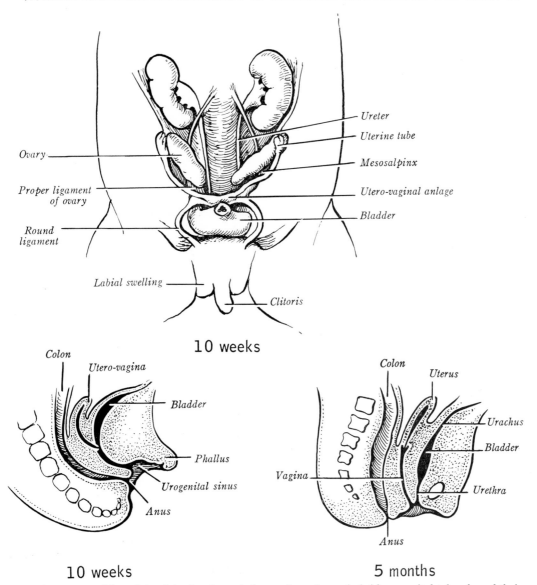

Fig. 2-3. The origin of the female genital tract from the genital ridges, genital tubercle and their derivatives, demonstrated in longitudinal and cross sections, at 6 and 8 weeks of embryonic development. At 10 weeks and beyond the definitive female differentiation of the müllerian ducts becomes evident, as shown in sagittal sections. (Modified from L. B. Arey: *Developmental Anatomy*.)

When the child's own estrogen begins to appear late in childhood, preceding adolescence, the vaginal epithelium is the first target organ to respond. Cornification can be seen in the vaginal smears before there is any clinically evident estrogenic response on the part of the epithelium grossly. The epithelial cells, in addition to showing increasing cornification, also appear to be larger, with medium-sized nuclei, and have lighter-staining protoplasm (Fig. 2–4, *B*). Gradually as the child approaches the menarche the vaginal epithelium reflects the estrogenic stimulation grossly and

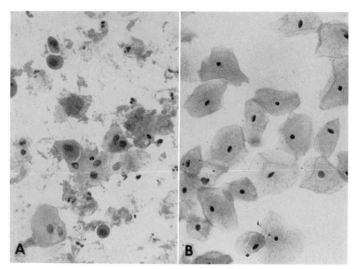

Fig. 2-4.   *A,* Inactive vaginal smear from an 8-year-old girl. The cells are rounded with prominent nuclei. *B,* Vaginal smear from a 12-year-old girl, manifesting estrogen effect. The cells are larger, paler-staining and polygonal, and the nuclei are smaller. Papanicolaou stain, × 125. (Courtesy of Dr. Priscilla Taft, Vincent Memorial Hospital.)

becomes thick and soft. The amount of vaginal fluid increases, and the pH becomes more acid. The degree of cornification in the cells increases, and more glycogen is present in them.

During early childhood the depth of the vagina changes very little. In general the growth of the vagina parallels over-all structural growth. No set pattern is observed, but the average depth of the vagina ranges from 1½ to 2 inches. Because of the inelasticity of the vaginal walls and the nature of the epithelium which tends to make it stick together, the distensibility of the vaginal canal is sharply restricted.

Under the influence of hormonal activity the vagina gradually increases in depth and ability to distend. This is partly due to the growth factor, but more to the change in the vaginal epithelium. The depth of the vagina approximately doubles from early childhood to the time of the menarche, when it averages 11 cm., the posterior length being greater. The development of the vaginal fornices awaits the full impact of the hormones (Fig. 2–5).

What Are the Anatomic Characteristics of the Uterus in Childhood?

As we noted in earlier discussion, the uterus is larger in proportion to body weight at birth because of the maternal hormones than it is at any other time until the premenarchal period. After the first few weeks when the influence of the maternal estrogen is withdrawn the uterus regresses to approximately the size of an olive (2 cm. in length) and grows no more until the child's own hormones take over by about the age of 9 or 10 years (Fig. 2–5).

At birth the cervix does not stand out as a vaginally discernible separate structure. Autopsy specimens, however, demonstrate a prominent cervix equal in size to the whole fundus. The epithelium of the upper part of the vagina merges with that of the cervix, so that no external os is seen and its boundaries cannot be defined. Not much change is noted in early childhood when the cervix is nothing more than a flat plate at the vaginal apex. Occasionally a vague external os can be seen, but there are no cervical secretions.

With the first evident activation of the feminizing hormones the cervix alters in size and shape. With the approach of the menarche it thus increases in size and begins to assume a conical shape. It feels rather like a flat coat button high up in the vagina. Until hormones change the epithelium of the upper part of the vagina it can be seen by speculum examination only with great difficulty.

Although the uterus can be palpated through the rectum at birth, the observations are less valid later in childhood. Schauffler makes the practical point that negative rectal findings are important in this age group. If all other factors appear to be normal and no pelvic tumor or tenderness is present, the fact that the uterus cannot be felt should be no cause for concern and the child may be considered normal. The reason the uterus and ovaries cannot be accurately outlined, unless tumors are

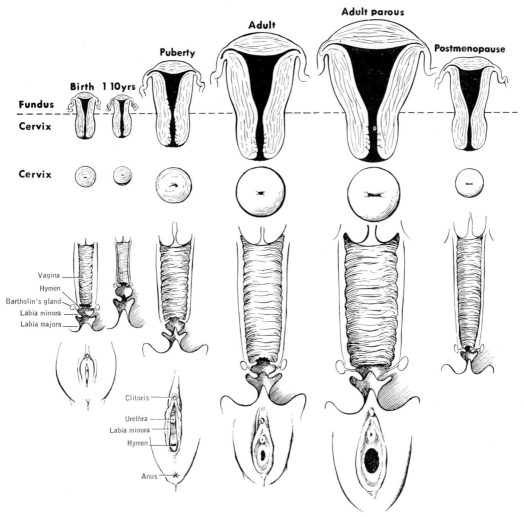

Fig. 2-5. Relative sizes of the uterus, vagina and external genitalia from birth through adult life. The growth of the uterine cervix, fundus and vagina at puberty is striking.

present, is partly that they are as yet underdeveloped, but the anatomic character-istics of the pelvic floor at this stage of the child's life are a greater reason. Not only are the organs small, but also the pelvic connective tissue and musculature are much more compact and inelastic than one normally finds in the adult.

As the child passes into the prepuberal stage the developing uterus, under the influence of the hormones, assumes a somewhat retroverted position in the long axis of the vagina. With continued growth the uterus tends to drop backward toward the sacrum with a greater angulation in relation to the cervix.

One of the most striking differences between the uterus of the premenarchal child and that of the adult is the relative length of the cervix compared with the fundal portion. At puberty approximately two thirds of the total bulk of the uterus is cervix. Under hormonal influence the fundus grows at the expense of the cervix. On occasion, however, the menarchal proportions persist into adult life to become a problem in fertility. The patient is then said to have a hypoplastic or infantile uterus.

What Are the Characteristics of the Child's Ovary and Tube?

The growth of the ovary and tube from birth to puberty occurs in an orderly fashion under normal conditions. Growth is not great until pituitary gonadotropic hormonal stimulation occurs. The ovary at birth is smaller than a kidney bean, and the tubes externally appear as simple strings. Progressive enlargement takes place from birth until puberty. Normally ovaries are so small they cannot be felt. If they can be palpated, one may say with reasonable assurance that a tumor of the ovary is present.

Parental Attitude toward Pelvic Examination in the Child

In this present era of medicine emphasis in all fields except pediatric gynecology has been placed on prevention. For one reason or another both the parents and the medical profession have adopted an overprotective attitude toward the young girl. Far too little attention has been paid to the wide variety of developmental conditions and congenital abnormalities that appear in infancy and childhood. Many of these are correctable, but go unrecognized until the child enters adolescence or contemplates matrimony. It has been said that 30 per cent of serious disease in women occurs in the organs of reproduction, yet little attention is paid to this important region during the most important phase of growth and development. It is only when the organs function badly or not at all that the parents and physician become concerned.

There is an overwhelming emphasis on the psychiatric overtones of all disease processes in present medical thinking, yet in the area where it is most needed the child is simply allowed to grow up. Interest is shown in the child's future reproductive possibilities only after pathologic conditions or developmental deviations from the normal have been permitted to become firmly established. The psychologic complications that arise when attempts are made to correct the underlying faults beyond the age of childhood have far more serious import then than they might have had if the defects were noted and treated in infancy and early childhood.

It is difficult to understand the reason for what appears to be a tragic lack of interest in or understanding of the child's development regarding anything other than skeletal growth. The family readily consults the physician if the child appears too tall or thin, or short and fat, but the same parents are unwilling, and physicians do not insist upon, a pelvic examination to determine whether the pelvic organs are present or likely to function normally if they are. The basic reason for this appears to be an archaic desire to protect the child's virginity. Both parents and physicians reflect their own prudishness by not wanting to have the child examined. They rationalize their attitude by saying that they do not want to focus the child's attention on the sexual organs because of the psychiatric implications. The psychiatrist, on the other hand, who has faced this problem suggests that psychic trauma is not created in the infant by examination of the genital organs, for the simple reason that the infant at birth and for the next two or three years has no sex consciousness. The training and education of the parents and physician should precede that of the child. The parents must be taught that more psychiatric difficulties are produced by not paying attention to genital development than can ever be created by pelvic examination. The physician must also be convinced that all concerned have much to gain by an intelligent attempt to evaluate the reproductive status of the young girl. Too often fatherly counsel is given without a pelvic examination, even in the girl who comes to the physician for premarital advice. The young girl approaching puberty is acutely aware of her sex and would like a few straight answers rather than fanciful explanations based on the flight of the bee or growth of the flower that do not satisfy either her interest or curiosity.

In most instances the reaction of the young girl in late childhood toward a pelvic examination will reflect the attitude of the mother or physician. Allen suggests that the child is more resentful of the fact that the examination may interfere with her planned trip to the movies than any aversion to the examination itself. He does suggest, however, that the child be indoctrinated slowly. To this end he recommends that the mother bring the daughter with her for examination at the time of her own regular checkup, beginning at the age of seven. In this manner the child comes to accept the examination as a regular part of her life and has no psychologic reaction to it. Perhaps the mere fact that the young girl becomes accustomed to the routine of a pelvic examination is more important than the finding of a developmental or pathologic lesion.

If the physician will routinely do a complete examination at birth and the mother will institute a program which calls for periodic yearly examinations after the age of seven, there will be far less sexual maladjustment in adult life with or without marriage. Many of our taboos and fears and much of our own false modesty stem from an unrealistic attitude toward sex on the part of the parents and physicians during the growth period of the child.

REFERENCES

Allan, F. D.: The Embryology of the Reproductive System; in J. T. Velardo, Ed.: *Endocrinology of Repro- duction.* New York, Oxford University Press, 1958, Chap. III, p. 21.

Fluhmann, C. F.: The Glandular Structures of the Cervix Uteri. *Surg., Gynec. & Obst.,* 106: 715, 1958.

Idem: The Developmental Anatomy of the Cervix Uteri. *Obst. & Gynec.,* 15: 62, 1960.

Hamperl, H., and Kaufmann, C.: The Cervix Uteri at Different Ages. *Obst. & Gynec.,* 14: 621, 1959.

Krantz, K. E.: The Gross and Microscopic Anatomy of the Human Vagina. *Ann. New York Acad. Sc.,* 83: 89, 1959.

Price, D.: Influence of Hormones on Sex Differentiation in Explanted Fetal Reproductive Tracts; in C. A. Villee, Ed.: *Gestation.* New York, Josiah Macy, Jr. Foundation, 1956, p. 173.

Schauffler, G. C.: The Female Genitals in Immaturity. *Pediat. Clin. N. Amer.,* 5: 3, 1958.

Wells, L. J.: Embryology and Anatomy of the Vagina. *Ann. New York Acad. Sc.,* 83: 80, 1959.

Willier, B. H.: The Embryonic Development of Sex; in E. Allen, Ed.: *Sex and Internal Secretions.* Baltimore, Williams & Wilkins Company, 1939, p. 64.

Chapter 3

Examination of the

Newborn Female Infant

What Developmental Abnormalities Can Be Detected at Birth and in Early Infancy?

Physical examination of the newborn, when carried out by the obstetrician, is all too frequently limited to a hasty inspection of the external genitalia. It is not surprising, therefore, that many congenital defects in the female genital tract are not recognized until growth or functional demand brings them sharply into focus. With proper recognition of anatomic development in the growing child it should be possible to detect some of the departures from the normal at birth or in early infancy. Some of the developmental defects have a genetic background or are secondary to disturbances in intrauterine environment, while others are due to overactivity on the part of the fetal adrenal cortex.

Most abnormalities are limited to the external genitalia, lower third of the vagina and the rectum. Thus we find such anatomic deviations as absence of the vagina, clitoral hypertrophy, labial fusion, partitioning of the vagina and imperforate hymen or anus. All these are recognizable at birth. Some of them will need immediate attention, while others should be corrected later. Early detection allows the physician to plan his future therapy intelligently.

The important thing to remember is that a wide variety of causes can produce the same defects in the external genitalia. For example, the external anatomic variations produced by congenital hyperplasia of the adrenal (the adrenogenital syndrome) are identical with those created by the nonhormonal forms of ambisexual development which have a genetic background.

There are some disorders of function in the child's own endocrine glands which are congenital in origin. Early recognition and treatment are essential if irreparable damage is to be prevented. A few of these can be spotted in the immediate neonatal period. The infant with a congenital failure of the thyroid is a prime example. If the malfunction is recognized early and there is no additional defect in the brain, the ingestion of thyroid extract may prevent the mental retardation and stunted structural development which are common in cretinism. Another example is the group of congenital anomalies associated with hyperplasia of the adrenal cortex. At times severe electrolyte imbalance occurs in the adrenogenital syndrome at birth which, if it is not recognized, may lead to the death of the child in the neonatal period.

Finally it is important to establish as early as possible the sex chromatin pattern in any child who has a congenital anomaly of the genital tract. Many children are reared as males who have the sex chromatin pattern of the female. Early recognition may prevent severe psychologic readjustment later in adolescence when the sex hormones become active.

What Information Can Be Gathered from the General Physical Examinations?

Certain basic observations should be made and recorded at the time of birth. They are useful in (a) detecting abnormalities or arousing suspicion of their presence, and (b) providing a base line for comparison with similar observations made in the future.

The *skeletal measurements* of height, weight and circumference of the head are basic requirements. In addition, the relative length of the trunk and extremities should be noted. We observed earlier that the pituitary dwarf was normal in length and weight at birth. Later in childhood it may be important to distinguish between the constitutional and the pituitary dwarf. The observations made at birth may prove useful in establishing the true diagnosis. Likewise the relative proportions of trunk to extremity are important in differentiation between the thyroid and the pituitary or constitutional dwarf. In the former the infant continues to have a long trunk and short legs. The circumference of the head is also a basic measurement. The infant may be mongoloid or perhaps microcephalic. The birth measurements compared with those taken later will aid in the diagnosis of cretinism, for we have previously noted that in thyroid deficiency there is an arrest in the normal development of the cranial and facial bones.

The *condition of the skin and its circulation* should be carefully inspected and recorded. Too much wrinkling may suggest malnutrition, while too smooth a skin points to edema. Mottling of the skin often occurs when the peripheral circulation is sluggish. If the extremities are also cold, thyroid insufficiency is suspected. When to these observations at birth are added indications of lethargy, constipation and a persistence of neonatal jaundice, cretinism is a real possibility.

Recent reports in the literature call attention to the fact that it is possible to suspect and actually make a diagnosis of *ovarian dysgenesis* at birth. The main physical findings which arouse suspicion are (a) pronounced edema of the hands and feet, (b) short neck with loose redundant skin, (c) a peculiar circular pattern to the growth of hair well down on the nape of the neck, (d) low-set ears and a high arched palate (Figs. 3–1, 3–2). The main characteristics, lymphedema in the extremities and a short neck, are not encountered in other pathologic entities in the newborn. Such a child should have her sex determined by buccal smear technique, for 80 per cent are said to have the chromatin negative pattern. Details of the determination of sex chromatin will be discussed later (p. 52). It is important to know the sex pattern as early in infancy as possible in order to avoid social and psychologic complications later in life.

All structural abnormalities that are obvious on direct examination should be measured and recorded for purposes of comparison with similar observations made later. It is possible that some of the skeletal deformities may be associated with genital defects in the female. So many of the congenital malformations are multiple that the presence of one should arouse suspicion that others, which are less obvious on direct inspection, may be present and manifest themselves at later stages in the child's development. This is particularly true of urinary tract anomalies.

It is not easy to detect *evidence of mental retardation* in a child at birth or in the

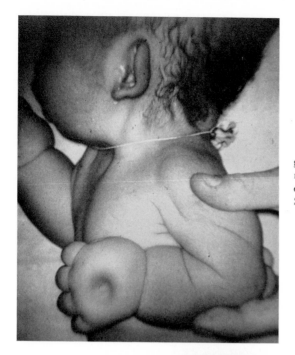

Fig. 3-1.   An infant with ovarian dysgenesis, showing the typical webbing of the neck, growth of hair on the nape, and pitting edema of the hand. (Courtesy of Dr. Sydney S. Gellis, Boston City Hospital.)

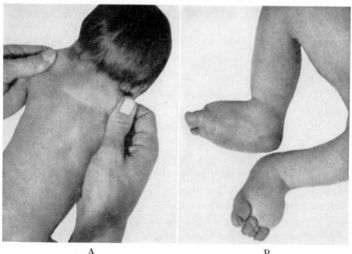

A   B

Fig. 3-2.   A, Infant with ovarian agenesis at birth, showing webbing of the neck. (Courtesy of the *Year Book of Pediatrics*, 1957–1958, edited by S. S. Gellis. Chicago, Year Book Publishers, Inc.) B, Lymphangiectatic edema of the feet. (Courtesy of H. K. Silver: *Pediatrics*, Vol. 17.)

immediate postnatal period. About all the physician has to go on are alertness and the quality of the baby's cry, together with its body measurements. When other congenital anomalies are present, particularly those of the skeletal system, one should be suspicious of brain damage, for the two often go hand in hand. It is important to remember that the newborn infant's entire existence depends on how well the spinal cord and lower levels of the brain function. Observations of the child's movements and reactions to external stimuli may be good indicators of any departure from the normal.

What Can Be Determined by Local Examination of the Genitalia?

Direct inspection and examination of the external genitalia at birth are essential. With the infant held in a modified knee-chest position both inspection and examination can be carried out with ease, because of the tendency of the vagina to distend with air.

CLITORAL ENLARGEMENT AND LABIAL FUSION.   With the infant in this position the size of the clitoris and development of the external genitalia are immediately apparent. Clitoral enlargement and fusion or maldevelopment of the labial folds may lead to early detection of the adrenogenital syndrome. If this syndrome is suspected, one should look for anomalies of the urinary tract which may show up as abnormal positions of the external urethral orifice.

In the presence of clitoral enlargement differentiation must be made between (*a*) congenital hyperplasia of the adrenal cortex (the adrenogenital syndrome), (*b*) the effect of hormone ingestion by the mother which may stimulate the fetal clitoris, and (*c*) variations in the infant's sex chromatin pattern (Fig. 3–3).

What Other Evidence Do We Have of the Effect of Maternal Hormones upon the Fetus?

We have previously noted that the maternal hormones may induce an engorgement of the breast in the newborn infant which persists for several weeks after birth. There may actually be secretion of milk from the engorged breast ("witch's milk"). In addition to the effect of the maternal hormones on the breast, the newborn infant occasionally experiences a sort of pseudomenstruation. The infant may bleed from actual proliferation of the uterine endometrial lining, or perhaps for the same reason that adults bleed when estrin stimulation is suddenly withdrawn. The effect of the maternal hormones rarely persists for more than three weeks.

The treatment of clitoral enlargement and labial fusion will be outlined in the discussion of the female pseudohermaphrodite (p. 59).

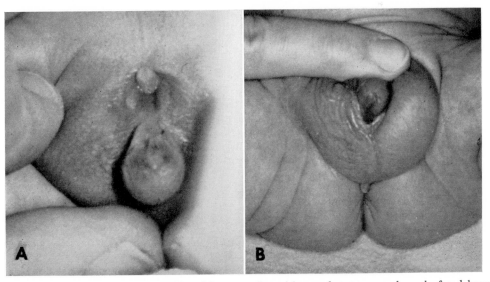

Fig. 3-3.   Two instances of clitoral hypertrophy with pseudoscrotum and partly fused hypertrophied labia in female infants whose mothers were treated with progesterone during pregnancy. These are iatrogenic instances of female pseudohermaphroditism. (Courtesy of Dr. Sydney S. Gellis, Boston City Hospital.)

IMPERFORATE HYMEN AND EVALUATION OF THE PATENCY OF THE VAGINAL CANAL

The state of the hymen and the patency of the vaginal canal can easily be determined with the child in the knee-chest position by inspection and by inserting a small probe. In this position it is also possible to carry out a bimanual abdominorectal examination with relative ease if a well lubricated little finger is inserted in the anal opening.

Although one may not choose to correct a congenital absence of the vagina or vaginal partitioning until puberty is imminent, it is important to discover the abnormality at birth. Since congenital absence of the vagina and other less severe vaginal anomalies are due to a failure in the development and fusion of the müllerian ducts, there may also be congenital absence or duplication of the uterus. In addition, anomalies also appear in the upper genitourinary tract, as well as bony defects in the lumbar spine and pelvis. Since the uterus at birth is still under the influence of the maternal hormones, it is often large enough to be felt on rectal examination. When duplication of the uterus is suspected, one may feel small buttons of tissue on either side of the pelvis with an intervening partition of fibrous tissue.

IMPERFORATE HYMEN.　　If the genital area is thoroughly examined with the child in the knee-chest position at birth, there is no reason why an imperforate hymen should be overlooked. Rarely, however, is it discovered before puberty and the onset of menstruation. Occasionally the newborn infant, because of the action of the maternal hormones, will trap a sizable collection of secretions behind an imperforate hymen. At this period of life the secretions are usually mucoid in nature, with some blood and desquamated epithelium when the stimulus from the mother's hormones has been sufficiently strong to activate the infant uterus and vagina. This condition

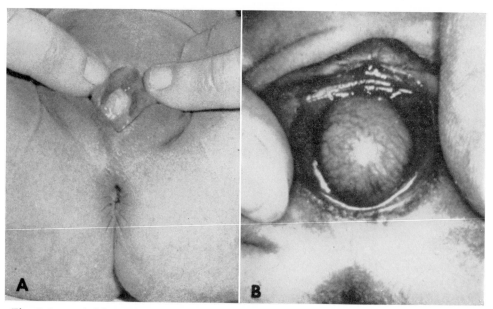

Fig. 3-4.　　*A*, Mucus had collected behind this newborn infant's imperforate hymen, which bulged like a tumor. *B*, The darker color of this protruding hymen suggests hematocolpos. (*B*, Courtesy of H. Ulfelder: *Clin. Obst. & Gynec.*, 1960.)

is known as hydrometrocolpos (Fig. 3–4). If there is a bleeding component, the term "hematometrocolpos" or "hematocolpos" is used.

The impatent hymen bulges outward, owing to the pressure of the secretions trapped behind it, and provides a typical picture on examination. On rare occasions the accumulation may be so extensive that the secretions distend the infant vagina and uterus and an abdominal mass develops. Unless one is aware of the possibility of hydrometrocolpos, the suprapubic mass may be confused with the presence of a pelvic neoplasm.

The protruding hymen should be incised as early as possible after its discovery, whatever the age. This should not be done casually, for the position of the urethra may be altered appreciably by the hymenal distention. Later in childhood the surgeon may prefer to excise, rather than incise, the hymen.

IMPERFORATE ANUS

It is important to remember that a female infant with an imperforate anus may also have a rectovaginal fistula. The fistula may occur anywhere in the lower vaginal canal, but in most instances appears near the fourchette. The actual opening may be difficult to find in a newborn child, for it is frequently occluded by mucoid secretions and meconium. The association of an imperforate anus with vaginointestinal fistulas, however, is so high that the physician should be on the alert. Frequently they can be demonstrated by gentle probing. Occasionally the female infant with an imperforate anus may also have a urethro-vesico-vaginal fistula, but the association appears less frequently than fistula into bowel. The treatment of imperforate anus falls in the province of the pediatric general surgeon.

DETECTION OF PELVIC TUMORS IN THE NEWBORN INFANT

It is important to remember that some congenital defects involve histologic as well as gross organic and skeletal structures.

One may detect genital tumor formation on abdominorectal examination. The majority of pelvic tumors in the preadolescent girl appear in the years immediately preceding puberty, but dermoids, teratomas and simple cysts of the ovary, as well as sarcoma botryoides arising from the vagina and cervix, have been discovered at birth or shortly thereafter. It must be kept in mind that the anatomic arrangement of the pelvic structures in infancy is such that intra-abdominal tumors, particularly those that arise from the ovary, tend to rise out of the pelvis and are best felt by abdominal examination.

The examination of the infant at birth is easier and more revealing than any performed from then on until the onset of puberty. The information obtained can serve as the basis for immediate investigation and treatment and form the background for observations made later in childhood.

HERNIAS IN THE NEWBORN INFANT

Most hernias that appear at birth or are noted in the immediate postnatal period are due to congenital defects. Aside from umbilical hernias, they are almost invariably inguinal, and simply are complications of processes of development present in fetal life. The processus vaginalis, which is nothing more than an outpocketing of the peritoneum that descends alongside the round ligament, normally is pinched off and atrophies. When this fails to take place, the funnel-like extension of the peritoneum remains open, and the child has a congenital indirect hernia communicating with the peritoneal cavity. The extent of the process varies, and the hernia may be long or short. This maldevelopment is far more common in boys than in girls, but approximately 10 per cent of all inguinal hernias will occur in the female infant. The hernia is usually located on the right side, with about a 15 per cent chance that there will be a bilateral defect.

The presence of the hernia may well be overlooked at the initial examination after birth, though the defect may be present at that time. The first indication of a hernia is usually the appearance of a bulge in the inguinal area when the child is two or three months old. The size of the hernia will vary widely, depending on the extent of the peritoneal prolongation along the round ligament. As the child becomes more active the intra-abdominal tension tends to increase and small intestine or intraperitoneal fluid is forced into the sac, keeping it open and at times distending it. Rarely does the omentum enter the hernial sac of a young infant, for it is rather underdeveloped at this age.

Symptoms and Physical Findings

The symptoms are minimal, for the sac is usually sufficiently wide to permit the intestine to slip in and out without bothering the infant to any extent. If this does not occur easily, the child may be restless and fretful and lose both appetite and weight. The diagnosis is usually made by seeing and feeling the bulge in the groin and obtaining a history of appearance and disappearance of the mass. If the middle finger is placed over the bulging mass and gently rotated from side to side, the sac can be felt, and the mass itself can usually be reduced when gentle pressure is applied locally with the child in the recumbent position.

In rare instances the contents of the inguinal sac may become incarcerated in young girls and infants. This is a far more common occurrence in the male. The intestine may get caught within the hernial sac, strangulate and produce symptoms of intestinal obstruction. In this case the patient will exhibit a tense, tender swelling, obviously be suffering from severe pain and frequently be vomiting. Not infrequently, perhaps one third of the time, the incarceration occurs without any previous indication that the child ever had a hernia. The hernia will not reduce, and immediate operation is indicated.

Differential Diagnosis of Inguinal Hernia

HYDROCELE.   The chief difficulty is in deciding whether the patient has a simple hydrocele of the round ligament (cyst of the canal of Nuck) or a true hernia. She may of course have both. It should be possible to transilluminate the mass and make the diagnosis, but unfortunately this does not work if the bowel is empty of fecal content and fluid, for if only gas is present, it too will transmit light.

The best method of distinguishing between the two is to try reducing the hernia. This must be done with care and entirely differently than in the adult. The physician should never try to insert a finger in the external inguinal ring, for this is very disturbing to the child. She should be placed in a recumbent position with the head down. Gentle palpation with a rolling motion to the tips of the fingers of the extended hand over the presenting mass will usually reduce the hernia. The intestine can be felt suddenly to slip back into the abdomen. If the swelling is due to encysted fluid, the mass cannot be reduced in size with any ease, and if it does decrease, the bulge does not do so suddenly. The patient then likely has a hydrocele of the round ligament.

INGUINAL MASS WITH AMBIGUOUS EXTERNAL GENITALIA.   In the presence of congenital abnormality in the external genitalia the infant's groins should be palpated. If the clitoris is enlarged, resembling a hypospadiac penis, and the external genitalia appear normal, the gonads may be felt in the groins. The first problem is to decide whether the child has simple inguinal hernias or whether gonads are included in the sacs (Fig. 3–5). If the masses appear to be gonadal, the next problem is whether they

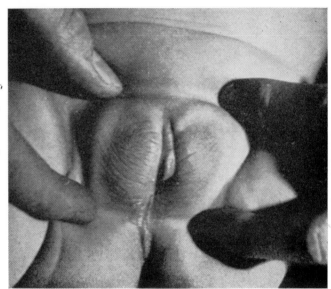

Fig. 3-5.   Close-up of the external genitalia of a child whose inguinal swellings were found to contain testes. The external genitalia were of female appearance, so that this represented male pseudohermaphroditism. (From M. R. Gaspar, J. H. Kimber and K. A. Berkaw: A.M.A. J. *Dis. Child.*, Vol. 91.)

are ovaries or testes. Although it is possible for tube and ovary to descend into a hernial sac, it is far more likely that the masses felt are testes. In general an inguinal mass of this sort that is easily reducible will prove to contain ovary, or ovary and tube, rather than testis.

REFERENCES

Genital Abnormalities

Richart, R. M., and Benirschke, K.: Diagnosis of Gonadal Dysgenesis in Newborn Infants. *Obst. & Gynec.*, 15: 621, 1960.

Rosenthal, A. H.: Symptomatic Genital Anomalies in Childhood. *Clin. Obst. & Gynec.*, 3:146, 1960.

Schauffler, G. C.: *Pediatric Gynecology, with Sections on Urology and Proctology.* 3rd Ed. Chicago, Year Book Publishers, Inc., 1953.

Silver, H. K.: Symmetric Form of Bonnevie-Ullrich Syndrome. (Webbing of Neck, Lymphangiectatic Edema, Shortness of Stature, Cubitus Valgus and Deformity of the Toes.) *Pediatrics*, 17: 725, 1956.

Wells, L. J., and van Wagenen, G.: Androgen-Induced Female Pseudohermaphroditism in Monkey (Macaca Mulatta): Anatomy of Reproductive Organs. *Carnegie Contrib. Embryol.*, 35: 93, 1954.

Witschi, E.: Etiology of Gonadal Agenesis and Sex Reversal; in C. A. Villee, Ed.: *Gestation*. New York, Josiah Macy, Jr. Foundation, 1957, p. 119.
Witschi, E., Nelson, W. O., and Segal, S. J.: Genetic, Developmental and Hormonal Aspects of Gonadal Dysgenesis and Sex Inversion in Man. *J. Clin. Endocrinol. & Metab.*, 17: 737, 1957.

Hernias in Infancy

Gaspar, M. R., Kimber, J. H., and Berkaw, K. A.: Children with Hernias, Testes and Female External Genitalia. A.M.A. *J. Dis. Child.*, 91: 542, 1956.
Nelson, W. E.: *Textbook of Pediatrics*. 7th Ed. Philadelphia, W. B. Saunders Company, 1959.

Chapter 4

Congenital Anomalies

THE MOST common disturbances in the growth pattern seen at childbirth and early infancy are congenital malformations. The manifestations are many and varied. Some are local, while others are widespread. We are primarily interested in the congenital anomalies that are associated with gynecologic problems in the growing period of the girl's life. Nevertheless many of the developmental abnormalities in the genital region occur in young female children who also have other anomalies which may be less obvious, or vice versa.

What Is the Incidence of Variation in the Normal Growth Pattern?

It is almost impossible to tell how frequently congenital anomalies appear. This is in part due to the fact that the definition of congenital defect has not been clearly established. Fortunately many embryos with serious congenital defects die during intrauterine life. Most of the pregnancies which end in abortion are defective, for example. Many more fetuses that survive to term die at birth or immediately thereafter. It has been said that 1 per cent of all fetuses that survive 20 weeks of intrauterine life have malformations that are either lethal or result in major interference in normal development. The fatal cases most often have a basic defect in the central nervous system. Congenital malformations in the cardiac, gastrointestinal and genitourinary systems follow in frequency in the order named.

The National Office of Vital Statistics in 1950 recorded 4.4 congenital anomalies for 1000 live births. This figure in all probability is too low. If one considers such relatively common findings as Mongolian spots, pigmented nevi, hemangiomas, inclusion cysts, undescended testes and polydactylism, the percentage of congenital deformity may well be in the neighborhood of 10 per cent of live births. Furthermore, many malformations are so minor that they are never reported.

Congenital malformations appeared by the time the child was 1 year old in 7 per cent of 5964 pregnancies studied at Columbia. It is interesting that only half of these were discovered at birth on direct inspection. The others were detected only after illness had developed. Complaints such as pyelitis, cystitis, malnutrition, vomiting and the symptom complex associated with hypothyroidism are often outward manifestations of a concealed congenital defect. Because of the tendency among physicians to classify congenital defects in such general terms as blindness, deafness, mental deficiency or endocrine disease, the true incidence of developmental abnormalities is not easily determined.

It is fortunate that although 10 per cent of live infants may have some sort of a deformity present if one includes such things as hemangiomas, only about 4 per cent have a deformity serious enough to require correction. The number is, nevertheless, disturbing, as one can easily confirm by checking the wards of a children's hospital. Nearly one third of the patients will be there for a correction of some congenital defect.

The total number of congenital defects recognized early will depend on the experience of the physician and the completeness of his examination. Many anomalies are completely compatible with normal health and only come to light years later when illness appears. Unless suspected, the underlying congenital defect may then be overlooked.

What Factors in the History Should Arouse Suspicion of the Presence of Congenital Anomalies at Birth?

Most malformations are not due to any single factor, but to a combination of many. Certain anomalies have a genetic background, but it is difficult to eliminate the possibility that intrauterine environmental factors may also be present. The number of malformations due to genetic causes alone probably total no more than 10 per cent of all the malformations encountered.

If one is to uncover congenital malformations in early infancy, there must be a high index of suspicion when one encounters a newborn baby who either does not look or act as one might expect. A number of factors in the history tend to increase the element of suspicion.

AGE OF THE PARENTS. It is well known, for example, that age, particularly of the mother, has a bearing on the likelihood of congenital deformity in the infant. The lowest frequency of growth abnormality appears in the age group between 25 and 30 years, in which it is placed at 6.4 per 1000 live births. In girls under 20, however, the incidence increases to 7.8, and to 22.5 for mothers under the age of 15. The reproductive system could be regarded as too immature to handle the intricacies of producing a normal full-term infant. The same factors are noted at the other end of the reproductive spectrum. Approximately 12.7 infants will have some congenital malformation per 1000 live births in women over 35. The incidence of mongolism, for example, rises sharply after the maternal age of thirty-five. The chance of having a mongoloid child is said to be forty times greater when it is born to a woman over forty-five than to a girl in the twenty- or thirty-year age group. The decline in ovarian function early in pregnancy may be such that in some older women the hazard of producing a malformed infant is increased. The older germ plasm of the father must also be considered, for a deterioration may appear that produces genetic changes which could result in malformations.

HEREDITY. Some congenital defects and pathologic conditions result from abnormalities in a pair of genes. If the abnormalities are genetically dominant, they may be traced back to an affected parent through many generations. They are kept in the population through new mutations and reproduction by affected persons. They are reduced in number by natural selection. Not infrequently the dominant trait may skip a generation. When the characteristics are recessive, it is harder to identify the inheritance factor, for the defect may not be present in the parents or any of the living collateral relatives. In many instances the infant simply inherits the tendency to develop congenital anomalies. Whether or not they do appear may depend on exposure to certain environmental stimuli. For example, a child may inherit a tendency to develop an allergy, but may never do so unless there is exposure and sensitization to a particular allergen.

Structurally, an infant may be found to have such anomalies as multiple exostoses, polydactylism, brachydactylia, syndactyly or chondrodystrophy. Pathologic neurologic conditions such as diabetes insipidus, Huntington's chorea, neurofibromatosis (von Recklinghausen's disease), Friedreich's ataxia, progressive muscular dystrophy and hereditary spastic paraplegia are thought to be inherited. A great many disorders of the optic pathways can be traced to transmitted pathologic traits. Thus cataracts, optic atrophy and night blindness are occasionally encountered in families.

The most common congenital defects such as harelip, cleft palate, spina bifida aperta and clubfoot tend to occur more often in relatives of the affected infant than one would expect to find in the general population. It is still uncertain whether these defects are entirely due to defective genes or whether environmental factors have not also played a contributing role. A hereditary influence may be suspected if the history reveals that similar defects have appeared in other members of the family.

FERTILITY. For some reason or another some women have great difficulty in getting pregnant. In many one finds a history of repeated abortions, stillbirths or neonatal deaths. As we have noted previously, many of these embryos have basic congenital defects. It is difficult to decide whether these malformations were the result of environmental factors, nutritional inadequacy, systemic disease or hormonal imbalance. As the woman with this kind of history grows older she often becomes more and more determined to have a living child. Unfortunately the woman with this kind of reproductive history not infrequently gives birth to a malformed child.

From the History What Specific Environmental Factors Appear to Influence the Production of Congenital Anomalies?

We have noted that genetic factors alone may be responsible for congenital anomalies in approximately 10 per cent of those who have such defects. It is also true that the factors which produce subtle changes in the intrauterine environment are many and varied. Rarely is there one predominant cause. A few patients with congenital malformations will have a definite major genetic cause and a few more have a specific environmental explanation. For the most part, however, a combination of factors is at work.

Many observations on the cause of a congenital anomaly seem to suggest that definite environmental factors are operating, but only a few can be said to be specific. Lead and ergot poisoning are two traditionally important situations that predispose to fetal wastage through toxic damage in utero, causing abnormal fetal development and death. Also, for example, anencephalus is said to be twenty times more common in Belfast, Ireland, than in Paris, not many miles away. This suggests a geographic variation. Dislocated hips appear as an anomaly twice as often in the winter months. Thus there appears to be a seasonal variation. The parents' social class seems to have something to do with it, for more anencephaly, spina bifida aperta and hydrocephalus are found in the poorer economic groups. Previously we noted that physiologic changes in the aging mother might be implicated in the development of deformities. All these observations are correct, but none is the sole precipitating cause.

THE ROLE OF NUTRITION. Although they are not an important cause of anomalies, there can be little doubt that nutritional disturbances in the mother, particularly deficiency in the vitamin B group, influence the developing embryo adversely. For the embryo to progress normally in its development it must be provided with and utilize properly the essential amino acids and vitamins.

Proof is available from statistics compiled after the last war in countries that suffered from dietary deficiencies. Infants born to mothers after a prolonged period of dietary inadequacy showed a definite reduction both in weight and length when compared to the normal. Statistics from elsewhere amply confirm the observation that more stillbirths and premature infants are born to mothers whose diet has been inadequate than to those whose food intake has been sufficient.

Experimentally, it has been practically impossible to produce malformations in animals by starvation. An inadequate diet will almost invariably produce a cessation of reproductive cycles. This same observation was made during the last war, when the conception rate was shown to fall sharply in women who lived in countries where the diet approached starvation levels. There would appear to be a narrow margin between the dietary factors that permit normal development and those that result in complete failure to develop at all.

What Specific Illnesses or Therapy May Alter the Intrauterine Environment and Produce Congenital Anomalies?

Congenital anomalies may arise as a direct result of changes in the intrauterine environment produced by (1) virus infections such as German measles (rubella) and parasitic diseases such as toxoplasmosis acquired by the mother in the early weeks of gestation; (2) certain drugs given to the mother to forestall a threatened abortion, such as progestin, androgen or estrin. In the same category are the antifolic acid drugs such as aminopterin, which are sometimes used to induce an abortion. (3) Ionizing radiation given over the pelvic region in the early months of pregnancy.

The physician should remember when he uses any of the drugs mentioned above or radiation in a pregnant woman early in pregnancy that the fetus may be injured by any of these noxious agents without in any way influencing the health of the mother.

The *time factor* during which these so-called noxious agents exert their influence on the fetus is of basic importance. Any one of the factors mentioned above, including the virus infections, may be relatively harmless at one stage of development, but very damaging at another. Thus radiation given to rats on the ninth day of pregnancy will produce ocular and cerebral defects, while only skeletal defects appear after the fourteenth day.

The most severe congenital anomalies involving both organ structure and function appear when the therapy is given or the infectious disease is acquired early in pregnancy, usually within the first two months. At this time the fetal organs are going through their most rapid phase of differentiation.

MULTIPLE DEFECTS.   Some defects are widespread and are not necessarily due to specific action of a single agent. Two reasons are advanced to explain the appearance of multiple defects. (1) Any organ going through the differentiation process at the same time would tend to be affected by the action of a deleterious agent; (2) the relative sensitivity of the organ will depend on its metabolic need of essential material. The action of the damaging agent is to create a deficiency. Some organs in their differentiation will have a greater requirement than others, but if the agent operates long enough and in sufficient doses, all organs will be affected.

For example, animals given a diet deficient in vitamins A and E will have progeny with many of the defects commonly produced in other animals by radiation. Both show ocular damage as well as anomalies in the cardiovascular system. Interventricular septal defects and abnormalities of the aortic arch occur along with developmental faults of the genitourinary system such as horseshoe kidney. On the other hand, radiation is more prone to damage the brain, while vitamin deficiency interferes more with the differentiation of the genital tract.

THE ROLE OF INFECTION.   One might expect that any serious illness in the mother during the early phases of pregnancy would so alter the intrauterine environment that malformation would be prone to occur. Actually, the mother is far more likely to abort than to give birth to a malformed child. In animal experimentation and human beings only a few virus infections have been implicated in the causation of congenital anomalies.

Mothers who have had *German measles* (rubella) during the first few months of pregnancy do have a tendency to produce infants with congenital defects in the eye (cataracts), auditory apparatus and brain. The association of this maternal measles and congenital maldevelopment is well documented. When this observation was first made, 90 per cent of mothers were supposed to produce infants with one or more of the defects. This led to many therapeutic abortions as a preventive measure. Statistics gathered from many sources throughout the world now place the incidence at a much lower figure (10 to 20 per cent). The fact that a high percentage of, but not all, infants born to mothers who have measles early in pregnancy are normal suggests that the fetus was either resistant or not susceptible at the time.

Prenatal *toxoplasmosis*, another type of virus infection, has been solidly linked to the creation of such congenital defects as chorioretinitis, hydrocephalus and microcephaly.

Systemic infections which manifest themselves later in fetal development after the period of rapid organ differentiation are unlikely to produce lethal malformations. Fetal measles, scarlet fever, smallpox, tuberculosis and syphilis have been reported as a result of placental transmission. The fetus may survive such uterine infection and simply manifest the same effects she might be expected to show if the infection were acquired after birth.

Of course untreated syphilis in the mother characteristically results in reproductive difficulties, typically abortions followed by stillbirths, and later by live born infants with the stigmata of congenital syphilis. Among the effects of syphilis on development are malformations of the teeth (Hutchinson's incisors, mulberry molars), the nose (saddle deformity) and bones (saber shin), all of which become evident later in childhood.

THE ROLE OF IONIZING RADIATION.   It is now well known that pelvic irradiation, either external or intrauterine, can produce malformations when given in heavy enough dosage over a limited time. A variety of defects occur, but the chief damage to the embryo appears in the eye and brain and takes the form of arrested development. The brain and eye damage is most likely to appear when the irradiation is given very early in pregnancy. Microcephaly and mental retardation are most frequently encountered.

Experimentally in animals microphthalmia and anophthalmia are the most common defects which appear when radiation is given between the ninth and eleventh days to rodents with pregnancy normally of twenty-one days' duration. One also notes mental retardation, brain damage and spina bifida when irradiation is

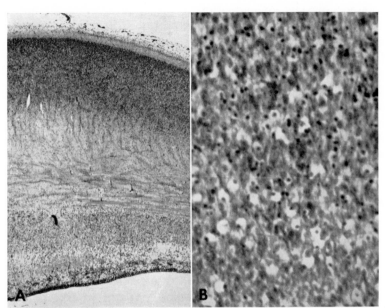

Fig. 4-1.   Radiation damage to the embryonic mouse brain is localized in the most rapidly developing cells. *A*, The moth-eaten appearance just above the ventricular ependyma, at the bottom, is due to radiation necrosis. *B*, The swollen brain cells with pyknotic nuclei were killed by irradiation. (Courtesy of Dr. Samuel P. Hicks, New England Deaconess Hospital.)

delivered at this time. Later on irradiation produces defects in the heart and a right-sided aortic arch. X-ray treatment given after the fourteenth day produces congenital skeletal defects, such as extra digits and club feet. Facial and palatal defects such as cleft palate and harelip less commonly occur. Rarely examination reveals situs inversus and a horseshoe kidney (Fig. 4–1).

The effects of radiation will be different, depending on the stage of development at the time it is administered.

FOLIC ACID DEFICIENCY.   It has been shown that folic acid antagonists such as aminopterin (4-aminopteroylglutamic acid) when given to induce abortion in the first trimester of pregnancy will eventually produce malformation if the attempt at abortion is unsuccessful and a child is born. Hydrocephalus, meningoencephalocele, cleft palate and harelip are the most common anomalies encountered. The majority of the defects created are apparently due to retardation in normal development. Animal experiments suggest that the type and number of abnormalities produced will depend on the time a deficiency in folic acid is produced, in relation to the stage of the developmental process. An animal in the earlier stages of development will be more severely affected by an equal period of deficiency than an older animal. For example, if a dietary deficiency in folic acid occurs on the seventh or eighth day, the majority of effects appear in the brain and eye. Multiple abnormalities involving the skeletal, cardiovascular and urogenital tracts appear when the deficiency begins on the ninth to the eleventh day. On the other hand, a predominance of urogenital anomalies appears when the deficiency operates during days ten to thirteen. Two thirds of the animals show abnormalities in position of the kidney or gonad. From the eleventh to the fourteenth day the defects appear in the skeleton.

Likewise, the various organs in the infant apparently differentiate on different time schedules. The type of response of any given organ to the deprivation of essential metabolic needs will depend on its sensitivity in relation to its growth pattern.

THE HORMONES.   Under normal conditions estrogenic hormones during pregnancy are present in large amounts and have no difficulty in crossing the placental barrier, as shown by the development of breast, vagina and uterus, and the occasional evidences of function such as postnatal vaginal bleeding and nipple secretion.

Hormonal stimulation may interfere with the proper development of the embryo if excessive masculinizing hormones are added to the normal complements through (a) a fetal adrenal cortex with congenital hyperplasia; (b) exogenous hormones provided to the mother in the early trimesters of pregnancy to prevent abortion; and (c) rare masculinizing tumors of the ovary such as the arrhenoblastoma. Because of the added hormonal stimulation at the specific point in the developmental time schedule, certain structures which would normally be expected to regress fail to do so, while other structures tend to overgrowth. In this manner congenital malformations occur. Masculinization of the female infant which manifests itself by enlargement of the clitoris and varying degrees of anatomic deviations from the normal such as labial fusion or persistence of the urogenital sinus provides an example. It is an interesting observation that the exogenous hormones, whether androgen, progesterone or estrin, tend to affect the external genitalia without a corresponding departure from the normal in the internal female genital organs (Fig. 4–2).

A possible explanation for this observation may be found in the timing of the development of the various structures in the embryo. In the normal course of events the male penis and urethra develop and scrotal fusion takes place under the influence of androgen, and the process is completed by the fourteenth week of pregnancy. On the other hand, the differentiation of the female genitalia and development of the vulvar vestibule which contains the orifices of the vagina and urethra are not complete before the twentieth week.

The hormones implicated are usually given to prevent abortion. By and large they are given before the tenth week when abortion is most imminent. Curiously

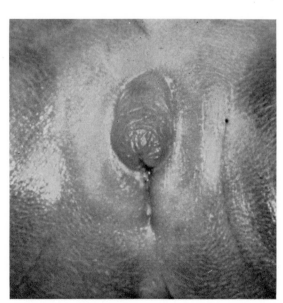

Fig. 4-2.   Clitoral hypertrophy of a newborn girl whose mother received synthetic progesterone type of hormone therapy during pregnancy. The internal genitalia were unaffected. (Courtesy of Dr. Kurt Benirschke, Boston Lying-In Hospital.)

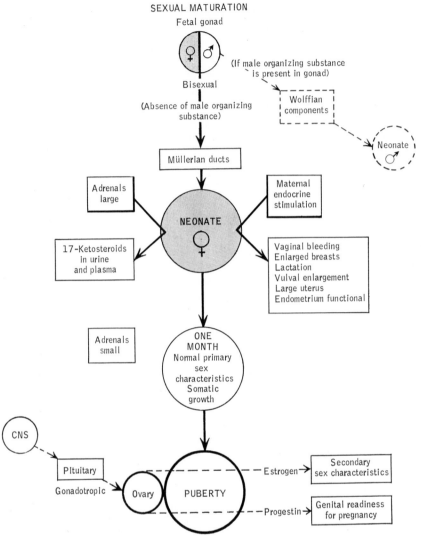

Fig. 4-3.   The normal endocrine stimuli influencing the fetal, neonatal and puberal development of the female genitalia. Administration of hormones to the mother or to the girl during childhood may upset the developmental process.

enough, oral preparations such as anhydrohydroxyprogesterone (Pranone, Progestoral, Lutocylol) seem to be much more likely to produce the masculinization than progesterone given as intramuscular injections. It is not surprising, then, that ambiguous external genitalia appear (Fig. 4–3). The male element, which appears earlier in developmental time, is stimulated, while the female component is suppressed.

When one encounters an infant with (1) an enlarged clitoris, perhaps somewhat smaller than one sees in the adrenogenital syndrome, but still large enough to be obvious, and (2) varying degrees of fusion of the labial-genital folds, one should be suspicious of the possibility that the effect may have been produced by the ingestion of either an androgen, estrin or progestin by the mother early in pregnancy.

This is not a universal response, for not every woman who has this sort of therapy produces an infant with an enlarged clitoris and fusion of the labial-scrotal folds. It appears only occasionally. Hormone therapy to prevent miscarriage is worthwhile, for many women with progestational deficiencies have borne babies who otherwise would not. Diabetic mothers have likewise been able to deliver normal children under the influence of intensive estrin therapy. A word of caution is offered, however, particularly in view of the advent of the newer progestational drugs (Norlutin, Delalutin), which are approximately five times as powerful as the old forms of progestin. One may expect that they will be used more frequently in the future in women who have infertility problems.

Why Do Progestin and Estrin Produce Masculinization?

One might expect male characteristics to appear in the female child as the result of testosterone ingestion by the mother. It is well known that phallic enlargement can be produced by androgenic stimulation at any time, either before or after birth. It is less easy to understand why an infant is masculinized by oral progestin or estrin.

As far as progestin is concerned, one must presuppose possibly an abnormal permeability of the placental membrane, for under normal conditions large amounts of progesterone are secreted by the corpus luteum and placenta. With this there must be an abnormal metabolism of the progesterone. The chemical structure of progestin and androgen is similar.

The mechanism of masculinization following the use of estrin is even less clear. One must postulate an increased production of androgen by the fetal adrenal as the result of increased estrin stimulation. There is some experimental evidence in rats, but none in the human being, that the size of the adrenal can be increased by the administration of estrogen. It has also been shown that estradiol given to pregnant rats will inhibit the development of the female genital system. There must, however, be a high degree of selection, for estrin has been given to diabetic mothers very early in pregnancy and in large doses without any evidence of masculinization in their infants.

Why Is It Important to Differentiate Masculinization Due to Hormone Therapy from the Adrenogenital Syndrome?

In most instances masculinization in the infant is due to the adrenogenital syndrome. In extremely rare instances the same picture can be produced by the presence of maternal arrhenoblastoma. These are rare tumors, and their association with pregnancy is even more remote. Pseudohermaphroditism, which is part of the adrenogenital syndrome, accounts for half of all cases of abnormal sex differentiation.

It is important to distinguish between the child who has an enlarged clitoris and abnormal external genitalia due to hormone ingestion by the mother, and the girl who has the same anatomic abnormalities due to congenital adrenal hyperplasia.

The important factor to remember is that the basic adrenal defect in adrenogenital hyperplasia is a lack in the proper enzyme mechanism to complete the synthesis of hydrocortisone. There is therefore instead a continual production of excess androgen after birth and up to adult life. Conversely, any androgenic effect from the ingestion of hormones by the mother took place during the embryonic developmental phase, but ceased after birth or when the therapeutic hormones were discontinued. Except for the obvious anatomic deviation the genital tract is entirely normal. If need be, surgical correction can be carried out to amputate the phallus and restore a functional vaginal outlet. Subsequently the child develops normally and may be expected to have children of her own. One does not have to be concerned with continuing production of androgen, as in the adrenogenital syndrome.

REFERENCES

Environmental Factors in Congenital Anomalies

Burke, B. S., Harding, V. V., and Stuart, H. C.: Nutrition Studies during Pregnancy—Relation of Protein Content of Mother's Diet during Pregnancy to Birth Length, Birth Weight, and Condition of Infant at Birth. *J. Pediat.*, 23: 506, 1943.

Collins, I. S.: Incidence of Congenital Malformations Following Maternal Rubella at Various Stages of Pregnancy. *M.J. Australia*, 2: 456, 1953.

Feldman, H. A.: Toxoplasmosis. *Pediatrics*, 22: 559, 1958.

Fraser, F. C.: Antenatal Factors in Congenital Defects; Problems and Pitfalls. *New York State J. Med.*, 59:1597, 1959.

Hicks, S. P.: Developmental Malformations Produced by Radiation: Timetable of Their Development. *Am. J. Roentgenol.*, 69: 272, 1953.

Hill, A. B., Doll, R., Galloway, McL., and Hughes, J. P.: Virus Diseases in Pregnancy and Congenital Defects. *Brit. J. Prev. & Soc. Med.*, 12: 1, 1958.

Ingalls, T. H.: Causes and Prevention of Developmental Defects. *J.A.M.A.*, 161: 1047, 1956.

Jackson, A. D., and Fisch, L.: Deafness Following Maternal Rubella—Results of Prospective Investigation. *Lancet*, 2: 1241, 1958.

Langman, J., Van Drunen, H., and Bouman, F.: Maternal Protein Metabolism and Embryonic Development in Human Beings. *Am. J. Obst. & Gynec.*, 77: 546, 1959.

Lock, F. R., Gatling, H. B., Mauzy, C. H., and Wells, H. B.: Incidence of Anomalous Development following Maternal Rubella. *Am. J. Obst. & Gynec.*, 81: 451, 1961.

Logan, W. P. D.: Incidence of Congenital Malformations and Their Relation to Virus Infections during Pregnancy. *Brit. M.J.*, 2: 641, 1951.

McDonald, A. D.: Maternal Health and Congenital Defect—A Prospective Investigation. *New England J. Med.*, 258: 767, 1958.

Murphy, D. P.: Ovarian Irradiation and Health of Subsequent Child—A Review of More than 200 Previously Unreported Pregnancies in Women Subjected to Pelvic Irradiation. *Surg., Gynec. & Obst.*, 48: 766, 1929.

Newcombe, H. B.: Detection of Genetic Trends in Public Health; in Effect of Radiation on Human Heredity. World Health Organization, Geneva, AEC Publ. No. 560, 1957, p. 157.

Pitt, D. B.: Congenital Malformations and Maternal Rubella. *M.J. Australia*, 1: 233, 1957.

Plummer, G.: Anomalies Occurring in Children Exposed in Utero to the Atomic Bomb in Hiroshima. *Pediatrics*, 10: 687, 1952.

Portmann, U. V., and McCullagh, E. P.: Developmental Defects Following Irradiation of Ovaries in Child. *J.A.M.A.*, 151: 736, 1953.

Record, R. G.: Environmental Influences in the Aetiology of Congenital Malformations. *Proc. Roy. Soc. Med.*, 51: 147, 1958.

Siegel, M., and Greenberg, M.: Poliomyelitis in Pregnancy—Effect on Fetus and Newborn Infant. *J. Pediat.*, 49: 280, 1956.

Idem: Virus Diseases in Pregnancy and Their Effects on the Fetus. Preliminary Report of a Controlled Prospective Study. *Am. J. Obst. & Gynec.*, 77: 620, 1959.

Idem: Fetal Death, Malformation and Prematurity after Maternal Rubella. *New England J. Med.*, 262: 389, 1960.

Smith, C. A.: Effects of Maternal Undernutrition upon Newborn Infant in Holland (1944–1945). *J. Pediat.*, 30: 229, 1947.

Warburton, D.: Factors in Etiology of Spontaneous Abortion. M.Sc. Thesis, McGill University, 1959.

Warkany, J., and Schraffenberger, E.: Congenital Malformation Induced in Rats by Roentgen Rays; Skeletal Changes in Offspring Following Single Irradiation of Mother. *Am. J. Roentgenol.*, 57: 455, 1947.

Wilson, J. G.: Differentiation and the Reaction of Rat Embryos to Radiation. *J. Cell. & Comp. Physiol.*, 43: (Suppl. 1) 11, 1954.

Idem: Experimental Studies on Congenital Malformations. *J. Chr. Dis.*, 10: 111, 1959.

Wilson, J. G., Roth, C. B., and Warkany, J.: Analysis of Syndrome of Malformations Induced by Maternal Vitamin A Deficiency. Effects of Restoration of Vitamin A at Various Times during Gestation. *Am. J. Anat.*, 92: 189, 1953.

Anomalies Produced by Antimetabolites and Hormones

Grunwaldt, E., and Bates, T.: Non-adrenal Female Pseudohermaphrodism after Administration of Testosterone to Mother during Pregnancy. *Pediatrics*, 20: 503, 1957.

Hayles, A. B., and Nolan, R. B.: Female Pseudohermaphroditism—Report of Case in an Infant Born of a Mother Receiving Methyl-Testosterone during Pregnancy. *Proc. Staff Meet., Mayo Clin.*, 32: 41, 1957.

Hillman, D. A.: Fetal Masculinization with Maternal Progesterone Therapy. *Canad. M.A.J.*, 80: 200, 1959.

Meltzer, H. J.: Congenital Anomalies Due to Attempted Abortion with 4-Aminopteroglutamic Acid. *J.A.M.A.*, 161: 1253, 1956.

Nellhaus, G. N.; Artificially Induced Female Pseudohermaphroditism. *New England J. Med.*, 258: 935, 1958.

Nelson, M. M., Asling, C. W., and Evans, H. M.: Production of Multiple Congenital Abnormalities in Young by Maternal Pteroylglutamic Acid Deficiency during Gestation. *J. Nutrition*, 48: 61, 1953.

Nelson, M. M., Baird, C. D. C., Wright, H. V., and Evans, H. M.: Multiple Congenital Abnormalities in the Rat Resulting from Riboflavin Deficiency Induced by the Antimetabolite Galactoflavin. *J. Nutrition*, 58: 125, 1956.

Nelson, M. M., Wright, H. V., Baird, C. D. C., and Evans, H. M.: Effect of Thirty-Six Hour Period of Pteroylglutamic Acid (PGA) Deficiency on Fetal Development in Rat. *Proc. Soc. Exper. Biol. & Med.*, 92: 554, 1956.

O'Dell, B. L., Whitley, J. R., and Hogan, A. G.: Vitamin B_{12} Factor in Prevention of Hydrocephalus in Infant Rats. *Proc. Soc. Exper. Biol. & Med.*, 76: 349, 1951.

Ray, E. W., Sterling, K., and Gardner, L. I.: Congenital Cretinism Associated with I^{131} Therapy of the Mother. A.M.A. *J. Dis. Child.*, 98: 506, 1959.

Warkany, J., Beaudry, P. H., and Hornstein, S.: Attempted Abortion with Aminopterin (4-Amino-Pteroylglutamic Acid). A.M.A. *J. Dis. Child.*, 97: 274, 1959.

Whitehouse, D. B., and McKeown, T.: Note on Significance of Attempted Abortion in Aetiology of Congenital Abnormalities. *J. Obst. & Gynaec. Brit. Emp.*, 63: 224, 1956.

Wilkins, L., Jones, H. W., Jr., Holman, G. H., and Stempfel, R. S.: Masculinization of the Female Fetus Associated with Administration of Oral and Intramuscular Progestins during Gestation: Non-adrenal Female Pseudohermaphrodism. *J. Clin. Endocrinol. & Metab.*, 18: 559, 1958.

Types of Genital Anomalies and Related Conditions

Arey, J. B.: Pathologic Findings in the Neonatal Period. *J. Pediat.*, 34: 44, 1949.

Bowman, J. A., Jr., and Scott, R. B.: Transverse Vaginal Septum. *Obst. & Gynec.*, 3: 441, 1954.

Brayton, D., and Norris, W. J.: Further Experiences with the Treatment of Imperforate Anus. *Surg., Gynec. & Obst.*, 107: 719, 1958.

Calvin, J. K., and Nichamin, S. J.: Hematocolpos Due to Imperforate Hymen. *Am. J. Dis. Child.*, 51: 832, 1936.

Cohen, H. J., Klein, M. D., and Laver, M. B.: Cysts of the Vagina in the Newborn Infant. A.M.A *J. Dis. Child.*, 94: 322, 1957.

Davis, M. E., and Potter, E. L.: Congenital Malformations and Obstetrics. *Pediatrics*, 19: 719, 1957.

Gross, R. E.: *The Surgery of Infancy and Childhood.* Philadelphia, W. B. Saunders Company, 1953.

Gruenwald, P.: Survey of Congenital Anomalies in 1131 Necropsies. *Illinois M.J.*, 79: 55, 1941.

Jones, H. W., Jr.: Female Hermaphroditism without Virilization. *Obst. & Gynec. Survey*, 12: 433, 1957.

Lide, T. N., and Coker, W. G.: Congenital Hydrometrocolpos: Review of the Literature and Report of a Case with Uterus Duplex and Incompletely Septate Vagina. *Am. J. Obst. & Gynec.*, 64: 1275, 1952.

McIntosh, R., Merritt, K. K., Richards, M. R., Samuels, M. H., and Bellows, M. T.: Incidence of Congenital Malformations: Study of 5964 Pregnancies. *Pediatrics*, 14: 505, 1954.

Malamud, N.: Recent Trends in Classification of Neuropathological Findings in Mental Deficiency. *Am. J. Ment. Defic.*, 58: 438, 1954.

Miller, N. F., and Stout, W.: Congenital Absence of the Vagina. *Obst. & Gynec.*, 9: 48, 1957.

Moore, T. C., and Lawrence, E. A.: Congenital Malformation of the Rectum and Anus; Clinical Features and Surgical Management in 120 Cases. *Surgery*, 32: 352, 1952.

Nalle, B. C., Jr., Crowell, J. A., and Lynch, K. M., Jr.: Solitary Pelvic Kidney with Vaginal Aplasia. *Obst. & Gynec. Survey*, 4: 874, 1949.

Neel, J. V.: A Study of Major Congenital Defects in Japanese Infants. *Am. J. Human Genet.*, 10: 398, 1958.

Nowlin, P., Adams, J. R., and Nalle, B. C., Jr.: Vulvar Fusion. *J. Urol.*, 62: 75, 1949.

Patten, B. M.: Varying Developmental Mechanisms in Teratology. *Pediatrics*, 19: 734, 1957.

Potts, W. J., Riker, W. L., and De Boer, A.: Imperforate Anus with Recto-vesical, -urethral, -vaginal and -perineal Fistula. *Ann. Surg.*, 140: 381, 1954.

Rosenthal, A. H.: Symptomatic Genital Anomalies in Childhood. *Clin. Obst. & Gynec.*, 3: 146, 1960.

Thomson, G. R.: Complete Congenital Absence of the Vagina Associated with Bilateral Herniae of Uterus, Tubes, and Ovaries. *Brit. J. Surg.*, 36: 99, 1948.

Warkany, J.: Role of Congenital Anomalies in Etiology of Chronic Disease. *J. Chr. Dis.*, 3: 46, 1956.

Warner, R. E., and Mann, R. M.: Hematocolpos with Imperforate Hymen; Report of Five Cases. *Obst. & Gynec.*, 6: 405, 1955.

Chapter 5

Genetic Sex:

The Sex Chromatin Pattern

THE ACTUAL pattern of genetic sex is determined at the time of fertilization of the ovum. Whether or not the child of this union develops normally or demonstrates abnormal structural, organic or mental traits depends on the composition of the fertilized egg (the zygote). If there are abnormalities in the zygote, one can expect a congenital defect to appear.

Over the past thirty years there has been universal acceptance of the presence within the human nuclear substance of forty-eight chromosomes, one half traceable to the maternal germ cell, the other half stemming from the paternal side. Recently there has been reported new, well documented evidence showing that the chromosomes actually are forty-six in number, rather than forty-eight.

In the natural process of formation of a germ cell each of the twenty-three paired chromosomes divides meiotically with only half of each pair entering the final germ cell. It seems to be largely a matter of chance whether chromosomes containing genes of maternal or paternal origin finally predominate. The final mature germ cell therefore is a composite of maternal and paternal genes, crossovers and mutant chromosomes. As a result all manner of combinations are possible. The twenty-two paired autosomal chromosomes are each responsible for some special phases of development. It may be structural growth or some special element in organ or system maturation. Thus every hereditary trait is determined by the action of single or multiple genes.

In addition to the twenty-two paired autosomes, the mature germ cell contains one of a pair of sex chromosomes, thus bringing the final total to twenty-three. The male differs from the female germ cell in the nature of these paired sex chromosomes or heterochromosomes. In the human female the mature germ cell normally always contains an X chromosome, while the male cell has either an X or a smaller Y chromosome.

Diagrammatically, one may plot the result to be anticipated (Fig. 5–1). Thus at fertilization 50 per cent of the eggs will be XX, or female, and 50 per cent XY, or male.

How Are the Numbers of Chromosomes Identified?

It has never been an easy problem to study chromosomes in the human being. Nevertheless, in recent years, significant investigative work has been done on (1)

45

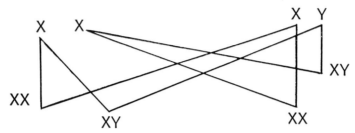

Fig. 5-1.   Diagram showing how an ovum with an X chromosome (at upper left), when fertilized by a sperm with either an X or a Y chromosome (at upper right), will result in a zygote with XY chromosomes (a male) or XX chromosomes (a female).

tissue obtained from testicular biopsy, (2) squashed cell preparations, and (3) tissue culture material. The true sex of some hermaphrodites, for example, was established after an intensive review of material from gonadal biopsies. Tissue cultures of dermal cells were helpful in identifying the Y chromosome.

Several recent advances have simplified the technique of evaluating human chromosomes. (1) In the field of tissue culture, short-term cultures of marrow cells obtained by sternal puncture have supplanted older methods which had the disadvantage of being both time-consuming and expensive. Moreover, the newer technique reduced the possibility of anomalies appearing because the material was left in tissue culture too long. (2) The specific Feulgen stain for desoxyribonucleic acid has been helpful in its power to sharpen the details involved in identifying the nuclear sex chromatin, which has always been hard to recognize. (3) The most important advance has been the utilization of the so-called squash technique used in the study of cells after the mitoses have been arrested by the addition of colchicine. Colchicine not only arrests mitotic division, but also tends to prevent the crowding of chromosomes on a spindle. Because there are more cells with identifiable chromosomes available, owing to the arrest in mitotic activity, and they are less crowded together, owing to the inhibition in spindle formation, the evaluation is greatly simplified.

THE SQUASH TECHNIQUE.   A wide variety of tissues may be used, but for the most part the cells for chromosome study have been obtained from the bone marrow by sternal puncture. The marrow cells are then suspended in a solution of glucose, saline and serum from the patient's own blood. The hypotonicity of the solution causes the cells to expand, so that the chromosomes can be separated out more easily. The cell suspension is then incubated and exposed to colchicine for one hour. The material is now fixed and stained with the Feulgen stain, which tends to sharpen the detail as well as being specific for chromosome detection. A drop of the stained material is placed on a glass slide and covered with a glass slip. The slip is then crushed against the slide by pressure of the thumb exerted through filter paper protection.

The technique of matching up chromosomes, despite the improvements, is not an easy one. It still requires a painstaking search and complete knowledge of the variations in chromosome patterns, particularly when they have been treated with colchicine.

In a recent study Court-Brown and co-workers noted three possible areas where variations might appear in chromosome counts of marrow cells: (*a*) artefacts, (*b*) mitotic abnormalities, and (*c*) mosaicism. In a large series they found 12 per cent with chromosome counts less than 46 (usually 45) and only 2 per cent with more than the

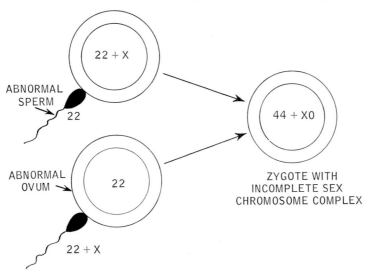

Fig. 5-2. Mechanisms that may lead to the production of a zygote with XO sex chromosomes. (Modified from M. L. Barr and D. H. Carr.)

modal number. They believe that by far the greatest number of departures from the normal expectancy are due to artefacts in preparation. The chromosomes seem to resist the trauma of crushing, but the nuclear membrane, made fragile by the hypotonic salt solution, is apt to fragment and disappear, carrying with it one or more chromosomes. It would appear, then, that the modal number is the true somatic number and that most variations are due to faulty preparation of the slide.

It is also apparent that some of the cells which show an atypical count do so because some of the chromosomes have split without being recognized. They may be widely separated and are counted as two chromosomes.

It is important to determine the true chromosome picture before classifying the patient as a mosaic (neither one sex nor the other). For example, a true case of gonadal dysgenesis or Turner's syndrome will have the chromosome arrangement XO with forty-five chromosomes. Many congenital abnormalities are noted in patients who have Turner's syndrome. They are probably due to a complete loss of a chromosome with all the genes responsible for a particular phase of development. In certain cases of Turner's the XO pattern is not found universally in all tissue. There may be patches of cells showing an XX pattern immediately adjacent to an XO. This patient may be a mosaic, or perhaps the odd picture is due to a mutation or partial loss of a chromosome (Fig. 5–2).

The differences noted in the counts are probably due more to persistent errors in tabulation than to the likelihood that there is any real variation in the number of chromosomes in individuals. There has been enough confirmatory evidence from laboratories throughout the world to accept the fact that man has forty-six chromosomes rather than forty-eight. It also seems likely that there are more clinically significant deviations from the normal number than we ever believed existed before.

Why Is It Important to Know the Number of Chromosomes?

Knowledge that the total chromosome component is not standard is of great importance in the understanding of some of the gynecologic problems of childhood and adolescence. In recent years many interesting and noteworthy contributions have been made as the result of attempts to determine the proper nuclear sex of an individual. For example, it is now known that patients with Klinefelter's syndrome, for the most part, are chromatin positive and therefore genetically female, while the patient with gonadal dysgenesis is chromatin negative and therefore genetically more like a male. To these interesting bits of information can now be added the observation that there is an actual alteration in the chromosomal pattern, for the Klinefelter's type will have an extra X and be XXY, while one of the sex chromosomes is missing in Turner's syndrome, so that the patient is XO.

Other defects appear in the autosomes. It is now well recognized that the mongoloid patient has an extra chromosome which is probably an autosome. These patients, then, have forty-seven chromosomes. The basis for the interest in the chromosome number of mongoloid patients came from a study of patients with leukemia in whom an abnormal number of chromosomes was found. The frequency of the association of mongolism with leukemia led to the discovery of an extra chromosome. Another reason for investigating the chromosomal pattern of the mongoloid stemmed from the observation that many patients with Klinefelter's syndrome, in which an extra chromosome is present, had mental defects. Recently a case has been reported in which Klinefelter's syndrome and mongolism coexisted. It is not surprising to find that this patient had forty-eight chromosomes, gaining one sex chromosome from Klinefelter's syndrome and one small autosome because of the mongolism. In mongolism the extra chromosome is generally believed to be due to tripling of the pairs. It would appear to be an autosome and not an extra small Y, which it closely resembles.

Finally, for the first time there has been reported a superfemale with an extra X chromosome and a chromosomal number of forty-seven. This patient is therefore XXX. One would expect such a patient to have all the feminine attributes in excess, but the one patient reported has underdeveloped external genitalia and breasts, secondary amenorrhea and deficient follicular development in the ovary.

How Do Genes Influence the Rate of Growth?

It is a well known clinical observation that girls grow in physical stature much faster during infancy and childhood and reach physical maturity much sooner than boys do. This is true not only of human beings, but also of such laboratory animals as the chimpanzee, rhesus monkey and rat.

The stimulus to skeletal growth apparently begins very early in intrauterine life with the appearance of certain ossification centers in the female, fully two weeks ahead of beginning bone development in the male. The increment of growth is progressive from then on until puberty, when the female sex hormones appear and epiphysial closure takes place. At the time of birth the female child has progressed several weeks in development over and above the growth rate of the male, and by the time the menarche appears girls may be fully two years ahead of the male. Similar differences are noted between the sexes when other indications of growth are considered, such as the date of eruption of teeth and the growth curve of physical measurements other than height alone. The reason for this phenomenon is not immediately apparent.

It would appear from recent studies made on patients with Klinefelter's syndrome, who have an XXY chromosome pattern, and Turner's syndrome (gonadal dysgenesis) in which an XO chromosome arrangement exists, that the genes in the

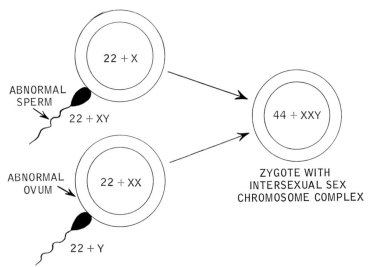

Fig. 5-3.   Mechanisms that may result in a zygote with XXY sex chromosome complex. Note also Figures 5–2 and 5–4.

Y chromosome are responsible for the retardation in skeletal maturation. This is an interesting development, for previously the Y chromosomes were believed to be inert. Evidently the genes in the Y chromosomes are responsible for the differentiation of the gonad. This begins early in fetal life, probably around the seventh week. It would seem, then, that as the gonad differentiates toward the male side retardation in the growth rate begins (Fig. 5–3).

. The reason why growth retardation of males persists through childhood is not well understood. We know little about the growth hormone of the human pituitary, for it has not yet been recovered in quantity. We do know that the thyroid is implicated and that its hypofunction is associated with deceleration in the growth rate generally. There appears to be some unknown factor in the tissues themselves that determines the rate of growth. For example, any debilitating illness will retard growth, but a pronounced acceleration is noted upon recovery. An automatic brake appears from somewhere, however, for the spurt in growth then ceases and does not go beyond the pattern previously set for that individual.

What about the Chromosomes and Body Build?

By and large the weight of the individual follows the pattern of height. As far as body build itself is concerned, the child with the sex chromatin pattern of the male is always more muscular than the female. In all probability the male habitus is not the result of the action of the Y chromosomes acting either directly on the muscle tissue or indirectly through the secretion of fetal androgen. For example, the Klinefelter children, who are XXY, do not resemble normal male children, who are XY. The difference seems to lie in the presence of the double X (XX) chromosome, which acts to inhibit the degree of muscular development one expects to find in the male.

It would appear, then, that the chromosomes do influence the rate of maturation in man. The Y chromosome, previously believed to be inert, does play a role in development, but largely through its power to influence the differentiation of the gonad along masculine lines.

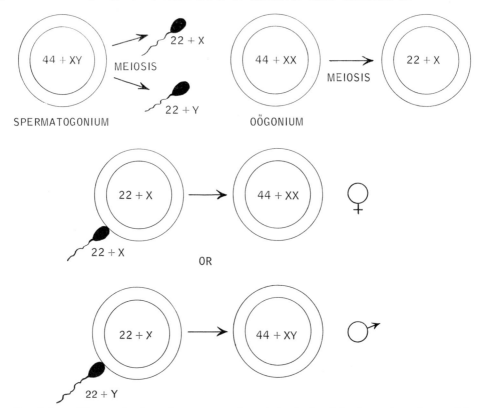

Fig. 5-4.   The mechanism of gametogenesis and the basis of the formation of normal human female and male zygotes illustrated diagrammatically for comparison with Figures 5–2 and 5–3.

How Do the Sex Chromosomes Act in Abnormal Differentiation of the Gonad?

The major deviations from the normal chromosomal pattern have almost all been in the sex chromosomes. The only exception to this to date is noted in mongolism, in which the extra chromosome is known to be an autosome. We recognize that the large X chromosome has a female connotation, while the smaller Y is found in the male. The female with two similar X chromosomes (XX) is homogenetic, while the male is heterogenetic, since the chromosomes are dissimilar (XY). It should be easy to recognize one to the exclusion of the other, but the geneticist must be well versed in the variables that may appear, particularly if the cells are in mitosis or the investigations are carried out in cell groups treated with colchicine to arrest mitoses, where many strange forms are encountered (Fig. 5-4).

The abnormal sex chromosomes can be responsible for many intersex problems. They seem to act in bringing about an abnormal differentiation in the gonad.

In the course of the normal embryologic development the primary gonad has both sex components up to about the seventh week of intrauterine life. The medullary portion of the gonad contains the male element, while the female potential rests in the cortex. The direction in which the cells develop is determined very early in the game by the sex hormones (XX, female, and XY, male). Under normal conditions if development starts in one direction, it will continue to progress along that line, while the other element is repressed. For progress to continue along the male line it is absolutely essential for the gonad to secrete a fetal androgen. Apparently the feminizing factor is not necessary to become a female. If for any reason the masculinizing factor is inhibited, development will occur along the female pattern, regardless of the genetic sex of the individual. This, then, is sex reversal.

How Important Is It to Determine the Sex Chromatin Pattern?

From a practical clinical point of view it is far more important to determine the sex chromatin pattern of the child than to know the number of the chromosomes. The chromosomes and known aberrations that result in deviations from the normal pattern of genital growth and function are fortunately few in number. In many instances, however, it is of the greatest clinical importance to determine the sex of the gonad. For example, the child with congenital hyperplasia of the adrenal, despite the fact that she demonstrates abnormalities in the external genitalia and lower part of the vagina, has in most instances a perfectly normal uterus and ovaries. The chromosome pattern is invariably female. Not only should such a child be reared as a female, but also with surgical correction of her anatomic anomaly she may expect to function normally and have a family of her own. The same thing may be said about the child who has clitoral enlargement and labial fusion because of the hormones ingested by the mother. On the other hand, the other nonhormonal types of ambisexual development may have either ovaries or testes or a combination of both and may have either the male or female sex chromatin pattern.

Before the physician decides upon the proper sex to rear the child he will need all the information he can get in these ambiguous cases. The sex chromatin pattern as determined by buccal smear, blood smear or skin biopsy is not as accurate as actual biopsy of the gonad. It does, however, provide useful information until such time as the physician wishes to have the abdomen explored. It should also be kept in mind that in a few of the most doubtful cases gonadal tissue may not be available for biopsy because it cannot be identified at operation (Fig. 5–5).

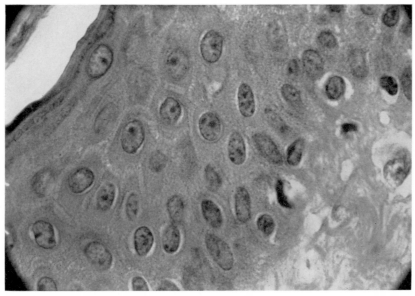

Fig. 5-5.   A skin biopsy was made to determine the genetic sex. Two epidermal cells in the center of the illustration have dark-stained chromatin masses attached to the nuclear membrane. These are the female sex chromatin bodies, indicating a genetic female. $\times$ 800.

For practical purposes it can be said that the sex chromatin determination as established by buccal smears will truly reflect the gonadal structure. There are a few exceptions. In Klinefelter's syndrome the child will have small, atrophic scrotal testes, vas deferens, prostate and penile urethra, yet often a female sex chromatin pattern. Apparently a complete sex reversal takes place in the embryonic ovary which permits the differentiation of the wolffian duct structures early in development. The reverse of this process is seen in Turner's syndrome (gonadal dysgenesis), in which the sex chromatin pattern is predominantly male, yet the patient has a uterus and vagina, but no ovaries. In this instance müllerian duct differentiation continued while the fetal testes regressed before they could adequately establish wolffian duct development.

In the presence of either of these two conditions, which fortunately are rare, the physician should determine the true sex by an actual biopsy of the gonad, but should treat the child according to the appearance of the external genitalia.

What Are the Common Methods of Determining the Sex Chromatin Pattern?

The sex chromatin pattern was originally identified by biopsy of the gonads. Later it became evident that almost any human tissue except the basal layer of the skin would provide enough nuclear detail to determine the chromosome arrangement. Biopsies are not in general use, but are of particular value to check the evidence provided by microscopic study of (*a*) blood smears or (*b*) cell scrapings from the buccal mucosa.

THE BLOOD SMEAR.   The extra mass of chromatin, which contains the two X heterochromosomes, appears in the form of a so-called drumstick attached to the nucleus of the polymorphonuclear leukocyte. Under oil immersion the "drumstick" appears as a hyperchromatic area approximately 1.5 microns in diameter and

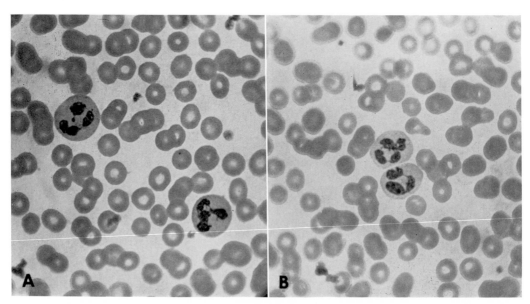

Fig. 5-6.   *A*, Blood smear from a woman, with a typical "drumstick" attached to the uppermost nuclear mass of the neutrophilic leukocyte at the upper left. *B*, Blood smear from a man, with small, nondiagnostic "clubs" attached to the nuclear chromatin of the upper neutrophil. Wright's stain, × 1200. (Courtesy of Dr. Charles P. Emerson.)

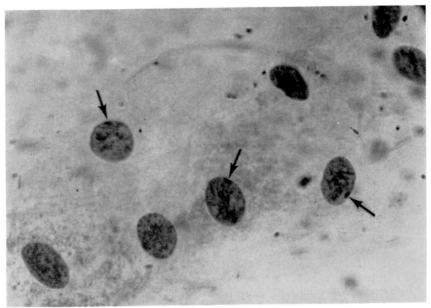

Fig. 5-7.   Buccal smear with female type of nuclear chromatin bodies indicated. Feulgen stain,
× 1200.

attached by a fine stem to the nucleus of the leukocyte (Fig. 5–6). Experience will differentiate "small clubs" or accessory lobes of the nucleus, which are simply morphologic variations and have nothing to do with the establishment of sex chromatin.

When 6 such drumsticks are noted in the examination of 200 or 300 cells, the patient is said to be chromatin positive, or female. If none are found after examination of 500 or more cells, the subject is said to be chromatin negative, or male.

THE BUCCAL SMEAR.   Barr and his co-workers developed a simple method of determining the sex chromatin pattern of an individual. Scrapings are taken from the inner surface of the mucosa of the cheek with the sharp edge of a tongue depressor. The material is then spread on a slide and immediately immersed in the same solution one applies for a vaginal smear, namely, equal parts of ether and 95 per cent alcohol. The smears are then stained with the Feulgen method, which is specific for nucleo-protein.

The difference in the cytologic appearance of the cell nucleus provides the clue to sex differentiation. In the female pattern many, sometimes at least 50 per cent of the cell nuclei counted, will show a distinct mass that stains deeply and assumes a round or biconvex shape lying beneath the nuclear membrane. It is rarely more than 1 micron in size (Fig. 5–7).

It is interesting that all cells and all tissues do not show the characteristic body of chromatin. For example, it is frequently not visible in the basal layer of the skin or in lymphocytes. The presence of two X chromosomes is necessary for the appearance of the sex chromatin body. There must be some other factor as yet unknown to explain the absence of the chromatin body in some normal female patients. The important point in the differentiation of male from female lies in the fact that only 3 to 4 per cent of the male cells show this mass. It is something of a mystery why any male cells should.

For all practical purposes the appearance of this concentration of nuclear material within the nucleus in many of the cells studied is a reliable indication of the feminine sex.

REFERENCES

Ashley, D. J. B., and Jones, C. H.: Discrepancies in the Diagnosis of Genetic Sex by Leucocyte Morphology. *Lancet,* 1: 240, 1958.

Barr, M. L.: The Skin Biopsy Test of Chromosomal Sex in Clinical Practice. *Anat. Rec.,* 121: 387, 1955.

Barr, M. L., and Carr, D. H.: Sex Chromatin, Sex Chromosomes and Sex Anomalies. *Canad. M.A.J.,* 83: 979, 1960.

Böök, J. A., and Reed, S. C.: Empiric Risk Figures in Mongolism. *J.A.M.A.,* 143: 730, 1950.

Bradbury, J., Bunge, R. G., and Boccabella, R. A.: Chromatin Test in Klinefelter's Syndrome. *J. Clin. Endocrinol. & Metab.,* 16: 689, 1956.

Briggs, D. K., and Kuppermann, H. S.: Sex Differentiation by Leukocyte Morphology. *J. Clin. Endocrinol.,* 16: 1163, 1956.

Bunge, R. G., and Bradbury, J. T.: Genetic Sex: Chromatin Test versus Gonadal Histology. *J. Clin. Endocrinol.,* 16: 1117, 1956.

Carpentier, P. J., and Potter, E. L.: Nuclear Sex and Genital Malformation in Forty-Eight Cases of Renal Agenesis, with Special Reference to Nonspecific Female Pseudohermaphroditism. *Am. J. Obst. & Gynec.,* 78: 235, 1959.

Court-Brown, W. M., Jacobs, P., and Doll, R.: Interpretation of Chromosome Counts Made on Bone-Marrow Cells. *Lancet,* 1: 160, 1960.

Davidson, W. M.: Sex Determination: Diagnostic Methods. *Brit. M.J.,* 1: 1901, 1960.

De Grouchy, J., Lamy, M., Frezal, J., and Ribier, J.: XX/XO Mosaics in Turner's Syndrome. *Lancet,* 1: 1369, 1961.

Ferguson-Smith, M. A.: The Prepubertal Testicular Lesion in Chromatin-Positive Klinefelter's Syndrome (Primary Microorchidism) as Seen in Mentally Handicapped Children. *Lancet,* 1: 219, 1959.

Idem: Cytogenetics in Man. *A.M.A. Arch. Int. Med.,* 105: 627, 1960.

Ford, C. E., and Hammerton, J. L.: Chromosomes of Man. *Nature,* 178: 1020, 1956.

Ford, C. E., Jacobs, P. A., and Lajtha, L. G.: Human Somatic Chromosomes. *Nature,* 181: 1565, 1958.

Ford, C. E., Jones, K. W., Polani, P. E., Almeida, J. C., and Briggs, J. H.: A Sex-Chromosome Anomaly in a Case of Gonadal Dysgenesis (Turner's Syndrome). *Lancet,* 1: 711, 1959.

Ford, C. E., and others: The Chromosomes in a Patient Showing Both Mongolism and the Klinefelter Syndrome. *Lancet,* 1: 4, 1959.

Fraser, F. C.: Medical Genetics in Pediatrics. *J. Pediat.,* 44: 85, 1954.

Idem: Genetic Counselling in Some Common Paediatric Diseases. *Pediat. Clin. N. Amer.,* 5: 475, 1958.

Gluecksohn-Waelsch, S.: Genetic Control of Embryonic Growth and Differentiation. *J. Nat. Cancer Inst.,* 15: 629, 1954.

Greenblatt, R. B.: Clinical Aspects of Sexual Abnormalities in Man. *Rec. Prog. Hormone Res.,* 14: 335, 1958.

Greenblatt, R. B., and Manautou, J. M.: A Simplified Staining Technique for the Study of Chromosomal Sex in Oral Mucosal and Peripheral Blood Smears. *Am. J. Obst. & Gynec.,* 74: 629, 1957.

Greene, R., Matthews, D., Hughesdon, P. E., and Howard, A.: Further Note on Cytological Findings in Case of True Hermaphroditism. *Brit. J. Surg.,* 41: 548, 1954.

Grumbach, M. M.: Chromosomal Sex and the Prepuberal Diagnosis of Gonadal Dysgenesis. *Pediatrics,* 20: 740, 1957.

Grumbach, M. M., and Barr, M. L.: Cytologic Tests of Chromosomal Sex in Relation to Sexual Anomalies in Man. *Rec. Prog. Hormone Res.,* 14: 255, 1958.

Grumbach, M. M., Blanc, W. A., and Engle, E. T.: Sex Chromatin Pattern in Seminiferous Tubule Dysgenesis and Other Testicular Disorders, with Relation to True Hermaphroditism and to Klinefelter's Syndrome. *J. Clin. Endocrinol. & Metab.,* 17: 703, 1957.

Haddad, H. M., and Wilkins, L.: Congenital Anomalies Associated with Gonadal Aplasia—Review of Fifty-Five Cases. *Pediatrics,* 23: 885, 1959.

Hamblen, E. C.: The Assignment of Sex to an Individual—Some Enigmas and Some Practical Clinical Criteria. *Am. J. Obst. & Gynec.,* 74: 1228, 1957.

Hayward, M. D.: Sex Chromatin Mosaicism in Man. *Heredity,* 15: 235, 1960.

Hsia, D. Yi-Yung: Medical Genetics. *New England J. Med.,* 262: 1172, 1960.

Hsu, T. C., Hooks, C. A., and Pomerat, C. M.: Opportunities for Determining Sex in Human Tissues. *Texas Rep. Biol. & Med.*, 11: 585, 1953.

Ingalls, T. H.: Causes and Prevention of Developmental Defects. *J.A.M.A.*, 161: 1047, 1956.

Jacobs, P. A., and Strong, J. A.: A Case of Human Intersexuality Having a Possible XXY Sex Determining Mechanism. *Nature*, 183: 302, 1959.

Jacobs, P. A., Baikie, A. G., Court-Brown, W. M., and Strong, J. A.: The Somatic Chromosomes in Mongolism. *Lancet*, 1: 710, 1959.

Jacobs, P. A., and others: The Evidence for the Existence of the Human "Super Female." *Lancet*, 2:423, 1959.

Idem: Use of the Term "Super Female." *Lancet*, 2: 1145, 1959.

Idem: Chromosomal Sex in the Syndrome of Testicular Feminization. *Lancet*, 2: 591, 1959.

Idem: Abnormalities Involving the X Chromosome in Women. *Lancet*, 1: 1213, 1960.

Klinefelter, H. F., Jr., Reifenstein, E. C., Jr., and Albright, F.: Syndrome Characterized by Gynecomastia, Aspermatogenesis without A-Leydigism, and Increased Excretion of Follicle Stimulating Hormone. *J. Clin. Endocrinol.*, 2: 615, 1942.

Krivit, W., and Good, R. A.: Simultaneous Occurrence of Leukemia and Mongolism; Report of 4 Cases. *A.M.A. J. Dis. Child.*, 91: 218, 1956.

LeJeune, J., Gauthier, M., and Turpin, R.: Les chromosomes humaines en culture de tissue. *Compt. Rend. Acad. de Sc.*, 248: 602, 1959.

Marberger, E., Boccabella, R. A., and Nelson, W. O.: Oral Smear as Method of Chromosomal Sex Detection. *Proc. Soc. Exper. Biol. & Med.*, 89: 488, 1955.

Naib, Z. M.: Nuclear Chromatin Sex Determination in Patients with Genital Abnormalities. *Obst. & Gynec.*, 18: 64, 1961.

Neel, J. V.: Some Applications of the Principles of Genetics to the Practice of Medicine. *M. Clin. N. Amer.*, 35: 519, 1951.

Idem: Genetics and Human Congenital Malformation. *Pediatrics*, 19: 749, 1957.

Nelson, W. O.: Sex Differences in Human Nuclei, with Particular Reference to "Klinefelter's Syndrome," Gonadal Agenesis and Other Types of Hermaphroditism. *Acta Endocrinol.*, 23: 227, 1956.

Nelson, W. O., and Boccabella, R. A.: Application of the Sex Chromatin Test. *Fertil. & Steril.*, 8: 333, 1957.

Patanelli, D. J., and Nelson, W. O.: Sex Chromatin and Chromosomes in Man. *Postgrad. Med.*, 29: 3, 1961.

Penrose, L. S.: Mongolian Idiocy (Mongolism) and Maternal Age. *Ann. New York Acad. Sc.*, 57: 494, 1954.

Idem: Parental Age and Mutation. *Lancet*, 2: 312, 1955.

Polani, P. E., Hunter, W. F., and Lennox, B.: Chromosomal Sex in Turner's Syndrome with Coarctation of Aorta. *Lancet*, 2: 120, 1954.

Reed, S. C.: *Counseling in Medical Genetics*. Philadelphia, W. B. Saunders Company, 1955.

Riis, P., Johnsen, S. G., and Mosbech, J.: Nuclear Sex in Klinefelter's Syndrome. *Lancet*, 1: 962, 1956.

Robertson-Smith, D., and Davidson, W. M.: *Symposium on Nuclear Sex*. New York, Interscience Publishers, Inc., 1958.

Severinghaus, A. E.: Sex Chromosomes in Human Intersex. *Am. J. Anat.*, 70: 73, 1942.

Sohval, A. R., Gaines, J. A., and Strauss, L.: Chromosomal Sex Detection in the Human Newborn and Fetus from Examination of the Umbilical Cord, Placental Tissue and Fetal Membranes. *Ann. New York Acad. Sc.*, 75: 905, 1959.

Stanton, E. F.: Pregnancy after Forty-Four. *Am. J. Obst. & Gynec.*, 71: 270, 1956.

Stewart, J. S. S., Ferguson-Smith, M. A., Lennox, B., and Mack, W. S.: Klinefelter's Syndrome: Genetic Studies. *Lancet*, 2: 117, 1958.

Sun, L. C. Y., and Rakoff, A. E.: Evaluation of Peripheral Blood Smear Test in Detection of Chromosomal Sex in Human. *J. Clin. Endocrinol.*, 16: 55, 1956.

Tanner, J. M., Prader, A., Habich, H., and Ferguson-Smith, M. A.: Genes on the Y Chromosome Influencing Rate of Maturation in Man—Skeletal Age Studies in Children with Klinefelter's (XXY) and Turner's (XO) Syndromes. *Lancet*, 2: 141, 1959.

Tjio, J. H., and Puck, T. T.: Somatic Chromosomes in Man. *Proc. Nat. Acad. Sc.*, 44: 1229, 1958.

Idem: Genetics of Somatic Mammalian Cells. II. Chromosomal Constitution of Cells in Tissue Culture. *J. Exper. Med.*, 108: 259, 1958.

Tristan, T. A., Eberlein, W. R., and Hope, J. W.: Roentgenologic Investigation of Patients with Heterosexual Development. *Am. J. Roentgenol.*, 76: 562, 1956.

Witschi, E.: Overripeness of Egg as Cause of Twinning and Teratogenesis. *Cancer Res.*, 12: 763, 1952.

Worcester, J., Stevenson, S. S., and Rice, R. G.: 677 Congenitally Malformed Infants and Associated Gestational Characteristics; Parental Factors. *Pediatrics*, 6: 208, 1950.

Chapter 6

Treatment of Congenital
Defects Found at Birth and in Infancy

WE HAVE stressed the fact that many of the genital defects, due to genetic cause, are similar to those noted when the explanation can be traced to the child's adrenal glands or appear in the infant because the mother has ingested hormones in the early months of her pregnancy. The former may have a female configuration with a male sex chromatin pattern, while the latter have normal internal genitalia and female sex chromatin pattern. It is important, then, to know the true sex pattern in an ambiguous case before attempting surgical correction. It is also essential that this information be made available as soon after birth as possible, so that surgical correction can be made within the first year of life to avoid the many complications that arise when the child has been reared in the wrong sex. This is true despite the fact that practical experience would suggest that it is wiser to convert the child into, and raise her as, a female regardless of the chromosomal sex, if the external genitalia have not developed sufficiently to permit them to function adequately as a male's in later life.

In addition to the use of buccal smears or skin biopsies (1) to determine the proper sex chromatin pattern, and (2) to distinguish the congenital anomalies due to genetic cause from those created by adrenal hyperplasia, the urinary assay of 17-ketosteroid excretion will help to decide whether or not the child has adrenal hyperplasia.

How Do 17-Ketosteroid Excretion Studies Establish the Diagnosis of Adrenal Hyperplasia?

After the first two weeks of age the child who is born with or without labial fusion, but with an enlarged clitoris, should have a twenty-four hour urinary assay to determine the level of the 17-ketosteroid excretion.

In the neonatal period the normal level should be less than 0.5 mg. per day. The child with adrenal hyperplasia will usually produce 2 to 6 mg. per day. Occasionally the values are borderline in the range of 1 to 2.5 mg. daily, and the diagnosis is in doubt. In this case the urine should be assayed for pregnanetriol by the method of Bongiovanni. Large amounts are recovered in patients with virilizing hyperplasia. The important factor in the differential diagnosis is the determination of the presence of excess amounts of androgen in the urine.

56

When Should the Child with Clitoral Enlargement and Labial Fusion Have Surgical Correction?

In general it may be said that the earlier the surgical correction is made, the better. If the diagnosis is clear, there is every reason to operate on the child before the age of two. The reason for this will be made clearer by the discussions on sex rearing.

If doubt exists, it will be better to postpone the surgical correction until the developmental pattern becomes less obscure. Although much information can be obtained from 17-ketosteroid determinations, pregnanetriol excretion studies and the reading of buccal smears or skin biopsies, one may prefer to perform a laparotomy to obtain actual biopsies of the gonads before deciding on the sex pattern.

The technique of the surgical procedure and the indications for operation are identical whether the underlying cause of the clitoral enlargement is adrenal hyperplasia or maternal ingestion of progesterone, androgen or estrin. Drug cause differs from the child with female pseudohermaphroditism largely in the fact that the androgenic effect is already complete and the damage done. No further virilizing activity may be expected, and it is not necessary to check the electrolyte balance or to support the infant with cortisone before, during or after the operation, as one must do when the basic problem is that of congenital hyperplasia of the adrenal cortex.

CONGENITAL ABSENCE OF THE VAGINA AND PARTITIONING

Congenital absence of the vagina is all too frequently discovered in adolescence when the girl consults the physician for the first time, because she has not had a period, or later in her life when she plans to get married. We have previously pointed out that congenital absence of the vagina can be identified at birth or in early childhood. Unfortunately the diagnosis is rarely made at this time, not so much because it is difficult to do, but more because the examination is either never done or it has been done inadequately. The fact that there may be other anomalies in the internal genital organs, genitourinary tract or bony defects in the pelvic bones makes the diagnosis important.

Before embarking on any corrective surgery it will be well to establish as far as possible the extent of the congenital abnormality. Even in the immediate neonatal period it is often possible to inject an opaque substance, such as Urokon 30 per cent, into the urogenital orifice in order that the cavity be outlined by roentgenograms. The injection may be made through a catheter or blunt-nosed syringe. The syringe is regarded as more useful. In this manner the extent and nature of the urogenital cavity can be determined. This may be a helpful diagnostic tool, particularly when the presence of labial adhesions leads to a mistaken diagnosis of vaginal atresia (Fig. 6–1).

The external genitalia in children with congenital absence of the vagina will usually appear normal, though the introitus is either lacking entirely or represented by a shallow depression. Less often a transverse partition at the upper and middle third of the vagina blocks the canal and is mistaken for congenital absence. Longitudinal partitioning may be either obvious or obscure, but the defect is far less serious than total absence of the vagina. Although early recognition of these anatomic

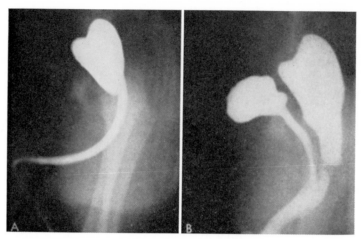

Fig. 6-1.   *A*, The first injection of Iodochloral by catheter into a single perineal orifice revealed a single structure thought to be bladder. *B*, On the second attempt, 2 weeks later, urinary bladder with urethra and vagina was demonstrated, so that vaginal atresia did not exist. (Courtesy of T. A. Tristan et al.: *Am. J. Roentgenol.*, Vol. 76.)

deviations from the normal vaginal anatomy is important, there is no immediate call for surgical correction. Since anomalies in the child's genital tract do not interfere with function, it will be well to leave them alone until puberty and the stimulus of ovarian hormonal activity make operation essential. This is particularly true when the adolescent girl has normal development of the uterus, tubes and ovaries, above the vaginal defect.

A reconstructive operation for complete absence of the vagina can be satisfactorily performed, but its chances of success are much greater if the procedure is carried out about the time of puberty, if the child has a functioning uterus and adnexa, or at the time of contemplated marriage if she has not. To be successful, the canal established surgically must be kept dilated, either by repeated coitus or by a vaginal obturator. Thus the existence of vaginal atresia should be detected in childhood, but may not be treated until years later.

IMPERFORATE HYMEN AND IMPERFORATE ANUS

The treatment of these conditions has been considered previously in the discussion of the early recognition of departures from the normal anatomy of the external genitalia (p. 29).

SEX REVERSAL

What Are the Common Examples of Sex Reversal?

The genetic implications of nuclear sex are apparent when one studies the most common examples of intersex phenomena: (*a*) the adrenogenital syndrome; (*b*) Klinefelter's syndrome; (*c*) ovarian dysgenesis (Bonnevie-Ullrich-Turner syndrome); (*d*) true hermaphroditism; (*e*) male hermaphroditism, including the testicular feminization syndrome.

Female Pseudohermaphroditism at Birth and in Infancy

The female pseudohermaphrodite presents a wide variety of developmental abnormalities in the external genitalia and vagina at birth. The most common deviation from the normal is apparent in the clitoris. This is usually enlarged and closely resembles a hypospadiac penis which has a firm fibrous cord running along the full length of its under surface. Along with it one finds fusion of the labioscrotal folds in varying patterns (Fig. 6–2). In some there may be no departure from the normal, and both the urethra and vagina have independent openings. In others the fusion is complete to the base of the enlarged clitoris. In this case the vaginal opening is obliterated and replaced by a solid partition with a median raphe resembling a scrotum. Behind it, in the midline, lies a narrow urogenital sinus which has as its only opening a narrow slitlike meatus at the base of the enlarged phallus. When lesser degrees of fusion are present, there is usually a shallow depression representing the vulva with a funnel-like opening at the posterior end into which the urethra and vagina open.

Congenital malformations of this sort, with all the variations, constitute the characteristic external picture of the child with female pseudohermaphroditism.

Why Do Congenital Anomalies Appear with Female Pseudohermaphroditism?

In most instances female pseudohermaphroditism is due to congenital hyperplasia of the adrenal gland. Rarely adrenocortical tumors are responsible. Far less often it is due to a defect in the genes. The basic underlying cause for the production of these congenital anomalies is the overproduction of androgen operating at a time in embryonic development when the müllerian ducts have completely differentiated to form the uterus and tubes, but labial fusion has not yet taken place.

In the adrenogenital syndrome (female pseudohermaphroditism) caused by congenital adrenocortical hyperplasia, the fetal adrenal apparently lacks the proper enzyme mechanism to complete the synthesis of hormones of hydrocortisone type. Hydrocortisone-type steroids normally control the output of the adrenocorticotropic

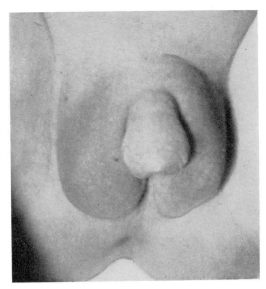

Fig. 6-2. A case of female pseudohermaphroditism characterized by the phallus-like clitoris and fused labial folds that resemble a scrotum. (Courtesy of Dr. Sydney S. Gellis, Boston City Hospital.)

hormone (ACTH) by the pituitary. When they are not produced, ACTH may be liberated in excess with the result that adrenal hyperplasia occurs and overproduction of androgen results. The fetal adrenal in this condition seems to be able to metabolize all the precursors up to hydroxyprogesterone, but something happens at this point so that other compounds than hydrocortisone are produced, among them pregnanetriol. This is why the finding of excessive quantities of urinary pregnanetriol is important in establishing the diagnosis of female pseudohermaphroditism.

What Entities Simulate the Adrenogenital Syndrome?

In earlier discussions we have noted that an enlarged clitoris with redundant foreskin and varying degrees of labial fusion are occasionally found in infants born to mothers who have received progesterone, estrogen or androgen to prevent abortion. To produce this train of events the medications had to be given early in pregnancy before anatomic development of the genitalia was complete. In a variety of ways these hormones were converted into or were responsible for an overproduction of androgen.

It is also possible to have a female pseudohermaphrodite or true hermaphrodite without hyperplasia of the adrenal gland. In some patients with defective genes the same external genital deformities are present, but these patients have either testes or ovotestes. Anatomically, they are indistinguishable. There is one important differential point. When the congenital anomalies are due to excessive androgen produced by adrenal hyperplasia, the virilization becomes more pronounced as the child continues to grow.

Congenital Hyperplasia of the Adrenal Associated with Pseudohermaphroditism and Electrolyte Imbalance

In addition to the congenital anomalies, the child with the adrenogenital syndrome may also have a severe electrolyte imbalance, particularly as it applies to sodium and potassium regulation. The clinical picture is not unlike that found in Addison's disease. Approximately one quarter of the infants who have this syndrome will lose so much sodium and potassium that death from dehydration or circulatory collapse will take place unless the condition is recognized and supportive therapy is given.

It is important, therefore, to determine at birth whether the child who has congenital anomalies of the external genitalia has hyperplasia of the adrenal gland or not. This may be done by determining the sex chromatin pattern and the level of 17-ketosteroid excretion. At the same time the infant's blood serum should be checked for sodium, potassium and carbon dioxide levels. If there is an electrolyte imbalance, the potassium level will be high and the other elements low. The chloride determinations are so variable that they may be of little value. The electrocardiogram, on the other hand, provides the quickest and most accurate method of detecting electrolyte imbalance. The variations in potassium levels produce characteristic and recognizable tracings.

How Should the Female Pseudohermaphrodite with Electrolyte Imbalance Be Treated?

Proper therapy for these infants can be a very exacting problem. There are two factors at work: (1) the tendency to lose salt and (2) the progressive virilization. The primary concern during the acute phase of dehydration is the regulation of the water and electrolyte imbalance. This can be done by replacing water and sodium chloride and giving desoxycorticosterone. The last is necessary, for an abnormal secretion of the adrenal hormones will tend to increase the sodium loss. Unless the adrenal cortical secretions are under proper control, the electrolyte imbalance may recur and become a serious problem under the stress of even a minor illness.

There still remains the problem of progressive virilization. Salt and fluid replacement and desoxycorticosterone will regulate the electrolyte imbalance, but they will do nothing to reduce the amount of excess androgen which is the cause of virilization. The best method of treatment is to combine salt replacement and desoxycorticosterone acetate with cortisone therapy. In this manner both androgen suppression and electrolyte regulation are achieved.

The doses of salt and cortisone needed vary with age, clinical condition, body weight, and so on. Some children with this problem can be satisfactorily managed at home on a daily regimen of oral cortisone, 15 to 20 mg., supplemented by 2 to 3 gm. of salt added to the diet. The parents should thoroughly understand that the daily dosage of cortisone must be increased and more salt must be added to the diet when any infection appears, however minor it may seem to be.

Treatment of the Female Pseudohermaphrodite Who Has No Electrolyte Imbalance

The most important factor in outlining proper therapy for the pseudohermaphrodite is the prior assurance that the underlying cause is congenital hyperplasia of the adrenal and that the girl does have a female sex chromatin pattern. Once the diagnosis is established the treatment can proceed along two lines: (1) suppression of the excess production of androgen and (2) surgical correction of the congenital anomalies.

CORTISONE THERAPY.   Since the basic defect in this syndrome is the inability of the child's adrenal to convert hydroprogesterone to cortisone-type steroids, they must be supplied in adequate amount, or androgen will produce progressive virilization. If the diagnosis is made at birth or before the age of two, cortisone therapy begun then is said to offer the greatest chance for the child to progress normally in growth and development.

The amount of cortisone required depends upon the ease with which the ketosteroids are depressed and maintained at a low level. The normal level for an infant is in the range of 2.5 mg. per day. The average daily maintenance dose of cortisone for a child under 2 years varies from 8 to 12 mg. when given intramuscularly. Oral medication is preferred, for the patient will have to be given cortisone for the rest of her life. The usual daily dose of cortisone administered orally is in the range of 15 to 20 mg.

SURGICAL CORRECTION.   Since the congenital anomalies in female pseudohermaphroditism are confined to the external genitalia and lower part of the vagina, and the uterus, tubes and ovaries are normal, surgical correction is possible and logical. After operation the girl has an opportunity to develop normally as a female with a perfectly good chance that she will marry and bear children. The earlier the required operative procedures are carried out, the better. If there are no problems in general health and the electrolytes are in balance, operation can be done satisfactorily any time within the first two years. When the operation is done at this age, the child will not remember it and all the psychologic hazards will be avoided, for she will never have been conscious of any defect.

The surgeon should keep firmly in mind that the child should receive twice the maintenance dose of cortisone before, during and after the operation whether she has electrolyte imbalance or not. After the seventh day the dose can be reduced to maintenance levels, provided there is no infection.

The operation chosen will depend on the degree of anatomic variation. It may be well to obtain a vaginogram to determine the type of anomaly before embarking on the surgical procedure. The majority of the operations found to be necessary are relatively easy to perform.

The overgrown clitoris may be resected if there is reason to believe that it will be a source of embarrassment in the future. This is better than partial surgical amputation, for it is less likely to be followed by a painful amputation stump. There need be no fear that the patient's libido will be jeopardized in later life. At the time this is performed the varying degrees of labioscrotal fusion can be divided, so that the urethral and vaginal orifices are exposed.

With androgen secretion therapeutically depressed and the vaginal anomalies corrected, the female child can look forward to a reasonably normal existence. The problems are more complicated when the diagnosis is made and treatment instituted later on in childhood.

Can an Adrenal or Ovarian Tumor Produce Virilization?

The masculinizing effects produced by congenital adrenal hyperplasia are obvious at birth and become more pronounced as the child grows older. This type of virilization must be distinguished from the acquired type of adrenocortical hyperplasia. The chief point in establishing the correct diagnosis of acquired hyperplasia rests in the observation that the child had perfectly normal external genitalia at birth and acquired the enlarged clitoris and hirsutism with a masculine distribution later. In both the congenital and the acquired types of adrenal hyperplasia the 17-keto-steroids will be elevated.

The most important factor to determine is whether the virilization which begins to appear in the postnatal period and has been noted as early as two months is due to acquired adrenocortical hyperplasia or to adrenocortical tumor. Fortunately the acquired type of masculinization is relatively rare, for it is most often due to malignant tumor of the adrenal cortex. A few benign tumors of the adrenal with associated virilism have been reported. It has been said that the appearance of virilizing signs up to the time of puberty, following the birth of a child with normal genital anatomy, is far more likely to be caused by tumor than hyperplasia. The chances are about equal after the menarche. The child with an adrenocortical tumor characteristically has an enlarged clitoris, demonstrates a pronounced tendency to accelerated skeletal growth and tends to exhibit early growth of axillary and pubic hair. As in the congenital and acquired types of adrenocortical hyperplasia, the child with adrenocortical tumor has an elevated 17-ketosteroid excretion.

How Is the Differential Diagnosis Established between Adrenal Hyperplasia and Adrenocortical Tumor?

The differential diagnosis is established by giving the child sufficient cortisone to suppress androgen excretion. If the elevated 17-ketosteroids are due to hyperplasia of the adrenal cortex, 100 mg. of cortisone given intramuscularly daily for one week will depress the excretion level appreciably, while no effect, or perhaps even a rise, will be noted in the presence of an adrenal tumor. The child who has a female sex chromatin pattern and elevated 17-ketosteroid excretion levels, which can be suppressed by cortisone, is considered to have adrenal hyperplasia, not adrenocortical adenoma or carcinoma. If the masculinizing signs are present at birth and normal development of the external genitalia is observed, then the child has pseudohermaphroditism and not acquired adrenal hyperplaia.

OVARIAN TUMOR. A functioning tumor of the ovary which produces virilization such as the arrhenoblastoma or an adrenal rest tumor appearing in the ovary could masculinize the external genitalia and simulate the adrenogenital syndrome or acquired adrenocortical hyperplasia.

It is theoretically possible for such tumors to appear in early childhood and to become large enough to be felt through the rectum. Gross has stated that any ovarian tumor in childhood which produces functional alteration in the external genitalia of a female infant is large enough to be felt. This theoretical possibility is unlikely to present as an actual problem, for adrenal rest tumors in the ovary are extremely rare, and only one case of arrhenoblastoma has been reported before the age of fifteen years.

TYPES OF SEXUAL DEVIATIONS ASSOCIATED WITH AN ABNORMAL SEX CHROMATIN AND CHROMOSOMAL PATTERN

KLINEFELTER'S SYNDROME

This is an example of complete sex reversal in that the child is brought up as a male because of fully developed scrotal testes, vasa deferentia, penile urethra and prostate. Microscopically, the testes typically show hyalinized seminiferous tubules and small clumps of Leydig cells, but otherwise they are atrophic. Less than 5 per cent show spermatogonia. Despite the fact that testicles are present, these patients have a female sex chromatin pattern.

The chromosomal component is also at variance with the normal, as already mentioned. Though the patient has testes, the basic genetic pattern of these patients is XX, or female, but in addition there is an extra Y chromosome, bringing the total number to forty-seven. The patient with Klinefelter's syndrome is therefore an XXY genetically.

It would seem that the basic gonad is sound, but that the genetic factor operating through the cell nuclei does one of two things: either weakens the potential which would permit development to proceed as an ovary, or strengthens the male differentiation, so that the gonad becomes a testis.

Clinical Findings

The development of the child follows the normal pattern of the male, and the entity is not suspected until after puberty, when a eunuchoid habitus or excessive bilateral enlargement of the breasts develops. There is nothing about this syndrome that can be detected at birth.

These patients develop normally both in muscular and skeletal structure through infancy and childhood. The external genitalia are perfectly formed, and descent of

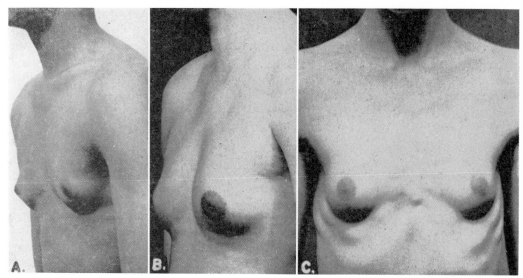

Fig. 6-3.   Gynecomastia of 3 adults with Klinefelter's syndrome. No normal hirsutism of the chest or prominence of the larynx occurs, as seen in virile adult males. (Courtesy of H. F. Klinefelter, Jr., from *Hermaphroditism, Genital Anomalies and Related Endocrine Disorders*, edited by H. W. Jones, Jr., and W. W. Scott. Baltimore, Williams & Wilkins Company.)

the testicle into the scrotum always occurs bilaterally at the proper time. The male phallus, although perhaps smaller than the normal, is perfectly adequate for satisfactory sexual intercourse, despite the fact that the ejaculate contains no sperm.

The first indication that all is not normal may be the gradual enlargement of the breasts, which begins to appear bilaterally some time after puberty. The enlargement is gradual and may not reach full development until several years have passed. Cases have also been reported which had all the other characteristics of Klinefelter's syndrome, but without the typical gynecomastia (Fig. 6-3).

The explanation for the gynecomastia is not clear. Normally one would expect to find ample laboratory evidence of ovarian hormone production, particularly estrin. To date no excessive estrin production has been encountered, and in fact hormone studies indicate conclusively that the patient with Klinefelter's syndrome secretes abundant quantities of the pituitary gonadotropin FSH, which would suggest that estrin production is low rather than high.

In the past psychosomatic symptoms that many of these patients are apt to exhibit were explained on the basis of embarrassment caused by the gynecomastia. This may well be true, but it is also well known that some of the patients with Klinefelter's syndrome are mentally deficient, despite the fact that no organic disease is found in the brain. A recent study in Glasgow of mentally retarded children in the prepuberal age revealed an incidence of 1.2 per cent of ostensibly male children with a chromatin-positive (female) sex pattern, when buccal smears were performed. It was the discovery of the extra Y chromosome in Klinefelter's syndrome (XXY), bringing the total number to forty-seven, which led to similar findings in patients with mongolism.

Treatment

Little can be done hormonally for the patient with Klinefelter's syndrome whose chief complaints are breast enlargement and infertility. The pituitary is already working overtime on a substrate which is poor, as shown by the elevated urinary levels of follicle-stimulating hormone (FSH). Hormone therapy will do nothing to decrease the size of the breasts.

If the enlarged breasts progress to the point at which the patient is embarrassed, they can be removed surgically.

Ovarian Agenesis or Turner's Syndrome

In contrast to the patient with Klinefelter's syndrome, the patient who has the characteristics of ovarian agenesis has less than the usual number of chromosomes (forty-five) and often a sex chromosome constitution of XO. Despite the fact that approximately 80 per cent of these patients are chromatin negative, there is really little reason to regard these patients socially as males, for psychologically and anatomically they are females. According to Guevin, Turner's syndrome is a spectrum of chromosomal disorders:

CLINICAL CLASSIFICATION	TEST FOR SEX CHROMATIN	KARYOTYPE	PHENOTYPE	OTHER ANOMALIES
Turner's	—	XO	Fertile	Yes
Turner's	—	XO	Immature Menstruating	Yes
Turner's (Classical)	—	XO	Immature	Yes
Turner's	+	XX,Xx		Yes
		XX,XO		
		XO	Immature	
Pure Gonadal Dysgenesis	—	XY	Immature	No
Turner's—Male	—	XO	Cryptorchid Hypospadiac	Yes
Turner's—Male	—	XY	Cryptorchid Dysgenetic	Yes

The reduction in the number of the chromosomes to forty-five comes about through loss of the Y chromosome. Such a patient then has no male component and only half the customary female component. It is hard to see how one can call such a patient a male despite the sex chromatin pattern.

The failure seems to rest in the actual development of the gonad itself in its embryonic beginnings. This could come about in one of two ways: either due to some environmental factor, as yet unknown, acting in utero to prevent gonadal development, or possible failure of the germ cell to invade the urogenital mesenchyma as it normally should. Since there is no masculinizing factor, the patient develops as a female despite the vestigial gonad and the male sex chromatin pattern.

It is increasingly evident that the Y chromosome, which has previously been thought to be inert, actually plays a decisive role in sex differentiation. If the Y chromosome is lacking, the patient has a female phenotype, such as we see in this syndrome. It is the genes that are wrong. The patient is still basically a female. In contrast, the additional X chromosome, which makes up the XXY chromosomal constitution in Klinefelter's syndrome, places these patients in the category of the male phenotype.

The Clinical Picture

At Birth.   Unlike Klinefelter's syndrome, it is possible to recognize Turner's syndrome (ovarian dysgenesis) at birth on the basis of the clinical findings. Whenever

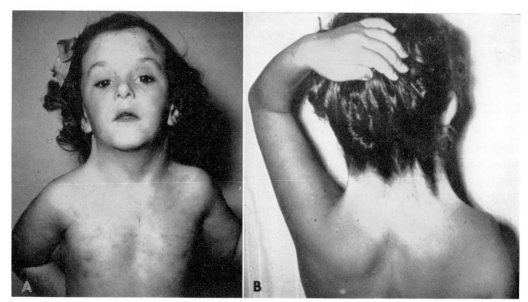

Fig. 6-4.   Child with the webbed neck and hair growth on the neck characteristic of Turner's syndrome. Her short stature is not apparent in these pictures. (Courtesy of Dr. Sydney S. Gellis, Boston City Hospital.)

one finds (*a*) extensive edema of both hands and feet, which may or may not pit, and (*b*) a short neck, low hanging ears, a high arched palate and a tendency for the hair to curl in a peculiar whorled fashion well down on the nape of the neck, one should be suspicious that the newborn child has ovarian agenesis (Fig. 6–4). The clinical features are enough to make the diagnosis, for competent observers fail to find this type of lymphedema of the extremities in other pathologic entities in the newborn. This is important, for approximately one fifth of the patients who have ovarian dysgenesis show the sex chromatin pattern of the female.

IN CHILDHOOD.   The main clinical characteristics of ovarian dysgenesis are (*a*) shortness of stature, (*b*) webbed neck, (*c*) cubitus valgus, and (*d*) complete absence of development of the breast and other secondary sex characteristics despite the presence of the barest minimum of sexual hair. In many instances other congenital abnormalities are present (Fig. 6–4).

The Growth Pattern in Ovarian Dysgenesis during Childhood

The growth pattern in ovarian dysgenesis closely resembles that of primordial dwarfism, which has no known endocrine background. The infant at birth rarely weighs over 5 pounds, and the growth rate is steady but slow throughout early childhood. The ossification centers appear at the usual time, and fusion finally does take place, but the time schedule does not conform to the normal pattern. In fact, the delay is so great that these children rarely attain a height above 58 inches before the epiphyses close permanently. The usual range is between 52 and 58 inches. It is this characteristic shortness of stature which has led to the descriptive term "ovarian dwarf."

Although the ovarian dwarf is without a gonad, the stunted growth cannot be attributed to lack of hormonal stimulation. The well known observation that girls who are castrated before puberty grow taller, not shorter, supports this contention.

How Does the Ovarian Dwarf Differ from the Hypothyroid and Hypopituitary Dwarf?

It is possible in many instances to distinguish between the hypothyroid and ovarian pituitary dwarf: (1) Like the infant with ovarian dysgenesis, the pituitary dwarf has normal bodily proportions at birth and grows normally for three or four years, while the hypothyroid infant maintains the infantile type of build as she grows older. (2) The untreated cretin (hypothyroid dwarf) has a characteristic facial appearance which is due to failure of the naso-orbital bones to develop properly. The pituitary dwarf has a well formed but juvenile type of face which persists into adulthood. In ovarian dysgenesis the facial appearance does not differ from that of the normal child, although there may be some underdevelopment of the lower portion of the face and chin. Despite this, there is no alteration in the schedule of dental development. (3) Although the time schedule for development of the ossification centers is behind the normal both in ovarian dysgenesis and pituitary insufficiency, one does not see the characteristic x-ray picture of epiphysial dysgenesis commonly found in the thyroid dwarf.

Differential Diagnosis between Ovarian Dysgenesis and Hypopituitarism

The chief points in the differential diagnosis between ovarian dysgenesis and hypopituitarism are as follows: (*a*) Despite the retardation in linear growth found in ovarian dysgenesis, the children are husky, well nourished and strong. This is in contrast to the pituitary dwarf, who tires easily and has little muscle tone. (*b*) The patient with ovarian dysgenesis has a high titer of FSH, which is completely lacking in panhypopituitarism. Moreover, since all pituitary gonadotropins are diminished or lacking in the patient with pituitary deficiency, urinary assays for 17-ketosteroids (stimulated by pituitary ACTH) show little or no excretion, in contrast to ovarian dysgenesis, in which they are diminished, but not absent. (*c*) The genetic factors are not operative in panhypopituitarism, and no congenital defects are noted. (*d*) The x-ray appearance of bone differs in the two entities: (1) Osteoporosis is common with ovarian agenesis, but rare in the pituitary dwarf. (2) The bone age is somewhat retarded, but the epiphyses eventually unite in the ovarian dwarf, while interference of growth together with continuing failure of epiphysial union is noted when the abnormality is centered in the pituitary. (*e*) Finally, the girl with ovarian agenesis who has no basic trouble with her adrenal gland, but only a depressed production of estrogen, eventually develops sexual hair on the labia, pubis and axilla. This does not occur in the hypopituitary dwarf.

What Congenital Anomalies Are Associated with Ovarian Agenesis?

The child with ovarian aplasia tends to have a wide variety of congenital anomalies along with the stunted growth. Such children are particularly prone to have a webbed neck and coarctation of the aorta. There are all degrees of webbing from the extreme case in which the skin web, containing no muscle, extends from the lobe of the ear to the midclavicular line to the less severe forms in which the neck appears to be simply shortened and triangular. With this deformity goes a lowering of the hairline and a tendency for the hair to grow down along the web onto the back of the neck. The skin is apt to hang loosely not only in the neck region (cutis laxa), but in other areas of the body as well. Occasionally the skin shows signs of premature senility with fine wrinkling. Coarctation of the aorta frequently accompanies webbing of the neck. This anomaly is often associated with a hypertension which is more evident in the upper extremities than in the lower. Among the other defects noted are a high arched palate, deep-set ears, deformity of the nails and cubitus valgus, an increased carrying angle between the forearm and upper arm.

How Does One Make the Diagnosis of Ovarian Agenesis before the Hormones Become Active?

It is no longer necessary to perform an exploratory laparotomy or wait until a child reaches puberty before making the diagnosis of ovarian agenesis. In the past the final diagnosis depended on the development or lack of development of the secondary sex characteristics, and laboratory evidence obtained by urinary assays of the gonadotropins.

The diagnosis should be suspected when (1) a young girl is stunted in growth with a bone age appreciably less than her chronologic age, and (2) accompanying this failure to grow and develop normally there are such congenital anomalies as webbing of the neck, coarctation of the aorta and the other malformations just recorded. These children look like girls and have female genitalia, yet approximately 80 per cent will have the sex chromatin pattern of the male when buccal smears or skin biopsies are done. There is a good chance that the child has ovarian aplasia when this combination is present. The diagnosis is not absolute, for 20 per cent do have the female sex chromatin arrangement. In them one can establish the diagnosis only by (*a*) surgical exploration or (*b*) waiting until the time when the sex hormones should become active.

How Is the Diagnosis Made in the Premenarchal Years?

One of the characteristics of ovarian agenesis is the lack of development of secondary sex characteristics and failure of the menarche to appear. These factors are dependent upon the presence of the pituitary gonadotropins and the secretion of sex hormones from the main target organ, the ovary. Rarely can they be detected before the eighth or ninth year.

Since the young girl without ovaries lacks the proper gonadal equipment, she never can develop any of the secondary sex characteristics for which estrin is responsible. The child tends to have a broad, shield-shaped chest with a conspicuous lack of breast development. Both breast and nipples are infantile. The external genitalia are feminine, but the labia, vagina and uterus are definitely immature. The vaginal epithelium shows no estrogen effect, for none is being produced. The girl with ovarian agenesis will eventually develop some sexual hair, though she may not do it until she is well along in adolescence. This is the function of the adrenal, not the ovary.

Further support for the diagnosis of ovarian agenesis can be obtained from the laboratory. By x-ray interpretation one notes that (*a*) there is late union of the epiphyses and retarded bone growth; (*b*) there may be osteoporosis as the result of estrogen lack; (*c*) coarctation of the aorta may be apparent on x-ray of the chest. Urinary assays provide useful information that will aid in the diagnosis. With ovarian agenesis one can expect to find (*a*) an increased titer of FSH and (*b*) a low titer of 17-ketosteroids.

These findings coupled with the stunting of growth and the presence of congenital anomalies are usually enough to make a diagnosis of ovarian agenesis. The final proof awaits abdominal exploration and tissue biopsy.

There is one minor exception to the established picture of the girl with ovarian agenesis. On rare occasions ovarian agenesis appears in girls of normal or slightly increased height. It would seem that arrest in ovarian development occurred after normal structural growth, but before the ovarian hormones became active, since these patients show pubic hair, but none of the other secondary sex characteristics. This form of ovarian agenesis does not have a genetic background, for the other congenital defects are absent.

What Does the Surgeon Find at Operation?

On abdominal exploration the vagina, uterus and tubes are present, though they are definitely infantile. In place of the ovary one often finds simply small, firm white streaks or ridges of tissue paralleling the tube and running out into the broad ligament (Fig. 6–5). Microscopically, the structures resemble those normally found in the

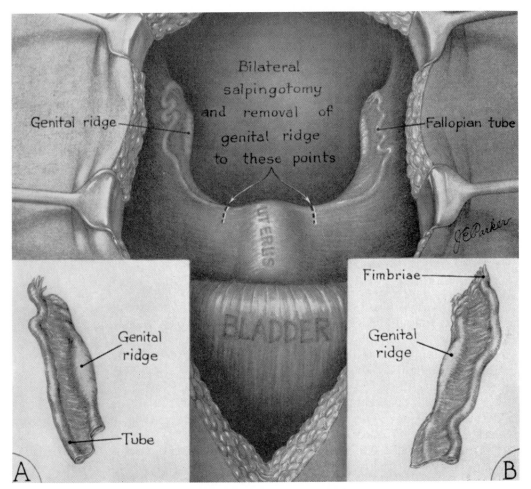

Fig. 6-5.   At operation in Turner's syndrome the ovaries are either absent, poorly formed or very small. The fallopian tubes and uterus are hypoplastic. (Courtesy of H. W. Jones, Jr., and W. W. Scott: *Hermaphroditism, Genital Anomalies and Related Endocrine Disorders.* Baltimore, Williams & Wilkins Company.)

ovarian hilus. There are a few rete tubules and rare clumps of cells that closely resemble Leydig cells, but the epithelial, stromal and germ cells that normally go to make up the ovarian cortex and follicles are totally absent.

What Treatment Can Be Offered the Girl with Gonadal Dysgenesis?

There is little that can be done to alter the basic underlying defect in these patients. If the epiphyses are still not united, some increase in bone growth may be obtained by giving estrin. The effect is indirect, operating probably through the release of LH and subsequent stimulation of the adrenal cortex.

Psychologically, much can be done by stimulating the growth of secondary sex characteristics by the use of oral estrogen. The breasts develop, and the growth of sexual hair increases. Along with these direct estrin effects it is also possible to produce growth of the uterus, vagina and external genitalia. When the uterus has developed sufficiently, artificial menstrual periods can be induced by providing estrin withdrawal bleeding. On a schedule of daily oral administration of any of the estrins such as Estinyl, 0.5 mg., Premarin, 2.5 mg., or diethylstilbestrol, 2 mg., for 3 weeks, followed by one week without medication, vaginal bleeding will occur. If one chooses, progestin may be added for its nitrogen-sparing effect and the sense of well-being that follows, but the patient and family should clearly understand that pregnancy is not possible. In general the patient's response to this disappointment is one of complete acceptance, mixed with gratitude that the substituted hormones have made it possible to conform outwardly to the appearance of her normal contemporaries.

TRUE HERMAPHRODITISM

This is a rare form of sex deviation in which both male and female elements are found in either the internal or external genitalia. The characteristic thing about this form of hermaphroditism is the fact that both ovary and testicle are present in the same patient. All combinations are possible. There may be an ovary on one side and a testis on the other, ovotestes on both sides or an ovary and a testis on each side. The chromosome pattern and the histologic picture of the testes do not conform.

What Is the Clinical Picture?

The diagnosis can only be suspected, for there is nothing characteristic about the clinical manifestations of the true hermaphrodite which will distinguish it from the other forms of hermaphroditism.

The external genitalia usually have such pronounced male characteristics that the child is brought up as a boy. Curiously enough, however, most of the true hermaphrodites will develop breasts at or about the time of puberty. A few will menstruate. This of course will depend on the extent of development of the uterus. If the uterus has developed to any extent, menstruation is likely to occur, even though the source of ovarian stimulation is buried in an ovotestis.

The final diagnosis awaits abdominal exploration and biopsy of the gonad (Fig. 6–6). This may not be easy, particularly if an ovotestis is present. There is nothing characteristic about the gross appearance of the gonad, and a small portion of ovary may exist within a gonad which is primarily testicular. If there is any doubt about the true sex of a young child, exploration should be carried out early before the

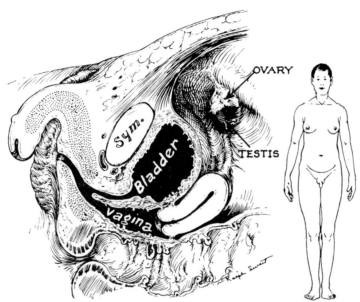

Fig. 6-6. Diagrammatic representation of a true hermaphrodite, who had a penis, gynecomastia, a uterus and vagina, testis and ovary. (Modified from F. Hinman, Jr.: *Pediat. Clin. N. Amer.*, Vol. 4.)

problems of management become confused by the impact of the hormones at the time of puberty.

Treatment

In general the pattern of treatment should concentrate on trying to make the child conform to the sex in which it seems best to rear it. These problems will be discussed later, for they apply in general to all deviations from the normal sex pattern. When possible, the gonad which is in conflict with the sex pattern should be removed and the external genitalia fashioned accordingly.

How Are Other Forms of Hermaphroditism Reflected in the Sex Chromatin Pattern?

Although the patient with true hermaphroditism has a normal complement of chromosomes, there is an obvious derangement, for the resulting types of sex deviation are so varied. The chromosome pattern and the histologic picture of the gonads may not conform. It is not surprising, then, to discover that the interpretation of buccal smears for sex chromatin is not very helpful, for one may reasonably find either the male or female type.

The two other forms of hermaphroditism, (*a*) the female pseudohermaphrodite and (*b*) the male hermaphrodite (often called male pseudohermaphrodite), have an ambiguous development of the genital organs, with different sex chromatin patterns, but no obvious variation in the genetic composition. One of the most fascinating facts about the recent discovery of abnormality in both chromosome number and constitution in the sex deviates represented by Klinefelter's and Turner's syndromes is the possibility that a more intense study of these chromosomes and their arrangement may provide a clue to explain some of the congenital anomalies which have hitherto been hard to understand.

FEMALE PSEUDOHERMAPHRODITE

Female pseudohermaphroditism associated with congenital hyperplasia of the adrenal is by far the most common type presenting congenital anomalies of the external genital apparatus. The female pseudohermaphrodite who has no adrenal hyperplasia is seen far less often. The adrenogenital syndrome has been discussed in detail earlier in this chapter.

In brief there does appear to be a genetic factor present, for there is a familial tendency. The sex chromatin pattern and development of the female gonad proceed normally, but further differentiation along anticipated lines does not follow.

THE MALE "HERMAPHRODITE" (MALE PSEUDOHERMAPHRODITE)

There is a small group of children who are born with mixed genital equipment. The majority have a true male sex chromatin pattern, but many female bodily characteristics in their development.

The possible explanation of these ambiguities in development may be found in experiments performed on laboratory animals. It would appear from experimental data that development will not occur along masculine pathways unless there is a strong male hormonal stimulus acting at the precise point in embryonic life when structures are beginning to differentiate into the male genital apparatus. If such a force is lacking or imperfect, there is a strong tendency for the infant to develop as a female, regardless of the sex chromatin pattern. The proper chromosomes then may be responsible for the development of the male gonad, but unless its gonadal function is adequate, the child will develop partly or wholly as a female, despite the fact that she may have a male sex chromatin arrangement.

The child with the male sex chromatin pattern should begin the differentiation into male structures between the sixth and twelfth weeks of embryonic life. If the male gonad functions properly, the wolffian duct structures develop at the expense of the müllerian duct derivatives, which undergo atrophy.

The male hermaphrodite, however, does not have testes that function normally. The strong stimulus to carry out development along male lines is lacking or varies in amount. Because of the deficient testicular function all manner of variations in male differentiation are found, depending on the extent of impairment.

The extent of development of the müllerian duct is also subject to wide variation. The larger group will have well formed müllerian duct derivatives to go with the equivocal development of the external genitalia. Somewhat less frequently one finds either a complete lack or, at the most, only vestigial remains of the uterus and tubes. In either case there is at least a rudimentary vagina present.

The growth patterns of the external genitalia are also dependent on the degree of the stimulus which directs development along masculine lines.

1. If the deficiency is minor, the child may have a simple hypospadias with a cleft scrotum and palpable gonads in the labia or inguinal region. This condition is present at birth. On examination there is always a vagina of some sort, but no cervix can be seen on endoscopic examination (Fig. 6–7).

2. When the testicular deficiency is more pronounced, the child at birth will tend to have a vagina of varying depth together with labial folds and phallus which would be considered large for a girl, but small for a man. This is enough to have the child raised as a girl, but unfortunately the müllerian duct derivatives are either

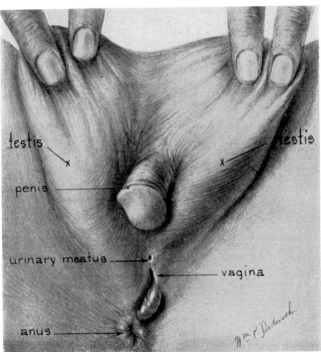

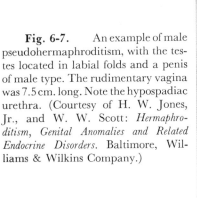

Fig. 6-7. An example of male pseudohermaphroditism, with the testes located in labial folds and a penis of male type. The rudimentary vagina was 7.5 cm. long. Note the hypospadiac urethra. (Courtesy of H. W. Jones, Jr., and W. W. Scott: *Hermaphroditism, Genital Anomalies and Related Endocrine Disorders.* Baltimore, Williams & Wilkins Company.)

rudimentary or absent. The gonads are testes which have not descended and are found either in the inguinal region or within the abdomen. This is probably the most common type of male pseudohermaphrodite.

3. One of the most interesting variants in the hermaphroditic pattern is the child who has feminine external genitalia in varying stages of development, but lacks normal development of the uterus and tubes. They may be entirely absent or exist only as vestigial remnants. In this situation, which has been called the "testicular feminization syndrome," the sex chromatin pattern is that of a male, yet the male gonad functions in a female medium. The testes function abnormally, and no masculinization occurs.

In this instance the gonad and its accessory attributes develop and function in the male pattern. Though androgen is present to provide the stimulation for masculinization, none appears, for the defect lies in the target organs. For some unexplained reason, perhaps chromosome aberration, they are unresponsive to androgenic stimulation from either the patient's own gonads or even any testosterone administered exogenously. For example, these patients have normal hair follicles, but no suggestion of hirsutism appears. Apparently the testes in this syndrome have the ability to produce both estrogen and androgen. That estrin is actually produced by these testes can be attested to, since (1) FSH determinations, which are usually in the range of premenopausal women before testes of this type are removed, rise to menopausal levels when the patient is castrated; (2) the patient complains of hot flashes after castration. On microscopic section of the undescended testes one finds the usual immature seminiferous tubules with little evidence of spermatogenesis, but there is a striking increase in the number of ripe Sertoli cells full of lipid material. This is believed by some to be the source of the estrin produced.

What Are the Clinical Manifestations of the Testicular Feminization Syndrome?

As a result of the estrogenic stimulation the person with this syndrome tends to full-scale breast development and female body habitus when she reaches the period of life when adolescence might be expected. Several curious factors appear. (*a*) The breasts are either normally developed or there is an actual increase in size. (*b*) The distribution of hair on the scalp follows the female pattern and does not recede at the temples. (*c*) Although the testicle is also secreting androgen, no hair appears on the face. (*d*) Conversely, although the testicle is secreting estrogen, minimal amounts of hair are seen over the pubis or in the axilla. As one might expect, these girls have the psychosexual adjustment of the female, despite the fact that they will never menstruate.

Other Types of Male Pseudohermaphroditism

Again, depending upon the degree of stimulus which directs the development along masculine lines, the child may have an enlarged clitoris, labial folds and only a dimple for a vagina. The testes are found within the abdomen.

The male pseudohermaphrodite can also have fully developed male genitalia, complete with hypospadiac penis and fully descended testicles, but in addition a cleft scrotum and a shallow vagina.

In contrast to the forms of male pseudohermaphroditism previously described, the child may have well developed male genitalia externally, but female structures such as uterus and tubes within the abdomen. The testes are always ectopically placed, but are usually found in the inguinal region.

All but those with the last form of male pseudohermaphroditism are commonly reared as girls because (*a*) the clitoris is hypospadiac and, though enlarged, does not have the full development or conformation of the true male penis, and (*b*) there is usually some suggestion of a vagina present, even though it be only a shallow recession with a urethral meatus at the base of the phallus. The possibility of male development is not considered, and the sex chromatin pattern is rarely established at birth or in childhood. The final discovery is made only when the pituitary gonadotropins become active.

REFERENCES

General Observations

Allen, E. D.: Examination of the Genital Organs in the Prepubescent and in the Adolescent Girl. *Pediat. Clin. N. Amer.*, 5: 19, 1958.

Rosenthal, A. H.: Symptomatic Genital Anomalies in Childhood. *Clin. Obst. & Gynec.*, 3: 146, 1960.

Segal, S. J., and Nelson, W. O.: Developmental Aspects of Human Hermaphroditism—The Significance of Sex Chromatin Patterns. *J. Clin. Endocrinol.*, 17: 676, 1957.

Straffon, R. A.: Diagnosis and Treatment of Ambisexualism in Children. *Urological Survey*, 11: 6, 1961.

Tristan, T. A., Eberlein, W. R., and Hope, J. W.: Roentgenologic Investigation of Patients with Heterosexual Development. *Am. J. Roentgenol.*, 76: 562, 1956.

Adrenogenital Syndrome (Female Pseudohermaphroditism)

Atkinson, W., and Masson, J. C.: Bicornuate Uterus; Atresia of Vulva with Double Vagina; Pseudohermaphroditism. *S. Clin. N. Amer.*, 14: 571, 1934.

Bartter, F. C., and others: Effects of Adrenocorticotropic Hormone and Cortisone in Adrenogenital Syndrome Associated with Congenital Adrenal Hyperplasia. *J. Clin. Invest.*, 30: 237, 1951.

Bastenie, P. A.: Cortisone Treatment in Adrenogenital Syndrome. *Lancet*, 1: 915, 1953.

Bierich, J. R., Bohe, E., and Voight, K. D.: New Aspects of Pathogenesis of Adrenogenital Syndrome. *Acta Endocrinol.*, 18: 512, 1955.

Blackman, S. S., Jr.: Concerning the Function and Origin of Reticular Zone of Adrenal Cortex; Hyperplasia in Adrenogenital Syndrome. *Bull. Johns Hopkins Hosp.*, 78: 180, 1946.

Bongiovanni, A. M., Eberlein, W. R., and Cara, J.: Studies on Metabolism of Adrenal Steroids in Adrenogenital Syndrome. *J. Clin. Endocrinol.*, 14: 409, 1954.

Bradbury, J. T.: Adrenogenital Syndrome and Adrenal Hyperplasia. *Clin. Obst. & Gynec.*, 1: 257, 1958.

Crigler, J. F., Jr., Silverman, S. H., and Wilkins, L.: Further Studies on Treatment of Congenital Adrenal Hyperplasia with Cortisone; Effect of Cortisone and Compound B in Infants with Disturbed Electrolyte Metabolism. *Pediatrics*, 10: 397, 1952.

Darrow, D. C.: Congenital Adrenal Cortical Insufficiency with Virilism. *Yale J. Biol. & Med.*, 16: 579, 1944.

Ely, R. S., Kelley, V. C., and Raile, R. B.: Studies of 17-Hydroxycorticosteroids in Children; Peripheral Blood Levels in Health and Disease. *J. Pediat.*, 42: 38, 1953.

Iversen, T.: Congenital Adrenocortical Hyperplasia with Disturbed Electrolyte Regulation; "Dysadrenocorticism." *Pediatrics*, 16: 875, 1955.

Jailer, J. W., Louchart, J. J., and Cahill, G. F.: Adrenal Virilism; Metabolic Studies. *J. Clin. Invest.*, 31: 880, 1952.

Jones, H. W., Jr., and Scott, W. W.: *Hermaphroditism, Genital Anomalies and Related Endocrine Disorders.* Baltimore, Williams & Wilkins Company, 1958.

Kyle, L. H., and Knop, C. Q.: Simulation of Cardiac Disease by Adrenocortical Failure in Infants. *New England J. Med.*, 243: 681, 1950.

Landing, B. H.: Studies on the Anatomy of the Human Adrenal Cortex in Various Functional States. *Ciba Foundation Colloquia on Endocrinology.* Boston, Little, Brown & Co., 1955, Vol. VIII, p. 52.

Migeon, C. J., and Gardner, L. I.: Urinary Estrogens in Hyperadrenocorticism—Influence of Cortisone, Compound F, Compound B, and ACTH. *J. Clin. Endocrinol.*, 12: 1513, 1952.

Rosenthal, I. M., Gellman, V., Hyde, J. S., and Bronstein, I. P.: The Effect of Stress on Patients with Congenital Virilizing Adrenocortical Hyperplasia. *Pediatrics*, 25: 598, 1960.

Sydnor, K. L., Kelley, V. C., Raile, R. B., Ely, R. S., and Sayers, G.: Blood Adrenocorticotropin in Children with Congenital Adrenal Hyperplasia. *Proc. Soc. Exper. Biol. & Med.*, 82: 695, 1953.

Wilkins, L.: Diagnosis and Treatment of Congenital Virilizing Adrenal Hyperplasia. *Postgrad. Med.*, 29: 31, 1961.

Würterle, A.: Therapy of the Adrenogenital Syndrome in Females. *Internat. Abstr. Surg.*, 108: 482, 1959.

Klinefelter's Syndrome

Bunge, R. G., and Bradbury, J. T.: Newer Concepts of the Klinefelter's Syndrome. *J. Urol.*, 76: 758, 1956.

del Castillo, E. B., Trabucco, A., and de la Balze, F. A.: Syndrome Produced by Absence of the Germinal Epithelium without Impairment of the Sertoli or Leydig Cells. *J. Clin. Endocrinol.*, 7: 493, 1947.

Heller, C. G., and Nelson, W. O.: Hyalinization of the Seminiferous Tubules Associated with Normal or Failing Leydig Cell Function. Discussion of Relationship to Eunuchoidism, Gynecomastia, Elevated Gonadotrophins, Depressed 17-Ketosteroids and Estrogens. *J. Clin. Endocrinol.*, 5: 1, 1945.

Klinefelter, H. F., Jr.; in H. W. Jones, Jr., and W. W. Scott, Eds.: *Hermaphroditism, Genital Anomalies and Related Endocrine Disorders.* Baltimore, Williams & Wilkins Company, 1958.

Klinefelter, H. F., Jr., Reifenstein, E. C., Jr., and Albright, F.: Syndrome Characterized by Gynecomastia, Aspermatogenesis without A-Leydigism, and Increased Excretion of Follicle-Stimulating Hormone. *J. Clin. Endocrinol.*, 2: 615, 1942.

Turner's Syndrome

Guevin, R.: Bio-science Seminar—Chromosomal Disorders in Man. *Henry Ford Hosp. Med. Bull.*, 9: 231, 1961.

Hamblen, E. C., Palma, E., and Poshyachinda, D.: Congenital Rudimentary Gonad Syndrome. *Clin. Obst. & Gynec.*, 3: 207, 1960.

Sosnowski, J. R.: Factors to Be Considered in the Treatment of Ovarian Agnesis. *Am. J. Obst. & Gynec.*, 78: 792, 1959.

True Hermaphroditism

Gresham, G. A., and Fairgrieve, J.: True Hermaphroditism. *Brit. J. Surg.*, 48: 235, 1960.
Jones, H. W., Jr.: Hermaphroditism; in J. V. Meigs and S. H. Sturgis, Eds.: *Progress in Gynecology*. New York, Grune & Stratton, Inc., 1957, Vol. III, p. 35.

Male Pseudohermaphroditism

Bradbury, J. T., and Bunge, R. G.: Male Intersex with Ambiguous External Genitals and Well Developed Müllerian Elements. *Am. J. Obst. & Gynec.*, 80: 76, 1960.
Teter, J., and Terlowski, R.: Tumors of the Gonads in Cases of Gonadal Dysgenesis and Male Pseudohermaphroditism. *Am. J. Obst. & Gynec.*, 79: 321, 1960.

Chapter 7

Sex Rearing in the
Child with an Intersex Problem

THE PROPER assignment of the child's true sex should be made at the time of birth. In most instances this is a relatively easy matter, for the sex assigned will in most instances correspond with the anatomic conformation of the external genitalia. If there are obvious doubts based on departures from the normal growth pattern, the physician should not be content to base his assignment of sex on the predominant characteristics of the genitalia without more thorough investigation. Too frequently the examination is less than adequate. Fortunately for him, the child in later life continues to adjust to a sex assignment which subsequently proves to be at variance with the true gonadal sex, provided no attempts are made to change the pattern. This is more a matter of good luck on the part of the physician than good management. The physician does a great disservice to the female pseudohermaphrodite who is assigned a male role because of a predominance of masculine characteristics in the genitalia. As we have noted, these patients have the female sex chromatin pattern and normal internal genitalia which are well developed and fully capable of normal function. A simple operative procedure will permit such a patient to live the normal life of a female, which indeed she is. The diagnosis of female pseudohermaphroditism should be established at birth.

If the obstetrician will routinely examine the infant at birth rather than

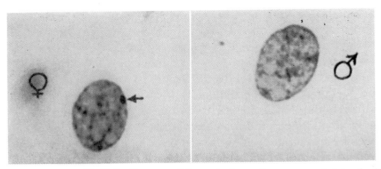

Fig. 7-1.   Nuclei of epithelial cells scraped from the buccal mucosa and stained with Cresyl echt violet. The so-called sex chromatin body, indicated by the arrow, is a characteristic of genetic females, and males show few nuclei that contain such chromatin bodies. (From M. M. Grumbach: *Pediatrics*, Vol. 20.)

cursorily inspect the external genitalia, the margin of error will be materially reduced. An infant at birth should have (1) a rectal examination to form some idea of whether or not the internal genitalia are present. Under the influence of the maternal hormones they are more prominent at birth than they will be any time before puberty. (2) If there are any ambiguous elements present on examination of the external or internal genitalia, a buccal smear for sex determination and a 17-ketosteroid urinary excretion study should be performed (Fig. 7–1). The combination of the buccal smear for sex determination and a 17-ketosteroid excretion is done to separate the pseudo-hermaphrodite, due to excess androgen production, from (a) the child whose mother received estrin or progestin therapy early in pregnancy, and (b) the true intersex problems such as the hermaphrodites. The history may rule out the former, leaving the physician with the problem of determining the proper sex in an intersex problem.

Why Should the True Sex Be Established in Early Infancy in Problems of Intersex?

Psychiatrists have shown conclusively that the true sex should be established, if at all possible, early in infancy and that the assigned sex should not be tampered with thereafter, other than in exceptional circumstances. This opinion stems from two important observations: (1) serious psychologic maladjustments follow any attempt to reverse the assignment of sex after the neonatal period. Conversely, no major difficulty was encountered when the sex was changed within the first year. (2) The child's adjustment to the sex assigned depends more on the gender role than on the anatomic characteristics of the gonad or the chromosomal arrangement. In most instances psychiatrists have found that the child learns to think, react, talk, play and dream in terms that are completely compatible with the assigned sex. Apparently there is no tendency on the part of the child to demonstrate any bizarre erotic behavior, either in the growing period or later. Even in the hermaphrodite it has been amply proved that the so-called gender role follows more closely the assigned sex than any other factor.

What Are the Common Pitfalls in Problems of Sex Rearing?

In the presence of obvious maldevelopment of the external genitalia the physician is apt to fall into one of two traps which tend to complicate subsequent management. (1) He either decides that the infant is a boy or a girl on inadequate evidence, or (2) he procrastinates or vacillates in his decision and tends to postpone the final assignment until later in childhood, when it is too late to change. Obviously these points of view are in error, for an attempt should be made to determine the true sex of the child at birth. The physician may be reluctant to have the child go through a surgical exploration, but it is a relatively simple matter to take a buccal smear and determine the genetic sex. In the majority of instances the sex in which the child is raised should correspond with the chromosomal sex. The obstetrician, should, however, exercise some judgment and may elect to assign a sex which does not correspond with either the chromosomal or gonadal sex. For example, it cannot lead to anything but frustration to attempt to construct a functioning penis out of an inadequate, hypospadiac type of clitoris. Regardless of the chromosomal or gonadal sex, the obstetrician should decide that the child should be raised as a female if an essentially normal penis cannot be constructed. It is a relatively easy matter to construct a vagina adequate for coitus which allows the girl to live happily as a female without ever knowing that she had testes instead of ovaries. To support the obstetrician in making such a decision is the well known observation that the male pseudohermaphrodite, who has feminine external genitalia and no clitoral enlargement, will feminize at puberty.

There are other problems in management that may appear later on or will require attention in anticipation of their appearance, but the obstetrician is aware of the possibilities. So informed, he can manage the parents and the patient far more intelligently and plan his subsequent moves far better.

Although there appears to be no great harm in assigning the wrong sex to an intersex infant, provided you do not try to change it, it makes far more sense to try to establish the sex in infancy before assigning one based solely on anatomic configuration.

THE PARENTAL ATTITUDE.   Faulty assignment of sex that becomes obvious later in childhood leads to the next pitfall, which concerns the attitude of the parent. It is confusing and embarrassing for the parents to learn that the child they thought was a girl actually is a boy, or vice versa. The mental turmoil increases if the physician vacillates in his decision and is further aggravated by ill-advised attempts to change the sex back and forth.

In their disturbed frame of mind the parents become hopelessly involved in attempts to explain to the rest of the family, neighbors, playmates and school associates just what is going on. If ill informed, they acquire many false concepts which influence their reaction and compound the difficulties of management. Some of this stems from misunderstanding of the terms used by the physician to explain the situation. For example, the layman has great difficulty in considering hermaphroditism as distinct from homosexuality. The parents live in great dread that this child, whom they consider to be part girl and part boy, will sometime in her life develop abnormally erotic sexual behavior or even become a sexual pervert. As a result the family tries to overprotect the child and throws so much secrecy over the situation that the child never has a chance to develop normally and becomes psychologically maladjusted.

The physician's role in this problem of sex determination is clear. Primarily he should obtain as much information as he can and come to a definite conclusion about the sex of the child, and then not deviate from it. The decision should consider all factors and take full cognizance of the fact that the child can be raised in a sex which is seemingly at variance with its chromosomal, gonadal or hormonal sex.

EDUCATION OF THE PARENTS.   Education of the parents is an important part of the program. The doctor should try to explain to them in simple terms what the problem is and what they may expect. For example, they should be told that the sexual organs are malformed rather than a bold statement that the young girl has testes. This is a less frightening approach and makes it easier to understand why corrective procedures may be necessary later on in childhood to allow the child to conform outwardly to the appearance of her contemporaries. Above all, neither the family nor the physician should be stampeded into ill-advised attempts to alter the sex of rearing to permit it to conform to the chromosomal or gonadal sex if the child gains little from the change.

REASSURING THE CHILD.   Obviously, children with an intersex problem who have been raised in the wrong sex will eventually become aware of the fact that their development differs from that of their contemporaries. Authorities vary in their thoughts about how much of this problem should be discussed with the child. Certainly she should be reassured and told that any development which is embarrassing to her can be corrected, but any attempt to discuss the gonadal sex pattern is definitely ill-advised. Every attempt should be made to further her adaptation to her gender role, rather than trying to modify it to conform to her gonadal sex pattern. When she reaches marital age, the problem can be discussed more freely and the patient reassured that a satisfactory sexual and marital life is possible despite the fact that she may not have children.

What Additional Support Can Be Given to Help the Child in Early Childhood to Adapt to Her Sex?

As far as possible, every effort should be made to permit adequate sexual function. The problem varies with the individual patient. We have previously noted that the masculinizing factor in the female pseudohermaphrodite is confined to the external genitalia, the vulva and lower third of the vagina. It is possible, then, to construct a vaginal outlet adequate for coitus and even for delivery. Any child who is reared as a girl, but has an embarrassingly large clitoris, should have it removed. This can be done with impunity, for the antiquated impression that all sexual sensation rests in the clitoris has been dissipated. It is better to make these surgical alterations in infancy or early childhood, to avoid an unnecessary focusing of attention on the genitalia. Although it is desirable to correct such anatomic abnormalities early in childhood, it is probably wise to delay construction of an artificial vagina in a child who has no clitoral enlargement until she is just about to be married. Up until this time there is little reason for performing any corrective surgery, for (a) girls with congenital absence of the vagina in most instances also lack normal development in the internal genitalia. There is no necessity then for an operation to avoid the complications that would follow menstruation into a blind cavity. (b) There is no reason for the girl to be embarrassed about her absent vagina, unless there is occasion to use it. Also there are practical reasons for the delay, since the newly constructed vagina remains open and functional far better if it is in regular use.

In general it is far easier to construct the external genitalia in the female mold than to try to construct a functioning penis, for reasons we have previously outlined. The prime object in corrective surgery should be (a) restoration of the external genitalia as far as is practicable, in the pattern that best meets with the established sex, and (b) removal of any embarrassing attributes that may appear and form a basis for poor psychiatric adjustment.

What about Corrective Procedures in Intersex Problems That May Be Done Later?

It is obvious in intersex problems, when the gonad is at variance with the outward appearance of the external genitalia and the sex of rearing, that psychologic situations will be bound to appear as the child approaches puberty and the sex hormones become active. It may be advisable to remove the structures, whether they be wolffian or müllerian, which act in opposition to the chosen pattern of sex.

For example, the female pseudohermaphrodite who has been reared as a boy should have the uterus and ovaries removed to try to help prevent the embarrassing secondary sexual development of the female body contour and particularly the breasts. The male pseudohermaphrodite raised as a girl should have the testes removed to avoid androgenic stimulation of the accessory sex and other target organs.

At puberty the testes tend to cause deepening of the voice, through enlargement of the larynx, and the appearance of hair generally over the body, but particularly on the face. There is little point in trying to do anything about the patient with ovotestes, but much can be done by way of prevention of contradictory sex characteristics in the true hermaphrodite who has both an ovary and a testis. In this case the gonad which does not conform to the sex pattern established for the individual should be removed.

After the removal of the gonad which functioned in opposition to the established sex, further support along the chosen line of development can be given by instituting hormonal substitution therapy.

What about Removal of the Testes in the Male Pseudohermaphrodite?

The decision as to how the child should be brought up should be reached as soon as possible after birth, preferably within the first year. In general, the more complete the feminine configuration of the external genitalia, the more likely that feminization will take place at the time of puberty. The converse is also true. Psychiatrists feel that the therapeutic aim should be directed toward improving whatever the child has in the way of feminine equipment if she is to grow up as a well adjusted adult, regardless of the sex chromatin. The chances of accomplishing this improve if surgical therapy and hormonal correction are carried out before androgenic stimulation creates a virilization that may be difficult to reverse.

Practically, there is another major consideration why a child should be reared as a female if it is at all feasible. Surgically, it is a far easier matter to remove the testicles and amputate the clitoris than to construct a functional penis adequate for coitus. The female body habitus and secondary sex characteristics can be acquired through the substitution of female sex hormones. Moreover, the testes in these patients are so defective in their basic elements that they will never be able to produce spermatozoa, however vigorous the stimulus applied to them is. It is, therefore, better that the testes be removed. Another strong argument for surgical excision of the intra-abdominal testes exists when one recalls that even a normal testicle in an ectopic position has a better chance than average of undergoing malignant change. There are two particular problems that arise: (1) the necessity for removal of the gonad, and (2) the timing of the orchidectomy.

In all probability the testes should be removed, for they can hardly be expected to function often enough to justify the risks involved in preserving them. The main reason for removal is that of possible malignant change. Testicular tumors are found in association with male pseudohermaphroditism in approximately 33 per cent. Of these, only one third will be malignant, but the degree of malignancy is so high and the outlook so poor that orchidectomy is the treatment of choice.

The timing of the orchidectomy is a subject for discussion. The male pseudo-hermaphrodite, for example, does not always respond in the same way to retention of the testes. For example, Wilkins notes that, contrary to what one might expect, patients who have genital organs which appear to be predominantly feminine usually masculinize at puberty, while the reaction may go one way or the other when only vestigial remains of female internal genital structures are present. One might then be tempted to leave the testes alone at the time of the original exploration, to determine the sex and wait to see what effects were produced by them on the external genitalia. At puberty this seems unwise, in view of the chance of masculinization combined with the risk of malignant change.

In the testicular feminization syndrome the testes should eventually be removed. Authorities disagree as to when this should be done. Morris feels that they should be left alone until puberty or shortly thereafter, in order that the child receive the benefit of estrin secreted by the testes both in this syndrome and in male pseudohermaphroditism. The decision must be made whether to perform an orchidectomy in early childhood and rely on substitution estrin therapy, or to wait until after puberty and run the risk of a malignant testicular transformation.

REFERENCES

Bromwich, A. F.: True Hermaphroditism. *Brit. M.J.*, 1: 395, 1955.

Cecil, A. B.: A True Hermaphrodite. *Tr. Am. A. Genito-Urinary Surgeons*, 45: 140, 1953.

Davis, D. M., and Scheffey, L. C.: A Case of True Hermaphroditism. *J. Urol.*, 56: 715, 1946.

del Castillo, E. B., de La Balze, F. A., and Argonz, J.: Syndrome of Rudimentary Ovaries with Estrogenic Insufficiency and Increase in Gonadotropins. *J. Clin. Endocrinol.*, 7: 385, 1947.

Ehenfeld, E. N., and Bromberg, Y. M.: Syndrome of Gonadal Dysgenesis with an Enlarged Clitoris in Chromosomal Males. *Acta Endocrinol.*, 28: 590, 1958.

Engle, E. T., Yeaw, R. C., and Lattimore, J. K.: True Hermaphroditism and Supplementary Report of a Case. *J. Urol.*, 56: 731, 1946.

Gaspar, M. R., Kimber, J. H., and Berkaw, K. A.: Children with Hernias or Testes and Female External Genitalia. *A.M.A. J. Dis. Child.*, 91: 542, 1956.

Gordon, G. S., Overstreet, E. W., Traut, H. F., and Winch, G. A.: Syndrome of Gonadal Dysgenesis—A Variety of Ovarian Agenesis with Androgenic Manifestation. *J. Clin. Endocrinol. & Metab.*, 15: 1, 1955.

Greenblatt, R. B.: Sex Reversal in Pseudohermaphroditism. *Am. J. Obst. & Gynec.*, 70: 1165, 1955.

Greenblatt, R. B., Carmona, N., and Higdon, L.: Gonadal Dysgenesis with Androgenic Manifestations in the Tall Eunuchoid Female. *J. Clin. Endocrinol. & Metab.*, 16: 235, 1956.

Greenblatt, R. B., Vasquez, E., and de Acosta, O. M.: Gonadal Dysgenesis—Report of Four Cases. *Obst. & Gynec.*, 9: 258, 1957.

Grumbach, M. M., Van Wyk, J. J., and Wilkins, L.: Chromosomal Sex in Gonadal Dysgenesis (Ovarian Agenesis); Relationship to Male Pseudohermaphroditism and Theories of Human Sex Differentiation. *J. Clin. Endocrinol. & Metab.*, 15: 1161, 1955.

Hamblen, E. C., Palma, E., and Poshyachinda, D.: Congenitally Rudimentary Gonad Syndrome. *Clin. Obst. & Gynec.*, 3: 207, 1960.

Hoffenberg, R., Jackson, W. P. U., and Muller, W. H.: Gonadal Dysgenesis with Menstruation—A Report of Two Cases. *J. Clin. Endocrinol. & Metab.*, 17: 902, 1957.

Howard, F. S., and Hinman, F.: Female Pseudohermaphrodite with Supplementary Phallic Urethra. Report of Two Cases. *J. Urol.*, 65: 439, 1951.

Jungck, E. C., Greenblatt, R. B., and Manautou, J. M.: Abnormal Sex Development in Children. *Pediat. Clin. N. Amer.*, 5: 137, 1958.

Marshall, V. F., Paquin, A. J., and Pierce, J. M.: True Hermaphroditism—A Conference on One Patient. *J. Urol.*, 72: 77, 1954.

McIver, R. B., Seabaugh, D. R., and Mangels, M., Jr.: True Hermaphroditism. Report of Two Cases. *J. Urol.*, 52: 67, 1944.

Moore, K. L.: Sex Reversal in Newborn Babies. *Lancet*, 1: 217, 1959.

Morris, J. M.: The Syndrome of Testicular Feminization in Male Pseudohermaphrodites. *Am. J. Obst. & Gynec.*, 65: 1192, 1953.

Morris, J. M., and Scully, R. E.: *Endocrine Pathology of the Ovary*. St. Louis, C. V. Mosby Company, 1958.

Perloff, W. H., Conger, K. B., and Levy, L. M.: Female Pseudohermaphroditism—Description of Two Unusual Cases. *J. Clin. Endocrinol.*, 13: 783, 1953.

Sargis, H. T., Wylie, B., Thomay, W. S., and Kalani, H.: Construction of a Functional Vagina. *Am. J. Obst. & Gynec.*, 79: 67, 1960.

Stern, O. N., and Vandervort, W. J.: Testicular Feminization in a Male Pseudohermaphrodite. *New England J. Med.*, 254: 787, 1956.

Taylor, E. S., and Snow, R. H.: Adrenal Virilism in the Female Child and Adult. *Am. J. Obst. & Gynec.*, 67: 1307, 1954.

Wilkins, L.: Masculinization of Female Fetus Due to Use of Orally Given Progesterone. *J.A.M.A.*, 172: 1028, 1960.

Wilkins, L., and Fleishmann, W.: Ovarian Agenesis: Pathology, Associated Clinical Symptoms and Bearing on the Theories of Sex Differentiation. *J. Clin. Endocrinol.*, 4: 357, 1944.

Wilkins, L., and Jones, H. W., Jr.: Masculinization of the Female Fetus. *Obst. & Gynec.*, 11: 355, 1958.

Williams, D. I.: The Diagnosis of Intersex. *Brit. M.J.*, 1: 1264, 1952.

Idem: The Intersexed Female. *Clin. Obst. & Gynec.*, 3: 220, 1960.

Witschi, E., Nelson, W. O., and Segal, S. J.: Genetic, Developmental and Hormonal Aspects of Gonadal Dysgenesis and Sex Inversion in Man. *J. Clin. Endocrinol. & Metab.*, 17: 737, 1957.

Young, H. H.: Mixed Sex. *Bull. Johns Hopkins Hosp.*, 35: 165, 1924.

Idem: *Genital Abnormalities, Hermaphroditism and Related Adrenal Disease.* Baltimore, Williams & Wilkins Company, 1937.

Chapter 8

Problems Affecting the
Genitalia in Early Childhood

AFTER the period of infancy, which comprises the first two years of the child's life, and until the hormones begin their activity, childhood problems are largely those concerned with somatic growth and development. The young girl is usually brought to the physician during this period for one of two reasons: (*a*) The child does not develop according to the parents' idea of the normal pattern, considered in Chapter 13, or (*b*) the child has specific symptoms that require attention.

What Gynecologic Conditions Produce Local Symptoms in a Growing Child?

The exposed position of the vulva in the child makes it particularly prone to trauma and infection. Despite the fact that most children seem to be able to mature in the genital area without infection, the great majority of children who appear in pediatric clinics for gynecologic complaints, between the ages of two and eight years, do so because of vulvovaginal discharge and inflammation. In most instances the cause can be traced to inadequate care or nutritional deficiency.

VULVITIS AND DERMATITIS

General Considerations

There are certain factors present in the skin of a newborn infant and young child that make the vulvar area particularly prone to specific types of infection. Many of them are simply manifestations of a generalized infection which localizes in the anogenital area because of anatomic considerations, such as fatty folds or creases which make it nearly impossible to keep the area dry. In the young infant protective diaper pads also tend to increase local heat and retain moisture. Actually there are few cutaneous diseases that are peculiar to children.

The skin of a young infant seems to be particularly vulnerable, however, to bacterial infection and oversensitive to the application of chemical agents. To a less degree viral infections and allergic manifestations appear.

The skin of the young child differs from that of the adult in several important particulars. Since the infant's skin is thinner and less cornified, it tends to be much

84

more permeable to secretions from both without and within. This, coupled with the fact that the infant's skin has an increased sensitivity to superficial bacterial infection, particularly by staphylococci, makes the skin in the vulvar region more vulnerable. The intact skin resists infection fairly well, but if the area is subjected to repeated minor trauma, superficial skin infections are apt to develop. Vulvar infections tend to be primary, and their course is not likely to be modified by any acquired sensitization or immunity. The infant simply has not had time or enough maturity to form antibodies.

The increased permeability and the fact that there is less cohesion at the dermal-epidermal junction may account for the observation that exudative lesions of the same etiology tend to ooze more and be wetter in children than in adults.

In addition to the fact that the skin is thinner in infants, there are also fewer sebaceous and sweat glands as well as less hair. For this reason such infections as folliculitis are rare in children. The child is not plagued with odoriferous sweating from the apocrine glands, which are prominent in the young adult, both in the vulvar and axillary regions, for they are not fully developed or do not function until sex hormonal activity appears on or about the time of puberty.

Basic Considerations in the Prevention of Vulvitis in the Infant or Child

It is obvious from the foregoing discussion that the most prominent feature in all the skin lesions that affect the infant or young child is the increased sensitivity to superficial bacterial infection. The basic aim in preventing such infection, until such time as the child has had an opportunity to establish its own antibodies and create its own immunity, is to keep the anogenital region clean, dry, cool, well aerated, and free from any element such as rubber pants that will cause friction or maceration of the skin.

The infant's skin is thin, but it is tough and will remain in good condition as long as it is kept clean and free from trauma. To accomplish this one has only to use the simplest methods to ensure skin hygiene. The most satisfactory agents are soap and water applied in the gentlest manner. The kind of soap used is of little importance, despite the fact that the popular literature is filled with advertisements about the merits of special soaps designed for the tender babies' skin. Actually babies' skin in this regard is little different from that of the adult. It has been said that the best soap to use is the one that provides the largest amount for the least money. Contrary to general impression, it is not necessary to bathe the infant repeatedly, nor to apply antibiotic ointments, powder, emulsions or other agents which are supposedly protective.

What Are Some of the Common Vulvar Infections?

There are many forms of infantile eczema that appear in the vulva or anogenital region. The most common types are diaper rash in the young baby and intertrigo in the growing child.

DIAPER RASH

Although there is a general belief that the beefy red, oozing erythematous rash is due to alteration of the pH of the skin by ammoniacal decomposition products of the urine, there is no proof that this is true. It is far more likely that the diaper itself is the chief culprit and that simple maceration of the skin plays the major role. It is a full-time job to keep a young baby dry. Unless great care is taken to diaper the child properly, the moist padding tends to soften and macerate the skin, and the wriggling motion of the unhappy baby produces trauma to the area through friction. It will only compound the difficulty to add rubber or plastic pants, for they simply increase the retained moisture, the heat and humidity, by cutting down on the aeration. In effect, you have applied a urinary poultice.

To prevent the development of diaper rash the mother should follow a simple regimen of (1) daily sponge or tub bath, using warm water and soap, (2) thorough drying with a soft towel, (3) powder with talc, (4) frequent changes of soiled diapers and outer garments. Soap, water and powder are far better than oils, and rubber or plastic pants should be avoided. In making up the diaper it will be well to fold it in two layers. The inner layer, lying next to the skin, should be made of a soft, rather closely woven cotton cloth; (b) the outer layer should be absorbent. This increases the amount of aeration and decreases the movement of the padding, which produces friction, for in a diaper so fashioned the outer layer moves, but the inner one does not.

INTERTRIGO

This is one of the more common forms of dermatologic infection that one finds in early infancy and childhood. It is particularly prone to appear at this age, for it tends to arise in parts of the body which by their anatomic location either bring skin surfaces in close apposition to other skin areas, such as the upper thigh, groin and vulva, or require that the region be constantly covered with clothing, such as the anogenital area and buttocks.

Thus we find intertrigo where the skin falls naturally together, such as in the axilla and umbilicus, as well as in the groin and gluteal creases. It is in these areas that sweat is retained, evaporation is less, mechanical cleansing is difficult, and debris accumulates. The moist, warm, less readily aerated body areas provide an excellent environment for the superficial bacteria which are always present.

How Does Intertrigo Develop?

Under the conditions mentioned above the outer layer of the infant's skin softens and macerates in the deep creases. At first it is beefy red, but later exudation appears. The already adequate culture medium is further fortified by the change in surface pH toward the alkaline side. It is small wonder, then, that superficial pyogenic and fungus infections are superimposed. In nearly every case of intertrigo there will be superimposed these elements: (a) bacterial infection and (b) fungus growth.

How Do You Prevent Intertrigo from Developing in the Older Child, and How Do You Treat It?

The primary principles for the prevention of intertrigo hold true for all ages, including childhood. A premium is placed on dryness, aeration and personal hygiene, such as porous clothing and cleansing after toilet. The local area should be maintained at both low temperature and humidity. This is perhaps most easily accomplished in the infant when the mother is responsible, but as the child grows older she must be taught the value of cleanliness as to bathing and toilet habits.

The treatment of intertrigo follows the regimen laid down for all acute infections of the vulva.

OTHER TYPES OF VULVITIS IN THE YOUNG CHILD

Vulvar inflammation varies all the way from a minor irritation which produces simple erythema and engorgement of the vulvar tissues to inflammations so severe that the labia become agglutinated. For the most part inflammation of the vulva occurs without any accompanying vaginal infection. Upon culture, the majority will grow out bacterial colonies of the coliform group. This again suggests that the primary cause of vulvitis is perineal contamination secondary to faulty hygiene. If the vagina is also involved, one should suspect (*a*) gonorrheal infection, (*b*) invasion of the vaginal canal by intestinal parasites, or (*c*) foreign body. In general, the infections which are primary in the vagina and affect the vulva secondarily are generalized infections which involve all the vaginal epithelium, while those that spread from an acute vulvitis to the vagina involve only the lower third.

Two relatively common vulvar infections of the young child are moniliasis and impetigo.

Monilia

Mycotic infections of the vulvar area are seen occasionally in young children. In most instances the infection is due to monilia, for *Trichomonas vaginalis* is rarely found before the premenarchal age. Mycotic vulvitis may appear in association with intertrigo or be a secondary manifestation of a primary lesion in the lower part of the vagina. On rare occasions mycotic infections may be traced to the use of antibiotics administered for a disease elsewhere in the body.

When moniliasis appears on the skin of the vulva, it produces a characteristic picture, made up of red, moist, granulomatous lesions which ooze at first, but later form crusts over the surface. It is common to see satellite lesions beyond the area of major involvement. Because the lesions create a pruritus, they frequently become ulcerated as the infant tries to relieve the discomfort by scratching or rubbing.

How Do You Treat Monilial Infections of the Vulvar Skin?

The diagnosis is readily made from wet smears taken from one of the oozing exudative lesions. One should be careful about treating the area too vigorously in the early acute phase. The treatment for this phase differs from that outlined for intertrigo, with emphasis on hot wet applications until the acute inflammation subsides. The main idea in therapy at this time is to soften the skin so that the affected areas can be peeled off. It is probably the shedding of the affected skin that is the most important part of therapy. When the infection passes into the subacute stage, the emphasis in therapy should shift to fungicides which promote keratolysis. Mycotic infections respond satisfactorily to ointments containing nystatin (Mycostatin).

IMPETIGO

Ulcerative impetigo is a common skin infection in infants and young children. In the older child it has a predilection for the face and both the upper and lower extremities, but in the infant and young child it may appear anywhere, including the anogenital area. The organism, which is usually either a streptococcus or a staphylococcus, is normally present in quantity on the unclean skin. It waits for a chance when the integrity of the skin is interrupted to penetrate and permeate just beneath the horny layer (stratum corneum). This may occur through the friction of a diaper, bite of an insect or any other factor that will cause a break in the skin. The infection does not penetrate deeply, but tends to spread laterally, paralleling the skin surface. This is why it tends to be so persistent and recurrent when once firmly established. It is unlike furunculosis or folliculitis (rare in young children), in which the infection descends along the hair follicles.

What Does Impetigo Look Like Clinically?

At the onset pinhead or pea-sized vesicles with a rather thin top covering appear beneath the horny layer of the skin. At first they are clear and transluscent vesicles, but rapidly become cloudy pustules. Since the epidermal-dermal junction in the young child is loosely coupled, the lesions in childhood tend to become bullous and rather extensive. They rupture with ease and spill their purulent discharge onto the surrounding skin. The ruptured pustule seals over and forms a tenacious crust. When this is removed, one sees an excoriated area bathed in pus overlying red oozing granulations. If the lesion is not treated, the crust will simply form again. The lesions become extensive, for the discharge sets up its own autoinoculation (Fig. 8–1).

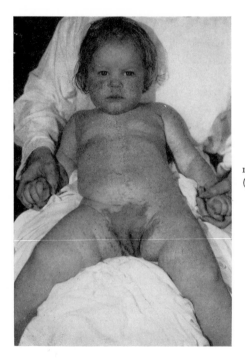

Fig. 8-1.   Vulvar and facial impetigo in an 8-month-old girl. Typically the lesions are bright red. (Courtesy of Dr. F. Ronchese, Providence, R.I.)

How Do You Treat Impetigo?

There are few dermatologic lesions that simulate the appearance of impetigo. Drug eruptions are usually seen in the deeper layers of the skin. Perhaps the two skin infections which are most likely to confuse the diagnosis are a fungus infection or herpes simplex that have become secondarily bacterially infected.

The best method of establishing a diagnosis is to treat the lesion. This consists simply in removing the crusts with a bland soap and warm water. In the acute phase hot applications of potassium permanganate 1:6000 or Burow's solution 1:20 are indicated. After a few days of this type of treatment, ointments such as ammoniated mercury 5 per cent or one of the antibiotic group should be applied. With proper attention the entire process can be cleared up in a week or ten days. Average attention to skin hygiene should prevent recurrence.

General Information about Impetigo

The contagiousness of impetigo has been exaggerated. This is certainly true of the older child. In the past these children were isolated from their playmates without adequate cause. The newborn child, however, is a different matter. Since it has no local immunity to skin infections, it is abnormally sensitive, and these infants need to be protected in the nursery, with particular attention paid to carrier personnel.

SOME SEQUELAE OF VULVAR INFECTIONS

There are two conditions, relatively common, that may arise from infection of the vulva secondary to improper hygiene: (*a*) labial adhesions and (*b*) the adherent clitoral prepuce.

Labial Adhesions

Labial adhesions are not uncommon in the young girl in early childhood, before the hormones become active. It has been said that somewhere between 10 and 20 per cent of all female infants will have labial adhesions during the first year of life. The great majority, however, appear between the ages of two and six years.

Almost invariably the adhesions of the labia, often severe enough to simulate labial fusion, are the result of infection. The infection need not be severe and is usually secondary to faulty hygiene. Rarely is there any severe vulvitis (Fig. 8–2).

At times the condition is so extreme that the child is suspected of having vaginal atresia. The cause, however, is neither congenital nor due to hormones ingested by the mother. At birth the child had normal genital development. In conversation with the mother one can usually obtain a history of vulvar infection followed by a gradual alteration in the appearance of the external genitalia.

As a result of the inflammation of the vulva, which produces superficial erosion and excoriation of the sensitive skin of the labia, thin adhesions form which lead to a fusion of the labia and complete blocking of the vaginal opening. In most instances the urethral orifice escapes, but in extreme cases it, too, may be trapped in the vaginal

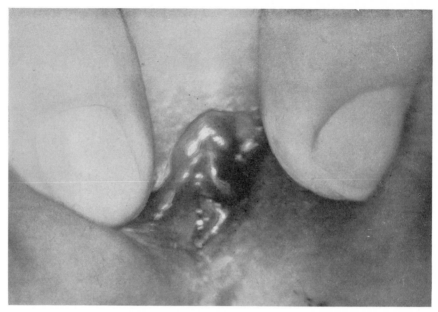

Fig. 8-2.   Labial adhesions in an infant, secondary to infection. (Courtesy of Dr. Sydney S. Gellis, Boston City Hospital.)

vestibule, and the inflammatory process becomes augmented by the vulvovaginitis which follows.

How Do You Distinguish between Labial Adhesions and Congenital Defects?

The most important points in the differential diagnosis between labial fusion due to inflammatory cause and a possible congenital defect are the observations that (a) genital development was normal at birth, and (b) there has been a history of previous vulvitis. The physical findings in labial fusion with an inflammatory background are fairly characteristic. Huffman has pointed out that these children will usually show a thin median raphe running in an anteroposterior direction, which suggests the line of adhesion. One can usually pass a probe with relative ease into the vestibule behind the adhesions if the urethral opening is in view and an opening appears below it. The diagnosis will eventually be made through natural developmental processes if nothing is done, for the appearance of the estrogenic hormones will automatically provide for separation of the labia. Labial adhesions are not found in the adolescent girl.

How Do You Treat Inflammatory Labial Fusion?

The most important part of therapy is to establish the cause, for actually nothing need be done, since the child has few symptoms from the condition. In many instances the labia can be teased apart very gently by manual separation of the labia. Once separated, a recurrence can be prevented by instructing the mother to bathe the area and keep it clean. There is no excuse for forceful or surgical separation, for the simple application of estrin ointment along the line of fusion will cause the labia to assume their normal position.

The Adherent Prepuce

The child may be born with adhesions between the prepuce and the glans clitoris. It is far more likely that the underlying cause is uncleanliness, for one commonly finds an accumulation of smegma beneath the adherent folds. In most instances the condition produces no symptoms, and the child is totally unaware of it. Occasionally, however, the underlying smegma may cause such an irritation that the child constantly rubs the area, an act which in turn so aggravates the inflammatory process that a local abscess may develop.

If there are no symptoms, bathing of the parts may be all that is necessary. When the symptoms are severe enough to warrant stripping back the prepuce, the separation had best be done under anesthesia. Since this condition usually disappears when the genital area comes under estrin stimulation, one may correct the situation earlier in childhood by simple local application of estrogenic ointment.

DERMATOLOGIC LESIONS IN THE ANOGENITAL REGION IN CHILDHOOD

There are a few dermatologic lesions which appear sufficiently often during childhood to warrant a brief discussion. Such entities as infectious granulomas and condylomata acuminata arise in association with a coexisting vulvovaginitis, while others such as lichen sclerosus et atrophicus, psoriasis and herpes simplex are true dermatologic lesions which occasionally manifest themselves in childhood.

Infectious Granuloma

In infectious granuloma the excoriation and maceration of the vulva are so extreme that shallow ulcers form as a result of the constant vaginal discharge. In most instances they are found in neglected children or those who have an obvious nutritional disturbance. If the cause is not clear, the ulcerated area should be biopsied and cultured to rule out the more specific disease processes which could serve as the explanation. Unfortunately infectious granulomas do not respond to antibiotic therapy. The greatest success will follow elimination of the activating cause, but some benefit can be obtained from the use of local applications of estrogenic ointment. Estrogenic substances seem to make the underlying tissue more mature and therefore less sensitive to secondary infection.

Condyloma Acuminatum

This is another relatively uncommon form of dermatologic lesion which appears on the vulva of young children. In this age group the lesions usually appear as warty, vegetative exfoliating proliferations of tissue rather than ulcerations. They may arise in isolated areas or fuse and cover the entire vulva. In most instances the child also has a moderate degree of vaginal discharge (Fig. 8–3). If the child is old enough to pay attention to instructions not to touch the affected area, successful elimination of the lesion can be accomplished by local application of 20 per cent podophyllin ointment. The young child, however, is apt to spread the ointment, which is caustic in action, to other parts of the body, and therefore the physician should try not to use it. He will do better if he first tries ammoniated mercury, 5 per cent, reserving

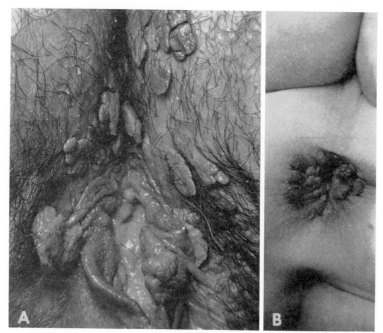

Fig. 8-3.   Vulvar condylomata acuminata in (*A*) mother and (*B*) her daughter, 4 years old. This may indicate their infectious nature. (Courtesy of Dr. F. Ronchese, Providence, R.I.)

electrocoagulation or the application of dry-ice pencils for the cases that fail to respond to simple therapy. The latter treatments had best be done under anesthesia.

LICHEN SCLEROSUS ET ATROPHICUS

Although we commonly associate the appearance of grayish, white, atrophic plaques and thinning of the skin which covers the external vulva with women in the adult age group, it may occur at any time of life and can appear in childhood. There is little difference in the gross appearance of the lesion in whatever age group it is encountered.

In the older patient the differential diagnosis between lichen sclerosus et atrophicus and both kraurosis and leukoplakia is important because of the precancerous connotation attached to the latter. In childhood one need have no such concern. In fact, when the condition has been seen in childhood, and the child is allowed to progress to adulthood without therapy, there appears to be a tendency toward regression to the normal state.

The typical lesion is an irregularly shaped flat-topped macule or papule, which has a rather characteristic mother-of-pearl color, surrounded by an erythematous zone. Within the center of each plaque one usually sees one or more dark comedo-like plugs which extend down into the corium. At times they may be replaced by a central depression on the flat-topped surface. Since the process is basically an atrophic one, there may be some wrinkling of the skin, for the normal elastic fibers have been lost. These plaques may be discrete or coalesce to form an uneven surface over a wide area. In most instances, however, the margins of the individual plaques are evident (Fig. 8-4). The characteristic histologic picture will be discussed in detail in the meno-

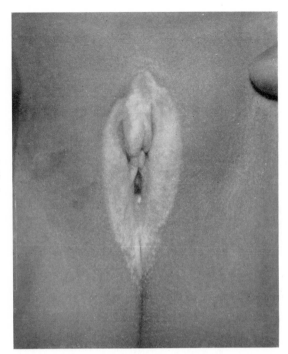

Fig. 8-4.   Vulvar leukoderma and lichen sclerosus et atrophicus, as shown by Wood's light, in a 4-year-old girl. (Courtesy of Dr. F. Ronchese, Providence, R.I.)

pausal age group, where it occurs more frequently and closely simulates the precancerous lesions, kraurosis and leukoplakia.

Like many of the dermatologic lesions of the vulva, lichen sclerosus et atrophicus tends to be extremely pruritic. It is not surprising, then, to find excoriation, maceration and fissuring in the atrophic areas, as secondary infection follows trauma produced by scratching. The diagnosis is relatively easy to establish, for the lesions are characteristic and are unlike any other dermatologic lesion in this area during childhood.

Since the etiology is unknown, the treatment is not very satisfactory. Despite the fact that the process has been known to regress with the onset of puberty, estrogenic substitution therapy has not helped to any extent. Although vitamin deficiency, particularly A and D, seems to contribute to the causation of vulvar atrophy in older women, supplements of these vitamins either systemically or as local ointments have not changed the appearance of the lesion in childhood. The greatest success will come from the use of antipruritic lotions or ointments, and prevention of trauma through friction. This regimen is far more likely to produce favorable results than hydrocortisone ointment.

PSORIASIS

Although this type of dermatologic lesion is most often found on the elbows, knees, lower portion of the back and scalp, it not infrequently is noted in the genital area, particularly on the labia majora and in the intergluteal cleft. Psoriasis is encountered in maximal incidence around the age of twenty and is rarely seen before the age of five years, yet occasional cases are seen in the older growing child. The etiology is unknown.

Psoriasis is one of the more common and disturbing skin lesions, for it is persistent, tends to flare up at periodicintervals and is resistant to treatment. The family should

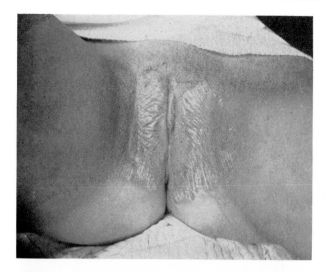

Fig. 8-5.   Psoriasis of the vulva in a $4\frac{1}{2}$-year-old girl whose mother also had psoriasis. (Courtesy of Dr. F. Ronchese, Providence, R.I.)

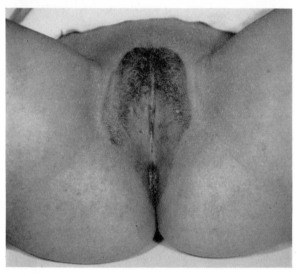

Fig. 8-6.   Vulvar and perianal psoriasis with secondary infection in a 10-year-old girl. (Courtesy of Dr. F. Ronchese, Providence, R.I.)

be reassured, however, and told that the lesions rarely carry any serious connotation as far as general health is concerned.

In the vulvar area one encounters both the acute form, in which minute, red scaly lesions are noted, and the more advanced stages showing circumscribed patches with silvery scales in layers. The lesions are confined to the skin of the vulva and never invade the vaginal epithelium (Fig. 8–5).

In the anogenital area where the skin surfaces are in apposition and irritation through friction is apt to occur, the psoriatic patches often become inflamed, and consequently oozing and crusting occur. The maceration and secondary infection in the groin lead to infection of the skin over the entire vulva, which then tends to become diffusely swollen and erythematous (Fig. 8–6).

Since the natural disease is marked by regression and exacerbation, one should not expect to achieve a permanent cure. Apparently the patient's general health is rarely impaired by psoriasis, and one may elect to do nothing about the lesions, provided they are minimal in extent and produce no symptoms.

By and large there is little to gain by systemic therapy. One may try diet, cortisone, vitamins or antibiotic therapy, but there is little evidence that they have any lasting effect or are any better than topical applications.

The most satisfactory therapy for psoriasis in the vulvar area takes the form of local applications of coal tar solution, 20 per cent, combined with hydrophilic ointment USP, which is designed to relieve the symptoms arising from the inflammation. This preparation is less messy than other crude coal tar ointments. It should be accompanied by ultraviolet light therapy, although it is the tar in all probability that does the most good. By using this combination the majority of exacerbations can be brought under complete control, though not exterminated, in ten to thirty days.

Herpes Simplex

It is fairly common to observe vesiculations on the lips, the mouth, or the labia of the vulva in the course of an acute febrile reaction to a systemic disease such as pneumonia. In some instances such reactions follow the use of drugs or may be attributed to food sensitivity. They may appear simply as the result of local trauma. At first the involved area becomes erythematous, and later a group of vesicles appears. Because they are painful, itch and burn, they are readily traumatized as the child seeks to obtain relief through scratching. This type of infection is particularly troublesome in the young child when it occurs on the genitalia. Secondary infection appears as the result of scratching, and tense umbilicated vesicles rupture and crust over (Fig. 8–7). Because of the infection, though it is largely confined to the dermis, the regional nodes become swollen, tender and painful. In most instances, unless the secondary infection has been severe, the lesions heal within a two-week period without scar formation.

The chief factor in treatment is protection from trauma, in order that secondary infection be avoided. To this end spirits of camphor are applied locally, not because of any specific action on the virus, but simply as a means of relieving, or at least cutting down, the pain and itching. With the same aim in view, one may choose to give an ointment containing zinc oxide 15, talc 15 and glycerin 10 parts.

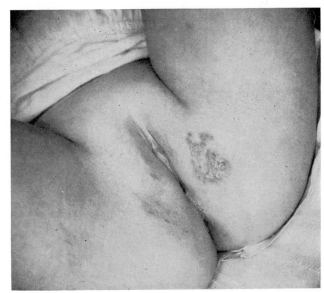

Fig. 8-7. Herpetic lesions of the vulva with crusting in a 2-year-old girl. They are caused by herpes simplex virus, which also produces the more common perioral "fever blisters." (Courtesy of Dr. F. Ronchese, Providence, R.I.)

It is an interesting observation that herpes simplex sometimes tends to recur at the time of puberty and periodically with each successive menstruation.

Herpes zoster is rare in childhood, but the viruses of chickenpox (varicella) and herpes zoster are closely allied and may coexist, with simultaneous manifestations of both types.

TRAUMA TO THE EXTERNAL GENITALIA

Since the deposits of subcutaneous fat within the labia are scanty in the young child, the external genitalia lie in an exposed position which can readily be traumatized. The great majority of injuries are caused by an accidental fall across some object, either blunt or sharp. Less often the vulvar trauma is self-inflicted or the result of sexual assault. Whatever the cause, the child is uncomfortable and the family apprehensive.

ACCIDENTAL INJURIES

Two anatomic factors are concerned in genital injuries produced by a fall across a solid bar or sharp penetrating object: (a) the subcutaneous tissue is loosely arranged, and (b) the area is very vascular. Direct blows of this sort then tend to produce contusions and hematomas rapidly. Since there is little underlying protective tissue, the vulvar area on the side of the trauma distends rather extensively with blood. Bleeding occurs promptly, but is usually self-limited, and with enough pressure from within the bleeding usually stops. Massive swelling of the vulva need not alarm the physician, for it will subside rapidly when cold packs and external pressure are applied. Only on rare occasions will it be necessary for the surgeon to evacuate the blood clot under anesthesia. The important factor is to relieve the child's discomfort and reassure the parents that no permanent damage will follow.

Lacerations may occur if the child has fallen on a sharp penetrating object. In this case the important fact to establish is the degree of penetration and whether or not the urethra, bladder, rectum and peritoneal cavity are intact. If there is evidence of any such perforation, immediate operation is indicated. When only external lacerations are present, the degree of injury will determine whether or not any suturing is necessary. It should be kept in mind that there is a tendency for the local tissues in this area to return to normal. Only rarely, then, are surgical procedures indicated.

SELF-INFLICTED INJURIES

The vulva and hymen can be traumatized by the child's attempts to insert objects into the vagina. Since this is not easily accomplished in the younger child, the manifestations of the effort usually appear as abrasions. Contusions may appear if the child has the habit of forceful masturbation. By and large, self-inflicted injuries are rare in the younger child.

FORCEFUL ASSAULT

When there has been an attempt at forceful penetration by sexual assault, the lacerations of the vulva, hymen and perineum assume a fairly characteristic picture.

It is not enough to find a patulous vaginal orifice to make a diagnosis of rape, for some children have this type of conformation of the vaginal orifice at birth. In general, if force has been applied to the immature vulva, the pressure of the penis will exert circumferential pressure which produces a stellate kind of laceration. The hymen will show several longitudinal splits. If the pressure is maintained and actual penetration occurs, it is possible to perforate the child's bladder or tear into the peritoneal cavity.

Before a diagnosis of rape can be substantiated, there must generally be other evidence of trauma in other parts of the body, in addition to the local signs in the genital region. When confronted with this situation, immediately after the fact, the physician should try to obtain smears or washings from the vagina and perineum so that they can be examined in the police laboratory for possible spermatozoa. It would be well also to confiscate the child's clothing for the same reason.

REFERENCES

Anderson, O. W.: Treatment of Labial Adhesions in Children. *J.A.M.A.*, 162: 951, 1956.

Callomon, F. T., and Wilson, J. F.: *Non-venereal Diseases of the Genitals. Etiology, Differential Diagnosis and Therapy.* Springfield, Ill., Charles C Thomas, 1956.

Ditowsky, S. P., Falk, A. B., Baker, N., and Schaffner, M.: Lichen Sclerosus et Atrophicus in Childhood. A.M.A. *J. Dis. Child.*, 91: 52, 1956.

Gray, L. A., and Kotcher, E.: Vulvovaginitis in Childhood. *Clin. Obst. & Gynec.*, 3: 165, 1960.

Huffman, J. W.: Vulvar Disorders in Premenarchal Children. *Clin. Obst. & Gynec.*, 3: 154, 1960.

Hunt, E.: *Diseases Affecting the Vulva.* 4th Ed. St. Louis, C. V. Mosby Company, 1959.

Leider, M.: *Practical Pediatric Dermatology.* St. Louis, C. V. Mosby Company, 1956.

Nowlin, P., Adams, J. R., and Nallie, B. C., Jr.: Vulvar Fusion. *J. Urol.*, 62: 75, 1949.

Schauffler, G. C.: Psychosomatic Factors and Masturbation. *Pediat. Clin. N. Amer.*, 5: 111, 1958.

Chapter 9

Tumors in Childhood

A few benign and, occasionally, true malignant genital neoplasms may appear in childhood. For the most part these tumors have ovarian origin. Some of this group are extremely malignant and carry a poor prognosis. Tumors of the uterus and vagina are extremely rare in childhood, but they occur often enough to alert the physician to the possibility of malignant disease when a young child is presented with a history of vaginal bleeding, spotting or hematuria. The same may be said of vulvar tumors.

OVARIAN TUMORS

In childhood these tend to fall into the same classifications that apply to neoplasms of the ovary in adult life. The cystic tumors tend to be benign, while practically all the solid tumors are malignant. Although ovarian neoplasms are infrequent, they are important because of their lethal potentialities. It has been said that 35 per cent of all ovarian tumors at this age are malignant. The malignant potential rises when solid tumors are found.

What Symptoms Are Produced by Ovarian Tumors?

The symptoms produced by ovarian tumors in childhood are often nearly completely masked, and their presence is frequently unsuspected. A bizarre event such as precocious menstrual bleeding may draw attention to the tumor, but otherwise the neoplasm goes unrecognized until either the patient has severe abdominal pain or a massive enlargement of the abdomen is noted.

The presenting symptoms tend to fall into three groups: those that have (*a*) acute abdominal pain, (*b*) chronic abdominal discomfort, and (*c*) remote symptoms or manifestations of endocrine activity. The last will be discussed in the consideration of functioning tumors of the ovary (Chap. 55).

Acute Abdominal Pain.   Approximately 65 per cent of all ovarian tumors in childhood are either simple cysts (15 per cent) or cystic teratomas ("dermoids") (50 per cent). Because these tumors in childhood tend to be unilateral and grow on a pedicle, they are prone to twist and obstruct their blood supply. The acute pain that follows the ischemia and hemorrhage into the cavity of the cyst often provides the first indication that a tumor is present. Too often the tumor is unsuspected, and a

98

diagnosis of appendicitis, intussusception, Meckel's diverticulum, pyelitis or mesenteric adenitis is entertained. This is not surprising, for the nature of the pain is similar, and the young child tends to localize the pain to the area around the umbilicus and lower part of the abdomen. The pain may be steady or colicky, as in appendicitis. In the infant the only expression of pain may be restlessness or crying. Because of the possibility of an incorrect diagnosis, a bimanual abdominal and rectal examination should be done on any child who has acute abdominal pain. Not to do so is to run the risk of encountering a large pelvic tumor which cannot be dealt with adequately through a small appendectomy incision. Any tumor large enough to produce symptoms in a child can be felt by rectum.

CHRONIC ABDOMINAL DISCOMFORT.   This is perhaps more common than acute pain in the young child who has an ovarian tumor. It may be just that and nothing more, for the final diagnosis is often suspected only when the mother notices that the child has an abdominal mass. Occasionally the child may experience intermittent episodes of fairly severe pain, associated with nausea and vomiting during the acute phase, but with prompt recovery. Pain of this sort is usually due to partial obstruction of the blood supply to the ovarian tumor pedicle, which may relieve itself promptly.

What Types of Ovarian Tumor Are Encountered in Childhood?

DERMOID CYST.   Benign cystic teratomas of the ovary (dermoid cysts) are the most common tumor type in this age group. The diagnosis is suspected when the mother notices abdominal enlargement in the child, and the physician palpates an abdominal tumor. Occasionally a cyst can be felt as a firm, tense, rounded mass on rectal examination, but the pelvic floor of the child is so constructed that the cyst usually rises out of, rather than descends into, the pelvis. X-ray films may show the presence of teeth or bone. There is nothing characteristic about the symptomatology, which may take the form of (*a*) acute pain, (*b*) chronic abdominal discomfort, or (*c*) pressure on some neighboring organ such as the bladder.

SIMPLE BENIGN CYSTS.   These cysts, full of clear serous fluid, have been encountered at birth and throughout childhood. Enlarged ovaries containing follicle cysts frequently are noted when a child is sexually precocious. They may cause abdominal enlargement but few other symptoms. Like the dermoids, they too grow on a pedicle which may twist and jeopardize the blood supply to the tumor.

SOLID TUMORS OF THE OVARY.   Carcinoma is the most common form of solid tumor in the young child. Embryonic in nature, it has lethal possibilities. Unfortunately the symptoms produced are no different from those caused by benign ovarian growths, with the possible exception of weight loss. The majority are discovered inadvertently when the family seeks an explanation for rapidly increasing abdominal girth in a young child.

Since the mass presents in the abdomen rather than in the lower pelvis, the solid tumor of ovarian origin must be differentiated from the other large abdominal tumors which are found in childhood.

There are three cancers which appear in children with sufficient frequency to be confused with malignant ovarian neoplasms: (*a*) embryoma (Wilms's tumor) of the kidney, (*b*) neuroblastoma, which arises from the adrenal, and (*c*) retroperitoneal sarcoma. All grow slowly in insidious fashion, and although they begin as laterally placed tumors, they are not usually discovered until they fill one side of the abdomen. Unfortunately they, too, produce little in the way of symptoms, except for the pressure they exert on other organs. The renal embryoma, like the neoplastic ovary, is smooth and round, while the neuroblastoma is more apt to have an irregular surface. X-ray films of the abdomen and the kidney, including an intravenous pyelogram, may be useful in differentiating the embryoma of the kidney from other entities.

Since the dermoid cyst is the predominant ovarian tumor in childhood, it is important to check carefully every dermoid cyst removed, with the possibility of malignancy in mind.

Among the malignant solid tumors of the ovary, carcinoma, teratocarcinoma and dysgerminoma are the most common and most lethal. Fortunately sarcoma (usually fibrosarcoma) is found infrequently, for it grows rapidly and metastasizes early. The *carcinomas* are predominantly solid, although they may have cystic components. In most instances the cystic element is due to necrosis within a solid tumor, but rarely malignant change within a solid area in the trabeculations of a serous cystadenoma may occur. The *solid teratocarcinoma*, which is a malignant counterpart of the benign dermoid cyst, has a particularly bad prognosis. Less than half of the children with this type of tumor survive for any appreciable time. The prognosis improves if the tumor is encapsulated.

The gross pathologic aspect of solid ovarian cancers is usually much alike, regardless of the microscopic pattern. The masses are rounded or multinodular and partly covered by a thin capsule. Most often they are locally or generally softer than might be expected of cancers generally. When cut, the tumor tissue is pale gray-white or tan, and often resembles brain. Typically, a teratocarcinoma will have both solid areas and cysts, perhaps with foci of gross cartilage and bone, but many examples are not so distinctive.

Microscopically, ovarian carcinoma in childhood ordinarily is rather undifferentiated, composed of epithelial cells of an indefinite origin. Carcinomas that arise in cystadenomas are described later. Dysgerminoma, microscopically, is characterized by sheets of large, pale, watery, anaplastic cells reminiscent of urogenital neoplasms such as renal hypernephromas. Foci of lymphocytes and other leukocytes provide a "lymphoid stroma," which is a characteristic common to the ovarian dysgerminoma and testicular embryonal carcinoma. Histologically, these two neoplasms are indistinguishable (Fig. 9–1, *A*).

Wilms's tumor, also called Wilms's embryoma or adenosarcoma, may be primary in the ovary, although the most common site of origin is in the kidney. Grossly, it forms a rather encephaloid solid mass containing small cysts. Microscopically, much of the neoplastic growth has an undifferentiated primitive sarcomatous pattern. Within this sarcoma foci are found of differentiation of some malignant cells into fibrous tissue, striated or smooth muscle, cartilage or other types of connective tissue. Scattered glands lined by primitive mesonephric epithelium are intermingled (Fig. 9–1, *B*).

Teratocarcinoma of the child's ovary is rare. Evidence of origin from a benign teratoma may be found in the form of masses of epithelium and also small cysts of squamous, mucous, respiratory or other types. The bulk of the tumor, microscopically, appears like an undifferentiated malignant neoplasm, with foci of differentiated connective tissue and epithelium. Some components of embryonal carcinoma or choriocarcinoma may be present (Fig. 9–2, *A*).

The theory that teratomas of childhood represent incomplete twinning is no longer popular. Instead, these tumors, either benign or malignant, are regarded as neoplasms arising in the germ cells of the host.

Not all solid tumors have the same malignant potential. The granulosa cell tumor of the ovary is occasionally found in prepuberal girls. Approximately 10 per cent of all such tumors appear at this time. In the older age groups the clinically malignant possibilities of the granulosa cell tumor run as high as 30 per cent, but in

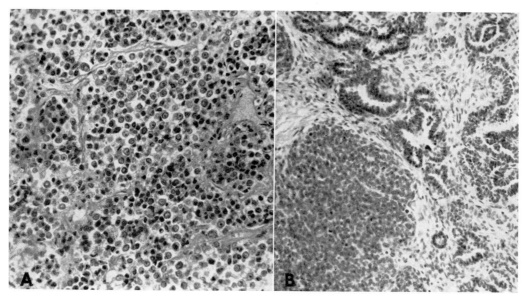

Fig. 9-1. *A*, The sheetlike growth of large cells with clear cytoplasm, prominent nuclei and nucleoli is characteristic of dysgerminoma. Some lymphocytes with dark-stained nuclei are intermingled. *B*, Wilms's tumor of the kidney or ovary is composed of solid foci of undifferentiated cancer, as shown at lower left, undifferentiated sarcoma, at upper right, and tubular neoplastic growths resembling primitive renal tubules.

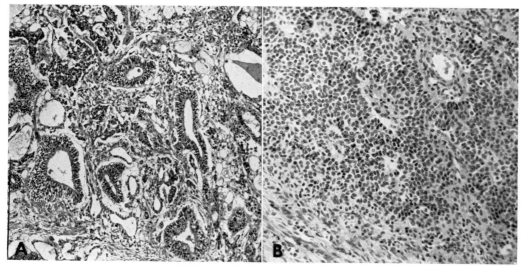

Fig. 9-2. *A*, Malignant ovarian teratoma, or teratocarcinoma, with cysts resembling the primitive neuroenteric canal and undifferentiated carcinoma, as shown at upper left. *B*, Granulosa cell tumor of ovary, with orderly growth of well differentiated small cells, benign in appearance.

childhood the tumor is less likely to metastasize or recur after adequate removal (Fig. 9–2, *B*).

The great majority of the solid tumors of the ovary are unilateral, grow on a pedicle and lie free in the abdominal cavity. The dysgerminoma, on the other hand, tends to be bilateral, though the other characteristics are similar. There seems to be a great concentration in the number of dysgerminomas encountered in the years immediately preceding puberty. Approximately one third of all the dysgerminomas found in any age group are discovered in childhood, yet they are rare before the age of ten years.

OVARIAN TUMORS WITH ENDOCRINE SYMPTOMS.   The diagnosis of a functioning tumor of the ovary is not difficult when the patient bleeds precociously and has obvious enlargement of the uterus and breasts. Both the granulosa cell and the theca cell tumors can produce feminization of a prepuberal child. Actually, it is the theca cell element within a granulosa cell tumor that is believed responsible for the production of estrin. The theca cell tumor as well as the granulosa cell type of neoplasm may occur at a very early age. One theca cell tumor has been reported at the age of one year, and we have personal knowledge of a thirteen-months-old child who had a granulosa cell tumor. In both there was evidence of uterine and breast enlargement, growth of the external genitalia and pubic hair, and cornification of the vaginal epithelium to accompany the appearance of cyclic menstrual bleeding. The bleeding is always anovulatory, in contrast to sexual precocity of the constitutional variety. The two must be distinguished, for while the child with granulosa or theca cell tumor cannot become pregnant, because she is not ovulating, the child who simply develops precociously can. It is fortunate that such tumors grow to appreciable size, since palpation by rectum of the unsuspected tumor will establish the true diagnosis. Gross, for example, has stated that any tumor of endocrine significance which is capable of producing feminization is large enough to be felt by rectum. After the discovery and surgical removal of the tumor all or most of the precocious femininity regresses to its normal childhood state, to reappear normally at puberty.

The masculinizing tumors of the ovary are rare. Only one instance of an arrhenoblastoma has been reported before the age of fifteen years. Masculinization of the external genitalia can, however, occur in rare instances from an adrenal tumor in this age group. It is more likely, however, that the male attributes will develop secondary to the more common hyperplasia of the adrenal cortex. The morphologic aspects of these functioning tumors are described later (p. 801).

It is important to remember that dysgerminomas are apt to be associated with female pseudohermaphroditism. The appearance of an enlarged clitoris, hypospadiac urethra and scrotal fusion along with palpation of bilateral solid ovarian masses may suggest that the ovarian tumors are responsible for the masculinization. This is in error, for the dysgerminoma is a neutral tumor and usually secretes no hormone. The developmental abnormalities observed are due to its association with pseudohermaphroditism.

The diagnosis of forms of ovarian tumor other than those with endocrine effect is less obvious when the symptoms do not focus on the abdomen and pelvis, but manifest themselves in more remote areas of the body. The first sign of primary malignant ovarian neoplasm, for example, may be cough, pain in the chest or the finding of an enlarged node in the left supraclavicular area. Teratocarcinomas of the ovary are prone to reveal themselves in this manner.

What Treatment Is Indicated?

The primary factor in treatment is a high index of suspicion that an ovarian tumor may be present in any child who has either chronic abdominal distress or acute pain. The presence of any tumor felt by rectum or abdominally is all that is required to demand prompt abdominal exploration. This is true whether the neoplasm is solid or cystic. Because the incidence of cancer is so high in ovarian tumors of childhood and the differential diagnosis so hard to establish, the surgeon should be extremely cautious in applying a benign diagnosis to such a growth.

Frequently the distinction between a benign and a malignant growth cannot be made at the time of operation by simple inspection and palpation of the tumor. The error will be less if the surgeon regards every solid tumor as malignant. Most cysts will be benign, but enough carry a malignant component to insist on the rule that after removal every cystic ovarian tumor should be opened in the operating room before the abdomen is closed. Any solid portion of a cystic tumor and all solid tumors should be presented to the pathologist for his opinion.

It is a difficult decision to carry out radical surgical procedures which call for removal of the genital equipment of a young girl. This, however, may be the only chance the child has to survive. Conservatism, however, should be practiced in removing all cystic structures whenever possible. Cysts may be excised out of the ovary in many instances. It is not necessary to remove the entire ovary. This is all that need be done if the opened cyst shows no suggestion of malignancy. If the cyst proves to be of dermoid type, it will be wise to split the other ovary and look at the interior, for dermoid tumors tend to be bilateral.

Although granulosa cell tumors and malignant teratomas have different degrees of malignancy associated with them, one may choose to take a calculated risk and remove only the single involved ovary. Teratocarcinomas are far more lethal than granulosa cell tumors, but if they are encapsulated, surgical excision of the single involved ovary may provide as good a chance of cure as total bilateral extirpation. The granulosa cell tumor in this age group is far less likely to recur than it is in the older age groups, and one ovary may be removed, leaving the uterus and other ovary. The same attitude expressed for the solid teratocarcinoma may be extended to include the dysgerminoma. In older women the index of malignancy is high, but the encapsulated dysgerminomatous tumor in childhood is less lethal. There is another factor that favors conservatism in the young child with dysgerminoma. The tumor is very radiosensitive. Thus one can afford to leave the other ovary and the uterus if the tumor is unilateral and encapsulated. Should the tumor progress despite surgical excision, x-ray treatment can be given.

There is nothing to be gained from conservative treatment in a young child who has a solid ovarian carcinoma, sarcoma or any other malignant tumor, such as a solid dysgerminoma, teratoma or a cystic serous cystadenocarcinoma that has broken through its restraining capsule. Total removal of the uterus and both tubes and ovaries is indicated.

TUMORS OF THE UTERUS

Fortunately, malignant tumors of the uterus in children are relatively rare, for the prognosis is usually poor.

CARCINOMA OF THE CERVIX

Benign growths such as polyps and erosions have been reported in young children, but rarely require any particular therapy. Rosenthal and Hellmann have reported the appearance of adenomatous hyperplasia and epidermidization of the cervix in young girls, with some of the growth characteristics of carcinoma in situ.

The carcinomas of the cervix in children reported in the literature have almost invariably either been undifferentiated or adenocarcinoma. Although there has usually been a history of vaginal bleeding, its significance has gone unrecognized for so long that the cancer has become too far advanced to offer anything but a poor prognosis. This observation further accentuates the need for earlier examinations of such young children. Radical surgery has proved of value in the child who has a uterine cancer that is sufficiently confined to warrant it.

SARCOMA BOTRYOIDES

The manifestations of this rare tumor are most dramatic. It is partly undifferentiated and in part a rhabdomyosarcoma that arises from the cervix and upper part of the vagina, rapidly involves the uterus and fills the vagina with pale, colorless, solid masses arranged in grapelike clusters. The first manifestation may be the appearance of tumor tissue at the vaginal outlet (Fig. 9–3).

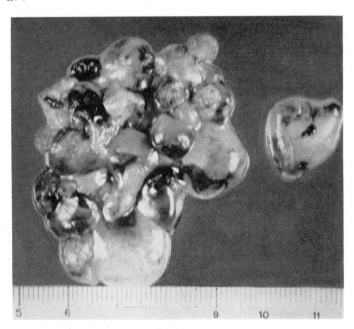

Fig. 9-3. Typical rounded, smooth masses of uterine sarcoma botryoides, with focal hemorrhage and necrosis. These grapelike tumors protruded into the vagina.

The tumor is apt to appear in very young children more often than in postmenopausal women, which is the other age group in which it is chiefly found. Sarcoma botryoides is a very malignant tumor which can be successfully treated only by radical surgical extirpation of all the pelvic viscera. X-ray therapy is completely ineffective, and anything short of extremely radical surgery is contraindicated. Few cures are reported.

TUMORS IN THE VULVAR AREA

Several benign and a few malignant tumors occur in the region of the vulva and vagina, though they are rare. Nevertheless, any unexplained swelling or ulceration in this region must be excised or biopsied to rule out a possible cancer, particularly if it is accompanied by vaginal discharge or bleeding. The majority of vulvar tumors appear in the form of indurated swellings, ulcerations or vegetative growths.

Although most malignant tumors of the vulva in young children are sarcomas, particularly sarcoma botryoides, carcinomas have been reported. Like the cervical neoplasms in children and in direct contrast to the type encountered in adults, the vulvar tumors are usually adenocarcinomas. In all probability they arise in embryonic rests of mesonephric or paramesonephric origin. The most common vascular tumors are hemangiomas and lymphangiomas. One need not be alarmed about the presence even of a sizable hemangioma, for they have a peculiar habit of disappearing without any therapy as the child grows older. They are usually asymptomatic, so that one can afford to await the passage of time (Fig. 9–4).

There have recently been reports in the literature of a number of granular cell myoblastomas. In most instances they appear as nontender swellings of no great size in and around the vulva. Sometimes they arouse a suspicion of malignant disease, particularly when the surface of the lump ulcerates. Since clinically they resemble basal cell or epidermoid carcinoma, they should be biopsied. The best way to biopsy the lesion is to excise it completely, with a wide margin around the growth, since they are rather poorly demarcated from the surrounding tissue.

On histologic examination the myoblastoma is composed of large rounded cells with a considerable amount of bright acidophilic cytoplasm and small nuclei. The appearance is reminiscent of striated muscle, but there are no cross-striations, and instead many fine granules occur in the cytoplasm (Fig. 9–5). The tumor cells usually appear orderly, but may recur locally or metastasize, and it is believed impossible to predict the outcome from pathologic examination. Some consider this a nerve-sheath tumor, and believe granular cell myoblastoma to be a misnomer.

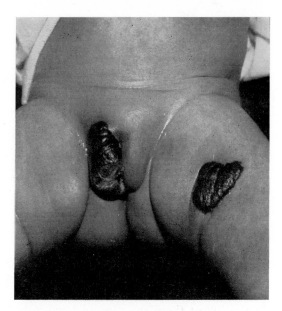

Fig. 9-4.   Hemangiomas of the vulva and thigh in an infant girl. (Courtesy of Dr. F. Ronchese, Providence, R.I.)

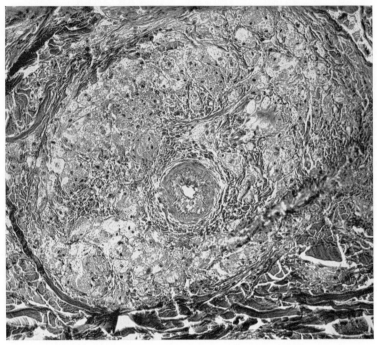

Fig. 9-5.   A granular cell myoblastoma, with the characteristic large cells forming a rounded
nodule in the midst of striated muscle.

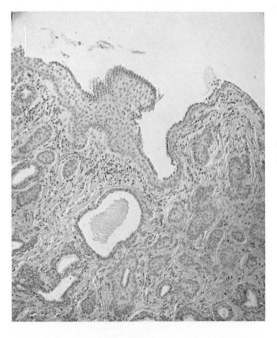

Fig. 9-6.   Vaginal cyst lined by duct
epithelium, evidently arising from a paravaginal
gland.

A number of varieties of vaginal cysts are seen in infancy and childhood. The
most important vaginal cyst to rule out is the hydrometrocolpos, secondary to the
presence of an imperforate hymen. Incision and drainage are indicated, for frequently
in the infant there may be an accumulation of mucus and serous fluid behind the
obstruction. This is good prophylactic surgery, for in this manner hematocolpos will

be avoided at the time of the menarche when the ovarian hormones have become active and menstrual bleeding begins.

Rarely one encounters vaginal cysts, such as inclusion or paraurethral cysts, which are usually incidental findings and rarely produce symptoms. If they are asymptomatic, they need not be biopsied, and no treatment is indicated. Occasionally a paraurethral duct cyst will be large enough to press on the urethra and interfere with micturition. In such a case the cyst should be excised in the interest of relieving symptoms and possibly preventing the development of a urethral diverticulum as the child passes into adulthood (Fig. 9–6).

REFERENCES

Ovarian Tumors

Bruk, I., Dancaster, C. P., and Jackson, W. P. U.: Granulosal Cell Tumours Causing Precocious Puberty. *Brit. M.J.*, 2: 26, 1960.

Butt, J. A.: Ovarian Tumors in Children. *Am. J. Obst. & Gynec.*, 69: 833, 1955.

Costlin, M. E., and Kennedy, R. L. J.: Ovarian Tumors in Infants and Children. *Am. J. Dis. Child.*, 76: 127, 1948.

Craig, J. M.: Tumors of Lower Genitourinary Tract. *Pediat. Clin. N. Amer.*, 6: 491, 1959.

Dargeon, H. W.: Ovarian Tumors in Childhood. *Pediatrics*, 3: 773, 1949.

Darte, J. M.: Ovarian Tumors in the Premenarchal Child. *Clin. Obst. & Gynec.*, 3: 187, 1960.

Gagner, S., and Sjövall, A.: Ovarian and Paraovarian Tumors in Children. *Acta Obst. & Gynec. Scandinav.*, 28: 110, 1948–49.

Gordon, V. H., and Marvin, H. N.: Theca Cell Tumor of Ovary in One Year Old. *J. Pediat.*, 39: 133, 1951.

Gross, R. E.: Neoplasms Producing Endocrine Disturbances in Childhood. *Am. J. Dis. Child.*, 59: 579, 1940.

Idem: *The Surgery of Infancy and Childhood.* Philadelphia, W. B. Saunders Company, 1953.

Guinn, G. H., and Gilbert, E. F.: Cushing's Syndrome in Children Associated with Adrenocortical Carcinoma—Review of Literature. *A.M.A. J. Dis. Child.*, 92: 297, 1956.

Huffman, J. W.: Tumors of the Female Genitalia; in I. M. Ariel and G. T. Pack: *Cancer and Allied Disease. of Infancy and Childhood.* Boston, Little, Brown & Company, 1959.

Huffman, J. W., and Wieczorowski, E.: Gynecology of Children and Adolescents. *Pediatrics*, 22: 395, 1958.

Kimmel, G. C.: Sexual Precocity and Accelerated Growth in a Child with a Follicular Cyst of the Ovary. *J. Pediat.*, 30: 686, 1947.

Knaus, W. E., Campos, J., and Rose, W.: Meigs Syndrome—Report of a Case in a Child. *F. Pediat.*, 43: 88, 1953.

Longino, L. A., and Martin, L. W.: Abdominal Masses in Newborn Infant. *Pediatrics*, 21: 596, 1958.

Meigs, J. V.: *Tumors of Female Pelvic Organs.* New York, Macmillan Company, 1934.

Neigus, I.: Ovarian Dysgerminoma with Chorionepithelioma. *Am. J. Obst. & Gynec.*, 69: 838, 1955.

Pedowitz, P., Felmus, L. B., and Mackles, A.: Precocious Pseudopuberty Due to Ovarian Tumors. *Obst. & Gynec. Survey*, 10: 633, 1955.

Radman, H. M., and Korman, W.: Ovarian Tumors in Children. *Am. J. Obst. & Gynec.*, 79: 989, 1960.

Scarpa, J. B., Beheran, H., Raices, A. A., and Bur, G. E.: Ovarian Tumor, Precocious Puberty and Adrenal Hyperfunction. *Am. J. Obst. & Gynec.*, 78: 821, 1959.

Schaeffer, G., and Verprovsky, E. C.: Ovarian Neoplasms in Children. *Am. J. Obst. & Gynec.*, 58: 718, 1949.

Sobel, E. H., Lee, C. M., Jr., Esselborn, V. M., and Clark, L. C., Jr.: Functioning Adrenal Tumors in Childhood—Consideration of Diagnosis, Surgical Approach, Postoperative Management. *Am. J. Dis. Child.*, 86: 733, 1953.

Taylor, E. S., and Snow, R. H.: Adrenal Virilism in Female Child and Adult. *Am. J. Obst. & Gynec.*, 67: 1307, 1954.

Zemke, E. E., and Hernell, W. G.: Bilateral Granulosal Cell Tumor—Successful Removal from a Child Fourteen Weeks of Age. *Am. J. Obst. & Gynec.*, 41: 704, 1941.

Uterine and Cervical Tumors

Boyes, D. A., Hardie, M., and Agnew, A. M.: Carcinoma of Cervix in an Infant. *Am. J. Obst. & Gynec.,* 72: 1353, 1956.

Creadick, R. N.: Sarcoma Botryoides. *Am. J. Obst. & Gynec.,* 68: 567, 1954.

Duncan, A. S., and Fahny, E. C.: Sarcoma Botryoides of Vagina and Cervix in Children. Report of Two Cases and Plea for Early Clinical Diagnosis. *J. Obst. & Gynaec. Brit. Emp.,* 60: 87, 1953.

James, T.: A Benign Polypoid Tumour of Cervix Uteri in a Girl Three Years Old. *J. Obst. & Gynaec. Brit. Emp.,* 58: 762, 1951.

Kamorowska, A., Liniecka, J., and Mazurkiewicz, M. R.: Carcinoma of the Cervix Uteri in a Nine Month Old Girl. *Gin. Polska,* 5: 539, 1957; *Internat. Abstr. Surg.,* Sept., 1958, p. 264.

Marcus, S. L.: Müllerian Mixed Sarcoma (Sarcoma Botryoides) of Cervix. *Obst. & Gynec.,* 15: 47, 1960.

Ober, W. B., and Edgecomb, J. H.: Sarcoma Botryoides in the Female Urogenital Tract. *Cancer,* 7: 75, 1954.

Pinkel, D., and Pickren, J.: Rhabdomyosarcoma in Children. *J.A.M.A.,* 175: 293, 1961.

Pollack, R. S., and Taylor, H. C.: Carcinoma of the Cervix during the First Two Decades of Life. *Am. J. Obst. & Gynec.,* 53: 135, 1947.

Rosenthal, A. H., and Hellmann, L. M.: Epithelial Changes in the Fetal Cervix, Including the Role of the "Reserve Cell." *Am. J. Obst. & Gynec.,* 64: 260, 1952.

Shackman, R.: Sarcoma Botryoides of the Genital Tract in Female Children. *Brit. J. Surg.,* 38: 26, 1950.

Speert, H.: Cervical Cancer in Young Girls. *Am. J. Obst. & Gynec.,* 54: 982, 1947.

Vaginal and Vulvar Tumors

Baldwin, L. G.: Primary Carcinoma of the Vagina in Girl Fourteen, with Consideration of Age Incidence of 905 Cases of Carcinoma of Uterus, Vagina and Vulva. *Am. J. Obst. & Gynec.,* 21: 728, 1931.

Bishop, H. C., and Wagner, B. M.: Granular Cell Myoblastoma in Childhood. *Pediatrics,* 19: 858, 1957.

Cohen, J. F., Klein, M. D., and Laver, M. B.: Cysts of the Vagina in the Newborn Infant. *Surg., Gynec. & Obst.,* 94: 322, 1957.

Daniel, W. W., Koss, L. C., and Brunschwig, A.: Sarcoma Botryoides of the Vagina. *Cancer,* 12: 74, 1959.

Dargeon, H., Eversole, J., and Del Duca, V.: Malignant Melanoma in Infant. *Cancer,* 3: 299, 1950.

Gerbie, A. B., Hirsch, M. R., and Greene, R. R.: Vascular Tumors of the Female Genital Tract. *Obst. & Gynec.,* 6: 499, 1955.

Hoge, R. H., and Benn, V. A.: Carcinoma of Vulva and Vagina in Infancy. *Am. J. Obst. & Gynec.,* 46: 286, 1943.

Huffman, J. W.: Disorders of the External Genitals and Vagina. *Pediat. Clin. N. Amer.,* 5: 35, 1958.

Idem: Vulvar Disorders in Premenarchal Children. *Clin. Obst. & Gynec.,* 3: 154, 1960.

Lash, A. F., and Davis, B. A.: Squamous Cell Carcinoma of the Vulva in Young Women. *Am. J. Obst. & Gynec.,* 78: 841, 1959.

McKay, D. C., Fowler, R., and Barett, J. S.: Pathogenesis and Treatment of Primary Hydrocele in Infancy and Childhood. *Australian & New Zealand J. Surg.,* Aug., 1958.

Ober, W. B., Smith, J. A., and Rouillard, F. C.: Congenital Sarcoma Botryoides of the Vagina. *Cancer,* 11: 620, 1958.

Ronchese, F.: Hemangiomas—Should Treatment Be Expectant or Active? *Rhode Island M.F.,* 29: 658, 1946.

Idem: The Spontaneous Involution of Cutaneous Vascular Tumors. *Am. J. Surg.,* 86: 376, 1953.

Rubin, A.: Granular Cell Myoblastoma of the Vulva. *Am. J. Obst. & Gynec.,* 77: 292, 1959.

Ulfelder, H., and Hendren, W. H., III: Vaginal and Uterine Tumors in Children. *Clin. Obst. & Gynec.,* 3: 175, 1960.

Ulfelder, H., and Quan, S. H.: Sarcoma Botryoides Vaginae—Complete Excision of Tumor in Infant by Combined Abdominal and Perineal Approach. *S. Clin. N. Amer.,* 27:1240, 1947.

Winkelstein, L. B., and Friedman, S.: Granular Cell Myoblastoma of the Vulva. *Am. J. Obst. & Gynec.,* 75: 325, 1958.

Chapter 10

Examination of
the Young Female Child

THERE appears to be a natural reluctance on the part of both physician and family to examine the young female. Yet there may be conditions in the premenarchal child that should be recognized before the advent of puberty. A few, such as vaginal bleeding, discharge, vulvovaginal infection and either local vulvar or intra-abdominal tumors, produce enough symptoms to bring the child to the physician. Unfortunately, other conditions are allowed to go unrecognized because of reluctance to have the child examined. These include abnormalities in the development of the external genitalia, disturbances in skeletal growth, abnormally early onset of puberty, delayed maturation and either precocious or delayed appearance of the secondary sex characteristics. The tendency is to explain them away rather than investigate the possible causes.

The local gynecologic examination, performed as part of the general physical examination, need not be any more of an ordeal for the physician or a cause of psychic trauma to the child than an ordinary examination of the nose and throat, provided certain basic principles are observed: (1) In the first place, the mother should be told that the child will not be hurt or the genitalia, particularly the hymen, damaged. She should be assured that any instruments used are specially designed to take care of the child's problem. (2) The child should be told that the examination will not hurt and that the doctor will stop examining her if she does feel pain. Most older children will submit readily to the examination if you tell them what you are going to do and why you have to do it.

A large part of the success of the surgeon's approach to the child, previous to actual examination, will depend on how he goes at it, and the degree of confidence he can instill in both the patient and the mother. The examiner should go about his work quietly in a relaxed atmosphere and can afford to spend some time in explaining to the child what he plans to do. The preliminary phase of the examination, however, should not be too prolonged, for overmuch indecisive delay may increase the apprehension of both child and mother. In the young child who has just begun to assert herself the physician may expect an automatic "No" to any request for cooperation, but this can usually be overcome by directing the child's attention elsewhere.

Little will be accomplished if the child becomes frightened or refractory before the examination begins. In many instances, however, the child reflects the mother's

109

concern. It is better to have the mother present, if at all possible, but at times the examination can be carried out with greater ease if the mother either does not come into the room at all or leaves the handling of the child to a sympathetic nurse.

Rarely is it necessary to have the child examined under anesthesia when the basic principles are followed. If, however, the child continues to be fearful or resentful, forceful persuasion can only result in frustration for the physician and psychic trauma to the child. In this case the physician should refrain from any further attempt to complete the examination and submit the child to investigation under anesthesia.

What about the Physical Examination Itself?

The technique of the examination varies with the age of the child. In infancy and early childhood the young female may resent being placed on her back on the examining table. The examination can easily be performed with the child held in the lap of the mother or nurse. All clothing should be removed, but the child must be kept warm. The examiner will be well advised to keep his hands warm also, or the examination will be less than satisfactory. The older child may resent having her panties removed at the beginning of the examination. In this case the physician should respect her feeling of reluctance and proceed with the general examination. By the time he is ready to do the pelvic portion of the examination the child usually has lost her apprehension and readily submits to the removal of the rest of her clothing. Elaborate draping of the child is not necessary and may actually defeat the purpose.

Older children of the preschool age can be examined on the table in most instances, but the initial move may frighten her. Practically, it is better to allow the child to sit on the edge of the table at the start of the examination; later on, as she loses her apprehension, the rest of the examination can be carried out with the patient in the lithotomy or knee-chest position. The latter is satisfactory in early infancy and in the cooperative girl at adolescence, but is apt to frighten the younger child. The Sims position is preferred for this age group. It provides an adequate opportunity for successful examination, since all areas are readily accessible, and the child with her face everted from the physician cannot see the actual moves he makes or the type of instrument he uses. The older girl, approaching the menarche, can perfectly well use the regular lithotomy position with her feet in stirrups.

The physician should remember that it is impossible to do a digital examination of the vagina in a prepuberal girl. The child's vaginal canal is too narrow and lacks the power to distend. All the necessary information can be obtained by a recto-abdominal examination with a well lubricated little finger in the rectum. If gentleness is used, the rectal examination need not be a traumatic experience for the child.

In evaluating the pelvic findings the examiner should keep in mind that the pelvic tissues are naturally condensed and the genital structures small. Any intrapelvic abnormality sufficient to produce symptoms can usually be felt. If no lesion can be felt to explain the symptoms, the mere finding of a negative examination should be reassuring. If the examination is performed with the idea of evaluating the state of development of the internal genital organs, the findings are variable. The uterus is usually not much more than a nub at this stage of development. It may not be palpable, therefore. In this case the vaginal canal should be inspected to see whether a tiny flat button can be seen at the vaginal apex. This is the infantile cervix, and one may assume that the child has a uterus. The ovaries are too small at this stage to be felt, unless they contain tumors.

What Do You Look for in the General Examination of the Girl?

One of the most important parts of the examination of the girl in childhood, both early and late, is simple inspection. In normal growth and development there are two major factors in action during this period. One has to do with skeletal and muscular growth, the other with sexual maturation. In early childhood, up to the age of approximately eight years, development occurs primarily along the lines of structural growth. In late childhood the sex hormones become active and stimulate

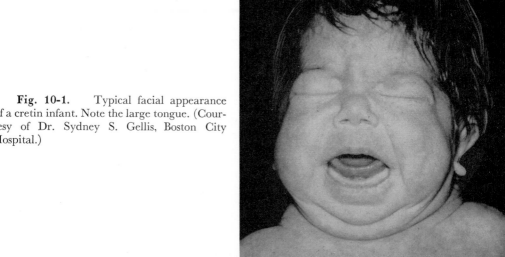

Fig. 10-1. Typical facial appearance of a cretin infant. Note the large tongue. (Courtesy of Dr. Sydney S. Gellis, Boston City Hospital.)

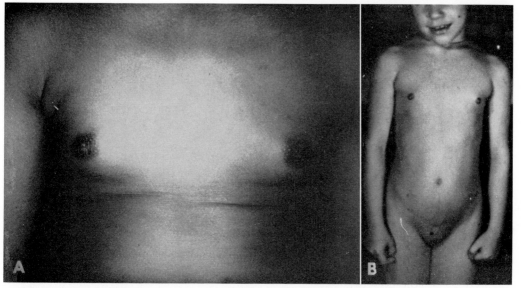

Fig. 10-2. *A*, Breast enlargement and pigmentation of the nipples in a young girl, developing after isoniazid hydrazide therapy. *B*, Stilbestrol intoxication, with breast development and nipple pigmentation. (Courtesy of Dr. Sydney S. Gellis, Boston City Hospital.)

the target organs. Hormonal changes are evident in the external genitalia, in the areas where secondary sex development can be expected and in body habitus.

Thus on general inspection we look for any variation from the normal pattern of skeletal growth in this age group. Observations are made on (*a*) linear growth in relation to the chronologic age; (*b*) span; (*c*) relative proportion of trunk to extremity; (*d*) size and development of the head; (*e*) development of the facial bones. Changes from the normal pattern may suggest thyroid deficiency, defective genes, gonadal agenesis, sexual precocity, primordial dwarfism or simple delay in the normal process of growth development (Fig. 10–1). If nutritional deficiencies are present in a child who does not develop normally, there will usually be other evidences of it on general examination.

Along with observations on the state of structural growth, one may obtain some suggestion of the pattern of mental development. Departures from normal may be detected by observing the degree of alertness, responsiveness, disinterest, apathy or excitability. Mental retardation may be accompanied by delay in structural growth, suggesting a basic developmental defect or possible endocrinopathy.

Signs of female sexual development should begin to be apparent normally at

Table 4.   Time of Appearance of Sexual Characteristics in American Girls

Pelvis. . . . . .Female contour assumed and fat deposition begins at 8 to 10 years
Breasts. . . . . .First hypertrophy or budding at 9 to 11 years. Further enlargement and pigmentation of nipple at 12 to 13 years. Full maturity at 16 to 18 years
Vagina. . . . . .Secretion begins and glycogen content of epithelium increases with change in cell type at 11 to 14 years
Pubic hair. . . . . .Initial appearance at 10 to 12 years. Abundant and curly at 11 to 15 years
Axillary hair. . . . . .Initial appearance at 12 to 14 years
Acne. . . . . .Varies considerably from 12 to 16 years

PUBIC HAIR STAGES

Four years are required, on the average, to go from stage II to V. This may occur in 2 years.
Stage
I. . . . . .No pubic hair
II. . . . . .Sparse growth of long, slightly pigmented, downy hair, usually straight or only slightly curled along labia
III. . . . . .Hair now darker, coarser, more curled; sparsely spread over pubis
IV. . . . . .Almost adult, but not as much as in adult; no spread to thighs
V. . . . . .Adult in quantity, quality and type. Horizontal escutcheon pattern. None on midline of abdomen. May spread to thighs

BREAST DEVELOPMENT

Stage
I. . . . . .The adolescent shows elevation of papilla only
II. . . . . .Breast bud stages with elevation of breast and papilla as small mound and enlargement of areolar diameter
III. . . . . .Further enlargement and elevation of breast and areola occurs, with no separation of their contours
IV. . . . . .Projection of the areola and papilla forms a secondary mound above the level of the breast
V. . . . . .Mature state
Most of the enlargement is due to fat deposit in connective tissue lobules

From Tanner, 1960.

approximately the age of eight years (Table 4). Diagnostic problems arise if signs of feminization or virilization appear before this time. Many girls menstruate by the age of ten, and most by the age of twelve years. If it appears earlier or is delayed longer than sixteen years, investigation is indicated. The secondary sex characteristics begin to appear around the age of eight years, as shown by the appearance of sexual hair and enlargement of the breasts. If these changes come abnormally early or fail to appear at the time expected, a diagnostic problem is involved (Fig. 10–2, *A*). Usually the skeleton matures before the secondary sex characteristics become evident, but on some occasions the timetable is reversed. As further evidence of ovarian activity, one anticipates the appearance of fatty deposits in specific body areas during the premenarchal and puberal periods. The child is said to have assumed the feminine body habitus (Fig. 10–2, *B*). Failure to do so suggests a constitutional delay in acquiring sexual maturity or a basic endocrine defect associated with an android body build.

What about the Local Inspection of the Vulvar Area?

Most congenital anomalies in the external genitalia are apparent at birth, but unfortunately, owing to the cursory examination too frequently given at that time, the true significance of the abnormality is not recognized. In far too many instances the child is reared in the wrong sex. If the child has not had an adequate examination at birth, the anatomic variations may first come to light on examination later in childhood.

We are therefore interested in the anatomic development of the external genitalia, specifically as it applies to the size of the clitoris, the condition of the hymen, the extent of labial development, the presence of labial adhesions and the depth of the vagina. These may be normal or represent variations from normal. Variations may be the result of hyperactivity on the part of the adrenal cortex, examples of abnormal

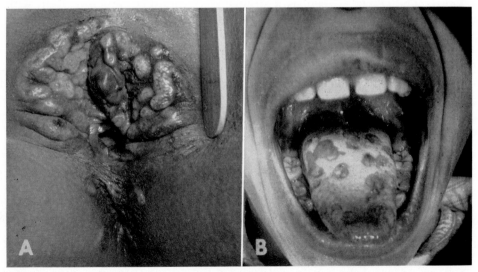

Fig. 10-3.   Severe condylomatous vulvitis (*A*) and glossitis (*B*) in a 10-year-old girl with secondary syphilis. (Courtesy of Dr. F. Ronchese, Providence, R.I.)

development in the hermaphrodite, manifestations of anatomic variation due to defective genes, or the simple aftermath of vaginal infection.

In the child who has dermatitis of the external vulva there may be varying degrees of inflammation (Fig. 10–3). The examiner will do well to remember that the presence of erythema is not enough to make a diagnosis of vulvitis, for the child's vulva is normally apt to be red, owing to the thin skin covering overlying an area of increased vascularity. The state of pudendal hygiene will be immediately apparent and give a clue to the source of the vulvovaginitis which may have brought the child in for examination.

By inspection of the external genitalia and vagina one can obtain an idea of the extent of estrinization. The appearance of the labial skin, the degree of fat deposit in the labial folds, the color of the tissues and the extent of fullness and swelling of the labia all afford evidence of estrogenic activity. If estrogen effects appear earlier than expected or are delayed in development, one may suspect variations in the normal progress of development, either too much or too little. The vulvar hair also offers confirmatory evidence of maturation.

What Information Can Be Gathered from Direct Inspection of the Vaginal Canal?

Although inspection of the vulva can be carried out with little trouble, examination of the vagina is less easily accomplished. As noted before, the immature vagina is narrow and does not distend easily. It therefore cannot be examined digitally. The most useful instrument for this purpose is a long thin vaginoscope containing a built-in light like a cystoscope, which can be gently inserted in the vaginal canal. This is a far better way of examining the vagina than with a nasal speculum or otoscope. These instruments either do not give enough light or cannot be introduced deeply enough to provide an adequate view of the upper portion of the vagina.

With proper lubrication the vaginoscope is gently inserted in the vaginal canal, with regard for the fact that in the young child the vaginal fornices have not yet developed. The cervix is seen as a dimple or button-like structure flush with the vaginal wall. The mere presence of this rudimentary cervix is circumstantial evidence that the rest of the internal genital organs at least are present. The vaginal walls are inspected as the instrument is withdrawn. Any vaginal ulceration should be biopsied, and smear and culture should be taken of any discharge. If infection is present, the cultures and smears should be taken so as to avoid contamination from the vulva, which may be the site of a variety of bacteria that have nothing to do with the specific vaginitis. A grasping instrument should be available for use if a foreign body is encountered.

REFERENCES

Brack, C. B., and Guild, H. G.: Urethral Obstruction in the Female Child. *Am. J. Obst. & Gynec.*, 76: 1105, 1958.

Carrington, E. R.: Gynecologic Problems in Infants and Prepubertal Girls. *S. Clin. N. Amer.*, 34: 1615, 1954.

Childs, B., and Sidbury, J. B.: A Survey of Genetics as It Applies to Problems in Medicine. *Pediatrics*, 20: 177, 1957.

Hertz, R.: Accidental Ingestion of Estrogens by Children. *Pediatrics*, 21: 203, 1958.

Huffman, J. W.: Gynecologic Examination of the Premenarchal Child. *Postgrad. Med.*, 25: 169, 1959.

Idem: Vulvar Disorders in Premenarchal Children. *Clin. Obst. & Gynec.*, 3: 154, 1960.

Palmer, C. E.: Growth and the Economic Depression. *Pub. Health Rep.*, No. 481277, 49: 1453, 1934.

Schauffler, G. C.: The Female Genitals in Immaturity. *Pediat. Clin. N. Amer.*, 5: 3, 1958.

Tanner, J. M.: *Growth at Adolescence*. Springfield, Ill., Charles C Thomas, 1955.

Idem: The Development of the Female Reproductive System during Adolescence. *Clin. Obst. & Gynec.*, 3: 135, 1960.

Turner, H. H.: Ovarian Dwarfism; in J. V. Meigs and S. Sturgis, Eds.: *Progress in Gynecology*, 1: 134, 1946.

Wagner, R.: Endocrine and Pseudo-Endocrine Problems in Childhood. *New England J. Med.*, 229: 737, 1943.

Washburn, A. H.: The Appraisal of Healthy Growth and Development from Birth to Adolescence; in J. Brennemann, Ed.: *Practice of Pediatrics*. Hagerstown, Md., W. F. Prior Company, 1945, Chap. 8.

Chapter 11

Factors Concerned
with Sexual Maturation

IN THE neonatal period and early childhood the gynecologic problems are largely concerned with congenital anomalies and structural growth. Except for the thyroid and the pituitary, the glands of internal secretion, which are implicated in sexual development, show little activity until later in childhood.

Although small amounts of both estrogen and androgen are produced during the early years, little difference in quantity is noted, whether the child be male or female, until around the age of eight years. It is possible that the small amounts produced may come from the adrenal gland rather than the ovary. Despite the fact that the pituitary gonadotropins are not detectable in the urine until shortly before puberty, the normally developing female will, by about the age of eight years, begin to secrete

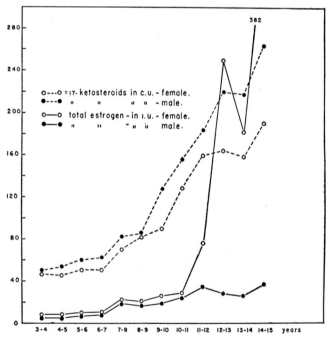

Fig. 11-1. Urinary excretion of 17-ketosteroids and estrogens in girls and boys of different ages. By newer techniques the rise in estrogen output is found in girls before 10 years of age. (From I. T. Nathanson, L. E. Towne and J. C. Aub: *Endocrinology*, Vol. 28.)

116

more estrogen than androgen (Fig. 11–1). Gradually a fluctuation appears in the amounts of urinary estrogen recovered, and the excretion begins to assume a cyclic pattern. This becomes more pronounced as puberty approaches.

Just what the mechanism is that touches off this sudden output of hormones in abundance at the time of puberty is not completely known. The hypothalamus, the pituitary gland and its gonadotropic hormones are definitely implicated. At this stage in the child's development, and from then on, the pituitary is more implicated in development of the body along lines of sexual maturity than in the promotion of growth.

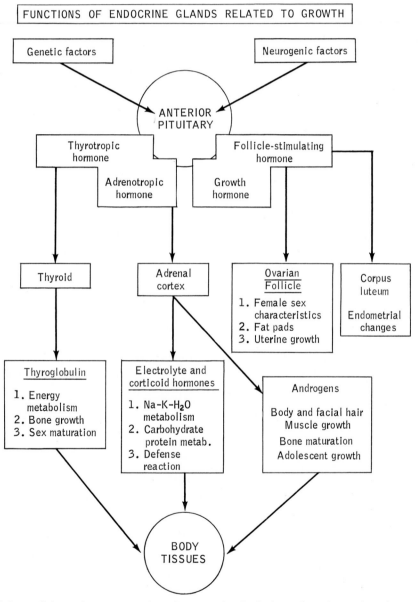

Fig. 11-2.   Schematic representation of some endocrinologic aspects of growth and maturation.

What Factors May Be Concerned with the Initiation of Puberty?

Although the actual mechanism that sets off the train of events which we call puberty is not clear, certain well known factors appear to play a role. We know, for example, that genetic aspects are involved, for a strong hereditary influence is noted which has both a familial and a racial pattern. We are well aware that the onset of puberty is linked to skeletal development and perhaps to the maturation of the central nervous system as well. The mechanism can be regarded as protective. Until the child has developed sufficiently in bone and organ structure, one may not expect the onset of adolescence. The observation has been repeatedly made that the onset of puberty goes hand in hand with the degree of development of the ossification centers in the epiphyses of long bones. If the bony skeleton and organ development are in abeyance, there undoubtedly is the same lack of maturity on the part of the central nervous system. In general, although complete proof is lacking, the trigger mechanisms which initiate puberty are neural or neurohumoral stimuli which come from the hypothalamus and either initiate the production of the gonadotropic hormones or their release from the anterior pituitary lobe. Before menstruation occurs, the ovary must be mature enough to respond to the stimulus offered by the pituitary hormones.

There are many factors that can disturb the mechanism, among them poor nutrition, debilitating constitutional disease, general lack of maturation in the individual, dysfunction of other endocrine glands such as the thyroid and adrenal, and finally genetic defects.

The physiology of menstruation, development of the secondary sex characteristics and the growth problems of adolescence will be discussed in more detail in Part II.

What Are the Main Problems in Late Childhood and the Premenarchal Age?

The main problems that appear in the premenarchal period are related to disturbances in the time schedule of the appearance of the sex hormones. If sexual maturity appears too early, we have the problem of sexual precocity. When puberty is delayed or the external evidence of hormonal activity is lacking, we must decide whether the child is simply slow in developing or whether there is a hormonal imbalance, either due to failure in development of the gonad or to some disturbance in the pituitary-ovarian-adrenal-uterine axis (Fig. 11–2).

REFERENCES

Clements, E. M. B., and Pickett, K. G.: Body Weight of Man Related to Stature, Age and Social Status. *Brit. J. Prev. & Soc. Med.*, 8: 99, 1954.

Dreizen, S., Stone, R. E., and Spies, T. D.: The Influence of Chronic Undernutrition on Bone Growth in Children. *Postgrad. Med.*, 29: 182, 1961.

Gesell, A., Ilg, F. L., and Ames, L. B.: *Youth—The Years from 10 to 16.* New York, Harper & Bros., 1956.

Hartmann, C. G.: *Carnegie Contrib. to Embryology*, 23: 1, 1932.

Johnston, J. A.: Nutritional Problems of Adolescence. *J.A.M.A.*, 137: 1587, 1948.

Jones, W. N.: Delayed Menarche. *Clin. Obst. & Gynec.*, 1: 252, 1958.

Michelson, N.: Studies in Physical Development of Negroes: Onset of Puberty. *Am. J. Phys. Anthropol.*, 2: 151, 1944.

Mills, C. A.: Temperature Influence on Human Growth and Development. *Human Biol.*, 22: 71, 1950.

Nathanson, I. T., Towne, L. E., and Aub, J. C.: Normal Excretion of Sex Hormones in Childhood. *Endocrinology*, 28: 851, 1941.

Nicholson, A. B., and Hardy, C.: Indices of Physiological Maturity and Deviation and Interrelationships. *Child Develop.*, 24: 3, 1953.

Randall, R. V., and Rynearson, E. H.: Clinical Aspects of Anterior Pituitary Failure. *Postgrad. Med.*, 29: 24, 1961.

Reynolds, E. L., and Wines, J. V.: Individual Difference in Physical Changes Associated with Adolescence in Girls. *Am. J. Dis. Child.*, 75: 329, 1948.

Shuttleworth, F. K.: Sexual Maturation and the Skeletal Growth of Girls, Age 6–19. *Monograph. Soc. Res. Child Develop.*, Washington, D.C., 1938, Vol. 3, No. 5, Series 18.

Simmons, K., and Greulich, W. W.: Menarchal Age and the Height, Weight and Skeletal Age of 7–17 Years. *J. Pediat.*, 22: 518, 1943.

Stuart, H. C.: Normal Growth and Development during Adolescence. *New England J. Med.*, 234: 666, 1946.

Tanner, J. M.: *Growth at Adolescence*. Springfield, Ill., Charles C Thomas, 1955.

Idem: The Development of the Female Reproductive System during Adolescence. *Clin. Obst. & Gynec.*, 3: 135, 1960.

Watson, E. H., and Lowrey, G. H.: *Growth and Development of Children*. 3rd Ed. Chicago, Year Book Publishers, Inc., 1959.

Wilkins, L.: Abnormalities and Variation of Sexual Development during Childhood and Adolescence; in *Advances in Pediatrics*. New York, Interscience Publishers, Inc., 1948, Vol. III, p. 159.

Idem: *The Diagnosis and Treatment of Endocrine Disorders in Childhood and Adolescence*. Springfield, Ill., Charles C Thomas, 1957.

Chapter 12

Sexual Precocity

THE APPEARANCE of secondary sex characteristics with or without vaginal bleeding before the time when they are normally expected has been called sexual precocity. It is not unusual for a female child to show signs of sexual development as early as eight to ten years. In some instances the only signs may be enlargement of the breasts or the growth of pubic hair, while in others the ovary matures early and true menstrual bleeding, complete with progestational phase, takes place much earlier than is normally expected. The latter is called precocious puberty, while the term "sexual precocity" includes both.

The two conditions occur much more commonly than is generally believed. Usually they are not reported, for these children mature normally except for their height, which is always less than that of the average girl. These children then are regarded as normal. Any appearance of the characteristics mentioned above, before the age of eight, should in contrast be considered abnormal.

What Are the Causes of Sexual Precocity?

There is a wide variety of causes that may explain the premature appearance of secondary feminine sex characteristics and vaginal bleeding.

In some instances the end-organ seems to be abnormally sensitive to minimal amounts of hormonal stimulation. For example, the breasts may develop very early in childhood. This condition has been called "premature thelarche" or "premature gynecomastia." We noted in earlier discussions that breast engorgement is often present in the newborn infant, undoubtedly owing to the influence of the maternal hormones. This effect does not last long, and the breast development rapidly regresses. It is not unusual, however, to find that a girl in early childhood will show enlargement of one or both breasts, usually both, without other secondary sex manifestations. There is no accompanying maturation of the labia, vagina or uterus. Not infrequently the gynecomastia is a transient phenomenon. No clear-cut explanation for early development of the breasts can be advanced. In all probability the breast tissue affected is more responsive to small doses of estrin or other hormones than any of the other target organs normally stimulated by them.

Another example of abnormal organ sensitivity is the condition known as "premature pubarche," which is simply the premature appearance of the sexual hair. This also may occur without any other secondary sexual development. It is not uncommon to find a light growth of hair on the vulva of a three-year-old child, which

120

tends to increase in abundance as age advances. Rarely the child develops axillary hair as well, but it is extremely rare to find any more widespread hirsutism. There are no other signs of virilization. Girls with this condition are usually somewhat taller than average for the same age. Bone development is often one to four years in advance, though some girls show little variation from the normal.

The explanation of this isolated secondary sex development in all probability lies in either (1) abnormal sensitivity of the hair follicles to the normal amount of androgen secreted at this age, or (2) an increased production of androgen on the part of the adrenal, despite the fact that pituitary gonadotropins are not yet active. It is interesting to note that the urinary 17-ketosteroid excretions range from 0.8 to 6 mg. per day, suggesting that more than one mechanism is at work.

Vaginal bleeding, except for the type noted at birth while the maternal hormones are acting, rarely occurs without other signs of secondary sexual development. Occasionally menstruation will appear as early as five or six years without breast development or the appearance of pubic hair, but invariably there will be some other evidence of sexual maturation such as estrogenic effect shown by vaginal smear or advanced bone age. Usually vaginal bleeding at an early age is evidence of precocious puberty. It is interesting that the girl who has precocious puberty has the menopause no earlier than her normal sisters.

What Is Precocious Puberty?

Under normal conditions the immature ovary awaits the appearance of gonadotropic stimulation from the pituitary before elaborating any hormones of its own. The gonadotropic hormones first appear in quantity by about the age of eight or nine years and are produced or released in increasing amounts thereafter. The exact mechanism which triggers the earlier release or production of the hormones is not known, but it is certainly mediated through the hypothalamus.

CONSTITUTIONAL PRECOCITY.   In the vast majority (over 90 per cent) the girl who undergoes premature sexual development and begins to menstruate at an early age has no organic disease. The pituitary-ovarian-adrenal axis is intact and functions normally in both childhood and adult life. No abnormality can be demonstrated in any of the target organs or in the nervous system. This is the so-called *constitutional type* of precocious puberty. It would seem that the premature activity of the pituitary gonadotropins is due to a genetic influence.

CEREBRAL TYPE.   Less often the explanation may be found in the presence of tumors or disease processes which arise or localize in the hypothalamus, floor of the third ventricle or base of the brain. The tumors are usually neoplastic and tend to invade the floor of the third ventricle. Their point of origin and pattern of growth vary. It is possible, then, to have a small, slowly growing tumor without any presenting sign other than the early appearance of puberty. The tumor need not be malignant, for a few cases of a benign hyperplastic growth or hamartoma have been found in children with precocious puberty. Pituitary adenomas are practically never seen. Most often an astrocytoma or other malignant glioma is responsible.

The mechanism by which the pituitary is activated to produce or release the gonadotropins is not clear, nor is the vulnerable area within the hypothalamus established. Wilkins suggests that a growing tumor may possibly produce some neurohumoral secretion which touches off the whole process. It is possible that nonspecific irritation of the hypothalamus from the mere presence of the tumor is all that is necessary.

A variety of disease processes which affect the cerebrum or the meninges can also evoke precocious puberty. It has been known to follow encephalitis caused by measles and miliary tuberculosis, for example.

Finally Albright has described an interesting syndrome wherein precocious puberty in girls is accompanied by unilateral brown pigmented spots on the skin and fibrous dysplastic degeneration in the long bones. In most instances the pigmentation and bone changes appear on the same side. The disease has been called "polyostotic fibrous dysplasia" because of these scattered areas of rarefaction seen on x-ray films of the long bones. Rarely are these changes seen in the skull. This combination of events may appear very early in the child's life, and the syndrome has been reported as early as five months.

The underlying abnormality may be an overgrowth of bone at the base of the skull which impinges on the hypothalamus. It may be extensive enough to encroach on the optic nerve, producing either alterations in the visual field or even atrophy of the nerve. Nearly half of the young girls who present this picture have precocious puberty.

What Is the Clinical Picture Associated with Precocious Puberty?

The clinical picture of precocious puberty is the same whether the underlying cause is idiopathic or intracranial disease. The only real difference is that in the constitutional type the child matures normally and may marry and have children. The child with the intracranial form develops similarly, but usually dies before she even has a chance to demonstrate whether she is fertile.

In early childhood the girls who develop precociously show an accelerated rate of skeletal growth. At the time when evidence of precocity first appears they are much taller than the average girl of the same age. The growth rate, however, is not maintained, for the pituitary gonadotropins stimulate the ovary to put out so much estrin that the epiphyses close and the growth period ceases before these girls ever achieve a normal adult stature. In the constitutional type of precocious puberty this is the only residuum or reminder that puberty began at an early age. All other factors are normal and remain so.

The sexual development keeps pace with the bone growth. Abnormal enlargement of the breasts, mature development of the external genitalia and actual menstruation have been noted as early as one month after birth, and repeated instances appear in the literature of similar development in two- or three-year-old children. The menstruation, once begun, continues regularly as in the adult.

As the result of premature activity on the part of the pituitary gonadotropins, the ovaries enlarge, owing to the development of the graafian follicles. At times the proliferation is so excessive that large follicle cysts are present which can be palpated on rectal examination. Biopsy of these ovaries reveals histologic evidence of follicular activity and may show luteinization in the theca layer of the follicle. Occasionally a regressing corpus luteum can be found.

In the very young girl, menstruation, though it occurs regularly, is probably anovulatory, but sooner or later ovulation will appear. Pregnancy is therefore possible. Vaginal bleeding in precocious puberty is not like that produced by functioning tumors of the granulosa cell or theca cell type, for in the latter, ovulation does not occur. The girl with sexual precocity must be protected against the possibilities of pregnancy, for it is an unfortunate fact that her psychologic progress does not keep up with her accelerated sexual and osseous development. The situation should be explained to the parents and by them to the child.

The chance of pregnancy is a very real one. There are instances in the literature of pregnancy in children under ten years of age. The most famous case is that of the young girl from Lima, Peru, who began to menstruate at eight months and delivered a 6-pound infant, by cesarean section, at the age of 5½ years.

What Entities Simulate Precocious Puberty?

A few ovarian tumors and a rare feminizing adrenal tumor may produce all the outward signs of precocious puberty. There is one distinct difference, however, for the estrin stimulation comes from the tumor itself and is not the result of pituitary gonadotropic stimulation. The portions of the ovaries not involved in tumor are normal for the child's age. There are no maturing follicles or any other suggestion of ovulation. The periods often occur at regular intervals, but are always anovulatory.

The ovarian tumors are of two types: (a) granulosa and theca cell tumors which produce their own estrin, and (b) teratomatous tumors such as the embryonal carcinoma and chorionepithelioma which secrete their own gonadotropins.

Whatever the cause, the excess production of estrin causes a rapid progression in development both in body build and bone age, while the mental processes lag behind. Any target organ normally stimulated by estrin undergoes hypertrophy. Thus we have (a) enlargement of the breasts, (b) development of the external genitalia, (c) uterine growth, and (d) glandular hyperplasia of the endometrium, but no secretory phase. These tumors often appear very early in childhood and have been reported as early as five months. We have knowledge of one granulosa cell tumor which produced sexual development at the age of eighteen months. The chorionepitheliomas tend to appear later in childhood, around the age of six or eight years.

Their malignant potentiality is different. The granulosa cell tumors in this age group are relatively benign, slowly growing tumors. The embryonic teratocarcinomas, on the other hand, are highly lethal.

How Can the Diagnosis Be Made?

Fortunately, any tumor which is large enough to produce estrin in a quantity sufficient to cause secondary sexual development and vaginal bleeding can be felt either abdominally or on rectal examination. If no tumor is palpable, true precocious puberty should be suspected.

Laboratory tests are helpful in making the differential diagnosis. The great majority of children with granulosa cell tumors will have large amounts of estrin in the urine. If one then finds a high urinary estrogen and a low assay for urinary gonadotropins, an ovarian tumor is probably present. In the presence of a chorionepithelioma a positive pregnancy test (Aschheim-Zondek, e.g.) may be expected.

It is an interesting fact that after removal of either a granulosa cell tumor, chorionepithelioma or malignant teratoma the signs of sexual precocity revert to the infantile state, and the urinary assays for both estrin and chorionic gonadotropin show complete disappearance of the hormones. On the other hand, they may reappear if the tumor appears in the opposite ovary or if metastases develop.

Treatment

Except for the types of precocious puberty which are due to tumor formation, the best form of treatment is to educate the parents and child, but otherwise leave her alone.

It would be ideal therapy to suppress pituitary activity and prevent ovulation until the time one would normally expect the menarche to take place, but unfortunately to date the ideal agent has not become available, unless synthetic progestins such as Norlutin should prove to be the answer. Unsuccessful attempts have been made to neutralize the effect of estrogen by giving the child androgen, for example. All this does is to provide for a temporary suppression of menstruation, but at the expense of virilization and accelerated growth of bone.

When precocious puberty is due to a brain lesion, an attempt should be made to remove it surgically, but the prognosis is poor, since most of the tumors are malignant and highly invasive. Ovarian tumors, however, can be removed with profit. If a granulosa cell tumor is present, it may be excised without disturbing the uterus and other ovary. They have a relatively low malignant potential and rarely recur or metastasize when they are found in this age group. Radical extirpation of the uterus and adnexa should be the treatment of choice when ovarian chorionepitheliomas are encountered. Fortunately they are extremely rare. The benign cystic ovaries should be left strictly alone.

What Do You Tell the Parent and the Child?

The family should be reassured and told that (*a*) the child is not a freak; (*b*) she is not a social menace, nor will she be one; (*c*) she will need instruction about the facts of life in terms that she will understand; (*d*) she should not be pushed beyond her capacity simply because she has the outward signs of a more mature child; (*e*) there need be no psychologic maladjustment if the parents maintain a normal sympathetic attitude toward the child's problems; (*f*) the child will grow up naturally and, except for her small stature, will be normal in every way, including the ability to have a family.

The child in turn should be told that because her breast development is very noticeable when compared with that of her contemporaries, she is in no sense an abnormal child. It would also be well to explain in simple terms what menstruation means so that she will not be frightened when it appears. The basic essential in therapy of the girl with precocious puberty is good common sense on the part of the physician and the parents.

REFERENCES

Albright, F.: Polyostotic Fibrous Dysplasia. Defense of an Entity. *J. Clin. Endocrinol.*, 7: 307, 1947.
Albright, F., Butler, A. M., Hampton, A. O., and Smith, P.: Syndrome Characterized by Osteitis Fibrosa Disseminata, Areas of Pigmentation and Endocrine Dysfunction with Precocious Puberty in Females. *New England J. Med.*, 216: 727, 1937.
Bauer, H. G.: Endocrine and Other Clinical Manifestations of Hypothalamic Disease. *J. Clin. Endocrinol.*, 14: 13, 1954.
Bronstein, I. P., Luhan, J. A., and Mavrelis, W. B.: Sexual Precocity Associated with Hyperplastic Abnormality of the Tuber Cinereum. *Am. J. Dis. Child.*, 64: 211, 1942.

Cook, C. D., McArthur, J. W., and Berenburgh, W.: Pseudoprecocious Puberty in Girls as a Result of Estrin Ingestion. *New England J. Med.*, 248: 671, 1953.

Escomel, E.: La plus jeune mère du monde. *Presse méd.*, 47: 875, 1939.

Freed, S. C., and Goldberg, M. B.: Constitutional Precocious Puberty in Female. Control by Androgen. *J. Clin. Endocrinol.*, 8: 1081, 1948.

Greenblatt, R. B., Barfield, W. E., Jungck, E. C., and Manautou, J. M.: Gynecologic Aspects of Sexual Precocity. *Pediat. Clin. N. Amer.*, 5: 71, 1958.

Hain, A. M.: Constitutional Type of Precocious Puberty. *J. Clin. Endocrinol.*, 7: 171, 1947.

Hampson, J. G., and Money, J.: Idiopathic Sexual Precocity in the Female. *Psychosom. Med.*, 17: 16, 1955.

Hoge, R. H.: Precocious Puberty in Girls. *Am. J. Obst. & Gynec.*, 57: 388, 1949.

Jacobsen, A. W., and Macklin, M. T.: Hereditary Sexual Precocity—Report of a Family with Twenty-Seven Affected Members. *Pediatrics*, 9: 682, 1952.

Jailer, J. W.: Virilism. *Bull. New York Acad. Med.*, 29: 377, 1953.

Jolly, H.: *Sexual Precocity.* Springfield, Ill., Charles C Thomas, 1955.

Idem: Female Isosexual Precocity. *Clin. Obst. & Gynec.*, 3: 197, 1960.

Lloyd, C. W.: Precocious Puberty of Female Type. *J. Clin. Endocrinol. & Metab.*, 13: 1518, 1955.

Loeb, M. J., and Levy, W.: Ovarian Cysts and Tumors in Children under Ten Years of Age. *Arch. Pediat.*, 49: 651, 1932.

Mason, L. W.: Precocious Puberty. *J. Pediat.*, 34: 730, 1949.

Novak, E.: The Constitutional Type of Female Precocious Puberty with Report of Nine Cases. *Am. J. Obst. & Gynec.*, 47: 20, 1944.

Parks, J.: Granulosal Cell Tumors of the Ovary with Precocious Puberty. *Am. J. Obst. & Gynec.*, 36: 674, 1938.

Pedowitz, P., Felmus, L. B., and Mackles, A.: Precocious Pseudopuberty Due to Ovarian Tumors. *Obst. & Gynec. Survey*, 10: 633, 1955.

Richter, R. B.: True Hamartoma of the Hypothalamus Associated with Pubertas Praecox. *J. Neuropath. & Exper. Neurol.*, 10: 368, 1951.

Rush, H. P., Bilderback, J. B., Slocum, D., and Rogers, A.: Pubertas Praecox (Macrogenitosomia). *Endocrinology*, 21: 404, 1937.

Scarpa, J. B., Beheran, H., Raices, A. A., and Bur, G. E.: Ovarian Tumor, Precocious Puberty and Adrenal Hyperfunction. *Am. J. Obst. & Gynec.*, 78: 821, 1959.

Seckel, H. P. G.: Precocious Sexual Development in Children. *M. Clin. N. Amer.*, 30: 183, 1946.

Idem: Six Examples of Precocious Sexual Development—Studies in Growth and Maturation. *Am. J. Dis. Child.*, 79: 278, 1950.

Seckel, H. P. G., Scott, W. W., and Benditt, E. P.: Six Examples of Precocious Sexual Development. I. Studies in Diagnosis and Pathogenesis. *Am. J. Dis. Child.*, 78: 484, 1949.

Silverman, S. H., Migeon, C. J., Rosemberg, E., and Wilkins, L.: Precocious Growth of Sexual Hair without Other Secondary Sexual Development, "Premature Pubarche"—A Constitutional Variation in Adolescence. *Pediatrics*, 10: 426, 1952.

Talbot, N. B., Sobel, E. H., MacArthur, J. W., and Crawford, J. D.: *Functional Endocrinology from Birth through Adolescence.* 2nd Ed. Cambridge, Harvard University Press, 1952.

Whittle, C. H., and Lyell, A.: Precocity in a Girl under Five Due to Stilbestrol Inunction. *Proc. Roy. Soc. Med.*, 41: 760, 1948.

Wilkins, L.: *The Diagnosis and Treatment of Endocrine Disorders in Childhood and Adolescence.* 2nd Ed. Springfield, Ill., Charles C Thomas, 1957.

Zemke, E. E., and Herrell, W. E.: Bilateral Granulosal Cell Tumor. Successful Removal from a Child Fourteen Weeks of Age. *Am. J. Obst. & Gynec.*, 41: 704, 1941.

Chapter 13

Delay in Normal Development

ONE OF the most perplexing problems in the growth period preceding puberty is that of trying to separate the child who is slow in developing because of genetic, constitutional or nutritional cause from the patient who has a basic endocrine disorder. The former requires no treatment, but the latter needs it.

The great majority of patients in the premenarchal period have no basic defect, but are simply slow in maturing. Their retardation in development is noticeable in comparative bone age, in which a delay of several years in epiphysial maturation is not uncommon (Table 5). Along with the deceleration in skeletal growth one also observes a slowing down in the development of the sex organs, both primary and secondary. Thus there seems to be a relation between somatic growth and sexual development. If puberty normally begins when the child's bone age is approximately twelve or thirteen years, one cannot expect a child of chronologic age twelve to menstruate if her bone age is only nine. The child is simply not ready for it. Eventually the child usually matures in a normal manner both physically and sexually.

Table 5.   Age at Onset of Fusion in Skeletal Regions Used as Index of Maturity during Adolescence

REGION OF EPIPHYSIAL CLOSURE	SKELETAL AGE IN YEARS
Elbow:	
Begins in humerus	11–11.5 years
Completed in ulna	12.5–13 years
Foot and ankle:	
Begins in great toe	12.5–13 years
Completed in tibia and fibula	14–14.5 years
Hand and wrist:	
Begins in distal phalanges	13–13.5 years
Completed in radius	16–16.5 years
Knee:	
Begins in tibial tuberosity	13.5–14 years
Completed in fibula	16–16.5 years
Hip and pelvis:	
Begins in greater trochanter of femur	14–14.5 years
Completed in symphysis pubis	17.5–18 years
Shoulder and shoulder girdle:	
Begins in greater tuberosity of humerus	14–14.5 years
Completed in clavicle	17.5–18 years

From Watson & Lowrey. See Chap. 11.

In too many instances the delay in sexual maturity is attributed to hormonal inadequacy. Rarely is this the sole cause. The age at menarche varies so widely in patients who subsequently prove to be completely normal that it is obvious that many factors are implicated other than hormonal cause alone. By and large the delay in development is due to some minor imbalance, secondary to a constitutional, nutritional or genetic cause.

For example, it is well known that children who are obese at or about the expected time of puberty tend to have a delayed onset of menstruation. Obesity could be due to endocrine cause, but it is far more likely that constitutional or environmental factors are at work, such as a familial tendency to obesity or the pattern of eating common to the family. At times it may be traced to a faulty psychologic adjustment to the environmental state. In only the rare case is it due to a hypothalamic or pituitary disorder.

Under normal conditions we assume that at the proper moment neural or neurohumoral stimuli from the hypothalamus will initiate the production or release of the gonadotropic hormones from the pituitary. The "proper moment," however, is conditioned by physiologic maturity of both the gonad and the tissues stimulated by its hormones. If they are not in the proper state of preparedness, one of three things may happen: either (1) the stimuli from the hypothalamus to the pituitary are not forthcoming; (2) the gonad fails to respond to the pituitary prodding; or (3) the tissues of the end-organs fail to receive or react to the ovarian hormones.

There are many factors which operate either to speed up or retard the production or release of the gonadotropic hormones. Thus we have the girl with sexual precocity on the one hand and the child with delayed adolescence on the other. The family or the physician should not rush to the assumption that because puberty is delayed the child will subsequently have difficulty in fulfilling her reproductive function. Delayed adolescence may well be a natural method of protecting the child who lacks sufficient maturity of tissues to cope with the problems of sex and reproduction.

A more detailed discussion of the factors involved in the problems of delayed adolescence will appear in Part II.

How Do You Distinguish the Various Types of Dwarfs from the Child with Delayed Adolescence?

Sexual maturity has been related to bone age, but one may have considerable difficulty in differentiating the child who seems to be retarded in somatic development from the child who has delayed adolescence.

The thyroid dwarf at birth and in early childhood can be recognized by the disproportion in the measurements of the trunk in relation to the extremities. In early childhood, however, it may be impossible to distinguish between the constitutional or primordial dwarf, who will develop normally in every way except size, and the pituitary dwarf, who will never mature sexually. In this case there are no variations in linear length. The distinction can be made only when the full impact of the hormones comes into play.

The constitutional or primordial dwarf has no endocrine defect. There is nothing retarded about the child. Because of the genetic influence, the girl was small at birth and grew at a somewhat slower rate than normal through childhood. The time schedule for the ossification centers and epiphysial closure is essentially normal. Sexual maturation may occur normally or be delayed, but eventually the constitutional or primordial dwarf has a normal sex life wherein she marries and has children, many

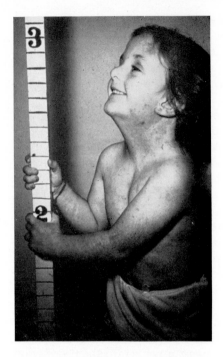

Fig. 13-1.   A child with Turner's syndrome of ovarian agenesis, showing dwarfism and webbed neck. (Courtesy of Dr. Sydney S. Gellis, Boston City Hospital.)

of whom may be entirely normal in size. The constitutional defect lies in the genes and in the tissues, not in the endocrine glands.

In contradistinction, the child with gonadal dysgenesis is dwarfed because of deficient gonadal development. In early childhood, up to the time when the sex hormones become active, the ovarian and primordial dwarf have the same growth pattern. Epiphysial ossification and fusion are only slightly delayed. The final differentiation awaits the appearance of the secondary sex characteristics. In the ovarian dwarf they are never found (Fig. 13–1).

As a guide and time schedule for the appearance of sexual characteristics in late childhood the following tabulation has interest (Table 6):

Table 6.   Age at Appearance of Manifestations of Sexual Development

Growth of the bony pelvis Budding of the nipples	9–10 years
Budding of the breasts Pubic hair	10–11 years
Changes in the vaginal smear and epithelium Growth of external and internal genitalia	11–12 years
Pigmentation of nipples Enlargement of breast	12–13 years
Axillary hair Menarche (anovulatory bleeding)	13–14 years
Deepening of voice	15–16 years
Arrest of skeletal growth	16–17 years

From Wilkins.

Treatment of the Child with Delayed Adolescence

In outlining therapy the physician should try to distinguish the normal child who is slow in maturing from the girl who has a basic endocrine defect, such as the pituitary, ovarian or thyroid dwarf.

Much can be accomplished by thyroid substitution in the girl with hypothyroidism, whether the defect is congenital or acquired. In the pituitary or ovarian dwarf one cannot hope to produce any alteration in the defective sexual development pattern, but with estrogen substitution the child may acquire several extra inches in linear growth as well as some of the outward signs of femininity. The estrogen must be given before the epiphyses close to have any effect on bone growth. The actual mechanism is not clear, but it probably operates through the pituitary to stimulate the adrenal to put out more androgen. The estrogen must be continued on a regular schedule if the secondary sex characteristics are to be preserved.

If there is no obvious deficiency in the endocrine glands, the physician will be well advised if he lets the patient alone and does not try any form of therapy to speed up the appearance of menstruation. Irreparable harm may be produced if overenthusiastic attempts are made to correct a simple constitutional variation in endocrine balance. A great deal can be accomplished, however, by regulating the diet, controlling the obesity and the proper substitution with thyroid extract when a deficiency exists.

REFERENCES

Arey, L. B.: Degree of Normal Menstrual Irregularity: Analysis of 20,000 Calendar Records from 1500 Individuals. *Am. J. Obst. & Gynec.*, 37: 12, 1939.

Blodgett, F. M., Burgin, L., Iezzoni, D., Gribetz, D., and Talbot, N. B.: Effects of Prolonged Cortisone Therapy on Statural Growth, Skeletal Maturation and Metabolic Status of Children. *New England J. Med.*, 254: 636, 1956.

Broch, H.: Physiologic and Psychologic Aspects of Food Intake of Obese Children. *Am. J. Dis. Child.*, 59: 739, 1940.

Collett, M. E., Wertenberger, G. E., and Fioke, V. M.: Effect of Age upon Pattern of Menstrual Cycle. *Fertil. & Steril.*, 5: 437, 1954.

Corner, G. W., and Csapo, A. I.: Action of Ovarian Hormones on Uterine Muscle. *Brit. M.J.*, 1: 687, 1953.

Cruickshank, R., and Scharman, A.: The Biology of the Vagina in the Human Subject. *J. Obst. & Gynaec. Brit. Emp.*, 41: 190, 1934.

Dupertuis, C. W., Atkinson, W. B., and Elftman, H.: Sex Difference in Pubic Hair Distribution. *Human Biol.*, 17: 137, 1945.

Engle, E. T., and Shelesnyak, M. C.: First Menstruation and Subsequent Menstrual Cycles of Pubertal Girls. *Human Biol.*, 6: 431, 1934.

Escamilla, R. F.: Stimulation of Growth in Short Children. *J. Clin. Endocrinol.*, 14: 255, 1954.

Fluhman, C. F.: *Management of Menstrual Disorders*. Philadelphia, W. B. Saunders Company, 1956.

Garn, S. N.: Changes in Areolar Size during the Steroid Growth Phase. *Child Develop.*, 23: 55, 1952.

Gordon, H. H.: A Summary of Some Clinical Aspects of Obesity. *Pediatrics*, 20: 556, 1957.

Greenblatt, R. B., and Nieburgs, H. E.: Some Endocrinologic Aspects of Retarded Growth and Dwarfism. *M. Clin. N. Amer.*, 31: 712, 1947.

Li, C. H.: Pituitary Growth Hormone as a Metabolic Hormone. *Science*, 123: 617, 1956.

Martin, M. M., and Wilkins, L.: Pituitary Dwarf. *J. Clin. Endocrinol. & Metab.*, 18: 679, 1958.

Mayer, J.: Correlation between Metabolism and Feeding Behavior and Multiple Etiology of Obesity. *Bull. New York Acad. Med.*, 33: 744, 1957.

Perloff, W. H.: Hirsutism—A Manifestation of Juvenile Hypothyroidism. *J.A.M.A.*, 157: 651, 1955.

Talbot, N. B.: Dwarfism in Children. *Bull. New England M. Center*, 7: 117, 1945.

Wilkins, L.: *Endocrine Disorders in Childhood and Adolescence*. 2nd Ed. Springfield, Ill., Charles C Thomas, 1957.

Chapter 14

Vaginitis

VAGINAL discharge is one of the most common problems that arise between birth and the onset of puberty. Since the anatomic development and the actual physiology of the vagina change with varying concentrations of the estrogenic hormones, it is not surprising that the cause of vaginitis and the laboratory findings will not be the same in early childhood and at the time of the menarche. We are aware of the fact that the maternal hormones persist for a short time after birth and actually produce changes in the infant external genitalia and vagina. This is the *neonatal period*.

In *early childhood* the maternal hormones are no longer active, and the child has not yet produced any of her own. This condition without estrinic stimuli is present during the period between one month and eight years of age, from the time when the action of the mother's hormones ceases until the child begins to manufacture her own. Gradually the ovary begins to put out small amounts of estrin on its own initiative and without evident stimulation by the pituitary gonadotropins. The concentration of the estrogenic hormones gradually increases, and cyclic fluctuations begin to appear in this period of the child's life which we may designate as *late childhood*. During this time the secondary sexual characteristics begin to appear, in proportion to the increase in estrin stimulation.

Finally, in the *premenarchal period*, which is usually the year immediately preceding the onset of the menarche, a tremendous increase in the output of the estrogenic hormones coincides with the appearance of gonadotropic stimulation from the pituitary. The anatomic characteristics of the external genitalia and the vagina, together with its epithelium, undergo major alterations in the direction of maturity and the final adult structure.

What Physiologic Variations Appear in Each Phase of Childhood?

The laboratory findings, upon investigation of the child's vaginal discharge, are completely different in each group.

THE NEONATAL PERIOD.   Previously we have commented on the anatomic changes. During the two to four weeks in which the maternal hormones continue their action the following factors are noted: (1) The vaginal pH at birth is in the range of 5.7 to 7.0. It is therefore acid, but becomes more so in the next twenty-four hours, owing to the appearance of the lactobacilli (Döderlein bacilli) which produce lactic acid. These organisms are not present at birth. Within the next four days the pH is in the range of 4.0 to 5.0. After approximately ten days the lactobacilli are

130

gradually replaced by other organisms such as cocci, gram-negative rods and diphtheroids. The acid reaction then slowly shifts toward the neutral side, where it remains until the child's own estrogenic hormones take over.

Directly after birth and for the next few days the vaginal smear resembles that of an adult, for the epithelial changes are similar and glycogen is present. As the influence of the hormone is withdrawn the vaginal epithelium thins out and the glycogen disappears. There is, therefore, no sign of estrogenic activity in the vaginal smear from shortly after birth until approximately the age of eight years if development proceeds along normal lines. The chief value of the Papanicolaou smear in childhood, aside from sex chromatin determinations, lies in its ability to reflect the state of ovarian activity. It is interesting, however, that the type of organism recovered from vaginal culture in the presence of a vaginitis varies with the degree of estrogenic effect.

What Are the Characteristics of the Discharge in the Neonatal Period? The healthy vagina at birth is free of any organisms, yet the child may have a gelatinous discharge, gray and rather sticky, which covers the entire vulvar area. It is made up almost entirely of desquamated epithelial cells mixed with serum, but does not contain mucus, for none is being produced. Occasionally white curds made up of the same desquamated cells are seen in the discharge. In the presence of an imperforate hymen there may be a large collection of this type of fluid discharge retained in the distended immature vaginal canal. Occasionally the discharge may be bloody. If it is actually blood, the cause can usually be found in the withdrawal of activity of the maternal hormones which have produced a temporary stimulation of the entire genital tract epithelium (Fig. 14–1). There may be some difficulty in distinguishing between actual blood and the so-called brick dust, which is nothing more than urate deposits from urinary spillage. Whatever the cause, it should ordinarily alarm no one.

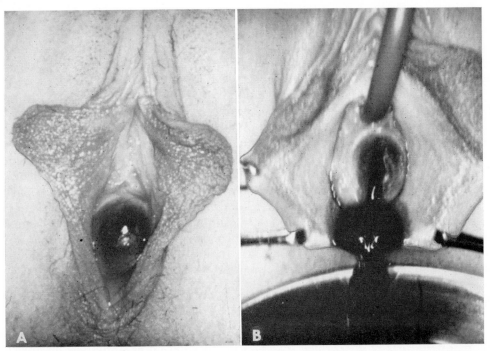

Fig. 14-1. Hematocolpos with imperforated hymen, before (*A*) and after (*B*) incision. (Courtesy of Dr. Sydney S. Gellis, Boston City Hospital.)

WHAT ARE THE CLINICAL EXPLANATIONS OF VAGINITIS FOUND IN EARLY CHILD-HOOD?   The important matter to remember in explaining the cause of vaginitis is the fact that the infant's vagina is no longer under the influence of hormones and takes part in somatic growth only to a minimal extent. Hence the vulvar and vaginal epithelium are thin and tend to be red, for the underlying vascular stroma shines through. The mere fact that the vulva is red does not signify that inflammation is present. The very thinness of the vulvovaginal epithelium in its exposed position, however, makes the area particularly vulnerable to trauma and infection. Since the child is not yet old enough to develop the habit of cleanliness, there is bound to be some element of fecal contamination. The vagina becomes involved in the spread of any infection from the external vulva. Since there are few bacteria in the vagina in early childhood under normal conditions, one should look to the gastrointestinal tract as the source of contamination when a nonspecific vaginitis appears in early childhood. The bacteria that are found by culture in young girls of this age group who have no obvious infection are, in addition to *E. coli*, chiefly diphtheroids, non-hemolytic streptococci and the micrococcus pyogenes. If great care is taken to avoid touching the vulva while taking the cultures, the vagina of children in this age group will be found to be relatively free of pathogenic bacteria.

It is perhaps more interesting to note one organism that does not appear and cannot, therefore, be implicated as a cause of vaginitis in the young child. *Trichomonas vaginalis* is not found in early childhood. This is in direct contrast to myocotic infec-tions, such as with *Candida albicans*, which may occur in any age group. The trichom-onad apparently awaits the effect of estrogen stimulation and the appearance of the lactobacillus. The majority of mycotic infections can be traced to the use of antibiotics.

GONORRHEAL VULVOVAGINITIS

In discussing the etiology of vaginitis it has become the custom to divide the causative factors into specific and nonspecific. Gonorrhea, which is not infrequent in young girls, is an example of a specific infection.

The incidence of gonorrheal inflammation in young children has dropped appreciably, paralleling the improved therapy of the adult, with the advent of the antibiotic and therapeutic drugs. It is unlikely that the child becomes infected through sexual intercourse, but is is easy to understand how the vulva might become contaminated by contact with her elders who do have the disease and are untreated. In the past, gonorrheal vulvovaginitis would spread with the speed and violence of a prairie fire through a children's ward. There being little resistance on the part of the inactive nonestrinized vaginal epithelium of the infant, the gonococcus rapidly spread from infant to infant, not through contamination from the bed linen, bedpans, towels or other utensils, but rather through personal contact. It might be possible for a young girl at home with an infected parent to become infected if any fresh discharge were left on a toilet seat or upon the towel or bed clothing.

What Are the Clinical Findings in Gonorrheal Vulvovaginitis in Childhood?

The clinical findings of gonorrheal vulvovaginitis are unlike those in the adult. The manifestations of gonorrheal infection in the internal genitalia are discussed in detail in Chapter 44. In the young child the disease tends to be confined to the vulva and lower third of the vagina. The cervix does not become infected and never serves as a focus of recurring infection. There appears to be an anatomic barrier at the cervix which prevents the spread of the gonorrhea to the uterine cavity and tube. One rarely encounters severe complications in gonococcal vulvovaginitis in children. Salpingitis, peritonitis, arthritis and septicemia rarely, if ever, occur.

The disease process is sharply limited to the lower recesses of the vaginal tract. From there it may spread to the rectum and produce a proctitis. Gonorrheal ophthalmia can be a distressing and serious complication, but it does not appear in the eye as part of the normal progress of the disease. It is carried there by the contaminated fingers of the child herself or whoever happens to attend her.

The nonestrinized vaginal epithelium has no resistance to the gonococcal infection, and characteristically both vulva and lower part of the vagina become involved in an acute inflammatory process which produces varying degrees of discharge. In the mild case it may appear as a moderately copious thin discharge, but as the severity of the infection increases the discharge becomes profuse and purulent. Engorgement and hyperemia of the vulva are present. The thick, yellow discharge bathes the external vulva, lower part of the vagina and urethral opening. The vestibular and paraurethral glands become involved, and the inflammation not infrequently spreads to the anus and lower portion of the rectum. The irritating effect of the discharge produces maceration of the thinned-out epithelium covering the vulva and vagina.

It is amazing how much inflammation may be present without particularly bothering the child. When the infection is severe and the maceration extreme, the child will naturally complain of pain in this area, which is aggravated by walking. Frequently the child has dysuria and urinary frequency. The symptoms are entirely local, and the general health of the child is unimpaired.

How Is the Diagnosis Made?

Although gonorrheal vulvovaginitis is less frequently found in the young child than was formerly true, it nevertheless occurs often enough so that one can accept a diagnosis of nonspecific cause only after ruling out the gonococcus.

The diagnosis is confirmed by vaginal smear and culture. The cultures are

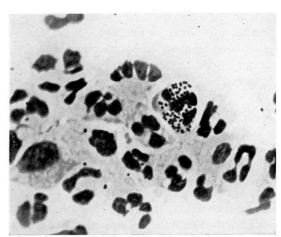

Fig. 14-2. A positive gonococcal smear showing the intracellular diplococci, which are gram-negative, in polymorphonuclear leukocytes of the exudate.

necessary, for other forms of intracellular gram-negative diplococci such as the *Neisseria sicca* can produce a similar type of vulvovaginitis. The clinical findings and smear characteristics are identical (Fig. 14–2). To be sure that the cultures are truly representative of the offending organism the material for the culture should be taken from the vagina, not from the external vulvar area. There is too much chance of nonspecific bacterial contamination with the latter.

What Treatment Can Be Offered the Child with Vulvovaginitis?

There are several forms of treatment that may be offered the child which will relieve the vulvar discomfort and produce a cure.

The genital area should be kept clean by gentle bathing several times daily. There is no indication for the use of douches, and in fact they should be avoided. Great care should be taken in handling anything that comes in contact with the child This applies equally well to thermometers, bedpans and bed as well as personal linen. The child may use the toilet seat and bathtub, but they must be thoroughly cleansed and scrubbed afterward. If there are other children in the family, the affected child must be isolated from them. Above all, the closest attention must be paid to cleansing the hands of both patient and attendants. The child must be warned not to put her hands to her eyes.

Estrin Therapy.   In the past the chief reliance in therapy was placed on the use of estrin designed to produce an adult type of epithelium. The rationale for this type of therapy was based on the observation that gonorrheal vaginitis in the young child ran a self-limited course and tended to disappear spontaneously at the time of puberty. Rarely does it become an ascending infection and a later cause of sterility.

Antibiotic Therapy and Chemotherapy.   With the advent of drugs such as sulfonamides and penicillin, which are far more effective, the enthusiasm for estrin has disappeared. Of the two drugs now in common use, penicillin is preferred, on a daily regimen of 300,000 units, given intramuscularly. The smears and cultures usually become negative in forty-eight hours. If one elects to use sulfonamides, the oral dose should not exceed 2 gm. a day. The response to therapy is not as dramatic as that following the use of penicillin, and it may take a week before the cultures and smears become negative.

To be sure that the child is entirely free of her infection the penicillin or sulfonamide in the doses mentioned should be repeated at monthly periods for at least three months. Only then, when the smears and cultures continue to be negative, can she be allowed to come in contact with the other children in the family. The physician cannot afford to be content with a single negative smear and culture. It must be repeated.

NONSPECIFIC VULVOVAGINITIS

The diagnosis of nonspecific vulvovaginitis is made only after gonorrheal infection has been excluded. Since the clinical findings in both are restricted to the external genitalia and lower part of the vagina, it is impossible to differentiate one from the other by attempting to evaluate the nature of the discharge or the appearance of the vulva and vagina. In either case the thin epithelium is swollen, red and frequently macerated. The external appearance, amount and nature of the discharge and the severity of the symptoms will depend on the virulence of the offending organism.

What Are the Possible Sources of Nonspecific Vaginitis?

There are a wide variety of causes of vulvovaginitis of nonspecific origin. They include (*a*) fecal contamination, (*b*) pinworm infections, (*c*) foreign bodies, (*d*) upper respiratory tract infections, (*e*) urinary tract infections, (*f*) diphtheria, and (*g*) mycotic infection.

FECAL CONTAMINATION.   There appears to be little doubt that the great majority of nonspecific vaginal infections in young children can be traced to the bacteria commonly found in the gastrointestinal tract. The vagina becomes contaminated because of unclean habits, improper anal cleansing after toilet and clothing soiled with fecal matter. Huffman finds that nearly 80 per cent of the bacteria recovered in young girls with nonspecific vaginitis grow out as *E. coli* on culture.

PINWORM INFECTIONS.   Under ordinary circumstances the pinworm (*Enterobius vermicularis*) is a harmless intestinal parasite. When the vagina becomes infested with the pinworms, an acute inflammatory process results. The source of the contamination is similar to that noted in fecal contamination. Pinworms are rarely found except in conditions of poor hygiene. It is of the utmost importance that their presence be ruled out, for the most intensive antibiotic or chemotherapy program will be useless until the parasites are eliminated from the gastrointestinal tract.

UPPER RESPIRATORY, URINARY AND DIPHTHERITIC INFECTIONS.   Vulvovaginitis is often noted after an acute infection in the upper respiratory tract or bladder. Less commonly one finds a membrane in the vagina in the course of the acute infection with diphtheria. Occasionally pneumococcal vaginal infections are seen during a pneumonia.

MYCOTIC INFECTIONS.   As we have previously noted, typical mycotic infections of the vagina may follow the use of antibiotic therapy for disease elsewhere in the body.

FOREIGN BODIES.   The unexplained appearance of a vaginal discharge which tends to recur and does not respond to treatment should make one suspicious of a foreign body in the vagina, particularly if the discharge is at all bloody. The discharge is usually heavy, purulent and often foul.

Almost any article of a proper size to permit entry through the hymenal opening has been recovered from the vagina. These range all the way from wads of paper and pieces of clothing to solid particles, such as portions of a rubber eraser or safety pins. There is little to be gained from asking the child whether she has ever inserted anything, for she will usually deny it and then promptly do it again.

The bacteria found when foreign bodies are present are variable. Naturally the vaginitis with its profuse discharge will persist until the foreign body is detected and removed.

What Tests Should Be Done to Determine the Cause of Nonspecific Vulvovaginitis in Young Children?

The most important thing to do in investigating the cause of vulvovaginitis is to rule out the gonococcus. Only then can one make the diagnosis of nonspecific vaginal infection. Since the causes are many and varied, a number of tests must be carried out in addition to the routine use of smears and cultures. For either, the material should be taken from the vaginal canal. It is not necessary to obtain cervical cultures or smears, for the cervix and upper part of the vagina rarely take part in the infectious process in this age group. Vaginal and perianal smears should be taken to rule out pinworms. Direct inspection of the vagina through a vaginoscope is necessary if the foreign bodies are nonmetallic. If the foreign body is metal, it can be seen by x-rays. If x-ray facilities are not easily available, it may be possible to detect a metallic foreign body by inserting a metal probe in the vagina, while one finger palpates the posterior vaginal wall. A metallic click suggests the presence of a metallic object, and its outline can be estimated by palpation.

Wet smears will help in detecting *Candida albicans* (Fig. 14–3). Finally, sensitivity tests should be done if the cultures produce pathogenic organisms.

How Are the Cultures To Be Taken?   Since much depends on the culture in specific as well as nonspecific vaginitis, it is important that the culture be taken properly. The main consideration is the source from which the material for smear or culture is taken. Great care should be exercised to take it from the vagina, while avoiding contamination from the vulvar area. Huffman insists that the collection of material *should not* be made by inserting a cotton-tipped probe through the hymen or by exerting pressure on the posterior vaginal wall with a finger in the rectum, but rather by gently inserting a small wire loop through a sterile vaginoscope. If a specific area in the canal can be seen, the secretion should be taken from that area, but if no suspicious areas are present, any spot in the lower part of the vagina will be satisfactory.

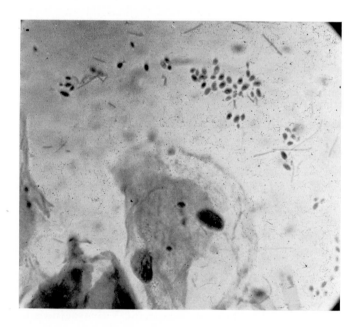

Fig. 14-3.   Stained yeasts in vaginitis due to *Candida albicans*. The long, threadlike bacilli suggest effects of antibiotic therapy, which may predispose to Candida infection.

How Do You Treat Nonspecific Vulvovaginitis?

The type of treatment used to cure nonspecific vulvovaginitis naturally depends on the cause and the severity of the infection. In general it may be said that the simpler types of therapy are more practical than antibiotic, chemotherapeutic or estrogenic drugs. Hormones are rarely effective, and the former should be reserved for the more stubborn cases. It should be kept in mind that pinworm infections of the vagina can be eradicated only by clearing the intestinal tract of the parasite, and infection caused by foreign bodies will continue until the object is removed.

The milder forms of infection will respond readily to hot sitz baths and gentle cleansing of the vulva with a bland soap, followed by thorough drying. Since the majority of infections seem to arise because of fecal contamination, absolute perineal cleanliness must be maintained. The child should also be instructed to wipe the anal opening with toilet tissue in the direction away from the vagina.

Occasionally it may be advisable to irrigate the vaginal canal with lactic acid or vinegar in mild solution (2 teaspoonfuls to a quart.) The mother should be taught to insert a small catheter in the vagina and inject the solution with a syringe while the child lies on her side. This should be done two or three times daily during the acute phases of the infection.

Recently Huffman has found that Nitrofurazone in the form of urethral suppositories can be easily inserted in the vaginal canal. When this is done nightly for several weeks, the nonspecific vaginitis disappears nearly 90 per cent of the time.

Technique of Removal of Foreign Bodies.   The best method of detecting and removing foreign bodies from the vagina is to insert a vaginoscope of small dimension. This is an instrument similar to a Kelly cystoscope. The child will frequently be cooperative if you spend some little time in getting her confidence and assuring her that it will not hurt. If at all possible, the examination should be carried out in the knee-chest position, but the lateral Sims position will be satisfactory if the child refuses to assume the other position. The instrument should be inserted gently, keeping in mind that the immature vagina is narrow, does not distend readily and has no fornices. If the child is too apprehensive or if there is any suggestion from the history that the removal may be prolonged or painful, the procedure should be carried out under anesthesia.

To remove the foreign body a long, narrow, grasping instrument should be used. There is no problem if the foreign bodies are nonmetallic, but if hairpins, safety pins or other solid objects are present, and they have been there any length of time, they may become imbedded. As a practical point, when the metallic object is a pin, the rounded or blunt end should be withdrawn first to prevent the sharp end from sticking into the vaginal epithelium.

REFERENCES

Boisvert, P. L., and Waldcher, D. N.: Hemolytic Streptococcus Vaginitis in Children. *Pediatrics*, 2: 24 1948.

Braid, F.: Vulvo-vaginitis in Children. *Clin. J.*, 66: 378, 1937.

Brewer, J. I., Halpern, B., and Thomas, G.: Hemophilus Vaginalis Vaginitis. *Am. J. Obst. & Gynec.*, 74: 834, 1957.

Butler, B. C., and Beakley, J. W.: Bacterial Flora in Vaginitis. *Am. J. Obst. & Gynec.*, 79: 432, 1960.

Carter, B., and Jones, C. P.: A Study of the Vaginal Flora in the Normal Female. *South. M.J.*, 30: 298, 1937.

Clarke, B. G., and Eisenberg, H. H.: Gonococcus Vaginitis in Children Treated with a Single Injection of Penicillin in Beeswax and Peanut Oil. *Am. J. Dis. Child.*, 74: 707, 1947.

Cruickshank, R., and Sharman, A.: Biology of Vagina in Human Subject. Bacterial Flora and Secretion of Vagina at Various Age Periods and Their Relation to Glycogen in Vaginal Epithelium. *J. Obst. & Gynaec. Brit. Emp.*, 41: 208, 1934.

De Bord, G. G.: Species of the Tribes Mimae Neisseriae and Streptococcae Which Confuse the Diagnosis of Gonorrhea by Smears. *J. Lab. & Clin. Med.*, 28: 710, 1943.

Englehard, C. F.: Candida Albicans Infection in Child. *J. Pediat.*, 32: 404, 1948.

Feo, L. G.: The Incidence of Trichomonas Vaginitis in the Various Age Groups. *Am. J. Trop. Med. & Hyg.*, 5: 786, 1956.

Gardner, H. L., and Dukes, C. D.: Haemophilus Vaginalis Vaginitis— A Newly Defined Specific Infection Previously Classified "Nonspecific Vaginitis." *Am. J. Obst. & Gynec.*, 69: 962, 1955.

Gray, L. A., and Kotcher, E.: Vulvovaginitis in Children. *Clin. Obst. & Gynec.*, 3: 165, 1960.

Hardy, G. C.: Vaginal Flora in Children. *Am. J. Dis. Child.*, 62: 939, 1941.

Hedlund, P.: Acute Vulvovaginitis in Streptococcal Infection. *Acta paediat.*, 42: 388, 1953.

Heltai, A., and Taleghamy, P.: Non-specific Vaginal Infections. *Am. J. Obst. & Gynec.*, 75: 865, 1958.

Hepp, J. A., and Everhardt, W. C.: Foreign Body in Immature Vagina. *Am. J. Surg.*, 79: 589, 1950.

Huffman, J. W.: The Structure and Bacteriology of the Premenarchal Vagina. *Ann. New York Acad. Sc.*, 83: 227, 1959.

Jones, C. P., Carter, B., Thomas, W. L., Ross, R. A., and Creadick, R. N.: Mycotic Vulvovaginitis and the Vaginal Fungi. *Am. J. Obst. & Gynec.*, 54: 738, 1947.

Kotcher, E., Keller, K., and Gray, L. A.: A Microbiological Study of Pediatric Vaginitis. *J. Pediat.*, 53: 210, 1958.

Lang, W. R.: Pediatric Vaginitis. *New England J. Med.*, 253: 1153, 1955.

Idem: Premenarchal Vaginitis. *Obst. & Gynec.*, 13: 727, 1959.

Lee, H. F., and Susman, W.: Penicillin Treatment of Childhood Gonorrhea. *J. Pediat.*, 28: 590, 1946.

Naegele, C. F.: Gonorrheal Vaginitis in Children. *Arch. Pediat.*, 62: 516, 1945.

Pettit, H., and Hitchcock, C. H.: Normal Flora in the Prepuberal Vagina. *J. Infect. Dis.*, 53: 372, 1933.

Reichert, J. L., Epstein, I. M., Jung, R., and Colwell, C. A.: Infection of Lower Part of Genital Tract in Girls. *Am. J. Dis. Child.*, 54: 459, 1937.

Schauffler, G. C.: Identity of Neisseria Other than Gonococcus Isolated from the Genitourinary Tract. *J. Ven. Dis. Inform.*, 31: 208, 1950.

Idem: Management of Vaginitis; in G. C. Schauffler: *Pediatric Gynecology*. 3rd Ed. Chicago, Year Book Publishers, Inc., 1953.

Schnoor, T. G.: The Occurrence of Monilia in Normal Stools. *Am. J. Trop. Med.*, 19: 163, 1939.

Streypt, R.: Importance of Vaginitis in Urinary Infection in Childhood. *J. Urol.*, 72: 963, 1954.

Weaver, J. D.: Non-gonorrheal Vulvovaginitis Due to Gram Negative Intracellular Diplococci. *Am. J. Obst. & Gynec.*, 60: 257, 1950.

Weinstein, L., Bogin, M., Howard, J. H., and Finkelstone, B. B.: Survey of Vaginal Flora at Various Ages, with Special Reference to Döderlein Bacillus. *Am. J. Obst. & Gynec.*, 32: 211, 1936.

PART II

Gynecologic Problems
of Puberty and Adolescence

Chapter 15

General Considerations

AT THIS stage in the child's life profound changes take place. The onset of menstruation, the so-called menarche, is but one manifestation of a series of developmental phases which have been going on quietly but progressively for several years. Until approximately the age of eight years limited amounts of both estrogen and androgen have been secreted. Gradually periodic variations begin to appear in the levels of measurable estrin excretion. The production of estrin begins to exceed the output of the male hormone in the female child, and a recognizable pattern is evolved which simulates that seen later in her established menstrual life. In the earlier years the source of both estrogen and androgen is probably predominantly the adrenal cortex. About the same time as the first appearance of measurable amounts of pituitary gonadotropic hormones in the urine, a change is noted in the appearance of the child. This usually takes place by about the age of eleven, with a range of nine to fifteen years.

Definitions

The following definitions may be of use:

Childhood . . . . Birth to menstruation or puberty
Prepuberty . . . . The accelerated growth period before the menarche
Puberty . . . . From the menarche to completion of somatic growth
Adolescence . . . . From puberty to somatic, sexual and psychologic maturity

Puberty is placed legally at twelve years in many states of the United States of America.

Skeletal Growth

Up to this point the growth rate has progressed in a leisurely linear manner. When the impact of the various pituitary hormones begins to be noted, an acceleration in growth occurs. The pituitary growth or somatotropic hormone, the thyroid and adrenal cortex are implicated. The pituitary acidophil cells of the anterior lobe are responsible for the production of the growth hormone (STH), the sparsely granulated basophil or amphophil cells secrete the thyroid-stimulating hormone (TSH), and cytologically as yet unidentified cells produce the adrenocorticotropic hormone (ACTH). In response to stimulation from their respective pituitary hormones, both the adrenal cortex and the thyroid gland also increase both in size and weight.

141

Each of the hormones plays a role in skeletal growth. They may not be in action at the same time, and some of the effects may be selective. For example, we know that the thyroid is concerned with linear growth, since in the presence of thyroid deficiency in the prepuberal age stunted growth occurs. Thyroid function is also concerned, however, with other features in the child's development, such as changes in the skull, the relation of the cranial and facial bones, the time of eruption of teeth, as well as with brain development.

Morphologic Changes in Fat and Muscle

Along with the increase in linear growth coincident with the first appearance of measurable gonadotropic hormones in the urine, there is an acceleration in both localized fat deposit and muscular development. All three pituitary hormones just mentioned (STH, TSH and ACTH) play an important part in muscle building, for all are known to increase nitrogen retention and indirectly contribute to protein synthesis. The adrenal sex hormones are perhaps also concerned, for a measurable increase in growth and muscularity is noted when testosterone is injected into a patient with panhypopituitary deficiency.

As far as the deposition of fat is concerned, it is clear that the secretion of either estrin or adrenal corticoids will stimulate it, but when excess fat is present, the urinary excretion of the adrenal corticoids is often high, while the estrin factors may be unchanged. Estrin has little to do with acceleration in growth or nitrogen retention. In fact, estrogen acts to encourage the epiphyses to close and thus limits the growth of girls.

The one major factor in the pronounced morphologic changes that take place in female adolescence must rest partly with the adrenal cortex and also with its androgenic-type hormones that are nonvirilizing, since the adrenal cortex is the major source of androgens in the female. The enlargement in the size of the adrenal gland before and at puberty is in part due to the increased number of androgen-secreting cells.

We are all familiar with the sudden alteration in the shape of the growing female child (see Fig. 1–1). This is due to an abrupt increase in fat deposits, which is synchronized with the first appearance of measurable pituitary gonadotropins in the urine. This obvious change in the child's appearance precedes the acceleration in bony growth by nearly a year. As growth continues, some of this fat is retained and the feminine contour is preserved, but the excess fat of childhood disappears when pituitary growth hormone and the nonvirilizing androgenic-type hormones of the adrenal cortex become increasingly active, and muscular development accelerated.

Age of Adolescence

The time of onset of the accelerated growth pattern is inconstant and subject to many variables. Heredity, for example, may play a part. It is not uncommon for a daughter to duplicate the mother's experience. There is some suggestion, however, that genetic factors may have a greater influence over the child's ultimate size than upon the rate of her growth or the age of entering adolescence. Seasonal factors are noted in all growth patterns. For some unexplained reason, linear as well as muscle growth usually takes place in the spring, while body weight is increased in the fall and winter months. It is a well substantiated fact that some children grow in spurts with intervening plateaus. They may grow more in one year than in another. This may be due to an alteration in the amount of hormone produced at any one time or the receptivity of the tissue to the changed stimulation. This in turn may be modified by malnutrition or severe illness. Certainly the growth pattern can be profoundly influenced by diet. Climate and race were formerly believed to have some effect upon the age of sexual maturity. More intensive study would seem to implicate social and economic conditions, genetic factors and malnutrition as the more important controlling factors. There are so many deviations from the generally accepted concept of the proper chronologic age for sexual maturity that it is surprising that we can maintain any standard of normality (Fig. 15–1).

Secondary Sex Characteristics and the Gonadal Hormones

A general maturation factor appears to be a prime requisite for the complete action of the pituitary gonadotropins, both in their production and the receptivity of target organs and body tissues. Gonadal development is preceded by accelerated structural growth in the normal progression toward maturity. Growth of bone and muscle has been going on for some time before the gonads become active. If for any of a number of reasons structural development is delayed, sexual growth will also be retarded. This is not the only factor in the maturing process. The central nervous system is also involved. We know that the production or release of hormones from the pituitary depends on neural or neurohumoral stimuli from the hypothalamus. If the hypothalamus has not ripened sufficiently, these stimuli will not occur. It is not enough to have a sound pituitary. When the proper degree of maturity has been acquired by the hypothalamus, the stimuli from it cause pituitary FSH and LH to be released, and the ovary and the adrenal cortex respond by putting out an increasing amount of their own hormones, which bring about sexual maturation. As these

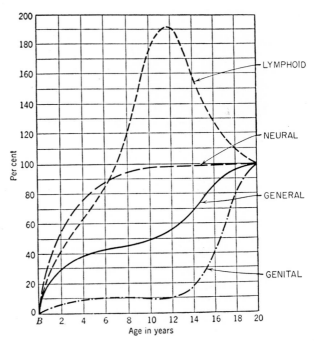

Fig. 15-1. Relative growth of various types of tissue at different ages indicates graphically how lymphoid tissue atrophy and active genital growth both accelerate by about 12 years of age. (Alma Nemir: *The School Health Program;* from R. E. Scammon: The Measurement of the Body in Childhood, in J. A. Harris and others: *The Measurement of Man.*)

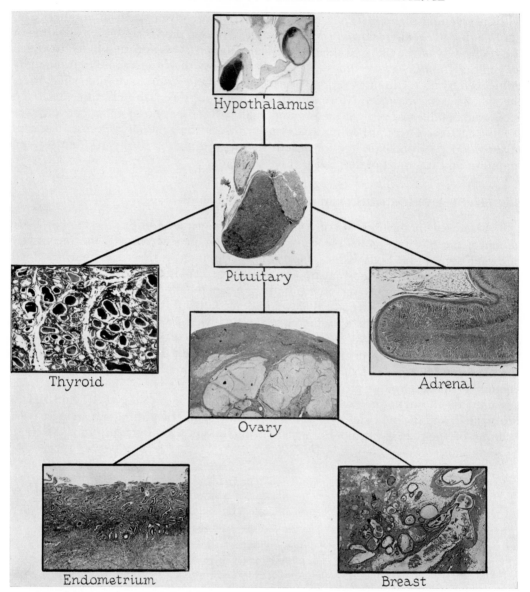

Fig. 15-2. The neuroendocrine control of the female genitalia involves the hypothalamus, anterior pituitary and, through it, the ovary and adrenal and thyroid glands.

hormones increase in quantity, and the target organs become adjusted to the stimulation, the response to growth hormone gradually declines, the epiphyses close, and linear growth ceases. The amount and constancy of the secretion of the hormones will also depend on how well the hypothalamus has developed (Fig. 15–2).

Temporary imbalances in hormone production are common in this age group, as the relative amounts of FSH and LH production wax and wane. This temporary imbalance is further influenced by variations in the response of the target organs and tissues. The hypothalamus in its newly acquired maturity is extremely sensitive to such variables as systemic disease, malnutrition and psychic unrest. Any of these may retard the normal progress of adolescence. It is obvious from the preceding discussion that there is a wide variation in the average time factor concerned with both structural development and gonadal function. Some girls will have established a recognizable menstrual pattern before others have entered the accelerated growth phase.

When the hormones are secreted either constantly or sporadically from the maturing hypothalamic-pituitary-ovarian-adrenal axis, the outward manifestations of their stimulating effects become obvious. Secondary sex characteristics develop in an orderly sequence, regardless of the chronologic age of maturity.

One of the first bits of clinical evidence we have that gonadal hormones have become active, after a sudden increase in height, is the development of the breast (Fig. 15–3). The first noticeable change is an elevation of the mammary papillae above the chest wall. These are the so-called breast buds. The areolae also develop and darken in color. Gradually this recedes, and the breast papilla again projects beyond the areola. The breast then increases in form and substance as it takes part in the general redistribution of fat under the first impact of the sex hormones. Fat is distributed through the connective tissue surrounding the immature mammary lobules. As yet the breast has not fully matured, for estrin stimulation provides mainly for the development of the duct system. Enlargement of the lobules awaits the action of progestin after complete maturation of the ovum and corpus luteal activity, which appears only after ovarian function has come to full ripening.

The development of the breast is closely followed by the first appearance of pubic hair. This is probably an adrenal rather than an estrin effect, for pubic hair has been known to appear in patients with congenital absence of the ovary. The effect of estrin may be indirect, however, through stimulation of the pituitary to put out more adrenocorticotropic hormone (ACTH). The adrenal cortex responds to such stimulation partly by secreting more androgenic-type corticoids. Under the influence of these, the deposits of hair first appear in the pubic area, beginning around the labia and gradually spreading up over the mons veneris, darkening in color and increasing in density as they proliferate. The growth pattern is specific for the female and forms a typical triangular arrangement with a horizontal upper border. Variables are noted in some women, who demonstrate some midline hair that extends in a pyramidal fashion toward the umbilicus, which is more typical of the male. Much of this variation may be attributed to an imbalance in the estrin-androgen ratio which may be normal for that person. Extreme variations in hirsutism should be regarded as pathologic. The amount of hair that appears depends more upon the level of androgen secretion and the different response of the hair follicles than upon secondary sexual differentiation.

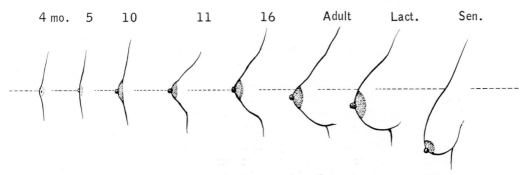

Fig. 15-3.   Diagrammatic representation of the prepuberal breast from 4 months to 11 years of age. The adolescent breast of 16 years and the fully developed adult breast undergo further alterations, as indicated, with lactation and senility.

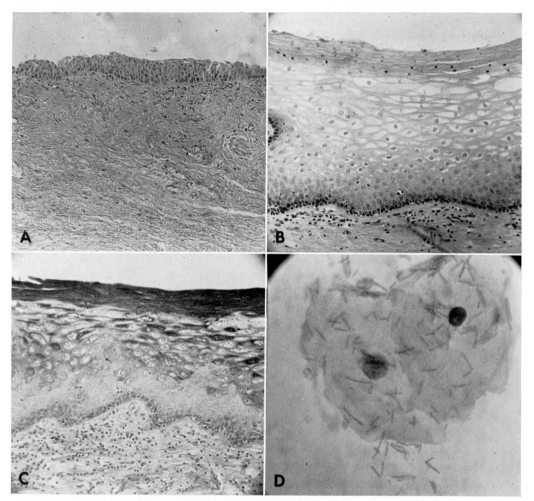

Fig. 15-4.   *A*, The thin vaginal mucosa of the child. *B*, The mature estrogenized vaginal epithelium. *C*, Periodic acid Schiff (PAS) stain colors the glycogen red-violet, shown as black. *A*, *B* and *C* at the same magnification. *D*, Portion of a vaginal smear, with rod-shaped Döderlein bacilli on and around the desquamated vaginal epithelial cells. High magnification.

It is the difference in the local threshold for androgenic stimulation that explains the initial appearance of hair around the pubis. Axillary hair is often not fully apparent until the menstrual cycles are established. The delay in growth of hair in these areas may be attributed either to a higher threshold for androgenic stimulation or to lessened sensitivity in the response of the hair follicles.

After the appearance of the breast buds and sexual hair one begins to observe a subtle change in the bodily contour. As part of the accelerated deposit of fat which follows directly upon the sudden impact of the gonadal hormones, the hips begin to broaden as fat is deposited on the sides and rear. The flat hips of the male or female child give way to the rounded form characteristic of the adult female. This is accompanied by a gradual widening of the bony pelvis (see Fig. 1–1).

The influence of increased estrin production is evident in the development of both the external and internal genitalia. The vulva changes in appearance as the labia majora develop, and fat is deposited in the subcutaneous tissue beneath them. This is also apparent over the pubic symphysis and mons veneris. The fine, soft baby hair covering the area becomes increased in density and texture. The clitoris becomes more prominent. Any abnormal enlargement should be regarded with suspicion, for it carries with it the stigma of masculinization.

The vagina takes part in the generalized increase in size of the genitalia. The prepuberal epithelium of the vagina, which is normally only three or four cell layers deep, changes, and many layers are seen, composed of cells which for the first time contain glycogen. The vaginal pH changes toward the acid side as lactic-acid producing Döderlein bacilli replace the mixed vaginal flora (Fig. 15–4).

The infantile uterus is characterized by an elongated cervix as compared with the size of the fundus. Under hormonal stimulation, largely estrogenic, both the cervix and fundus enlarge, but the major change is noted in the fundus, which increases in bulk in all directions, so that it eventually makes up fully three quarters of the entire uterine size (see Fig. 2–5). The endometrium proliferates in response to estrin stimulation. The progestational phase appears later when the ovary has fully matured.

The ovary and tube take part in the generalized development of the genitalia, but grow rather more slowly. The tubes enlarge and lose some of their tortuosity. The ovaries increase progressively in size, but reach their final stage of development only after they are capable of reacting to both the follicle-stimulating and luteinizing hormones. A decided increase in ovarian weight is said to take place between the ages of seventeen and twenty years.

Menarche

The first menstrual period, or menarche, appears only after the body, central nervous system and endocrine glands have reached the proper degree of maturity. The actual date of onset varies widely and is dependent on the same factors that influenced structural growth.

As in structural development, heredity plays a role, for the pattern of the young girl's menarche likely will closely simulate that of her mother and sisters. In recent years girls have tended to begin menstruating earlier in life than their mothers did,

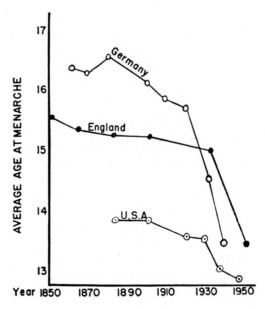

Fig. 15-5. The progressively younger age of the menarche during the past century is evident in 3 representative countries. (C. F. Fluhmann: *The Management of Menstrual Disorders.*)

but since sexual function is related to structural development as well as genetic influences, this may be due to the fact that girls of the present era are larger (Fig. 15–5). Physical condition, as modified by economic status and diet, also influences the time of onset of the first menstruation. In a depleted state created by malnutrition or anxiety the pituitary gonadotropins are hindered either in production or in release through hypothalamic inhibition. Social custom and perhaps psychic stimulation may have a bearing upon the date of the first menstrual cycle. Early maturity, for example, is the rule among savage tribes where sexual promiscuity is less well controlled. It also seems to be true that girls brought up in the city are more likely to have an earlier menarche than those in the country. Geographic and racial factors are hard to evaluate. Their influence may be more socio-economic and have a direct relation to the adequacy of the diet. It is also difficult to determine what part climate plays in the initiation of the menstrual cycle. We know that more girls begin their menstrual periods in the cooler months from September to June. It is also true that the Eskimo girl menstruates at a somewhat earlier age than the average, but the same tendency is noted among girls in tropical climates. The influence of climate upon the menarche is obscure. Considering all the factors involved, one may place the average age of the menarche, at least in temperate zones, to be somewhere between twelve and fourteen years.

When the uterus and ovaries are sufficiently mature, the first menstrual cycle is experienced. The bleeding becomes cyclic, but the complete pattern and rhythm have not yet been established. These may take as long as three years to acquire. For a year or more after the first menstrual period the interval between the periods often varies widely. The second period may not appear again for six months or may recur after three weeks. Irregularity in the time of onset may be regarded as normal during this maturing process. The average intermenstrual interval is about thirty-three days. The variability decreases with repetition, and the patient's interval pattern is usually set after about forty cycles, or between three and four years.

Menstrual bleeding at the menarche is considered usually to be *anovulatory in type* and may continue so for several months or years. The maturing ovary accepts the stimulation of the pituitary gonadotropin, FSH, elaborates a mature follicle that in turn produces estrin, which creates a proliferative type of endometrium in the uterine cavity. The ovary has perhaps not matured sufficiently to allow full maturation of the ova. When the estrin effect upon the endometrium, proliferative in type, has been built up, menstrual desquamation occurs as the estrogen blood level drops, and estrogen withdrawal bleeding occurs.

How long a pattern of anovulatory bleeding persists depends upon how rapidly the immature ovary becomes fully sensitized to the pituitary gonadotropins. There may be an anatomic explanation for ovarian immaturity. If the ovarian follicle is to respond to FSH stimulation, the vascular system of the young ovary must be sufficiently well established to transport the stimulus to the follicle cells. In early adolescence the vascular system is only in the developmental stage. Small amounts of FSH reach the follicle and produce estrin in proportion to the stimulus offered. The vascular elements respond to estrogenic stimulation with gradual and progressive proliferation. With fully developed vascular channels the full impact of the gonadotropins is felt on the follicle, and maturation of the ova occurs. It is a well known fact that the ovarian bulk increases sharply when true ovulatory cycles are established. This may take months or years after the menarche.

Not only must the ovary be mature enough to respond to the pituitary gonadotropins, in order that ovulation occur, but the central nervous system and the hypothalamus must also have reached maturity. The two hormones, in addition to FSH, that are concerned with ovulation and the development of the corpus luteum are the luteinizing hormone (LH or, in the male, ICSH) and the luteotropic hormone (LTH).

Luteotropic hormone is responsible for the release of the luteinizing hormone. Without it ovulation allegedly does not occur. Moreover, the corpus luteum will not develop without the stimulation of the luteotropic hormone, even though ovulation has occurred. This may theoretically serve as an explanation of the observation that the menstrual cycle is perhaps more aluteal than anovulatory. The degree of maturity in ovary and central nervous system (hypothalamus) varies from individual to individual in the same age group.

It is also evident that the same maturing factor must be present in the response of the target organs to hormonal stimulation before any regular cyclic ovulatory patterns can be established. Much of this information comes from animal experimentation, since laboratory methods for detection of minor fluctuations in hormonal output may not be sufficiently sensitive as yet. It is known that it is impossible to make the immature mouse uterus grow by giving estrin until it is ready to do so, regardless of whether the ovaries are present or not. When the uterus is sufficiently mature, hormonally stimulated growth will follow. In the immature monkey which has had both ovaries removed larger amounts of estrin are necessary to induce withdrawal bleeding than in the older, more mature animal.

The ovaries and uterus develop a full response to hormonal stimulation in a progressive manner. At first the stimulation is sporadic. The ovarian follicles start to grow, but regress and become atretic as the pituitary stimulus varies. Lacking proper constant cyclic pituitary stimulation, the estrin level also wavers, and the endometrium upon which it depends for growth and maintenance undergoes withdrawal desquamation and is sloughed off. Gradually the estrin stimulation becomes constant, and finally enough estrin is produced to trigger the release of the pituitary luteotropic and luteinizing hormones, and the ovulatory cycle is established. There is some evidence that the endometrium responds to progesterone in similar steplike fashion. Monkey experiments would suggest that there is a steady progression from amenorrhea through varying degrees of anovulatory bleeding to the final establishment of the complete ovulatory cycle.

Certainly full maturity is not acquired with the menarche, regardless of whether the periods are anovulatory as commonly believed, or aluteal as some investigators suggest. Some girls establish the adult pattern within a year or more of the first menstrual cycle, while in others it is delayed until later.

Fertility at Puberty

Because of the tendency to have anovulatory cycles at the onset of the periods, pregnancy is a rare event. It may occur early, because of individual variations in the length of time for the reproductive system to reach maturity, but even in the races among which child marriages are common or social customs permit promiscuous and unrestrained intercourse, pregnancies rarely occur until roughly three years after adequate sexual relations have been established. The fertility curve gradually rises after the menarche to reach its peak about the age of nineteen years. This rising curve parallels the full growth and maturation of the endocrine glands, central nervous system and target organs. This may be one of nature's protective devices, for the obstetrical history of the young adolescent is replete with unhappy complications. The incidence of toxemia runs as high as 20 per cent, and the younger the patient, the higher the incidence. Eclampsia is said to occur seven times and pre-eclampsia two and one-half times more frequently in the adolescent mother, as compared with pregnancy in the adult.

General Observations on the Management of the Girl during Puberty and Adolescence

Since some girls mature early, while others are late, chronologic age cannot be used as a working guide in the interpretation of the adolescent behavior pattern, nor as an indication of need for therapy. Because a child does not menstruate at the age when the parents think she should, there is no reason to consider an endocrine problem. Variations in hormonal balance are common to this age group. Most of these will be corrected by time, diet and a sensible regimen of living, and they do not require meddlesome hormone therapy which does not help and may be detrimental both functionally and psychologically. The maturing process cannot be forced. There are certain variations from the normal pattern which do represent major endocrine disorders, but in most instances they carry their own stigmata that allow them to be differentiated from the minor imbalances which are self-corrective. Intelligent observation, patience and understanding are the keynotes in bringing the young girl to maturity.

When one considers the massive impact of all the factors simultaneously at work on the unsuspecting child, it is small wonder that this developmental phase of existence is so perilous. The endocrine problem alone is enough to upset the mature woman at the menopause. It is but one of a series of powerful elements in the developing child. With the sharp increase in hormonal stimulation come powerful sex urges to plague the young girl, who has had no experience in coping with such demands. Interest in the opposite sex shows a decided change. With it comes an alteration in the behavior pattern. More attention is placed on personal appearance. Emotional outbursts are not uncommon. The child in her recently acquired awareness of the opposite sex becomes overmodest, blushes easily and is often highly critical of her parents' behavior. She is convinced that her parents do not understand her, and she wishes to be independent of their direction. Common to this age group is great interest in humanity and the downtrodden. She has a great drive to express her personality, but a high degree of uncertainty as to what sort of person she is.

All these factors are in full force at a time when a large portion of the child's energy is being consumed in the simple process of growth. The parent must be careful that too great demands are not placed on the child at this time. The father may want his daughter to take a greater interest in athletics. If the child is late in developing, she also is behind her age group in strength and does not have the ability to compete with a mature child of the same age.

It takes great patience and understanding to cope with an adolescent child. Too frequently the child is left to struggle with her own problems, because parents, particularly the mother, feel inadequate to deal with the complicated situation. Not infrequently the child is sent away to school, where more experienced advisors may or may not be present. We will be more effective in our management of the adolescent problem if we will take the time to consider the powerful stimuli that are in action during this growth period.

There are specific things that the parents can suggest to the growing child. Since a major portion of the child's energy is being used up in growth, in addition to being a little more tolerant of her lackadaisical and seemingly disinterested attitude, the parents should insist on a regimen which will provide adequate food, sunshine and exercise, but above all plenty of sleep. The school work schedule should be reviewed, and the child encouraged not to work beyond her capacity simply for the sake of getting better marks. This is particularly important at the present time, when competition for college education is so violent. If the parents will try to understand that girls in this age group are highly romantic, imaginative and impressionable, there will be less emotional strain on all concerned, particularly the child.

The mother can be of immeasurable help if she will take the trouble to sit down with the child and explain about the anticipated first menstrual period. The approach should be intelligent and objective. Stress should be laid on the fact that this is a naturally occurring phenomenon, completely devoid of dire consequences. It is a normal occurrence that should not be shunned or labeled with such appellations as the "curse" or being "unwell." There is no reason why the menstrual period should interfere with her normal existence in any way. The child should be encouraged to play tennis or golf and need not refrain from bathing or swimming. Moderation is in order, but a program of life as usual is much to be preferred to one of retirement from the world on a recurring monthly schedule.

Whether the patient utilizes the sanitary napkin or the vaginal tampon for protection is a matter of individual preference and facility of use. In many patients the hymenal ring will not permit the introduction of a tampon. If tampons can be inserted in the vaginal canal, no harm comes from their use, provided there is no indication of cervical or vaginal infection.

REVIEW OF ENDOCRINE PHYSIOLOGY WITH PARTICULAR REFERENCE TO MENSTRUATION

The menstrual cycle depends on the interlocking relations in function of the hypothalamus, pituitary, ovaries, uterus, thyroid, and adrenals. In order that menstrual bleeding occur it is essential that the patient have (1) a mature hypothalamus capable of receiving and transmitting stimuli from the rest of the central nervous system, (2) an anterior pituitary lobe capable of producing the pituitary gonadotropic hormones which act upon the ovary, (3) an ovary able to respond to such stimulation and in turn to elaborate its own estrogenic hormones, (4) a uterus with an endometrium sensitive enough to react to the stimulating effect of the ovarian hormones, (5) a thyroid gland to ensure maintenance of a sound bodily metabolism and proper utilization of the various other hormones produced, (6) adrenocortical tissue sufficient to control salt, water, protein and glucose metabolism, and to contribute some sex steroids.

All these factors are present in the patient who has normal, regular menstrual cycles. In the girl who does not there is an additional possible weak link, namely, adrenal dysfunction, that is frequently suspected. Any defect in this chain may result in the failure of menstruation, either in its initiation or in maintenance of a regular cyclic pattern.

THE ANTERIOR PITUITARY

The anterior lobe of the pituitary is the main regulating center for control of production of the hormones concerned with the menstrual cycle. The *acidophil cells* ("alpha" cells) are believed to produce (*a*) growth hormone and (*b*) luteotropic or

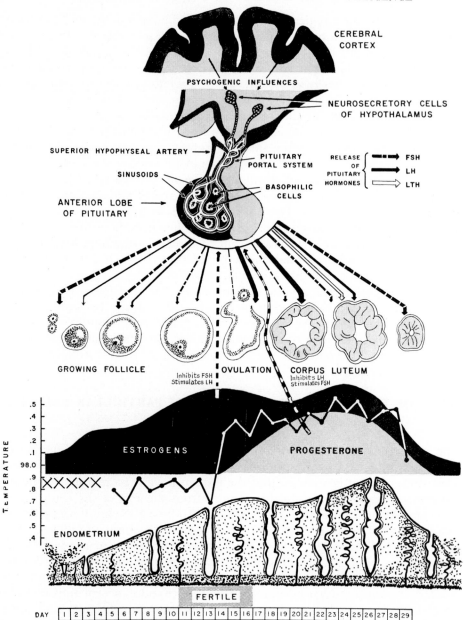

Fig. 15-6.   Cerebral, hypothalamic, pituitary, ovarian and endometrial interrelations of the menstrual cycle. Note the correlation of basal body temperature with other aspects of the cycle, including the period of fertility. (Courtesy of F. Netter: The Reproductive System. Ciba Med. Illustrations, 1954.)

lactogenic hormone (LTH). The basophil cells ("beta" cells) produce the gonadotropic hormones (*a*) follicle-stimulating hormone (FSH) and (*b*) luteinizing hormone (LH). Amphophil cells ("sparsely granulated basophils") produce thyrotropic hormone (TSH) and perhaps adrenocorticotropic hormone (ACTH). The hypothalamus is connected by neurohormonal pathways to the pituitary, and is thought to be concerned with the release of the various anterior lobe hormones. The degree of sensitivity of the hypothalamus may determine whether the afferent stimuli will increase or decrease the pituitary hormonal output.

The action of tropic hormones may make the target organ either release the hormone already stored in the organ, as in the thyroid, or stimulate the gland to produce its own hormone and release it immediately. Since pituitary overstimulation may result in target gland exhaustion and subsequent atrophy, a brake is provided, in that the presence of a hormone concentration adequate for proper function reflexly inhibits the pituitary stimulation by "feedback control," and balance is restored.

In the presence of disease or imbalance there may be (1) a loss of this feedback inhibition and a continued production of excess amounts of hormones, which will produce an abnormal response in the tissues normally affected by that particular hormone; or (2) the production of the hormone may be normal, but its metabolism may be so altered that relatively minor changes in its chemical structure result in an unaccustomed biologic response in the target tissue or end-organ. The latter situation is noted not infrequently experimentally with the hormones of estrogen, androgen, adrenocorticoid and progestin types.

When the anterior pituitary lobe and hypothalamus reach a sufficient degree of maturity, usually by about the age of eleven years, the "beta" cells of the anterior lobe begin to secrete the follicle-stimulating hormone (FSH). Apparently it is utilized in the same form that it is produced and gradually increases in amount as the child grows. Under the influence of this hormone a number of follicles within the ovary increase in size. Though the follicles grow, they are believed incapable of producing estrin unless they also receive some stimulation from the interstitial cell stimulating hormone (ICSH) of the male which we commonly call in gynecology LH (luteinizing hormone). The combined actions of FSH and LH stimulate the ovarian stromal and theca interna cells to secrete estrin.

As more ovarian estrin is produced, less pituitary follicle-stimulating hormone is needed. The feedback braking effect comes into play, and the FSH production is inhibited, while the basophil cells are stimulated to put out relatively more LH (ICSH). This hormone produces growth among the granulosa cells of the follicle. Many follicles have been stimulated to grow, but usually only one is destined to ovulate monthly. The luteinizing hormone aids in the selection and provides the stimulus for the one follicle to migrate from its position within the ovary toward the surface, where ovulation can occur more readily. The remaining follicles rest or become atretic, but continue to produce estrin.

The final stimulus to ovulation occurs when enough LH has been produced to overbalance the gradually declining amount of FSH. A small residual amount of the follicle-stimulating hormone is apparently essential. Ovulation then occurs, and the two hormones combine to bring about the formation and growth of the corpus luteum. The luteinizing hormone is responsible for the storage within the ovarian granulosa and theca interna cells of substances, such as cholesterol, which will subsequently be used to produce progestin, when the corpus luteum develops and functions.

The responsibility for the further growth and function of the corpus luteum rests in animals and possibly in women with the luteotropic hormone (LTH). This hormone is a product of the acidophil, or "alpha," cells of the anterior pituitary and is released by stimuli from the hypothalamus. Under the stimulating action of LTH the granulosa and theca interna cells, previously prepared by the luteinizing hormone, become luteal cells and secrete progestin. The braking effect is again in evidence as progesterone in sufficient quantity suppresses the pituitary output of LH and LTH. This again throws the balance in favor of production of the follicle-stimulating hormone, which begins to prepare the ovarian follicles for the next cycle, provided pregnancy does not intervene (Fig. 15–6).

THE ADRENAL

The effects of the pituitary hormones are also apparent on adrenal function and indirectly involve the menstrual cycle. Both the luteotropic hormone and the luteinizing hormone stimulate the adrenal cortex experimentally to secrete *androgens*. These are produced in the zona reticularis of the adrenal gland. This is a direct form of stimulation. Primarily androgen is concerned with protein synthesis, but it also has an inhibitory or neutralizing action on the circulating estrogen, in its effect upon both end-organs and tissues in general.

The adrenocorticotropic hormone (ACTH) is not gonadotropic, but is indirectly active, through its stimulating effect on the adrenal cortex, in producing hormones which are concerned with menstruation. Basically it is active in the production and release in adults of hydrocortisone, which is responsible for the conversion of protein and fat into carbohydrate. Cortisone-type hormone is produced in the zona fasciculata of the adrenal. When there is normal and adequate production of hydrocortisone, the feedback brake effect is again noted, and the secretion of pituitary ACTH is inhibited. If there is some defect in production or metabolism of hydrocortisone, as may take place in the adrenogenital syndrome, or if an increase in body need calls for a greater utilization, a deficiency of cortisone may arise. The reciprocal arrangement between adrenal cortex and pituitary is again evident, for the pituitary responds by elaborating more ACTH. Practically, the overactivity on the part of ACTH can be inhibited by the therapeutic use of cortisone-type steroids. The pituitary ACTH stimulates both the zona fasciculata and zona reticularis, but in certain diseases such as the adrenogenital syndrome there is a basic defect in the zona fasciculata, where cortisone is synthesized. The unbalanced excess of ACTH then excessively stimulates the zona reticularis where the sex steroids such as androgen and estrogen are produced. As a result the production of both LH and FSH may be inhibited, and ovarian dysfunction may result.

In addition, the outermost zone of the adrenal cortex, the zona glomerulosa, is concerned with menstrual function through variations in the control of the electrolytes which have to do with the storage of water in tissue, and particularly by the action of aldosterone upon renal tubules. With normal tissue hydration, high sodium and low potassium levels, there is less stimulus for aldosterone production. In reverse, with high potassium and low sodium levels an increased production of aldosterone is required. Cyclic alterations in fluid and electrolyte storage are a part of the menstrual picture.

THE THYROID

A normally functioning thyroid gland is essential to proper gonadal function. The sparsely granulated amphophil, or thyrotropic basophil, cells of the anterior lobe of the pituitary are responsible for the elaboration of the thyroid-stimulating hormone (TSH), which causes the thyroid gland to produce, store and release hormones such as triiodothyronine and thyroxin. The thyroid hormone is directly involved in the maintenance of general body homeostasis. It has been shown to be necessary for growth and is essential in metabolic regulation of all living cells. These factors bear directly on menstruation, both in its initiation and in its normal course. The activity of the thyroid gland is closely linked to gonadotropic activity. It is a well known fact that women are more prone than men to have both hyperthyroidism and myxedema.

Not infrequently, thyroid malfunctions manifest themselves at puberty, pregnancy or the menopause, when the maximal variations in general hormonal activity are apparent.

The effect of the thyroid on the ovary is in all probability influenced through the pituitary, but there is some experimental evidence that this may take place as a result of direct action. If thyroid hormone is in excess, increased catabolism of tissue takes place, and disturbed nutrition follows and with it an increase in emotional sensitivity. As a result of the excessive thyroid secretion the brake is again in operation, and the pituitary TSH production is inhibited. In addition, the output of gonadotropic hormones is diminished, either because of the effect on the pituitary or because of alteration in the sensitivity of the hypothalamus. If thyroid hormone is being produced in inadequate quantity, the pituitary is stimulated to increase the output of the thyrotropic hormone. This increased demand on the part of the anterior pituitary is accompanied by a diminished output of the follicle-stimulating hormone. As a result insufficient estrin is produced, resulting in ovarian atrophy and, if extreme, uterine atrophy.

Animal experiments have suggested that there may be a direct thyroid action on the ovary, for thyroid hormone seems to decrease the response of the ovary to gonadotropic hormone stimulation, when given to mice which have had the pituitary removed. Conversely, more estrin is produced when pituitary hormones are given to mice which have had a thyroidectomy.

Whatever the mechanism of its action, the thyroid gland is largely responsible for some of the most common manifestations of malfunction of the endocrine glands in puberty and adolescence. In the older patient faulty functions of the thyroid may be responsible for either excessive bleeding or amenorrhea. Largely this takes place through a pathologic reciprocal interplay in the pituitary-thyroid-ovarian axis, but it may be secondary to faulty metabolism of thyroid hormone at the tissue level. The final end-product of the thyroid is considered to be triiodothyronine. In certain hypometabolic states the function of the thyroid gland may be adequate, as measured by the common laboratory procedures, such as the basal metabolic rate, serum protein-bound iodine determinations and the extent of uptake by the gland of radioactive iodine. The patient, however, continues to have typical symptoms of thyroid lack, because the final breakdown of thyroxin to triiodothyronine does not occur, and the target organs reflect the loss of proper stimulation.

The Ovary

The ovary is the target organ for the pituitary gonadotropic hormones. The thyroid and adrenal hormones affect its function indirectly through the production of its pituitary stimulating hormones or by neutralizing the hormones it produces. This relation is reciprocal. The mature ovary in normal function elaborates two major types of hormones, estrins and progestins.

Estrin

The basic function of estrin is to prepare the growing girl for reproduction. In the course of the normal progress of growth during puberty and adolescence the effect of estrin in this maturing process has been obvious, through its selective action on the genital tract, the vulva, vagina, uterus and increase in breast size. In its absence,

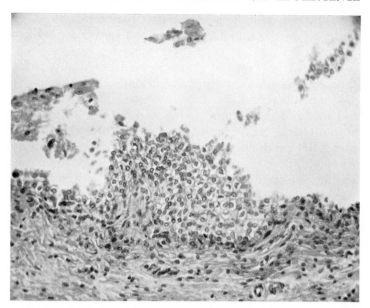

Fig. 15-7.   Glycogen-rich clear cells lining the bladder are responsive to estrogenic stimulation. This reactivity is also found in the cloacogenic zone between the anal skin and mucous membrane of the rectum.

development does not occur in these areas or, if estrin secretion is withdrawn, atrophy follows. The degree of estrin stimulation is often measured by the extent of cornification of the cells of the vaginal epithelium. Though estrin has no direct action in promoting linear growth of bone, it is intimately connected with its metabolism, for it stimulates osteoblastic activity and bone formation. Withdrawal will result in osteoporosis.

Estrin does have an effect on linear growth of bone, indirectly through the pituitary, by bringing about epiphysial closure, thereby restricting the height of girls. Its influence on the actions of pituitary growth hormone is manifest both at puberty and the menopause. Gigantism seen at puberty occurs usually in the presence of a relative failure in sexual maturity. Since there is estrin lack, the normal depressant action of estrin on the growth hormone is lacking. It is also noted at the menopause when estrin depletion is evident. Changes in facial appearance then, with some tendency toward acromegaly, are not uncommon.

Though it has so far been impossible to measure the estrin concentration in skin, it is obvious from animal experiments and clinical appraisal in human beings that estrin does have an effect on skin metabolism in general, with particular reference to the pubic area. One has only to observe the dramatic changes in the perineal area of the baboon during estrus or the pigment changes in women during pregnancy to realize that these color alterations are most evident when estrin secretion is at its peak. When estrin is withdrawn after castration or is depleted at the time of the menopause, atrophy of the vulva and perineal skin becomes obvious. The same effect, though to a less extent, is noted in skin throughout the body. The loss seems to be in subcutaneous fat and elastic tissue fibers.

The same effects are apparent in the mucous membranes of the genitourinary tract. The changes in the vaginal epithelium are the most dramatic, but they are also evident in the cells lining the urethra and bladder neck. These are maintained by estrin in preparation for and during active menstrual life, but atrophy is apparent when the estrin level falls (Fig. 15–7).

Estrin also has an effect on the other endocrine glands, such as the thyroid, adrenals and pancreas. It is most obvious in the thyroid, which can be seen or felt. Thyroid enlargement at puberty is common. This is perhaps nature's response to need, for the body is being groomed for maturity, and full metabolism of the growing cells is important to the process. Here the effect is exerted on the thyroid indirectly through the pituitary, in the same manner that estrin stimulates the adrenals. There is also convincing evidence of a direct effect of estrin on both these glands. Again acting through the pituitary, the pancreas is stimulated by estrin to put out more insulin. In combination with LH, estrin causes cholesterol and like substances to be deposited in both the ovary and the adrenal to aid in the elaboration of both progesterone and androgen.

The primary purpose of estrogen, to which all other factors contribute, is the creation of an endometrium suitable to receive the fertilized ovum in anticipation of successful pregnancy. To this end estrin suppresses the follicle-stimulating hormone so that the luteinizing hormone can aid in bringing about ovulation. Within the ovary it has stimulated the theca cells and interstitial stromal cells to proliferate. It has somehow selected the follicle destined to mature and with the help of LH brought about its migration to the surface of the ovary, where the ovum can be given off. It has caused cholesterol to be stored in the ovarian granulosa and thecal cells, so that progesterone can be produced. Within the endometrium the cells lining the glands are encouraged to grow in size and number. The glands and stroma likewise take part in the growth phase. Alkaline phosphatases and beta glucuronidase, under the influence of estrin, assist in the storage and mobilization of glycogen, which will help to nourish the ovum if it becomes impregnated. Estrin combines with progestin to maintain growth of the endometrium suitable for the lodging of the ovum, while progestin provides for its sustenance. If pregnancy does not occur, the estrin level falls and the endometrium breaks down and is discarded at menstruation.

The entire process is another example of the reciprocal relations of ovary and pituitary. In the presence of need the pituitary is stimulated to produce more folliclestimulating hormone, while estrin in excess causes its suppression. Clinical application is found in the use of estrin to inhibit the increased activity of the follicle-stimulating hormone at the time of the menopause, when the normal estrin is produced in decreasing amounts. Another example can be found in the use of estrin, given in excess quantity, to prevent ovulation by inhibiting FSH production to such an extent that FSH is not present in sufficient quantity to initiate the ovulatory process.

METABOLISM OF ESTRIN. Since only about 10 per cent of estrin injected into human beings can be recovered in the urine, it has been difficult to refine the laboratory tests so that minor fluctuations in amount can be detected. Apparently estrin is bound to protein elements in the blood, and attempts are now being made to determine which of the protein fractions carries the biologically active factor in estrin metabolism. Estrin is found in the blood and urine mainly in the form of estradiol, estrone and estriol. The final product in the breakdown of the estradiol, produced by the theca interna and stromal interstitial cells, seems to be estrone. The biologically active factor has not been determined, but the most important would appear to be estradiol. Since large amounts of estrin can be found in the bile and feces, there is a suggestion that estrin in its passage through the liver is inactivated and by enzymatic action converted from estradiol to estrone. Experiments designed to bypass the liver by placing an estrogenic source within the spleen tend to confirm these observations.

Progesterone

This product of the lutein cells of the functioning corpus luteum is solely concerned with the maintenance of pregnancy when fertilization of the ovum has been accomplished. Its effect is manifest solely on the endometrium and the breast.

Progesterone is produced when the ovary has matured sufficiently to accept the pituitary stimulation offered by the luteinizing hormone (LH) and the luteotropic hormone (LTH). The latter is essential to maintenance and normal function of the corpus luteum, whose lutein cells produce progestin and create the secretory endometrium. The fully mature endometrium is now conditioned to receive and nourish the impregnated ovum. If impregnation does not occur, the luteinizing hormone is inhibited, and endometrial regression is followed by menstruation. This is another example of the feedback brake effect. If pregnancy does occur, progestin is essential in maintaining the pregnancy until the placenta can mature sufficiently to produce enough chorionic gonadotropin and to take over the role of progestin production. This is believed to take approximately three months. Clinically it is known that about one third of the patients will abort if the corpus luteum is removed surgically before two months after the first missed period. The remaining patients have developed a placenta mature enough to sustain the pregnancy without help from the corpus luteum of pregnancy. The production of progestin continues through the first trimester of pregnancy, but in gradually decreasing amount. The progestational changes in the endometrium will be discussed in Chapter 16.

In order that there be functioning progestational endometrium, it is essential that estrin be present. This is used as a test for ovarian function. The injection of progestin in a patient whose endometrium has been previously conditioned by estrin administration will cause bleeding three or four days after the last injection of progestin. This is called "progesterone withdrawal bleeding." This will not occur without the estrin priming. We have noted that estrin has been responsible for the deposition of cholesterol within the granulosa and theca cells of the ripening follicle. These cells become the lutein cells, and the cholesterol assists in their synthesis of progestin. The alkaline phosphatase and beta-glucuronidase have mobilized glycogen under the influence of estrin. Progestin provides for its utilization in the nourishment of the fertilized ovum. Without sufficient glycogen secretion the free-floating fertilized ovum does not receive adequate nourishment and either never implants or does so reluctantly, and early abortion is inevitable.

The same factors are noted in the breast. In early puberty the duct system develops under the influence of estrin, before the ductular elements respond to the stimulation of progestin. Cyclic variations are noted in the breast during the menstrual cycle under the combined influence of estrin and progestin.

Progestin has another important effect on menstrual activity. Alterations in electrolyte balance and water storage occur cyclically with menstruation. Progestin acts upon the renal tubules, just as aldosterone does, to prevent the excretion of water, sodium and chloride, while potassium loss is encouraged. This increase in the water content of the cerebral cortex tends to produce a transient ischemia, which may explain the increased sensitivity and irritability that some women experience before and during menstruation. Some sedative effect is noted both on the central nervous system and on uterine motility when large amounts of progestin are given· This may be another example of the brake effect.

METABOLISM OF PROGESTERONE. Progesterone is formed by the granulosa and theca cells of the maturing follicle, which become lutein cells as the corpus luteum develops. The cholesterol mobilized by estrin and the luteinizing hormone is utilized in the formation of progesterone. When the precursor substances are exhausted, the corpus luteum degenerates. The biologically active progesterone breaks down and is excreted as sodium pregnanediol glucuronide. The conversion takes place largely in the liver. Though some progesterone is produced by the adrenal, the excretion values of pregnanediol are a fair index of the amount of progesterone present. Approximately 20 per cent of the amount of progesterone injected is recovered in the urine.

GENERAL OBSERVATIONS ON ENDOCRINE FUNCTION

Abnormal function of the endocrine glands may result either from too much or too little stimulation. The need of body tissue for a regular supply of hormones may provide the impetus. Any alteration in tissue requirements created by trauma, disease or local resistance to the hormone will call for an increased production. Primary proliferations, either tumor or hyperplasia, in the hypothalamus, pituitary, ovary, thyroid or adrenals may cause hyperactivity on the part of the gland and excess production of its hormone. Either neoplasm or nonfunctional hyperplasia can lead to eventual atrophy through decreased hormone production. The tumor may grow to such proportions that the normal gland is destroyed. Prolonged stimulation which leads to hyperplasia produces an excessive tissue and end-organ response. If the feedback control mechanism does not function properly, "exhaustion" atrophy of the remaining glandular tissue may result. Moreover, if the hormone supply is in excess, the target organ may not be able to metabolize it properly, so that the effect on the tissues normally affected becomes bizarre.

DIAGNOSTIC PROCEDURES TO DETECT THE EFFECT OF THE SEX HORMONES IN THE FEMALE

Although the methods of detecting the various hormones implicated in both normal and abnormal endocrine function in the female are constantly being revised, improved and simplified, it would be well to give a brief outline of the analytical recourses now in vogue, as well as a workable idea of what the results mean in terms of diagnosis and treatment. Many of the tests now used simply record the presence or absence of the hormone and give no indication of the relative amounts present. The problem is further complicated by the fact that the hormone may have several components, only one of which may be biologically active. Furthermore, under certain conditions conversion may take place from one hormone to another, such as testosterone to estrone, estradiol to estriol, pregnanetriol to pregnanediol, progesterone to estrin, and so on (Fig. 15–8). Present investigations are directed toward the partitioning of the hormones and the determination of the active biological element. For example, we recognize three basic partitions of estrin, (a) estrone, (b) estradiol, (c) estriol, but there are many more departures from the basic pattern.

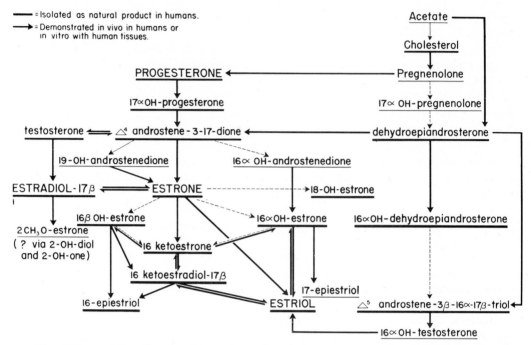

Fig. 15-8. A flow diagram of the major pathways of progesterone and estrogen metabolism. The underlined compounds occur normally in women. The reactions with dotted lines are the theoretically possible sources of some hormones isolated. (See Dorfman and Ungar, 1953.)

For practical purposes, however, we will attempt to record the present methods of detection.

Clinical Evaluation

Much information can be obtained about the activity of the hormones simply by observing and then examining the patient. The tests for the hormones are both time-consuming and expensive, and they are frequently impossible to obtain in the geographic area in which the physician must practice. He must then rely on his clinical acumen.

The secondary sex characteristics reflect the activity of estrin. With the onset of puberty one would expect to note the appearance of sexual hair in the normal feminine pattern, development of the breasts and external genitalia and the female habitus, as well as cornification in the vaginal epithelium. Any departure from this pattern would indicate either that there is a decrease in or relative absence of the secretion of estrogen or a disturbance in balance of the androgen-estrogen ratio. If, for example, hair appears on the face, chin and areola of the breast, and the patient has a male pubic hair escutcheon, then one may assume that some androgenic factor is present, though the actual source may remain in doubt. It may well be adrenal in origin, although some clinicopathologic entities suggest that the hilar cells in the ovary are producing the androgen. When the scalp and body hair distribution is that of the male, the breasts are atrophied, the hips flattened and the patient has enlargement of the clitoris, then virilizing elements are present which are directly traceable to increased androgen production. If a pelvic tumor is palpable, one might suspect the presence of a masculinizing tumor of the ovary. In the absence of such a tumor the adrenal would be suspect.

Complete absence of ovarian activity may also be suspected from clinical observation. The classic picture of ovarian aplasia is frequently sufficiently obvious for one to make a diagnosis without laboratory confirmation. There are too many variables to rely on the clinical evaluation completely, but the physician has a working background on which to base therapy. The clinical picture has already been described (p. 128).

Cushing's syndrome and Sheehan's syndrome provide classic pictures which are immediately evident on physical examination. Likewise one gets a fair idea of whether a patient is pregnant by observing the changes in the vaginal epithelium, which reflect the increased output of the ovarian hormones. A lack of hormonal activity may also be apparent on inspection of the vaginal epithelium. In the absence of estrin activity the vaginal epithelium is less soft and succulent. These observations have practical value. For example, carcinoma of the endometrium rarely appears in a patient with an atrophic vaginal epithelium.

These are but a few examples, but they point out the practical value of observation. When this is coupled with pelvic examination and proper evaluation of the condition of the pelvic organs, much information can be obtained. Chemical and biological assays are needed only to confirm, and at times to measure, the relative degrees of hormone excess or deficiency.

Methods of Determining the Presence of the Hormones

The hormones may be detected and quantitative differences determined by (a) bio-assays on urine and blood, (b) chemical assays based on urinary excretion, (c) chemical measurements of the concentration in the plasma.

Whenever possible, chemical analyses should supplant bio-assays. Unfortunately, certain of the hormones such as the pituitary gonadotropins can be assayed only on laboratory animals. The partitioning and separate identification of the biologically active component within a group of chemically structurally similar hormones cannot be achieved readily, but in many instances this is of little practical value.

Chemical analyses of twenty-four-hour urine specimens have as their chief value the estimation of the total amount of hormonal secretion over that period of time. Minor variations or fluctuations in amount and the biological activity of the individual components cannot be detected by this method. Evaluation of the amount of the steroid hormones in the plasma is useful in determining the hormonal concentration at a given time.

BIO-ASSAYS FOR THE PITUITARY GONADOTROPINS. Since chemical determinations are not available for the evaluation of pituitary gonadotropins, bio-assays on laboratory animals are essential. They are available for the determinations of (a) chorionic gonadotropin, as in pregnancy, (b) follicle-stimulating hormone (FSH), (c) luteinizing hormone (LH), synonymous with male interstitial cell stimulating hormone (ICSH), (d) thyroid-stimulating hormone (TSH), (e) adrenocorticotropic hormone (ACTH). It is possible to detect other pituitary hormones with specific actions, but those listed above are our chief concern.

PREGNANCY. The *Aschheim-Zondek* test for pregnancy, based on the assay of placental gonadotropin, depends on the injection of a sample of the urine of a pregnant woman into immature female mice. If the patient is pregnant, corpora lutea develop in the ovaries, and typical corpora hemorrhagica appear grossly. The *Friedman* test uses the immature female rabbit rather than the mouse. The *frog* test, which is currently popular because of the low cost of laboratory operation and the speed with which the results are known (four to eighteen hours), depends on the increased urinary excretion of chorionic gonadotropin that is found in the first half of pregnancy to stimulate the female South African frog (*Xenopus laevis*) to extrude eggs. At present sperm discharge from domestic male frogs (*Rana pipiens*) is utilized more commonly. In addition to their value in establishing the presence or absence of pregnancy, these tests are important in detecting abnormalities of conception and related neoplasms, since chorionic gonadotropin is excreted in large amounts by hydatidiform moles and chorionepitheliomas. The chief disadvantage in the use of frogs is the variation in sensitivity of the animals, which seems to follow a seasonal pattern. For example, in the spring of the year falsely positive tests may appear.

THE FOLLICLE-STIMULATING HORMONE.   The test for FSH has widespread clinical application, despite the fact that it does not provide a true scientific evaluation of the hormone. There are many investigators who believe that the follicular stimulating hormone itself is a combination of both FSH and the luteinizing hormone. We have previously noted that FSH depends on the presence of LH for the initiation of ovulation. Nevertheless the detection of the amount of FSH, whether normal, excessive or diminished, does have practical value.

Before the urine can be injected into an infantile or hypophysectomized albino mouse it must first be concentrated and the protein elements precipitated. The concentrate is then injected and the response sought in both ovary and uterus. The graafian follicle in the ovary is stimulated to put out estrin, which in turn causes the uterus to enlarge and increase in weight.

What Is the Normal Value?   The numerical value of the FSH is calculated from the determination of the uterine weight. The normal value for the adult woman in the reproductive years ranges from 6 to values slightly in excess of 50 mouse units per 24 hours. The actual daily values vary in accordance with the cyclic pattern of menstruation. Follicle-stimulating hormone does not make its appearance in any quantity until about the time of puberty or shortly before.

Under normal conditions with an intact and functioning endocrine axis the FSH stimulates the graafian follicle to produce estrin, which in turn acts as a brake on the anterior pituitary and inhibits the production of excess FSH. If the ovary is absent or unresponsive because of immaturity or advanced age, no estrin is produced, and the braking effect is lacking. The pituitary then puts out more FSH. When the pituitary is deficient, either from disease, destruction by tumor, malnutrition or psychogenic influence, little or no FSH may be recovered in the urine. The pituitary deficiency may be transitory if the last two factors are operating.

The test, then, is of great value at both ends of the reproductive spectrum. It will help in determining whether the primary amenorrhea of the adolescent girl is due to a basic defect in the pituitary or whether the ovary is at fault. In older women, when ovarian activity is on the wane, an increase in the amount of FSH is noted before, during and after the menopause, and is usually present when the patient complains of hot flashes. It must be noted, however, that the intensity of the symptoms has no relation to the amount of FSH being produced. Moreover, in many instances the exogenous administration of estrin, particularly diethylstilbestrol, relieves symptoms without altering the level of circulating FSH. This may be because synthetic estrogen does not produce the same braking effect on the pituitary as natural estrogens.

THE LUTEINIZING HORMONE (LH OR ICSH).   As previously noted, the total FSH value may include measurement of the LH factor, as well as FSH. McArthur has attempted to isolate the LH element by injecting the same concentrate used in FSH determinations into hypophysectomized or immature rats. Luteinizing hormone values are determined by weighing the ventral prostate of these animals after the injection. In this manner it is possible to isolate the LH factor.

THYROTROPIC HORMONE (TSH).   Attempts to measure the amount of thyroid-stimulating hormone by assay of blood or urine have been too cumbersome to have any practical value. Clinical estimates of pituitary control of thyroid function are still best obtained indirectly, by the radioactive uptake studies of I^{131} after the injection of thyrotropic hormone or by the determination of protein-bound iodine in the serum.

ADRENOCORTICOTROPIC HORMONE (ACTH).   A variety of methods are available for measuring pituitary ACTH. The latest method is concerned with the measurement of compound B (Corticosterone) in the blood of the adrenal vein of the hypophysectomized rat.

What Tests Do We Have to Measure Estrin Activity?

In addition to the observations that are clinically obvious, such as the secondary sex characteristics and gross appearance of the vaginal epithelium, one may evaluate the degree of estrogenic activity by (a) interpretation of the vaginal smears, (b) bioassay of estrin in twenty-four-hour urine specimens, (c) chemical determinations of estrin in blood and urine, (d) endometrial biopsy, (e) electropotential differences in the vaginal epithelium.

VAGINAL SMEARS.   The interpretation of the estrogen effect in vaginal smears depends on the recognition and the relative composition of the cells which make up the various layers of the vaginal epithelium. Since the amount of estrin produced varies at the two ends of the reproductive age spectrum, the vaginal smears reflect the sharp difference. Likewise, the estrogen activity fluctuates in the normal menstrual cycle of the adult woman. Cyclic variations, then, are noted in the cell pattern, but the changes are too gradual to provide an end-point which might be used to determine the day of ovulation.

The vaginal epithelium has three distinct layers, each characterized by a different type of cell (Fig. 15–9, B). The deepest, the basal cell layer, is composed of small rounded cells which have large basophil nuclei and stain strongly with the Papanicolaou stain. As the basal cells mature and migrate toward the surface an intermediate layer, made up of precornified cells, is noted. These cells are larger with rounded or oval shapes and more cytoplasm that stains green with Papanicolaou stain; too, they tend to have a centrally placed vesicular nucleus. Approaching the surface, the superficial layers contain large cornified cells, which have flattened shapes that tend to lie parallel with the surface. The nuclei are either absent or pyknotic. The cytoplasm tends to be acidophilic, clear or foamy, and the cells take the orange-pink Papanicolaou stain rather poorly. These are the fully cornified cells, rich in cytoplasmic glycogen, which one sees only in the presence of estrogenic activity.

Tracing the changes in smears of the vaginal epithelium in different age groups, we note that shortly after birth the cells reflect the influence of maternal estrin, for cornified cells are present (Fig. 15–9, A). This rapidly disappears, and one then sees

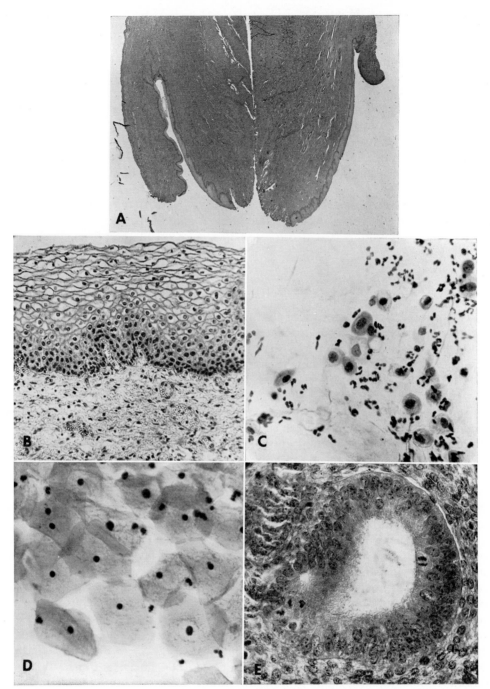

Fig. 15-9.   *A,* Microscopic section of the uterine cervix of the newborn, with estrogenized cervical and vaginal epithelium normally present, owing to maternal and placental hormones. *B,* Section at medium magnification of the mature pars vaginalis epithelium, showing the basal, precornified and fully cornified cell layers. *C,* Vaginal smear that shows no estrogen effect. The cells are of basal and parabasal types. *D,* Fully estrogenized vaginal smear (at same magnification as *C*)composed of cornified polygonal epithelial cells. *E,* Field from an endometrial biopsy. Mitotic figures in the glandular epithelium indicate proliferative activity due to estrogenic stimulation.

largely cells derived from the deeper layers. They are usually round or oval, have prominent basophil nuclei and take a deeper dark stain (Fig. 15–9, *C*). As puberty approaches, the cells resemble those seen in the intermediate or precornified, rather than the basal layers, although some of the latter linger on. The precornified cells are larger and irregular in shape with large, deeply staining nuclei. The cytoplasm takes on a bluish green stain. The cells tend to arrange themselves in clumps and are now surrounded by more leukocytes and debris made up of the cytoplasm of disintegrating cells. At puberty the increase in estrogen activity is shown by the appearance of pinkish stained cells with pyknotic nuclei. These cornified cells come from the superficial layer and are large, flat and polygonal (Fig. 15–9, *D*). The white blood cells, debris and nonspecific bacteria disappear, in favor of large, rod-shaped Döderlein's bacilli.

The epithelial changes in vaginal smears reflect the fluctuation in estrin activity during the cycles of the normal adult. Early in the cycle the cells tend to be clumped and appear as a mixture of cells from both the intermediate and superficial layers. As one approaches the midpoint of the cycle, when estrogenic activity is high, the cells are mostly large and polygonal and have pyknotic nuclei. They are about equally divided between cornified and precornified cells. They tend to be disseminated rather than clumped together. The leukocytes and debris seen earlier in the cycle are absent. As the cycle progresses into the luteal phase and the estrin effect falls off, the fully cornified cells become fewer. More precornified cells are seen. Degenerative changes are noted with cells of wrinkled outline surrounded by leukocytes and bacteria. The majority of cells take a deep blue-green rather than a red or pinkish stain with the Papanicolaou method.

Finally, in the premenopausal and menopausal years, as estrogenic activity falls off, the epithelial layers become thinned out, and both cyclic activity and cornification disappear. Most cells in vaginal smears are basal and parabasal in appearance, with prominent nuclei, scanty cytoplasm and degenerative changes.

ESTROGEN BY BIO-ASSAY.   The most common method now in use is the bio-assay method proposed by Allen and Doisy, in which the degree of estrogenic activity is determined by the minimal amount of test material required to induce cornification in the atrophic vaginal epithelium of the castrated mouse or rat. Vaginal smears of these animals are read to evaluate the degree of cornification of the cells of the vaginal epithelium. Complete cornification of the cells is taken as the end-point, while anything less suggests reduced estrogen activity.

The Astwood six-hour test measures the increase in wet weight of uterine tissue from immature rats injected with different concentrations of estrogens in samples of urine. Ratios between different individual estrogens also may be determined by a modification of this method.

ESTROGEN BY CHEMICAL DETERMINATION.   With use of twenty-four-hour urine specimens, preferably collected over an entire cycle, it is possible on a research basis to determine total estrogen excretion or the output of individual estrogens. In the normal cycle there are so-called ovulation and luteal peaks. In pregnancy urine estriol, believed to be of placental origin, is greatly increased. By chemical analysis of ovarian stromal biosynthetic activity, some estrogen production is evident up to sixty-five years of age.

The latest method (Brown) uses chromatography for the separation of methyl esters of major estrogenic metabolites. At present, investigators are working with gas vapor chromatographic methods designed to simplify and speed up the analyses

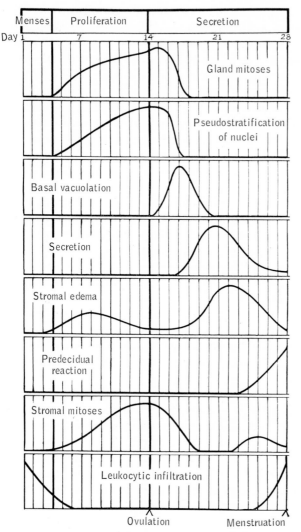

Fig. 15-10. Representation of the major changes in the endometrium during a normal 28-day menstrual cycle. Gland mitoses are the most useful diagnostic criterion of the proliferative phase. Glandular vacuoles and secretory discharge characterize the early secretory phase, and predecidual reaction of the endometrial stroma typifies the late secretory phase. (Redrawn from R. W. Noyes, A. T. Hertig and J. Rock: *Fertil. & Steril.*, Vol. 1.)

ENDOMETRIAL BIOPSY.   The endometrial biopsy is useful in evaluating the effect of estrogenic secretion. The changes found throughout the cycle may be illustrated in graphic form (Fig. 15–10). One expects to find proliferation of the endometrium during the early phases of the menstrual cycle. Whenever anovulatory cycles appear in women of menstrual age, a proliferative phase will be noted from biopsy material obtained anywhere in the cycle (Fig. 15–9, *E*). The cells will be abnormally crowded and palisaded in the gland linings, owing to uninterrupted proliferation. Such cycles are common in bleeding patterns encountered at puberty and again in the menopause, but may appear sporadically at any time.

ABDOMINOVAGINAL ELECTROPOTENTIALS.   This is a relatively new method of measuring the effect of estrogenic activity upon the vaginal epithelium. Acid epithelial surfaces generate minute electropotentials under the influence of hormonal activity. The exact mechanism is not known, but it has something to do with the transport of sodium across a semipermeable membrane, such as the vaginal epithelium. The electropotentials are captured by glass electrodes filled with saline solution in contact with the vaginal epithelium. The electrolyte transfer is captured, passed into a saline column which leads through a calomel half-cell unit and thence through a highly sensitive resistance unit. The potential differences are recorded on graph paper in much the same manner as an electrocardiogram. The recordings are made in both the positive and negative ranges, the latter expressing electronegativity.

The electropotential recordings have been balanced against simultaneous studies of total urinary estrogen assays (Brown method) and vaginal smear studies, both taken throughout the cycle. The correlation between the three elements is close. The electropotential recording, then, can be considered to be an accurate measure of estrogen production and release. It is far more sensitive than the vaginal smears in its ability to pinpoint the day of ovulation.

What Methods Do We Have to Estimate Progesterone Production?

When ovulatory cycles are established, cyclic variation is noted in the endometrial pattern. As the corpus luteum appears and progesterone is produced, the endometrium responds and becomes secretory in action. In many gynecologic con-

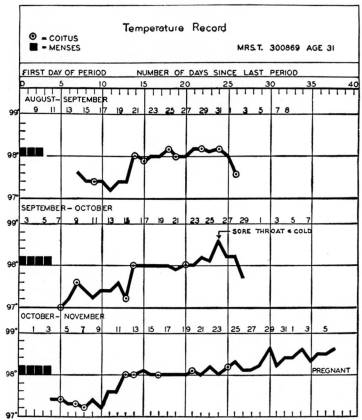

Fig. 15-11. Basal temperature record of a patient that covers 3 monthly cycles. In August the temperature remained under 97.6° until the twelfth day after the beginning of menstruation, when it suddenly began to rise, reaching the plateau on the thirteenth day. It remained elevated until day 25, when it began to drop, followed by menstruation 36 hours later. The rise in temperature is indicative of the rupture of a mature follicle and the formation of a corpus luteum. In October no drop in temperature occurred. The continued elevation indicated that the patient was pregnant. (From Davis and Scheckler: *Obstetrics for Nurses.* 17th ed.)

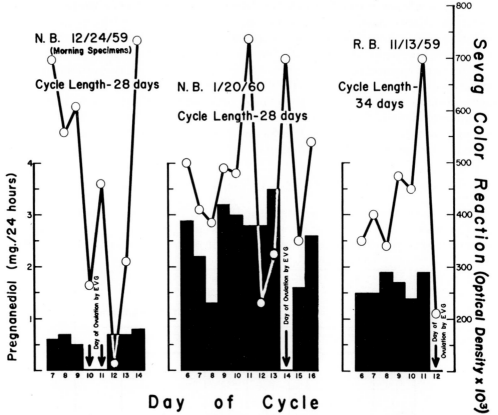

Fig. 15-12.   Excretion of pregnanediol in the urine is indicated by black blocks during 3 cycles of 2 patients. The absence of measurable pregnanediol and the electrovaginal potential indication of ovulation day coincided.

ditions it is essential that the presence or absence of ovulation be established. It is of basic importance when infertility problems are present. Abnormal bleeding is rarely encountered in menstrual cycles which are ovulatory, and the source of irregular vaginal bleeding is far more likely to be an organic rather than a functional abnormality. Measurements of body temperature, the analysis of endometrial morphology and estimations of progesterone chemically are of valuable assistance, aside from the investigations of vaginal cytology and electropotential just discussed.

BASAL TEMPERATURE CURVE.   This is a common method of determining whether or not ovulation has taken place. In the first part of the menstrual cycle the resting morning body temperature is consistently low. After ovulation the basal temperature rises and never returns to the previous low until menstruation again appears. If pregnancy occurs, the temperature remains elevated (Fig. 15–11). This test has been used in fertility studies to indicate the day of ovulation, but the readings are often too complicated to interpret accurately. There is also considerable evidence that it measures ovulation only after it has occurred. This is too late for the patient with a fertility problem. It is, however, an excellent indication of the secretion of progesterone and the establishment of an ovulatory cycle.

ENDOMETRIAL BIOPSY.   The presence of a secretory endometrium is definite evidence of ovulation, the development of a corpus luteum and the secretion of progesterone. The secretory endometrium may be imperfect in its development, and an irregular bleeding pattern may result, but in most instances bleeding from a secretory endometrium has an organic explanation.

CHEMICAL MEASUREMENT OF PREGNANEDIOL AND PREGNANETRIOL.   Until recently the measurement of progesterone excretion has not been accurate enough to be of any great clinical value. The chief problem seemed to be that the methods used recorded both pregnanediol, a metabolite of progesterone, and pregnanetriol, secreted by the adrenal. The method of Bongiovanni and Clayton using enzymatic rather than acid hydrolysis provides for separation of the two and recording of individual values for each. Clinically, pregnanediol values are important in fertility problems. Thus pregnanediol determinations are valuable in providing evidence that ovulation has occurred and that the corpus luteum has formed. In some instances ovulation may take place, but progesterone production may be inadequate.

One of the standard methods of evaluating corpus luteum function is to measure the urinary output of pregnanediol. It is not surprising that levels as high as 15 mg. per 24 hours have been recorded in the postovulatory phase, for this is the time when the endometrium has its greatest need for progesterone, as it prepares to nourish a potential impregnated ovum. For many years there has been general agreement that pregnanediol could be detected only in the postovulatory phase of the cycle when corpus luteum activity is in full play.

Recently reports have appeared in the literature to suggest that this observation, though generally accepted, may not be entirely accurate. With more refined methods of laboratory analysis such as paper and gas vapor chromatography, significant levels of pregnanediol have been found in the preovulatory phase of the cycle. Recent publications by Klopper, Loraine and their coauthors, as well as by Wotiz, report pregnanediol values in the range of 0.75 to 1.5 mg. per 24 hours in the follicular phase.

One can only speculate on the source, but in all probability it is basically from adrenal cortex, with an assist from the ovary. The actual mechanism of production, as well as its source, awaits the appearance of more sensitive laboratory techniques for determining the metabolites in the urine.

Concomitant electro-abdomino-vaginal potential studies have suggested that on the day the potential readings record ovulation the pregnanediol values fall quite sharply. This may be of real importance in detecting the true ovulatory date. The patient who has an anovulatory cycle continues to show the flat excretion curve throughout the cycle and fails to demonstrate the drop in pregnanediol noted in the woman who is ovulating normally (Fig. 15–12).

In addition to their value in sterility, pregnanediol determinations are also useful in the diagnosis of an adrenal hyperplasia which produces virilizing symptoms. In this pathologic entity the normal progression in biosynthesis of progesterone and 17-hydroxyprogesterone to 17-hydroxycorticosterone (compound F) is blocked. Large amounts of pregnanetriol appear in the urine and disappear when cortisone is given to combat the excess production.

What Tests Do We Have to Measure Androgen?

Excessive production of the male androgenic hormone may manifest itself in two ways. The lesser manifestation might be the development of hirsutism, such as one sees in the Stein-Leventhal syndrome; or the greater effect would be actual virilization, as seen in masculinizing ovarian tumors such as the arrhenoblastoma. The measure of androgen activity is directly related to the growth of hair. One may obtain a fair clinical estimate of androgenic activity by observing changes in the growth pattern of axillary hair during the course of therapy.

Androgenic activity is measured in two ways: (1) bio-assays for total androgen in the twenty-four-hour urine specimen and (2) clinical evaluations of the 17-ketosteroids.

EVALUATION OF ANDROGENIC ACTIVITY BY BIO-ASSAY OF URINE.   The measurement of total androgens, which most accurately records their activity, is made by extracting them from the urine and testing the effect of injections of the steroids on the comb of the immature chicken or capon, or upon the size of the prostate and seminal vesicle of rats.

DETERMINATION OF THE 17-KETOSTEROIDS BY CHEMICAL ANALYSIS.   The measurement of the total 17-ketosteroid excretion includes many steroids which have closely related chemical structures, but are actually biologically inactive. Various modifications in the testing technique described by Zimmerman have been used by different laboratories. For practical purposes the evaluation of the total urinary neutral 17-ketosteroids, without attempting to break them down into the various components, is sufficient.

The normal values (using the Zimmerman method) for daily urinary excretion of the 17-ketosteroids in women range between 5 and 14 mg., produced apparently by the adrenal.

What Is the Clinical Significance?   The estimation of the 17-ketosteroids is helpful in establishing a correct diagnosis in obscure endocrine disorders. For example, any disease or constitutional state such as chronic illness or starvation which interferes with normal pituitary function will result in a lowering of the urinary excretion of the 17-ketosteroids. They may even be absent in true panhypopituitarism. Tuberculosis of the adrenal gland (Addison's disease) may seriously interfere with the production of the steroids. We have noted that some women may have hirsutism without virilization. In these instances the 17-ketosteroid levels may be normal or only slightly elevated, like values in the polycystic ovary syndrome.

The 17-ketosteroids are of particular value in the maldevelopment problems of infancy and adolescence. The differentiation between the adrenogenital syndrome, adrenocortical tumors and other forms of disordered sex development should be made as early as possible after birth. Since it is impossible to make an accurate diagnosis on the basis of clinical examination of the anatomy of the external genitalia, reliance must be placed on the chemical analysis of the urine for both 17-ketosteroids and pregnanetriol.

In the interpretation of the relative amounts of urinary excretion it should be kept in mind that the values vary with the age of the infant. Thus a level of 2.0 mg. would represent a significant increase in a 6-month-old child, when the normal expectancy is less than 0.5 mg. Directly after birth the 17-ketosteroids will normally range to 2.6 mg. per day, in contrast with the normal infant value of 0.5 mg.

In the next 2 or 3 years, if these values increase to 6 to 15 mg. per 24 hours, such abnormal findings would usually be accompanied by an increase in the normal growth rate, appearance of sexual hair and ossification of the epiphyses. In the adolescent period, if the diagnosis of the adrenogenital syndrome has not been established and corrected earlier, the urinary 17-ketosteroids might reach levels far in excess of those recorded in the adult female (5 to 14 mg. per 24 hours).

If the 17-ketosteroids remain consistently low, yet the anatomic configuration suggests pseudohermaphroditism, other causes for the altered sex development should be sought. Sex chromatin studies would help in making the distinction.

Whenever there is a decided increase in the production of 17-ketosteroids, one may suspect overactivity on the part of the adrenal gland, due to either tumor or hyperplasia. The differentiation is made between adrenocortical tumor and a bilateral virilizing hyperplasia which results in pseudohermaphroditism (adrenogenital syndrome) by giving the patient cortisone. If the urinary 17-ketosteroids drop sharply after continuous therapy, adrenal tumor is usually ruled out.

The same technique used for the measurement of total 17-ketosteroids, with modification, also permits an evaluation of dehydroepiandrosterone. This is another adrenal gland product that suggests the presence of a virilizing adrenocortical tumor when the urinary excretion levels are in excess of the usual 30 per cent that this compound makes up of the total 17-ketosteroid output. Virilizing hyperplasias will increase the amount to a certain extent, but not to the high levels noted in adrenocortical tumors.

The foregoing methods of determining the 17-ketosteroids are practical for most of the common endocrine problems, but fractionation technique will be required in the more obscure malfunctions, in order to isolate the active biological component.

REFERENCES

Growth and Puberty, and Their Management

Ellis, R. W. B.: Age of Puberty in the Tropics. *Brit. M.J.*, 1: 85, 1950.
Goldzieher, M. A.: Treatment of Excessive Growth in the Adolescent Female. *J. Clin. Endocrinol. & Metab.*, 16: 249, 1956.
Johnston, J. A.: Nutritional Problems of Adolescence. *J.A.M.A.*, 137: 1587, 1948.
Mills, C. A., and Ogle, C.: Physiologic Sterility of Adolescence. *Human Biol.*, 8: 607, 1936.
Peters, H., and Shrikande, S. M.: Age at Menarche in Indian Women. *Fertil. & Steril.*, 8: 355, 1957.
Simmons, K., and Greulich, W. W.: Menarchal Age and the Height, Weight and Skeletal Age of Girls 7 to 17 Years. *J. Pediat.*, 22: 518, 1943.
Sutherland, A. M.: Functional Uterine Haemorrhage in Puberty and Adolescence. *Glasgow M.J.*, 34: 496, 1953.
Wilson, D. C., and Sutherland, I.: The Age of the Menarche in the Tropics. *Brit. M.J.*, 2: 607, 1953.
Idem: The Present Age of the Menarche in Southern England. *J. Obst. & Gynaec. Brit. Emp.*, 67: 320, 1960.
Young, W. C., and Yerkes, R. M.: Factors Influencing the Reproductive Cycle in the Chimpanzee; The Period of Adolescent Sterility and Related Problems. *Endocrinology*, 33: 121, 1943.

Pituitary, Adrenal and Thyroid

Astwood, E. B.: Symposium on the Thyroid. *Metabolism*, 5: 623, 1956; 6: 1, 1957.
Bennett, L. L., and others: Failure of Hypophyseal Growth Hormone to Produce Nitrogen Storage in a Girl with Hypophyseal Dwarfism. *J. Clin. Endocrinol.*, 10: 492, 1950.
Carballeira, A., Elvick, H., Mackenzie, K. R., and Browne, J. S. L.: Effects of Single Intravenous Injections of Pituitary Growth Hormone to Normal Adult Men. *Proc. Soc. Exper. Biol. & Med.*, 81: 15, 1952.
Chu, J. P., and You, S. S.: Role of Thyroid Gland and Estrogen in the Regulation of Gonadotropic Activity of the Anterior Pituitary. *J. Endocrinol.*, 4: 115, 1945.
Comminos, A. C.: Thyroid Function and Therapy in Reproductive Disturbances. *Obst. & Gynec.*, 7: 260, 1956.
Council on Pharmacy and Chemistry of the American Medical Association: *Glandular Physiology and Therapy.* 5th ed. Chicago, American Medical Association, 1954, Chaps. 2, 3, 6–8.

Editorial: The Adrenogenital Syndrome. *J.A.M.A.*, 173: 1358, 1960.

Emmens, C. W.: *Hormone Assay*. New York, Academic Press, 1950.

Fevold, H. L.: Extraction and Standardization of Pituitary FSH and LH. *Endocrinology*, 24: 435, 1939.

Goldzieher, J. W., and Woolley, H. L.: Gonadotrophins; in J. V. Meigs and S. H. Sturgis, eds.: *Progress in Gynecology*. New York, Grune & Stratton, Inc., 1957, Vol. III, p. 253.

Jailer, J. W., and Longson, D.: Hormonal Changes during Pregnancy. *S. Clin. North America*, 37: 341, 1957.

Velardo, J. T., ed.: *The Endocrinology of Reproduction*. New York, Oxford University Press, 1958.

Ovary

Dorfman, R. I., and Ungar, F.: *Metabolism of Steroid Hormones*. Minneapolis, Burgess Publishing Co., 1953.

Hisaw, F. L.: Development of the Graafian Follicle and Ovulation. *Physiol. Rev.*, 27: 95, 1947.

McKay, D. G., and Robinson, D.: Observations on the Fluorescence, Birefringence and Histochemistry of the Human Ovary during the Menstrual Cycle. *Endocrinology*, 41: 378, 1947.

Morris, J. McL., and Scully, R. E.: *Endocrine Pathology of the Ovary*. St. Louis, C. V. Mosby Company, 1958.

Smith, G. V.: The Ovaries; in R. H. Williams: *Textbook of Endocrinology*. Philadelphia, W. B. Saunders Company, 1955, Chap. 6.

Hormone Estimations

Antoniades, H. N., and others: Distribution of Infused Estrone in Human Plasma. *Am. J. Physiol.*, 189: 455, 1957.

Astwood, E. B., and Jones, G. E.: A Simple Method for the Quantitative Determination of Pregnanediol in Human Urine. *J. Biol. Chem.*, 137: 397, 1941.

Bongiovanni, A. M., and Clayton, G. W., Jr.: A Simplified Method for the Routine Determination of Pregnanediol and Pregnanetriol in Urine. *Bull. Johns Hopkins Hosp.*, 94: 180, 1954.

Brown, J. B.: A Chemical Method for the Determination of Oestriol, Oestrone and Oestradiol in Human Urine. *Biochem. J.*, 60: 185, 1955.

Davis, M. E., Plotz, E. J., LeRoy, G. V., Gould, R. G., and Werbin, H.: Hormones in Human Reproduction; Metabolism of Progesterone. *Am. J. Obst. & Gynec.*, 72: 740, 1956.

Holyoke, J. B., and Hoag, E. E.: Seasonal Variation in Pregnancy Test Using Rana Pipiens. *Am. J. Clin. Path.*, 21: 1121, 1951.

Jailer, J. W.: Metabolism of Estrogens. *J. Clin. Endocrinol.*, 9: 557, 1949.

Klopper, A. I.: Excretion of Pregnanediol in the Normal Menstrual Cycle. *J. Obst. & Gynaec. Brit. Emp.*, 64: 504, 1957.

Loraine, J. A.: *Clinical Applications of Hormone Assay*. Baltimore, Williams & Wilkins Company, 1958.

McArthur, J. W.: The Bioassay of Pituitary Interstitial Cell Stimulating Hormone (ICSH) in Human Urine. Preliminary Report. *J. Clin. Endocrinol.*, 12: 914, 1952.

Parsons, L., Lemon, H. M., and Whittaker, J.: Abdomino-vaginal Electropotential Differences in the Menstrual Cycle. *Ann. New York Acad. Sc.*, 83: 237, 1959.

Pearlman, W. H., and Cerceo, E.: Isolation of Progesterone from Human Placenta. *J. Biol. Chem.*, 198: 79, 1952.

Reifenstein, E. C., Jr.: 17-Alpha-Hydroxyprogesterone and the Virilism of the Adrenogenital Syndrome Associated with Congenital Adrenocortical Hyperplasia. *J. Clin. Endocrinol. & Metab.*, 16: 1262, 1956.

Smith, O. W., Smith, G. V., and Gavian, A. B.: Urinary Estrogens in Women. *Am. J. Obst. & Gynec.*, 78: 1028, 1959.

Sommers, S. C., and Verendia, J. B.: An Appraisal of Laboratory Determinations of Estrogens. *Am. J. Clin. Path.*, 35: 319, 1961.

Sommerville, I. F.: Methods of Hormone Assay; in R. H. S. Thompson and E. J. King, eds.: *Biochemical Disorders in Human Disease*. New York, Academic Press, 1957, p. 773.

Chapter 16

The Menstrual Cycle

THE ROLE of the endocrine glands in preparing the female for the phenomena of reproduction has been outlined. The preparations are elaborate, affecting the ovary and all its target organs, such as the uterus with its fallopian tubes, endometrium and blood vessels as well as the vagina, vulva and breasts. The preparations are on behalf of the possible implantation of an embryo and thus are reproductive in intent.

After menstruation, and even in the course of it, there are evident preparations for the next developmental cycle. The pituitary stimulates the growth of the graafian follicle within the ovary as the initial cyclic event. An attempt will be made to outline the series of events that lead up to the time either of the establishment of pregnancy or of failure to do so and menstruation.

THE GROWTH PHASE

The first portion of the menstrual cycle is concerned with the growth phase. Within the *ovary* the follicle is stimulated to grow and liberate its ovum. In addition, the ovary elaborates a combination of hormones, estrogenic and progestinic, which complement each other in providing adequate housing and nourishment for the ovum, should it become fertilized. In the growth or proliferative phase we are mainly concerned with the estrogenic hormones. The *endometrium* proliferates under the stimulus of estrogens in anticipation of the receipt of the fertilized egg and the hope for its successful nidation. The *spiral arterioles* supplying the upper layers of endometrium proliferate to provide adequate nourishment for the growing endometrium. The muscle cells within the *myometrium* enlarge, elongate and become narrower in anticipation of uterine growth. The submucosal layer of muscle is still dense and firm, but gradually softens as the cycle continues. The contractions of the uterine musculature are spontaneous and rapid, but of low amplitude under the influence of estrin. The *fallopian tubes* increase their rate of rhythmic contractions to speed the passage of the ovum into the uterus. In the *cervix* the mucus alters its characteristics as the time of ovulation approaches. This mechanism is obviously designed to enhance the passage of sperm upward into the uterus. The *vaginal changes* parallel those of the endometrium. Under the influence of estrin, progressive growth of the epithelial cell layers occurs, together with an increasing concentration of glycogen within the cornified vaginal cells. The *mammary glands* respond to estrin stimulation by proliferation and dilatation of the smaller ducts and growth of the cells lining the ductules of the lobules. These changes occur in anticipation of possible pregnancy (Fig. 16–1).

173

THE MENSTRUAL CYCLE – Growth Phase

I.

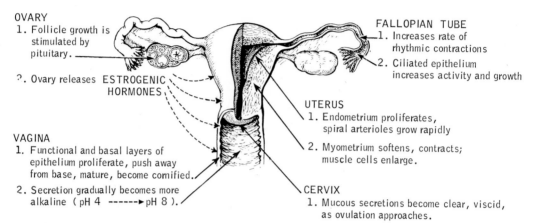

OVARY
1. Follicle growth is stimulated by pituitary.
2. Ovary releases ESTROGENIC HORMONES

VAGINA
1. Functional and basal layers of epithelium proliferate, push away from base, mature, become cornified.
2. Secretion gradually becomes more alkaline (pH 4 ------► pH 8).

FALLOPIAN TUBE
1. Increases rate of rhythmic contractions
2. Ciliated epithelium increases activity and growth

UTERUS
1. Endometrium proliferates, spiral arterioles grow rapidly
2. Myometrium softens, contracts; muscle cells enlarge.

CERVIX
1. Mucous secretions become clear, viscid, as ovulation approaches.

Fig. 16-1.   The growth phase of the menstrual cycle is initiated by the pituitary when it stimulates the growth of the graafian follicle. The ovary then releases estrogenic hormones which cause growth in other parts of the female reproductive organs.

Growth Phase in the Ovary

After menstruation a number of primary ovarian follicles begin to develop in the inner cortical zone of the ovary as a result of stimulation from the pituitary by the gonadotropin FSH. A variable number, from two to thirty-two such follicles, respond to the stimulating agent. With rare exceptions all but one of these follicles cease growing or undergo atresia, leaving but one or rarely two per month that continue on to full maturity.

The reason why one follicle persists and the others regress is not known. There are two ovaries. One might expect that one follicle in each ovary might reach maturity in each menstrual cycle. The number of follicles that ripen to their full extent appears to be about evenly divided between the two gonads, and for the most part a pattern of alternate development in successive cycles appears to be the rule. Patients frequently are convinced that ovulation occurs on one side or the other. Occasionally ovulations occur in sequence from the same side, though this is by no means the expected.

WHAT HAPPENS IN THE FOLLICLE THAT IS DESTINED TO GO ON TO FULL MATURITY?   The original primordial ova exist as primary infantile equipment in numbers estimated as ranging from 40,000 to 400,000. The follicles are initially each composed of an ovum surrounded by a layer of granulosa cells. Under the stimulus of the pituitary gonadotropin FSH the granulosa cell layers begin to proliferate, and they gradually differentiate. This produces the graafian follicle. Fluid, "liquor folliculi," accumulates in an eccentrically placed cavity lined by small undistinguished granulosa cells, which go to make up the *membrana granulosa*. Within the cavity the cells of the membrana granulosa tend to concentrate in a heap near one side of the cavity to form the discus proligerus, or *cumulus oophorus*. Within this mound of cells the ovum rests surrounded by the cells of the membrana granulosa. There is an outer envelope of the ovum called the *vitelline membrane*. The *perivitelline* space lies just external to it and is simply a thin narrow space lying adjacent to the transparent refractile zone of ovum called the *zona pellucida*. This rests in close apposition to a ring of granulosa cells in radial arrangement called the corona radiata. The cells of the inner stromal layer, the *theca interna*, are important cells, for they have definite hormonal function and produce estrin. Under the growth stimulus this layer of cells, which is at first poorly developed,, enlarges, and the cells take on a polyhedral shape. The *theca externa* is made up of relatively ordinary connective tissue cells derived from the ovarian stroma. This particular layer has little part to play in the continued existence of the follicle.

As the time of ovulation approaches, the ovarian follicle continues to develop. The increased size is due to actual proliferation of the granulosa cells and distention of the cavity with more fluid, which is at first clear, but later becomes viscous as it is mixed with fibrin and the estrogenic hormones. The theca interna takes part in the development, as shown by hypertrophy and hyperplasia of its cells. Thin-walled, fine capillaries may ramify through the theca interna, providing nourishment for the granulosa cell layer. Gradually the maturing follicle comes to occupy a more superficial position near the surface of the ovary.

The mechanism involved in the assumption of this external position has not been completely established, but it has been suggested that the proliferating cells of the theca interna form a wedge which penetrates into the stroma. In this accessible position rupture of the follicle is more readily accomplished.

Elaboration of the Estrogenic Hormone

ESTRIN PRODUCTION IN THE GROWTH PHASE.   As the graafian follicle continues its growth, increasing amounts of estrin are produced from the cells of the granulosa layers and theca interna. The level of estrin in the blood can be determined by both chemical and biological means, using blood or urine. Urinary excretion fairly accurately measures the level of actively circulating estrin in the blood. Bioassay is a cheaper, less time-consuming and often a more accurate clinical method of measuring estrin, but it has been supplanted by chemical methods as a laboratory research tool. Recently attempts have been made again to work with blood, in the hope that the active biological principle, which seems to be bound to protein, can be isolated. There is considerable evidence that in pathologic states the form of estrin excreted is perhaps more important than the amount.

Estrin appears in three common forms, estrone, estriol and estradiol. These three normally occurring estrogens differ in the potency of their biological action. Estradiol appears to be the most powerful. Laboratory interpretation of the quantity of circulating estrogens has been handicapped by the fact that the amounts to be measured are relatively small and the laboratory methods too gross to pick up minor fluctuations under normal physiologic conditions or pathologic states. The levels vary considerably from patient to patient and even in the same patient from month to month. In interpreting results the values must then be individualized and related to the phase of the cycle and the symptoms presented.

Part of the reason why true values of estrogens are hard to determine lies in the fact that they are so rapidly destroyed. Minor concentrations are found in the bile and gastrointestinal tract. The amount of a test dose that is not destroyed in the liver is recovered in the urine, but this accounts for only about 10 per cent of the amount of estrin injected. The role of the liver in estrogen metabolism has been pointed up in experiments by implanting ovarian material or estrogen pellets in the spleen. The estrin enters the portal circulation, and lesser amounts of urinary estrin are recovered.

Despite many drawbacks in determining the amounts of biologically active estrin circulating in the blood at any given phase of the menstrual cycle, it is nevertheless well substantiated that the amount of estrin gradually rises in the growth phase until it reaches a peak at or about the time of ovulation.

Uterine Changes in the Growth Phase

The effects of the newly elaborated estrin produced by the granulosa and theca cells of the growing follicle have their most profound and most easily recognizable influence upon the endometrium. Nevertheless both myometrium and cervix respond to the action of the estrogenic hormones in preparation for the receipt of the anticipated fertilized ovum.

MYOMETRIUM.   After menstruation the uterine muscle, which underwent enlargement and softening at that time, becomes firm or hard and exhibits little in the way of spontaneous contraction. The uterus remains in this state from approximately the fifth to the ninth day of the normal cycle. As the amount of estrin elaborated by the growing follicle rises, the muscle cells respond by a gradual increase in size, particularly in length. The uterine musculature becomes progressively softer. Under the influence of estrogenic stimulation the uterine musculature ceases its inactivity, and a series of contractions begins on approximately the ninth day after the onset of menstruation. These contractions, followed by periods of relaxation, begin at the tubal isthmuses and progress toward the cervix. The frequency of the contractions steadily mounts until they reach their height about the time of ovulation and continue for a few days thereafter, corresponding to the time when progestin becomes active. This mechanism is designed to speed the passage of the fertilized egg into the uterine cavity.

CERVIX.   Unlike the endometrium, there appears to be no universal agreement that the epithelium of either the external portion of the cervix or the endocervix responds cyclically to ovarian hormonal stimulation. It is apparent that functional activity does occur in the latter part of the growth phase, as the time of ovulation approaches. The chief evidence for this observation rests with the changes noted in the cervical mucus. In the earlier part of the growth cycle the cervical mucus is heavy, thick, dense and jelly-like. In anticipation of ovulation, in the few days immediately preceding it, the mucus increases in amount and becomes clear, viscid and sticky. As a clinical test of ovulation the mucus can be stretched out into thin, stringy strands (*Spinnbarkeit*) and placed on a glass slide, where it crystallizes and forms a fernlike pattern. This change is noted only at this time and is peculiar to estrogenic action, for it disappears in the presence of progestin. This mechanism is obviously designed to permit an easier upward passage of the sperm into the endometrial cavity.

FALLOPIAN TUBES.   Since the ovum must proceed from the ovary down through the tube to be impregnated either there or perhaps in the uterine cavity, it is not surprising to observe cyclical changes in the tubal epithelium and in the action of the tubal musculature. Three types of cells are normally present in the tubal epithelium. In the growth phase, under the influence of estrogenic activity, the broad-based ciliated cells, which are tall columnar with round nuclei situated near their bases, increase in number and size. They reach their maximum development at the approximate time of ovulation. The nonciliated cells are secretory in type and are most active after ovulation. Another type of cell is noted, the "peg" cell. This is commonly found, but appears to be either a reserve cell or simply a transition form from the ciliated to the nonciliated type. It is present in greatest concentration during the early growth phase.

It takes several days for the fertilized ovum to pass from the ovary to the endometrial cavity. The downward passage of the ovum is expedited by the action of the ciliated cells of the tubal epithelium and the peristaltic movement of the tubal musculature. Both are under the influence of estrogenic activity. To initiate this movement, the ciliated cells are found alone at the fimbriated end of the tube. The midportion of the tubal epithelium presents a mixture of ciliated and nonciliated cells.

The action of the cilia of the tubal epithelial cells tends to create a current moving peritoneal fluid in the direction of the tube, thereby creating a fluid transport medium for passage of the ovum. To augment the progress of the ovum, spontaneous rhythmic contractions of the tubal musculature occur which alter the intratubal pressure, creating a peristaltic movement. As the time of ovulation approaches, late in the proliferative phase, these tubal contractions increase in frequency and amplitude, reaching their maximum of some four to eight contractions per minute in the few days before ovulation and continuing for one or two days thereafter.

THE ENDOMETRIUM.   The regeneration of endometrium after menstruation proceeds somewhat erratically and covers a varying period of time, as some portions of the endometrium continue to break down, while others have already entered the growth phase. The tissue lost in menstruation is confined to the superficial layers of the endometrium, without destruction in the basal layer. Regeneration begins as the interstitial tissue grows out from the basal endometrium. The cells of the glands torn in the course of desquamation at menstruation proliferate and rapidly re-epithelialize the ragged surface epithelium left after menstruation. This period of re-epithelialization covers a period of two or three days.

As the ovarian follicle continues in its development and more estrin is produced, a recognizable pattern of endometrial growth begins to emerge. It is in the endometrium that the ovarian hormones produce their most readily recognized effect. Toward the end of the first week, as the ovarian follicle grows and produces more estrin, the functional layer of endometrium begins to proliferate rapidly and to increase in thickness. A threefold increase of endometrial height will be noted before ovulation occurs.

Evidence of the rapidity of epithelial growth is noted in the number of mitotic figures seen in the cells of the stroma and glandular epithelium. The endometrial glands in the earlier portion of the growth phase are short and straight with round regular lumens lined with cylindrical cells of medium height. These cells show acid-staining cytoplasm and nuclei which occupy a basal position. There is as yet no evidence of secretion, for glycogen and mucin are absent. Granules are noted in both nucleus and cytoplasm, a circumstance which probably denotes enzyme activity.

Earlier in the cycle the interstitial tissue of the endometrium is made up of a dense stroma composed of packed spindle and stellate cells. Under the progressive estrogenic stimulation this layer gradually loosens up, owing to the accumulation of intercellular fluid within a reticular network. The glands, which were originally straight and narrow, gradually become twisted and tortuous as estrogenic stimulation causes the epithelial lining to proliferate faster than the surrounding stroma.

Arteriolar and Venous Changes Noted in the Growth Phase

It is axiomatic that with proliferation and growth in the functional parenchyma of the endometrium the vascular supply must keep pace. Under the influence of estrin the blood supply to the endometrium expands through progressive development and growth of the spiral arterioles. These arterial branches spring from the radial arteries, which arise from branches of the uterine artery and run at right angles to the surface of the endometrial cavity at the border between the myometrium and endometrium. Separate basilar branches supply the bottom portions of the endometrial glands, which lie in the basal layer and are totally unaffected by hormonal action. They represent the living tissue bank from which epithelial regeneration occurs after the desquamation of menstruation. The spiral arterioles are the terminal branches which supply the superficial two thirds or functioning layer of the endometrium, which is responsive to estrogenic stimulation. The growth in this spiral arteriolar system is accelerated as the estrin influence becomes increasingly manifest and the major spurt in endometrial growth is noted. During the proliferative phase the spiral arterioles increase greatly in length, so that they have to twist and coil to adapt themselves to the lesser extent of endometrial growth. Usually this progressive extension into the endometrium begins about the tenth day and continues as long as there is a chance of reproduction. Along with the growth of the arterioles the thin-walled veins and capillaries develop and form a plexus surrounding the endometrial glands in the form of a widespread network paralleling the surface epithelium. The collecting veins, small in the earlier phases of the growth cycle, increase in number as their walls become thicker. The arrangement of blood vessels within the growing endometrium must be flexible enough to provide for the ultimate aim, which is pregnancy.

Histochemical Changes during the Growth Phase

Studies of the histochemical changes which occur cyclically in the ovary and endometrium in relation to the ovarian hormones are just beginning. Changes appear to be linked to enzymes which seem to be under hormonal control. The actual mechanism by which the estrogens act upon tissues is not known, but it appears that they seem to catalyze and regulate cellular growth, rather than contributing material for tissue metabolism. Since the chief aim of endometrial growth is to provide bed and board for the impregnated ovum, it is not surprising that glycogen production by the cells of the endometrial glands is an important factor (Fig. 16–2). Glycogen metabolism seems to be partly under the control of the enzyme alkaline phosphatase. Relatively little glycogen can be found in the endometrial cells during the early part of the growth phase. Alkaline phosphatase content, however, is high during this period. The amount present seems to be linked to the concentration of estrogen, for it diminishes as progestin appears, while the glycogen content rises. The increase in glycogen is nature's response to possible need, for the impregnated unimplanted ovum must be nourished largely by carbohydrate. The role of alkaline phosphatase would appear to be that of a regulator of endometrial cell growth, as well as fat and glycogen metabolism. The source of the alkaline phosphatase apparently resides in the endothelial cells of the arterioles and capillaries.

Among the many other chemical and enzymatic reactions that correlate with the rise and fall in estrin production are endometrial ribonucleic acid, which increases

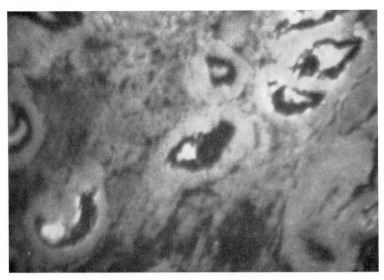

Fig. 16-2.   Fluorescence staining of human secretory endometrium with periodic acid-auramine O-Schiff stain (PAOS method) demonstrates bright patches of glycogen both in epithelium lining the glands and in their lumens. (Courtesy of Dr. Anthony Betts, Massachusetts Memorial Hospitals.)

in quantity during the proliferative phase of the cycle and is found in diminishing quantity thereafter, and beta-glucuronidase, which is found early and in increasing amounts as long as a chance of pregnancy exists. Both are linked to estrogen activity. Much new and important information may be expected from continued research in these fields of investigation.

Vaginal Changes during the Growth Phase

Examinations of microscopic sections and smears of vaginal secretions have been instructive in determining the action of the ovarian hormones upon vaginal epithelium. There appears to be a definite vaginal cycle.

The interpretation of daily vaginal smears indicates that there is a progressive increase in the growth of the vaginal epithelium as the reproductive cycle develops. There are three layers in the vaginal epithelium: basal, intermediate or functional, and cornified. Directly after menstruation, on about the fifth day, when the effect of estrin first becomes apparent, an increase is noted in the functional layer, together with a proliferation of the basal layer, whose cells show numerous mitoses. As the cycle continues, the intermediate and cornified layers become many cell layers thick. They are at the greatest thickness at the time of ovulation, when basal cell mitoses are also seen in greatest concentration. As the cells proliferate and the epithelial layers become thicker, the superficial cells are pushed further from the base from which they derive their blood supply. As a result, they mature, degenerate and are cast off as fully cornified cells. As the time of ovulation approaches, the number of desquamated cornified cells increases.

The cyclic changes noted in the vaginal epithelium apparently may also take place within the bladder, for examination of the urinary sediment shows similar cyclic cytologic variation with a preponderance of desquamated cells at the time of ovulation.

The variation in hydrogen ion concentration in the vaginal epithelium parallels the epithelial changes, which have been shown to be under hormonal control. The reaction of the vagina is normally acid. In the earlier portion of the growth cycle the acidity is approximately at pH 4.0. A gradual progression toward alkalinity is noted until, at the time of ovulation, the vaginal reaction approaches a pH of 7 or 8. With this swing toward the alkaline side there is also an increasing concentration of glycogen within the cells of the vaginal epithelium. The change in the pH follows the pattern of change noted in the cervical mucosa. Both mechanisms prepare a fertile ground and easier passage for the spermatozoa at the approximate time of ovulation.

The Mammary Glands during the Growth Phase

Since the mammary glands must prepare for nourishment of the product of conception, it is not surprising that their function is intimately linked to that of the ovary. There is ample clinical evidence that this is so, for patients complain of painful,

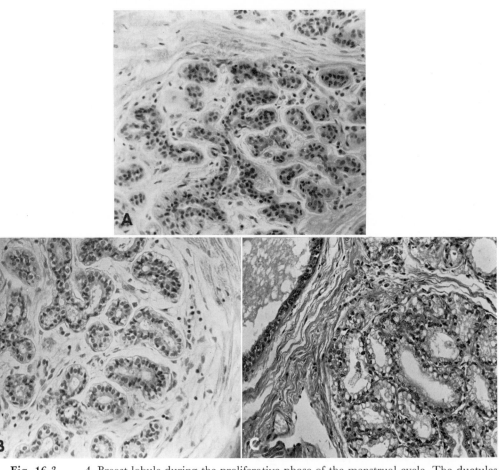

Fig. 16-3.   *A,* Breast lobule during the proliferative phase of the menstrual cycle. The ductules are narrow, epithelial nuclei stain darkly, and the adjacent intrinsic stroma is compact. Mitoses may be evident. *B,* Lobule during the secretory endometrial phase. Now the mammary ductules are open, with larger epithelial cells. Secretion is seen as cytoplasmic vacuoles and within ductules. The intrinsic breast stroma is edematous. *C,* The lobule during pregnancy shows mammary acini with physiologic hyperplasia and active secretion. The intrinsic stroma is stretched and tenuous.

tender, swollen breasts in the ten-day interval before the menstrual period. There is incomplete histologic evidence that cyclic changes take place in the epithelium of the ductules in breast tissue.

Reasonably good evidence exists that during the latter part of the growth phase, when the concentration of estrin is high, in anticipation of ovulation, the epithelium of the small ducts and lining cells of the ductules actually undergo proliferation and then become filled with secretions. During the premenstrual and menstrual phases these alterations regress. Breast acini in women are found chiefly late in pregnancy and during lactation. These observations of cyclic changes are backed by animal experiments and routine pathologic studies of patients who have received estrin, indicating that the administration of estrogens does stimulate the mammary epithelium (Fig. 16–3).

OVULATION PHASE

Ovulation

The entire intricate pattern of reproduction is directed toward building an endometrium that will provide adequate lodging and nutritional support for an ovum that may or may not become fertilized. The point at which the egg reaches full maturity and bursts onto the surface of the ovary is called ovulation (Fig. 16–4).

Despite the fact that many follicles are frustrated in their desire to be the one chosen for maturation of its ovum, they continue to function hormonally in support of the development of the follicle of election. The theca interna cells of the follicles destined to become atretic undergo some hypertrophy. Since predominantly estrin is believed to arise from this layer, the augmented supply of estrin from these sources just before ovulation is the catalytic agent that stimulates the pituitary to secrete the luteinizing hormone, thereby initiating ovulation.

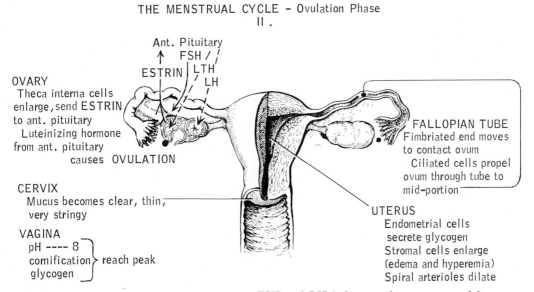

Fig. 16-4. The normal interplay of pituitary FSH and LH induces ovulatory rupture of the ovum, which is then attracted into the fimbriated tubal ostium.

Changes in the Ovary Noted during Ovulation

Immediately preceding rupture of the follicle and extrusion of the ovum definite changes are observed in the gross and microscopic pictures of the ovary. Grossly, when seen through a pelviscope, the unruptured follicle presents as a hemispherical, transparent protuberance on the surface of the ovary. Observed consecutively, a perifollicular hemorrhage develops which dissects into the theca externa layer of the cortex, before the actual rupture occurs. Within a short time thereafter hemorrhage occurs into the follicle. Ovulation is not always an explosive event, though it may occur in this fashion and produce severe pelvic pain (*Mittelschmerz*) which the patient recognizes as ovulatory pain. More often the process takes place slowly, as the liquor folliculi escapes into the peritoneal cavity from a small round opening on the surface of the follicle, which is then promptly sealed over by connective tissue from the ovarian cortex. The liquid content of the ruptured mature follicle carries the ovum, which has separated from the granulosa layer, onto the surface of the ovary.

Microscopically, definite changes are noted in the mature follicle about to rupture. Chiefly these are found in the cells of the theca interna, which surround or wall off the follicle. The cells themselves become larger, clearer and less like connective tissue cells as they tend to proliferate on the side of the follicle nearest the ovarian surface. Here they form a wedge into the supporting tissue to provide an escape for the fully developed ovum.

Why the follicle ruptures and the mechanism of its search for the peripheral position are not clearly understood. A number of different theories are advanced to explain the trigger mechanism in ovulation. Of all the theories evolved, including (1) increased osmotic pressure within the follicular fluid secondary to disintegration of the Call-Exner bodies, (2) rhythmic contraction of smooth muscle in the ovarian stroma, (3) enzymatic destruction of the lining of the follicle, the role of the endocrine system in initiating ovulation is the most logical. Other possible explanations for the initiation of ovulation will be discussed under sterility (p. 314).

Behavior of the Fallopian Tube at Ovulation

At ovulation the ovum separates from the granulosa layer and is deposited with its corona radiata upon the surface of the ovary, where it sticks, owing to the adhesive action of the liquor folliculi. Just before ovulation, owing to estrin activation, the ovarian ligaments and tubal musculature have been seen to contract in such a way that the fimbriated end of the tube is brought in contact with the ovum as it lies on the ovarian surface. Erectile tissue at the fimbriated end of the tube keeps its ostium open. With the extrusion of the ovum from the follicle varying amounts of fluid, up to 60 cc., have been recorded as escaping into the peritoneal cavity. This fluid acts as the transport medium for the ovum, and the action of the cilia of the tubal epithelial cells provides the motivating force to propel the ovum down the lumen of the tube. The passage through the tube is interrupted at its midportion owing to (1) contraction of the musculature at the isthmic end of the tube and (2) because the concentration of ciliated cells is less in the midportion. During the three or four days after ovulation, before tubal relaxation occurs and the passage of the ovum is resumed, it is nourished by the secretion of the nonciliated cells. The relaxation of the uterine end of the tube usually takes place about the seventh day after follicle rupture. All told, then, it takes nearly a week for the ovum to pass through the tube to meet the spermatozoa in either the tube or endometrial cavity.

This mechanism may explain the observation that the ciliated cells after ovulation tend to diminish and to be replaced by the nonciliated or secretory type of cell.

Effect of Ovulation upon the Endometrium

A gradual transition in the uterine lining takes place preceding the time of ovulation and continues until the progestational effect becomes operative. In the earlier period of the growth phases the glandular cells of cuboidal type simply proliferate, as shown by the numerous mitotic figures present. There is no evidence of any secretion. Progressively, the cells of the endometrial glands become taller and more columnar in type, and the number of mitotic figures decreases sharply. The cells are about to assume the function for which they were designed, namely, to provide nourishment for the ovum should it become impregnated. The first evidence of the functional maturity of these glands is in the increased amount of glycogen present, and the alteration of its position within the epithelial cells. By differential staining methods considerable numbers of glycogen granules and fat can be seen in the glandular epithelium. In the four days immediately following ovulation some glycogen granules can be seen to bulge out into the gland lumens, giving a ragged appearance to the cell outlines. As the movement of glycogen within the cells increases, it escapes and is recoverable in the lumens of the glands. Obviously this secretory process is designed to provide nutrition for the fertilized ovum.

Other evidence of secretory activity within the cell is migration of the nucleus of the cell toward the lumen and the beginning appearance of subnuclear glycogen-filled vacuoles. These changes are noted two to four days after ovulation has occurred, and supranuclear vacuoles can be observed until about the twenty-first day of a normal twenty-eight-day cycle (Fig. 16–5).

Thus the mobilization of glycogen, and the subnuclear and later supranuclear vacuolization in endometrial glands go hand in hand. The cells are still under the influence of estrin and have not yet become mucin-secreting. When the glandular secretion comes under the influence of progestin, some mucin replaces the glycogenic secretion, which tends to disappear.

The endometrial glands and stroma undergo further morphologic change in anticipation of alterations in function. The glandular changes are noted first in the deeper portion of the functional layer. Though the deeper portions of glands tend to become increasingly enlarged, coiled and tortuous, the necks of the gland near the surface remain straight and narrow, and here there is less evidence of secretion.

The stroma at this stage enters a growth phase, increasing in quantity as the cells enlarge, and soon assume the polyhedral shape characteristic of predecidual cells. The first clear evidence of predecidua is seen on the twenty-third day, and two days later much of the superficial stroma has undergone a predecidual change. Edema and hyperemia are noted, as the blood vessels present show a sharp increase in number and size. This phase in the endometrial cycle might rightly be called that of prepregnancy or pseudopregnancy, for these elaborate preparations have been made to accommodate the fertilized egg.

Vascular Changes in the Uterus at Ovulation

During the early part of the growth phase the spiral arterioles which supply the functioning layer of the endometrium extend only about halfway through the

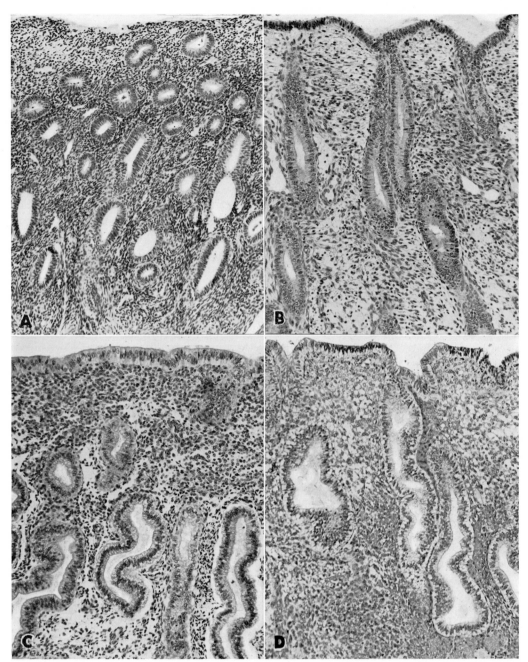

Fig. 16-5. *A*, Early proliferative endometrium is demonstrated about the tenth day of the normal menstrual cycle. The glands are straight and cylindrical, with mitotic figures and without any obvious secretion. The entire endometrial thickness, which measures less than 1 mm., is illustrated. *B*, Later stage of the normal proliferative endometrium. The glands now have a spiral shape, with numerous epithelial mitoses. There is no secretory activity. About half of the endometrial thickness, which measures more than 1 mm., is included. *C*, Two days after ovulation a characteristic early secretory endometrium of the sixteenth day of the normal menstrual cycle is present. Note that a few clear vacuoles are present beneath the nuclei of some glandular epithelial cells. A little foamy mucoid secretion is present in the lumens of the glands. *D*, Active early secretory endometrium, characteristic of the seventeenth day of the normal menstrual cycle, demonstrates many more subnuclear vacuoles in the glands than were present on the previous day. Foamy secretion is being delivered into the lumens of the tortuous glands. The endometrium has grown and now measures 2 mm. in thickness.

184

endometrium. With continued growth of the endometrium the spiral arterioles grow in length out of proportion to the increase in endometrial proliferation. Accordingly the vessels must accommodate themselves to the thickness of the endometrium. They can do this only by increased coiling.

The spiral arterioles go through alternate phases of contraction and dilatation throughout the growth period, as seen in the transplants of endometrium in the monkey eye. Rhythmic contractions take place every sixty to ninety seconds, producing a blushing-blanching appearance in the transplant. This process continues up to the time of menstruation, except that contraction of the spiral arterioles gives way to one of vasodilatation in the twenty-four-hour period in which ovulation occurs. The alternate contraction-dilatation process resumes on the following day and continues until shortly before menstruation.

Changes in the Cervix at the Time of Ovulation

The epithelial changes occurring in either cervical or endocervical epithelium show no consistent histologic pattern that can be said to be indicative of ovulation, though such changes are observed in pregnancy.

Definite alteration in the function of the endocervical glands is apparent at the time of ovulation. The thick, heavy, gelatinous mucus becomes clear, thin and stringy. At ovulation it crystallizes when placed on a glass slide to form a characteristic "fern" pattern. The composition of the mucus alters, and there is a recognizable increase in the number of epithelial cells as well as a greater content of water, carbohydrate and amino acids. The vaginal acidity, which in the first part of the cycle has been in the range of pH 4, sharply increases to a pH of 7 or 8.

The changes in mucus composition and consistency, together with the swing of the vaginal pH toward the alkaline side, facilitate the adaptation of the spermatozoa toward the mucin secretion and speed sperm passage into the uterus.

Changes in the Vaginal Epithelium with Ovulation

The growth of the vaginal epithelium has paralleled the growth phase of the endometrium throughout the early part of the menstrual cycle. At the midinterval, corresponding to the time of ovulation, the vaginal epithelium has reached its greatest thickness, and the number of mitoses noted is maximal. About this time a new layer of cells appears between the basal and functional layers. This is called the intraepithelial zone of cornification. At ovulation epithelial growth, mitoses, cornification and glycogen content of the vaginal cells are at their peak. There are few signs of degeneration in the vaginal epithelium. The vaginal pH parallels that noted in the cervix.

Time of Ovulation

The complex and intricate mechanism of the early phases of the menstrual cycle is directed toward the all-important point of rupture of the mature follicle and release of the ovum. To understand the normal and better to interpret the abnormal menstrual cycle, it is important that the day of ovulation be pinpointed as far as possible. Great variables exist. Usually ovulation is expected to occur any time between the twelfth and fifteenth days of a normal twenty-eight- or thirty-day cycle, but there is ample evidence in otherwise normal cycles that ovulation may take place any time from the seventh to the twenty-first day. In shorter or longer cycles the actual day of ovulation is harder to determine. In common usage the variable appears to be in the growth phase, for the duration of the progestational phase is considered to be constant at fourteen days plus or minus two. There is an increasing mass of evidence that this is not always the case. Recent observations by investigators in a number of different laboratories have provided circumstantial evidence that the progestational phase may be prolonged to approximately twenty days, at least in the nonfertile woman. If this is true, ovulation is occurring earlier in the cycle than we have formerly believed. These findings have not been generally accepted, for much confirmation is needed. For example, it has been repeatedly claimed that ovulation may take place at any time during the course of the menstrual cycle, or even twice within the same cycle. It has also been said that ovulation may occur at any time, independent of the regular changes of the current cycle.

In the usual twenty-eight-day cycle, for practical purposes, ovulation may be said to occur on or about the fourteenth day. The clinical observations and laboratory evidence for dating ovulation will be discussed in greater detail when we come to consideration of the problem of sterility.

THE LUTEAL OR SECRETORY PHASE

The level of estrin circulating in the blood rises and reaches its peak on or about the time of ovulation. An adequate bed has been prepared for receipt of the ovum, and the growth phase of the endometrial cycle is complete. Obviously there is no further physiologic need for the follicle to be stimulated.

Since there is no further need for follicle stimulation, the brake phenomena come into play, and FSH production is inhibited. This in turn stimulates the basophil cells of the anterior pituitary to put out the luteinizing hormone in anticipation of final rupture of the follicle and release of the ovum. Small amounts of FSH are necessary,

THE MENSTRUAL CYCLE – Secretory Phase
III.

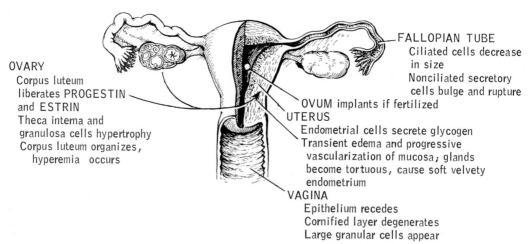

OVARY
Corpus luteum
liberates PROGESTIN
and ESTRIN
Theca interna and
granulosa cells hypertrophy
Corpus luteum organizes,
hyperemia occurs

FALLOPIAN TUBE
Ciliated cells decrease
in size
Nonciliated secretory
cells bulge and rupture
OVUM implants if fertilized
UTERUS
Endometrial cells secrete glycogen
Transient edema and progressive
vascularization of mucosa; glands
become tortuous, cause soft velvety
endometrium
VAGINA
Epithelium recedes
Cornified layer degenerates
Large granular cells appear

Fig. 16-6.   After ovulation, establishment of the corpus luteum affects the appearance and activity of other parts of the genital tract through the secretion of progesterone.

together with estrin, to bring about the release of LH, which will be responsible for the development of the corpus luteum. Ovulation does not occur, and the corpus luteum does not function unless the hypothalamus also releases the luteotropic hormone, which is responsible for the maintenance of the corpus luteum and the production of progestin.

The final impetus for follicle rupture and ovulation apparently comes from the sudden increase in the amount of estrin produced by the cells of the hypertrophied theca interna of the secondary follicles which become atretic as the single follicle matures. The luteinizing hormone, then, is responsible for the development of the corpus luteum. The luteotropic hormone (LTH) initiates ovulation and is responsible for corpus luteum function and the production of progesterone. Overproduction of LH and LTH is prevented by the inhibiting action of progesterone (Fig. 16–6).

Changes in the Ovary during the Luteal or Secretory Phase

The growth phase of the cycle has prepared a mature endometrium to receive and nourish the impregnated ovum. The principal concern of the corpus luteum in the second half of the menstrual cycle is to provide nutrition by elaborating the hormone progestin, which is responsible for bringing out the secretory and pro-gestational functions of the endometrial cells. To maintain the endometrium in a healthy state it is also necessary for the corpus luteum to secrete large amounts of estrin, in addition to progestin. Unless the cells of the endometrial glands are properly maintained, the secretory function induced by progestin will be absent or ineffective. It is a well recognized clinical observation that progestin therapy is successful only in the presence of estrin.

After ovulation the corpus luteum develops under the influence of both estrin and LH, while the luteinization is maintained by the luteotropic hormone. The secretory phase of corpus luteum activity, in the absence of pregnancy, operates over a limited period after ovulation has taken place.

In the gradual formation of the corpus luteum the pattern of development initiated in the preovulatory phase continues. The cells of the theca interna increase further in size and number, largely owing to the accumulation of fat droplets. The granulosa cells proliferate at an accelerated rate as evidenced by the increased number of mitotic figures, and the entire layer hypertrophies to such an extent that cells pile upon themselves and the entire granulosa layer is thrown into folds. The granulosa cells alter their configuration and gradually assume polyhedral shapes as they are converted into lutein cells.

At present, in human beings, the more active functional cells of the corpus luteum are believed by some to be formed from luteinized theca cells. The cells of the theca interna assume an epithelial-like appearance and tend to collect in small nests in the angles created by the folds produced by the expansion of the granulosa cell layers. As the development of the corpus luteum continues, the theca interna and the layer of newly formed peripheral lutein cells merge, and the line of demarcation between the two becomes indefinite. To support the expansion in cell size and growth an increase in vascularization takes place to provide adequate nourishment (Fig. 16–7).

An extreme degree of hyperemia of the theca interna becomes apparent, and the peripheral blood vessels follow the wedge and penetrate progressively into the inner layers of the young corpus luteum. Eventually the widespread capillary net-

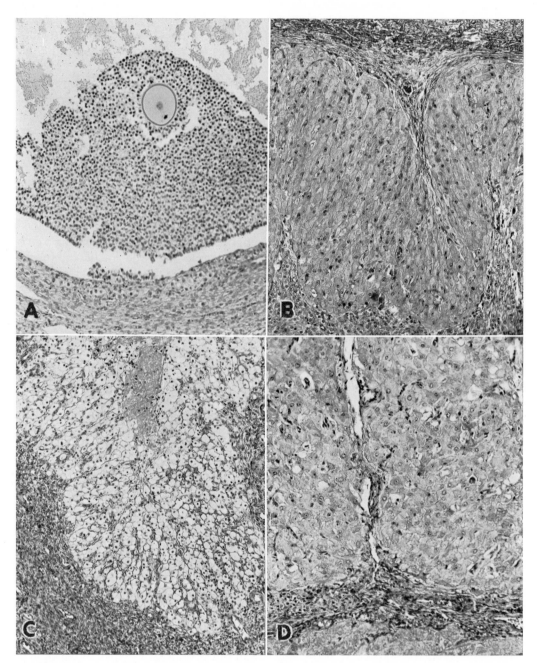

Fig. 16-7.   *A*, Mature ovum surrounded by the cumulus oophorus of granulosa cells. The dark spot below the nucleus may be a polar body. The granulosa cell layer is artefactually torn loose from the theca interna cells. *B*, A corpus luteum in active stage of secretion, 7 days after ovulation. At the top, fibroblasts are growing into the central hemorrhagic cavity. Aside from the polygonal cells in the corpus luteum, there are some elongated elements called K cells that are histochemically active. *C*, Degenerated corpus luteum with shrinkage and fatty degeneration, belonging to a cycle 1 or 2 months past. *D*, Part of the wall of a corpus luteum of pregnancy, with large luteal cells and more vascularity.

work develops into a vascularized connective tissue with fibroblasts in layers lying along the inside of the central cavity. This fibroblastic layer is sharply outlined and distinct from the blood and fibrin found in the cavity of the corpus luteum. Fibroblasts begin to line the cavity seven days after ovulation.

At the height of its development, on completion of the stage of vascularization, the corpus luteum measures from 1 to 2 cm. in diameter. Most often it can be seen projecting above the surface of the ovary as a dark red mound. At its summit there may be a hemorrhagic spot, the "stigma" of ovulation. At other times it may be found entirely within the substance of the ovary. There is a characteristic picture to the cut section. The festooned edges have a bright yellow color which is brighter by contrast with the blood clot that fills the cavity.

At this point, about seven days after ovulation, the corpus luteum reaches its maximum in secretory function, unless pregnancy ensues. Older authors believed that the peak production of progestin was achieved only after the stage of vascularization was completed. There is ample reason at present to believe that this is not so. The phospholipid content of the lutein cells, which imparts the yellow color to the maturing corpus luteum, increases in amount until approximately the twenty-fourth day. Likewise the excretion of sodium pregnanediol glucuronide, which is the end-product of luteal metabolism, reaches its height on the twenty-first day. This train of events occupies about the same length of time that it takes for the egg to pass through the tube into the endometrial cavity, where, if it is impregnated, it implants and must be maintained.

Elaboration of Progesterone in the Luteal Phase of the Cycle

All these changes have taken place in the ovary so that the corpus luteum may produce sufficient progesterone to sensitize the endometrial mucosa for the maintenance and nourishment of the impregnated ovum. The corpus luteum then must produce both estrogen and progesterone. Production of a healthy secretory endometrium, which is the ultimate aim, can be achieved only by balancing the action of estrogen with that of progestins.

It is difficult to measure accurately the amount of progesterone circulating in the blood. Apparently it is produced continuously in large quantity and is promptly metabolized. The end-product, detected in the urine by chemical extraction, is sodium pregnanediol glucuronide. Its presence in the urine is indicative of a functioning corpus luteum, but gives incomplete evidence of how well it functions. Since the pregnanediol is recoverable in small quantities, tests devised for its detection to date have not been sufficiently refined to distinguish minor fluctuations in amount. These may be important in malfunctioning conditions or pathologic states. We know that large quantities are produced, for it takes a large amount of progesterone to produce a progestational endometrium in a properly primed estrogenized endometrium. Yet only small amounts are recovered. The interpretations of variations in the amounts of circulating progesterone are further complicated by the fact that pregnanediol is also a metabolic end-product of some other steroid hormones, such as desoxycorticosterone of adrenal origin. Since only a small fraction of the pregnanediol is derived from the metabolism of steroids other than progestin, the amount recovered can mostly be attributed to the corpus luteal source.

We know that pregnanediol can be recovered in urine one or two days after ovulation has occurred. The maximum excretion occurs about the twenty-first day

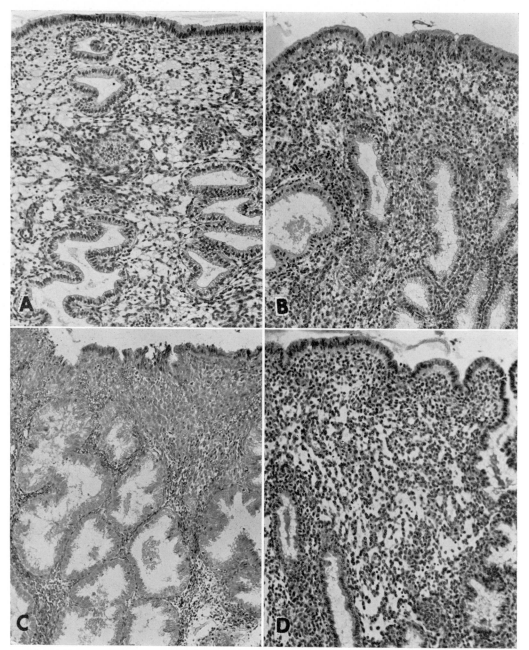

Fig. 16-8.   *A,* The fourth postovulatory day is characterized by both supranuclear and infranuclear epithelial vacuoles, and flocculent secretion is visible in the gland lumens. Inconstant stromal edema shown here begins in this so-called 18-day endometrium. *B,* The next day of the cycle (fifth postovulatory day) shows practically all supranuclear epithelial vacuoles. *C,* Two days later (seventh postovulatory day) the glands have a more saw-tooth outline, and the secretion is more stringy in their lumens. *D,* On the ninth postovulatory day, or so-called 23-day endometrium, definitely saw-tooth glands are present that contain inspissated secretion. Stromal edema is subsiding.

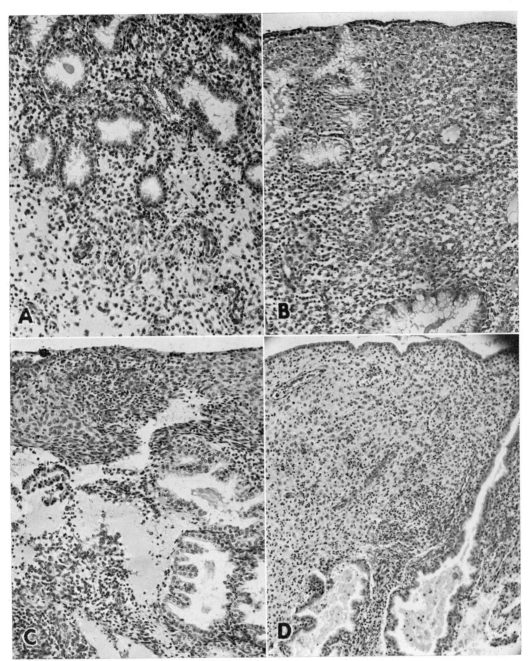

Fig. 16-9.   *A*, On the tenth postovulatory day cellular aggregates appear around the spiral arterioles seen near the bottom of the illustration, with mitoses here indicative of the onset of the predecidual reaction. *B*, Two days later, the so-called 26-day endometrium, or 2 days premenstrual, is recognized by a diffuse infiltrate of lymphocytes and macrophages into the endometrial stroma. The spiral arteriole that crosses the middle of the illustration horizontally is collapsed contracted and sagging. *C*, Premenstrual or so-called 28-day endometrium is infiltrated with neutrophils and shows hemorrhages dissecting through the necrotic endometrium. Menstrual vaginal flow begins the next day. *D*, So-called progestational hyperplasia, characterized by abundant predecidua, continued active glandular secretion and vascular dilatation. There may be a pregnancy under way, but often abundant progesterone secretion in the nonpregnant woman is responsible.

of the cycle, when some 5 to 8 mg. is recoverable. The range in the total amount excreted in the course of a menstrual cycle will vary from 3 to 54 mg., depending on the method of urine collection and the techniques used for chemical extraction.

Evaluations of the amount of circulating progesterone by blood determination and bio-assay have recently been made. The variations in amount are estimated, based on microscopic study of histologic changes occurring in the injected rat. Such readings are subject to error in individual interpretations, but those that have been made would seem to bear out the observations made by chemical extraction of the urine. Relative lack of progesterone occurs in the cyclic growth phase and peak excretion approximately one week after ovulation.

Effect of Progestin Secretion upon the Endometrium

The endometrial changes perpetuate those begun after the completion of the growth phase and the establishment of ovulation. Just before ovulation occurred we noted that the cuboidal cells in the endometrial glands of the growth phase became increasingly taller and more columnar. In preparation for secretory function increasing amounts of glycogen were noted within the cells. As the postovulatory phase progressed, the glycogen granules migrated to the surface of the cells and finally were extruded into the gland lumens and uterine cavity. This corresponded in time with the appearance of the subnuclear vacuoles, which pushed the nuclei from the basal location in the cells. This process reached its culmination about the twenty-first day. To this point the endometrial function had largely been under the influence of estrin (Fig. 16–8).

Now the role of delivery of secretion comes into play as progestin secretion approaches its maximum. This is the normal expectancy, for the ovum has passed through the tube and entered the endometrial cavity, where it needs to be nourished. The evidence for secretion is apparent in both epithelial cells and stroma. As the cells of the endometrial glands hypertrophy, the glands themselves become increasingly "sawtoothed," coiled, elongated and tortuous, with their epithelium thrown into papillary folds. The individual cells increase in size, intracellular vacuoles appear, and the nuclei gradually recede nearly to the basilar position. The cell outline alters and presents a ragged or wavy appearance, due to the disruption of the cell surface by accumulated secretion. Glycogen disappears from the cells to be replaced by mucin.

The stromal changes are marked by transient edema and progressive increase in vascularization within all three layers of the endometrial mucosa. The basal layer is not under hormonal control and persists unchanged. The two more superficial layers, however, are functional in nature and respond to the progestational stimulation. The superficial layer of the stroma is most abundant and contains the rather straight necks of the tortuous glands lying beneath it. This layer is full of engorged venules, between which are large polyhedral stromal cells, now with ample cytoplasm and large round nuclei, in contradistinction to the earlier phases of the cycle when little cytoplasm was seen. Predecidual cells form by mitotic cell divisions first visible around spiral arterioles on the twenty-third day of a twenty-eight-day cycle (Fig. 16–9).

In the middle layer, or stratum spongiosa, one finds the greatest degree of tortuosity of the glands. The stroma is less abundant, but is rich in arteriolar branches of the spiral arteries. Narrow bridges of the stroma, containing decidua-like cells, extend down in between the glands.

Changes in the Vascular Supply to the Endometrium

Although the most rapid proliferation of the endometrium occurred during the early growth phase, thickening of endometrium becomes even more pronounced during the period following the development of the corpus luteum under the influence of both estrin and progestin. Increased fluid content, cell size and vascularity are responsible, rather than cell division. At this phase the mucosa is succulent, soft and velvety, measuring from 3 to 8 mm. in thickness, depending on individual differences of response to progestin. On gross inspection it appears pale and succulent, though chemical determinations seem to suggest that the greatest concentration of free water is in the stage of proliferation rather than that of secretion.

One of the most striking changes noted in the stroma during the phase of secretory activity is the increased prominence of arterioles, branches of the spiral arteries. This is not surprising, for the spiral arterioles respond to hormonal stimulation and try to keep pace with the increasing abundance of endometrium. As they grow in length they become progressively more tortuous and coiled. Growing out from the myometrium, muscle fibers extend beneath the "intima" of the arterioles, forming the so-called contraction cones around the base of the spiral arteries. These are under hormonal control. Contraction of these cones under hormonal stimulation accounts for the blushing-blanching effect as the terminal branches of the spiral arterioles contract.

Histochemical Changes in the Endometrium during the Secretory Phase

In order that the impregnated ovum be sustained it is important that it not only have a proper housing in an adequate endometrium, but also that it be properly nourished. The endometrium must produce adequate amounts of carbohydrates, such as glycogen and vitamin C, and also enzymes such as alkaline phosphatase, which is linked to the metabolism of glycogen. In the absence of these vital elements, pregnancy cannot be maintained, and abortion may occur.

Alkaline phosphatase is found in the earlier phases of the growth cycle and gradually disappears after ovulation has occurred. It seems to have useful function in the maintaining of endometrial growth and the synthesis of glycogen as well as in fat metabolism. It can be found in the endometrium as long as chance for pregnancy exists. Two other enzymes, phosphorylase and amylase, are also found during the secretory phase of the endometrial cycle. Phosphorylase is concerned with the synthesis of glycogen, while amylase mobilizes the glycogen stored in the cells. The glycogen, under its influence, is converted into sugar, which diffuses through the cell membranes and is utilized by the newly implanted ovum. Only by receiving such nourishment for glycolysis can the ovum hope to survive.

Still another enzyme, beta-glucuronidase, may be found as long as there exists a need for maintenance of a healthy endometrium. It is found during the growth phase and continues throughout the period of progestational stimulation, to disappear when regression of the endometrium sets in.

Staining of preparations of endometrial cells with Sudan black B confirms the histologic impression that there is an increased concentration of fatty substances at this phase of the cycle. There is some question as to what the presence of fat actually means. The majority of investigators agree that fat in the cells indicates functional activity rather than degeneration.

Changes in the Tubal Epithelium during the Secretory Phase

After ovulation the ciliated cells, which were prominent during the time when they were most needed to propel the ovum along the tube into the uterus, gradually diminish in size. The nonciliated cells, which are secretory in nature, become more prominent and project above the surface to give the mucosa a ragged, uneven appearance. The cells themselves bulge, and some tend to rupture into the tubal lumen, carrying the nuclei with them. This mechanism is designed to nourish the egg while in transit through the tube.

Changes in the Vaginal Epithelium during the Secretory Phase

The height of growth and cornification of the vaginal epithelium occurred at the time of ovulation. In the postovulatory phase there is a gradual recession in growth of the vaginal epithelium, and fewer cornified cells are found in smears. They show some degeneration, become folded and are found exfoliated in clumps. The acidophil cells prominent in the growth phase are fewer in number. Instead, epithelial cells with large vesicular nuclei and granular cytoplasm are found.

Changes in the Mammary Glands

Though many investigators deny that there is any cyclic variation in breast epithelium, there is a substantial body of evidence that it does proliferate under the influence of progestin stimulation. This is notable in the smaller ducts and the lining of the ductules of the lobules. Droplets of secretion are seen in ductular cells and in the ducts. It may be that the distention of the lobules and accumulation of secretion within the dilated ducts explain in part the engorgement of the breast and discomfort experienced by some women in the ten-day period preceding menstruation. Progestin has the known quality of promoting fluid storage. It is possible that the breast enlargement may be mostly due to increased hyperemia and edema of the interstitial breast tissue. In one or both ways progestin influences the mammary glands at this phase of the menstrual cycle.

The Corpus Luteum of Pregnancy

If the ovum becomes impregnated and has received sufficient nutritional support from the endometrium to be finally implanted, the corpus luteum continues to enlarge. The lutein and paralutein cells derived from the theca interna layer become both large and numerous. No endocrine function has been assigned to the paralutein cells, but the function of the lutein cells is well recognized. K-cells, narrow stellate cells seen best by special stains, become numerous (Fig. 16–7, *D*).

Later on in pregnancy the functions of the corpus luteum are taken over by the trophoblasts in the young placenta. The hormone elaborated by it, the chorionic gonadotropic hormone, produces enough estrin and has sufficient luteinizing effect to maintain the pregnancy. It is recoverable as early as the twenty-third day and is the basis for the Aschheim-Zondek and similar tests for pregnancy. Nevertheless it is not sufficiently powerful to maintain the impregnated ovum in the very early phases of pregnancy. For this reason the corpus luteum of pregnancy secretes for two or three months in order that adequate quantities of progestin be produced

Surgeons have learned to postpone any contemplated operation on the ovary of a pregnant patient until after the placenta has assumed full responsibility for continuation of the pregnancy. This is commonly placed at three months. When emergency surgical intervention is required, progestin replacement in adequate quantity is given parenterally.

The corpus luteum of pregnancy is up to twice the size of a corpus luteum in a nonpregnant woman. It is spherical, not convoluted, and has a central smooth-walled cavity that contains clear fluid. The central cyst is lined by layers of fibroblasts. The wall is perhaps 5 mm. thick, bright yellow and well vascularized. Microscopically, the individual corpus luteum cells in pregnancy are much enlarged and can be recognized by their size. Research studies show functionally active K-cells.

THE PHASE OF REGRESSION

If pregnancy does not take place, the elaborate endometrial bed, for which there is no longer a need, must be discarded, in order to prepare for the new cycle and a subsequent ovulation. Regressive changes begin as early as the twenty-third day and coincide with the end of the period of secretory activity. When pregnancy is no longer possible, the growth factors, estrin and progestin, begin to diminish in concentration. Not all authors agree that regressive changes begin this early in the cycle, and some tend to place the onset of regression within two or three days of the time of menstruation. The observations in human beings, however, seem to parallel those seen in the endometrium transplanted in the eye of the monkey, where cessation in growth is apparent four or five days before the onset of menstruation. The difference in point of view may be traced to the fact that the obvious effect of change in functional activity of the corpus luteum is not immediately apparent on the target endometrium, or even by histologic interpretation of the corpus luteum itself (Fig. 16–10).

THE MENSTRUAL CYCLE – Regression Phase
IV.

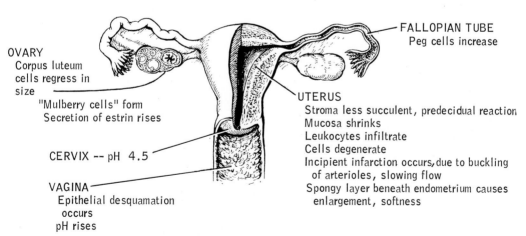

OVARY
Corpus luteum cells regress in size

"Mulberry cells" form
Secretion of estrin rises

CERVIX -- pH 4.5

VAGINA
Epithelial desquamation occurs
pH rises

FALLOPIAN TUBE
Peg cells increase

UTERUS
Stroma less succulent, predecidual reaction
Mucosa shrinks
Leukocytes infiltrate
Cells degenerate
Incipient infarction occurs, due to buckling of arterioles, slowing flow
Spongy layer beneath endometrium causes enlargement, softness

Fig. 16-10. Beyond the ninth day after ovulation, if impregnation has not occurred, the corpus luteal function declines, and with it preparations for menstruation ensue.

Changes in the Ovary in the Period of Regression

The corpus luteum has reached the height of its usefulness and gradually begins to lose its endocrine function. To gross observation the mature corpus luteum usually protrudes above the surface of the ovary as a red molded dome. On occasion the pronounced yellow color characteristic of the interior of the corpus luteum, when sectioned, may reflect through the cyst wall. Since the cavity contains varying amounts of fluid, the size is not always constant, but customarily the cavity is large, measuring between 1.0 and 1.5 cm. in total diameter. As the nodule matures, the fluid within the cavity gradually resorbs, and a definite connective tissue is deposited along the luminal edge of the lutein zone which tends to wall off the lutein cells from the central lumen. When this process is completed and a definite division appears, about the twenty-first or twenty-second day, the corpus luteum has reached full maturity. On cut section the broad, convoluted, festooned band of lutein cells stands out with a characteristic carrot-yellow color. This is due to the pigment carotene within the cells.

The process of retrogression is a gradual one. It first manifests itself in the shrinking size of the peripheral luteinized cells. Nests of rounded cells with centrally placed nuclei and coarse cytoplasmic vacuoles all around the outside develop at the periphery of the corpus luteum. These are so-called mulberry cells, believed to be inactive. They first appear by the twenty-third day and increase progressively. As the luteinized cells undergo fatty degeneration and gradually disintegrate, they finally become hyalinized (Fig. 16–7, *C*).

Hemorrhagic infarction also ensues at the time of menstruation. The corpus luteum normally is now dead. The convoluted outline of the hyalinized lutein cells is recognizable, together with the yellowish-white central core. This is the *corpus albicans*.

Variations in Hormonal Secretion in the Regressive Phase

After the peak production of estrin at the time of ovulation and that of pregnanediol on the twenty-first day, there is a decline in recoverable estrin and progestin through most of the regressive phase. In order to prepare the endometrium for the oncoming cycle, in face of rapid destruction of the old one, a secondary rise in estrin production occurs in the few days preceding menstruation. This may be due to the reduction of progestin which has had an antagonistic effect as well as a synergistic action on estrin production. The impetus could come from the pituitary, as it receives stimulation from the cells of the disintegrating endometrium, and begins to affect the ovarian follicles and stroma.

Changes in the Endometrium in the Regressive Phase

The culmination of the secretory effect in the endometrium becomes apparent about the twenty-third day. At that time the stroma was loose and edematous. Proliferation in cellular growth that had occurred within the glands gave them a tortuous outline. The glandular cells themselves appeared ragged, showed evidence of secretion and contained glycogen and fat droplets. There was evidence of increase in vascularity of the endometrium.

The growth and secretory phases cease as the phase of regression begins. This can be seen in the endometrium implanted in the monkey eye, where endometrial growth stops some five days before the onset of menstruation.

The most striking changes which forecast gradual disintegration and beginning menstruation appear in the stroma. In the face of a declining corpus luteum, with accompanying diminution in estrin and progestin stimulation, the stroma becomes less succulent. Shrinking in the mucosal layer begins. The predecidual cells become prominent, as do the spiral arterioles supplying the contracting endometrium. The other notable feature in the stroma is the sharp increase in the distribution of leukocytic infiltration. It is first evident on the twenty-fifth day. This is secondary to the extensive cellular degeneration and eventual destruction that now ensue. The cells show a progressive loss of secretion and gradually lose their cell outline as they undergo disintegration. The nuclei become pyknotic (Fig. 16–9, B).

The leukocytic infiltration and evidence of cell destruction might be thought to simulate the picture of endometritis. The changes are those of incipient infarction, however, not infection. Lymphocytes appear scattered in small numbers through the predecidual cells on the twenty-fifth day. By the next day many macrophages are also present. One day before menstruation, the twenty-seventh day, neutrophils also appear in the stroma.

The sum total of this process results in a progressive reduction in the thickness of the endometrial mucosa. As menstruation approaches, the decrease amounts to nearly 50 per cent.

VASCULAR CHANGES IN THE ENDOMETRIUM IN THE REGRESSIVE PHASE. Whether the reduction in endometrial thickness is the result of dehydration and absorption of edema or is due to the arteriovenous shunts which appear in the vascular network in anticipation of menstruation is not clear. The spiral arterioles and venous network which have expanded to nourish the growing endometrium now find themselves with nothing to do and nowhere to go. With further recession of the endometrium they become increasingly evident in the histologic picture. Throughout the greater part of the cycle the alternate dilatation and contraction of the spiral arterioles have caused a blanching and blushing phenomenon which occurs every thirty to ninety seconds. This now disappears, and the endometrium remains pale as the blood flow through the spiral arterioles slows down appreciably. This is essential, for the spiral arterioles have to buckle their coiled portions to accommodate themselves to the sharply curtailed endometrium.

Histologic study on or after the twenty-fifth day shows the muscular walls of the spiral arterioles to be abnormally overlapped and their lumens to be progressively narrowed. This spastic contraction, which is generalized by the twenty-seventh day, is so severe that the arteriolar lumens become too narrowed to permit the passage of a single red blood cell.

Other Changes Noted in the Regressive Phase

The only change observed in the fallopian tubes is the increased number of the so-called peg cells, which appear to be an intermediate stage between the nonciliated and the ciliated varieties. The *uterus* becomes softer and increases slightly in size, owing to the development of a spongy layer beneath the endometrium as menstruation approaches. The *cervix* shows no recognizable change, though the pH of its secretion reverts to the acid side at pH 4.5. The *vaginal epithelium* shows further desquamation, and the secretion is mixed with white blood cells, histiocytes and a few red blood cells. For some unexplained reason the vaginal pH rises slightly just before the onset of the menstrual period. The interstitial portion and lobules of the *breast* undergo regression, and the premenstrual engorgement disappears.

MENSTRUATION

Menstruation (or catamenia) has been defined as physiologic bleeding from the endometrium that occurs periodically in a regularly recurring pattern. It is more than an isolated physiologic phenomenon. The elaborate preparation for possible pregnancy that has been initiated by endocrine stimulation to provide for local tissue growth and blood vessel alteration as well as histochemical changes within the genital tract also produces effects that are manifest throughout the whole organism. The primary aim is nidation of the ovum. Menstruation is nature's way of expressing her frustration, as well as her persistence. Failing to establish a pregnancy in one cycle, the elaborate preparations are discarded in anticipation of the possibilities in the next cycle. Since the primary aim is pregnancy, anovulatory bleeding should be regarded as a functional derangement rather than as true menstruation.

Probable Exciting Cause in the Initiation of Menstruation

The actual stimulus to the initiation of menstruation is not known, but it appears to follow withdrawal of a hormone that has been instrumental in the preparations for pregnancy. The combined action of estrin and progestin has provided for adequate growth of the endometrium and proper means to sustain the fertilized ovum. When pregnancy does not supervene, the corpus luteum somehow is notified, loses interest in a lost cause and begins to degenerate. As a result its hormones are no longer produced in adequate quantity, and the hormonal levels drop to a point at which the endometrium breaks down and bleeding appears. The key to the whole picture is the function of the corpus luteum.

Both types of female sex hormones are implicated. It is well known from both animal studies and human experience that a decrease in the amount of estrin circulating in the blood will produce uterine bleeding. For example, withdrawal of estrin, used to bring about the development of endometrium in a castrate monkey or a woman with her uterus intact, but no ovaries, will result in bleeding in approximately two to eight days. This can be prevented by supplying more estrin either orally or parenterally. Bleeding in the anovulatory cycle is another excellent example.

It has also been shown that the withdrawal of progesterone will result in uterine bleeding. It forms the basis of a test to determine the sensitivity of the endometrium to hormonal stimulation. In the presence of an endometrium properly primed by estrin, bleeding will occur after the last injection of progesterone. Estrin and progesterone deficiencies then act together to produce menstrual bleeding. We have noted that estrin-withdrawal bleeding can be prevented by giving more estrin. But when progesterone is administered parenterally during the course of estrin therapy, in order to create a secretory endometrium, bleeding will follow within two or three days after the last injection, whether estrin is given to prevent it or not. On the clinical side, pregnanediol excretion studies show a pronounced fall, roughly two days before the onset of menstruation. The key to the initiation of menstruation seems to be progesterone withdrawal. The withdrawal of hormonal support explains reasonably satisfactorily why menstruation begins, but how it occurs still requires further elaboration.

The Mechanism of Menstruation

As part of the complex preparation of the uterus and endometrium for pregnancy, under the influence of the ovarian hormones, an elaborate system of arteriovenous channels develops within the functioning endometrium. The classic experiments of Markee provide the most logical explanation of the progress of events leading up to menstruation. These have to do with the vascular changes in the endometrium and were observed directly from endometrium implanted in the anterior chamber of the eyes of Macaque monkeys.

In order that the endometrial proliferation produced by the action of the ovarian hormones be continued and maintained in preparation for possible pregnancy, it is essential that there be an adequate blood supply. The blood supply is provided by the radial artery and its branches. The basal artery supplies the basal layers of the endometrium close to the myometrium. The spiral arterioles are the terminal branches of the radial artery and service the upper two thirds or functioning layer of the endometrium. It is this layer, together with the spiral arterioles, that responds to hormonal stimulation. The basal layer is not influenced. During the proliferative growth phase the spiral arterioles keep pace with the growing endometrium. Likewise there develops a network of veins and capillaries which form a bed around the proliferating endometrial glands. This bed runs parallel to the endometrial surface to empty into longitudinal collecting channels. These too take part in the growing phase, for they gradually increase in number and thickness of wall as the endometrial cycle progresses.

When ovulation occurs, the impetus to further growth increases in anticipation of possible need. The endometrium continues to grow under the influence of estrogens and becomes secretory under the stimulus of progestin in anticipation of its role in sustaining the impregnated ovum. The blood supply keeps pace with the increase in rate of endometrial growth. The arrangement of blood vessels within the endometrium must be flexible enough to provide for any contingency, for the ultimate aim is nidation of the ovum. The spiral arterioles respond by overproduction and increase their length as much as tenfold over the depth of the endometrium. They can do this only by creating bends and coils in their course through the endometrium. The venous and capillary beds likewise undergo expansion, and the distended veins give the appearance of "lakes" beneath the endometrial surface. At this point also arteriovenous anastomoses appear in the superficial layer of the functional endometrium. The endometrium of the uterus is prepared for pregnancy.

When the ovum is not impregnated, the corpus luteum regresses, and the hormonal stimulus to the endometrium recedes. The endometrium now enters the phase of regression. In the course of the next two days it may lose as much as two thirds of its substance. In the twenty-four hours immediately preceding menstruation some unknown chemical factor appears which seems to be a powerful vasoconstrictor with selective affinity for the spiral arterioles. These are now far too well developed for the needs of a shrinking endometrium. They become more tortuous, coiled and kinked, thereby producing a slowing of blood flow. This results in tissue damage through anoxia and eventually to complete stagnation of blood in the superficial

THE MENSTRUAL CYCLE – Menstruation Phase
V .

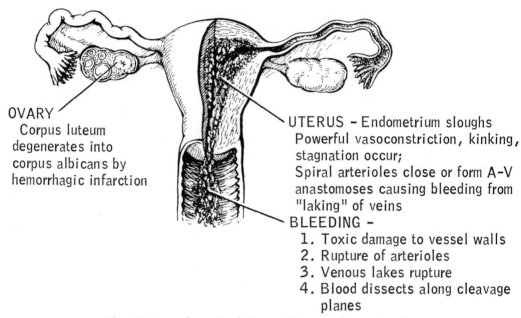

OVARY
  Corpus luteum
degenerates into
corpus albicans by
hemorrhagic infarction

UTERUS – Endometrium sloughs
Powerful vasoconstriction, kinking,
stagnation occur;
Spiral arterioles close or form A-V
anastomoses causing bleeding from
"laking" of veins
BLEEDING –
  1. Toxic damage to vessel walls
  2. Rupture of arterioles
  3. Venous lakes rupture
  4. Blood dissects along cleavage
     planes

Fig. 16-11.   Synopsis of changes that occur in menstruation.

layers. A blanching of the ocular implant in the monkey's eye is noted at this point, as the vasoconstricting agent is liberated from the necrosing endometrium.

Bleeding occurs in a number of different ways: (1) Toxic damage to the vessel walls as the result of tissue ischemia may permit escape of blood through diapedesis. (2) The arteriole ruptures after a period of constriction. The blood either escapes directly or a subepithelial hematoma forms as leakage occurs into the surrounding tissue. (3) Subsequently this lake of blood ruptures, and the blood escapes into the uterine cavity. (4) Dissection of the escaping blood into the depths of the endometrium establishes a cleavage plane, and fragments of endometrium are cast off. This results in tearing of the vein walls and more bleeding (Fig. 16–9, *C*).

This same process of gradual, irregular shedding of patches of endometrium begins microscopically on the twenty-eighth day and continues over the next three or four days until the entire surface is denuded. Bleeding finally ceases as the vaso-constricting agent clamps down on the ruptured spiral arterioles and clogs their open ends with cell debris. The endometrial surface is restored by migration of cells from the edges of the torn endometrial glands. The endometrium begins to regenerate through renewed activity on the part of the hormones and becomes revascularized from the stumps of the old coiled arteries. The basal layer of the endometrium with its basal arteries has remained essentially undisturbed throughout the period of menstruation (Fig. 16–11).

The actual identity of the vasoconstricting agent has never been established. Smith and Smith speak of a menstrual toxin which is produced by the disintegration of the endometrium as it regresses. This seems to have a specific action on the spiral arterioles. Other investigators, notably Menkin, have observed a similar toxic agent.

Not all experimenters are agreed that changes in the spiral arterioles are essential for menstruation. Apparently some forms of monkey, notably the Rhesus monkey, menstruate when there are no spiral arterioles present. Nevertheless the observations of Markee seem to be well substantiated by anatomic studies on human patients, notably those of Brewer and Okkels.

LYMPHATIC DRAINAGE. Because not all are in agreement about the role of the spiral arterioles in the mechanism of menstruation, another explanation has been advanced. This has to do with the adequacy of lymphatic drainage. Because there is an insufficiency of lymphatic channels within the endometrium, the breakdown products that follow hormonal withdrawal cannot be extruded rapidly enough. Continued production of this necrotizing material remaining in situ from the degenerating cell produces progressive destruction until the basal layer is reached. Experimentally, in animals it has been possible to produce a complete transition from full-blown functional endometrium to the resting stage without necrosis, desquamation or hemorrhage by slow withdrawal of estrin. Practically all mammals except primates have this type of endometrial regression. In theory, adequate time has been given to absorb the products of tissue degeneration.

The exciting cause is provided by the withdrawal of hormonal support and implemented by a progressive series of quick alterations in the specialized vascular arrangement within the endometrium. These changes may be due to the coiled spiral arterioles, arteriovenous shunts or inadequate lymphatic drainage.

Duration of the Menstrual Cycle

Though most women believe that their menstrual periods occur at regularly recurring intervals measured in days, some departure from the normal time interval may be expected if accurate records are kept. It is a common belief that the menstrual cycle, measured from the first day of one to the beginning of the other, consumes twenty-eight days. When attempts are made to confirm this impression by review of calendar records of any large number of women, it is apparent that their memory is not infallible. Approximately one third may be expected to show departures from the normal, up to two or more days either way. There are perhaps more shorter cycles than there are longer, and this tendency seems to increase with age in the ratio of one day in every five or six years.

The adolescent girl who has not fully established cyclic function shows the greatest variation, with an average interval of about 33.6 days. A twenty-seven-day cycle occurs most commonly in the adult woman, but the average is about 29.5 days. This variation in length appears to be independent of season, occupation or the length of the previous cycle. There is some evidence that amenorrhea is prone to occur during the warmer months in the adolescent, but no variation is seen in the adult.

With the adult woman ovulating normally one may reasonably expect to find variations in the length of the cycle, ranging from twenty-four to thirty-two days. Should the menstrual interval depart from this range consistently, then the possibility of abnormality in function or underlying disease should be considered.

RELATIVE LENGTHS OF THE GROWTH AND SECRETORY PHASES. Since the entire explanation of the menstrual cycle and menstruation itself is linked to the development of the ovum, the length of the cycle may depend on the date of ovulation. The constant factor, until recently, has been considered to be the length of the postovulatory phase, which remained at fourteen days after ovulation had occurred. The variation in the length of the cycle has always been traced to the difference in time necessary to complete the proliferative or growth phase.

There is some reason to believe that this may not be true and that both the preovulatory and postovulatory phases may vary within a wider range. It has been said in the regular twenty-eight-day cycle that as one phase lengthens, the other shortens. This observation may also be questioned. It is still possible that variations in length of either the preovulatory or postovulatory phase may influence the duration of the menstrual cycle.

This problem will be reviewed in greater detail in the discussion of sterility, where it has increased practical value.

Duration of Menstruation

The length of the menstrual period follows a fairly constant pattern for any given woman. There is such a wide variable among women in general that it is difficult to establish a normal duration of flow. The number of women who keep an accurate menstrual calendar is relatively few. A compilation of the experience of 76 women by the Stanford Medical School through 823 periods placed the average at 4.6 days. Approximately one third menstruated four days and an equal number five days. The remaining third either flowed less than four days or continued longer than six. The average, then, was 4.6 days with variations from 2 to 8 days.

Blood Loss during Menstruation

The amount of blood loss during menstruation again varies from woman to woman and often within the same woman. It is subject to many different factors that influence endometrial degeneration. General physical well-being, psychic causes, exposure to unfavorable conditions, and degree of progestational stimulation all play a part and may either increase the amount of flow or suppress it for hours or even days.

The endometrium is cast off piecemeal, and ordinarily it takes four or five days to complete full desquamation. One observes areas of regeneration within the endometrium at the same time that desquamation is taking place. There is some reason to believe that only that part of the endometrium influenced by progestin is cast off, and not the entire functional layer down to the basal layer. This will influence the amount of blood lost.

Menstrual blood leaves the uterus spasmodically in spurts, as the uterus contracts somewhat irregularly, but approximately every one to fifteen minutes, gradually decreasing in frequency as menstruation continues. In the nonpathologic state there is no steady stream of blood expelled.

The actual amount of blood lost is hard to estimate. Women commonly measure this by the number of sanitary napkins used, the degree of saturation and the frequency of change, usually three times daily. Attempts have been made to evaluate the degree of loss by collecting the discharge in cups applied to the cervix or inserted in the vagina. The most accurate method of measuring blood loss has been by chemical determination of the iron content in blood extracted from the napkins. On this basis the loss is placed at 30 to 150 ml., some women showing more or less flow.

The Nature of the Menstrual Discharge

The composition of the menstrual discharge is chiefly blood, but the discharge also contains products of endometrial desquamation in varying stages of degeneration, some of them viable, cervical mucus, degenerated vaginal epithelium and a variety of bacteria. The amount of epithelial desquamation recovered is highest during the second day of flow. The menstrual discharge is characteristically dark red, for 75 per cent of it is blood. It is stringy and viscid, owing to the accompanying cervical mucus. There is a characteristic odor, which is probably due to the decomposing action of bacteria upon the blood elements which takes place within the vagina. Degenerating epithelium is not enough to explain it, for when taken from the endometrial cavity, the discharge is odorless.

Though occasional small clots are seen in the menstrual discharge, there is a surprising disinclination on the part of menstrual blood to clot. A variety of explanations has been offered as to the possible mechanism. Chief among them have been suggestions either that an anticoagulant factor has been added by the degenerating endometrial or cervical epithelium or that the normal clotting factor has been altered by the passage of the systemic blood through this endometrium.

There is general agreement now that menstruating blood does clot within the endometrial cavity, but undergoes liquefaction or fibrinolysis as the result of the action of a fibrinolytic or proteolytic enzyme closely akin to trypsin. Such an enzyme has been recovered in the menstrual discharge in both the vagina and the endometrial cavity. Recent studies have shown that menstrual fluid recovered from the vagina is not whole blood, but serum, which lacks the essential ingredients for clotting, namely, prothrombin and fibrinogen.

Though much has been said about the presence of a toxin in menstrual discharge, no such element has been isolated to date.

The Systemic Effects of Menstruation

Although it may be difficult to find laboratory confirmation of some of the subjective symptoms, menstruation does have an influence on general well-being. Most women get by with a minimal amount of discomfort and no curtailment of activity. Others, apparently normal in all other respects, experience lower abdominal discomfort and heaviness in the pelvis which extends to the upper thighs. Urinary frequency is common, as well as change in bowel habit, which may alter either toward constipation or more frequent movements.

The fact that the blood contains less hemoglobin and iron, as well as a diminished number of red blood corpuscles, may explain why some women do not feel up to par during menstruation. One would expect to find a low basal metabolism at this time. Though no consistently low levels are found, it is common clinical practice to avoid testing the basal metabolism during menstruation, for the values obtained are notoriously unreliable.

One of the most striking features of menstruation is the change in emotional stability. Most women exhibit increased nervousness at this time. It is an interesting fact that some 80 per cent of crimes of violence committed by women are performed in the week preceding the menstrual period. A drop in serum protein and sodium chloride occurs at this time. One may speculate that increased water storage, which is known to occur in the breast and gastrointestinal tract, may also take place in the brain. This factor has been advanced as an explanation of dysmenorrhea. The increased sensitivity of the cerebral cortex may be due to local ischemia and to the increased fluid accumulation.

Severe allergic reactions tend to occur with menstruation. Laboratory evidence confirms the clinical observation, for the highest titers of antibodies have been found at this time. A clinical impression also exists that the body has less resistance to infection during menstruation. This may have something to do with the fact that the number of white blood cells is reduced, and the sedimentation rate is high. Not only does this seem to be true, but also there are several other clinical observations about this decreased resistance that are worth mentioning. Scarlet fever, furunculosis and herpes simplex tend to be more common at the time of the period. Diphtheria is also prone to begin at this time. Because there seems to be some increase in (1) storage of water in the skin and (2) the susceptibility to capillary poisons, the reaction of the Schick test may be delayed, and the response to diphtheria toxin may be over-severe.

REFERENCES

Menstrual Cycle

Bradbury, J. T., Brown, W. E., and Gray, L. A.: Maintenance of Corpus Luteum and Physiologic Actions of Progesterone; in G. Pincus, ed.: *Recent Progress in Hormone Research*. New York, Academic Press, 1950, Vol. 5, p. 151.

Brewer, J. I.: Studies of the Human Corpus Luteum. Evidence for Early Onset of the Corpus Luteum of Menstruation. *Am. J. Obst. & Gynec.*, 44: 1048, 1942.

Engle, E. T.: Endometrium of Monkey and Estrone-Progesterone Balance. *Am. J. Anat.*, 63: 349, 1938.

Gillman, J., and Stein, H. B.: Human Corpus Luteum of Pregnancy. *Surg., Gynec. & Obst.*, 72: 129, 1941.

Goldberg, B., and Jones, H. W., Jr.: Acid Phosphatase of the Endometrium. *Obst. & Gynec.*, 1: 542, 1956.

Goldzieher, J. W., Henkin, A. E., and Hamblen, E. C.: Characteristics of the Normal Menstrual Cycle. *Am. J. Obst. & Gynec.*, 54: 668, 1947.

McKay, D. G., Hertig, A. T., Bardawil, W. A., and Velardo, J. T.: Histochemical Observations on the Endometrium. *Obst. & Gynec.*, 8: 22, 140, 1956.

Markee, J. E.: Morphological Basis for Menstrual Bleeding. *Bull. New York Acad. Med.*, 24: 253, 1948.

Idem: The Morphological and Endocrine Basis for Menstrual Bleeding; in J. V. Meigs and S. H. Sturgis, eds.: *Progress in Gynecology*. New York, Grune & Stratton, Inc., 1950, Vol. II, p. 63.

Noyes, R. W., Hertig, A. T., and Rock, J.: Dating the Endometrial Biopsy. *Fertil. & Steril.*, 1: 3, 1950.

Papanicolaou, G. N.: Sexual Cycle in Human Female as Revealed by Vaginal Smears. *Am. J. Anat.*, 52 (Suppl.): 519, 1933.

Phelps, D. H.: Physiology of Menstruation and Ovulation; in *Glandular Physiology and Therapy*. 5th ed. Philadelphia, J. B. Lippincott Company, 1954, p. 162.

Reece, R. P.: Mammary Gland Development and Function; in J. T. Velardo, ed.: *The Endocrinology of Reproduction*. New York, Oxford University Press, 1958, p. 213.

Smith, O. W.: Menstrual Toxin. Experimental Studies. *Am. J. Obst. & Gynec.*, 54: 201, 1947.

Turner, C. W.: The Mammary Glands; in E. Allen, C. H. Danforth and E. A. Doisy, eds.: *Sex and Internal Secretions*. 2nd ed. Baltimore, Williams & Wilkins Company, 1939, p. 740.

Velardo, J. T.: The Anatomy and Endocrine Physiology of the Female Reproductive System; in *The Endocrinology of Reproduction*. New York, Oxford University Press, 1958, p. 101.

Idem: *Essentials of Human Reproduction*. New York, Oxford University Press, 1958.

Mechanism of Menstruation

Bartelmez, G. W.: Menstruation. *J.A.M.A.*, 116: 702, 1941.

Corner, G. W.: Nature of Menstrual Cycle. *Medicine*, 12: 61, 1933.

Engle, E. T., ed. *Menstruation and Its Disorders*. Springfield, Ill., Charles C Thomas, 1950.

Goldzieher, J. W.: Present Concepts of Menstrual Physiology: A Critical Appraisal. *Fertil. & Steril.*, 6: 1, 1955.

Okkels, H.: Histophysiology of Human Endometrium; in E. T. Engle, ed.: *Menstruation and Its Disorders*. Springfield, Ill., Charles C Thomas, 1950, p. 139.

Rock, J., Garcia, C.-R., and Menkin, M. F.: A Theory of Menstruation. *Ann. New York Acad. Sc.*, 75: 831, 1958.

Smith, O. W., and Smith, G. V.: Studies Concerning the Cause and Purpose of Menstruation. *J. Clin. Endocrinol.*, 6: 483, 1946.

Swyer, G. I. M.: Hormones and Human Fertility. *Brit. M. Bull.*, 11: 161, 1955.

Chapter 17

Anovulatory Bleeding

AN IRREGULAR bleeding pattern at the start of menstrual activity constitutes one of the chief gynecologic problems in the puberal age group. The adolescent patient may bleed irregularly, excessively, persistently or not at all. For varying periods ranging from months to years after the menarche, bleeding may occur intermittently from a proliferative type of endometrium. Such bleeding is called anovulatory bleeding. It is not uncommon for normal women to have one or two anovulatory cycles annually. This type of bleeding, however, is most often encountered at puberty and again near the time of the menopause.

What Is the Microscopic Picture of an Anovulatory Endometrium?

This endometrium is recognizable microscopically by a tendency for the glandular nuclei to become layered and compressed together to form two, three or more irregularly palisaded strata in the glands. Some glands are of the usual tortuosity, while others demonstrate dilatation locally, and still others have small, finger-like outpouchings. There is glandular epithelial mitotic activity. The stroma is compact and composed of spindly cells. It is this microscopic picture that gives rise to the diagnosis of "proliferative endometrium, consistent with an anovulatory cycle (or cycles)." The longer the endometrium continues to proliferate without an interruption by ovulation or menstruation, the more hyperplastic it becomes. There is no suggestion of any secretory activity (Fig. 17–1).

What Is the Mechanism of Anovulatory Bleeding?

In order for menstruation to occur at puberty there must be (1) a pituitary capable of stimulating the ovary through its gonadotropins, (2) an ovary able to respond to such stimulation and in turn to elaborate its own hormones, (3) a uterus with an endometrium capable of reacting to the stimulating effect of the ovarian hormones. All these factors are normally present in the young girl who bleeds at puberty. There is no basic defect.

The primary difficulty in the irregular bleeding pattern which appears at puberty is the fact that ovulation does not occur. There is enough estrin present to stimulate the endometrium to proliferate, but it is unbalanced by progestin. If ovulation does not take place, no corpus luteum is formed and no progesterone is elaborated. The bleeding occurs from a proliferative endometrium, and the primary defect is the lack of progestins (Fig. 17–2).

206

Though progestin lack is usually responsible for the irregular bleeding, which is occasionally troublesome, often prolonged and excessive, uterine bleeding may come from an atrophic or inactive, rather than a proliferative, endometrium.

The explanation of this type of bleeding from an inactive or atrophic endometrium is not clear. It is possible that the immature ovary may be refractory to pituitary stimulation and responds with a minimum output of estrin. The endometrium may be capable of responding to the ovarian hormone, but receives inadequate stimulation. Individual patients are known to bleed periodically from a lowered estrin level in the blood, so that the endometrium never has a chance to develop. Though there is no obvious evidence of uterine abnormality, some part of the odd bleeding pattern may be traced to a disturbance in the blood supply to the endometrium, secondary to an imbalance in sympathetic and parasympathetic nervous control, or to an actual disorder in the spiral arteriolar system itself. Rarely blood platelet or other clotting defects are also implicated. The full answer to these perplexing problems will not be forthcoming until we have a more complete understanding of uterine physiology in relation to minor fluctuations in hormonal production. To date the laboratory has not been able to make such fine differentiations in quantitative analyses of the ovarian hormones.

Why Does Ovulation Not Occur?

There is a wide variety of reasons why anovulatory periods occur at puberty and throughout the menstrual life of women. Anovulatory periods are common to the menarche and the menopause.

The reason for the failure to ovulate at puberty can be traced to immaturity of the ovary. Enough follicle-stimulating hormone is elaborated to initiate the development of the primary follicle and produce adequate amounts of estrin, but the vascular network within the ovary has not developed sufficiently to allow the anterior pituitary to deliver enough LH to induce ovulation. In a sense the mechanism is protective, for the child is not yet ready for pregnancy. Under the influence of estrin the vascularity improves progressively, so that after several months enough LH reaches the

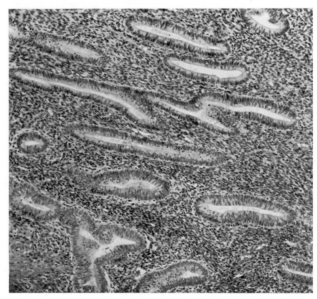

Fig. 17-1.   Endometrium with a proliferative glandular pattern and mitotic figures, but with excessive layering of epithelial nuclei, is characteristic of an anovulatory growth pattern.

MECHANISM OF ANOVULATORY BLEEDING

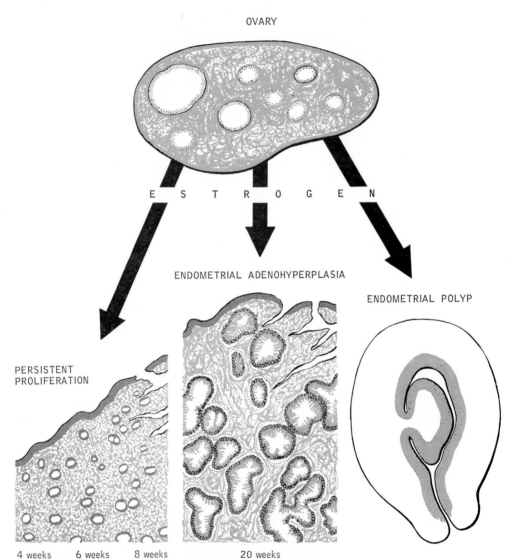

OVARY

E S T R O G E N

ENDOMETRIAL ADENOHYPERPLASIA

ENDOMETRIAL POLYP

PERSISTENT
PROLIFERATION

4 weeks   6 weeks   8 weeks   20 weeks

Fig. 17-2.   Continued ovarian estrogenic stimulation results in endometrial overgrowth that eventually assumes adenomatous or polypoid hyperplastic forms.

follicle to promote full maturation of the ova, ovulation and development of a corpus luteum.

At the menopause the pituitary tries to stimulate an exhausted and aging ovary. The result in both cases is anovulatory or functional bleeding secondary to progestin lack.

What Other Factors Contribute to Anovulatory Bleeding?

For practical purposes, however, the great majority of cases of abnormal vaginal bleeding at the time of the menarche can be laid directly to an imbalance between the estrogenic and luteal ovarian hormones. Other factors influence this imbalance. Malnutrition, emotional unrest, obesity, diminished thyroid function and systemic diseases all may affect the endocrine imbalance, either by inhibiting the functions of the ovary and pituitary or by nullifying the normal action of the hormones on the uterus or endometrium. The presence of one or any combination of these elements will modify a menstrual pattern, inducing either excessive bleeding or amenorrhea.

Malnutrition, improper diet, systemic disease and psychologic disturbances exert their effect through either the pituitary or the hypothalamus. Nutrition is definitely related to endocrine function. Observations on animals have shown that a diet deficient in protein and vitamin B will result in a diminished output of FSH by the pituitary and a secondary atrophy of the ovary. The same thing is noted in human beings subjected to protracted illness with resultant debilitation. The effect is mediated through the pituitary. Starvation and chronic wasting conditions induce a secondary pituitary hypofunction. Many young girls in puberty and adolescence go on bizarre diets in a misguided effort to improve the girlish figure. Frequently these diets are deficient in protein and vitamin B.

Psychologic factors must be considered. Emotional shock, intense worry, depression states or apprehension and stress of school work all may influence the menstrual pattern. Amenorrhea is the most common response, but not infrequently abnormal bleeding may be traced to these factors. The explanation offered concerns the hypothalamus and its effects upon release of the luteinizing hormone. The pituitary FSH cannot bring about full maturation of the ova without the luteinizing hormone. The release of LH in turn depends on the luteotropic hormone. Any malfunction or external influences such as psychic stimuli affecting the hypothalamus may block the liberation of the pituitary LH. An imbalance in the hormones may explain the abnormal bleeding or total absence of menstruation.

Obesity and hypofunction of the thyroid go hand in hand. Deficiency in thyroid function parallels the state of bodily nutrition. Again, hypothyroid states are implicated in both excessive bleeding and amenorrhea.

TREATMENT

General Observations on the Management of Irregular Vaginal Bleeding at Puberty and Adolescence

The great majority of girls at puberty will establish a normal balance between estrin and progestin after a few periods of anovulatory bleeding. Other girls are slow to reach a proper equilibrium in hormonal balance and may not acquire it for a year or more, owing to variations in sensitivity of the immature ovary to pituitary stimulation. When imbalance persists, the patient complains of (1) too frequent periods interspersed with occasional amenorrhea or (2) irregular spotting before the menstrual period begins.

Anovulatory vaginal bleeding which accounts for the "too frequent" periods (the foreshortened interval between periods) usually corrects itself in a short time. Such bleeding, unless it becomes excessive, is of no particular significance. It is of far greater concern to the mother than the child. Occasionally the young girl may become overemotional about the fact that she seems to be having periods twice in a month. It is often advisable to ask her how she measures the interval. Frequently she numbers the days from the end of one period to the beginning of another. If the menstrual phase is five days to a week in duration, the intermenstrual interval is actually about three weeks. This is not uncommon. Such patients may subsequently change to a twenty-eight-day cycle or continue through the rest of the menstrual life on a three-week pattern.

Before concluding that abnormal vaginal bleeding at puberty is primarily due to ovarian dysfunction, it is important to exclude other possible sources of bleeding. Granulosa cell tumors, dysgerminomas, dermoid cysts and serous cystadenomas have been found in this age group. The likelihood of these is not great, but the possibility of their presence should not be overlooked. There are two other elements that frequently first manifest themselves at the time of puberty and are intimately concerned with abnormal bleeding. They are (1) the hypothyroid state and (2) idiopathic thrombocytopenic purpura.

Patients with a low basal metabolic function bleed profusely in a gushing manner, similar to that produced by the submucous fibroid in older women. Thrombocytopenic purpura frequently first appears in the form of vaginal bleeding. Normally one becomes suspicious of its presence from the appearance of purpuric skin spots, confirmed by various laboratory studies of the bleeding time, the capillary fragility, clot retraction and platelet count. Remissions are common, and both obvious signs and laboratory support for the correct diagnosis may be absent. Tragic or unnecessary hysterectomies have been performed for excessive uncontrolled vaginal bleeding when the diagnosis of idiopathic thrombocytopenic purpura had not been considered.

Specific Recommendations for Therapy

Basically, one should always keep in mind that anovulatory bleeding will usually cure itself if left alone. Time becomes an important element in therapy. Unless the vaginal bleeding is excessive to the point at which the general health is impaired or the child has to remain home from school, only simple supportive measures combined with maternal reassurance are indicated in therapy.

NUTRITION.   One of the simplest forms of treatment will be to correct any evidence of faulty nutrition in the adolescent child. Abnormal vaginal bleeding is common in "run down" girls. Many of these children are either too fat or too thin, or have undergone too sudden weight loss on ill-advised diets deficient in the necessary requirements of protein and vitamins. The ovary has never had a proper chance to function normally. Not infrequently simple regulation of the eating and living habits will be all that is necessary to overcome the bleeding problem. Many young girls have an anemia which tends to produce a vicious circle. The child may bleed because of bodily depletion caused by the anemia. This in turn increases the degree of secondary anemia and the amount of vaginal bleeding. Daily doses of iron, commensurate with the degree of anemia, should be added to the balanced diet. Vitamins C, B complex and K seem to be intimately linked to the bleeding problem. Preparations containing these vitamins should supplement the regimen of iron and diet.

THYROID AND OBESITY.   Hypofunction of the thyroid and obesity are common to this age group. Many problems can be solved by a simple, well supervised weight reduction diet with the addition of thyroid extract. Although the basal metabolism, serum protein-bound iodine, cholesterol and radioactive iodine uptake studies do not always adequately reflect the state of thyroid function, these tests are indicated. Patients with basal metabolic rates in the range of −15 to −20 menstrually bleed excessively in uncontrolled bursts of gushing and flooding. The patients with true myxedema usually do not bleed. In many instances satisfactory results can be obtained from the empiric use of thyroid extract, using the patient's pulse rate and general response as indicators of the proper dose. Clinically, one gets a fair idea of the patient's need for thyroid supplement by asking the girl about (1) her response to cold, (2) her reaction to hot weather and the extent to which she perspires, (3) the difficulty in keeping her weight down, (4) the degree of fatigue, and (5) her ability to stay awake and concentrate. Thyroid extract in 1- or 2-grain doses daily will accomplish a great deal in the patient with these symptoms who is bleeding irregularly or excessively. A properly functioning thyroid and sound state of bodily nutrition are essential if the hormones are to function normally. This is true whether the patient tries to get along on her own hormones or whether you supplement them.

Hormone therapy should be reserved for the girl who is bleeding really excessively, even though progestin lack appears to be the obvious explanation. It is far better to support the child as outlined above and allow her to regulate herself, as she will do in most instances.

Specific Therapy for Excessive Vaginal Bleeding

Rarely, bleeding becomes so excessive that definitive rather than supportive measures are indicated. Fatal hemorrhages have been reported, though the likelihood is not great. The child's health as well as her normal existence and education program may be seriously jeopardized. Both mother and child become emotionally and physically exhausted.

The aim in therapy is (1) to stop the bleeding in such a way that the child's reproductive possibilities are not compromised, and (2) to create a proper background which will ensure the establishment of a normal cycle. It is ordinarily possible to accomplish this by use of hormones.

IMMEDIATE CONTROL OF BLEEDING. (1) Estrin given intravenously in the form of Premarin, 5 ml. (i.e. 20 mg.), for three or four doses has been used effectively to stop the severe vaginal bleeding phase, and will usually do so in twelve to twenty-four hours. Supposedly it is effective through raising the estrin level above the critical bleeding point. Oral administration of diethylstilbestrol or Premarin in daily dosage ranging from 6 to 10 mg. has been recommended by a number of advocates. Should the bleeding continue excessively or be prolonged two or three days, the dosage is doubled.

(2) The male sex hormone has its champions. Doses of 25 to 30 mg. of testosterone propionate may be given intramuscularly daily for four or five days until the bleeding stops. Why this is effective is not clearly understood. It may act through neutralizing any excess in the amount of the circulatory estrogens, or its effect may be directly on the uterine musculature or via constricting muscle fibers of the coiled spiral arterioles within the endometrium. Testosterone is not dissimilar in action to progesterone. Relaxation of the uterine muscle may take place, by continuing the effect of estrin, while at the same time the blood supply is reduced through constriction of the spiral arterioles.

(3) It would appear far more logical to use progesterone rather than estrin, if one is to use hormones for the purpose of stopping excessive vaginal bleeding. Though there is a suggestion of progestin lack, there is no corresponding evidence of hyperestrinism. There seems little reason for using testosterone, therefore. In the face of

adequate if not superfluous estrin, there seems to be small excuse for giving more, unless the dosage schedules, which are many times the physiologic doses, are aimed at suppressing pituitary function. By giving progestin one simply hopes to replace a known deficiency. Since all hormone therapy is pure substitution, the rationale for the use of progesterone appears more reasonable.

How Is Progesterone Administered for the Control of Hemorrhage? Intramuscular injections of progesterone in oil in 50-mg. doses daily for three days provide the most effective method of controlling hemorrhage by the use of hormones. At least 100 mg. of progesterone are necessary to arrest hemorrhage. If you choose, and the amount of hemorrhage is not alarming, you may elect to spread the injections out over a longer period in 25-mg. daily doses for 5 or 6 days.

There has been some enthusiasm for the combined use of intramuscular injection and vaginal suppositories of progesterone. In the past, attempts were made to supplement the injections by buccal tablets of anhydrohydroxyprogesterone (Pranone), but the vaginal suppositories with their absorbable base have been more effective. The dosage schedule for the combined treatment in the control of hemorrhage is (*a*) 25 mg. of progesterone daily by intramuscular injection for 4 to 6 doses, or 50 mg. every other day for 3 doses; (*b*) vaginal suppositories containing 50 mg. of progesterone nightly for 4 to 6 nights.

Recently newer agents have become available.

Injectable Progestational Agents.   A long-acting injectable progesterone such as 17-alpha-hydroxyprogesterone caproate (Delalutin) has proved an effective and convenient means of giving progesterone for the patient whose acute hemorrhage has stopped, when the physician wishes to supplement progesterone to prevent any further recurrence of excessive bleeding. Unfortunately, it does not act rapidly enough to control hemorrhage.

Oral Progestational Agents.   There is increasing enthusiasm, however, for the new oral medications. The progestational activity of the new compounds such as (*a*) 17-alpha-ethinyl-19-nortestosterone (Norlutin), (*b*) 17-alpha-methyl-19-nortestosterone (Methalutin), (*c*) 17-alpha-ethinyl-5 (10)-estranolene (Enovid) and (*d*) medroxyprogesterone (Provera) is roughly five times as great as the old buccal tablets of anhydrohydroxyprogesterone (Pranone). The response is far more predictable, for older types of progesterone had a variable rate of absorption from the gastrointestinal tract. The effect of the newer agents appears to be directly upon the endometrium.

The dosage schedule recommended for the control of hemorrhage is 10 to 20 mg. every 3 hours for 5 doses. In most instances this will cause a cessation of active endometrial bleeding within twelve to twenty-four hours. There may be some slight staining for several days, but the acute blood loss subsides promptly. One may choose to continue with the oral progestational agents for 1 to 2 weeks thereafter on a dosage regimen of 10 mg. daily, simply to prevent any recurrence of bleeding and give the patient time to recover from the effect of the hemorrhage.

What Is the Best Method of Arresting Hemorrhage?   Of all the treatments suggested for the immediate control of excessive uterine bleeding at this age, curettage is by far the best. Two things are accomplished: (1) The bleeding is immediately controlled, and (2) histologic examination of the endometrium will provide a sound rational basis for the management of any abnormal bleeding that may reappear in later months. In most instances curettage will produce a definite arrest of the disturbed bleeding pattern, as well as control the immediate hemorrhage. It rarely fails to check the bleeding, at least temporarily.

Failure to control the vaginal bleeding permanently may be due to the fact that the patient is bleeding from an inactive endometrium. Curettage will provide evidence for this (Fig. 17–3). These patients bleed profusely and over a long period. Curettage is less effective, and progestin therapy fails, for there is inadequate estrin present. Such a uterus must be "primed" with a continual daily oral administration of estrin over a period of two or three months before adding progestin to the therapy. If the bleeding is excessive, one may wish to give estrin parenterally to raise the level of estrin and control the immediate bleeding. With bleeding arrested, the estrin may be continued by mouth in a daily dosage equivalent to 3 to 5 mg. of stilbestrol.

Such therapy accomplishes two things: (1) It raises the estrin level to control the immediate hemorrhage, and (2) it builds up and sensitizes the uterus to the subsequent administration of progestin, so that there is some continuity about therapy for the future. The rationale of the therapy is based on the hope that the pituitary and the ovary will be rested. The pituitary FSH is inhibited. There is less stimulation of the ovarian follicles, which become static. Since the hormone is being substituted, there is no occasion for either the pituitary or the ovary to exert its secretory functions. As the hormone is withdrawn, a sudden demand is placed on the resting pituitary and ovary to go into effective activity. One hopes that the rebound will be sufficiently strong to produce a more normal pituitary-ovarian stimulation.

Continued Therapy after the Arrest of Hemorrhage

If one elects to try hormone therapy before or instead of curettage, the treatment must be empiric, based on the assumption that there is a progestin lack. Endometrial biopsies taken at intervals are impractical in this age group, and the laboratory studies are protracted, expensive and not very revealing. When one curettage has been done, an examination of the curettings will provide a more adequate basis for prolonged therapy.

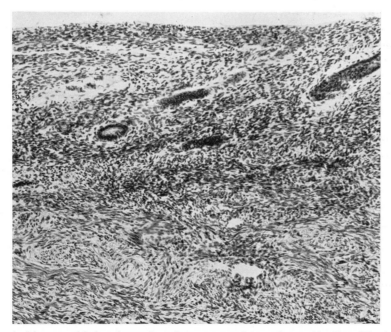

Fig. 17-3.   A thin, atrophied endometrium from a case of anovulatory bleeding. The lower half of the tissue shown is myometrium.

With any recurrence in vaginal bleeding after curettage one may safely carry out future therapy with hormones. Unless the bleeding is again excessive, one is reluctant to subject the younger patient to the emotional trauma of a second curettement. The emotional element is prominent in girls in this age group who present recurring menstrual bleeding problems. One may accomplish a great deal by explaining to the patient that her present problem will eventually straighten out and encouraging her cooperation for however long it takes to accomplish it.

PROGESTIN THERAPY.   When the irregular vaginal bleeding is the result of progestin deficiency, the substitution of progesterone in some form either parenterally or orally is by far the most logical treatment for a girl in this age group. In older women, when the cause of the vaginal bleeding is less obvious and bleeding seems to occur from almost any kind of endometrium, the results of hormone therapy are often disappointing. In adolescent girls excellent results may be anticipated. The aim of any form of hormone therapy is the establishment of a normal estrogen-progestin balance without the support of administered hormones. Since these girls frequently do this without any help at all, their future is brightened by conservative management.

A dosage schedule of intramuscularly administered progesterone, 10 mg. daily for 6 days, is usually given on or about the eighteenth day of the cycle. When vaginal bleeding has been continuous and no cyclic activity can be made out, the injections can be given while the patient is bleeding. Though the vaginal bleeding may slow down in the course of the progesterone series or even stop, the full number of injections should be given. Three or four days later the uterus extrudes the endometrium in toto, rather than in areas of patchy desquamation. The flow may be heavy, but it should cease in the normal four or five days. This has been called a "medical curettage." In planning therapy it is advisable to repeat the series of injections eighteen days after the first day of withdrawal bleeding for the next three months. The patient thereafter should be allowed to get along on her own without hormonal support.

This is an expensive, time-consuming therapy and often inconvenient, for the injections must be given on continuous days that frequently include the weekend. Recently a longer-acting progesterone has been produced in the hope that a single injection may take the place of multiple treatments.

For the same reason oral progestin has been tried, using the same dosage schedule used in the injection method. Anhydrohydroxyprogesterone in doses ranging from 50 to 80 mg. a day has been given, but with less satisfactory results. Buccal tablets of progestin in the same dosage and on the same schedule have also been tried. Results are less predictable when progestin is given by the oral route, for some of the effective principle appears to be lost in its passage through the gastrointestinal tract.

Though one may elect to use testosterone or estrin in the older patient with abnormal vaginal bleeding problems, progestin is the hormone of choice in the adolescent girl.

Injectable Progestational Agents.   The new long-acting form of progesterone, 17-alpha-hydroxyprogesterone (Delalutin) is now available as an effective agent for supplementary progesterone therapy. It has the advantage of convenience, in that only a single injection is required, for its action is exerted over a period of time. The older forms of progesterone had to be given repeatedly on continuous days that frequently involved the weekend. The maintenance dose recommended is 250 to 500 mg. injected intramuscularly on roughly the eighteenth day of the cycle.

Oral Progestational Agents.   For the same reasons—to avoid multiple injections and to counteract the inconvenient time schedule—the new oral progesterone agents have had increasing use. The dosage schedule of such oral progesterone preparations as Norlutin, Nilevar, Methalutin, Enovid or Provera for use in regulating the menstrual cycle after the excessive bleeding has been controlled is 10 mg. daily, beginning on the fifth and continuing through the twenty-first day. If there is any suggestion of breakthrough bleeding under therapy, the dosage should be increased to 20 mg. daily. Upon withdrawal of the progestational agent vaginal bleeding will reappear within two days and usually lasts for four. The bleeding is often heavy and may be painful, for decidual casts are sometimes formed.

New Progestational Agents and Medical Curettage. These preparations are effective in changing a persistent proliferative endometrium into one that is progestational. It takes longer to do this than with older forms of progestin (Proluton). Ten milligrams of Proluton given intramuscularly every day for five days would usually produce complete endometrial shedding within four days after withdrawal of the hormone. When the newer progestational agents are given, the 10-mg. dose must be given daily for at least 2 weeks. It is more practical, then, to give the usual progesterone medication rather than the more recent progestational agents if you wish to do a so-called medical curettage.

Summary of Treatment

The treatment of irregular menstrual bleeding in the young girl at puberty or in adolescence should be marked by intelligent observation and procrastination. A moderate degree of success will follow improvement in the nutritional state and the degree of thyroid activity. If hormone therapy is to be used, a corrective program is a basic consideration. When it is used disregarding expense and inconvenience, progesterone is the hormone of choice. If the gynecologist's hand is forced, and the vaginal bleeding is both profuse and prolonged, a curettage will often prove curative, at the same time providing information which will guide the physician in the more intelligent use of hormones should bleeding recur after curettage. After the arrest of hemorrhage a plan for supplementing the deficient endogenous supply of progesterone should be carried out for three or four months before the patient is allowed to menstruate without hormonal support.

VICARIOUS MENSTRUATION

In certain rare instances bleeding may occur periodically from extragenital sources at the time one would normally expect a menstrual period. The great majority of cases in which this kind of bleeding is noted are in the puberal and adolescent age groups. It may occur with or in the absence of ordinary menstruation. The most common source of the bleeding appears in the nasal mucous membrane, but it may appear from almost any mucous membrane surface, particularly if any pre-existing ulceration is present. The vascular organ of Rosenmueller in the nasal mucosa has long been considered a secondary sex organ responsive to hormonal action. Also one may occasionally note rhythmic discharge of blood at monthly intervals from the lung, skin or breast, with similar bleeding phenomena noted less frequently from the stomach, mouth, bladder, eyes, ears or larynx. The amount of blood loss is not great, nor is it constant, for it may occur at some menstrual periods and not with others. At times the bleeding is profuse and may be an adequate explanation of secondary anemia. Vicarious menstrual bleeding is not uncommon in the patient who has amenorrhea. This may be related to the observation that it is most likely to appear in the girl who has other stigmata of underdevelopment, such as uterine aplasia.

The appearance of bleeding from the nasal mucous membrane, a uterine fistula or from an open sore or any mucous membrane surface suggests that somewhere in the background there may be an element of generally increased capillary permeability related to the menstrual cycle, and it is probably concerned with estrin production and metabolism. Estrin is a vasodilator, and the variation in the amount of this circulating hormone may initiate bleeding from extragenital sources.

This supposition gains further support from the well substantiated observation that the mucous membranes of the nose and uterus respond to the same stimuli from the ovarian hormones. The older observers speak of "genital spots" which seem to appear on the inferior turbinates or the tuberculum of the nasal passages. Some women show a definite swelling and erythema of the nasal mucous membrane, which leads to a troublesome rhinorrhea preceding the onset of the menstrual flow. This condition can be produced expermentally by the injection of estrin and has led to the use of estrin therapy for atrophic rhinitis.

The breasts also seem to be activated in this same manner. Cyclic mastodynia is common in many menstrual cycles, and occasionally vicarious bleeding is noted from the nipple.

Before one can fully accept the concept of extragenital bleeding occurring with or replacing the menstrual cycle it is important to establish the relation definitely by careful history, after ruling out blood dyscrasias by careful blood studies. In the presence of other organic lesions it is perhaps more logical to attribute the bleeding to the basic disease, such as pulmonary tuberculosis, ulcers of the gastrointestinal tract or malignant tumors.

Since the bleeding is not of paramount importance in most instances, nothing need be done about it. The bleeding is generally from the nasal mucous membrane, and the local genital spots may be cauterized if the bleeding is troublesome or alarming. With severe bleeding from any other source the real explanation of its cause should be thoroughly investigated and the treatment individualized.

REFERENCES

Anovulatory Bleeding

Allen, W. M.: Functional Bleeding. *South. M.J.*, 44: 817, 1951.

Arey, L. B.: Degree of Normal Menstrual Irregularity. *Am. J. Obst. & Gynec.*, 37: 12, 1939.

Collett, M. E., Wertenberger, G. E., and Fiske, V. N.: The Effect of Age upon the Pattern of the Menstrual Cycle. *Fertil. & Steril.*, 5: 437, 1954

Engel, E. T., and Shelesnyak, M. C.: First Menstruation and Subsequent Menstrual Cycles of Pubertal Girls. *Human Biol.*, 6: 431, 1934.

McArthur, J. W.: Adolescent Menstrual Disorders; in J. V. Meigs and S. H. Sturgis, eds.: *Progress in Gynecology*. New York, Grune & Stratton, Inc., 1957, Vol. III, p. 153.

Rogers, J.: Disorders of Menstruation. *Disease of the Month*. Chicago, Year Book Publishers, Inc., April, 1957.

Southam, A. L.: The Natural History of Menstrual Disorders. *Ann. New York Acad. Sc.*, 75: 840, 1959.

Sutherland, A. M.: Functional Uterine Bleeding; in J. V. Meigs and S. H. Sturgis, eds.: *Progress in Gynecology*. New York, Grune & Stratton, Inc., 1957, Vol. III, p. 167.

Thyroid Dysfunction

Goldsmith, R. E., Sturgis, S. H., Lerman, J., and Stanbury, J. B.: The Menstrual Pattern in Thyroid Disease. *J. Clin. Endocrinol.*, 12: 846, 1952.

Hamolsky, M. W., and Freedberg, A. S.: The Thyroid Gland. (Medical Progress.) *New England J. Med.*, 262: 23, 1960.

Tyler, E. T.: The Thyroid Myth in Infertility. *Fertil. & Steril.*, 4: 218, 1953.

Blood Dyscrasias

Barnes, A. C.: The Relationship between the Hemorrhagic Blood Dyscrasias and Hypermenorrhea. *Am. J. Obst. & Gynec.*, 58: 570, 1949.

Buxton, C. L.: Menorrhagia as a Primary Factor in Various Blood Dyscrasias. *Am. J. Obst. & Gynec.*, 42: 502, 1941.

Dameshek, W., and Rheingold, J. J.: Idiopathic Thrombocytopenic Purpura and Menorrhagia Mistakenly Treated for Local Disease. *J.A.M.A.*, 139: 993, 1949.

Radman, H. M.: Blood Dyscrasia as a Causative Factor in Abnormal Uterine Bleeding. *Am. J. Obst. & Gynec.*, 79: 1, 1960.

Therapy

Buxton, C. L., and Hermann, W. L.: Effect of Thyroid Therapy on Menstrual Disorders and Sterility *J.A.M.A.*, 155: 1035, 1954.

Fluhmann, C. F.: *The Management of Menstrual Disorders.* Philadelphia, W. B. Saunders Company, 1957.

Gray, L. A.: Induced Menstruation for Metrorrhagia and Amenorrhea. *Am. J. Obst. & Gynec.*, 58: 1169, 1949.

Greenblatt, R. B., and Barfield, W. E.: The Effect of Intravenous Estrogen in Uterine Bleeding. *J. Clin. Endocrinol.*, 11: 821, 1951.

Taymor, M. L., and Sturgis, S. H.: Clinical and Laboratory Effects of Nortestosterone: The Management of Anovulatory Dysfunctional Uterine Bleeding. *Am. J. Obst. & Gynec.*, 79: 316, 1960.

Thomas, H. H.: Dysfunctional Uterine Bleeding. A Simplified One-Injection Treatment Using Long-Acting Ovarian Steroids. *South. M.J.*, 51: 1266, 1958.

Chapter 18

Amenorrhea

ONE OF THE most distressing, if not the most common, problems in the adolescent period is that of the girl who for one reason or another fails to establish a normal bleeding pattern within the time limit commonly regarded as normal. In the previous discussion it has been pointed out that the chronologic age at which menstruation may be expected varies widely. The parent and the physician should be alert, but not overapprehensive, if menstruation does not occur by the age of fourteen years. Evidence of severe endocrine imbalances will begin to be apparent at this time and should be investigated. If none appears, and the child simply develops slowly, the intelligent policy to pursue is one of watchful waiting. If the girl has not menstruated by the age of eighteen, however, it is imperative that the waiting program give way to one of thorough investigation. Although procrastination in therapy is the part of wisdom in the early years of adolescence, it may lead to irrevocable damage if carried too far. Practically, it is advisable that the cause for the menstrual delay be found before the girl enters the highly competitive field of secondary education, for she then has little time to devote to investigative studies of her own functional failure and fails to appreciate how important it is that the cause be found.

The failure to menstruate has been called amenorrhea. For discussion, amenorrhea has been given two main classifications: (1) primary amenorrhea and (2) secondary amenorrhea. In primary amenorrhea the girl has never menstruated. When the patient has had menstrual bleeding either rhythmically or sporadically, but then ceases to menstruate, the amenorrhea is called secondary. Any defects in the hypothalamic-pituitary-ovarian-uterine axis may result in failure of menstruation. In primary amenorrhea this defect may be basic. It is less so in secondary amenorrhea, for by definition the patient has menstruated at some time. The division of amenorrheic patients into the two classifications is of little help in establishing etiology, but it is of considerable practical importance in therapy (Fig. 18–1).

Since the all-important biologic event of menstruation may be influenced by a wide variety of factors other than physiologic disturbance in the endocrine glands, it is important to consider causative factors outside the field of the endocrines. One of the primary considerations should be the presence or absence of anatomic defects. The other nonendocrine factors to consider are those that affect the endocrines either directly by inhibiting the function of the ovary and the pituitary, or indirectly by nullifying the normal action of the hormones on the target organs. Obesity, disturbances in thyroid function, malnutrition, disease and psychic orders all play a role in

218

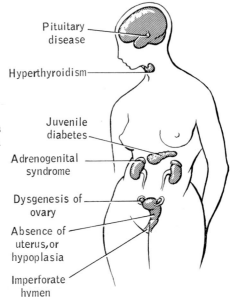

Pituitary disease

Hyperthyroidism

Juvenile diabetes

Adrenogenital syndrome

Dysgenesis of ovary

Absence of uterus, or hypoplasia

Imperforate hymen

Fig. 18-1. Endocrine dysfunctional conditions and genital abnormalities commonly associated with amenorrhea.

the explanation of why the patient either never menstruates, is delayed or ceases to have further menstrual periods after she has once started.

Anatomic Defects

The obvious point of departure in investigation as to the reason why a girl has not menstruated by the age of sixteen years should be a complete examination. This would appear to be axiomatic, but all too frequently the history reveals that these patients have received several series of hormone treatments without ever having been examined. One obvious explanation may be that the patient has an anatomic defect which makes menstruation impossible. If, for example, the child on physical examination appears adequate in structural growth and secondary sex characteristics are evident, the explanation of her failure to menstruate may be a simple imperforate hymen with hematocolpos. On the other hand, the anatomic variation may be basic. In either case physical examination is imperative. Delay in determining the cause of primary amenorrhea can only compound the problems of its correction, for the longer the genitalia remain underdeveloped, the more refractory they become to any sort of therapy. The great majority of congenital defects can be discovered in the simple routine gynecologic examination, provided the physician will take the trouble to look at the patient. Some of the defects are apparent in infancy or the prepuberal age group, but many are unrecognized until the time when menstruation is expected.

Imperforate Hymen

This is the most obvious explanation of why the menstrual period is delayed at puberty. The normally developing child at regularly recurring intervals experiences lower abdominal discomfort, loss of appetite, restlessness, backache and other menstrual molimina. The pain may be severe and cramplike. After a few days the symptoms disappear, only to reappear a month later, gradually increasing in severity as the months go by and menstruation does not appear.

On examination the explanation is often apparent immediately, for the vaginal canal is found to be completely closed. If there has been an accumulation of menstrual secretion behind the intact hymenal barrier, the hymen can be seen to bulge outward. This is called hematocolpos. If sufficient pressure is present, the blood may back up into the uterus, fill the tubes and spill into the general peritoneal cavity, producing first a hematometra, then a hematosalpinx and hemoperitoneum. The periodic discomfort experienced by the girl may be due to distention of the uterus or tubes or spillage of blood from the tubes onto the peritoneal surface.

This is the simplest form of congenital obstruction to the vaginal outlet and is readily corrected by simple excision. This is a hospital procedure, for the accumulated blood is an excellent culture medium for pathogenic bacteria. Infection may carry serious implications. Complete evacuation is important. If this cannot be achieved by simple vaginal incision, it may be necessary to supplement vaginal exploration by combined abdominal exploration and drainage of the retained blood.

CONGENITAL ABSENCE OF THE VAGINA: ATRESIA

This may be either total or partial. In both instances other anomalies in the genitourinary tract are common findings. Complete urologic studies are needed. In partial absence of the vagina the vaginal obstruction may occur higher up in the canal behind a normal-appearing hymen.

The lower part of the vagina is usually completely absent, while there is rudimentary development of the upper portion of the canal. A uterus and cervix may or may not be present. If the uterus is present and functioning, the escape of blood can only be back into the uterus. A hematometra develops, but there is no bulging of the hymen, since the obstruction is higher up in the canal.

In most instances when there is complete atresia of the vaginal tract, there is also complete absence or, at the most, an incomplete development of the uterus. In the rare instance in which the uterus does preserve some function, the situation is akin to partial atresia. In complete absence of the vagina, dimpling of several centimeters may be apparent in the lower portion of what should be the vaginal canal. This lower portion of the canal does not have a müllerian origin. It has been suggested that the vagina does not develop, because the adjacent vaginal segments of the müllerian duct are completely arrested.

Where there is evidence of uterine function, one may elect to create a vaginal canal, provided the child is mature enough to carry out the repeated vaginal dilatations which are an essential part of the reconstructive program.

UTERINE MALFORMATIONS

There are many types of maldevelopment of the uterus itself. Some of these manifest themselves at puberty, while others are not apparent until pregnancy intervenes or seems to be impossible. At puberty we are chiefly concerned with the uterus which is either absent or shows evidence of hypoplasia. The range of maldevelopments extends from a total absence of the uterus through the rudimentary type and the infantile uterine state to that of the uterus only slightly smaller than normal.

The uterus is rarely completely absent, but clinical evidence of its presence can hardly be determined on rectal examination. When viewed from within the abdomen, there is usually a rudimentary vestigial remnant which might one day have become a

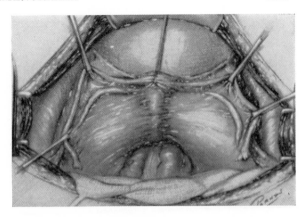

Fig. 18-2. Hypoplastic uterus, tubes and ovaries are outlined by instruments attached to the fundus and fallopian tubes. (From E. C. Jungck, R. B. Greenblatt and J. M. Manautou: Abnormal Sexual Development in Children. *Pediat. Clin. N. Amer.*, Vol. 5.)

uterus. This may be nothing more than a thickened midline strand of tissue resembling a ribbon strung between two cordlike structures with blind ends which are the rudimentary tubes. The true rudimentary uterus is simply a solid mass of muscle and fibrous tissue with varying degrees of abortive canalization. The entire block of tissue is not much more than 1 or 1½ inches in total bulk. At times the uterus does not develop beyond the size noted in the prepuberal state. The fundus and the cervix are of approximately equal length, and the tubes and ovaries are likewise undersized and maldeveloped (Fig. 18–2).

Treatment

Little can be accomplished by estrin therapy in the more severe forms of maldevelopment. There are varying degrees of the type of immature uterus designated as uterus pubescens. Although amenorrhea and sterility are common in girls with this kind of uterus, therapy is worth while, provided the condition is recognized early and the treatment is vigorous and persistent. The longer the hypoplasia is allowed, the more refractory it becomes to hormonal stimulation. The smaller the uterus, the less chance of achieving any lasting improvement.

Occasionally partial and, rarely, complete atresia of the cervix is found. Owing to the varying degrees of canalization, ranging from complete closure to partial block in the region of the isthmus, a hematometra or hematosalpinx may develop. Such conditions usually go unrecognized until the anticipated time of the menarche. The success from surgical intervention varies, depending on the severity of the underlying malformation.

OVARIAN AGENESIS

Disturbances in ovarian function resulting in amenorrhea vary in severity, depending on (1) basic alterations in the development of the ovary, or (2) how the other sexual hormones stimulate the ovary or balance the hormones secreted by it. The most extreme congenital maldevelopment is a complete absence of the ovaries (ovarian agenesis).

In common usage the term "ovarian agenesis," which, strictly interpreted, means total lack of anything resembling an ovary, is used interchangeably with "ovarian aplasia," which means failure of development of the ovarian anlage. On

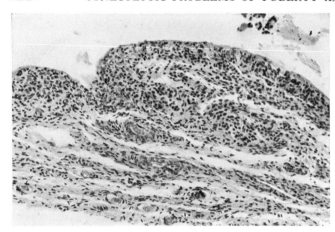

Fig. 18-3.   Ovarian aplasia in an infant, with connective tissue stroma devoid of cortical stroma, primordial ova or follicles.

abdominal exploration the uterus and tubes are present, though their appearance is infantile. In place of the ovary one often finds simply bilateral small, firm white streaks or ridges of tissue running out into the broad ligaments. Microscopically, the structures within this pseudo-ovary resemble those normally found in the ovarian hilus, but the stromal, granulosa and germ cells that combine to form the ovarian follicles are totally absent. Practically, we would appear, then, to be dealing with aplasia rather than agenesis (Fig. 18–3).

The main clinical characteristics of ovarian aplasia or agenesis are shortness of stature, accompanied by complete absence of development of the breasts and other secondary sex characteristics, despite the presence of the barest minimum of sexual hair. This is sometimes called ovarian dwarfism.

In many instances other congenital abnormalities are present. The combination of dwarfism with failure of genital development and amenorrhea and with the following defects, some of them congenital, comprises *Turner's syndrome:* (1) shortening of the neck and lowering of the hair line, with the appearance of a web extending from the bases of the ears to the midclavicular lines; (2) an increase in the normal carrying angle between the forearm and upper arm (cubitus valgus); (3) a broad, deep, shield-shaped chest with conspicuous lack of breast development; (4) late union of the epiphyses and retarded bone growth; (5) coarctation of the aorta and occasionally hypertension; (6) osteoporosis, secondary to estrogen lack; (7) precocious senility with fine wrinkling of the skin. (8) Sex chromatin studies now are claimed to show that at least half of the patients are genetic males.

The explanation of the main characteristic, shortness of stature, is not understood. In general these patients are remarkably uniform in height, with a range between 50 and 58 inches. This may be due to genetic or germ plasm defects; on the other hand, it is possible that the dwarfism may be related directly to estrin lack in the absence of functioning ovarian tissue. Estrin itself, except in certain cases in which the epiphyses have not united, has little effect on linear growth of bone. Estrin lack in this syndrome, however, may be the basic mechanism of failure of bone growth. If there is no estrin brake, the follicle-stimulating hormone either will be uninhibited and continue to be produced in excessive quantities or, as seems more likely from recent work, may be inadequately destroyed or metabolized. The excess of FSH is maintained at the expense of the luteinizing hormone. Because of the lack of the luteinizing hormone, the adrenal cortex receives inadequate stimulation, and fewer normal androgenic hormones, which are implicated in linear bone growth, are produced. The ketosteroid level is low, but not absent, while the FSH titer is abnormally high in ovarian aplasia.

Rarely, ovarian agenesis occurs in persons of normal or slightly increased height. It would appear that an arrest in ovarian development had occurred after normal structural growth, but that, except for the appearance of pubic hair, secondary sex characteristics are absent. The genetic influence is less apparent, for other congenital defects are not present.

Differential Diagnosis between the Ovarian and Hypopituitary Dwarf

Though these patients with ovarian aplasia are for the most part retarded in linear growth, they are husky, well nourished and strong, in contrast to the pituitary dwarf, who presents many of the other characteristics. The chief point in differential diagnosis between the ovarian and the pituitary dwarf is the presence of a high titer of FSH in ovarian agenesis and its complete absence in panhypopituitarism. Since all the pituitary gonadotropins are diminished or absent in the patient with pituitary deficiency, urinary assays for 17-ketosteroids show little or no excretion, in contrast to ovarian agenesis, in which they are diminished, but not absent. The same observations may be made from the insulin tolerance tests. In pituitary deficiency a failure to develop a hypoglycemic responsiveness is present, while insulin tolerance is normal in ovarian agenesis. Genetic factors are not operative in panhypopituitarism, and no associated congenital defects are noted. The x-ray appearance of bone differs in the two entities: (1) Osteoporosis is common with ovarian agenesis, but rare in the pituitary dwarf, (2) The bone age is somewhat retarded, and the epiphyses eventually unite in the ovarian dwarf, while interference of growth together with continuing failure of epiphysial union is noted when the abnormality is centered in the pituitary.

Treatment

Little can be done to alter the basic underlying difficulty in these patients. If the epiphyses are still ununited, some increase in bone growth may be obtained by giving estrin. The effect is an indirect one through pituitary release of LH and subsequent stimulation of the adrenal cortex. Psychologically, much can be done by stimulating the growth of secondary sex characteristics with the use of oral estrogen. The breasts develop, and growth of sexual hair increases. Along with these direct estrin effects, it is also possible to produce growth of the uterus, vagina and external genitalia. When the uterus has developed sufficiently, simulated menstrual periods can be produced by providing estrin-withdrawal bleeding. On a schedule of daily oral administration of any of the estrins, such as Estinyl, 0.5 mg., Premarin, 2.5 mg., or diethylstilbestrol, 2.0 mg., for 3 weeks, followed by one week without medication, bleeding will occur. If one chooses, progestin may be added for its nitrogen-sparing effect and the sense of well-being that follows, but the patient and her family should be informed that pregnancy is not possible. In general, the patient's response to this disappointment is one of complete acceptance, mixed with gratitude that the substituted hormones have made it possible to conform outwardly to the appearance of her normal contemporaries.

THE POLYCYSTIC OVARY AND THE STEIN-LEVENTHAL SYNDROME

This syndrome is gradually being recognized as one of the more common causes of either primary or secondary amenorrhea. Characteristically, the patient who has this syndrome has (1) increasing periods of amenorrhea, (2) on occasion excessive or prolonged flow of the anovulatory type, (3) obesity, (4) moderately severe hirsutism without virilization, (5) sterility, and finally (6) enlarged and polycystic ovaries. There are many variables, however, which are secondary to disturbances in endocrine function. Not all are true examples of the Stein-Leventhal type. It is important to pinpoint the basic defect, for successful therapy depends on the accuracy of the diagnosis.

What Information Do We Gather from the History?

Characteristically, either the adolescent girl has never menstruated, or secondary amenorrhea develops gradually. The usual history is that of a girl who, after a series of normal periods, begins to bleed excessively. As time goes on the periods become scanty and increasingly far apart. Commonly the scanty periods occur only two or three times a year. The amenorrheic phase progresses from two- to three- to six-month intervals and to complete cessation. When menstrual bleeding occurs, it is anovulatory.

In approximately 15 per cent the menstrual history is marked not by amenorrhea, but by irregular cycles, both in interval and duration, from the very onset. This bleeding is also anovulatory.

Unfortunately the adolescent girl, her family or her physician appears to have little concern about the abnormal menstrual pattern. The patients are usually so occupied by the demands for an education that they think little about it until they contemplate marriage or become married and are unable to have children. Sterility is therefore a major factor in bringing the patient to the physician. Relative infertility or actual sterility is a profound problem in patients who have this syndrome. If they have not been able to have children, they rapidly exhibit psychosomatic symptoms in the intensity of their desire to establish their femininity and to demonstrate their reproductive ability.

Finally, abdominal pain may be a symptom of the polycystic ovary syndrome. Because the follicles are prevented from developing normally, owing to the firm, thick capsule which surrounds the ovary in this condition, these patients have lower abdominal grinding pain in the earlier part of the cycle as the expanding follicles exert pressure against the ovarian capsule.

What Are the Typical Physical Findings?

In many instances the secondary amenorrhea is accompanied by obesity, the male type of hirsutism, retarded breast development and hypoplasia of the uterus (Fig. 18–4). The *sine qua non* for the diagnosis of the Stein-Leventhal type of ovary is the presence of bilateral ovarian enlargement. The obesity factor may interfere with an accurate estimation of ovarian size, but in the nonobese woman the enlarged ovaries are readily felt. Since the girls are frequently virginal as well as obese, it is possible to palpate the ovaries by rectum in only 50 per cent of cases when the syndrome is suspected. When felt, the ovaries are firm, oval, nontender and freely movable, lying adjacent to a small, underdeveloped uterus, which is usually in anterior position.

Not all patients who have the Stein-Leventhal syndrome show certain changes such as obesity, flat breasts or hirsutism, but polycystic ovaries are found in all cases.

The patient may be entirely feminine in appearance with only slightly under-developed breasts. In fact frequently the only thing that distinguishes this girl from her sister is the fact that she either has never menstruated or now has secondary amenorrhea. When classic symptoms are present, the diagnosis is immediately suspected. It should be considered in the completely feminine woman who has never menstruated. Since there is a high degree of infertility in patients with this syndrome, it is of the utmost importance to make the diagnosis and treat the girl early in her menstrual life. Hypoplasia of the uterus occurs in three quarters of the girls who have the Stein-Leventhal type of ovaries. If the condition is allowed to go untreated, the uterus will become increasingly more refractory to hormonal stimulation.

What Do the Ovaries Look Like at Operation or on Culdoscopy?

When seen at operation or through culdoscopy, the ovaries are symmetrically enlarged. In the true Stein-Leventhal syndrome they may be 3 or 4 times normal size, but rarely are they larger than 6.0 cm. in diameter. In patients who have moderate degrees of the polycystic ovary syndrome the ovaries are not greatly increased in size. Characteristically, they simulate the picture of an oyster with a smooth surface, grayish white in color, which is punctuated with small translucent areas that reflect the presence of small cysts lying beneath. No suggestion of corpora lutea, either new or old, can usually be found.

On cut section the observer is immediately impressed by the thick, heavy fibrous capsule of the ovary. Multiple small follicle cysts are seen lying directly beneath the

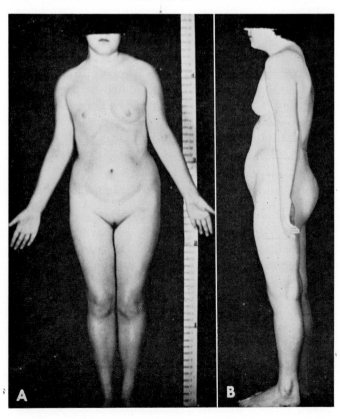

Fig. 18-4. A young woman with the Stein-Leventhal syndrome proved at operation. The deficiency in body hair, obesity about the hips, small breasts and underdeveloped secondary sex characteristics are seen in this condition, but are not in themselves diagnostic of it.

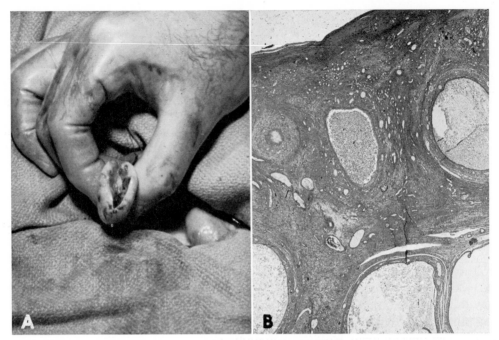

Fig. 18-5.   *A*, Polycystic ovary split longitudinally at operation. The thickened, smooth capsule is evident, as well as the numerous, clear fluid-filled cysts beneath. *B*, Under the thickened, superficial layer of ovarian cortical stroma are numerous follicle cysts lined by granulosa cells. One small cyst at the left margin has luteinized stroma. Excessive luteinization occurs in about 10 per cent of polycystic ovaries.

capsule, as well as throughout the deeper substance of the ovary (Fig. 18–5, *A*). Thorough search of the ovary reveals little evidence that any of these follicles ever went on to normal maturation. Apparently the life cycle of the follicle is thwarted by the thick capsule, and the follicle is prevented from developing normally and ovulating. Occasionally one finds evidence of stromal luteinization on microscopic examination, but only rarely is there an involuted corpus luteum (Fig. 18–5, *B*). Progestational activity is infrequently demonstrated in the endometrium, for the same reasons which prevent luteinization or corpus luteum formation in the ovary.

What Theories Are Advanced to Explain This Syndrome?

The actual cause of this syndrome is not known. In all probability it is not a congenital defect, although polycystic ovaries have been reported in newborn infants of diabetic mothers and in children with precocious puberty. It is unlikely that the thickened capsule is the result of inflammatory or degenerative changes in the ovary. There has been a suggestion in the literature that the thickening of the capsule is actually due to the presence of the multiple follicular cysts rather than being the cause of them. It should be noted that ovarian growth occurs, as well as cyst formation, and there is uniformly hyperplasia or fibrosis, or both, of the ovarian cortical stroma. It is this superficial thickening of cortical stroma which makes up the mechanical barrier that interferes with complete maturation of the ova.

Premenopausal women, or children who have primordial ova, develop polycystic ovaries upon excessive stimulation from the pituitary gonadotropins. On the other hand, women who are postmenopausal lack ova, and they respond to an analogous pituitary stimulation by forming solid nodular masses of hyperplastic stroma without any follicular cysts. Thus it would seem that polycystic ovaries in the young woman are akin to cortical stromal hyperplasia in the postmenopausal woman.

There appears, therefore, to be ample evidence, both clinical and laboratory, that the ovarian changes are due to disorders or *excess of pituitary gonadotropic hormone secretion.* Pituitary basophilism, polycystic ovaries and fibrocystic disease of the breast go hand in hand. In both animals and man the basophilic cells of the pituitary, which are considered to be the source of gonadotropic hormone production, are increased in polycystic disease of the ovary. Experimentally, it has been observed repeatedly that adult women treated with gonadotropins of pituitary origin, chorionic gonadotropin or pregnant mares' serum (largely containing FSH) in attempts to produce ovulation fail to ovulate, but they do form large and multiple ovarian follicular cysts.

Recently investigators have put forth the theory that it is the LH or ICSH fraction in the pituitary gonadotropins that produces the multiple follicular cysts and ovarian enlargement. They postulate that a continuous production of ICSH stimulates the ovarian medulla to form and secrete androgen. This in turn prevents the pituitary either from elaborating or releasing FSH, thereby preventing normal gonadotropic stimulation of the ovary.

Several other theories have been advanced to explain the ovarian enlargement and follicle development without ovulation. It has been said that the circulatory pattern in and around the developing follicles differs from the normal. It is also possible that the basic defect may lie in the ovary itself. The trigger mechanism for normal ovulation may rest in the ovary and not in the pituitary, or the ovary may simply be so responsive to pituitary gonadotropic stimulation that it responds excessively by increasing its bulk. Along the same line it has been suggested that ovulation failure occurs because the theca cone does not function properly. This would help to explain why the patient does not ovulate in the presence of apparently normal pituitary gonadotropic levels.

Finally, one must consider the possibility that the adrenal may be implicated. The hirsutism observed in about half of the patients who have the polycystic ovary syndrome may be due to the androgen secreted by the cells of the ovarian medulla, but it may also be due to hyperactivity of the adrenal cortex. In all probability, however, patients who have adrenal dysfunction associated with ovarian enlargement and who are improved by therapy designed to suppress adrenal activity are cases of a hormonal imbalance that closely simulates, but is not truly that of, the polycystic ovary syndrome.

All these theories are interesting, but most of them are unconfirmed. The theoretical concepts receive no particular help from laboratory hormonal studies, for in the majority of cases of the polycystic ovary syndrome the urinary FSH, 17-ketosteroids, pregnanediol and pregnanetriol excretions are normal, and the LH studies are difficult to perform and evaluate.

What Is the Differential Diagnosis?

It is of the utmost importance that the diagnosis of polycystic ovary syndrome be firmly established. There are a wide variety of endocrinologic entities that closely simulate it. The important thing to remember is that a simple operation, which removes wedge-shaped sections from the ovary, will restore normal ovarian function, complete with ovulation and the chance for reproduction. It will not be effective if the operation is performed for other than the polycystic ovary syndrome.

HISTORY AND PHYSICAL EXAMINATION.   The history and physical findings provide useful information. For example, the most common condition which is apt to be confused with the polycystic ovary complex is *metropathia haemorrhagica*. This functional disorder of menstruation, associated with anovulatory bleeding, is extremely common in the late teens and early twenties. This is also the age when the polycystic ovary syndrome is commonly found. In both, we find obese young girls who are either amenorrheic or have spells of profuse and prolonged periods after a preliminary phase of amenorrhea or oligomenorrhea. Approximately 15 per cent of patients who have the clinical history and some of the findings commonly associated with the Stein-Leventhal syndrome will have excessive bleeding rather than amenorrhea.

The history is helpful in distinguishing between the two, because the patient with the functional metropathic disorder has usually had a normal menstrual pattern in the past. Not infrequently the amenorrhea follows episodes of emotional unrest or other stress situations. The physical examination will show a normal-sized uterus and ovaries, in contrast to the polycystic ovary syndrome, in which the uterus is on the small side and the ovaries are palpably enlarged. Simple hormone substitution, giving estrin and progestin in cyclic fashion, will usually correct the abnormal vaginal bleeding pattern if it is due to functional cause. In fact, the correction will probably occur automatically if nothing is done. It is this very fact, however, that makes it necessary to distinguish between the functional vaginal bleeder and the girl who bleeds with the polycystic ovary syndrome. There is a tendency upon the part of the family and the local physician to let nature take its course and try not to interfere. This may be a serious error.

When the process is permitted to continue, there appears to be a progressive tendency toward increasing hirsutism and atrophy of the breast and uterus. The ovarian changes in the polycystic ovary syndrome continue and may reach such a state as to be irreversible unless some attempt is made to restore the ovary to normal function. The problem of restoring normal ovulatory cycles and fertility to such a neglected patient is formidable. To delay diagnosis and the institution of treatment in girls who are suspected of having this syndrome, whether it is accompanied by menorrhagia or amenorrhea, is therefore unwise and may result in irreparable damage.

LABORATORY TESTS.   The laboratory can be most helpful in pinpointing the diagnosis. The majority of cases will show normal urinary values for 17-ketosteroids, pregnanediol, pregnanetriol and gonadotropic hormone excretions. The 17-hydroxycorticoids are either normal or slightly depressed. There is an absence of diurnal shifts in the basal body temperature recordings, as well as a lack of endometrial secretory phase on biopsy studies. The endometrium is almost invariably in the proliferative phase. The vaginal smears show estrogen effect. Further help may be attained by (1) a scout film of the abdomen to detect ovarian enlargement, (2) pneumoperitoneum to sharpen the detail of the ovarian cysts seen by x-ray, (3) culdoscopy or peritoneoscopy for direct views of the ovary, (4) x-ray studies of the sella turcica to rule out a possible pituitary adenoma.

Recently another laboratory test has been introduced that may prove to be useful in detecting the proper candidates for wedge resection of the ovary. Electrovaginal potential readings suggest that a normally menstruating woman shows cyclic fluctuations at varying times during the cycle. These fluctuations are absent in the patient who has the polycystic ovary syndrome.

One should not neglect to rule out the thyroid as the cause of amenorrhea and sterility. Many women with thyroid dysfunction are obese and have varying degrees of hirsutism. A basal metabolism, serum protein-bound iodine or radio-iodine uptake study should be a regular part of the laboratory investigation. If the basic malfunction is ovarian, the tests will give normal results. There are obviously wide variations in the degree of ovarian change, both gross and microscopic. The microscopic changes are discussed in Part III. The large cysts noted by Stein are relatively rare, while the oyster-like ovaries showing moderate enlargement and multiple small follicle cysts are fairly common.

OVARIAN VERSUS ADRENAL PATHOGENESIS. The chief source of difficulty in the differential diagnosis is the distinction that must be made between pathologic alterations that are primarily ovarian and the simulated conditions which are due to adrenal dysfunction. The mere fact that approximately half of all the patients with the polycystic ovary syndrome have hirsutism points up the need for distinguishing between the two.

The typical picture of the Stein-Leventhal syndrome combines the male type of hirsutism and amenorrhea in an unmarried adolescent girl who either has never menstruated or does so only once or twice a year. She may or may not be obese. The hirsutism may come from adrenal hyperfunction or stem from the hilar or medullary cells in the ovary. It is possible, however, for the girl to have the male type of hirsutism and amenorrhea with a perfect feminine figure, and breast and uterine development. The diagnosis of Stein-Leventhal syndrome depends upon the findings of enlarged polycystic ovaries, but unfortunately they can be felt only about 50 per cent of the time. In the other 50 per cent one would have to be suspicious of adrenocortical hyperactivity.

The differential diagnosis is established by (*a*) laboratory evidence of elevation of the urinary 17-ketosteroids, (*b*) administration of 50 mg. of cortisone daily for 4 to 6 weeks. If the condition is due to adrenal hyperplasia, the ketosteroid excretion level returns to normal, and ovulatory periods return. In the true Stein-Leventhal syndrome the urinary 17-ketosteroid levels are normal, and the menstrual pattern is not altered by cortisone.

VIRILISM. It should be noted that hirsutism is not synonymous with virilism or masculinization. The patient may have underdeveloped breasts, some of the male habitus, hirsutism and amenorrhea in the polycystic ovary syndrome, but she does not have the male musculature or clitoral enlargement. The hirsutism may be due to genetic cause without abnormality in either the ovary or the adrenal. It is also possible for the girl to have moderate adrenal hyperplasia, enough to produce elevated urinary 17-ketosteroid levels and create anovulatory bleeding or amenorrhea without any of the other signs of virilism.

ADRENOGENITAL SYNDROME AND ADRENAL TUMOR. When the girl has enlargement of the clitoris or congenital maldevelopment of the external genitalia together with the other signs of polycystic ovary syndrome, she has either pseudo-hermaphroditism or adrenal tumor. The ovaries, if they can be felt, will not be enlarged. Differentiation between the congenital or acquired type of adrenal hyperplasia, changes due to an adrenal tumor, and the polycystic ovary syndrome is best established by laboratory tests and a clinical trial of cortisone.

The urinary 17-ketosteroid levels will be elevated in both the adrenogenital syndrome and adrenal hyperfunction due to hyperplasia or tumor, but will be normal in the polycystic ovary syndrome. The pregnanetriol excretion will be elevated in adrenocortical tumor, but this abnormality will be absent in pseudohermaphroditism and the Stein-Leventhal syndrome. The final differential point comes after the administration of cortisone. With adrenal tumor, cortisone will not lower the level of the urinary 17-ketosteroid excretion.

CUSHING'S DISEASE AND PITUITARY ADENOMA.   The obese, hirsute, amenorrheic or infertile female may also have either Cushing's disease, Cushing's syndrome or a functioning basophilic adenoma of the pituitary. The clinical characteristics and laboratory findings are discussed elsewhere (Chap. 19). They are mentioned here simply to be sure that they are considered and ruled out by appropriate means.

OVARIAN TUMORS AND HYPERTHECOSIS.   Finally, hirsutism may be caused by ovarian tumors, such as hilar cell tumors, adrenal rest tumors and arrhenoblastomas. All are rare, and all are associated with virilization as well as hirsutism. Arrhenoblastomas, in addition to being unusual tumors, are infrequently found in adolescence. Hilar cell tumors usually appear after the age of forty years. In any case they should either be felt on pelvic examination or be seen by culdoscopy. Hyperplasia with excessive luteinization of the ovary (hyperthecosis) can cause hirsutism, and this will be discussed later in Part III, since it would seem to be a more advanced phase in the evolution of the polycystic ovary.

The Final Diagnosis

Since many endocrine abnormalities will produce the same gross and microscopic pathologic picture in the ovary, it is obvious that there is nothing pathognomonic about the finding of polycystic ovaries. This means that polycystic ovaries occur in the absence of other aspects of the Stein-Leventhal syndrome. Endocrine dysfunction may accompany polycystic ovaries and also produce obesity, hirsutism, hypoplasia of the uterus and retarded breast development. The diagnosis of the Stein-Leventhal syndrome is achieved by exclusion of other possible causes and by noting a combination of elements that increases the likelihood of this being the correct evaluation.

The adolescent girl or young woman in her early twenties who has the polycystic ovary syndrome will frequently have a mild degree of hirsutism, hypoplasia of the uterus and bilaterally enlarged polycystic ovaries. If the patient does have menstrual periods at all, the bleeding will be anovulatory, and if she is married, sterility may be one of the major complaints. The basic fault in this respect appears to be ovarian, for the urinary FSH, 17-ketosteroid levels and the basal metabolism are normal. Lateral x-ray films of the skull are negative.

The diagnosis is therefore suspected from the history and physical findings, but must be confirmed by culdoscopy, special roentgenography or abdominal exploration.

What Is the Treatment of Polycystic Ovary Syndrome?

The basic aim in therapy is the restoration of a normal ovulatory menstrual cycle which will allow the young girl to menstruate and to become pregnant. This can satisfactorily be accomplished by wedge resection of the ovary if the patient actually has the syndrome. If the urinary ketosteroids are not elevated, all other endocrine dysfunctional causes are ruled out and culdoscopy reveals the typical picture of bilaterally enlarged ovaries, abdominal exploration may eventually be indicated. Nevertheless there appear to be enough patients with this syndrome, particularly those that have widely separated but still ovulatory menstrual periods, who respond to corticosteroid therapy by a restoration of cyclic bleeding to warrant a six-month trial period before resorting to abdominal exploration.

The following corticosteroid drugs may be used: (*a*) Prednisone, 5 to 10 mg. per day; (*b*) hydrocortisone, 25 to 40 mg. per day; (*c*) cortisone, 37.5 to 50 mg. per day. Along with this type of therapy it will be advisable to put the patient on a low salt, high protein, low carbohydrate diet. In any endocrine abnormality, thyroid hormone supplementation to improve the end-organs' metabolic response is always a helpful adjunct to therapy.

If the patient does not respond to corticoid therapy, abdominal exploration is indicated, particularly if the culdoscopic examination shows bilaterally enlarged ovaries. When cyclic bleeding reappears and continues under corticoid substitution, the therapeutic regimen can be extended for a year or more. At the end of that time the patient should be allowed to get along on her own, without help from the corticoid hormones.

WEDGE RESECTION.   This is a simple operation which calls for incision into the ovary with removal of a wedge-shaped section of ovarian tissue down into the hilar region. The incision may be placed longitudinally or transversely. Multiple small follicular cysts within the substance of the ovary are punctured. The ovarian capsule is then restored with interrupted catgut sutures (Fig. 18–6).

Why Is the Operation Effective?   Why this simple operation is effective generally is not known. Reducing the tension within the ovarian substance is perhaps one reason, but one would expect the situation to recur if this were the case. Once the normal balance has been restored and ovulatory cycles return, recurrences are unusual. It seems most likely that it is actually the reduction in ovarian bulk that is

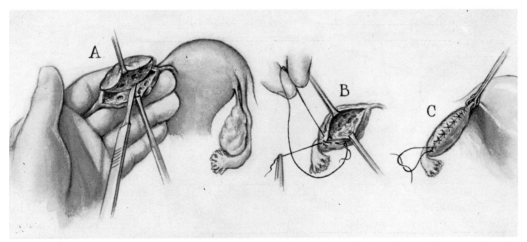

Fig. 18-6.   Wedge resection of the ovary for the Stein-Leventhal syndrome. The ovary has the characteristic appearance of multiple small follicular cysts and a heavy, thick cortical covering. Reduction of the bulk of the ovarian substance may correct the condition. *A*, The wedge-shaped section is excised. *B*, A Babcock clamp steadies the ovarian ligament medially, and the edges of the cavity are held apart with Allis forceps while the raw edges of the ovary are approximated by a suture which includes the base of the cavity. *C*, The running suture is completed by returning to its point of origin. Since the pathologic state is always bilateral, the procedure must be repeated on the opposite side.

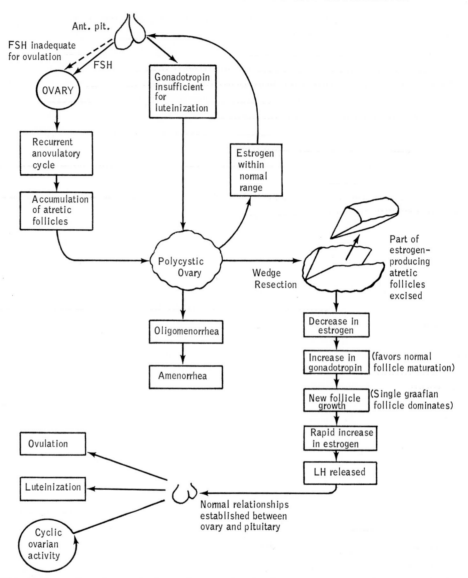

Fig. 18-7. One theory of why wedge resection is effective in the restoration of ovulatory cycles implicates an inadequacy or imbalance of pituitary FSH and LH. Present hormone studies do not refute this explanation, among various possibilities suggested.

the important factor, particularly if one assumes that the ovaries of these patients are abnormally responsive to the pituitary gonadotropins. The proponents of this theory point to the fact that (*a*) the reduction of the total ovarian mass by wedge resection of only one of the polycystic ovaries will frequently result in the reappearance of cyclic ovulatory bleeding; (*b*) corticosteroid therapy will sometimes restore normal cycles, in the absence of elevated urinary 17-ketosteroid excretion or wedge resection of the restricting ovarian capsule. This would seem to suggest that the ovary is abnormally sensitive to normal pituitary gonadotropic secretion (Fig. 18–7).

Recently there have been suggestions that the medullary portion of the ovary should receive the attention of the surgeon, with less emphasis on excision of the restraining capsule. It is suggested that the enlarged medullary portion of the ovary explains the increase in ovarian size, and it is pointed out that this tissue is most likely to contain remnants of testicle left behind in the differentiation of the embryonic gonad. Such tissue might then elaborate androgen and serve to inhibit the normal stimulating effect of the pituitary gonadotropins as well as contributing to the production of hirsutism. Some postulate that the embryonic testicular rests are genetic in origin, and in fact the ovary in the Stein-Leventhal syndrome is a form of ovotestis.

Against both theories—(*a*) abnormal sensitivity of ovarian tissue to gonadotropic stimulation and (*b*) embryonic testicular remnants in the medullary portion of the ovary—is the fact that in the past satisfactory results were obtained by splitting the ovary and turning the halves back to back without removing any tissue at all.

Whatever the basic cause and however the procedure is done, there are few surgical operations that produce such gratifying results from such a minor procedure, provided the patient has been properly selected. One can afford to take the time to perform the essential tests, for the success of the operation is closely linked to the accuracy of the diagnosis. Excellent results may be expected in at least 75 per cent of patients operated on, with a chance of pregnancy in 50 per cent of those who are married and desire children. In addition to the restoration of the ovulatory cycle, there is improvement in feminization in the group in which retardation in breast development has been noted. The uterus becomes of normal size, and obesity and acne disappear. The hirsutism, on the other hand, remains essentially unchanged, but does not increase. The improvement in mental attitude is dramatic, and there is far less frustration and depression.

It should be noted in the 25 per cent who have less than satisfactory results that some further improvement may be forthcoming from the use of corticosteroid therapy.

Causative Factors in Amenorrhea Outside the Endocrine Field

Before attempting to attribute the cause to endocrine malfunction and instituting therapy for either primary or secondary amenorrhea, we must consider such factors as obesity, disturbances in thyroid function, malnutrition and psychic disorders, all of which may play a role. These considerations are of prime importance, for endocrine therapy will be ineffective until they have been corrected, whatever the type of amenorrhea.

OBESITY

The adolescent girl who fails to develop a normal menstrual cycle at puberal age is frequently overweight. Too often both the physician and the parent attribute obesity to a disturbance in glandular function. Rarely is excess body fat believed due to any abnormality in the secretion of the pituitary hormones. Cushing's disease is one rare exception.

It must be kept in mind that a sudden alteration in the deposition of fat is one of the earliest manifestations of puberty, preceding the acceleration of growth of bone and muscle by nearly a year. It follows rapidly on the first appearance of the gonadotropic hormones in the urine, which customarily takes place at approximately eleven years. The responsible factor has not been clearly determined. Estrin and the adrenal corticoids have both been implicated. When excessive fat deposits are evident, the fault seems to lie with the adrenal corticoids, for urinary assays of the corticoids are elevated without any corresponding elevation in the estrogens. The important fact to remember is that a tendency to increased deposition of fat is normal for a girl at this age.

The young girl who is excessively overweight in the great majority of instances does not have glandular imbalance, but simply takes in an excess of calories over and above the requirements for growth and energy. To be sure, the growing child needs protein to build both muscles and bone, but calories in excess of need will be stored as fat whether they are ingested as carbohydrate or protein. The child should be encouraged to eat, but not to excess. The overeating habit is too easily acquired and too hard to break. As the child becomes more overweight, she becomes increasingly disinclined to burn off the excess caloric intake through exercise and takes a greater interest in the sedentary life. As a result less energy is expended, and a vicious circle develops. The fact that fewer, rather than more, calories are needed is not apparent to her.

Constitutional factors, which may be inherited, do appear to play a role, for obesity seems to occur with regularity in certain families. It is hard to decide whether the obesity is due to the fact that the child may have inherited a large appetite and an appreciation of high caloric foods or whether she is conditioned by the eating habits set by her parents. The basic fact remains the same, for these patients take in more calories than they need for energy or growth.

It is a well known fact that some people, including adolescent girls, tend to put on weight more easily on the same diet than others, but this fact cannot be attributed to any definite abnormality in fat metabolism. The cause has not been traced to a hormonal imbalance. It is true that the obese patient may maintain her weight for some time after being placed on a low caloric intake. The exact mechanism is not clear, but it seems to have something to do with an increased tendency to store water in the tissues.

The fact that the adolescent child may overeat because she is unhappy or maladjusted should not be overlooked. A difficult home situation may create conflicts, frustrations or jealousies. She may feel that she is unpopular with her contemporaries at school or play. Failing to find emotional outlet in normal fields of expression, she seeks and receives gratification by eating to excess. This in turn creates a vicious cycle, for lack of coordination and strength, together with an awkwardness, makes participation in sports increasingly difficult and distasteful. She retreats further into a sedentary life which requires less expenditure of energy. Much can be done for this patient if the cause of her unhappiness can be discovered and the conflicts eliminated. Flattery may be a more successful approach than any attempts to coerce the patient into eating less. The measure of success will be determined by the degree of cooperation she shows in following a balanced reducing diet.

The probable explanation of why the obese adolescent girl has a delayed menarche or subsequently has amenorrhea may be that the gonadal hormones are soluble in fat. The girl is producing normal amounts of hormones for her age, but they are somewhat taken up and stored in excess body fat. So trapped, they do not have an opportunity to assume their normal role in stimulating the growth of the genital organs and the development of secondary sex characteristics.

As soon as the girl begins to lose weight she develops sexually at a much faster rate. To the hormones she is producing regularly are now added those released by the loss of fat, and a rapid acceleration in sexual maturation takes place.

The essential consideration in treatment is a sensible weight reduction program rather than one of hormone substitutes. Clinically, this has proved a highly effective form of therapy. It is a basic element as a preliminary to other forms of therapy.

REFERENCES

Amenorrhea

Kuhlen, R. G.: *The Psychology of Adolescent Development.* New York, Harper & Brothers, 1952.
Rakoff, A. E.: Studies on High Dosage Progesterone Therapy of Amenorrhea. *Am. J. Obst. & Gynec.,* 51: 480, 1946.
Wilkins, L., and Fleischmann, W.: Sexual Infantilism in Females. *J. Clin. Endocrinol.,* 4: 306, 1944.

Stein-Leventhal Syndrome

Allen, W. M., and Woolf, R. B.: Medullary Resection of the Ovaries in the Stein-Leventhal Syndrome *Am. J. Obst. & Gynec.,* 77: 826, 1959.
Evans, T. N., and Riley, G. M.: Polycystic Ovarian Disease (Stein-Leventhal Syndrome). *Obst. & Gynec.,* 12: 168, 1958.
Ingersoll, F. M., and McArthur, J. W.: Longitudinal Studies of Gonodatropin Excretion in the Stein-Leventhal Syndrome. *Am. J. Obst. & Gynec.,* 77: 795, 1959.
Kaufman, R. H., Abbott, J. P., and Wall, J. A.: The Endometrium before and after Wedge Resection of the Ovaries in the Stein-Leventhal Syndrome. *Am. J. Obst. & Gynec.,* 77: 1271, 1959.
Keettel, W. C., Bradbury, J. T., and Stoddard, F. J.: Observations on the Polycystic Ovary Syndrome. *Am. J. Obst. & Gynec.,* 73: 954, 1957.
Leventhal, M. L.: The Stein-Leventhal Syndrome. *Am. J. Obst. & Gynec.,* 76: 825, 1958.
Sommers, S. C., and Wadman, P. J. : Pathogenesis of Polycystic Ovaries. *Am. J. Obst. & Gynec.,* 72: 160, 1956.
Stein, I. F.: Ultimate Results of Bilateral Ovarian Wedge Resections: 25 Year Follow up. *Internat. J. Fertil.,* 1: 333, 1956.
Idem: The Stein-Leventhal Syndrome. *New England J. Med.,* 259: 420, 1958.

Chapter 19

Common Endocrine
Causes of Amenorrhea

DISTURBANCES IN THYROID FUNCTION

DISTURBANCES in thyroid function are frequent in the patient with amenorrhea in the adolescent period. The most common association occurs with a decrease in thyroid activity. The hyperthyroid state, which may explain secondary amenorrhea in the older age group, appears in only 1 per cent of patients in adolescence and has little practical significance in evaluating the immediate problem.

THYROID HYPOFUNCTION AND OBESITY

On the mistaken impression that the obese child suffers from some glandular disturbance, it has become a common error to attribute excess weight to malfunction of the thyroid gland. This impression derives false support from the fact that the basal metabolism, figured by surface area standards calculated from the patient's actual weight and height, is often found to be low in the obese patient. Calculation of the basal metabolic rate on such a basis is bound to give an erroneously low reading. The reason for this is that, as the weight increases, the surface area does not increase in proportion to the increase in body tissue mass. As much as 30 per cent of the total body weight may be made up of fat, which has a notoriously low metabcli turnover. It is far better to calculate the basal metabolic rate of these obese adolescent girls on the basis of standard height tables. If the findings do not coincide with the clinical impression, the extent of thyroid deficiency can always be checked with the determination of the protein-bound iodine level as well as serum cholesterol. Since hypothyroidism in adolescence is intimately connected with bone growth, any deficiency may be evident in x-ray studies of the hand and wrist. Retarded skeletal development, when compared to chronologic age, should be regarded with suspicion. There is general agreement among the investigators that thyroid and pituitary deficiency are not commonly the causes of obesity.

Though the clinician seems to have firmly entrenched in his mind the fact that thyroid deficiency and obesity go hand in hand, he fails to recognize that the cold-skinned, thin, slowly maturing adolescent may also have thyroid deficiency. Such patients often have, in addition, such signs and findings as short stature with a minimal amount of subcutaneous tissue, intolerance to cold, poor appetite, retarded sex development, thin eyebrows and retarded structural growth, as evidenced by a bone age two or three years behind the chronologic age. The deficiency in thyroid activity is confirmed by a low protein-bound iodine level and elevated serum cholesterol. Such patients should be given a therapeutic trial with thyroid extract.

The truly hypothyroid adolescent may appear to be obese, but the increased weight is sometimes due to myxedematous fluid and not to deposit of fat. The subcutaneous tissues are loose and flabby, and the skin has a characteristic pallor. The hypothyroid child is stunted in growth, as shown by the failure of the long bones and skull to develop. This is accompanied by a delay in eruption of teeth and maturation of the epiphyses.

When the obese pubescent girl responds to a sensible weight reduction program, but fails to menstruate, thyroid substitution therapy is a rational form of treatment. We have pointed out that a normally functioning thyroid gland is essential to proper gonadal function. Thyroid deficiency may arise in two ways: (1) It may be due to failure of the anterior pituitary to release enough TSH to stimulate the thyroid gland to produce, store or release thyroxin or triiodothyronine. (2) Proper peripheral metabolism of thyroxin at the cellular level is essential for cell growth and survival. This metabolism may be incomplete.

Treatment

Dramatic results can be expected in the treatment of amenorrhea from thyroid replacement therapy when there is a true thyroid deficiency or hypothyroid state. In the presence of the clinical criteria for thyroid deficiency, such as lethargy, intolerance to cold weather, dryness of the skin and hair, loss of hair from the pubic area, axilla or lateral aspects of the eyebrows, the indications for thyroid therapy are present. When the clinical suspicion is backed by the laboratory findings of a low basal metabolic rate, protein-bound iodine or radioactive iodine uptake, together with a slightly elevated serum cholesterol level and a flat glucose tolerance curve (increased tolerance to glucose), the diagnosis of true hypothyroidism is established.

The true hypothyroid patient is very sensitive to thyroid replacement. To gain the optimal benefit the dose should be slightly below that of the tolerance or toxic dose for that person. It is usually given in the form of USP thyroid extract or thyroglobin. Recently a crystalline preparation of thyroid, L-triiodothyronine, has been made available, which seems to have qualities superior to those offered by either of the older medications. The chemical composition of the synthetic preparation is so constant that more predictable results can be obtained. It achieves its maximum clinical effect in forty-eight to seventy-two hours, in contrast to USP thyroid or thyroglobin, which may take two or three weeks. Moreover it is rapidly eliminated, thereby minimizing the toxic effect of possible overdosage. This is important, for the girl with true thyroid deficiency is extremely sensitive to the administration of thyroid. To produce the same effect that one may expect from 100 mg. of USP thyroid or thyroglobin, one would use 100 gammas of triiodothyronine.

THE HYPOMETABOLIC STATE

Varying degrees of thyroid deficiency are apparent in adolescence as well as in later years. Some of the clinical features are often lacking, and the patients seem simply tired and sluggish. Frequently thyroid is given without proper clinical or laboratory confirmation of any deficiency. The results may or may not be rewarding. Probably no drastic change is produced by thyroid given in this manner. At most the normal production of thyroxin is suppressed in proportion to the amount substituted. Thyroid extract should not, however, be used indiscriminately.

Occasionally the patient who has a few but not all of the symptoms of true thyroid lack simply reflects a generally lowered metabolic state, which affects all the endocrine glands. The laboratory findings will show a low 17-ketosteroid excretion as well as a low basal metabolic rate, elevated serum cholesterol level and flat glucose tolerance test curve. Not infrequently the protein-bound iodine and the radioactive uptake studies are normal. In this generalized hypometabolic state the final breakdown from thyroxin to the end-product triiodothyronine does not occur. Triiodothyronine is the basic thyroid hormone which is thought responsible for accelerating the metabolism of various living cells. For this reason the standard preparations, such as USP thyroid, may not be as successful as they are in the patient with true thyroid deficiency. In the adolescent girl with generally low metabolism the best results are obtained by the use of triiodothyronine.

In the adolescent with amenorrhea one may wish to try a combination of USP thyroid and L-triiodothyronine to reduce the toxic side effects from either hormone and improve the therapeutic response. A combination of two thirds the tolerated dose of each drug has been recommended.

DISTURBANCES IN FUNCTION OF THE ADRENAL GLAND

Evidence of combined ovarian and adrenal dysfunction may be traced to disease, congenital malformation or tumor of either the pituitary or the hypothalamus, but certain syndromes are known in which the primary abnormality lies in the adrenal cortex itself. The syndromes which manifest themselves by symptoms of dysfunction of the adrenal hormones are (1) the adrenogenital syndrome, (2) virilizing tumors of the adrenal cortex, and (3) Cushing's syndrome.

The Adrenogenital Syndrome

This syndrome is caused by hyperactive secretion of the adrenal cortex, due either to hyperplasia of this portion of the gland or tumor in this region.

The basic underlying pathologic physiology of the adrenogenital syndrome, aside from the genetic factor, is the lack of cortisone. For some reason the synthesis of 17-alpha-hydroxyprogesterone into hydrocortisone is blocked. Since it is not used to form cortisone, it is excreted in the form of pregnanetriol. As a result of cortisone lack, the anterior pituitary puts out more ACTH. The luteinizing hormone is also produced in excess, while the FSH remains normal. Both the LH and ACTH stimulate the adrenal cortex to put out an excess of the masculinizing hormones. The body tissues and end-organs respond to the adrenogenic stimulation by masculinization. The excessive androgen is metabolized and excreted as urinary 17-ketosteroids. The excretion is usually high in this syndrome, running from two to ten times the normal amount.

Congenital versus the Acquired Type of Adrenogenital Syndrome

Although the adrenogenital syndrome may be acquired, it is in most instances associated with a congenital defect. This is frequently recognizable at birth and in very early childhood and has been described in Chapter 6. The diagnosis of the congenital form is based on the presence of developmental abnormalities, together with clinical evidence and laboratory proof of an overproduction of androgen. In the immediate postnatal period there may be profound disturbances in electrolyte balance, associated with insufficient production of the salt- and water-controlling adrenal hormones.

The congenital type of the adrenogenital syndrome produces a classic picture which is readily recognized. The acquired forms of the symptom complex are less obvious.

CONGENITAL TYPE.   With androgen in excess from the prenatal state on, the external evidence of its activity is increasingly apparent. The congenital defects are obvious at once, particularly the clitoral enlargement and fusion of the labial folds. At approximately the age of five years the child begins to develop pubic hair, and later, axillary hair. The voice deepens and acne appears, but except for these obvious departures from the normal the child seems reasonably feminine in childhood.

As adolescence approaches, the full effect of overproduction of androgen is increasingly apparent. The male characteristics then predominate. The breasts never develop, and the menstrual periods fail to appear. The epiphyses, however, fuse, and these patients are usually strong and muscular, as well as short in stature. The male distribution of hair is noted in abundance on the thighs, legs, abdomen, breast and face. The shift toward the masculine side is completed as the patient's voice becomes increasingly deep and she develops a male aggressiveness of manner.

HOW DOES THE ACQUIRED TYPE OF ADRENOGENITAL SYNDROME DIFFER FROM THE CONGENITAL TYPE?   The signs and symptoms of the adrenogenital syndrome vary, depending on the degree of abnormal stimulation of the adrenal cortex and the need for cortisone production. The child who develops hyperactivity of the adrenal cortex after birth (acquired type) commonly has a much milder form, and full recognition may be in abeyance until the onset of puberty.

After puberty the adolescent child may develop hirsutism, acne and seborrhea, together with scanty or delayed menstruation. The secondary sex characteristics are present, but with diminished development of breasts and hips. The urinary 17-ketosteroid levels may be elevated, but at times they are within normal limits. These girls either have mild degrees of adrenocortical hyperplasia or are potential candidates to develop the adrenogenital syndrome later. Since they are borderline cases, one should be suspicious of the girl with mild degrees of acne and hirsutism, who is infertile and continues to have anovulatory cycles, though with only minor variations in the timing of the periods.

What Is the Treatment of the Adrenogenital Syndrome?

The problems of therapy in the congenital type discovered at birth have been discussed in Section I. When the diagnosis is made late in childhood or early adolescence, treatment should be directed along two lines: (1) the surgical correction of any anatomic defects, and (2) the suppression of the androgenic effects.

Although these girls have some of the male attributes, they are genetically

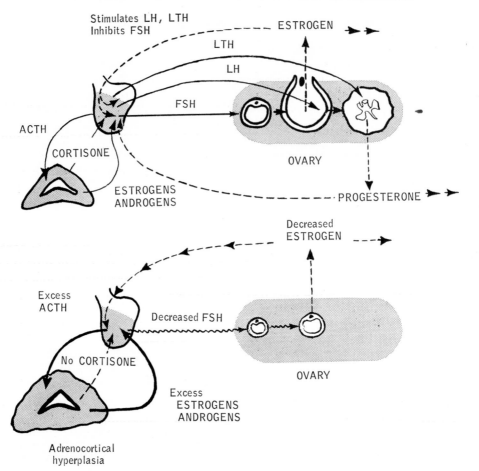

Fig. 19-1.   The abnormal endocrine metabolism of the adrenogenital type of adrenocortical hyperplasia (*lower*) compared to the normal interrelations of pituitary, ovary and adrenal cortex (*above*). In the absence of cortisone secretion pituitary ACTH is increased. One consequence is excessive adrenocortical production of androgens and estrogens. Another result is reduced FSH secretion and ovarian stimulation to secrete estrogen.

female. Simple surgical measures, such as excision of the clitoris and reconstruction of the vagina, are readily accomplished. After the plastic surgery the attention in therapy should be directed toward depression of function of the overactive adrenal cortex (Fig. 19–1).

This may be done by giving corticoid therapy in the form of cortisone, 12.5 mg. 3 times daily, hydrocortisone, 10 mg., also 3 times daily, or Prednisone, 2.5 mg., 4 times a day, as oral medication. There are few side effects, and in most instances restriction of salt intake is not essential. The actual size of the dose depends on how readily the 17-ketosteroids are suppressed or how rapidly menstruation and ovulation return. The choice of the individual drug to be given matters little. Prednisone is the choice if there is any tendency to store fluid, for it is said to increase salt excretion.

After the suppression of adrenocorticoid activity, oral estrogens should be given to help the girl in developing the secondary sex characteristics, which have been held in abeyance by the action of excessive androgen. The success of cortisone therapy in suppressing the androgenic effects can be measured by urinary assay of 17-ketosteroids and pregnanetriol excretion.

CUSHING'S SYNDROME

Since Cushing's syndrome is associated with either a tumor or hyperplasia of the adrenal cortex, the presenting symptoms may closely simulate those of the adreno-genital syndrome of the acquired type. For the most part, however, Cushing's syndrome is rare in early childhood. When a suspicious train of symptoms appears, in children it is far more likely to be due to an adrenal tumor than to hyperplasia. After the age of twelve years the symptoms are usually due to adrenal hyperplasia. Beyond childhood Cushing's syndrome produces 50 to 60 per cent of cases with the symptoms of adrenocortical hyperfunction.

[handwritten marginal note: Overproduction of Cortisone]

The basic fault in Cushing's syndrome lies in the overproduction of the cortisone family of corticosteroids. In addition to the structural changes noted in the adrenal cortex, the steroids produced bring about a typical degenerative degranulation of some of the pituitary basophils that normally produce gonadotropic hormones. These hyaline basophilic cells are the so-called Crooke cells, found in the anterior lobe of the pituitary in this syndrome. It is still unsettled whether the changes are a cause or an effect of the syndrome—probably an effect. As a result, however, the production of the pituitary gonadotropins is altered in varying degrees.

What Symptoms Are Traceable to Overproduction of the Glycogenic Hormone?

By and large the adrenocortical hormones, hydrocortisone and cortisone, concerned particularly with glycogenesis are secreted in overabundance, a fact which explains most of the symptoms of Cushing's syndrome. As a result of their increased secretion, increased amounts of amino acids are converted into carbohydrates. Since this takes place at the expense of protein synthesis, protein depletion occurs, thereby partly accounting for the increased capillary fragility and the typical thin skin that bruises easily. Purplish-red striae appear on the trunk and, to a lesser extent, on the extremities as characteristics of girls with Cushing's syndrome.

Since the secretion of hormones of the cortisone type is in excess and carbohydrate production is increased, a mild diabetes mellitus results that is relatively resistant to insulin. The increase in glycogenesis accounts for the rapid development of obesity. The obesity is said to be of the "buffalo" type and is concentrated about the face, neck, trunk and proximal portion of the limbs. The degree of obesity and the extent of protein deficiency vary within wide limits.

What Symptoms Are Due to Increased Androgen Production?

The chief symptoms in Cushing's syndrome attributable to an increase in the amount of circulating androgens are hirsutism and diminished ovarian function. Amenorrhea is nearly a constant finding. The hirsutism is excessive and appears with a typical male distribution. Virilism does not regularly accompany hirsutism, and the clitoris is not necessarily enlarged. Ovarian function is depressed, and the normal development of breast, labia, vagina and uterus may be held in abeyance. Despite these signs of genital atrophy, sexual hair appears in abundance.

One should become suspicious of the presence of Cushing's syndrome when an

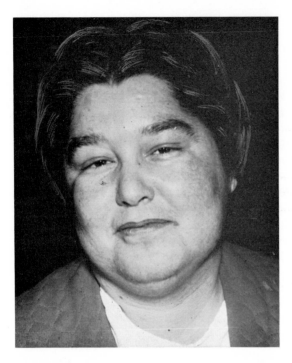

Fig. 19-2.   A young woman with Cushing's syndrome who has the characteristic plethoric, moon-shaped facies. Hirsutism is a variable sign, not present in this case. The ruddy complexion in Cushing's syndrome may reflect polycythemia, which is frequent.

adolescent girl, previously thin, becomes amenorrheic, and begins to gain weight and to have a ruddy complexion and a moon-shaped face (Fig. 19–2). Suspicion of the syndrome heightens if purplish streaks appear on the trunk and the girl begins to complain of pain in the back. The pain is traceable to osteoporosis due to protein deficiency and secondarily to disturbances in electrolyte balance with calcium loss.

What Is the Differential Diagnosis in Cushing's Syndrome?

Cushing's syndrome is rare in early childhood. Symptoms suggesting the possibility of the syndrome are apt to be due to adrenocortical tumors in this age group, as mentioned. Later in adolescence adrenocortical hyperfunction is far more likely to be due to adrenal hyperplasia. One must then differentiate between adrenal tumor and hyperplasia.

ADRENAL TUMOR OR HYPERPLASIA.   A common method of establishing the differential diagnosis is to give the patient cortisone in the same dosage used in the adrenogenital syndrome. Although this test is not infallible, in most instances one can expect an immediate reduction in the level of the urinary 17-ketosteroids when the primary disease is due to adrenal hyperplasia, in contrast to unaltered excretion when a tumor is present.

Another method of localizing the endocrine effect to the adrenal, although it does little to differentiate between a tumor and hyperplasia, is to evaluate enlargement of the adrenal glands by x-ray techniques. This may be done in one of two ways: (a) after air injection of the perirenal spaces; (b) x-ray study of the adrenal region by laminography. In either case the investigator looks for enlargement of the adrenal glands, with downward and forward displacement of the adjacent kidney.

The best method of measuring the functional capacity of the adrenal is to estimate the urinary excretion of 17-hydroxycorticosteroids and 17-ketosteroids after

ACTH stimulation. Twenty-five units of ACTH are given intravenously in 500 cc., either 5 per cent glucose in saline or normal saline, over an 8-hour period. This should be repeated on two successive days. Concomitant tests are made on 24-hour urine specimens for 17-ketosteroids and 17-hydroxycorticosteroids. If the basic problem is hyperplasia, the level of the 17-hydroxycorticosteroids will increase. When carcinoma is present, the 17-hydroxycorticosteroids are always abundant, and little increase can be expected after ACTH stimulation. Some increase in the output of this steroid appears after ACTH stimulation when the abnormality is an adenoma, but the increase is far greater in adrenal hyperplasia associated with Cushing's syndrome.

PITUITARY ADENOMA.   It is important to keep in mind that Cushing's syndrome and Cushing's disease are not one and the same, although both are associated with amenorrhea. The much less common condition is Cushing's disease, which has as the basic endocrine abnormality a basophilic pituitary adenoma. Sometimes a chromophobe cell adenoma may occur in the anterior pituitary lobe in Cushing's syndrome. It is thus possible to have adenomatous abnormalities, then, both in the adrenal and the pituitary in Cushing's syndrome. Abnormal stimulation of the region of the hypothalamus also can cause either an increased pituitary production or release of the adrenocorticotropic hormones. The basic difficulty is far more likely to be located in the adrenal, however.

To rule out a possible pituitary source in Cushing's syndrome x-ray pictures should be taken of the skull. The lack of any evidence of an expanded sella turcica will tend to support the contention that the problem is primarily one of adrenal function, particularly if the air injection studies show an enlarged adrenal.

OBESITY.   Some girls inherit a tendency to obesity and often have hypertension along with a full face of ruddy color. There are, however, no other signs of Cushing's syndrome, and the laboratory findings are essentially normal.

ADRENOGENITAL SYNDROME.   In making the differential diagnosis of Cushing's syndrome from the adrenogenital syndrome it is important to remember that the latter is five times more common than Cushing's syndrome in girls in this younger age group. The laboratory findings may be helpful, though the amount of urinary hormone excretion varies. The chief difference lies in the glycogenic factor. The diabetic glucose tolerance curve and the diminished response to insulin are common to Cushing's syndrome. The excretion of 17-hydroxycorticosteroids and 17-ketosteroids may be increased in both. Occasionally, altered electrolyte balance is noted in Cushing's syndrome. Then there is some increase in excretion of sodium, carbon dioxide and calcium, while the chlorides and the potassium are decreased.

What Is the Treatment of Cushing's Syndrome?

The basic consideration in outlining therapy for Cushing's syndrome depends on the age of the patient, and whether or not the physician believes that the underlying condition is due to tumor or hyperplasia of the adrenal cortex, or perhaps to a tumor of the pituitary or hypothalamus.

At times it may be difficult to distinguish adrenal tumor from adrenal cortical hyperplasia. If this is true, surgical exploration is warranted, provided there is no evidence of metastases in remote areas. Some adrenal adenomas are benign, but the majority have a highly malignant potential. Metastases occur frequently, and recurrence of the tumor after surgical removal is noted all too often. Surgical exploration is preferred to irradiation therapy, since the results of radiation for either hyperplasia or tumor of the adrenal have not been very rewarding.

If preliminary studies localize the tumor to the pituitary region, surgical exploration is warranted. In some instances radiation directed toward the pituitary has been helpful in improving the patient's general condition.

Medical therapy to support the patient's general condition takes the form of oral administration of testosterone, 10 to 25 mg. daily. In this manner some of the muscular weakness secondary to protein depletion is relieved. Although excess androgen in this condition is responsible for the hirsutism and amenorrhea, it may be advisable to give even more for *(a)* its protein-sparing effect and *(b)* its ability to combat the glucogenesis, thereby preventing further destruction of protein. In the effective range of 25 mg. of testosterone, given intramuscularly 3 times a week, there is a real chance that hirsutism will increase, but the gain measured in terms of increased protein anabolism, outweighs this obvious disadvantage.

Estrin is frequently given to counteract the osteoporosis, and in combination with oral testosterone may prove of value in recalcification and bone repair.

Surgery is by all odds the therapy of choice. Long-term suppressive therapy is not very successful, largely because of the inability of patients to tolerate large doses of androgen over a prolonged period. The child with adrenal hyperplasia associated with the adrenogenital syndrome apparently can tolerate cortisone therapy, but the patient with Cushing's syndrome gets into trouble in the long run because of sodium retention and the development of hypertension, as well as occasionally psychoses.

REFERENCES

Thyroid Hypofunction

Cassidy, C. E., and Vanderlaan, W. P.: Laboratory Aids to Diagnosis in Thyroid Disease. *New England J. Med.*, 258: 828, 1958.

Hamblen, E. C.: *Endocrinology of Woman.* Springfield, Ill., Charles C Thomas, 1945.

Heald, F. P., Masland, R. P., Jr., Renold, A. E., and Gallagher, J. R.: Hypothyroidism in the Adolescent. *J.A.M.A.*, 162: 161, 1956.

Adrenogenital Syndrome

Biggs, A. D., and Wied, D. M.: Management of Congenital Adrenogenital Syndrome. *Am. J. Obst. & Gynec.*, 74: 200, 1957.

Bongiovanni, A. M., and Eberlein, W. R.: Defective Steroidal Biogenesis in Congenital Adrenal Hyperplasia. *Pediatrics*, 21: 661, 1958.

Goldzieher, J. W.: Lack of Androgenicity of 17-Hydroxyprogesterone or Its 17-Caproate Ester. *J. Clin. Endocrinol. & Metab.*, 17: 323, 1957.

Jailer, J. W., Gold, J. J., Vande Wiele, R., and Liebermann, S.: 17-α-Hydroxyprogesterone and 21-Desoxyhydrocortisone, Their Metabolism and Possible Role in Congenital Adrenal Virilism. *J. Clin. Invest.*, 34: 1639, 1955.

Laidlaw, J. C., and others: Advances in the Diagnosis of Altered States of Adrenocortical Function. *New England J. Med.*, 253: 747, 1955.

Taylor, E. S., and Snow, R. H.: Adrenal Virilism in the Female Child and Adult. *Am. J. Obst. & Gynec.*, 67: 1307, 1954.

Wilkins, L.: Diagnosis of Adrenogenital Syndrome and Its Treatment with Cortisone. *J. Pediat.*, 41: 860, 1952.

Cushing's Syndrome

Cope, O., and Raker, J. W.: Cushing's Disease; The Surgical Experience in the Care of 46 Cases. *New England J. Med.*, 253: 119, 1955.

Dohan, F. C., Raventos, A., Boucot, N., and Rose, E.: Roentgen Therapy in ¡Cushing's Syndrome without Adrenocortical Tumor. *J. Clin. Endocrinol. & Metab.*, 17: 8, 1957.

Forbes, A. P., and Albright, F.: A Comparison of the 17-Ketosteroid Excretion in Cushing's Syndrome Associated with Adrenal Tumor and with Adrenal Hyperplasia. *J. Clin. Endocrinol.*, 11: 926, 1951.

Hechter, O., and Pincus, G.: Genesis of the Adrenocortical Secretion. *Physiol. Rev.*, 34: 459, 1954.

Heinbecker, P.; Pathogenesis of Cushing's Syndrome. *Medicine*, 23: 225, 1944.

Iannaccone, A., Gabrilove, J. L., Sohval, A. R., and Soffer, L. J.: The Ovaries in Cushing's Syndrome. *New England J. Med.*, 261: 775, 1959.

Munson, P. L., and Briggs, F. N.: The Mechanism of Stimulation of ACTH Secretion. *Recent Progress in Hormone Research*, 11: 83, 1955.

Plotz, C. M., Knowlton, A. I., and Ragan, C.: The Natural History of Cushing's Syndrome. *Am. J. Med.*, 13: 597, 1952.

Soffer, L. J., Eisenberg, J., Iannaccone, A., and Gabrilove, J. L.: Cushing's Syndrome; in G. E. W. Wolstenholme and M. P. Cameron, eds.: *The Human Adrenal Cortex*. Ciba Foundation Colloquia. Boston, Little, Brown and Company, 1955, p. 487.

West, C. D., Damast, B., and Pearson, O. H.: Urinary Estrogen Excretion in Cushing's Syndrome. *J. Clin. Endocrinol.*, 18: 15, 1958.

Chapter 20

Unusual Causes of Amenorrhea

GENETIC constitutional differences are common in the growing child. When development does not proceed along the pathway regarded by the parents as normal, the child is often considered to be a glandular problem. There may be nothing wrong with such a child, for the outstanding tomboy may become a ravishing feminine beauty. Beyond a point, however, it may become obvious as development proceeds or fails to occur that glandular deficiency or functional derangements are present.

Before attempting to treat the girl who is delayed in her menarche the physician must rule out basic endocrine abnormalities, due either to congenital defect, tumor formation or unbalanced hyperfunction. The locale may be either pituitary, thyroid, adrenal or ovary.

PITUITARY GONADOTROPIC INSUFFICIENCY

Since the main source of production and release of the gonadotropins concerned with menstrual function is the anterior pituitary lobe and adjacent hypothalamus, any tumor or congenital anomaly in this area may reflect on gonadal development. Depending on the age of the patient at the time the disturbance manifests itself, somatic growth may or may not be disturbed. Tumors of the pituitary are rare in childhood and adolescence.

Chromophobe pituitary adenomas are the most common. They are usually nonfunctioning space-occupying tumors that displace normal anterior lobe cells and thus reduce pituitary activity. As they enlarge, gonadotropic hormonal secretion is most commonly the first endocrine function to be affected. Amenorrhea, with inactivity of ovaries and uterus, is frequent. Later other hormonal activities may be interfered with. As the tumor grows, it typically presses on the optic nerves and produces headache and defects in vision, which more frequently bring the patient to the physician than do endocrine deficiencies.

Other space-occupying, nonfunctional lesions in this region may have the same endocrinologic effects. Cysts and cystic or solid craniopharyngiomas are among the more common, and tuberculous or syphilitic granulomas among the rarer conditions found here.

Perhaps the next most common pituitary tumor is the *acidophil* or *eosinophilic adenoma*, which produces gigantism, a condition not common in women. Gigantism is the result of overproduction of the pituitary somatotropic or growth hormone

246

before or at the time of puberty, when acceleration in structural growth is noted. The epiphyses in such cases remain open into the twenties, and as a result the trunk becomes long and slim, while the feet and hands are excessively large. This is a source of acute embarrassment to the adolescent girl. The facial characteristics are unaltered in adolescence. Acromegaly develops only after the epiphyses have united, in adult life.

At first there is little to distinguish the patient with an eosinophilic adenoma from the girl who is extremely tall because of hereditary influence. The tumor has not yet progressed or does not grow in size to the point at which the visual fields are impaired or pressure is exerted on the optic chiasm. Sexual development may be perfectly normal or even precocious, in keeping with the increase in structural growth. In this case the condition must be distinguished from other situations such as (1) the adrenogenital syndrome, in which advanced bone age is accompanied by virilization, or (2) Albright's syndrome, in which pigmentation of the skin and radiologic polycystic areas are noted in bone, besides precocious puberty. Also there may be little to distinguish incipient gigantism from the overstimulation of bone growth provided by hyperfunction of the thyroid.

As the tumor enlarges and involves more of the anterior lobe, signs of partial pituitary deficiency begin to appear. Muscular weakness becomes apparent, and thyrotropic and gonadotropic functions begin to fail as pituitary stimulation lessens.

The other pituitary tumor seen in the adolescent child is the *basophilic adenoma.* Cushing's disease, not Cushing's syndrome, which is basically adrenal in origin, is present in a high percentage of such cases. Since there is also a large component of secondary adrenal pathology present in this entity, it has been discussed under that heading. *Pineal gland tumors* produce disturbances in sexual development, but predominantly in males.

Pituitary dysfunction may be present as a congenital defect without the presence of tumor or any destructive lesion in the anterior lobe. There are wide variations in the extent of the pituitary deficiency. If the defect is serious, all the other tropic hormones as well as the growth hormone are deficient or lacking. In this case we have a hypopituitary dwarf. Because of the lack of growth hormone the patient is short in stature, while the facial features continue to be immature. The entire development is in proportion, but in miniature. This is the so-called Levi-Lorain type of dwarf. The gonadotropins are also absent. The urinary FSH drops to less than 6 rat units per 24 hours, and the ovary produces no estrin. As a result the breast fails to develop, and no pubic hair appears, while the vaginal smear shows a complete lack of cornified cells. The uterus is small, and menstruation is impossible. Adrenal function is deficient, for no adrenocortical stimulation is to be had either from ACTH or the luteinizing hormones, and axillary hair fails to appear. Both the glucocorticoid and sex-type hormones of the adrenal cortex are deficient. Urinary assays for both androgen and 17-ketosteroids show minimal values or total absence of excretion. The patients may have hypoglycemia, and thyroid function is minimal.

With minor degrees of functional impairment it may be difficult to differentiate between panhypopituitary disease and delayed adolescence. The pituitary gonadotropins are apt to be the first hormones adversely affected. Not infrequently, then, we see retarded sexual development without serious impairment of the growth hormone output or that of any of the other tropic hormones of the anterior lobe. The stature may be only slightly below normal, and adrenal function as measured by the 17-ketosteroid and androgen excretion may be entirely adequate. The response of

[handwritten: pituitary Defect - ↓ FSH / ovarian defect - ↑ FSH]

the blood sugar to insulin is not unusual. The extent of ovarian functional damage varies widely. It may be temporary and functional, subject to the various factors that affect hypothalamic release, such as malnutrition, debilitating disease or psychic unrest. On the other hand, the defect may be more basic. In this case the urinary FSH is depressed or absent, and the uterus remains in the infantile state. To distinguish between primary ovarian failure and a lack of pituitary stimulation one has only to measure the urinary output of FSH. It will be elevated in ovarian atrophy or agenesis and depressed or absent when the defect is primarily in the pituitary or hypothalamus.

HYPOTHALAMIC LESIONS

Serious malformation or any tumor that arises in the region of the hypothalamus or in the midbrain, causing pressure on or invasion of the hypothalamus, will likely produce disturbances in growth and endocrine function, due to alterations in secretion of the hormones by the anterior lobe of the pituitary. To a less extent the posterior pituitary is involved. Thus we may expect to see retarded structural growth and gonadal underdevelopment when the lesion creates inhibition of hormonal release from the pituitary, or sexual precocity if the tumor causes stimulation of the anterior lobe.

The most common tumors found in this region are the *craniopharyngioma or the suprasellar cyst*. Approximately 50 per cent are noted before the age of 15 years. These originate from a congenital anomaly arising above the sella turcica from the ectoderm in Rathke's pouch, originally found in the roof of the mouth. As they grow, they press on and eventually invade the hypothalamus and the third ventricle. Depending on their size and location, varying amounts of pressure are exerted on the optic nerves. Thus the patient may have optic atrophy, papilledema, diplopia or visual field defects. Also, depending on the degree and time of involvement of the hypothalamus, a variety of endocrine effects appear. If both the growth hormone and pituitary gonadotropins are inhibited in their production or release, the patient may resemble a hypopituitary dwarf. If only the gonadotropins are affected, the patient may be normal in structural growth, but retarded in sexual development. In any disturbance of the hypothalamus, obesity and frequently diabetes insipidus are also likely to be present. Disturbances in fluid balance are not uncommon. These may be due to involvement of the posterior pituitary, for a hormonal product of the posterior lobe has a known antidiuretic action and acts on the kidney tubules, inducing tubular water reabsorption. Other symptoms, perhaps traceable to hypothalamic damage, are somnolence and disturbances in the normal temperature regulation.

The obesity associated with craniopharyngiomas calls for special comment. When obesity is present and a true tumor can be demonstrated, the patient is said to have *Froehlich's syndrome*. Such lesions stimulate the child's appetite. Too many fat children are thought to have Froehlich's syndrome. The mere fact that the obese female child fails to menstruate at the expected time and has some evidence of gonadal underdevelopment is not enough to make a diagnosis of Froehlich's adiposity. The great majority of these girls will become completely normal as soon as they lose weight. The diagnosis of Froehlich's syndrome must be restricted to those patients who have a definite tumor in the hypothalamus which interrupts or destroys the neurohumoral pathways to the anterior pituitary. Only the gonadotropins are concerned, for such patients continue to secrete both the thyrotropic (TSH) and adreno-corticotropic hormones (ACTH). Thus Froehlich's syndrome differs from panhypo-pituitarism. Characteristically, these patients are short in stature with small hands and feet of delicate bone structure. The oval face resembles that of a child. The excess fat is heavily concentrated over the thighs, buttocks and lower part of the abdomen. In proportion the waist seems small.

The suspicion of the presence of a suprasellar cyst or craniopharyngioma may be confirmed by x-ray. The diagnostic points to observe are (1) destruction of the clinoid processes, (2) a flattening of the sella turcica, and (3) the presence of abnormal radiopaque shadows within the cyst due to calcification in its wall. These findings contrast with those noted in pituitary adenoma, in which the sella turcica may appear to be expanded.

Other tumors of the midbrain which may encroach upon or penetrate into the hypothalamus and produce the same symptoms and findings are gliomas, teratomas and cysts.

Congenital defects and lesions in the hypothalamus give rise to three other syndromes which have many symptoms in common, but with distinctive features which differentiate one from the other. The symptoms of obesity, sexual under-development and diabetes insipidus are common to them all.

The Laurence-Moon-Biedl syndrome also has (a) stunted growth, (b) retinitis pigmentosa, (c) mental deficiency, and (d) either syndactylism or polydactylism. Hand-Schüller-Christian disease has, in addition, stunted growth and xanthogranulo-matous lesions spread widely over the body. As a differential point in diagnosis, the syndrome may have a characteristic appearance on x-ray study of the skull, with punched-out areas seen in the cranial vaults. In Albright's syndrome the adolescent girl is apt to be tall for her age, rather than stunted. Sexual precocity is often present. In addition, *cafe-au-lait* geographic pigmentation of the skin and cystic disease in bone are often noted and frequently appear together, unilaterally.

OVARIAN TUMORS WITH ENDOCRINE SIGNIFICANCE

There are two types of unusual tumor in this age group that may produce hor-mones and are associated with menstrual dysfunction, for the most part amenorrhea.

THE ARRHENOBLASTOMA

This rare tumor is masculinizing, and its prominent functional symptom is amenorrhea. The tumor is particularly rare in childhood. The majority of cases reported have occurred after the age of fifteen, and find their greatest incidence between twenty and thirty years. The adolescent child has therefore reached full maturity before the masculinizing hormone exerts its effect. Consequently there are no developmental defects. The most prominent and earliest symptom is amenorrhea. Since the tumor secretes the male hormones, masculinization and virilization are present. The body contour takes on the habitus of the male. Atrophy of the breasts is apparent, together with male muscularity, hypertrophy of the clitoris, deepening of the voice and abnormal hirsutism.

All these manifestations are reversible, except for change in size of the larynx, which is responsible for the voice changes. Removal of the tumor restores femininity,

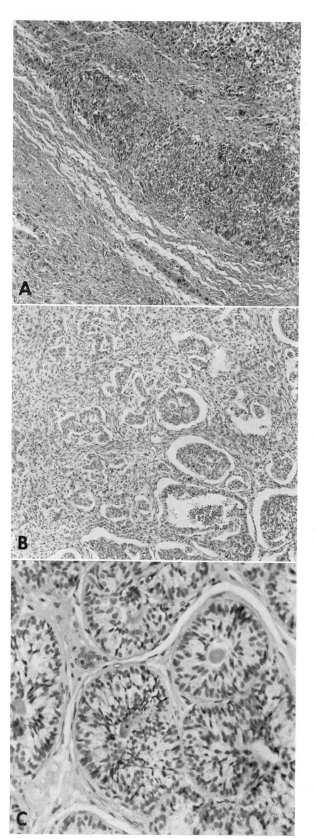

Fig. 20-1.   *A*, Portion of an undifferentiated arrhenoblastoma. Masses of cells not clearly recognizable as either carcinoma or sarcoma are seen mingled with fibrous stroma. *B*, The more common intermediate type of arrhenoblastoma (at same magnification). Some cells growing in cords simulate the embryonic testis. Nests of cells in the intervening stroma resemble immature Leydig cells. *C*, Part of a Pick's adenoma (at much higher magnification). The appearance of developing testicular tubules is closely imitated in this form of benign neoplasm. This tumor was not virilizing, so that the small nests of interstitial cells shown evidently were nonfunctioning.

250

with the return of menstruation as the initial evidence. A few instances of pregnancy have been recorded after excision of the tumor growth.

Grossly, arrhenoblastomas are not usually invasive or destructive and consist of a smooth-surfaced lobulated mass, partly gray-yellow and solid, partly cystic with clear fluid in smooth-walled locules. Histologically, the more active tumors functionally are the least well differentiated. The undifferentiated arrhenoblastoma is ordinarily malignant and consists of a sarcomatous spindle cell pattern of rather wild appearance, due to the lack of any organization. Some foci resemble poorly organized epithelium, but this type of arrhenoblastoma would often be called an undifferentiated malignant neoplasm or possibly ovarian sarcoma if the surgeon did not provide the helpful information that it was virilizing (Fig. 20–1, A). Although malignant, such arrhenoblastomas often do not metastasize or prove fatal.

The intermediate arrhenoblastoma is perhaps more common, and may be recognized microscopically. In the spindle cell stroma, with its rather loose myxomatous structure, are found nests of epithelium that locally form hollowed cords or tubules. These are lined with tall cells and are recognizable as resembling the spermatogenic tubules of the infant's testis. Between the tubules, if one searches, are found nests of polygonal cells with abundant eosinophilic cytoplasm, reminiscent of adrenal cortex (Fig. 20–1, B). These are the interstitial cells of Leydig that are responsible for testosterone production. In fact, crystalline male hormone may rarely be visible in the form of the capsule-shaped intracellular Reinke crystalloids.

The well differentiated Pick's adenoma type of arrhenoblastoma consists almost wholly of well formed infantile testicular tubules. It is a rare form of benign ovarian tumor, usually devoid of masculinizing activity, since it lacks Leydig cells (Fig. 20–1, C). Conversely, this type of neoplasm is rather common in the undescended testis.

Treatment

Since the majority of these tumors are found in the younger age group, conservatism is indicated, provided the tumor is small and encapsulated. The malignant potential is high, however, and any suggestion of recurrence should be followed by secondary exploration and radical extirpation of the uterus and adnexa. If the tumor has broken through its capsule and has either invaded or become adherent to other organs, radical surgery is performed at the time of the initial exploration.

The Dysgerminoma

This uncommon solid epithelial tumor, which is akin to the embryonal carcinoma of the male testis, is concerned with endocrine dysfunction more by association than by any influence the tumor may have in its production. Actually, the tumor itself does not usually secrete any known hormone. Since it occurs frequently in patients who have evidence of sexual and gonadal underdevelopment and are sexually neuters, with manifestations such as amenorrhea and pseudohermaphroditism, it has been erroneously believed to have endocrine significance (Fig. 20–2, A).

No change is noted in endocrine function or in the anatomic manfestations of pseudohermaphroditism after removal of the tumor. The patient later miay menstruate normally and even deliver a normal child. The growth pattern is insidious, and discovery is often made only when a pelvic mass is found. On the other hand,

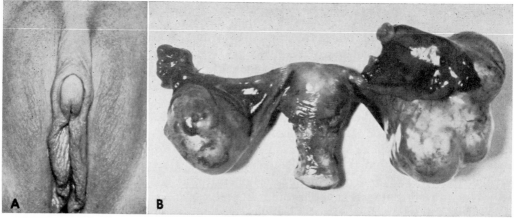

Fig. 20-2.   *A*, External genitalia of a female pseudohermaphrodite who had bilateral ovarian tumors. *B*, Bilateral ovarian dysgerminomas removed at operation, together with the uterus, from this woman.

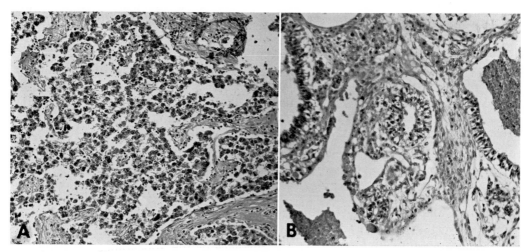

Fig. 20-3.   *A*, Loosely arranged cords of cells, some with watery cytoplasm, mingled with lymphocytes, are typical of the ovarian dysgerminoma microscopically. *B*, In the center of the illustration are 3 small spaces surrounded by dysgerminoma cells. These somewhat resemble a primitive neural canal, body cavity and gut, reading from below upward. Such a structure is fancifully called a homunculus.

enlargement of the clitoris and other stigmata of the pseudohermaphrodite may be present in the girl with amenorrhea. The presence of a pelvic mass in such a patient would point to the possible presence of a dysgerminoma.

The tumor may occur at any age, but is most common in the younger age groups.

Most dysgerminomas are rather large, poorly encapsulated masses of soft white tissue, partly degenerated and colored yellow, red or brown, owing to necrosis and hemorrhage (Fig. 20–2, *B*). Microscopically, the viable tumor consists of sheets and demarcated cords of cuboidal or polygonal cells with unusually clear cytoplasm and large, centrally placed nuclei that are rather poor in chromatin. Mitoses are abundant. Necrosis is obvious, and the stroma of the dysgerminoma is characteristically infiltrated with many lymphocytes, as well as some plasma cells, macrophages and even foreign body giant cells or foci of granulomatous inflammation. This gives the designation "embryonal carcinoma with lymphoid stroma" to the analogous testicular tumor (Fig. 20–3, *A*).

Robert Meyer originally called this tumor disgerminoma, meaning a tumor of the germ cell of both sexes that was so undifferentiated as to be of either sex. Study of the nuclear chromatin allegedly has indicated that all ovarian dysgerminomas have the genetic sex of the host, while analogous neoplasms of testis do not.

Dysgerminoma shades off in some cases into foci of teratoma, and there is discussion as to whether the portions that are dysgerminomatous matured into the teratomatous foci or arose from a primary teratoma by dedifferentiation. Sometimes foci simulating early embryos (homunculi) occur mixed with dysgerminoma, embryonal carcinoma of testis or teratocarcinoma (Fig. 20–3, *B*).

Treatment

Though the degree of malignancy varies, the malignant potential is high. There appears to be general agreement that an encapsulated tumor of the ovary in the younger age group should be treated conservatively by removal of the tube and ovary. Since the tumor may metastasize to the retroperitoneal lymph nodes in the absence of capsular invasion, and since dysgerminoma is extremely radiosensitive, many clinics now advocate external radiation therapy for the retroperitoneal nodes as adjuvant therapy. When the uterus and contralateral ovary are screened from the effect of the radiation and approximately 1000 r are given to 4 fields, anteriorly and posteriorly, a cure rate as high as 80 per cent has been reported. Moreover, subsequent pregnancy has been achieved in approximately 20 per cent of patients.

If postoperative x-ray therapy is not given to the patient with an encapsulated tumor, close supervision is essential in the years subsequent to conservative surgery. In general the cure rate is favorable and recurrence is uncommon in the early phase of growth. The surgeon may reasonably then defer the use of x-ray therapy until recurrence develops after conservative therapy.

When the tumor has broken through its capsule at the time of exploration, total removal of the uterus and adnexa is indicated. This should be supplemented by x-ray therapy. With any suggestion of recurrence or the appearance of ascites, re-exploration is essential, provided the extent of recurrence is not too great.

Metastases occur by way of the lymphatic system and through direct extension into the pelvic connective tissue. When cancer has grown to this extent, the recurrence rate has been as high as 33 per cent. Postoperative x-ray treatment should be given as adjuvant therapy.

REFERENCES

Pituitary and Hypothalamic Changes

Bauer, H. G.: Endocrine and Other Clinical Manifestations of Hypothalamic Disease. *J. Clin. Endocrinol. & Metab.*, 14: 13, 1954.

Franke, C.: Type of Hypogonadism in Laurence-Moon-Biedl Syndrome. *Nederl. Tijdschr. v. Geneesk.*, 93: 3261, 1949.

Friedgood, H. B.: Endocrine Function of the Hypophysis; in *Oxford Loose-Leaf Medicine*. New York, Oxford University Press, 1946, Vol. III, Part III.

German, W. J.: The Endocrine Effects of Pituitary Tumors. *Surgery*, 16: 47, 1944.

Israel, S. L., and Conston, A. S.: Sheehan's Syndrome. *J.A.M.A.*, 148: 189, 1952.

Russfield, A. B., Reiner, L., and Klaus, H.: The Endocrine Significance of Hypophyseal Tumors in Man. *Am. J. Path.*, 32: 1055, 1956.

Schnitker, M. T., Cutler, E. C., Bailey, O. T., and Vaghan, W. W.: Chromophobe Adenomas of Pituitary. *Am. J. Roentgenol.*, 40: 645, 1938.

Sommers, S. C.: The Pituitary and Hypothalamus; in J. T. Velardo, ed.: *The Endocrinology of Reproduction.* New York, Oxford University Press, 1958, p. 59.

Younghusband, O. Z., Horrax, G., Hurxthal, L. M., Hare, H. F., and Poppen, J. L.: Chromophobe Pituitary Tumors. I. Diagnosis. *J. Clin. Endocrinol. & Metab.*, 12: 611, 1952.

Arrhenoblastoma

Dockerty, M. B., and MacCarty, W. C.: Arrhenoblastoma. *Surg., Gynec. & Obst.*, 68: 767, 1939.

Hertig, A. T., and Gore, H.: Tumors of the Ovary and Fallopian Tube; in *Tumors of the Female Sex Organs.* Washington, D.C., Armed Forces Institute of Pathology, 1961, p. 33.

Hughesdon, P. E., and Fraser, I. T.: Arrhenoblastoma of the Ovary. *Acta obst. et gynec. Scandinav.*, 32 (Suppl. 4): 1, 1953.

Langley, F. A.: "Sertoli" and "Leydig" Cells in Relation to Ovarian Tumors. *J. Clin. Path.*, 7: 10, 1954.

Morris, J. M., and Scully, R. E.: Sertoli-Leydig Cell Tumors; in *Endocrine Pathology of the Ovary.* St. Louis, C. V. Mosby Company, 1958, p. 82.

Teilum, G.: Classification of Ovarian Tumours. *Acta obst. et gynec. Scandinav.*, 31: 292, 1952.

Thomas, C. Y., Jr., Fisher, E. R., Turnbull, R. B., and Krieger, J. S.: Arrhenoblastoma of the Ovary. *Ann. Surg.*, 135: 543, 1952.

Dysgerminoma

Blocksma, R.: Bilateral Dysgerminoma of the Ovary with Pseudohermaphroditism. *Am. J. Obst. & Gynec.*, 69: 874, 1955.

Burge, E. S.: Dysgerminoma Ovarii. *Am. J. Obst. & Gynec.*, 57: 1014, 1949.

Kottmeier, H. L.: Radiotherapy in the Treatment of Ovarian Carcinoma. *Clin. Obst. & Gynec.*, 3: 865, 1961.

Pedowitz, P., Felmus, L. B., and Grayzel, D. M.: Dysgerminoma of the Ovary. Prognosis and Treatment. *Am. J. Obst. & Gynec.*, 70: 1284, 1955.

Plate, W. P.: Dysgerminoma of the Ovary in a Patient with Virilism. *Acta endocrinol.*, 14: 227, 1953.

Scully, R. E.: Gonadoblastoma. A Gonadal Tumor Related to the Dysgerminoma (Seminoma) and Capable of Sex-Hormone Production. *Cancer*, 6: 455, 1953.

Thoeny, R. H., Dockerty, M. B., Hunt, A. B., and Childs, D. S., Jr.: A Study of Ovarian Dysgerminomas, with Emphasis on the Role of Radiation Therapy. *Surg., Gynec. & Obst.*, 113: 692, 1961.

Chapter 21

Treatment of Amenorrhea

PRIMARY AMENORRHEA

FROM the previous discussion it is evident that there is a variety of explanations as to why the developing girl either is delayed in or never establishes a menstrual cycle. One of the first things we must decide is whether the delay in the appearance of menstruation is part of the normal growth pattern or whether there is some basic anatomic or functional reason why menstruation has not taken place.

At what age do we decide that the policy of watchful waiting should be abandoned and investigations be started? Recent studies have shown that somewhere between 5 and 8 per cent of girls menstruate after the age of 16 years, while less than 1 per cent begin after the age of 18. Provided there are no stigmata of underdevelopment, there would appear to be a rational basis for procrastination in investigation and therapy until the age of eighteen years. Practically, however, it is advisable that the cause for the menstrual delay be found before the girl enters the highly competitive field of industry or secondary education, for she has little time afterward to devote to investigative studies of her functional failure and does not appreciate how important it is that the cause be found. Early investigative studies are important, for the longer any basic defect is allowed to exist, the harder it becomes to correct it. Since the end-organs apparently become increasingly refractory to hormonal stimulation, delay in determining the cause may lead to continuing faulty menstrual function and consequent infertility.

If we have ruled out delayed maturity, maldevelopment of the pituitary gonadotropic cells, the causative factors outside the endocrine field and organic disease within the endocrine glands concerned with menstruation, we may then assume that we are dealing with a functional defect somewhere in the pituitary-ovarian-uterine axis. We are still uncertain as to the defect in the trigger mechanisms which set off menstruation. After thorough physical examination we may turn to the evaluation of the circulating pituitary and ovarian hormones, through chemical and bio-assay laboratory studies, to pinpoint the defective link in the axis.

In general we can say that one may suspect that the basic fault is ovarian if there is an increase in urinary FSH in the presence of genital atrophy. If genital atrophy is present and the urinary FSH is minimal or lacking, the pituitary is probably defective. When the urinary 17-ketosteroid levels are elevated, the adrenal is suspect. Laboratory studies are important and helpful, but unfortunately from a practical point of view their usefulness is restricted by the fact that (1) they are not always available,

255

(2) many determinations are necessary if true evaluations are to be made, and (3) they are too costly for the average patient. We then tend to fall back upon our interpretation of the vaginal smear or endometrial samplings. These are also not always available. In many such instances it is hard to know whether minimal estrin or no estrin is present.

There is a practical test available to all which gives the maximum amount of information with the minimal expenditure of time and money. It is most helpful in determining whether the glandular axis is intact. This test is called the *progesterone withdrawal test*. Progesterone, 25 mg., is injected intramuscularly daily for 4 days. Uterine bleeding will appear within a few days, provided estrin is present. Since estrin must be present if we are to have withdrawal bleeding, we then know that there is (1) a uterus capable of response, (2) a functioning pituitary, and (3) an ovary responsive to pituitary stimulation and functioning well enough to produce estrin. The degree of response may be subnormal, but the essential ingredients of menstruation are present. This test is extremely practical. There are many cases of amenorrhea with borderline stigmata of underdevelopment. The obese girl with underdeveloped secondary sex characteristics frequently has amenorrhea and is too often thought to have Froehlich's syndrome. Menstruation may or may not be restored by a weight reduction program. If she really has Froehlich's syndrome, she has a basic irreversible pituitary defect. Progesterone-withdrawal bleeding is evidence for an intact and functioning pituitary gland, and the diagnosis of Froehlich's syndrome thus would not be substantiated.

If no bleeding follows progesterone withdrawal, either the uterus, ovary or pituitary may be at fault. The uterus may be intact, but functionless, either because it is not receiving estrin stimulation or because it has been without stimulation so long that it has become atrophic, or insensitive to hormonal stimulation. This is one of the reasons why an early investigation of the underlying cause of amenorrhea is important. The responsiveness of the uterus may be checked by giving oral estrin in whatever form one elects: Estinyl, 0.5 mg., diethylstilbestrol, 1 to 2 mg., or Premarin, 2.5 mg., daily for 3 weeks. If the girl does not bleed after estrogen withdrawal, the uterus is at fault. In the absence of any cervical stenosis or endometrial disease such as tuberculosis, the uterus in such cases must be seriously inadequate. One may attempt to build up the size of the uterus and the responsiveness of the endometrium by large doses of estrin over a six-month period, but the likelihood of success is not great for either the appearance of menstruation or subsequent pregnancy.

If estrin withdrawal bleeding does occur, then the fault must lie in the ovary or pituitary. One may check the pituitary by urinary assay for FSH. If it is present or in excess, the fault may lie in the ovary. When no FSH is recovered, the deficiency rests in the pituitary. If FSH is present, but in diminished amounts, and the urinary 17-ketosteroid excretion is high, adrenal cortical hyperplasia should be suspected. One may rule out the adrenal factor by giving cortisone, 12.5 mg., 3 times daily. If adrenal hyperfunction is the cause of the imbalance, the 17-ketosteroid excretion should fall and menstruation return.

Some investigators have been enthusiastic about the use of administered pregnant mares' serum in differentiating between pituitary and ovarian causes of primary amenorrhea. In daily injected doses of 500 international units, given 3 times weekly for 3 weeks, pregnant mares' serum will produce ovarian stimulation, provided the ovaries are capable of responding. As a result of successful stimulation the observer notes (1) increased breast development and (2) changes in the vaginal secretion, both in the increased amount of discharge and in the number of cornified cells seen.

If progesterone, 100 mg., is then given to the patient, uterine bleeding will follow 1 to 2 weeks later. From this sequence of events one may reasonably infer that the ovaries are capable of responding to stimulation, but since they normally are evidently receiving none, the pituitary thus must be at fault.

Once the source of the defect has been pinpointed, therapy may be directed at the specific glandular deficiency.

If the defect is basically in the pituitary, little can be done to create a normal menstrual cycle. The pituitary gonadotropins should provide ideal therapy, for they will stimulate and develop the ovary. Unfortunately they are largely ineffective in establishing a cycle and are dangerous to use. As yet the products are impure and contain so much foreign protein that serious anaphylactic incidents have followed their continued use.

Substitution therapy with the ovarian hormones, using both estrin and progesterone, may be of therapeutic as well as psychologic benefit to the patient with primary amenorrhea. The establishment of a simulated menstrual cycle does a great deal for the psyche of the girl who feels that her amenorrhea sets her apart from her contemporaries as an oddity. Moreover, the development of the secondary sex characteristics makes the departure from normal less obvious to others. These girls may marry and the union be a happy one, though pregnancy is impossible.

It is also possible that the interpretation of the investigative studies may be in error. The cyclic use of estrin and progestin may keep the uterus in a responsive state. After a trial regimen, consisting of oral estrin daily for 3 weeks, followed by 25 mg. of progesterone intramuscularly for 4 days with resultant bleeding, the therapy should be continued for another 6 months. The constant substitution may give nature a chance spontaneously to correct any temporary imbalance that is blocking the production or release of the pituitary hormones. After six months the therapy may be temporarily discontinued to see whether any normal rebound phenomenon occurs. Occasionally cycles may be restored in this manner.

When the laboratory tests have indicated that the primary difficulty lies with the ovary, while the pituitary and adrenal appear to be normal, one may also elect to use cyclic estrin and progesterone therapy.

There is a definite place for *abdominal exploration* in the patient with primary amenorrhea. Exploration is indicated when the adolescent child has been given every chance with adjuvant therapy to develop her own menstrual cycles and has failed. When the uterus is present and responsive, though underdeveloped because of deficiency elsewhere in the axis, one may choose to investigate the extent of the defect in the ovary by direct inspection. This is particularly true when the investigator places the blame on congenital maldevelopment. The diagnosis of inferred abnormality in the ovary or pituitary may be in error, especially when there is equivocal clinical confirmation. Before committing the patient to a life of endocrine substitution, it seems logical that the full extent of the ovarian or genital maldevelopment should be appraised by direct examination at the time of surgical exploration of the abdomen. For example, a recent case presenting all the clinical criteria and laboratory findings of ovarian agenesis proved to have the Stein-Leventhal syndrome.

SECONDARY AMENORRHEA

The problem in therapy of the patient with secondary amenorrhea differs materially from that in primary amenorrhea. Obviously, the defect in the pituitary-ovarian-uterine axis is not so basic, since this patient has menstruated at one time. For one of a variety of reasons the patient's catamenia has now ceased. If one can identify the source of the difficulty, treatment has a far greater chance of success than in primary amenorrhea. The degree of success will depend upon the duration of the amenorrhea and the nature of the deficiency or blocking agent. The longer the amenorrhea has persisted, the more refractory the uterus becomes, and the harder it is to bring about a restoration in the menstrual flow.

The primary cause of the amenorrhea may be dysfunction in any one of the elements that make up the axis, but more often the source of the disturbance will be found in some factor that has either interfered with her normal good health or has upset her mental equilibrium. The menstrual cycle is a sensitive indicator of the general state of health and may give the first indication that the patient's physical well-being is in jeopardy.

The appearance of amenorrhea after one or two normal cycles should not be regarded with too much concern in the adolescent child unless the menstrual pattern has previously been fully established. Not infrequently anovulatory bleeding, which is common in menstrual cycles at the menarche, will be accompanied by phases of amenorrhea.

History

Any persistence or prolongation of the amenorrheic pattern should be regarded with suspicion. Much can be learned by a careful history and physical examination. One of the most common causes of secondary amenorrhea in the adolescent virgin is tuberculosis. The primary source is probably pulmonary, but genital tuberculosis, though uncommon in childhood, is found with increasing incidence as ovarian activity speeds up.

Any prolonged illness can produce anemia and malnutrition. The presence of anemia alone may be enough to explain amenorrhea. It is frequently seen in the patient who has had either a sudden gain or loss in weight. When debilitating disease or malnutrition is present, none of the endocrine glands in the axis function normally, but the hypothalamus is particularly sensitive. A reduction in the normal intake of protein and vitamin B, common to malnutritional states, adversely affects the hypothalamus and blocks either the production or release of the pituitary gonado-tropins. In establishing a cure for secondary amenorrhea, careful search should be made to rule out any present or recent generalized infection.

The second factor to be investigated is the emotional aspect, which may have upset the normal balance. These factors also operate through the hypothalamus in the same manner as chronic disease and malnutrition. It has been said that half the cases of secondary amenorrhea are due to emotional disturbances. Sudden shock, fright, environmental dislocation or any element that will produce emotional stress may cause cessation of the normal periods. Unhappiness in the home has been shown to produce obesity and amenorrhea. Conversely, profound and prolonged depressions and anxiety states can bring about a distaste for food with amenorrhea as the result of both malnutrition and psychic stimulation of the hypothalamus.

Anorexia nervosa is an excellent example of what may be expected to follow prolonged mental unrest. When this disorder is encountered in adolescence, it is frequently misdiagnosed as panhypopituitarism or Simmonds's disease. This is a definite error, for anorexia nervosa in the young can be reversed, while Simmonds's disease, because it represents underlying irreversible pituitary disease, cannot be corrected. The difficulty lies in the fact that the wasting aspects of Simmonds's disease may not be apparent in the adolescent girl. Since the basic pituitary defect creates a deficiency in all the other glands of internal secretion, these patients have myxedema because of thyroid inadequacy. They may then appear obese, partly because of the accumulation of myxedematous fluid in the tissues, with masking of the muscle wasting which is a common sequel of panhypopituitarism. The patient with anorexia nervosa may faint easily because of hypoglycemia and have a low blood pressure, basal metabolic rate and pulse.

The history is helpful in distinguishing between the two conditions, for sudden aversion to food, characteristic of anorexia nervosa, may be traced to a definite train of circumstances that produced the emotional upset. Moreover, these girls are prone to be hyperactive, in contrast to the apathy and mental sluggishness commonly found in Simmonds's disease. If further proof is needed, one should look for evidence of deficiency in other endocrine glands. The urinary 17-ketosteroid levels, basal metabolism and hypoglycemic response to insulin should all be reduced. Since some estrin is present in anorexia nervosa, but absent in Simmonds's disease, the progesterone withdrawal test will provide a quick differential diagnostic guide.

When the source of the emotional conflict can be discovered and eliminated, the adolescent girl with anorexia nervosa may return completely to normal.

Physical Examination

The physical examination is important. The obvious thing to look for is evidence of estrin lack. Since this patient menstruated at one time, the ovaries must be present. Estrin deprivation suggests that some block, defect or disease has affected either the target organs or initiating glands. Either the ovary is not getting sufficient stimulation, or it has become refractory to such stimulation. The degree of estrin lack can be determined by vaginal smear and endometrial biopsy. An ovarian tumor may be felt. A tumor of the pituitary or hypothalamus may be suspected from the history of impairment of vision or the presence of headache and confirmed by ophthalmologic examination of the eyegrounds and evaluation of the visual fields. This can be further checked by neurologic examination for other cranial nerve disturbances and by x-ray studies of the skull.

Finally, despite the fact that pregnancy is uncommon in the adolescent girl, we must be assured that this is not the physiologic explanation of the secondary amenorrhea.

Therapeutic Procedures

It is obvious from the foregoing discussion that the treatment of secondary amenorrhea is that of the underlying condition that caused it. Amenorrhea is a symptom, not a disease (Fig. 21–1).

The progesterone withdrawal test is the quickest and least expensive way of determining whether the basic fault lies in the ovary. Withdrawal bleeding is an indication of the presence of estrin. This can be confirmed by a urinary FSH test. If FSH is normal or low, the ovary is functioning, and certainly some estrin is being produced. Because of the variable rate of FSH excretion, it is often hard to distinguish between a low and a normal rate. When the FSH is high, the ovary is definitely

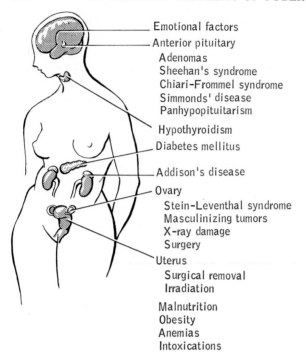

Emotional factors
Anterior pituitary
  Adenomas
  Sheehan's syndrome
  Chiari–Frommel syndrome
  Simmonds' disease
  Panhypopituitarism
Hypothyroidism
Diabetes mellitus
Addison's disease
Ovary
  Stein-Leventhal syndrome
  Masculinizing tumors
  X-ray damage
  Surgery
Uterus
  Surgical removal
  Irradiation
Malnutrition
Obesity
Anemias
Intoxications

Fig. 21-1.   Some functional and organic causes of secondary amenorrhea. Generalized functional changes of the body are more often responsible than the individual endocrine diseases listed.

at fault. The adrenal is sometimes implicated when there is evidence of estrin lack. If these suspicions are confirmed by finding a high level of 17-ketosteroid excretion, cortisone should be given in 12.5-mg. doses 3 times weekly. If 17-ketosteroid levels remain unchanged, tumor rather than hyperplasia is likely present in the adrenal cortex.

Our primary concern in therapy is to restore a sound state of general physical and mental health, so that the hormones will have a chance to act normally. This is a basic consideration in hormone therapy. To this end we must first correct any obesity and be sure that the diet is adequate in protein and vitamin B. A normal regimen of living must be established which will ensure plenty of sleep and exercise, combined with emotional stability at school, work and play. Emotional stability is important, since the majority of cases of secondary amenorrhea are thought to be due to disturbed emotional balance. During the adjustment period sedatives or even tranquilizing drugs are justified, provided one keeps in mind that drug addiction may itself contribute to amenorrhea. Acute and chronic disease should be ruled out or treated and any anemia corrected before embarking on a schedule of hormone substitution. Thyroid therapy in 1- or 2-grain daily dosages may be given empirically or increased if there is evidence of genuine thyroid deficiency. We must also assure ourselves that there is no organic disease in the endocrine glands concerned with menstruation before resorting to hormone therapy.

Little can be accomplished if the secondary amenorrhea is due to a basic defect in the pituitary or hypothalamus, unless a tumor can be removed. The remaining portion of the pituitary might then undergo hypertrophy and function be restored. At least 50 per cent of the pituitary gland must be damaged before normal function is disturbed. Early diagnosis is therefore important. When the secondary amenorrhea is due to hyperfunction or malfunction in one of the pituitary target organs, such as adrenal hyperplasia, which reflexly affects the normal production and release of the pituitary gonadotropins, removal of the basic cause will permit normal pituitary function. When a pituitary disease has involved 95 per cent of the gland, severe symptoms will result from lack of stimulation of all its target glands. Nothing can be done to restore normal function, but the patient can be made to feel better by giving (1) testosterone propionate, 25 mg., 3 times weekly intramuscularly, for its nitrogen-retaining effect; (2) cortisone, 12.5 mg. orally, 3 times weekly, for muscular weakness; (3) oral estrin to maintain the development of the breasts and the secondary sex characteristics in an adolescent girl.

The greatest chance of success in the treatment of secondary amenorrhea for the adolescent girl who has only partial ovarian failure and no obvious estrin lack, aside from the elimination of emotional conflicts, lies in hormone therapy. The success of such therapy will depend on how long the amenorrhea has been present. Under two years there is an excellent chance that progestin therapy alone may restore menstrual function. If the patient responds by withdrawal bleeding to a test dose of 25 mg. of progesterone given intramuscularly for 4 days, the therapy should be continued in reduced dosage for 3 to 6 months. The progesterone should be given intramuscularly in 10-mg. doses daily for 5 days, approximately 18 days after the last onset of withdrawal bleeding.

If the amenorrhea has been present more than two years, the uterus may have become refractory to estrin stimulation. In this instance it may become resensitized by larger doses of oral estrin, Estinyl, 0.5 mg., or Premarin, 2.5 mg., daily for 3 weeks out of the month, for a period of 6 months. At the end of this time, or earlier if the uterus responds by withdrawal bleeding from estrin therapy, combined cyclic estrogen and progestin therapy should be initiated. Estrin in the same dosage should be given daily for three weeks. Progestin intramuscularly, in 10-mg. doses for 5 days, is started on the eighteenth day. This program most closely corresponds to the normal secretion of the hormones. Thyroid extract, 1 or 2 grains daily, is a useful supplementary hormone in these cases.

The physician may choose to give the newer long-acting progestational agents, such as hydroxyprogesterone caproate (Delalutin), as a single intramuscular injection (250 mg.) on the eighteenth day of a simulated cycle. The action is too slow to be useful as a withdrawal test, but these hormonal agents are effective in the production of a progestational type of endometrium. For the same purpose, norethynodrel with ethynylestradiol-3-methyl ether (Enovid) can be given by mouth in 10-mg. doses from the fifteenth to twenty-fifth day of the cycle.

PITUITARY GONADOTROPINS.   When the ovary is in partial failure due to inadequate pituitary stimulation, the logical substitute in hormone therapy should be a gonadotropin of pituitary origin. Unfortunately, such hormones—whether they are equine, chorionic gonadotropin or extracts of the pituitary—are not only impure, but also ordinarily ineffective. Stimulation is possible, for these substances are known to produce ovarian cysts, but they do little to correct the basic defect. When they have been said to produce ovulation, the observations are open to question, for spontaneous ovulation has been known to occur without hormone therapy of any sort. Preliminary desensitization tests are essential if the pituitary gonadotropins are to be used, for severe anaphylactic reactions have occurred. Pregnant mares' serum has been used in combination with either estrin or chorionic gonadotropin by several competent observers, who believe the therapy to be rational. In the present state of their development gonadotropins can hardly be regarded as useful therapeutic tools when dealing with the problem of secondary amenorrhea.

Recently some interesting observations have appeared in the literature which hold some hope for the future. By giving purified extracts of human pituitary material in combination with intramuscular injections of chorionic gonadotropin, Buxton has been able to stimulate the ovary to such an extent that not one, but several ovulatory points have appeared. Gemzell, who has pioneered these investigations in Sweden, has produced one twin pregnancy by this method. In contrast to the anaphylactic reactions which followed the use of extracts of sheep or other animal pituitary, no adverse side effects of any amount have appeared. This may prove to be a useful adjuvant to the therapy of amenorrhea in the future, but it is obviously not yet ready for general clinical use.

X-RAY TREATMENT. Radiation therapy of ovary, pituitary and adrenal has been recommended for the restoration of the menstrual cycle in secondary amenorrhea, and several large series of successfully treated cases have been reported in the literature. A light dose of x-ray treatment is recommended. Since the basic effect of irradiation is destruction of tissue, it is difficult to see how x-rays can be selective in their attack on the cells in any gland that are primarily responsible for the dysfunction. In the very recent literature, as an aftermath to our fears of atomic radiation, there has been increasing interest in the possibilities of the damaging effects of radiation upon the embryonic cell. Warnings have been issued by radiologists as well as geneticists that x-ray therapy is not without its hazards. For example, the incidence of lymphoma in children is appreciably higher when they have been subjected to radiation, given for a variety of reasons. The use of x-ray treatment in secondary amenorrhea should be avoided, and if given at all, it ought to be reserved for those cases in which all other types of therapy have failed and the return of menstruation is of the utmost importance to the patient. If the patient does not care to menstruate, nothing need be done, for the general well-being is not dependent upon cyclic menstruation. Many women lead satisfactory lives who have never menstruated.

SURGERY. There is a place for surgery in the treatment of secondary amenorrhea. Some benign tumors of the adrenal and pituitary may be removed by surgical intervention, and menstrual function thus be restored.

The most satisfactory results from surgical therapy come in the patients who have the Stein-Leventhal syndrome. Why this simplest of all operations, the removal of a wedge-shaped section of tissue from both ovaries, should prove so effective is not known. Those who have followed up these patients subsequently claim that there is no recurrence of the original underlying abnormality after operation. This is important, for many of these patients have normal ovulatory cycles and become pregnant later. Early recognition and operation are important, for if left unoperated upon, many of these girls become sterility problems. The process becomes eventually irreversible as the uterine atrophy continues and the uterus becomes more refractory to ovarian stimulation.

One may be reluctant to operate on a young girl, but if she has not menstruated by the time she is of college age, or if she has periods only once in every six months to one year, exploration is indicated, provided there are no other obvious explanations of her amenorrhea and all other methods of therapy have been tried and have failed. It is reason enough to explore the abdomen that one can thereby come to know exactly the state of genital development. If the patient has never menstruated, she has the right to know whether she can ever menstruate and have children. Since there is a reasonable chance she may have the Stein-Leventhal syndrome, for which there is a simple, dramatic cure, there is ordinarily no excuse for not advising abdominal exploration. The operation is comparable in risk and time spent in convalescence to that of appendectomy, which may usually be performed incidentally. There is another element to consider, namely, that polycystic ovaries or a related change, like that of stromal hyperplasia, is commonly associated in later life with carcinoma of the endometrium and the breast. Since the polycystic process does not recur after operation, the operator can provide excellent cancer prophylaxis at an early age.

REFERENCES

Primary Amenorrhea

Cleghorn, R. A.: The Hypothalamic-Endocrine System. *Psychosom. Med.*, 17: 367, 1955.

Comninos, A. C.: Thyroid Function and Therapy in Reproductive Disturbances. *Obst. & Gynec.*, 7: 260, 1956.

Greer, M. A.: Studies on the Influence of the Central Nervous System on Anterior Pituitary Function. *Recent Progress in Hormone Research*, 13: 67, 1957.

Harris, G. W.: *The Neural Control of the Pituitary Gland*. London, E. Arnold, 1955.

Jöel, C. A., and Lancet, M.: The Question of a Psychogenic Factor in Some Cases of Primary Amenorrhea. *J. Clin. Endocrinol. & Metab.*, 16: 909, 1956.

Secondary Amenorrhea

Bickers, W.: Menstrual Arrhythmias. Oral Estrogen and Progesterone Therapy. *Am. J. Obst. & Gynec.*, 64: 148, 1952.

Bradbury, J. T., Brown, W. E., and Gray, C. A.: Maintenance of the Corpus Luteum. Physiologic Actions of Progesterone. *Recent Progress in Hormone Research*, 5: 151, 1950.

Buxton, C. L., and Herrmann, W.: Effect of Thyroid Therapy on Menstrual Disorders and Sterility. *J.A.M.A.*, 155: 1035, 1954.

Idem: Induction of Ovulation in the Human with Human Gonadotropins. *Am. J. Obst. & Gynec.*, 81: 584, 1961.

Frank, R., and Guterman, H. S.: Comparison of Progesterone Preparations in Secondary Amenorrhea. *Fertil. & Steril.*, 5: 374, 1954.

Gemzell, C. A.: Human Pituitary Follicle Stimulating Hormone. I. Clinical Effect of a Partially Purified Preparation; in *Colloquia on Endocrinology*. Ciba Foundation. London, J. & A. Churchill, 1960, Vol. XIII, p. 191.

Goldzieher, M. A., and Goldzieher, J. W.: Hormone Resistant Psychogenic Amenorrhea. *J. Clin. Endocrinol.*, 12: 42, 1952.

Greenblatt, R. B., Scarpa-Smith, C., and Metts, J. C.: Endocrinopathies and Infertility. II. Cushing's Syndrome and Pregnancy. *Fertil. & Steril.*, 10: 323, 1959.

Israel, S. L.: The Empiric Usage of Low-Dosage Irradiation in Amenorrhea. *Am. J. Obst. & Gynec.*, 64: 971, 1952.

Jones, H. W., Jr., and Jones, G. E. S.: Gynecological Aspects of Adrenal Hyperplasia and Allied Disorders. *Am. J. Obst. & Gynec.*, 68: 1330, 1954.

Kaplan, I. I.: The Treatment of Female Sterility with X-ray Therapy Directed to the Pituitary and Ovaries. *Am. J. Obst. & Gynec.*, 76: 447, 1958.

Kelly, K., Daniels, G. E., Poe, J., Easser, R., and Munroe, R.: Psychological Correlations with Secondary Amenorrhea. *Psychosom. Med.*, 16: 129, 1954.

Krosnick, A., and Kalser, M.: Differential Diagnosis of Functional Hypopituitarism Due to Malnutrition (Idiopathic Steatorrhea) and Organic Pituitary Insufficiency in the Puerperium. *Metabolism*, 5: 710, 1956.

Kupperman, H. S., and Lefkovics, S. C.: Progesterone in Problems of Sterility. Diagnostic and Therapeutic Use. *Fertil. & Steril.*, 8: 131, 1957.

Loeser, A. A.: Effect of Emotional Shock on Hormone Release and Endometrial Development. *Lancet*, 1: 518, 1943.

Perloff, W. H., and others: The Starvation State and Functional Hypopituitarism. *J.A.M.A.*, 155: 1307, 1954.

Raykoff, A. E.: The Endocrine Effects of Low-Dose Radiation to the Ovaries and Pituitary of Anovulatory Women. *J. Clin. Endocrinol. & Metab.*, 16: 969, 1956.

Reifenstein, E. C., Jr.: Psychogenic or Hypothalamic Amenorrhea. *M. Clin. N. Amer.*, 30: 1103, 1946.

Richter, C. P.: Ovulation Cycles and Stress; in C. A. Villee, ed.: *Gestation*. New York, Josiah Macy Jr., Foundation, 1957.

Stroink, J. A.: Kriegsamenorrhoe. *Gynecologia*, 124: 160, 1947.

Sydenham, A.: Amenorrhoea at Stanley Camp, Hong Kong, during Internement. *Brit. M.J.*, 2: 159, 1946.

Whitacre, F. E., and Barrera, B.: War Amenorrhea. Clinical and Laboratory Study. *J.A.M.A.*, 124: 399, 1944.

Zander, J.: The Chemical Estimation of Progesterone and Its Metabolites in Body Fluids and Target Organs; in A. C. Barnes, ed.: *Progesterone*. Augusta, Mich., Brook Lodge Press, 1961.

Chapter 22

Primary Dysmenorrhea

ONE OF the most common gynecologic complaints in women of all ages is painful menstruation, or dysmenorrhea. As with amenorrhea, dysmenorrhea is a symptom complex rather than a disease process. It too can be divided into primary and secondary types. In the adolescent group we are chiefly concerned with primary dysmenorrhea, when there is no palpable evidence of any organic disease to explain the cramplike pain which accompanies the menstrual cycle. Secondary dysmenorrhea appears later in life and is invariably associated with any number of pelvic reactive or inflammatory processes, which are more readily demonstrable.

Primary dysmenorrhea usually appears one or two years after the menarche, when the ovary has matured sufficiently to become sensitized to the action of the pituitary hormones. The anovulatory type of bleeding common in the menarche occurs for the most part without painful cramps. Occasionally one finds a puberal girl who has dysmenorrhea in the absence of ovulation, but this is certainly the exception and not the rule. These girls have lower abdominal discomfort and heavy bearing-down pain, but not colicky cramps. Cramps appear in the menses when the ovary comes to full development, maturation of the ova occurs, and progestin is secreted. Whether progestin actually produces the dysmenorrhea may be debatable. The fact remains that essential or intrinsic dysmenorrhea tends to be self-limiting in its duration and is most commonly found in the age groups in which the ovary is reaching maturity in function.

The etiology of dysmenorrhea is complicated by many factors, but one of the most constant observations is the fact that cramps do not appear in the adolescent girl who is having anovulatory cycles.

The basic complaint of dysmenorrhea is pain which appears either as (1) sharp, griping, cramplike pain, not unlike that of intestinal colic or abortion, or (2) a steady, dull ache accompanied by a bearing-down sensation which refers pain down the legs and to the suprapubic area. Approximately 60 per cent of adolescent girls will have cramps, while the remainder will complain of pelvic ache and discomfort. If cramps and bearing-down pain were the only symptoms of primary dysmenorrhea, the percentage of cures from modern therapy would be much higher than they are. Unfortunately, in addition to the pain, these patients complain of (a) abdominal distention, (b) painful breasts, (c) nausea and vomiting, (d) premenstrual tension, (e) depression, (f) irritability, and many other complaints. At times these associated symptoms may precede the actual onset of the cramps by a week or ten days, and are commonly designated as the "menstrual molimina." Characteristically, the pain comes on twenty-four to forty-eight hours before the appearance of the menstrual flow and persists for a varying time thereafter. The severe cramps usually disappear within the first twelve hours. Occasionally only vague discomfort is noted, the pain increasing as the flow increases in amount.

With such a wide spectrum of symptomatology it is not surprising that no one etiologic theory is sufficiently all-encompassing to explain all the varied manifestations of primary dysmenorrhea, much less cure them. This symptom complex has been cloaked in theoretical interpretations as to cause for many hundred years. "Hysteria" originally referred to the uterus, or hysteros. We are inclined now to think that the adolescent girl with her painful cramps is a product of the high-pressure age in which we live. Actually, dysmenorrhea was a recognized entity before the Christian era. Modern therapists can hardly improve on the regimen of rest, massage, hot baths and remedial exercises which were advocated at that time for the relief of dysmenorrhea.

What Is the Mechanism of Pain?

Though more than one hundred years of investigation have not produced a satisfactory explanation of dysmenorrhea, nevertheless certain pertinent observations have been made which serve as the basis for modern therapy.

CERVICAL OBSTRUCTION.   One of the earliest and most persistent theories advanced to explain the cramplike pain was cervical obstruction, particularly if the uterus seemed to be in the position of anteflexion. Certainly not all girls who have anteflexed uteri have cramps, nor do they have cervical stenosis. It is a well substantiated clinical observation that a probe can be introduced into the fundus at the height of the uterine contraction. It is true that some girls do appear to have more severe cramps when the flow is slow in getting under way and are relieved once it has reached its climax. These girls are also cured by dilatation of the cervix. It is probable, however, that this is due more to the forcible stretching of the sympathetic nerve fibers than to correction of any obstructive element in the cervical canal.

MEMBRANOUS DYSMENORRHEA.   Sometimes the endometrium is cast off in large pieces or as an entire castlike lining. Mechanical obstruction of such fragments in the cervical canal produces pain through stimulating tetanic uterine contractions. Membranous dysmenorrhea is not infrequently seen in patients who have had a bilateral tubal ligation.

HYPOPLASIA OF THE UTERUS.   Underdevelopment of the uterus is noted in a fair number of adolescent girls with dysmenorrhea. The cramps were thought to be due to the preponderance of fibrous tissue over muscle which produced irregular contractions. Not all girls who have uterine hypoplasia have cramps, and many healthy girls with normal healthy uteri are prostrated with their periods. Dysmenorrhea in the presence of a hypoplastic uterus may simply reflect a poor nutritional state or a nervously unstable patient who, because of these factors, has either deficient stimulation or utilization of the ovarian hormones.

HYPERCONTRACTILITY OF THE UTERUS.   The cramplike nature of the pain suggests hypermotility. The contractions are believed to be under hormonal control. Originally estrin was considered to be the factor responsible for the contraction, while progestin produced relaxation. Much of the earlier hormone therapy was based on this conception of hormonal action. There can be no doubt that normal uterine motility varies with the cyclic output of the ovarian hormones. Uterine contractions under the stimulus of estrin have been tested with intrauterine balloons attached to a pressure-recording kymograph.

In the preovulatory phase, under the influence of estrin, the contractions are low in amplitude, increasing in frequency and reaching a peak at the time of ovulation. In the postovulatory phase of the cycle, when progestin is present, the contractions become less frequent and more regular, but with a higher degree of amplitude. In dysmenorrhea there appears to be an imbalance between estrin and progestin. The uterine tone is high, and the contractions are not only irregular, but also appear to arise in isolated muscle groups. The exciting agent seems to be progestin. Dysmenorrhea of this type occurs only in ovulatory cycles, when progestin is present.

VASOCONSTRICTION.   An increasing amount of evidence shows that dysmenorrhea may be due more to vasoconstriction in the spiral arteriolar mechanism in the endometrium than to abnormal contractions of the uterine muscle. Observations on the endometrium planted in the anterior chamber of the rabbit's eye may produce the clue to the mechanism. The endometrium is normally supplied with an abundance of spiral arterioles in its functional layer. These coiled arteries lie in a spongy tissue layer and are far in excess of need unless pregnancy occurs. If pregnancy does not ensue, withdrawal of the growth stimulus causes the corpus luteum to degenerate, and a rapid regression in the thickness of the endometrium occurs, approximately one to five days before the period. With the regressive shrinkage of the endometrium a disproportion occurs between it and the length of the coiled arteries supplying the endometrium. The arterioles kink and contract, producing a slowing down of the circulation and a relative stasis of blood. As this process progresses, injury to the endometrium occurs, and the necrosis of menstruation appears. The necrosing endometrium tends to cause further vasoconstriction in the coiled arteries, perhaps by elaborating some toxic substance (menstrual toxin). Progestin seems to prolong this vasoconstriction by nullifying the dilating effect of estrin. As a result of the vasoconstriction, areas of ischemia also develop within the myometrium. The spasm resulting from contraction of muscle in the presence of the ischemic area explains the pain. This mechanism is not unlike that of toxic separation of the placenta, in which a similar type of pain arises when the uterus contracts. The explanation for the mechanism of pain in angina pectoris is not dissimilar.

PATHOLOGY WITHIN THE SACRAL NERVES.   Pathologic alteration in the fibers and ganglia of the presacral nerves is a frequent observation when the nerves are resected for incapacitating dysmenorrhea and examined pathologically. It cannot be determined preoperatively. At operation one may note that the nerve with all its widely ramifying branches is more than ordinarily firm, fibrous and adherent to the iliac vessels and the bony sacrum. The degree of fixation appears to correspond to the severity of the symptomatology. Pathologic alterations therefore vary in their extent. The sympathetic nerves and ganglia may appear normal or may show evidence of degeneration of the ganglion cells and chronic inflammatory changes of the fibers (Fig. 22–1). Subacute or chronic neuritis is not present in all resected presacral nerves, but over 70 per cent will show some variation from the normal. When such is present, it is logical to suggest that the pain may be due to the modification of the impulses passing along a nerve damaged by an inflammatory or degenerative process.

PSYCHOGENIC AND CONSTITUTIONAL FACTORS.   The threshold of pain in girls with the dysmenorrhea syndrome varies widely. This depends in part on the sensitiveness of the cerebral cortex to painful stimuli. The pain in nerve endings may be constant, but the patient's reaction varies, depending on this sensitivity. Trauma and disease lower the threshold for pain. The nutritional state is also important, for proper function of the hormones is directly dependent on it. The cause of the increased

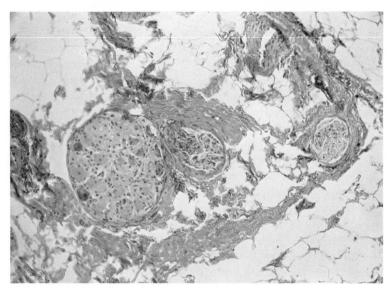

Fig. 22-1.   A nerve ganglion and nerve fibers from a presacral neurectomy performed for dysmenorrhea. The nerves and ganglion are enclosed in excessive fibrous scar tissue that might develop after a neuritis healed. Slight edema is present with dilated perineural spaces.

sensitivity in the healthy patient is not completely understood. Sensitivity may be influenced by the absorption of toxic products from disintegration of the endometrium. It is more likely, however, that the depression and irritability noted at the time of the period are due to the action of progestin. Progesterone is a vasoconstrictor with a known propensity for inducing water and salt retention in the extracellular tissues. Edema and ischemia of the brain cortex may then be the explanation of the increased sensitivity.

There can be little doubt that the mother's attitude toward the recurring phenomena of menstruation may condition the child's mind and influence her response. If the mother has had a bad time with her menstrual periods, she may attempt to coddle and protect her daughter from the same experiences which have plagued her. Under the misguided efforts of the mother, menstruation becomes the "curse" rather than a "friend." What was originally moderate discomfort becomes pain of varying severity, depending on the sensitivity of the girl.

One cannot discuss the mechanism of pain in primary dysmenorrhea without considering the psychogenic element. Since the cause of pain is incompletely understood and the physical findings are negative, it is not surprising that the complaints associated with the period are often attributed to psychiatric causes.

Many reports are appearing in the literature suggesting that psychotherapy is the sole answer to the problem of essential dysmenorrhea. There is no denying the fact that some of these patients present psychosomatic tendencies with perhaps a lowered threshold for pain. Many girls with severe dysmenorrhea are perfectly well adjusted to their environment through the rest of the month and rarely seek medical support for other cause. They appear perfectly well poised and adjusted after specific therapy, but are not improved by placebos. Apprehensions expressed at the time of the menstrual period may be the result, not the cause, of dysmenorrhea. Those who believe that psychic trauma is the basic cause of monthly pain are still unable to determine which comes first, the pain or the psychogenic response.

Dysmenorrhea would seem to be a somatic disorder with a psychogenic element superimposed. In extremely rare instances the psychiatrist may trace the underlying cause to fear or rejection of the feminine role, competition with the mother for the father's attention, or some disturbance in the relationship with the mother that brings out a feeling of guilt or hostility, which makes her want to be either totally disassociated from her mother or, if emotionally immature, more attached to her. By and large, common-sense psychology should apply. This is the premise of the family physician.

Because of these factors the proper management of the patient with dysmenorrhea provides an excellent test of our capacities as physicians. As much depends on our knowledge of human beings as of hormonology, neurology and pharmacology. We must have the patience to deal with the regularly occurring vagaries in disposition of both girl and mother. Our enthusiasm for any given form of therapy must be tempered by common sense. In outlining a plan of treatment for primary dysmenorrhea we must constantly keep in mind that we are dealing with a self-limited disease. Since there is a large element of psychogenic overlay, either as the cause or the result of pain, it is important to know the degree of severity of the pain and the extent of incapacity produced. Many girls have discomfort and pain; relatively few are incapacitated.

Management of a Mild Case

A sympathetic attitude on the part of the physician will do much to gain the confidence of the girl. In many instances the mother will have overstressed the rigors of the "curse" to the point at which the patient has regularly retired from the world to bed. Many young girls experience discomfort with the period, but under mother's influence it is an easy transition from discomfort to pain. The child should be told that such discomfort can be expected and regarded as normal. It will be advisable to have a heart-to-heart talk with the mother along the same lines. Many girls with intelligent handling, supplemented by simple analgesic drugs, can be talked out of their troubles.

Specifically, the patient should be kept on her feet, and encouraged to exercise instead of retiring to bed. Faulty posture may produce a pelvic tilt and compression of the ilio-inguinal and hypogastric nerves, thereby contributing to pelvic discomfort. Stretching exercises are helpful in reducing the pain which radiates to the groin and down the legs. Any moderate exercise is preferable to lying in bed. Fatigue, however, should be avoided, for it contributes to a lowered threshold for pain. Improvement in general well-being will improve the mental outlook toward the recurring phenomenon of menstruation. Trauma and disease lower the threshold for pain. Proper hygiene, regular hours and diet should be stressed. To minimize the nausea, vomiting and abdominal distention, a light diet, low in carbohydrates, combined with a mild cathartic should be taken at the time of the period. Ammonium chloride, 3 to 4 gm. daily, a mercurial diuretic such as Neohydrin, 2 to 4 capsules daily, or Diuril (chlorothiazide), 500 mg., with a low salt diet for 10 days before the period are helpful adjuncts. The drugs are harmless, widely available and useful. Since there are many mechanisms at work in dysmenorrhea, there is no reason why combination drug therapy should not be used.

Supplemental drug therapy should be in the nature of an analgesic, sedative or mild antispasmodic. Drugs such as Midol, Edrisal or Lutrexin may be given every six hours with the onset of the cramps. Atropine, belladonna and phenobarbital may be given in moderate doses. Empirin, phenacetin or aspirin may be used, either alone or in combination with ½ grain of codeine.

When the pain is severe enough to call for stronger doses of narcotics, we are no longer dealing with a mild case of dysmenorrhea.

Management of Severe Dysmenorrhea

As the symptoms become more severe, each month presents an increasing problem, since the simpler methods of therapy are less successful. The patient finally comes for help because the pain is incompatible with her plan of life for two or three days out of the month. There may be an element of psychoneurosis, but this pain is severe and increasing and bound to recur rhythmically on a monthly schedule.

To refer such a patient to the psychiatrist or resort to radical surgical intervention at this time is a mistake. This is the sort of patient in whom hormone therapy should be given as a trial. Since ovulation is a primary requisite, its suppression should be the aim of therapy. Once the follicle-stimulating hormone activates the ovary and the follicle begins to develop, nothing can normally be done to prevent it from maturing. Thus it is mandatory in this form of treatment that the estrin be given early enough in the cycle and in sufficient dosage to prevent ovulation. The oral route is preferred, for it avoids the use of repeated injections in a symptom complex that already has a large psychogenic element.

Therapy should begin on the first day of the cycle. Diethylstilbestrol, 1.0 mg., Estinyl, 0.05 mg., or 1.25 mg. of the conjugated estrins such as Premarin may be tried. Daily doses, usually at bedtime for twenty days, should begin with the first day of the period. About six days after the last dose estrin-withdrawal bleeding usually occurs. With the onset of bleeding the oral therapy is resumed, and the series is repeated monthly for three months. The patient should then be allowed to ovulate in the normal manner. If pain has been relieved and recurs when medication is withdrawn, a presacral neurectomy, if the symptoms are severe enough to consider it, will be successful in a high percentage of cases. This is an excellent screening test. Dysmenorrhea with anovulatory bleeding points to the likelihood of a fixed psychoneurosis.

The effect of estrin in suppression of ovulation is not always predictable. Often a dose adequate to suppress pain in one month may not produce the same effect in the following month. One can be sure that when ovulation is suppressed, pain will not appear. Some clinicians, therefore, prefer to give 5 mg. of diethylstilbestrol, 0.1 mg. of Estinyl or 3.75 mg. of Premarin to increase the chances of preventing ovulation. It is also true that estrin loses its power to prevent ovulation when given over a period of time. Pregnancies have been reported during therapy with estrin designed to suppress ovulation.

The enthusiasm for testosterone has diminished. It has been given in the form of methyltestosterone orally in 10-mg. doses beginning on the eighth day and continued through the sixteenth day of the cycle. The drug is given too late to prevent ovulation, and pregnancy has occurred during its use. Successful reports in the alleviation of pain are available, but the rationale of this therapy is questionable. To give doses large enough to suppress ovulation is to run the risk of masculinization. The risk outweighs the advantages.

Progesterone in large doses is said to be effective. On the basis of what we know, there seems to be little reason for its use, and the price to the average patient is prohibitive at this time. Norethynodrel with ethynylestradiol-3-methyl-ether (Enovid), one of the new synthetic steroids, however, has proved to be effective in suppressing ovulation when given orally in 10-mg. doses from day 5 through 25.

Estrin seems to be the hormone of choice, either because of its action in relaxing vascular spasm or because of its suppression of ovulation.

In addition to hormonal therapy, one should consider the advisability of a dilatation and curettage before advocating intra-abdominal surgery and presacral neurectomy. The curettage provides a clean base for the hormones to work upon, and the disruption of nerve supply through cervical dilatation may be sufficient to produce a cure. Fifty per cent of the patients will be relieved.

Management of Incapacitating Dysmenorrhea

The more drastic forms of therapy are reserved for the girl who is totally incapacitated for at least twenty-four hours out of each month. Since patients with dysmenorrhea of this degree exhibit a large psychosomatic element and a variable response to pain, it is a difficult decision as to whether the patient should be referred for psychiatric evaluation or be subjected to surgical intervention. Though no disease can be demonstrated, it is important to remember that 15 per cent will have unsuspected endometriosis at the time of exploration. It is unfair to label these patients as psychoneurotics. All forms of therapy should be tried before resorting to either psychiatry or presacral neurectomy. The number of candidates for either one is sharply limited. Of the two, presacral neurectomy seems more logical, but only 5 or 10 per cent of patients with dysmenorrhea are suitable candidates.

Some help in selection may be obtained by emphasizing the test of suppressing ovulation through the use of estrin. It is also true that patients who respond with cramplike pain to the introduction and rotation of a probe within the endometrial cavity are excellent candidates for presacral nerve resection. Mature judgment, however, is necessary in making the proper selection for or against surgery or psychiatry.

If presacral neurectomy is to be done, there is a further selection. It should not be offered to the patient who has lateral pain or backache. Experience has shown that it will be ineffective in these cases. Division of the infundibulopelvic ligaments containing the ovarian vessels in combination with presacral neurectomy has been advocated in foreign clinics, but has had little support in this country.

Presacral neurectomy is a satisfactory operation for the girl who has sufficient pain to warrant it, provided the patient is properly selected and an adequate operation is performed. Resection of the nerves does not interfere with satisfactory completion of the sexual act and permits labor to continue to the stage of perineal dilatation before pain is evident.

The success of presacral nerve resection is probably based on (1) the interruption of painful impulses passing from the uterus along nerve pathways to the higher centers and (2) upon the improvement in vascular flow to the uterus, by providing release of vasoconstriction. When the divided distal ends of the presacral nerves are stimulated electrically, the uterus does not contract, but undergoes alternate blanching and flushing, suggesting that the effect of presacral neurectomy is upon the vascular mechanism. There is further clinical evidence that such a mechanism is operative, from the observation that patients who have had presacral neurectomy invariably bleed vaginally three or four days after operation, regardless of the stage of the menstrual cycle. One may also postulate that better utilization of the hormones is thereby possible. Conversely, when the base of the broad ligament is stimulated, the uterus contracts violently, but shows none of the vascular changes. One may theorize that the patient who had cramplike pain might do well with presacral neurectomy, while the patient who has bearing-down pain would be improved by resection of Frankenhauser's plexus, which lies at the level of the internal cervical os and the upper part of the vagina, the uterosacral ligaments representing the lateral boundaries.

If presacral neurectomy is to be successful, it must be done adequately. Too many times in the past simple excision of a small section of nerve at the promontory of the sacrum was the extent of the operation. Many of the unsuccessful or equivocal results reported followed this procedure. The ramifications of the nerve are so widespread as they course on the under surface of the peritoneum and downward along the iliac and hypogastric vessels that interruption of all nerve fibers can be accomplished only by dissection of all pathways. It is important that a dissection, not excision, be done, since the nerve cannot be removed otherwise.

Psychiatry and hypnosis should be considered carefully for a certain number of patients, again relatively few, who are poor candidates for anything else.

Conclusion

Therapy of dysmenorrhea must be based on an understanding of the possible etiologic factors and on an intelligent appraisal of their application to the individual patient. No two cases are produced by the same mechanism, or respond in the same way if they are. We must individualize in the therapy of dysmenorrhea if we are to be successful.

INTERMENSTRUAL PAIN AND BLEEDING

Abdominal pain occurring at the midinterval in the cycle is a phenomenon common to the adolescent who has fully matured, but is rare at the menarche. Approximately 70 per cent of patients who complain of intermenstrual pain are in the adolescent age group. One of the most striking features of this midmenstrual pain is its regularity, for it tends to recur about the same time month after month. In some patients with regular cycles the pain is precisely midmenstrual, while in others it may precede or follow the midpoint in the cycle. The actual menstrual period itself seems to be unaltered, although many of these patients have dysmenorrhea. The timing and the dysmenorrhea lend support to the contention that the pain and bleeding that often accompany it are secondary to ovulation (*Mittelschmerz*). While these patients are experiencing this type of midmenstrual pain, however, there appears to be an element of relative infertility. This paradox may be explained by the fact that the patient becomes disinterested in intercourse, because of the pain at her most fertile point in the cycle.

There appears to be no solid explanation of the mechanism of the pain. Rupture of the follicle sometimes occurs explosively, as seen in certain moving pictures taken at the time of ovulation. The distention of the capsule of the ovary by the developing follicle may explain part of the pain, which is increased when free bleeding from the site of the follicle rupture spills onto the parietal peritoneum. The parietal peritoneum is sensitive to trauma of this sort, and the mechanism of pain in follicle rupture is not unlike that of ectopic pregnancy. Direct observation of the ovary and the finding of free blood in the cul-de-sac at the time of operation give some support to this explanation. Certain observers have sought to explain the pain on the basis of abnormal contractions of either tube or uterus, but this interpretation can hardly be classed as anything but speculation.

Menstrual spotting (*kleiner Regen*) and at times more pronounced bleeding may accompany the abdominal pain at the midmenstrual period. Though the pain tends to recur at regular intervals in succeeding months, the intermenstrual bleeding may be absent in one or two cycles, only to reappear in subsequent cycles. The amount of bleeding varies within wide ranges and usually disappears in a few hours or days. Sometimes the adolescent girl simply notes midmenstrual spotting, while others complain of a brownish discharge. At times the vaginal bleeding is active enough to simulate the menstrual period, and the patients not infrequently claim to be having two periods each month. Bleeding of this sort could come from a variety of pathologic entities such as a cervical or endometrial polyp, but a careful history will usually bring out the periodic nature of the bleeding. If the more important explanations of midmenstrual bleeding such as polyp or cancer can be ruled out, one can reassure the patient that such bleeding is of no particular consequence. When there is any element of doubt, serious pelvic disease should be excluded by a diagnostic curettage.

The treatment of midmenstrual bleeding is rather unsatisfactory. Buccal tablets of the new progesterone preparations such as Enovid or Provera, in 10-mg. doses daily for 14 days, are rational therapy, for the endometrium is usually found to be in the proliferative phase. The bleeding is probably due to an overabundant proliferative endometrium which has locally outrun its blood supply, rather than to any pronounced drop in the level of circulating estrogens.

Midmenstrual pain, or *Mittelschmerz*, with or without intermenstrual bleeding, is usually cramplike and at times severe enough for one to entertain the diagnosis of acute appendicitis. Not infrequently the pain is unilateral and accompanied by malaise, nausea and headache. The differential diagnosis between this kind of pain and that of appendicitis is not an easy one, for the symptoms and signs are similar, and the differential white blood cell count may show elevations as high as 18,000 per cubic millimeter, with a pronounced shift to the left. If there is any doubt, good judgment would favor the diagnosis of appendicitis.

The actual treatment of periodic pain of this sort is not very satisfactory, nor can one give an accurate prognosis of how long the pain is apt to continue. Many girls have midmenstrual pain throughout the rest of their menstrual life, while others have spontaneous relief either permanently or sporadically. When the pain bothers the patient sufficiently to require medication, it is better to rely on simple analgesic drugs or progestin-like hormones. Surgery offers nothing unless the ovaries are removed, and radical treatment of this magnitude would be inexcusable. Dilatation and curettage and presacral neurectomy have been tried unsuccessfully. Since spontaneous cures occur, and no pathologic sequence of events follows repeated incidents of midmenstrual pain, reassurance and simple drugs such as aspirin and codeine combined with hot baths and rest represent the optimum in therapy.

REFERENCES

Allen, E.: Pelvic Examination of the Preadolescent and Adolescent Girl. *Am. J. Obst. & Gynec.*, 68: 1311, 1954.

Bickers, W.: *Menorrhagia; Menstrual Distress.* Springfield, Ill., Charles C Thomas, 1954.

Billig, H. E., Jr.: Dysmenorrhea: The Result of a Postural Defect. *Arch. Surg.*, 46: 611, 1943.

Cotte, G.: Resection of the Presacral Nerve in the Treatment of Obstinate Dysmenorrhea. *Am. J. Obst. & Gynec.*, 33: 1034, 1937.

Curtis, A. H., Anson, B. J., Ashley, F. L., and Jones, T.: The Anatomy of the Pelvic Autonomic Nerves in Relation to Gynecology. *Surg., Gynec. & Obst.*, 75: 743, 1942.

Davis, A. A.: *Dysmenorrhoea. Its Aetiology, Pathology and Treatment.* London, Oxford University Press, 1938.

Diehl, W. K., and Hundley, J. M., Jr.: The Role of Uterine Motility in Essential Dysmenorrhea. *Am. J. Obst. & Gynec.*, 56: 281, 1948.

Dignam, W. J., Wortham, J. T., and Hamblem, E. C.: Estrogen Therapy of Functional Dysmenorrhea: Analysis of Clinical Results *Am. J. Obst. & Gynec.*, 59: 1124, 1950.

Duncan, C. J.: Surgical Treatment of Dysmenorrhea. *New York State M.J.*, 46: 2757, 1946.

Filler, W.: Preovulatory Administration of Methyltestosterone in Refractory Functional Dysmenorrhea. *J.A.M.A.*, 143: 1235, 1950.

Freeman, A.: The Distribution of the Nerves to the Adult Human Uterus. *Am. J. Clin. Path.*, 16: 117, 1946.

Gallagher, J. R.: Dysmenorrhea and Menorrhagia in Adolescence. *Connecticut M.J.*, 19: 469, 1955.

Golub, L. J., Lang, W. R., Menduke, H., and Gordon, H. C.: Teen-Age Dysmenorrhea. *Am. J. Obst. & Gynec.*, 74: 591, 1957.

Haman, J. O.: Pain Threshold in Dysmenorrhea. *Am. J. Obst. & Gynec.*, 47: 686, 1944.

Hayden, G. E.: Relief of Primary Dysmenorrhea. An Evaluation of the Newer Therapeutic Agents. *Obst. & Gynec.*, 16: 730, 1960.

Heald, F. P., Jr., Masland, R. P., Jr., Sturgis, S. H., and Gallagher, J. R.: Dysmenorrhea in Adolescence. *Pediatrics*, 20: 121, 1957.

Henry, J. S., Browne, J. S. L., and Venning, E. H.: Some Observations on the Relations of Estrogens and Progesterone to the Contractions of the Nonpregnant and Pregnant Human Uterus. *Am. J. Obst. & Gynec.*, 60: 471, 1950.

Hirsch, E. F., and Martin, M. E.: The Distribution of Nerves in the Adult Human Myometrium. *Surg., Gynec. & Obst.*, 76: 697, 1943.

Ibarra, J. D., Jr., and Higginbotham, W. H.: Endocrine Therapy of Amenorrhea, Dysfunctional Uterine Bleeding and Dysmenorrhea. *M. Clin. N. Amer.*, 39: 1189, 1955.

Ingersoll, F. M., and Meigs, J. V.: Presacral Neurectomy for Dysmenorrhea. *New England J. Med.*, 238: 357, 1948.

Jeffcoate, T. N. A., and Lerer, S.: Hypoplasia of Uterus, with Special Reference to Spasmodic Dysmenorrhoea. *J. Obst. & Gynaec. Brit. Emp.*, 52: 97, 1945.

Krantz, K. E.: Innervation of the Human Uterus. *Ann. New York Acad. Sc.*, 75: 770, 1959.

Kupperman, H. S., Rosenberg, D., and Cutler, A.: Relaxin in Dysmenorrhea and Its Effect in Vitro upon Muscular Contraction. *Ann. New York Acad. Sc.*, 75: 1003, 1959.

Lowe, C. R., and Ferguson, R. L.: Age Incidence of Dysmenorrhoea. *Brit. J. Social Med.*, 5: 193, 1951.

Lyon, R. A.: Relief of Essential Dysmenorrhea with Ethinyl Estradiol. *Surg., Gynec. & Obst.*, 77: 657, 1943.

Markee, J. E.: Menstruation in Intraocular Endometrial Transplants in the Rhesus Monkey. *Contrib. to Embryol.*, Carnegie Inst. Wash., 28: 223, 1940.

Meigs, J. V.: Excision of the Superior Hypogastric Plexus (Presacral Nerve) for Primary Dysmenorrhea. *Surg., Gynec. & Obst.*, 68: 723, 1939.

Miller, N. F., and Behrman, S. J.: Dysmenorrhea. *Am. J. Obst. & Gynec.*, 65: 505, 1953.

Parsons, L.: Dysmenorrhea, Its Causes and Treatment. *M. Clin. N. Amer.*, 38: 1419, 1954.

Paul, W. M., Glickman, B. I., Cushner, I. M., and Reynolds, S. R. M.: Cervical Tone and Pain Thresholds. (Study in the Non-gravid Uterus.) *Obst. & Gynec.*, 7: 511, 1956.

Pemberton, F. A.: Resection of the Presacral Nerve in Gynecology. *New England J. Med.*, 213: 710, 1935.

Schuck, F.: Pain and Relief in Essential Dysmenorrhea. *Am. J. Obst. & Gynec.*, 62: 559, 1951.

Sturgis, S. H.: The Use of Stilbestrol in the Relief of Essential Dysmenorrhea. *New England J. Med.*, 226: 371, 1942.

Sturgis, S. H., and Albright, F.: The Mechanism of Estrin Therapy in the Relief of Dysmenorrhea. *Endocrinology*, 26: 68, 1940.

Torpin, R., Woodbury, R. A., and Child, G. P.: The Nature of Dysmenorrhea. *Am. J. Obst. & Gynec.*, 54: 766, 1947.

White, J. C.: Conduction of Visceral Pain. *New England J. Med.*, 246: 686, 1952.

Winther, N.: Menorrheal Problems in College Women. *Am. J. Obst. & Gynec.*, 52: 803, 1946.

Chapter 23

Breast during

Puberty and Adolescence

THE PROBLEMS involving the breast in the prepuberal, puberal and adolescent age groups are (1) abnormalities in the development of the breasts and (2) circumscribed tumor growths, which in the great majority of instances are fibroadenomas.

It has been noted in earlier discussions that alteration in the appearance of the breasts is one of the earliest signs of genital development. This change commonly occurs at approximately the age of eleven years, when the pituitary gonadotropic hormones first really become active.

Should the female child present evidence of the constitutional type of precocious puberty or harbor one of the rare forms of tumor of the ovary, adrenal or third ventricle, there may be a rapid development of the breasts at a very early age. Occasionally this occurs within the first two years, and it has been reported as early as six months of age. The association of abnormal breast development with ovarian tumors can occur, but certainly the instances are rare. Since the primary factor in the growth of breast tissue is the presence of estrin, one might expect to find that with a granulosa cell tumor in an adolescent or prepuberal child there might also be present evidence of breast enlargement, for such tumors are known to secrete large amounts of estrin. Lutein cysts of the ovary have also been reported in association with abnormal breast development.

Actually, the female breast can enlarge at any age without demonstrable evidence of a physiologic imbalance or abnormal stimulation. This has been observed after hysterectomy and even after the menopause. Though abnormal secretion of estrin has been suspected, laboratory studies of urinary estrin excretion have been unable to demonstrate any constant excretory pattern, either high or low. One might suspect the pituitary, but our laboratory methods for detection of the pituitary gonadotropins have not been sensitive enough to demonstrate any appreciable change, and study of the so-called pituitary mammotropic hormone is as yet mostly experimental.

ABNORMAL DEVELOPMENT OF THE BREAST AT PUBERTY

This may take one of two forms: underdevelopment or hypertrophy (Fig. 23–1).

275

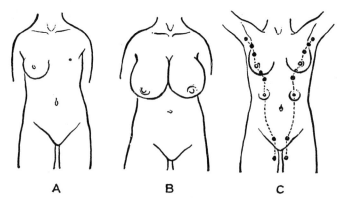

Fig. 23-1.   Anomalous developmental breast lesions. *A*, Failure of one breast to form, aside from a rudimentary nipple (amastia). *B*, Overdevelopment (macromastia). *C*, Accessory nipples, breast, or both. These are found along the "milk lines," which are potential mammogenic zones indicated by the dotted lines.

UNDERDEVELOPMENT

One expects to observe a gradual increase in the size of the breasts at puberty in the normally developing young girl. Failure in development immediately raises the question of whether or not there are any underlying deficient endocrine factors, the most extreme instance being ovarian agenesis. In most cases lack of breast development is but one of a series of stigmata which tend to point to endocrine abnormalities or disturbances in endocrine function. Many girls who are otherwise completely normal are simply flat-chested and never do develop adequate breast tissue. This is a continual source of annoyance throughout life and particularly tends to make the adolescent girl abnormally sensitive about her figure.

Failure of breast development in an otherwise normal girl has never been adequately explained. In certain animals at least five hormones are required for complete breast development. The true cause seems to lie less in a deficiency in hormone production and more in a lack of sensitivity of the target organ, which fails to respond to estrin stimulation in the normal fashion. This apparent fact receives support from the attempt to bring about enlargement of the breast artificially by giving estrin either orally, parenterally or as a local ointment. Rarely is this successful, and if so the effect is noticeable only so long as the estrin is administered or applied. When there is an absolute lack of estrin, as in ovarian agenesis, it may be possible to produce and maintain breast enlargement by the continuous use of estrogenic substances.

The breast tissues of some women appear to be refractory to normal estrin stimulation. This is in direct contrast to the breast with normal sensitivity in which the response to estrogen hormone therapy is immediate and dramatic. It is also an observed fact that the female breast may not respond uniformly in equal measure to the same amount of hormonal stimulation. Frequently a disproportion is observed in the size of one breast, as compared to the opposite one, in mature women who may or may not have borne or nursed children. When questioned, they frequently state that one breast, usually the left, has always been larger than its mate.

Treatment of the underdeveloped breast is not very rewarding to either patient or physician. Since the breast tissue seems abnormally refractory to estrin stimulation, such therapy, though rational, often fails to produce the enlargement so eagerly sought by the distraught patient. It is possible that she may acquire equally satis-factory results by simple and repeated massage of the breasts and use of ointments that do not contain estrin preparations. Attempts to improve the breast contour by grafting of fat pads should be considered a surgical stunt fraught with potential danger, for infection is not uncommon, and injection of oils or waxes or use of Ivalon sponge is to be heartily condemned.

ADOLESCENT HYPERTROPHY OF BREAST

The most frequent type of abnormal breast development is the massive hyper-trophy that sometimes occurs at the time of puberty and continues into adolescence. It is more often found in stocky, dark-skinned girls with a tendency toward hirsutism. Usually both breasts are equally involved, though occasionally the hypertrophy is unilateral, and the opposite breast develops normally. Exaggerated enlargement of the breast at the time of puberty is to be expected, but in the girl with abnormal hypertrophy the breasts continue to develop beyond the normal pattern. As exagger-

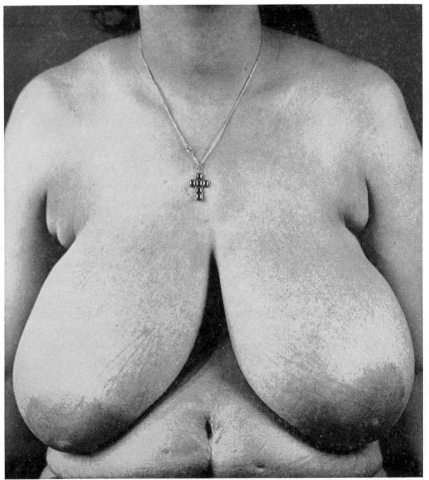

Fig. 23-2.   Adolescent hypertrophy of the breasts. Quantitatively, the excessive tissue is largely fibro-fatty. (Courtesy of C. D. Haagensen: *Diseases of the Breast.*)

ated growth continues, they become a source of constant embarrassment and not inconsiderable discomfort (Fig. 23–2). The growing girl tends to become round-shouldered for two reasons: (1) she is so acutely aware of the gross abnormality that she tries to hide it by letting her shoulders droop forward, and (2) the extra weight may actually produce a continuous drag on her shoulder girdle to the point of such discomfort that it is relieved only by the recumbent position.

Normal growth activity in the breast at the time of puberty is without doubt largely due to estrin stimulation. It is possible that excessive growth beyond the normal limits may be due to an abnormal sensitivity of the breast tissue to estrin stimulation. Laboratory studies fail to produce any evidence of overproduction of estrin. When the tissue from the hypertrophied breast is examined microscopically, there is little departure from the normal. In most instances the evidence for excessive growth is found as a hyperplasia in the duct system, involving both epithelium and intrinsic stroma, with some increase in the amount of periductal connective tissue and fat. The acini and lobular elements remain undeveloped, as in the normal breast, awaiting the stimulus of the luteinizing and lactogenic hormones.

Treatment

Since there appears to be little evidence that the breasts become smaller once the impact of estrin stimulation abates in the years immediately following puberty, the patient is confronted with a constant problem. If the discomfort is sufficiently great, it is possible to obtain relief from the constant dragging sensation and improvement in feminine configuration by resorting to plastic surgery, which removes the excess tissue while preserving the nipple.

FIBROADENOMA

Discrete lumps are commonly present in the adolescent breast. The most constant finding is a rounded, firm, lobulated nodule, varying in size from 1 to 5 cm., and occurring anywhere in the young female breast, but usually in the upper half, either along the outer quadrant or in relation to the nipple. This is in all probability fibroadenoma. This sharply demarcated tumor, made up of variable amounts of epithelial and stromal elements, is the most frequent growth seen in the puberal or adolescent breast (Fig. 23–3). At any age it is the most common benign tumor of the breast and is exceeded in frequency only by the more diffuse disease conditions, chronic fibrocystic disease and cancer. In the young woman this nodule, which is movable and does not retract the skin, for it sets up no fibroblastic reaction in the surrounding stroma, may be difficult to differentiate from a tense cyst. Since it produces no symptoms and is nontender, it is usually discovered by accident. A solitary nodule is the rule, but in some 15 per cent multiple tumors are present. There appears to be some racial factor, for they are found more commonly in the Negro race and at an earlier age than one notes in the white population. This tumor may be called either fibroadenoma or adenofibroma, but the first term is preferred, to avoid possible confusion with adenofibrosis, a diffuse fibrosis of breast tissue.

Etiology

The etiologic factor in the development of the fibroadenoma in the adolescent breast is closely linked to that of breast hypertrophy, for both are prone to appear during the accelerated growth period at puberty. The intense estrin stimulation may either cause the entire breast to enlarge, in which case there is breast hypertrophy, or to be confined to a localized area within the breast tissue, when fibroadenomas appear. Fibroadenomas are known to increase in size and to lactate during pregnancy and the puerperium. They have been shown to enlarge after estrin administration.

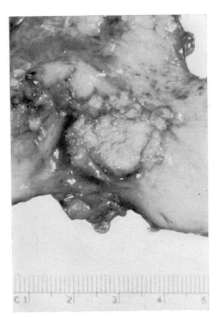

Fig. 23-3.   Cross section of a fibroadenoma, the pale, firm, granular rounded mass that appears sharply demarcated from the surrounding, smooth-surfaced breast stroma.

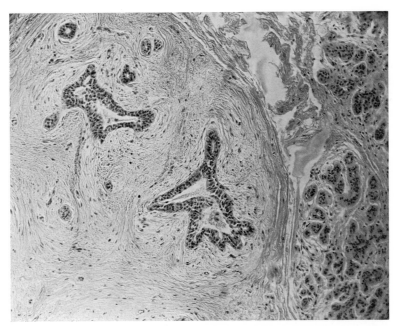

Fig. 23-4.   A fibroadenoma with its surrounding capsule is shown compressing an adjacent uninvolved breast lobule. As the name indicates, it is partly fibrous, owing to proliferation of the fibrillar intrinsic estrogen-responsive connective tissue stroma. It is also in part an adenoma, as shown by participation of ducts in this benign neoplastic growth.

Histologic studies of the excised nodules after estrogen therapy show largely increased edema and hyperemia of the lobules and proliferation of ductules (Fig. 23–4). With the termination of pregnancy or the withdrawal of estrin medication the tumors shrink.

The etiology of the fibroadenoma has not been clearly established. This benign neoplasm is similar enough functionally to normal breast to go through the usual cyclic changes accompanying the menses and to lactate.

Treatment

There appears to be no significant association of fibroadenoma with malignant disease. One can sometimes, therefore, afford to observe its rate of growth in the adolescent girl and to defer operation. This is particularly true when there is a soft discoid-shaped mass of tissue noted beneath the nipple, usually on one side, but occasionally bilateral, a common finding in the immature breast at puberty or in the years immediately preceding it. This might prove on excision to be adenofibrosis, not fibroadenoma. Overconcern on the part of the mother and the physician as to the possibility of malignant disease often leads to ill-advised attempts to biopsy or excise the mass. Such surgery may interfere with the normal development of the breast.

In the adolescent girl these tumors can take on an accelerated rate of growth and enlarge in 6 months to 3 or 5 cm., but usually they grow slowly or remain stationary. If there is evidence of rapid growth, it is wise to excise the lesion together with a margin of normal breast tissue. It is also possible that the more rapidly growing tumor is a cystosarcoma phylloides, which is usually a sinister name for a giant fibroadenoma. Commonly this large benign tumor occurs about the age of forty years, but it has been reported as early as fifteen years. In 98 or 99 per cent of cases cystosarcoma phylloides is nonmalignant.

Actual cancer of the breast is rare before the age of 25 years, with an incidence in this age group of approximately 0.4 per cent of all breast cancer. If there are any disquieting factors in the appearance of the growth pattern, excision of the breast nodule is advisable. Should it prove to be fibroadenoma, which is to be expected, the family and the patient need have no unusual concern about the subsequent development of malignant disease. If another tumor develops in youth after a previous excision, one is justified in watching it, provided the initial diagnosis was fibroadenoma. It may stay the same size or even regress.

Watchful expectant observation and surgical excision are the only logical forms of treatment. There is no place for hormone therapy or radiation.

REFERENCES

Cholnoky, T. de: Supernumerary Breast. *Arch. Surg.*, 39: 926, 1939.
Geschickter, C. F., and Lewis, D.: Pregnancy and Lactation Changes in Fibro-adenoma of the Breast. *Brit. M.J.*, 1: 499, 1938.
Haagensen, C. D.: *Diseases of the Breast*. Philadelphia, W. B. Saunders Company, 1956, Chap. 3.
Ingleby, H.: Relation of Fibro-adenoma and Chronic Mastitis to Sexual Cycle Changes in the Breast. *Arch. Path.*, 14: 21, 1932.
Keyser. L. D.: Massive Hypertrophy of the Breast. *Surg., Gynec. & Obst.*, 33: 607, 1921.

McDonald, J., and Harrington, S. W.: Giant Fibro-adenoma of the Breast—"Cystosarcoma Phyllodes."
   Ann. Surg., 131: 243, 1950.
Nathanson, I. T.: The Relationship of Hormones to Diseases of the Breast; in *Endocrinology of Neoplastic
   Diseases*. New York, Oxford University Press, 1947, p. 138.
Schauffler, G. C.: The Immature Breast. *Pediat. Clin. N. Amer.*, 5: 63, 1958.
Wulsin, J. H.: Large Breast Tumors in Adolescent Females. *Ann. Surg.*, 152: 151, 1960.

Chapter 24

Vaginal Discharge

SINCE the most common cause of vaginal discharge in children is gonorrheal in origin, one immediately suspects it when dealing with the pubescent or adolescent girl. Certainly gonorrhea should be ruled out by smear and culture before accepting a more banal explanation in any adolescent who has either a persistent vaginal discharge or an inflamed vulva. There are other responsible agents, however, and when gonorrhea has been excluded, one should think of such things as unrecognized foreign bodies, *Trichomonas vaginalis*, fungus infections and diabetes mellitus. In the absence of specific cause one must also look to improper hygiene or tissue hypersensitivity to underclothing, which may be either too tight or made from material to which the patient is allergic, e.g. nylon.

GONORRHEAL VULVOVAGINITIS IN THE ADOLESCENT

Primarily one expects to encounter gonorrheal vaginitis in the younger child, owing to the lack of local protection afforded by the immature, thin vaginal epithelium. As the estrogenic factor appears in the child's development at puberty, the cells of the vaginal epithelium approach the mature state. Nevertheless mature women are subject to gonorrheal infection, and there is no reason not to suspect it in the adolescent. The infection is usually caused by direct contact with an infected person in one way or another. The theory that this infection is contracted from such things as contaminated toilet seats cannot be supported by experimental observation. Epidemics do occur in institutional populations among children, although it has been impossible experimentally to implicate the bed linen. Despite the fact that the sole means of acquiring the disease appears to be bodily or sexual contact, cleanliness and common-sense protective measures, in the presence of a known carrier, cannot be stressed too strongly. It has been shown, for example, that during epidemics within a hospital the disease can spread from rectum to vagina by the careless use of rectal thermometers or enema tubes.

In addition to the foregoing means of acquiring the disease, one should keep in mind that the adolescent girl may herself be a carrier, based on infection acquired in late childhood, treated and believed to be cured. Before deciding whether the causative agent is gonorrheal in origin, one should place more reliance on bacteriologic culture methods than on Gram stains of vaginal spreads, in which false negatives are too frequently found.

282

The management of gonorrhea in the young child carries its own special problems (see Chap. 14), but the treatment of the adolescent does not vary appreciably from that of the adult woman. (The diagnosis and treatment will be discussed in Chapter 44.)

FOREIGN BODIES IN THE VAGINA

After eliminating gonorrhea as an etiologic possibility in adolescent vaginitis and before accepting nonspecific explanations, the presence of a foreign body within the vagina must be ruled out. This is not an uncommon source of vaginal discharge in any age group, but it is particularly prone to occur in children and adolescents. This discharge is copious, purulent, occasionally bloodstained and so irritating that the vulva is often red and swollen.

If gonorrhea is excluded and the symptoms and findings do not improve with rational therapy in a reasonable period, a foreign body should be suspected. There is little point in trying to obtain a history of inserting a foreign object into the vagina, for in most instances the girl either will deny it or will have forgotten that she has done it. Perhaps the most significant factor in the history is the bloody discharge.

Too frequently the possibility of a foreign body has not been considered, and unsuccessful attempts at treatment have been instituted, using douches, estrin therapy and chemotherapy without seeking the underlying cause. All manner of different objects have been recovered from the vagina, including pins of all sorts, e.g. safety pins, bobby pins, hairpins and even portions of a bed spring, coins and crayons. Not only is it important to discover the foreign body and remove it, but also it is imperative that the girl should not be labeled as a suspected case of gonorrhea resistant to therapy. The reasons why such objects are inserted may be important. Some are introduced through sheer curiosity and, once inserted, have been forgotten. Others are linked to the common habit of masturbation. Perhaps the most common

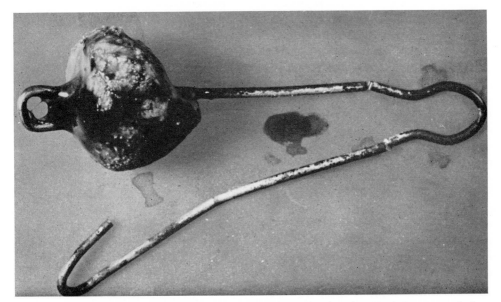

Fig. 24-1.   A wire foreign body with a concretion that developed around it, removed from a child's vagina. Allegedly a relative inserted the wire to render her sterile.

foreign body one now finds in the adolescent girl is the intravaginal type of tampon used instead of the vaginal napkin during menstruation.

The suspicion of the presence of a foreign body within the vagina may be confirmed in a number of different ways. (1) If the object is metallic, it can be detected by x-ray examination, but may not be localized accurately. The foreign body could be lodged in the urethra, bladder or cervix, as well as in the vagina. Moreover, not all such objects are radiopaque. (2) When distention of the hymenal ring permits and the girl cooperates, direct inspection of the vagina can be made with the patient in the knee-chest position, using a Kelly cystoscope, size 8 or 10, or a urethroscope, as an office procedure. This position allows the vagina to fill with air, so that the entire vaginal cavity can be seen. If the foreign body is accessible and not imbedded, it may be removed with a long blunt-nosed forceps passed through the scope. An open pin can be manipulated, using the same kind of forceps, into a position where the blunt nose of the pin faces the operator and can then be removed without injuring the patient. (3) If no type of endoscope is available or if the patient refuses to co-operate, it is still possible to carry out an office examination without too much physical or emotional distress. In nearly every instance, regardless of the size of the hymenal opening, a dull probe can be inserted into the vagina. If the object is metallic, it should produce a clicking sound when coming in contact with the probe. If it is soft and gelatinous, some portion of the material may stick to the probe. This maneuver will be greatly facilitated by introducing a finger into the rectum. If the patient is uncooperative through fear or disinclination, or when the foreign body seems to be firmly lodged in tissue, the patient should be hospitalized and the examination carried out under an anesthetic.

The practical point to remember is that vaginal discharge of no apparent etiology may be due to the unexplained finding of foreign bodies within the vagina, placed there deliberately and forgotten or found to be nonrecoverable and ignored.

NONSPECIFIC VAGINITIS

A not uncommon form of vaginitis manifests itself at the time of puberty and early adolescence as the result of the impact of estrin stimulation upon the immature vaginal epithelium. On smear examination no cytologic or bacteriologic suggestion of gonorrhea can be found, but an excessive exfoliation of vaginal cells without leukocytes is apparent. The patient is distressed by the persistence of the discharge and the fact that it may produce an odor, particularly if a tight hymen does not permit free drainage. Little can be done except to let it run its course, which is self-limited as the vaginal epithelium becomes more mature and estrin stimulation lessens. Attempts have been made to relieve the symptoms without affecting the causes by giving alkaline douches or suppositories.

Conversely, vaginal discharge occasionally occurs in the puberal girl when insufficient amounts of estrin are present to bring about the cornifying cell transformation in the vaginal epithelium. As in senile vaginitis, such undeveloped or atrophic epithelium is prone to become infected by such organisms as the colon bacillus, streptococcus or pneumococcus and to produce varying degrees of vaginal inflammation. One rarely sees diphtheria today in this age group, but, like the pneumococcus, it may be the responsible agent.

TRICHOMONAS VAGINALIS AND MONILIAL INFECTIONS

Although the protozoan *Trichomonas vaginalis* rarely occurs in the infant or puberal age group, it may be the etiologic factor in vaginal discharge in the older adolescent. The diagnosis is made on the basis of the symptomatology, the nature of the discharge and the finding of the organism in the wet smear preparation. The details of diagnosis and treatment will be discussed in greater detail in Chapter 40.

Monilia is not a common cause of vaginal infection in this age group. The older adolescent girl, however, does get pregnant. Also most girls of this age may have received a variety of forms of antibiotic chemotherapy for one reason or the other. Both factors may be instrumental in encouraging monilial infection in the vaginal canal.

DIABETES MELLITUS

One of the characteristic symptoms produced by diabetes in any age group is a troublesome irritation of the vulva. When this is advanced, the vulva becomes red, swollen and the center of intense itching.

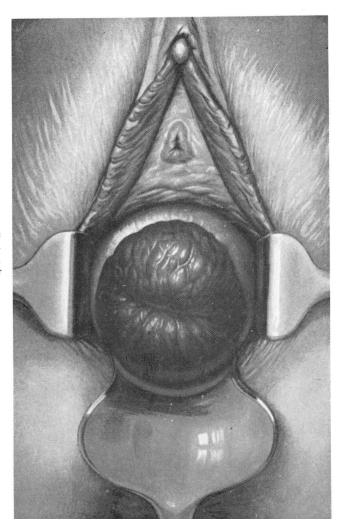

Fig. 24-2. Eversion of the endocervical mucosa, which produces the so-called congenital erosion. (From T. S. Cullen: *Cancer of the Uterus.*)

CONGENITAL EROSION OF THE CERVIX

Grossly, this appears as a circular ring of red-pink mucous membrane around what appears to be the external cervical os (Fig. 24–1). Actually, it is a prolapse downward or ectropion of the endocervical glandular mucosa, a congenital anomaly which should not be confused with true erosion. Biopsies are sometimes taken under the misapprehension that this is a true erosion, partly since the mucus-producing endocervical epithelium does not take up and stain with Schiller's iodine solution.

True erosions may be acquired after an infection within the endometrium cavity, as the result of the denuding effect of the discharge and a weakening of supporting tissues. Infection of the exposed glandular epithelium is prone to recur and frequently results in genuine ulceration and a profuse leukorrhea. The treatment of genuine erosions depends on the severity of the symptoms. Some help may be gained by increasing the acidity of the vaginal epithelium by using white vinegar douches. This often hastens squamous epithelial repair of the denuded surface. Cauterization and coagulation therapy will be discussed in detail in Chapter 40.

REFERENCES

Bedoya, J. M., Rico, L. R., and Rios, G.: Genital Trichomoniasis, a Venereal Disease; Incidence in Prostitutes and in Virgins. *Geburts. u. Frauenh.*, 18: 994, 1958 (*Internat. Abstr. Surg.*, 108: 481, 1959).

Chernosky, M. E., Derbes, V. J., and Burks, J. W.: Lichen Sclerosus et Atrophicus in Children. A.M.A. *Arch. Dermat.*, 75: 647, 1957.

Cockerell, E. G., Knox, J. M., and Rogers, S. F., Jr.: Lichen Sclerosus et Atrophicus. *Obst. & Gynec.* 15: 554, 1960.

Gardner, H. L., and Dukes, C. D.: Hemophilus Vaginalis Vaginitis. *Ann. New York Acad. Sc.*, 83: 280, 1959.

Hammond, D. O.: A New Pediatric Gynecologic Examining Instrument for Use in Diagnosis of Pediatric Vaginitis. *Am. J. Obst. & Gynec.*, 80: 85, 1960.

Heltai, A.: Hemophilus Vaginalis and Nonspecific Vaginitis. *Ann. New York Acad. Sc.*, 83: 290, 1959.

Huffman, J. W.: Disorders of the External Genitals and Vagina. *Pediat. Clin. N. Amer.*, 5: 35, 1958.

Idem: The Structure and Bacteriology of the Premenarchal Vagina. *Ann. New York Acad. Sc.*, 83: 227, 1959.

Hunter, C. A., Jr., and Nicholas, H. J.: A Study of Vaginal Acids. *Am. J. Obst. & Gynec.*: 78: 282, 1959.

Lang, W. R.: Genital Infections in Female Children. *Clin. Obst. & Gynec.*, 2: 428, 1959.

Silver, H. K.: Cytology of Urinary Sediment in Childhood. *Pediatrics*, 26: 255, 1960.

Weinstock, H. L., and Keesal, S.: Lymphogranuloma Venereum—Report of a Case in a Child. *Urol. & Cutan. Rev.*, 50: 520, 1946.

Chapter 25

Acne and Hirsutism

A DISCUSSION of acne vulgaris and hirsutism under ordinary circumstances would not appear in a gynecologic text. When one attempts to evaluate the problems of the adolescent girl, it can hardly be left out.

ACNE VULGARIS

This is one of the most common distressing problems confronting the growing girl from the prepuberal years well along into adolescence. Because it tends to undergo spontaneous cure at approximately the age of sixteen years, the etiology has been closely linked to endocrine dysfunction. The fact that the condition tends to suffer exacerbations at the time of the menstrual periods lends further support to this contention. Moreover, there is clinical evidence in abundance to suggest that acne and hirsutism may result from a disproportion between the male and female hormones.

The disease is so common that in its mildest form it can almost be regarded as physiologic and normal. Treatment, however, is indicated, for its normal habit is to progress and in slow stages to become more severe. In order that permanent scarring of the skin be avoided, it is important that the beginning manifestations be treated early.

The first evidence of acne vulgaris is manifested just before puberty, when comedones appear on the chin, nose, forehead and occasionally the cheeks. The child is accused of uncleanliness, but the pores are actually not plugged with dirt, but with cornified cells and secretions of the sebaceous glands. Ordinary soap and water is of little help in removing the comedones, and it may be necessary to resort to milder abrasive soaps such as Lava, which is effective without producing too much trauma. As the disease progresses, the skin becomes oily, and papules and pustules appear. Gradually the process becomes more extensive and severe. There is some tendency for the disease to become worse at the time of the menstrual period, but in this stage it does not disappear in the intermenstrual cycle. Later the acne spreads to the chest and back and on rare occasions to the extremities. Occasionally cystic comedones appear in the skin, which are extremely unsightly because of the pronounced redness of the skin overlying them. The more the complicating pyogenic infectious element appears, the greater the danger of permanent pitting and scarring.

Scarring and pitting of the face, chest and shoulders in a young girl can be a tragedy both cosmetically and psychologically. This process is reversible if treatment is carried out vigorously early in its development. Before instituting treatment one should be sure that there is no basic endocrine defect. Acne, seborrhea and hirsutism are common to the various conditions that result from increased corticoid secretion and androgen production, such as Cushing's syndrome.

Treatment

This can only be outlined in general terms. Though the disease may undergo spontaneous cure in adolescence, it is unwise to pursue a *laissez-faire* policy in therapy. As in all problems of this age group, diet, adequate sleep, exercise and a relaxed attitude are important, but it is not always easy for the patient to understand the point of such therapy. Diet particularly should be stressed. Plenty of energy foods should be provided in the form of milk and protein. Fresh vegetables, fruit and vitamins are necessary supplementary items. Certain foods seem to make the acne worse, particularly chocolate. Chocolate in any form should be strictly condemned. Rich carbohydrates and fatty foods, including bacon, should be also avoided. In further general support one may wish to resort to the antibacterial drugs in the presence of a predominantly pustular skin eruption. Procaine penicillin, 600,000 units 3 times daily, has been used in some cases. It must be given with other supportive treatment to have any effect.

Generally, treatment also should be directed toward relieving the constipation habit and correcting any existing anemia with iron. The girl should be advised not to pinch or squeeze the pustules, for trauma can only aggravate the condition. There has been a tendency to use estrogens in the latter half of the monthly cycle, when exacerbations are known to occur with the menstrual period. They certainly should not be used indiscriminately, but may be useful when this association is present. Because the disease tends to improve during the summer months with exposure to the sun, ultraviolet radiation therapy has been helpful. Neither ultraviolet nor x-ray therapy should be administered without the advice and supervision of a trained dermatologist.

HIRSUTISM

The problem of superfluous hair is common to the adolescent age group. Although it is closely associated with malfunction of the adrenal gland, most of the patients who present this complaint are perfectly normal women with adequate endocrine function. Most women on close inspection have a fine growth of hair, particularly on the upper lip and chin, but frequently it has a generalized bodily distribution as well. It is never a problem until it becomes conspicuous, either because it grows longer or changes in color and texture. Then it becomes a source of acute embarrassment to the adolescent and a constant nuisance to the older woman. There seems to be a genetic or constitutional factor involved, for it is often a family trait. Racial factors are evident, as one sees in the dark-skinned Mediterranean peoples, in whom facial hair is commonly present together with an excessive growth on the thighs.

The most common place for superfluous hair to appear is on the upper lip, chin and sides of the face. In most cases this can be treated by epilation, using electrolysis or high frequency current. This should preferably be done by a dermatologist rather than an operator in a beauty parlor. Each separate hair follicle must be destroyed with the minimum amount of current. With the unskilled there is the danger of infection and subsequent scarring. Girls frequently resort to plucking and bleaching where the facial hair growth is mild and not too extensive. The next most common hair sites are the extremities, particularly the thighs and lower legs. It is common practice for girls to shave their legs, even though a certain amount of hair growth on the legs is entirely normal. Some girls prefer to use pumice stone or depilatory pastes rather than shave.

When there is a glandular component or suspicion of endocrine dysfunction, the distribution of hair begins to assume the male pattern to a greater or less degree. The growth of facial hair becomes more abundant, darker in color and coarser in texture. Many women have to resort to shaving, for the growth is too extensive for electrolysis. Along with the increase in facial hair, more or less hair appears around the areola and over the manubrium between the breasts. Midline hirsutism is noted on the abdominal wall, bearing all the characteristics of the male escutcheon. Likewise an overgrowth of hair is noted on the lower extremities, with somewhat less on the forearms.

Such a distribution of hair is not an uncommon finding in pituitary dysfunctions such as the basophil adenoma of Cushing. Some of these patients have no other signs of Cushing's disease except that the menses may be irregular or absent. The urinary 17-ketosteroid levels are only moderately elevated. A moderate degree of hirsutism of this type is seen at times in the adrenogenital syndrome. Nearly half of the patients with the Stein-Leventhal syndrome have varying degrees of the male pattern of hair distribution. Whenever there is adrenal dysfunction as the result of hyperplasia or tumor, there is hypertrichosis with or without other signs of virilization.

Before one can safely disregard the masculine type of hirsutism as a normal finding, one should be alert to the possibility that there may be a basic endocrine cause. If the evidence is strong, x-ray films of the skull should be taken to rule out enlargement of the sella turcica or suprasellar cyst. Physical examination may disclose an adrenal or ovarian tumor. With an elevation of the urinary 17-ketosteroid excretion, cortisone therapy may distinguish between tumor and hyperplasia of the adrenal. Air injection of the retroperitoneal space and exploration of the adrenal are often unsatisfactory, for frequently they reveal neither tumor nor hyperplasia. It must constantly be kept in mind that certain patients will have an elevation of the urinary 17-ketosteroid level without adrenal hyperplasia, due in all probability to certain poorly understood genetic or constitutional characteristics.

If a tumor of ovary, pituitary or adrenal can be discovered and removed, the hirsutism may regress, but hormone therapy in general, including estrin, has little lasting effect.

REFERENCES

Behrman, H. T.: Diagnosis and Management of Hirsutism. *J.A.M.A.*, 172: 1924, 1960

Benson, R. C., Kolb, F. O., and Traut, H. F.: Hirsutism, Defeminization and Virilization. *Obst. & Gynec.*, 5: 307, 1955.

Bluefarb, S.: The Treatment of Acne Vulgaris. *M. Clin. N. Amer.*, 45: 869, 1961.

Brooks, R. V., and Prunty, F. T. G.: Patterns of Steroid Excretion in Three Types of Post-pubertal Hirsutism. *J. Endocrinol.*, 21: 263, 1960.

Edelstein, A. J.: Premenstrual Acne; A New Therapeutic Approach. *Pennsylvania Med.*, 63: 1503, 1960.

Epstein, J. A., Levinson, C. J., and Kupperman, H. S.: Ovarian Adrenal Rest Tumor (Masculinovo-blastoma) Simulating Adrenal Virilism. *Am. J. Obst. & Gynec.*, 74: 982, 1957.

Gemzell, C. A., Tillinger, K. G., and Westman, A.: Hirsutism: A Clinical Study of the Ovarian Pathology and Urinary Excretion of 17-Ketosteroids. *Acta Endocrinol.*, 30: 387, 1959.

Greenblatt, R. B.: Cortisone in Treatment of the Hirsute Woman. *Am. J. Obst. & Gynec.*, 66: 700, 1953.

Herrmann, W., Buckner, F., and Morris, J. McL.: The Problem of Mild Adrenal Hyperplasia. *Fertil. & Steril.*, 11: 74, 1960.

Jailer, J. W.: Virilism. *Bull. New York Acad. Med.*, 29: 377, 1953.

Jailer, J. W., Gold, J. J., and Cahill, G. F.: Hirsutism as the Only Clinical Manifestation of an Adrenal Adenoma. *Am. J. Obst. & Gynec.*, 67: 201, 1954.

Kappas, A., Pearson, O. H., West, C. D., and Gallagher, T. F.: A Study of "Idiopathic" Hirsutism, a Transitional Adrenal Abnormality. *J. Clin. Endocrinol.*, 16: 517, 1956.

Mescon, H. G., Moretti, G., and O'Connor, S. C.: Hypertrichosis: A Physiologic Approach to Etiology and Treatment. *Boston Med. Quart.*, 5: 7, 1954.

Perloff, W. H., Channick, B. J., Suplick, B., and Carrington, E. R.: Clinical Management of Idiopathic Hirsutism (Adrenal Virilism). *J.A.M.A.*, 167: 2041, 1958.

Strauss, J. S., and Kligman, A. M.: The Pathologic Dynamics of Acne Vulgaris. *A.M.A. Arch. Dermat.*, 82: 779, 1960.

Tompkins, M. G., Morse, W. I., Brennan, C. F., and Stewart, L.: Adrenal Function in Amenorrhea—Infertility and Hirsutism—Effect of Prednisone Therapy. *Canad. M.A.J.*, 81: 714, 1959.

Vesell, M.: Hirsutism: Report of Four Unusual Cases. *Obst. & Gynec.*, 3: 307, 1954.

Chapter 26

Pelvic Pain

THERE are three main symptoms in all gynecologic problems which appear in every age group: (1) abnormalities in the bleeding pattern, (2) vaginal discharge, and (3) pelvic pain. The physical findings in gynecology are also limited in scope. We are primarily interested in (*a*) palpation and inspection of the external genitalia, (*b*) the size, contour, mobility and sensitivity of the uterus, (*c*) the degree of fixation, extent of local tenderness of the pelvic floor and whether or not enlargement of the adnexa is present. A wide variety of pathologic entities and functional disorders provides the explanation for the findings. One may have pelvic pain with or without tumor or abnormal bleeding. Many patients complain of pelvic pain who have no disease that can be demonstrated by inspection or palpation.

Of the three main symptoms, pelvic pain presents the most confusing yet practical problem in the entire gynecologic field. Search for the true explanation is made no easier by the fact that women tend to focus their attention on the uterus and adnexa and attribute the majority of their ills to this source, yet they are wrong approximately 50 per cent of the time. Proper evaluation of the basic cause for the patient's pain in her pelvis taxes the medical intelligence and understanding to the utmost.

Many conditions that cause pelvic pain are rarer in adolescence than in adult life, but since pelvic pain first becomes a problem in adolescent patients, the causes are considered here for purposes of unity.

Why Is It So Difficult to Pinpoint the Cause of Pelvic Pain?

Women have great difficulty in localizing and describing pelvic pain. In all probability the explanation lies in the fact there are no great concentrations of sensory nerve ganglia in the pelvis, such as one encounters in the periosteum, the conjunctiva or the skin. Thus it is difficult for the brain to make a sharp differentiation as to the location of the pain, or its type and severity. If one injects an irritating solution, experimentally, into periosteum or skeletal muscle, there is also a difference in the patient's response to pain. The variation in the severity of the reactions and the accuracy of location of pain depend upon the concentration of pain receptors. They are densely concentrated in periosteum, but widely separated in muscle.

It is also a difficult task to localize visceral pain. Nerve endings extend into all internal pelvic organs, but they are relatively few in number. It requires a summation of stimuli over a wide area to produce pain. For example, bowel can be crushed with a clamp without producing pain, but as soon as the intestine becomes distended the pain can be definitely felt.

The intensity of the response to pain has wide variables in different persons or in the same person under different circumstances. For example, war and athletic injuries of the same magnitude are apt to be less painful than those suffered in one's ordinary existence, because of the elements of stress and excitement. Anxiety and fear may reverse the patient's normal response. Thus a healthy person who suddenly finds herself ill becomes frightened and may have more pain from the same degree of damage than the chronic invalid who has learned to live with her complaint. Furthermore, exaggeration and introspection often provide a neurotic superstructure, at times out of proportion to the intensity of the stimulus. The individual variation in the response to painful stimuli appears when stimuli reach the brain and is rarely due to any difference in the local skin pain threshold.

The threshold for pain in the higher centers is lowered by a number of factors, such as the patient's general condition, the degree of anemia or fatigue. The pain threshold is definitely reduced by acute inflammatory processes. For example, the normal skeletal muscle, relatively insensitive because of its few pain receptors, reacts only slightly to the introduction of a needle. Once infected, however, even the injection of Novocain produces pain.

Since women incorrectly attribute much of their lower abdominal discomfort to the genital organs, it is obvious that pain, believed by the patient to be visceral, actually may have somatic origin. Somatic pain usually results from irritation of the roots, ganglia or trunks of the spinal nerves. The point of origin is either in or close to the vertebrae. It may be caused by any disease process, toxic absorption or mechanical disturbance that irritates the spinal nerves. The fundamental difference between pain of visceral origin and that due to somatic cause is the wide segmental distribution produced by the latter. One of the main characteristics of somatic pain is its tendency to produce tender parietes. Thus such a patient has deep tenderness on palpation of the abdominal wall. The distinction lies in the fact that there is only localized tenderness when the abnormality is in a viscus, while the somatic cause produces, in addition to the local area of sensitivity, widespread segmental pain with tenderness in the paravertebral area as well as along the rib borders. The distribution of pain follows the pathways of the nerve supply to the anterior abdominal wall.

When we take into account all the variables noted above and realize that, in addition, there are other organs and other systems in the pelvis, as well as somatic sources, it is not surprising that both patient and physician experience difficulty in locating and evaluating the degree of pelvic pain.

What Are the Extragenital Causes of Pelvic Pain?

Any one of a variety of disease processes, either alone or in combination, can provide the explanation for pelvic pain. The gynecologist will be sorely disappointed at the number of incorrect diagnoses if he attributes the symptomatology entirely to the genital organs, without ruling out the possible extragenital sources. In addition to the various entities that fall within the scope of orthopedic interest, one must also consider the gastrointestinal and urinary tracts (Fig. 26–1). The female pelvis has been called the "melting pot" of the surgical specialists. A careful history will do much toward assigning the symptoms to their rightful area.

WHAT ARE THE ORTHOPEDIC CAUSES OF BACKACHE AND PELVIC PAIN?   A chronic pain in the back, located in the lumbosacral area, is a common complaint among women. Facetiously, woman has been described as a constipated biped with a pain in her back. Rarely, however, is this type of backache or pelvic pain due to disease or malposition of the genital organs. In the old days far too many uterine suspension operations were done for low sacral backache believed to be due to a retroverted uterus. Unless the uterus is fixed in this position by other abnormal conditions, the operation is rarely done today. In general one may say that backache is rarely an important symptom, even when known disease is present, such as pelvic inflammation, endometriosis, fibroids, ovarian tumors or even malignant disease.

A detailed history and thorough physical examination will usually localize the trigger point of pain to the back, despite palpable evidence of pelvic disease. Pelvic pain or backache which is brought on by movements of the spine, such as stooping, bending over or heavy lifting, is in all probability due to some disorder in the vertebrae or muscles of the back which produces stretching or pressure on the nerves. This is especially true if the pain is not relieved by bed rest. Pain that radiates down the back of the leg is far more often due to skeletal cause than to genital disease. In many instances the patient who complains of a constant pain in the back which is aggra-

EXTRAGENITAL CAUSES OF PELVIC PAIN

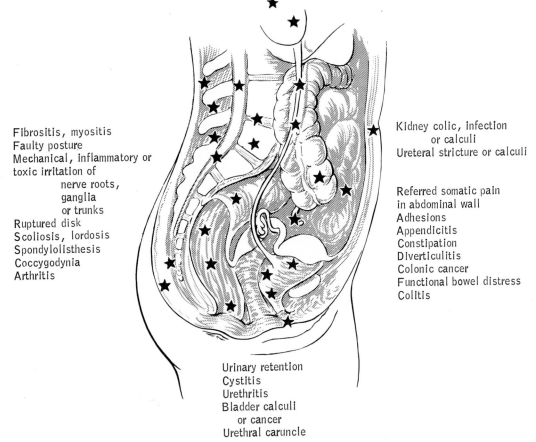

Fibrositis, myositis
Faulty posture
Mechanical, inflammatory or
toxic irritation of
nerve roots,
ganglia
or trunks
Ruptured disk
Scoliosis, lordosis
Spondylolisthesis
Coccygodynia
Arthritis

Kidney colic, infection
or calculi
Ureteral stricture or calculi

Referred somatic pain
in abdominal wall
Adhesions
Appendicitis
Constipation
Diverticulitis
Colonic cancer
Functional bowel distress
Colitis

Urinary retention
Cystitis
Urethritis
Bladder calculi
or cancer
Urethral caruncle

Fig. 26-1.   Possible nongenital etiologic factors in pelvic pain. Muscles, nerves, bones, joints, kidney and lower urinary tract, appendix and large intestine are included as sources of pain.

vated at times by increased activity will have symptoms of general fatigue and aching pain in the shoulders and upper back as well. The low back pain then is not due to genital cause, but is only one manifestation of a general lack in body tone.

Certain well recognized orthopedic entities may appear in a woman who also has pelvic pathology and are far more likely to be the cause of the backache. For example, there are a number of congenital deformities which result in an unstable spine and can be the cause of pelvic pain and backache. Most of them are evident by x-ray study, such as *spina bifida, spondylolisthesis, lordosis, scoliosis* and *kyphosis*. The amount of discomfort in the back will depend on the adequacy of muscle support. If it is poor, the patient will have chronic back pain. Poor posture, often accompanied by lordosis and obesity, is a frequent cause of backache in a woman who has to sit at her work for long hours, just as anatomic defects in the feet produce faulty posture and backache in a woman who has to stand up at her work.

Any disease in the spine or inflammatory process which irritates the spinal nerves will produce pain with abdominal reference. Thus *osteoarthritis of the spine*, evident by x-ray film, is a frequent cause of low pelvic pain referable to the back. Inflammatory processes along the spine or in the region of the sacroiliac joints, such as *fibromyositis* or *tuberculosis*, may produce pelvic pain which extends down the leg in a sciatic distribution. One of the most common causes today is the *herniation of an intervertebral disk*. Too many disk operations have been done ill advisedly for back pain of an indefinite nature. The true symptoms of a herniated disk are fairly characteristic. Along with a history of trauma the patient complains of low back pain with radiation down the leg. The pain is usually made worse by coughing or sneezing and is frequently accompanied by a loss of muscle substance in the lower leg, as well as absence of knee and ankle jerks. Tumors of the spine which exert pressure on the spinal nerves are prone to produce pelvic pain. They may be primary in the spine or metastatic from a source elsewhere in the body.

WHAT ARE SOME OF THE FUNCTIONAL OR PATHOLOGIC PROCESSES OF GASTRO-INTESTINAL NATURE THAT PRODUCE PELVIC PAIN?   The mechanisms of pain production, excluding the somatic sources, are similar, whether the cause be found in the genital, gastrointestinal or urinary tract. Pain is produced by pelvic abnormalities in the following manner: (*a*) sudden distention of a hollow viscus, (*b*) vigorous contraction of a hollow viscus, (*c*) rapid distention of the capsule of a solid organ, (*d*) anoxia of functioning muscle tissue, (*e*) crushing or stretching of blood vessels, (*f*) peritoneal contamination by blood, pus or inflammatory exudate, and (*g*) impingement on nerves by fibrosis or inflammation.

The most common gastrointestinal entities that produce pelvic pain are appendicitis and diverticulitis. In appendicitis the initial pain, without much localization, but with a tendency to center around the umbilicus, comes from distention of the lumen of the appendix by inflammatory exudate. As the disease process spreads to involve the parietal peritoneum, the pain travels along the pathways of the segmental nerves and localizes to the area on the anterior abdominal wall supplied by them. Thus we have low anterior wall pelvic pain concentrated on the right side. The same train of symptoms could be due to an ectopic pregnancy or early pelvic inflammation confined to the tube in a patient who has a pelvic tumor. The tumor, unless a vascular accident has occurred in it, is probably an incidental finding that has little to do with the explanation of the pain. If the appendix ruptures, an abscess may form which can be felt as a tender mass on vaginal or rectal examination.

Acute diverticulitis produces a train of symptoms which closely parallel those of appendicitis, but with a tendency to localize on the left. Since diverticulitis always occurs in the redundant loop of sigmoid, the low abdominal pain may concentrate in the midabdomen or right side. Because of its location in the redundant loop the inflamed diverticula may readily be felt on pelvic or rectal examination. If the diverticulum ruptures and forms an abscess, the parietal peritoneum is involved, and the pain localizes. Some of the symptoms are due to bowel distention, since there is always some element of intestinal obstruction in diverticulitis. The process is apt to be progressive, and the symptoms of constipation, alternating with diarrhea and lower abdominal pain, are apt to be chronic rather than acute and colicky. Any relation of pelvic pain to changes in bowel habit should call attention to the possibility that the intestine rather than the genital organs may be the cause.

The history, then, is of basic importance in evaluating the source of pelvic pain. For example, a history of alternating constipation and diarrhea, small ribbon-like stools and bloody defecation accompanied by colicky pain would suggest that the pain might be due to malignant disease in the sigmoid colon or rectum. Other factors appear in the history which operate in reverse. Pain on defecation may be due to extensive pelvic disease such as endometriosis or pelvic inflammation rather than lesions in the intestinal tract. Ulcerative colitis or functional diseases of the colon, the so-called irritable or spastic colon, may be the cause of pelvic pain. In many instances these entities are associated with pelvic disease, and the relation must be evaluated before attributing the pelvic pain to gynecologic cause alone.

The history will also be helpful in distinguishing pain due to varying degrees of small bowel obstruction from that due to pelvic disease. One can have a knuckle of small intestine caught at the site of a previous pelvic operation and have all the symptoms localized in the pelvis. The adherent loop of bowel produces chronic pain as it distends, the pain becoming increasingly severe and colicky as the obstruction becomes more complete. Should the distention become extensive enough to interfere with the circulation of the bowel, the other mechanisms of pain begin to operate, and the intensity of the pain in its pelvic location increases. It may be difficult on physical examination to differentiate an acutely obstructed and distended loop of intestine from a twisted ovarian cyst with damaged blood supply.

A high index of suspicion, based on facts obtained from the history, will usually direct the attention away from genital abnormalities to the true source in the intestinal tract. Appropriate diagnostic tests, such as x-ray examination by scout film or barium study, proctoscopic inspection and laboratory examination of stool specimens for blood, pus and parasites, are therefore indicated before abdominal exploration is attempted. The cause of the pain may prove to be truly intestinal, but functional rather than organic.

It is impossible to outline in detail all the symptoms or to establish a differential diagnosis for all the conditions within the intestinal tract that give rise to pelvic pain. The point to be made is that gastrointestinal disease should be regarded as one possible explanation before accepting gynecologic conditions as the sole cause of pain in the lower part of the abdomen and in the pelvis.

WHAT UROLOGIC CONDITIONS PRODUCE PAIN SIMULATING THAT CAUSED BY GYNECOLOGIC CONDITIONS? Any organ or malfunction in the urinary tract may be responsible for pelvic pain. Although located at a distance from the pelvis, the kidney may refer pain to the lower part of the abdomen and to the groin. It is usually dull and indefinite, but tends to localize on one side of the pelvis. Usually it extends upward along the course of the ureter to the lumbar region. Hydronephrosis, renal infection and renal calculi produce pelvic pain. Infection and calculi, together with urethral and ureteral stricture and inflammatory lesions, provide classic examples of urologic entities that produce pelvic pain. A ptosed kidney, like a uterine retroversion, may be a rare cause of pelvic pain, but like the uterine suspension operation, nephropexy should never be done unless all other causes have been ruled out and the therapeutic indications are definite.

The urologic lesions which most typically produce pelvic pain occur in the bladder and urethra. The most frequent lesion is *cystitis*. Suprapubic pain is elicited when the inflamed bladder becomes distended with urine. In acute cystitis the pains are severe and present almost constantly. In chronic infection the pain may be mild or absent. If infection is present, it should be evident on examination of the catheter specimen of bladder content. The same kind of pain noted in acute cystitis may be present in the condition known as *interstitial fibrosis of the bladder*. In this entity there is a decreased bladder capacity, and thus the mechanism of distention of a hollow viscus comes into play so that the patient has pelvic pain. The symptoms in the absence of infection may be due to fibrosis, contracture of the vesical neck and urethral stricture. In lesions of the vesical neck the pain is usually located along the course of the urethra or deep in the bony pelvis. This distribution of pain is common to *trigonitis, vesical calculi, stone in the lower ureter, stenosis of the vesical neck* or *neoplasm* involving the neck of the bladder.

The urethra itself provides the most frequent source of obscure pelvic pain, and lesions located here are likely to escape detection. On vaginal examination the gynecologist should routinely examine the external urethra for discharge, caruncle or tumor and palpate the course of the urethra to bring out any thickening or abnormal mass. In the course of this examination one may encounter a *urethral diverticulum*. This may be the source of vague pelvic pain. Gentle pressure may express urine or pus, and the diagnosis is made.

It is important to know whether the patient carries residual urine in the bladder. This may be the source of obscure pelvic pain, even when the other findings on cystoscopy are negative and infection is absent. Cystoscopy is always indicated when urinary disease is suspected as the cause of pelvic pain. Not only should the interior of the bladder be observed, but the urethra should also be thoroughly inspected. Too frequently this is not done. Many patients with no obvious urologic disease obtain complete relief of obscure pelvic pain by dilating the urethra with graduated Hank dilators or by bladder irrigation.

Chronic urethritis may be present without much to indicate it except the possible presence of a caruncle. In these cases the use of oral estrin may be rewarding, particularly in the postmenopausal patient whose ovarian secretion is on the low side or absent. Recently investigators have noted that the mucous membrane of the urethra atrophies and becomes easily infected when the ovary fails to produce estrin. Lymphocytic infiltration of the subepithelial layers indicating a degenerative or chronic inflammatory response of the tissue can be seen microscopically. By supplying estrin the urethral epithelium is reactivated, and inflammation disappears. *Urethral caruncles* are also said to vanish in the course of estrin therapy. This is the same mechanism we observe in gonorrheal vaginitis in children, in whom the infection disappears as the epithelium becomes mature under estrin therapy.

What about Pelvic Pain Originating in the Genital Tract?

All the mechanisms for the production of pelvic pain can be found in abnormal conditions or functions of the organs of the reproductive tract. If more than one condition exists or no palpable disease is present, the problem of proper interpretation of the pain is compounded. It is possible to have organic disease in the pelvis without demonstrable evidence on physical examination. The basic cause of the pain may be overlooked. For example, 15 per cent of patients who have endometriosis show no clinical evidence of its presence. Far more often, however, the physician attempts to attribute the cause of pain to an entity he suspects from a too casual evaluation of the symptoms, when actually there is no lesion present. Moreover, the true explanation may be functional in a patient who has a coexisting disease in the genital organs.

A careful history is therefore of basic importance. The intensity, duration, nature and relation of the pain to past events and other systems should be carefully evaluated. For example, a severe colicky pain coming in waves which appears suddenly suggests that acute disease has developed within the pelvic organs. In most instances the basic cause will be a serious one, such as intraperitoneal bleeding, accident within a pelvic tumor secondary to loss of its blood supply or infection, acute pelvic infection or a number of other entities referable to the urologic or gastrointestinal tract, such as ureteral stone or intestinal obstruction. A review of the past history, as it applies to both the genital tract and other systems, is most helpful in pinpointing the source of the pain (Fig. 26–2).

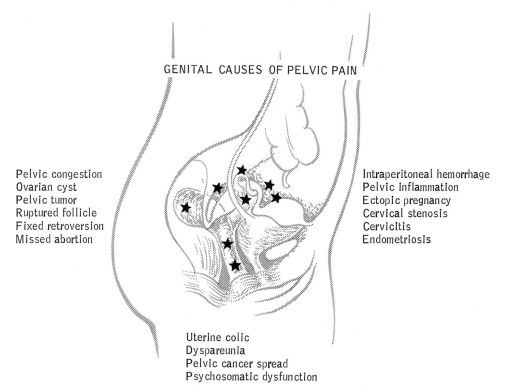

GENITAL CAUSES OF PELVIC PAIN

Pelvic congestion
Ovarian cyst
Pelvic tumor
Ruptured follicle
Fixed retroversion
Missed abortion

Intraperitoneal hemorrhage
Pelvic inflammation
Ectopic pregnancy
Cervical stenosis
Cervicitis
Endometriosis

Uterine colic
Dyspareunia
Pelvic cancer spread
Psychosomatic dysfunction

Fig. 26-2. Salient gynecologic causes of pelvic pain arising from the ovary, tube, uterus, cervix, vagina or the adjacent connective tissues and serous membranes.

For example: (*a*) if the patient's periods have ceased, when her previous menstrual history has been regular, the appearance of pain suggests that something has happened to a pregnancy either inside or outside the uterus. It could be either a missed abortion or an ectopic pregnancy. (*b*) An immediate past history of gonorrheal infection, abortion or cauterization of the cervix suggests that tubal infection or pelvic peritonitis in acute form is the cause of the pain. On examination one may find only tenderness on the pelvic floor. If the pain is less acute, and pelvic masses are felt, the same history from the more distant past may be elicited and provide a lead for the explanation of pain. (*c*) A history of previous pelvic surgery, the known existence of a hernia, or malfunction of either the gastrointestinal or urinary tract should focus attention on the other systems as the possible source. One can have pelvic pain due to genital disease or malfunction concomitantly with complaints referable to the other symptoms. Conversely, when the pain appears only during menstruation, one may concentrate on the uterus as the source of pain when the true cause is intestinal malfunction.

In obtaining the history the gynecologist should concentrate on the events that preceded the onset of pain. Pelvic discomfort or varying degrees of pain may follow sexual intercourse. It can be minor, such as is noted in dyspareunia, when pain may arise as a result of disproportion in size of the sexual organs, too tight a hymen or fixation of the uterus and pelvic floor. One of us has witnessed a fatal instance of intraperitoneal hemorrhage from an ectopic pregnancy which ruptured during intercourse.

The pain is not always acute and may be chronic or intermittent. For example, an ovarian cyst is prone to twist on its pedicle and produce pain. It may revert promptly to its previous position, however, with prompt disappearance of the pain. Ectopic pregnancies, tubal abortions or ruptured ovarian follicles produce varying degrees of pain, as blood drips onto the pelvic peritoneum. The insult may be transient and the pain intermittent. The same train of events would follow early tubal infection when pus is extruded from the open tubal ostia onto the pelvic floor. A chronic grinding pain may be secondary to cervical infection which has fixed the pelvic tissues through lymphatic infiltration.

The pelvic pains of psychogenic background are difficult to evaluate. In primary dysmenorrhea, which may produce incapacitating pain at the time of the menstrual periods, by definition there are no associated abnormalities that can be demonstrated on physical examination. Such dysmenorrhea is known to have overtones which are in the realm of the psychosomatic, but there is also an element of physiologic dysfunction. The so-called pelvic congestion syndrome falls into the category of the psychosomatic with a component of underlying but rarely detectable pathology.

It is thus abundantly evident that the evaluation of pelvic pain can be extremely difficult. Though we cannot be accurate all the time, we do know a few things. We know that pain of ovarian origin differs from that produced by lesions in the uterus. This is not surprising, since the sensory nerve fibers from the ovary emerge from the spinal cord at the tenth, eleventh and twelfth thoracic segments, higher up than those associated with uterine pain.

WHAT DO WE KNOW ABOUT PELVIC PAIN CAUSED BY ADNEXAL PATHOLOGY? As in all structures covered with visceral peritoneum, adnexal pain results from either stretching and distention of smooth muscle fibers or circulatory disturbances within the ovary itself. For example, the twisted ovarian cyst produces severe pelvic pain because of (1) the interference with its blood supply secondary to the torsion of the pedicle, and (2) the sudden hemorrhage that occurs within the cyst cavity. Since there are few nerve endings present, the hemorrhage within the cyst must be sudden and extensive enough to distend the cavity. Slow stretching of the capsule rarely produces pain. Thus one can have a large ovarian cyst and never know it, provided the enlargement takes place over a long time. This is why carcinoma of the ovary has such an insidious onset. Pelvic pain may occur in the ovary in the absence of any large cyst formation. For instance, the steady "dull stone ache" of the ovary in the Stein-Leventhal syndrome is due to the pressure exerted by multiple follicles of minute size expanding within the ovary. Since there is a heavy restraining capsule, the follicles cannot break out, pressure is exerted against the restricting cover, and the patient has pain.

Mittelschmerz, or rupture of the ovarian follicle, produces pain in a different manner. We know that the parietal peritoneum and underlying pelvic connective tissue are sensitive to irritation or trauma of any sort. As in ectopic pregnancy or rupture of an endometrial implant, the pain is produced by intraperitoneal hemorrhage. Except for the mild cramplike pain that comes from distention of the outer end of the tube, which has the same innervation as the ovary, there is little to distinguish ectopic pregnancy before rupture has occurred. The symptoms from all these entities are due to intraperitoneal hemorrhage and peritoneal irritation.

Patients who have endometriosis demonstrate several of the mechanisms at work in the production of pelvic pain. We have mentioned that pain results from spillage or hemorrhage of either an endometrial implant located on the pelvic floor or uterosacral ligaments, or from an endometrial cyst in the ovary. One can have large endometrial cysts in the ovary and have no suggestive symptoms, unless they leak or unless hemorrhage occurs within them to produce a sudden increase in size. Pain, seemingly out of proportion to the amount of disease found, may occur in an endometrial implant as the ovarian hormones stimulate the endometrial lining and cause swelling. Since the endometrial implant is always surrounded by a protective cover, it cannot rupture, and the pain can be severe. It coincides with the menstrual period and tends to disappear when the period is over and the ovarian stimulation subsides.

Pelvic inflammatory disease is due to either inflammation within the tubal lumen or infiltration of the pelvic connective tissue from a central focus of infection within the cervix or uterus. Various kinds of pain result, depending on the lesion.

Tubal Inflammation. An acutely infected tube can produce pelvic pain (1) through distention of the tube by exudate, early in the course of the disease; (2) by pus dripping onto the pelvic peritoneum and causing irritation; (3) by extension of the inflammation within the tube onto the adjacent parietal peritoneum. The more extensively the inflammatory process is in contact with the peritoneum, the greater the degree of pain. One can have considerable visceral disease, but unless the viscus becomes distended or inflammatory disease implicates the adjacent peritoneum, one may have little pain.

Chronic Pelvic Inflammation. The pain of the more chronic phases of pelvic inflammation differs in type and mechanism of production from that found in the acute phases. Lymphatic invasion of the paracervical and parametrial areas, secondary to chronic cervicitis, septic abortion or pelvic streptococcal infection, produces a deep pelvic "toothache," grinding in nature, because of the implication of the nerve fibers in the base of the broad ligaments by the fibrosis. Large inflammatory masses in the adnexa in contact with peritoneum add to the discomfort, which is increased by the fact that infection always lowers the threshold for pain. Any pathologic condition that produces pelvic congestion is apt to bring on the same sort of pelvic pain and discomfort.

How Can the Pain of Pelvic Inflammation Be Differentiated from Pain of Somatic Origin?

In many instances, particularly when palpable evidence of disease is not outstanding, it may be a difficult matter to distinguish between pelvic inflammation and diseases or structural abnormalities in and around the vertebral column. At times the pains of somatic and visceral origin have the same quality and segmental distribution.

There is, however, one major characteristic of pain produced by somatic cause. It almost invariably creates peritoneal tenderness. Thus any pressure of the peritoneum against any bony structure, contracted muscle or the abdominal wall will elicit tenderness. In many instances there will also be tenderness along the vertebral column or rib border.

By taking advantage of this fact one can use a simple maneuver suggested by Burch which will help in distinguishing between pain of skeletal origin and that due to pelvic cause. When the examining hand is placed on the abdominal wall, the patient complains of pain. The source of the pain may be either in the genital tract or in the back. The examining finger is then introduced into the vagina, anterior to the cervix, and gentle pressure is applied by both the abdominal hand and the vaginal finger. The pressure on the abdominal wall is gradually released. If the pain diminishes, and the uterus, adnexa and bladder are felt without pain, then the somatic origin is suspected. Too frequently in examining a patient the normal uterus is pressed against a tender abdominal wall.

What Mechanisms Are Involved in the Radiation of Pain of Uterine Origin?

There are several factors that bear on the mechanisms for production of pelvic pain of uterine origin. The uterus as a whole is poorly supplied with nerve endings. There is, however, a great concentration of nerve fibers from both the sympathetic and parasympathetic systems which coalesce in the region of the cervix on its posterior aspect in the area between the two uterosacral ligaments (Frankenhauser's plexus). This is the pain center of the uterus. Any trauma to, or infection of, this region will result in pain. The nature and distribution of the pain will depend on the intensity of the stimulus. For example, stimulation of the uterine cervix with an electric current will produce pain over the suprapubic area. If the stimulation is relatively mild, injection of saline solution into the skin overlying the pubis will relieve the pain, but when the intensity of the stimulation is increased, even the injection of Novocain has no effect. There is another factor concerned with uterine pain. The uterus is constantly subject to trauma. Repeated infection or trauma may either lower the threshold for pain at the local level or establish a pattern in the higher centers.

There are two main types of pain we associate with a uterine source: (*a*) acute colicky pain, and (*b*) dull grinding or bearing-down pain with radiation down the leg. All gynecologists are familar with uterine colic, which is secondary to powerful contractions of the uterine muscle as it attempts to rid itself of a foreign body such as a polyp, submucous fibroid or placental remnant. The more stenosed the cervix, the more severe the cramps, for the pain center is localized at the cervix. Any element that causes infection or stretching of the nerve fibers in this region will produce pain.

The colicky pain of essential dysmenorrhea has another mechanism. This has been discussed in detail elsewhere (Chap. 22). The contraction of muscle which has been rendered ischemic through anoxia, secondary to interference with the blood supply, always produces some pain.

In addition to the colicky cramplike pain, patients with uterine disease also complain of bearing-down pain with radiation down the leg. This may be due to irritation of the nerve endings through lymphatic permeation of the regional channels from such entities as chronic cervicitis, or it may be due to pulling on these nerves from prolapse or procidentia. For example, irritation of the nerves in Frankenhauser's plexus is the mechanism of pain in secondary dysmenorrhea. Retroversion, if it is fixed in the pelvis by other diseases or if there is congestion of the blood supply, may produce this bearing-down sensation. As we noted previously, however, low sacral backache is far more often due to posture, particularly in a woman over forty years, than to retroversion per se. Unless there is an element of uterine fixation, one should be careful about attributing the cause of pelvic backache to retroversion of the uterus.

Does Pelvic Cancer Produce Pain?

Unless an accident has occurred within a tumor or unless it has involved other structures, has extended out into the deep pelvic connective tissues or onto the peritoneal surface, the patient may harbor malignant disease in the pelvis without having any pain. This is true of primary sites in the bladder and the rectum, as well as ovary, endometrium and cervix. The same may be said of benign tumors within the uterus. The fibroid, for example, rarely produces pain. If a tumor is pedunculated and subject to torsion of the pedicle which will cut off its blood supply, or if it outgrows its blood supply and degenerates, then the patient may have exquisite pain. Large or strategically placed fibroids may cause discomfort through the pressure of increasing size, but not pain. The submucous fibroid at times may cause colicky pain as the uterus tries to get rid of it.

Cancer of the cervix, endometrium or ovary rarely produces pain in the early stages of growth. Only when it has left the primary site does it produce pelvic pain that can be identified clinically. Ovarian neoplasms not infrequently are the cause of pelvic pain, but the pain is not due to malignancy of the tumor. It is simply an indication that an accident has happened within the neoplasm. Ovarian tumors in the earlier phases of their growth may lie free in the abdominal cavity and grow on a pedicle. Like the pedunculated fibroid, they may undergo torsion of the pedicle, interfere with the blood supply and produce pain.

Pelvic Pain Due to Extension of the Cancer.   Patients who have extensive malignant disease do have severe, constant and often agonizing pelvic pain. Pain is a frightening thing, and once started, it tends to maintain itself. A vicious circle is established. Pain produces vasoconstriction, which may produce more pain. Total incapacity and physical deterioration may follow rapidly. It is our obligation as physicians to relieve pain and make the patient's life as tolerable as possible through its full span. We cannot dodge our obligation when all hope of curing the patient is lost.

The Value of Surgery versus Drug Therapy.   There is a natural reluctance to suggest surgery to a patient who has only a short time to live, but it may be preferable to asking the patient to get along as best she can with opiates. The kind of operation that will do most for the incurable patient is cordotomy. Symptomatic therapy for cancer of the pelvic viscera has little to offer. Cordotomy, when done early enough in the patient who has intolerable pain and a limited life expectancy, has much to recommend it. A well performed cordotomy creates little residual disability. The number of patients who have incisional pain, bladder dysfunction or difficulty in locomotion following cordotomy is increasingly few. When cordotomy is properly done before drug addiction or introspective depression has all but destroyed the patient through their distressing side effects, rehabilitation is possible and the results are gratifying. The course of the disease remains unchanged, but the pathway to the end has fewer horrors.

Pelvic Pain with Psychosomatic Overtones

The problem of interpreting pelvic pain and assigning it to the proper pelvic organ is less complicated when there are obvious physical findings and supporting laboratory evidence, but it can be extremely perplexing if no departures from the normal are found. Even when definite organic disease is present, there may be a large psychic component. Not only is it important to pinpoint the organic system that produces the pain, but also a distinction must be made between functional and organic cause.

Many women complain bitterly of severe, persistent lower abdominal pelvic pain, which is completely out of proportion to the physical findings. The pain is real to the patient, but she is totally unable to convey to the gynecologist any clear-cut description of its nature, its point of origin or its path of radiation. When asked to locate the area of the pain, she will almost invariably run her hand over the entire lower part of the abdomen with a tendency to localize the discomfort to the right lower quadrant. In many instances the pain seems to be aggravated by the menstrual cycle. The gynecologist becomes exasperated by the vagueness of the description of her difficulties. It is almost impossible to pin the patient down to a precise account of her pain. Usually when questioned further, the patient either becomes more dramatic in her recital of symptoms, but no more definite, or she begins to talk about something totally unrelated to her present complaint.

Although the major portion of her symptomatology is directed toward the pelvis and the genital organs, she will almost invariably have a wide variety of associated symptoms. Thus we may expect to learn that the patient has dyspareunia, vaginismus, abnormal bleeding patterns, urinary frequency and backache, but she will also have dizziness, fainting, palpitation, nausea and vomiting, weakness and fatigue, headaches and depression. Because she focuses so intensely on her pelvic difficulties, however, the gynecologist often, through sheer desperation, is trapped into performing some sort of gynecologic operation. Unfortunately, he can usually demonstrate some degree of pelvic tenderness or alteration in the size, shape or position of the uterus, especially when the patient keeps insisting that the pelvic organs are at fault. It is a well known fact that patients who have this train of symptoms are prone to have multiple operations. The incidence of operations, when compared to the normal, is reported in the range of seven to one.

What Are Some of the Underlying Causes of Functional Pelvic Pain?

It is a difficult matter to pinpoint the trigger mechanism for the production of pelvic pain due to functional cause. In general, there seems to be agreement that this kind of pain is related to some form of emotional disorder. The actual cause of the pain is similar to that noted in patients who suffer from hysteria. Such patients also have far more hospitalizations, operations and marital difficulties than the normal woman. Characteristically, they too cannot be specific about their complaints. They tend to have many and varied symptoms which they recount at length in dramatic fashion. The patient with hysteria, like the patient with atypical pelvic pain and no evident disease, tends to focus her attention on the pelvis. Moreover, they are strikingly similar in their personalities and attitude toward life. As a rule these patients are conscious of sex and go to considerable length to encourage it, but when confronted by the actual act, they are notoriously unresponsive. By and large they are emotionally immature, vain and egocentric and are prone to express their unhappiness in a highly dramatic, often fanciful fashion.

When psychologic and psychiatric interviews have been carried out, the patients with atypical functional pelvic pain all seem to present the same type of emotional background: (1) The patient's early childhood has almost invariably been unhappy and marked by lack of security. There has seemed to be a complete lack of affection on the part of both father and mother. In most instances the father had been either disinterested or ineffectual. Most of the resentment, however, has seemed to be directed toward the mother, who was always cold, lacking in affection, highly critical, complaining, dominating and given to expressing openly a hostility to sex and all it implied. As a result the patient's childhood has been full of discord and unhappiness. In many instances the unhappy woman has left home to get married at an early age, not because she was interested in having her own family, but simply to get away from her parents.

2. The patient's husband was usually a patient, kindly, understanding, dependable type without much drive or virility. Although the husbands have not resented their wives' disinterest in sex or the obligation of marriage, the marital existence has largely been based on passive acceptance rather than hearty cooperation. The marital relation, therefore, has been unsatisfactory to both.

3. The patient herself is lacking in sexual drive and interest in reproduction. Her deficiencies are augmented by the attitude toward sex inculcated in her by her mother, who taught her that everything to do with sex was unnatural and unclean. She frequently complains that her mother has not instructed her properly. The major defect, however, lies in the patient, who is basically immature, frightened by the sex act and fearful that she might get pregnant. If she becomes a mother, she is totally unable to cope with the responsibilities of bringing up one child, much less several children. Since she is basically insecure and dependent, she becomes easily upset, confused and baffled by the obligation that life thrusts upon her and is apt to react by being generally unhappy and dissatisfied with everything. As a result she focuses all her troubles on her pelvis.

It is possible that the patient's reactions may be conditioned as much by what she hears as by what she experiences if she is neurotically inclined. It has been said that anticipation, fear and sensory conditioning can provide the explanation for pelvic pain in the absence of disease. If these impressions are implanted deeply enough in the mind of the patient, she may well react by having pelvic pain without apparent adequate causation. Thus the patient who has been conditioned by her mother to abhor sex in all its implications may complain of menstrual difficulty, dyspareunia and vaginismus and do everything she can to avoid both intercourse and the possibility of pregnancy.

What about the Pelvic Congestion Syndrome?

All that has been said about the psychosomatic element in patients who have indefinable pelvic pain in the absence of pelvic disease is applicable to the so-called pelvic congestion syndrome. There is only one fundamental difference. Although no definite abnormality can be felt, there is one characteristic finding that appears almost invariably, namely, tenderness on palpation of the vaults and motion of the cervix. There are certain other physical findings which suggest that the pelvic tenderness is due to vascular congestion in the pelvic area. Thus one finds definite circulatory changes in the vaginal wall and cervix, which appear blue and congested. The cervix is often eroded and enlarged with abundant secretion. The fundus is frequently felt in retroversion and seems soft, boggy and definitely enlarged.

It is not easy to be certain that the tenderness is due to vascular congestion per se. One can have a tender pelvic peritoneum in the presence of a lesion in the back, as we have noted previously. The examiner could be palpating disease in the ovary or tube. By ruling out these two possibilities it is possible to say that the tenderness is due to increased vascularity. In favor of this explanation is the well known observation that the normal cervix can be moved freely in the healthy woman without producing pain.

Why these patients have pelvic congestion is another matter. Those who believe strongly in pelvic congestion as an entity feel that the increased blood supply to the area is a "bodily reaction to stressful life experiences." It is possible, then, that emotional crises may precipitate alterations in the normal vascular physiology and trigger the mechanism of pelvic pain. As supporting evidence investigators report intermittent color changes in the appearance of the vaginal epithelium in response to questioning of the patient on subjects that disturb her emotionally. There can be little doubt that the psychic factor plays an important role in the creation of vascular congestion, but many other factors are involved in the production of pelvic pain.

WHAT OTHER FACTORS CONTRIBUTE TO PELVIC CONGESTION? There are obvious anatomic factors which contribute to pelvic congestion. The main support to the vast vascular network in and around the uterus in the broad ligament comes from muscular and fascial structures. Any factor which will influence muscle tone or disturb the fascial support will interfere with the vascular channels, chiefly venous. Thus we often observe clinically an extensively dilated venous plexus with stasis in patients who have a relaxed pelvic floor or a uterus impacted in the cul-de-sac. That postural factors are also present is shown by the fact that, characteristically, the low backache in these patients increases as the day progresses.

It is also a well documented clinical observation that the patient's symptoms are more pronounced immediately before the onset of menstruation or the time when there is apt to be the greatest tissue edema. The edema is not confined to the pelvis. Patients with the pelvic congestion syndrome are apt to have extragenital symptoms as well. Tenderness in the breasts, headaches, frequent urination, watery bowel movements and increased irritability are frequently noted in the week immediately preceding the period. Hormonal imbalance, which manifests itself by storage of fluid in tissue spaces, is the reason commonly advanced to explain the symptom complex, which is much like that of premenstrual tension.

It is difficult to say just what influence the emotional state has on the sympathetic and parasympathetic nerve control of the blood vessels, but there is ample physiologic evidence that the blood supply to any given region is influenced by the emotional conditioning.

Whatever the mechanism of pain production, the mere fact that pelvic tenderness exists in patients who are unstable emotionally makes it easier to understand why (*a*) the patient with pelvic congestion syndrome complains of a low abdominal pain or low backache which is made worse by menstruation, fatigue or emotional trauma. (*b*) Some of these women have dyspareunia with pain felt not at the vaginal outlet, but deep in the pelvis. Motion of the cervix or contact with the tender vaginal vault would be enought to bring on the pain.

TREATMENT.   The gynecologist should be cautious about operating on any patient for pelvic pain in the absence of demonstrable pelvic disease. Too frequently no adequate explanation of the cause can be found, and all too often ill-advised operations are performed which bring little satisfaction to either patient or surgeon.

What about Adhesions as a Cause of Pelvic Pain?

The attitude toward pelvic surgery for functional symptoms alone can best be summarized by considering pelvic surgery for adhesions. In most instances operations performed for the sole purpose of relieving pain when no abnormality can be felt are usually most unsatisfactory. Even in the presence of known disease one should be cautious about attributing pain to the adhesions. There can be no doubt that the patient can have pelvic pain as a result of adhesions after an operation, infection or peritonitis from a variety of causes. The adhesions may be thin and filmy or dense and unyielding. The mere presence of adhesions, however, is not enough to explain abdominal pain or provide the indication for surgical exploration. Some patients seem to have a lot of pain from a moderate amount of adhesions, while others have no discomfort and more lesions. It makes some difference where the adhesions arise and to what they adhere.

For example, extensive matting together of loops of small bowel by adhesions, formed by a previous attack of peritonitis, may be present without the patient being aware of it. Likewise the omentum may adhere to the anterior abdominal wall or other viscera over a wide area and produce no symptoms. On the other hand, the intestine may twist around a single adhesive band and obstruct completely. Adhesions of bowel to pelvic viscera, such as uterus, tube or ovary, are far more likely to produce pelvic pain than other conditions in which the bowel is adherent to itself. Unless there is definite evidence of lesions which can be determined by physical or x-ray examination, the surgeon will do well to withold operative intervention for relief of a pain that he attributes to adhesions alone.

What about the Treatment of the Pelvic Congestion Syndrome?

Although many of the complaints and much of the etiology can be traced to the psychosomatic, the patient should be referred to the psychiatrist only after the simpler methods of therapy have been exhausted. There may even be a place for surgery in therapy when obvious contributory factors exist.

Much can be accomplished through reassurance and education. A sympathetic understanding of the patient's problems and an obvious desire on the part of the physician to help the patient overcome her problem are basic elements in any therapy. The patient is unaware of the underlying cause of her complaints, which are real to her. She always believes that the pain has visceral origin, and uncertainty as to what it might be brings her to the physician. Her fears will be minimized if she can be told that she does not need an operation, that there is no cancer present and that her fertility is not in jeopardy. The surgeon should be careful not to fall into the trap of conveying to the patient the idea that he thinks her pain is all a figment of her imagination. She must be carefully told the difference between organic and functional pain. Many automobile motors are perfectly sound structurally, but are relatively useless if for some simple reason, easily corrected, they cannot function. The analogy of the recurrent headache is an excellent one. Most women have experienced headache for which they have no explanation, but they do not become unduly alarmed because they do not know the cause. They recognize that it may appear during times of tension.

It is reasonable, then, to inquire about the patient's work, home and marital life, as well as sexual adaptation. The mere fact that the patient will discuss her maladjustments and feelings of emotional instability may be enough to straighten her out. In the course of these discussions it often becomes obvious to the gynecologist that the patient has a basic psychiatric defect. The help of a psychiatrist should be obtained only after simple remedial therapy has been tried or has been recognized as inadequate to deal with the individual situation.

Relief of many of the symptoms, both pelvic and extragenital, can often be obtained by simple medical therapy. Premenstrual congestion is frequently alleviated by drugs such as ammonium chloride, Neohydrin, or Diuril, designed to increase the fluid output and decrease tissue edema. If the patient has a uterine prolapse or obvious pelvic relaxation, she may benefit from the use of a pessary. The patients whose complaints are made worse by being on their feet should be encouraged to take periodic rest periods to relieve the pelvic congestion due to venous stasis. If the pelvic pain is aggravated by intercourse, the couple should be instructed to refrain from any sexual act that might increase the pelvic vascularity.

Finally, in a few selected instances, surgery may provide relief. The large, boggy, retroverted uterus can either be suspended or removed if the patient has passed the childbearing age. Occasionally nerve resection, either presacral neurectomy or resection of the uterosacral ligaments and Frankenhauser's plexus, may be indicated. Surgery is the last resort, and satisfactory results can be obtained only if the patient and her symptoms have been completely evaluated.

REFERENCES

Allbutt, T. C.: Neuroses of the Viscera. *Lancet,* 1: 459, 506, 1884.
Benson, R. C., Hanson, K. H., and Matarazzo, J. D.: Atypical Pelvic Pain in Women: Gynecologic and Psychiatric Considerations. *Am. J. Obst. & Gynec.,* 77: 806, 1959.
Breuer, J., and Freud, S.: *Studies on Hysteria.* New York, Basic Books Co., 1957.
Burch, J. C., Chalfant, R. L., and Lavely, H. T., Jr.: Somatic Pain; in L. D. Davis, ed.: *Christopher's Textbook of Surgery.* 7th ed. Philadelphia, W. B. Saunders Company, 1960, p. 931.
Cohen, M. E., Robins, E., Purtell, J. J., Altmann, M. W., and Reid, D. E.: Excessive Surgery in Hysteria. *J.A.M.A.,* 151: 977, 1953.
Chodoff, P., and Lyons, H.: Hysteria, the Hysterical Personality and Hysterical Conversion. *Am. J. Psychiat.,* 114: 734, 1958.
Deutsch, H.: Psychiatric Component in Gynecology; in J. V. Meigs and S. H. Sturgis, eds.: *Progress in Gynecology.* New York, Grune & Stratton, Inc., 1950, Vol. II, p. 207.

Duncan, C. H., and Taylor, H. C., Jr.: A Psychosomatic Study of Pelvic Congestion. *Am. J. Obst. & Gynec.*, 64: 1, 1952.

Gidro-Frank, L., and Gordon, T.: Reproductive Performance of Women with Pelvic Pain of Long Duration. *Fertil. & Steril.*, 7: 440, 1956.

Gidro-Frank, L., Gordon, T., and Taylor, H. C., Jr.: Pelvic Pain and Female Identity. *Am. J. Obst. & Gynec.*, 79: 1184, 1960.

Heckel, G. P., Leahy, M. F., Rose, A. L., and Strain, W. H.: Pelvic Pain and Autosensitivity. *Fertil. & Steril.*, 10: 596, 1959.

Hoagland, H.: Some Considerations of Adrenocortical Physiology in Relation to the Psychoses. *Internat. Rec. Med.*, 166: 183, 1953.

Hunter, W. E.: Psychic Component of Pain. *Am. J. Obst. & Gynec.*, 54: 848, 1947.

Landry, W. J., Bierre, J. T., and Hunt, N. S.: Radiological Evaluation of Low Back Pain. *J. Louisiana M. Soc.*, 107: 484, 1955.

Motley, L.: Neurogenic Pain Simulating Visceral Disease. *Am. J. Med.*, 4: 539, 1948.

Parsons, L.: Pelvic Pain. *Postgrad. Med.*, 23: 252, 1958.

Purtell, J. J., Robins, E., and Cohen, M. E.: Observations on Clinical Aspects of Hysteria. *J.A.M.A.*, 146: 902, 1951.

Taylor, H. C., Jr.: Pelvic Pain Based on Vascular and Autonomic Nervous System Disorder. *Am. J. Obst. & Gynec.*, 67: 1177, 1954.

Idem: The Pelvic Pain Syndrome. *J. Obst. & Gynaec. Brit. Emp.*, 66: 781, 1959.

Taylor, J. A.: A Personality Scale of Manifest Anxiety. *J. Abnorm. & Social Psychol.*, 48: 285, 1953.

Young, J.: Broad Ligament Neuritis. *Tr. Edinburg. Obst. Soc.*, 92: 165, 1933.

Idem: Lower Abdominal Pains of Cervical Origin, Their Genesis and Treatment. *Brit. M.J.*, 1: 105, 1938.

PART III

Gynecologic Problems of the Young Woman (Age 20 to 30)

Chapter 27

Sterility:

General Considerations,

and Physiology of Conception

A DISCUSSION of the all-important problem of sterility is a natural sequence to the review of normal development, physiology and endocrinology of the period from infancy through adolescence. The menstrual cycle has been developed with one purpose in mind, namely, reproduction. The fertility curve reaches its peak, and marriage and childbirth are common to the age group between twenty and thirty years. Unfortunately, not all marriages are fruitful, for approximately 10 per cent of marital couples are involuntarily sterile. This is a low estimate, for many sterile couples fail to consult a physician to make their plight known. Add to this another 10 per cent of pregnancies that end in spontaneous abortions, and the problem of infertility becomes a formidable one. There are myriad causes for reproductive failure, but some may be traced to conditions present in puberty and adolescence. Approximately one third of adult sterility cases can be traced to abnormal conditions existing at this time. The failure may lie in an inability to produce either sperm or ova. It is important, then, to pay attention to the testicular development of the young boy or the persistence of amenorrhea in the teen-age girl. Treatment carried out at this time may be successful. If the condition of delayed maturation is allowed to persist, under the mistaken impression that time will correct the defect, treatment in the young adult stage may be more difficult or even impossible.

What Do We Mean by Sterility?

It is important primarily to define the term "sterility." Sterility in women is the inability to become pregnant. It may be *absolute* if pregnancy is obviously impossible through a fundamental lack of equipment such as congenital absence of uterus or ovaries. *Relative* sterility exists when the patient fails to conceive, yet has all essential physical requirements. The basic cause of failure may be in a faulty function or organic disease. Though pregnancy may be difficult to achieve under these conditions, many defects can be corrected and a successful outcome anticipated in proportion to the extent of the underlying cause of failure.

311

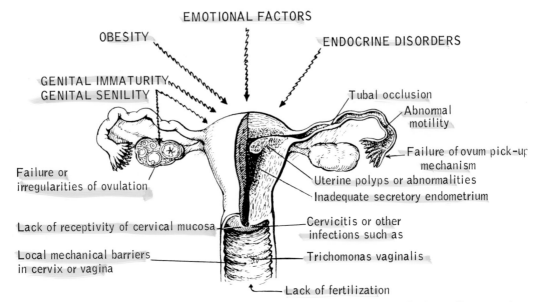

Fig. 27-1.   Some of the causes of sterility are localized in the genital tract, and others affect reproduction incidentally.

One may choose to break down the classification of sterility still further into primary and secondary (or acquired) sterility. In the former the patient has never become pregnant, while in the latter pregnancy has been achieved once or twice, but persistent attempts to repeat the initial success have not been forthcoming. The term "one child" sterility is in common usage. In the past the failure was usually blamed on gonorrhea. Today one or both partners would be considered subfertile, provided no other cause was found. More than likely the reason would be sought in the field of psychosomatics.

It is important at this juncture to point out the difference between sterility and infertility. We have noted that the *sterile* male or female patient never fertilizes an ovum or gets a pregnancy started. The *infertile* patient may be able to initiate a pregnancy, but a live baby is never forthcoming, for a variety of reasons.

When Does the Patient Become a Sterility Problem?

In the great majority of cases pregnancy occurs within the first year of married life, usually in the first six or seven months, in fertile couples who have regular intercourse, provided contraception is not practiced. Ninety per cent of all pregnancies occur within two years in this same group. One may say, then, that if pregnancy is earnestly desired and attempts at reproduction have failed after a two-year period, such a patient has a fertility problem. Some patients may be successful later (from personal experience we have known it to occur after seventeen years of marriage), but the chances are not great, and if a favorable result is sought, investigation as to the cause of failure should begin after two years of unsuccessful effort. The longer the investigation and reparative therapy are delayed, the less likely is the chance of pregnancy (Fig. 27–1).

What Are the Basic Essentials for Fertilization of an Ovum?

If pregnancy is to be initiated, the male must produce sperm capable of fertilizing the ova developed by the ovary. This presupposes that (1) the male testis produces an adequate quantity of viable sperm normal in morphology and motility, and that (2) the ovary on its part develops a healthy ovum and launches it from the surface of the ovary. In this connection it is interesting to keep in mind that many millions of sperm must be produced in order that one sperm may fertilize the single ovum predestined to be available for fertilization.

The next problem is that of transport of the sperm and ova to the point of fertilization. To accomplish this (1) the sperm must pass from the testis and be deposited in or about the vagina. In nearly every instance, after satisfactory intercourse, the sperm will be left in proximity to the cervical os. This presupposes that there is no block in the male conductive system. The spermatozoa must then, through their own motile power, perhaps aided by uterine muscular contractions, pass through the cervical os and endometrial cavity to enter the tube and make contact with the ovum. To accomplish this the sperm must encounter no interruption in transport from (a) mechanical obstructions in cervix, uterine cavity or tube or (b) from the presence of secretion that may enmesh the sperm or impair either their viability or motility. (2) The ovum must pass from the surface of the ovary through the tubal fimbriated end into the interior of the tube. This presupposes that there is no mechanical block or interference with the motility of the fimbriated end of the tube. Tubal functional activity is responsible for the passage of the ovum into its lumen. While there, it must encounter no hostile influence and acquire sufficient sustenance to survive. (3) Finally, the impregnated ovum must traverse the tube to become implanted in the endometrium, derive nourishment from it and survive. The tubal lumen must then be open to the passage of the egg and suitable conditions exist within the endometrial cavity so that the egg may implant and grow.

THE PHYSIOLOGY OF CONCEPTION

What General Conditions Influence both Male and Female Fertility?

There is a wide variety of factors outside the reproductive system which bear on the problem of sterility in both male and female. In many instances there is no evidence of organic disease or faulty function. Failure to fertilize an ovum cannot regularly be attributed to the ovum alone.

Age, general body health, state of nutrition, hormone production and utilization, psychic and emotional problems and genetic factors all come up for consideration in the subject of sterility.

Though we now recognize that the male factor in sterility is of far greater importance than originally believed, nevertheless the female must produce the ovum and incubate it after impregnation. The spermatozoa are essential to fertilization of the egg in the human species. In the invertebrates and in some animals, however, there is some evidence that segmentation and development may occur in the ova in the absence of spermatozoa. Instances of artificial fertilization of vertebrate eggs are on record.

The Role of the Ovary in Fertility

What Is the Source of the Ova?

The primary purpose of the ovary is to produce an ovum capable of being fertilized and to deliver it on the surface of the ovary. In all probability the monthly egg or eggs are drawn from a store previously provided in embryonic life. It is unlikely that the human ovary functions like the testis in being able to produce an ovum from the local germinal epithelial tissue within it. Normal human ovarian physiology ordinarily calls for the maturation of but one ovum, though many follicles are stimulated by the pituitary hormone FSH at the onset of the cycle. The mechanism has been discussed under the physiology of the menstrual cycle (Chap. 16). There are many unanswered questions. We would, for example, like to know whether the ovum is discharged from the same ovary each month, or whether there is a shift from side to side. The patient will frequently tell you that she ovulated on one side or the other and is often convinced of alternation from one side to the other.

What about the Ovary Itself?

There is a myriad of reasons why the ova may not develop normally. Some of these are anatomic, while others fall in the field of genetics and embryology. The relation of constitutional factors, nutrition and psychic unrest to endocrine function will be discussed later.

The basic difficulty in the production of ova may lie within the ovary itself. Some of these factors can be traced to puberty and adolescence. In the discussion on anovulatory bleeding of adolescence (Chap. 17) it was noted that the full response of the ovary to pituitary stimulation depended on the development of an adequate supply of arteries under the influence of estrin stimulation. Some part of ovarian failure may be traced to a faulty vascular development. The presence of a thick fibrous tunica around the ovary, as seen in the Stein-Leventhal syndrome, may also play an important role in denying normal development and maturation to the ova. Infectious diseases such as mumps might produce a secondary oophoritis similar to orchitis in males. General systemic infections cause changes within the ovary and interfere with its normal physiologic function. Likewise fibrous perioophoritis secondary to peritonitis from an appendicitis, abortion or salpingitis can prevent normal extrusion of the egg and result in sterility. Previous pelvic surgery often produces adhesions in and around the ovary and tube. Normal physiologic activity may not be possible under such conditions.

What Questionable Factors Are Present in the Mechanism of Ovulation?

In the discussion of the menstrual cycle we noted that the endocrine system was involved in the process of ovulation. Actually, we know little of what triggers the discharge of the ovum. Is ovulation due to hormonal stimulation or to growth of the follicle and changes in the liquor folliculi? It is possible that the follicle simply ruptures because of the accumulation of follicular fluid within it. As yet we are uncertain of the origin of this fluid. It has been suggested that estrin conditions the follicle and sensitizes it to the action of the pituitary hormones. We know that many follicles develop and then become atretic when the final selection of the one ovum destined to reach maturity has been made. Little is known of the process of selection of the individual follicle. Monkey experiments suggest that the atretic follicles augment the production of estrin at a time when it is needed both for ovulation and for luteinization of the follicle destined to rupture. We know clinically how sensitive the delicate mechanism of ovulation is to outside influences. It can be profoundly influenced by various factors such as psychic unrest or nutritional inadequacy. There is another factor about which little is known. Some animals apparently ovulate after copulation, and there is some clinical suggestion that the same thing may be true in women.

What about the Timing of Ovulation?

There is considerable evidence from experiments in the monkey and from limited clinical observation that impregnation is possible only within a twelve- to twenty-four-hour period. It is therefore of prime importance for successful fertilization to know the exact timing of ovulation. Actually, the means at hand for determining the precise moment of discharge of the ovum are not very accurate. The tests we now use do not indicate the release of a ripe ovum, but simply the physiologic changes associated with ovulation. These tests will be discussed in detail later.

We have some evidence in the human being when eggs have been recovered from the ovary and tube that ovulation occurs on the fourteenth day of a twenty-eight-day cycle. Many women, however, vary widely in the length of the cycles. Attempts to pinpoint ovulation in the girl who has completely irregular cycles have been most unsatisfactory. The timing of ovulation in such cases is highly theoretical, based on the assumption that the progestational phase of the menstrual cycle is constant at fourteen days, while the preovulatory stage varies widely. A girl with a thirty-five-day cycle would thus be expected to ovulate on the twenty-first day. There is some recent evidence that patients may ovulate earlier than previously thought and that the progestational portion of the cycle may be prolonged. Retroactive timing of ovulation is further complicated by the fact that the girl with the irregular cycle may not ovulate on the same day each month. If we are to be successful in our therapy of the infertile patient, it is of basic importance that the exact timing of ovulation be known.

How Viable Is the Ovum?

One of the factors in fertilization is concerned with the quality and viability of the ova. The life span of the free ovum is short. During a very small portion of this time (possibly only twelve hours) impregnation is possible, and normal development can be anticipated. Unfortunately we have no way of knowing whether the ovum is a healthy egg capable of being fertilized and developing normally, short of the test of actual pregnancy. We are aware that not all ova can be fertilized, and even if they are good, pregnancies do not invariably follow. Most miscarriages are now believed to be due to the so-called blighted ova that nature wants to eliminate. There may be defects due to genetic cause in either ova or spermatozoa in addition to chemical antagonism or temporary hormonal imbalance.

How Does the Ovum Get into the Tube?

Under normal conditions the ovum destined to be impregnated will arise in the ovary on the same side of the uterus as the tube it enters. This is not invariable, for in pathologic conditions of either the tube or ovary it is possible for the ovum to take origin from the opposite ovary, migrate across the pelvic cavity and enter the tube on the opposite side. Observations made on the location of corpora lutea in patients with ectopic pregnancies suggest that this may occur as often as once in ten times.

The outer, fimbriated end of the fallopian tube and the ovary normally lie in close proximity. From experiments performed in rabbits and monkeys and evidence provided by x-rays and cinematography in women, it would appear that at the time of ovulation the tubal musculature and that of the suspensory ligament of the ovary become increasingly active and tend to draw the ovary and the wide flaring end of the tube together. The sucking action produced by the tubal contractions causes the flaring open end of the tube with its ciliated epithelium actually to embrace the ovary. It is this sucking action, combined with the aspirating movement of the moving cilia, that draws the cumulus oophorus and the liquor folliculi from the ruptured follicle into the tube.

Tubal motility is therefore as important in infertility problems as actual patency of the tube. Since tubal function is believed to be under nerve and hormonal control, it is obvious that any disruption in balance between the two may interfere with the transport of the ovum in the tube. Its function will also be influenced by any pathologic process, present or past, which will interfere with normal tubal peristalsis. Tubal patency of course is basically important, for the ovum is the largest single cell in the human body except for the megakaryocyte, and the tubal lumen must be sufficiently patent to permit the migration of both sperm and ovum if impregnation is to occur.

What Happens to the Ovum While in the Tube?

The ovum, after entering the tube, is slowly propelled along the tubal lumen by the peristaltic action of the tubal musculature and finally passes into the uterine cavity. In addition to the sucking action produced by tubal contraction, the ciliated epithelium of the tube plays a part in separating the ovum from the cumulus cells which surround it, thus making impregnation easier. The progress along the tube is slow as the tubal peristaltic contractions occur in sequential fashion in response to the increasing bulk within the tube. Gradually as each portion of the tube becomes sensitized and contracts, the ovum and accompanying fluid are pushed along into the isthmic portion and, finally, into the endometrial cavity. The leisurely passage of the ovum from the ampulla of the tube into the uterus usually takes place over a period of three to four days.

This slow rate of passage allows time for progesterone to prepare the uterus for implantation and nourishment of the fertilized ovum. The biochemistry of the tubal fluid is not well known, but there is good evidence that it serves to condition the spermatozoa as well as the ovum so that impregnation may occur more readily.

Where and How Does Impregnation Occur?

Impregnation normally occurs in the outer end of the tube. For successful fertilization it is essential that a large concentration of sperm be present in anticipation of extrusion of the ovum, for there is a limited time when penetration of the ovum is possible. Aging of either sperm or ova is important in inhibiting fertilization. Aging ova will resist sperm penetration. If fertilization does occur, developmental defects are all too common. In order that penetration of the ovum by the sperm be made as easy as possible, something is needed to dissolve the cumulus of the ovum. This may well be the property of the tubal fluid. It is also more than likely that a high concentration of sperm serves a useful purpose. Numbers seem to be more important than the degree of motility or aggression. Though many are present, only one spermatozoon impregnates an ovum. The remainder apparently secrete an enzyme, hyaluronidase, which attacks and dissolves the cumulus and facilitates penetration of the egg.

What Is the Mechanism of Penetration of the Ovum?

After the cumulus of the ovum has been dissolved the egg is left with an inner exposed layer called the zona pellucida. Some protein substance on or within this layer seems to react with the sperm, and penetration is made easier. If this substance is washed away, penetration does not occur. Once the ovum is prepared for impregnation, tubal contractions and action of its cilia may determine the angle at which the sperm enters the ovary.

The Role of the Testis in the Physiology of Fertility

Before discussing the implantation of the impregnated ovum upon the endometrium we must now consider how the spermatozoa are produced and transported to the site of fertilization in the tube, as well as the factors that may influence the normal physiology adversely.

What Are the Functions of the Testes?

Like the ovary, the testis plays a dual role, in that it elaborates its own hormones and produces spermatozoa. For complete testicular function it is essential (1) that the testes secrete the male hormone, testosterone, from the interstitial cells (cells of Leydig), and (2) that the testes produce spermatozoa from the germinal epithelium of the seminiferous tubules. Both functions are under control of the basophil cells in the anterior pituitary, which are responsible for the essential stimulation of the germinal epithelium, while the luteinizing function of pituitary ICSH provides the impetus for the formation of testosterone from the mature interstitial cells.

Any factor which tends to interfere with the normal function of the anterior lobe of the pituitary will directly affect testicular function. Indirectly the testis may be modified by other glands of internal secretion such as the thyroid and adrenal. It is possible to have one element of testicular function present without the other. For example, adequate androgen production may be present while spermatogenesis is deficient or lacking.

In normal function the two elements complement one another. Fertilization cannot take place without the sperm, nor can the sperm be properly conditioned unless the androgenic component is present and functions properly. Testosterone production is also necessary for the development and maintenance of the accessory sex organs such as penis, scrotum, seminal vesicles and prostate. The viability and motility of the sperm depend on proper function of the seminal vesicles and prostate.

How Are the Sperm Produced?

Under proper stimulation from FSH the germinal cells lining the seminiferous tubules produce spermatogonia, which undergo mitotic cell division and become primary spermatocytes. Further miotic cell divisions take place, and secondary spermatocytes develop. These divide into spermatids, which gradually alter their cytoplasm and become the immature spermatozoa, complete with tails. Further development is essential before the sperm can function properly. Full maturation takes place in the Sertoli cells in the testicular tubules, in the epididymis and through the action of the secretions of seminal vesicles and prostate. This function will be discussed later.

What Factors Acting on the Testes Influence Spermatogenesis?

There are many causes for deficient sperm production, oligospermia, and its total absence, azoospermia. Some of these are basic endocrine disorders, while other factors such as debilitating disease, malnutrition, emotional and psychic disorders modify endocrine function and lead to diminished testicular function. When deficient spermatogenesis is due to a diminished gonadotropic activity of the pituitary, the disturbance may be due to a temporary functional imbalance and is therefore reversible. These gonadotropic factors that affect both male and female will be discussed later.

THE PART PLAYED BY FAULTY DEVELOPMENT.   In some instances failure to produce adequate sperm of sufficient quality and number to initiate fertilization may be traced to a developmental cause.

PRIMARY DEFECTS IN THE TESTES.   Lack of adequate pituitary stimulation will usually reveal itself by the extent of gonadal development, but in some males there is a basic defect in the testicle itself. The gonadotropins are present in increased quantity, but because of testicular inadequacy testosterone production is low and the 17-ketosteroids are diminished. In the majority of instances a basic defect of this extent will be recognizable in adolescence. The testes are small and often can be found in the inguinal canal rather than the scrotum. The secondary sex characteristics are in abeyance, and the distribution of the body fat in the breast and on the hips follows the feminine pattern. Often there is a mild to moderate eunuchoid overgrowth of the long bones.

In many males in whom the primary testicular defect is minimal the size of the testes and accessory sex organs shows little variation from the normal. There may be no alteration in body habitus, and the secondary sex characteristics are normal. The only evidence for faulty testicular function, except for the high FSH and low 17-ketosteroid excretion, is the presence of azospermia and infertility. In approximately 50 per cent of men who have azospermia the cause can be traced to a failure in normal testicular development.

HYPOGONADISM DUE TO FAULTY PITUITARY STIMULATION.   In some instances the lack of gonadal development is secondary to inadequate pituitary stimulation. The most obvious but rather rare example is Froehlich's syndrome. In the adult male this condition is readily recognized, for the lack of development is noted in all the male sex organs. In the adolescent the diagnosis is not so easy, for obesity, sluggish development of the genitals and secondary sex characteristics are common to the growing phase. Because both pituitary and testes are involved, the FSH will be diminished along with the 17-ketosteroids.

What Factors Produce Degenerative Changes in the Testes and Influence the Pituitary?

INFECTION.　　　Any acute infection, particularly those occurring in childhood, may affect the testes directly by creating interstitial damage. The prime example is mumps, but other systemic infections may do the same thing. The extent of damage to the germinal epithelium of the tubules depends on the degree of suppuration produced by the infection. If it is severe, the testicle may actually become entirely atrophic. Milder degrees of infection may damage the tubular epithelium and be responsible for oligospermia without leaving obvious stigmata (Fig. 27–2, *A*). Other chronic diseases such as syphilis, gonorrhea or tuberculosis tend to affect the epididymis, prostate and seminal vesicles rather than the testes. They modify the subsequent reproductive history, but do not interfere with spermatogenesis.

TRAUMA.　　　Degenerative changes in the testes may be set up by anything that will interfere with the external or intrinsic blood supply to the testes. Hemorrhage into the testes may follow direct trauma or torsion of the spermatic cord and its vessels. If the hemorrhage is extensive enough, atrophy may result. The same factors are occasionally noted following repair of a hernia or a varicocele. Pressure may produce atrophy if a hernia, varicocele or hydrocele is sufficiently large to interfere with the normal circulation to the testes.

EXPOSURE TO RADIATION.　　　It has been said that "small doses of irradiation either to testes or pituitary are stimulating," but the over-all effect actually is damag-

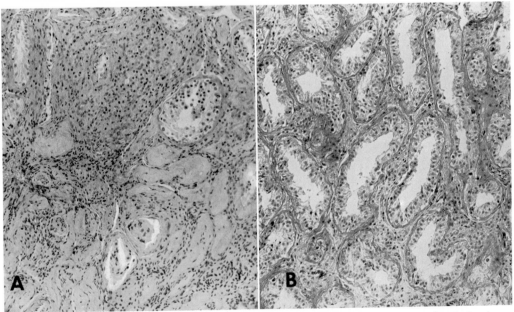

Fig. 27-2.　　*A*, Part of a testicular biopsy after orchitis. Most of the spermatogenic tubules shown are atrophied and either partially or completely hyalinized. Interstitial inflammation and fibrosis are present. *B*, Postirradiation atrophy of testis in a young man. Most of the testicular tubules are lined by Sertoli cells, and the spermatogenic elements have largely disappeared. The Leydig interstitial cells are practically unaffected by irradiation.

ing to the germinal epithelium. The action more clearly affects immature cells such as spermatocytes than the mature spermatozoa. The extent of damage produced seems to vary with the individual. Nevertheless, even in the smaller dose range irradiation should be avoided. Its deleterious effect on spermatogenesis should be kept in mind when advising roentgen therapy for dermatitis in the genital area or for pruritus ani (Fig. 27–2, *B*). Men who work with x-rays or handle radiation emanations should have adequate protection and spaced release from their work.

Exposure to High Temperatures. The testes, when exposed to high temperature, tend to undergo degeneration of the seminiferous tubules. We have noted this previously in severe, acute infections, but it may also become an occupational hazard. Stokers working on blast furnaces or in the holds of ships have a high incidence of defective spermatogenesis. Truck drivers are notoriously infertile. Their masculinity is unquestioned, but long hours in the engine cab over a hot engine definitely impair their ability to put out adequate quantities of normal sperm. The cremasteric reflex in males is nature's protective device. If the weather is cold, contraction of these muscles tends to pull the testes out of the scrotum toward the inguinal canals. Conversely, the testes descend into the bottom of the scrotum during warm weather. If the testes are continually compressed by tight jockey-type underwear or athletic supports, the increased warmth of body temperature will definitely impair the function of the seminiferous tubules and diminish the output of sperm.

Cryptorchidism. Failure of the testes to descend into the scrotum from their embryologic position within the abdomen or inguinal canal is called cryptorchidism. Normally, descent takes place in the last month of fetal life, but it may be delayed until puberty. The condition is usually unilateral, but it can occur on both sides. The testes fail to descend either because of a basic endocrine disorder or because of anatomic reasons such as a defective gubernaculum or tight inguinal ring.

The problem of what should be done and when depends on the likelihood of permanent damage to the testicle because of the increased temperature within the abdomen or inguinal canal. The undescended testicle is associated with a high degree of deficient spermatogenesis. There is no doubt that cryptorchid testes present evidence of persistent immaturity, and there is pathologic evidence that they later undergo degeneration. If there is no tumor present or other obvious danger, there is little reason to perform an operation before puberty, since the testis may descend at that time if left undisturbed. The operation carries with it a risk of damage to the circulation and subsequent atrophy. For this reason many prefer to try to accomplish the descent by the administration of gonadotropins, reserving surgery for the failures. The results in any case are not very rewarding. Late treatment is undertaken in the hope that the few normal tubules remaining will be sufficiently active to produce adequate amounts of viable sperm.

Other factors such as the technique and frequency of intercourse, the influence of the other endocrine glands, the role of malnutrition, chronic disease, psychic and emotional problems will be discussed later.

What about the Role of the Epididymis, Seminal Vesicles and Prostate?

Before we can discuss the volume of sperm, motility, abnormal forms, concentration and quality in relation to the power to fertilize, it is necessary to consider the part played by the accessory sex organs.

The Epididymis. The immature spermatozoa come to full maturation within the epididymis. This important accessory organ may be congenitally absent, obstructed or severely damaged by trauma, chronic disease such as syphilis, gonorrhea, tuberculosis or other nonspecific infections. Any damage to the epididymis may interfere with either the full development of the spermatozoa or their transport to the prostatic urethra.

THE SEMINAL VESICLES. The secretions of the seminal vesicles and prostate obviously serve as a vehicle for the transport of the spermatozoa, and they make up a large portion (95 per cent) of the ejaculate. It is also probable that they have an important role in nourishing and conditioning the sperm. The fertilizing capacity of the spermatozoa evidently does not depend on the seminal fluid, but on the energy of the sperm, their motility and ability to survive until they get to the point of fertilization. The energy for sperm motility seems to come from the glycolysis or fermentative breakdown of some sugar in the semen. This is believed to be fructose. Its source is thought to be the seminal vesicle, for none is found in the epididymis or testes, where the sperm are immobile. The *height of motility* comes when the sperm are in contact with the seminal fluid. This has a high concentration of fructose, which is subsequently broken down into lactic acid. The chemical composition of seminal fluid would appear too complex to constitute merely a simple vehicle for the transport of sperm. Since it contains amino acids, phosphorus, calcium, sugar, urea, enzymes and ascorbic acid, among other things, it would seem that the seminal fluid plays a definite role in the *nutrition of the sperm*. Alteration in the chemical structure of the seminal fluid may result in abnormal forms of spermatozoa. Nutrition continues both within the vesicle and after discharge of the semen into the vagina. The alkalinity of seminal fluid protects the sperm against any hostile acid pH factor in the vaginal canal before the sperm have a chance to enter the endocervical canal.

THE PROSTATE. To a less extent this gland may be considered a source of the all-important fructose, but its chief function seems to be to render the fluid less viscous and to increase the volume of the semen. When the seminal fluid is too viscous, the sperm become trapped and lose their motility in the struggle to escape. Any infection in the prostate or seminal vesicles which tends to increase the amount of mucus in the fluid will definitely interfere with sperm activity. The recovery of pus in the ejaculate is an indication that infection is present in either the prostate or seminal vesicles. Pus of itself does not interfere with the fertilizing capacity of the sperm, but it points to alterations in the seminal and prostatic fluids which do affect sperm adversely. This is independent of any damage to the ejaculatory ducts themselves.

What about Abnormal Forms Found in the Sperm?

A number of abnormal forms of spermatozoa found in the ejaculated specimen have long been considered one factor in sterility problems. This is difficult to assess. So much depends on the method of collection, staining technique, and the experience of the examiner in interpreting the findings. Since we do not know, after studying the specimen, whether the abnormal forms are due to defective spermatogenesis or inadequate maturation or simply represent degenerated forms of normal mature sperm, it is hard to evaluate the role they may play in an individual case.

The role of abnormal morphology of spermatozoa should not be evaluated on the basis of the examination of a single ejaculated specimen, but if more than 30 to 40 per cent of abnormal forms are noted after examining repeated specimens, the

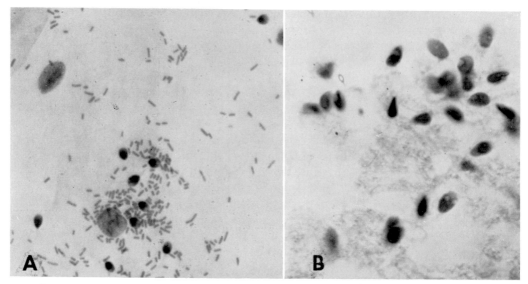

Fig. 27-3. *A*, Normal sperm found mixed with bacteria and cellular debris in a postcoital Papanicolaou vaginal smear. *B*, At higher magnification, a variety of abnormal sperm, some swollen, others shrunken or vacuolated. Special staining is often needed to demonstrate spermatozoal tails.

patient's fertility is regarded as definitely impaired. The normal sperm has a single head and tail. The head is oval in shape. The abnormal sperm heads vary in size and shape from minute to large and from round to tapering (Fig. 27–3). It is assumed, if a high percentage of abnormal forms are present, that the remaining spermatozoa, though they appear normal, may be physiologically abnormal. This does not mean that fertilization is impossible, for abnormal patterns of germinal epithelium maturation may be present in otherwise apparently normal men. Moreover, a small percentage of men who show more than 50 per cent of abnormal forms have been highly fertile. By and large, the higher the percentage of abnormal sperm morphologically, the less the chance of fertilization and the greater the likelihood of an abnormal pregnancy should impregnation occur. This is particularly true when the sperm count is also low.

What about the Motility of the Sperm?

Motility of the sperm is an important but not the sole criterion for determining the fertilizing potential of spermatozoa. Some may be nonmotile, yet be capable of fertilization, while others are aggressively motile, yet lack the power to penetrate the ovum. In evaluating motility of spermatozoa there are several things we want to know: (1) What percentage of the total sperm shows activity? (2) What is the extent of the motility? (3) How long does it last? For example, rabbit sperm may remain motile from two to five weeks, yet lose their power to fertilize after a week or ten days. By and large a specimen from a normally fertile male will show 70 to 80 per cent actively motile sperm after 2 hours. Examinations at four-hour intervals up to twenty-four hours are necessary to determine the over-all range of viability and the duration of motility. Between 25 and 40 per cent will be active at 24 hours. The great majority of sperm will demonstrate aggregation and vertical progression during this period.

If motility and viability are obviously impaired, either there is a basic defect in spermatogenesis or the sperm have been altered by changes in the secretions of the seminal vesicles and prostate. If, in addition, too many abnormal forms are present, the fault usually lies in the germinal epithelium.

What about the Volume of the Sperm?

The total number, measured in millions, of spermatozoa per cubic centimeter is the most popular method of evaluating the fertilizing potential. In the past the requisite minimum was believed to be 60 million per cubic centimeter or about 240 million spermatozoa per ejaculate, if we consider that the average volume of the total is 4 cc. The amount may be materially reduced by a disease in the prostate or seminal vesicles which alters the viscosity of the seminal fluid, entraps spermatozoa and interferes with the normal transmission through the ejaculating duct system. It may be reduced further by too frequent intercourse or the general state of health, among other factors.

The total volume of seminal discharge may be of great importance, for the concentration of sperm may prove to have greater significance than mere numbers. Experimentally, an undiluted specimen of rabbit's sperm produced ten times as many satisfactory impregnations as a diluted insemination.

It is also important to consider how many of the total are active, healthy spermatozoa. The requisite minimum for such a specimen has been placed at 85 million motile sperm per cubic centimeter. Other factors must be considered, for there are recorded many instances of pregnancy when the count was less than 20 million and a few isolated cases when the count was one million or less per cubic centimeter. The only thing of which we can really be sure is that pregnancy is impossible in the face of azospermia. Unless the azospermia has been determined on repeated specimens, it is unwise to make any absolute statement. If, however, the total number of active sperm is considered in relation both to the number of abnormal spermatozoa and to the fertility index of the female partner, a fair idea can be obtained of the likelihood of pregnancy for a given couple, provided no block exists to the transport of sperm to the site of fertilization in the tube.

The Transmission of Spermatozoa to Ovum

The problem of fertilization is not solved by the mere production of an ovum and spermatozoa. Fertilization occurs in the outer end of the fallopian tube. The spermatozoa must then pass from the primary source of production in the testicle through the ejaculating system into the vaginal canal. After this they must traverse the endocervical canal and endometrial cavity. Finally the spermatozoa must enter the lumen of the fallopian tube. Hostile mechanical, chemical and enzymatic influences may be present all along the line.

What Obstructive Factors May Be Present in the Male Generative Tract?

By and large, obstruction to the output of sperm in the male is due to inflammation. This may have its primary source in the epididymis, vas deferens, seminal vesicle or prostate. The obstruction results either from edema or actual stenosis of the vas deferens or ejaculatory ducts. Seminal vesiculitis is a great offender. Infection here spreads downward to involve the ejaculatory ducts. In acute infection the ducts are blocked by edema leading to stenosis as the infection becomes chronic. When the prostate is infected, the transporting seminal fluid becomes altered. In addition to chemical changes which influence the nutrition of the sperm, the viscosity of the fluid is affected. As a result the ejaculate in the presence of genital infection may be deficient in volume as well as quality.

Other causes of obstruction to the output of semen are congenital in origin. These include spermatocele, congenital stenosis and absence of the epididymis or vas deferens.

IMPREGNATION AND IMPLANTATION

What Role Does the Cervix Play in Transmission of Sperm?

The greatest barrier to adequate insemination is the delivery of an insufficient number of active, healthy motile sperm at the cervical os. The technique of coitus may be satisfactory and all other factors favorable, but if the sperm are deficient, the chance of fertilization is materially reduced. This is not surprising when we consider what the spermatozoa have to overcome to get to the ovum in the tube. To survive the long journey from vagina to tube in a state healthy enough to fertilize an ovum the spermatozoa must (1) overcome the hostile influence of an acid vagina, (2) pass through a cervix where conditions may be favorable or inimical, depending on the pH, amount and sterility of its secretions, and where mechanical obstruction from cervical polyps may also be present, (3) enter the endometrial cavity, where the environment may or may not be favorable. Under the best of conditions only a few spermatozoa survive to pass into the tube, and (4) overcome spasm and peristalsis in the interstitial portion of the tube.

All these impediments must be overcome and the spermatozoa delivered to the outer end of the tube in a relatively short time. It has been estimated that it takes the spermatozoa three hours to complete the entire journey. The more vigorous of the spermatozoa pass through the tube within one-half hour of the time of insemination. The majority take approximately twenty-seven minutes to cross the uterus and forty-two minutes to traverse the tube. The actual time in transport and the motility and aggressiveness of the sperm are influenced materially by structural, functional and metabolic factors encountered in the uterus.

It is small wonder, then, that only the most vigorous of the spermatozoa survive the journey in good enough physical shape to accomplish fertilization. Of the half billion of spermatozoa that may be produced in the ejaculate, only a few hundred are potential candidates for impregnation. Only one is destined to survive, but the concentration of the remainder is essential to prepare the ovum for final penetration.

When these factors are added to the observation that ova are receptive to impregnation for a period limited to twelve to twenty-four hours after discharge, it is overwhelmingly evident that *the nature of the semen is of basic importance if fertilization is to occur*.

How Do the Spermatozoa Overcome Vaginal Hostility?

Though the vaginal pH changes toward the alkaline side under the influence of hormonal activity at the approximate time of ovulation, it remains acid in relation to the alkaline secretions of the male ejaculate. Apparently the spermatozoa are protected from the destructive effect of the acid vaginal secretions by the piston-like action of the penis during the act of coitus. This tends to mix the alkaline seminal secretion with those drawn from the cervix and spread the alkaline medium over the cervix and upper part of the vagina. The protection lasts for a few hours, during which the healthy motile sperm enter the cervical canal. Under normal conditions thirty to a few hundred active spermatozoa per microscopic high-power field are found in the cervical canal within one-half hour of intercourse. Those that fail to enter the cervical canal and remain in the vagina lose their motile power and are destroyed.

What Factors Must the Sperm Overcome in the Cervical Canal?

Under normal physiologic conditions the cervical mucus is prepared for the receipt of the spermatozoa. This is under the control of the ovarian hormones. At the time of ovulation and for a few days thereafter the cervical mucus becomes abundant, thin, acellular, elastic and of low viscosity. The cervical mucus contains many carbohydrates such as glucose, maltose and glycogen. In addition, an enzyme, diastase, is present which augments the breakdown of glycogen into the more readily utilizable glucose and maltose. These factors contribute to the ease of transit as well as the nourishment of the spermatozoa in their passage through the cervical canal.

Abnormal cervical mucus will explain between 15 and 20 per cent of failures to accomplish fertilization. If infection is present or if the cervical glands have been improperly prepared by estrin stimulation, conditions are unfavorable to the passage of sperm. The change in type of cervical secretion may be obvious. If it is grossly purulent, the cervical glands are infected and must be treated either by chemotherapeutic drugs or surgical conization before one may reasonably expect the spermatozoa to survive. Failure to provide an adequate cervical secretion may be due to *faulty hormonal stimulation*. The alteration of secretion may be in the direction of overproduction or of paucity. At times the cervical secretion may be heavy, tenacious and viscous, forming a mucous plug which provides a mechanical block as well as a trap that enmeshes and destroys the sperm. On the other hand, inadequate hormonal stimulation may fail to provide an adequate amount of cervical secretion.

Other mechanical factors such as endocervical polyps or a long conical juvenile cervix with a pinpoint os may deny passage to the spermatozoa. A tumor such as a fibroid, malposition of the uterus or a pathologic process may be responsible through alteration of anatomic relations.

At times no apparent cause can be found. The cervical mucus may be clear, transparent, acellular and of normal viscosity, yet be hostile to fertile spermatozoa. Approximately 5 per cent of infertile women are in this category. Seemingly the fault is of endocrine origin. Adequate estrin stimulation is present, but the cervical glands fail to utilize it normally.

What Happens to the Sperm in the Endometrial Cavity?

Little is known of the fate of the spermatozoa in the endometrial cavity. The transport medium continues to be the same alkaline secretion produced in the cervical glands, augmented by the endometrial glands under the stimulation of estrin. We know that many spermatozoa die in the endometrial cavity, but we are uncertain whether this is due to faulty nutrition, hostile secretions or mere exhaustion.

The Role of Mechanical Obstruction in the Interstitial Portion of the Tube

Obstruction of the uterine end of the fallopian tube provides a double block. It prevents the spermatozoa from getting to the ovum in the tube and inhibits the passage of the ovum into the endometrial cavity if it has become impregnated.

The patency of this portion of the tube is usually tested by injection of carbon dioxide or radiopaque media into the uterine cavity. The passage of either one gives recognizable signs. These factors will be discussed later. Closure of this portion of the tube is a basic defect for which little can be done. It is therefore essential that the evidence for complete obstruction be absolute. Not infrequently the presence of a mucoid plug containing cellular debris or a localized spasm of the tube may deny passage to injected gas or oil. It is a well known observation that an abnormal test result may be obtained after several negative examinations.

What Is the Mechanism of Implantation of the Impregnated Ovum upon the Endometrium?

The passage of the impregnated ovum through the tube normally takes about three or four days. During this time the ovum is being nourished by tubal fluid and the endometrium is being prepared for its receipt. Implantation usually occurs about six or seven days after the ovum has been extruded from the ovary. The role of the endocrines in developing an endometrium that will provide both an adequate bed and nourishment has been discussed under the physiology of menstruation (Chap. 16). There are many variables which may influence the survival of the fertilized ovum adversely.

The optimal place within the endometrial cavity for the impregnated egg to implant is on the posterior wall of the uterus. The reason for this is not clear, but there may be greater concentration of glycogen in these areas. Whatever the cause, it is a well known observation that the pregnancy is more likely to be abnormal if implantation occurs on the anterior wall.

The actual mechanism of implantation has not been entirely established. The question seems to be whether the embryo elaborates a chemical agent or cytolytic enzyme which conditions the endometrium and favors implantation or whether the endometrium alone prepares the soil. Undoubtedly the coiled spiral arterioles which have been so elaborately developed with each menstrual cycle play a part in providing a rapid delivery of blood to the growing placental villi once implantation is assured.

The hostile influences upon the continued life of the impregnated ovum will be discussed under Ectopic Pregnancy (Chap. 32), miscarriage and threatened abortion (Chap. 31).

REFERENCES

General Considerations

Bartelmez, G. W.: The Phases of the Menstrual Cycle and Their Interpretation in Terms of the Pregnancy Cycle. *Am. J. Obst. & Gynec.*, 74: 931, 1957.
Buxton, C. L.: Human Infertility. *Am. J. M. Sc.*, 231: 694, 1956.
Curtin, R. R., and Ulfelder, H.: Gynecology; Medical Progress. *New England J. Med.*, 261: 849, 1959.

Glass, S. J., and Lazarus, M. L.: Improved Fertility and Prevention of Abortion after Nutritional Hormonal Therapy. *J.A.M.A.*, 154: 908, 1954.

Hartman, C. G.: Physiological Mechanisms of Conception—An Inventory of Unanswered Questions. *Perspectives in Biol. & Med.*, 4: 77, 1960.

Rock, J.: Causes and Relief of Infertility; in J. V. Meigs and S. H. Sturgis, eds.: *Progress in Gynecology*. New York, Grune & Stratton, Inc., 1946, Vol. I, p. 239.

Runner, M. N., and Gates, A.: Sterile Obese Mothers. *J. Hered.*, 45: 51, 1954.

Stanton, E. F.: Pregnancy after Forty-Four. *Am. J. Obst. & Gynec.*, 71: 270, 1956.

Velardo, J. T.: The Anatomy and Endocrine Physiology of the Female Reproductive System; in *The Endocrinology of Reproduction*. New York, Oxford University Press, 1958, p. 101.

Role of Ovary

Allende, I. de: Anovulatory Cycles in Women. *Am. J. Anat.*, 98: 293, 1956.

Brewer, J. I.: Studies of the Human Corpus Luteum. Evidence for Early Onset of Regression of the Corpus Luteum of Menstruation. *Am. J. Obst. & Gynec.*, 44: 1048, 1942.

Corner, G. W.: Development, Organization and Breakdown of the Corpus Luteum in the Rhesus Monkey. *Carnegie Contrib. to Embryol.*, 31: 117, 1945.

Doyle, J. B.: Cervical Tampon—Synchronous Test for Ovulation. Simultaneous Assay of Glucose from Cervix and Follicular Fluid from Cul-de-Sac and Ovary by Culdotomy. *J.A.M.A.*, 167: 1464, 1958.

Hammond, J.: The Fertilization of Rabbit Ova in Relation to Time. A Method of Controlling the Litter Size, Duration of Pregnancy and the Weight of the Young at Birth. *J. Exper. Biol.*, 11: 140, 1934.

Igarashi, M., and Matsumoto, S.: Induction of Human Ovulation by Individualized Gonadotrophin Therapy in Two Phases. *Am. J. Obst. & Gynec.*, 73: 1294, 1957.

Joel, R. V., and Foraker, A. G.: Fate of Corpus Albicans. A Quantitative Approach. *Am. J. Obst. & Gynec.*, 78: 1272, 1959.

Kalant, N., Patee, C. J., Simpson, G. W., and Hendelman, M.: Timing of Ovulation. *Fertil. & Steril.*, 7: 57, 1956.

Kurzrok, R., Wilson, L., and Birnberg, C.: Follicular Fluid. Its Possible Role in Human Fertility and Infertility. *Fertil. & Steril.*, 4: 479, 1953.

Sturgis, S. H.: Present Status of Measures for Detecting Ovulation; in *Progress in Gynecology*. New York, Grune & Stratton, Inc., 1957, Vol. III, p. 301.

Role of Testis

Brown, R. L.: Rate of Transport of Spermia in the Human Uterus and Tubes. *Am. J. Obst. & Gynec.*, 47: 407, 1944.

Hartman, G. G.: How Do Sperm Get into the Uterus? *Fertil. & Steril.*, 8: 403, 1957.

MacLeod, J., Gold, R. Z., and McLane, C. M.: Correlation of the Male and Female Factors in Human Infertility. *Fertil. & Steril.*, 6: 112, 1955.

Noyes, R. W., Adams, C. E., and Walton, A.: Transport of Spermatozoa into the Uterus of the Rabbit. *Fertil. & Steril.*, 9: 288, 1958.

Sohval, A. R.: The Anatomy and Endocrine Physiology of the Male Reproductive System; in J. T. Velardo, ed.: *The Endocrinology of Reproduction*. New York, Oxford University Press, 1958, p. 243.

Impregnation and Implantation

Böving, B. G.: Implantation. *Ann. New York Acad. Sc.*, 75: 700, 1959.

Burdick, H. O., Whitney, R., and Emerson, B.: Observations on Transport of Tubal Ova. *Endocrinology*, 31: 100, 1942.

Cohen, M. R., Stein, I. F., Sr., and Kaye, B. M.: Spinnbarkeit. A Characteristic of Cervical Mucus. Significance at Ovulation Time. *Fertil & Steril.*, 3: 201, 1952.

Fluhmann, C. F.: The Glandular Structure of the Cervix Uteri during Pregnancy. *Am. J. Obst. & Gynec.*, 78: 990, 1959.

Hertig, A. T., Rock, J., Adams, E. C., and Mulligan, W. J.: On the Pre-implantation Stages of the Human Ovum. A Description of Four Normal and Four Abnormal Specimens Ranging from the Second to the Fifth Day of Development. *Carnegie Contrib. to Embryol.*, 35: 199, 1954.

Lowi, R. N. P.: Uterine Tube Physiology—A Review of the Literature. *Obst. & Gynec.*, 16: 322, 1960.

Rock, J., and Hertig, A. T.: The Human Conceptus during the First Two Weeks of Gestation. *Am. J. Obst. & Gynec.*, 55: 6, 1948.

Shettles, L. B.: The Living Human Ovum. *Am. J. Obst. & Gynec.*, 76: 398, 1958.

Tyler, E. T.: The Vagina and Infertility. *Ann. New York Acad. Sc.*, 83: 294, 1959.

Westman, A.: Investigations into Transit of Ova in Man. *J. Obst. & Gynaec. Brit. Emp.*, 44: 821, 1937.

Zondek, B.: Functional Significance of the Cervical Mucus. *Internat. J. Fertil.*, 1: 225, 1956.

Chapter 28

Investigation and
Treatment of the Sterile Woman

THERE is a whole gamut of factors which bear on the problem of sterility in both the male and the female. In the past the blame was customarily placed on the female. Today we recognize that the male is often the defective partner. Since his contribution is largely that of producing healthy, active sperm in adequate quantity and delivering them at the cervical os, it should be relatively easy to assess. The investigation logically should begin with the male. The male ego is such, however, that it is usually the female who first consults the physician for help. Rarely do we encounter a male who will voluntarily undergo examination until repeated studies of his wife fail to demonstrate any deficiency on her part.

For practical purposes, then, the investigation of the sterile partnership will begin with a consideration of the problems in the female. Many of the diagnostic tests are complicated, time-consuming and expensive. Before making specific diagnostic tests the possibilities of interrogation and general physical examination should be explored. Much basic information may be uncovered which will aid immeasurably in determining the extent and direction of the subsequent examinations. It has been stated and confirmed by competent authority that more successful pregnancies stem from informative discussion of the problem coupled with a complete physical examination than from any other form of therapy for sterility.

What Can Be Accomplished by Conversation with the Patient?

The girl who consults her physician because of failure to conceive has an emotional problem, however well adjusted she may appear at the first examination. The measure of success in helping the infertile girl to become pregnant is in direct proportion to the physician's ability to bring about a release from her emotional tension through a sympathetic understanding of her problem. A great deal can be accomplished by thoughtful interrogations and instructions. Many women have but the scantiest knowledge of the physiology of conception. Some have no concept at all.

AGE: It is important to know the age of the marital partners. Woman is most fertile between the ages of twenty and twenty-four. There is a gradual decline to the age of forty and a precipitous one from then on. This is less true of the male. Apparently male fertility is unimpaired up to the age of forty-five, with less evidence

329

that the index declines after that age. Many men of seventy have normal active sperm.

In the discussion of the bleeding pattern during adolescence (Chap. 17) it was obvious that nature tends to provide a protective period of infertility. Until the ovary has matured sufficiently to respond in normal fashion to the stimulation of pituitary gonadotropin, ovulation does not occur. Maturity is acquired gradually. Though maturation of the ova occurs and pregnancy may take place in early adolescence, the percentages of stillbirths and abnormal pregnancies are high. The complications of pregnancy are also greater in this group.

Abnormalities of this sort seem to occur at both ends of the age spectrum of ovarian function, for they appear again in women pregnant for the first time after the age of forty. The percentage of patients experiencing stillbirths and the production of mongoloids is greater after forty than at other periods in woman's menstrual life. It is apparent that nature tries to provide protection for the patient who is either too young or too old from becoming reproductive. This problem is not confined to females alone, for stillbirth is also common when the male partner falls in these categories, regardless of the age of the mother.

2.   HOW LONG HAS THE COUPLE BEEN MARRIED?   It is of basic importance to know how long the patient has been married to the present husband, if this is her first marriage, and whether she has ever been pregnant if previously married. When the patient's confidence has been obtained, it may be well to question whether she has ever been pregnant before, whether married or not. Such information may be useful, but one should not attempt to elicit it on the first visit.

Some women become oversolicitous about their inability to conceive after only a few months of married life. Though it is true that the majority of first pregnancies occur within the first six months of marriage when no attempt is made at prevention, nevertheless a year or two may pass without success. Such a patient should be reassured, but she should not be sent home without hearing her story and advising her to have a complete physical examination. Every consideration should be given to her problem. A real defect may become evident which could be an excellent reason why she cannot or should not become pregnant.

3.   HAS CONTRACEPTION BEEN PRACTICED?   Many women will declare that they have been unable to become pregnant despite the fact that they have been married for several years. It is important to know for how much of that period they have actually tried to conceive. For a variety of reasons, usually economic, contraception may have been practiced, and the actual trial period may be a matter of months rather than years. Further investigation of the duration of the effort to conceive may reveal that the husband's occupation keeps him from home during his wife's most fertile period.

4.   WHAT DOES THE PATIENT KNOW ABOUT THE TIMING OF INTERCOURSE?   Many married couples are ignorant of the optimum time for fertilization. Some of the information they have acquired is often erroneous. The most likely time for conception may well have been studiously avoided. Since the most propitious time for successful impregnation is probably limited to the twenty-four-hour span associated with ovulation, it is particularly important to the sterile couple that the maximum effort should be concentrated on the day of ovulation. There are many methods designed to pinpoint this day. These will be discussed under special diagnostic procedures (p. 345). Considerable help can be offered the patient who has no idea of the timing of her fertile period by offering information on the approximate dating. Thus it is important to know the patient's menstrual history from the time of puberty on. Did

the patient begin to menstruate at the age of fourteen, or was the menarche postponed until some years later? What were the periods like at the onset? If irregular, how long before they followed a regular pattern? Has this pattern been maintained, and does she have short cycles of less than the usual twenty-eight-day interval, or are they constantly or sporadically delayed? Does she have localized lower abdominal pain midway between the periods or at the time of menstruation to suggest that ovulation has occurred and its possible date?

From information gathered in taking the history it may be possible to tell the patient when she is most likely to conceive and to advise her to concentrate on the approximate date of ovulation. If this is unsuccessful, the same facts will help in directing the investigative studies.

There can be no doubt that the timing of intercourse is of basic importance, but the overanxious wife must be careful that she does not subjugate the act of coitus to the desire to conceive. If she is completely occupied with the timing of intercourse and the appearance of the orgasm, she may so increase her anxieties and tensions that she unconsciously erects a psychologic barrier to conception.

5. FREQUENCY OF INTERCOURSE.   In the earlier enthusiastic years of marital life the sexual act may be indulged in to excess. To the highly fertile couple the frequency of intercourse may be of little importance. If one or both partners to the marriage are subfertile, it can be paramount. The infertile male should practice sexual abstinence for five days before the optimum time for fertilization. The fertile male who has a count of 200 million sperm per cubic centimeter will still have approximately 80 million at the date of ovulation if intercourse is practiced daily and not carried to excess, but the subfertile male may exhaust his quota and be totally inadequate on the optimal day.

Through ignorance or habit many couples practice intercourse once weekly or less. Usually it is the fault of the wife, who is so intent on her desire to become pregnant that she loses all interest in the marital act, particularly if it does not produce results. The normal healthy male maintains his highly fertile state by coitus twice weekly. When intercourse is practiced daily or on alternate days, even the fertile male becomes relatively subfertile. It has been suggested that, after a five-day abstinence, intercourse twice within a period of six to eight hours on the day of ovulation increases the chance of pregnancy.

6. WHAT ABOUT COITAL TECHNIQUE?   Since it is basically important that the male ejaculate be deposited on or near the cervix if maximal results are to be obtained, the patient should be questioned about the position assumed during the act of coitus. Most instances of failure to deliver the semen where it will do the most good result from faulty technique in the act of intercourse.

The most successful position is that of the woman on her back (supine) with her thighs flexed. Not infrequently questioning will show that this position has been reversed or the lateral position employed. It is also important to advise the male partner to delay withdrawal of the organ until it is in a flaccid state to minimize the loss of semen from the vagina. The female partner should remain on her back with the thighs acutely flexed and the pelvis tilted forward for at least one hour after completion of coitus. The position suggested will keep the cervix bathed in the pool of ejaculate deposited in the posterior vaginal fornix. Unless there is urgent reason, she should remain in bed for at least four hours thereafter. There are other factors involved in the technique of intercourse which are concerned with the anatomy of the respective partners. This will be discussed under the section devoted to the physical examination.

What Roles Do Constitutional and Nutritional Factors Play?

The chances of successful fertilization are improved when both partners are in good general health, both physical and mental. A debilitated couple who are highly fertile may still fertilize an ovum, as evidenced by the number of pregnant couples with pulmonary tuberculosis, but in general systemic disease or nutritional deficiency will obviously impair both the quantity and quality of either spermatozoa or ova. Chronic debilitating diseases such as diabetes, nephritis, hepatitis, long-standing anemias and chronic alcoholism tend to interfere with spermatogenesis and ovulation.

This is why it is important to know the past history as well as the present state of health. For example, it will be helpful to know whether there has been any history of constitutional disease or nutritional disturbance in the past. We would like to know not only the present nutritional state, but also if possible what it was at the time of puberty. Disturbances at that time may profoundly influence ovarian function at a later date. Was the girl skinny and scrawny at this time or obese? Were the periods delayed? Did she ever have painful periods? From the viewpoint of constitutional disease we would like to know whether she ever had any suggestion of tuberculosis, diabetes, nephritis, rheumatic fever or anemia. Were any of the childhood diseases such as mumps or scarlet fever particularly severe? Has she ever had any suggestion of pelvic inflammatory disease or pelvic peritonitis from acute appendicitis?

Some of the facts brought out may make pregnancy undesirable for the patient or serve as a possible explanation for her present failure to become pregnant.

The part played by systemic disease may be linked to malnutrition, vitamin deficiency and hormonal function. Both clinically and from animal experiments it is known that vitamins, proteins and minerals are essential requirements to normal hormone production and utilization. If vitamins are absent or in deficient supply, the hormones simply do not function normally. In the *female*, diets deficient in calories, protein and vitamins will result in ovarian atrophy. This is particularly true of vitamin A. Inadequate vitamin B in the diet tends to inhibit both ovarian and pituitary activity. This effect on ovarian function may be direct or mediated through interference in the production of pituitary hormones. In the *male*, animal experiments indicate that testicular spermatogenesis is influenced by vitamins A, B and E. In the female, vitamin E appears to be more directly concerned with survival of the impregnated ovum. Diets deficient in protein will produce ovarian atrophy in experimental animals, while the metabolism of spermatozoa in the male is directly dependent on an adequate supply of the amino acids lysine, arginine, tyrosine and tryptophan.

Systemic disease may influence fertilization by disturbing the normal utilization of hormones, as well as by inhibiting the production of pituitary gonadotropins. This may operate through the metabolism of either estrin or androgen by the liver, in the face of vitamin deficiency, particularly vitamin B. Enzyme activity dependent on parts of the vitamin B complex such as thiamine or riboflavin is thought to be a basic factor. It is assumed that the liver is the main organ in the breakdown of the hormones into various biologically inactive components, but other organs in the body may exert similar action. It is also probable that systemic disease and nutritional deficiency are detrimental to the normal action of the hormones at the cell level of the target organs.

What about Anxiety and Mental Fatigue?

The patient's emotional background can be as important as her physical health. Has her home life, both present and past, been free of tension and strife? Does she play the role of the housewife or does she also have a job? What is the nature of the job? Does it involve long hours of physical work, or is it one requiring a large expenditure of nervous energy? Does she have any sense of security or is she constantly harrassed by worries, economic or otherwise? What does she do about vacations? If she does not have a job, how does she occupy herself through the day? The same questions may be asked about the husband. His occupation may also be one of the determining factors. Are his habits or mode of life compatible with a restful state of mind for his wife, or do they contribute to her uncertainties?

Though it is difficult to prove because of the many factors concerned with fertility, it is clinically evident that the patient's mental health is of utmost importance in the sterility problem. This applies to both man and woman. In the present age both parties may live under conditions of stress and tension. In many instances both are employed in work that produces strain and mental fatigue. Such work is far more likely to make a subfertile couple than occupations which simply exhaust the patients physically.

Once a married couple has decided to have a family, it is the wife who seems to become increasingly apprehensive about her reproductive incapacity with each monthly period. Concern over her continued inability to become pregnant may prove to be a major deterent to pregnancy. We are aware that stress and apprehension as well as fright produce amenorrhea. The same factors and the same mechanisms seem to explain pregnancy failures. The actual mechanism is not entirely clear, but in all probability it is mediated through the hypothalamus and is concerned with normal production and release of the pituitary gonadotropins.

Release from worry and concern about the problems of daily living may trigger the onset of pregnancy in a patient who has allowed such anxieties to interfere subconsciously with conception. Clinically, all gynecologists are familiar with the patient who has tried persistently and intelligently to become pregnant, but does so only after she has adopted children. When the wife's desire for increased financial security or a career has subconsciously battled with her eagerness to become a mother, pregnancy may be possible only after she has elected to give up her professional career. A change to more satisfactory living conditions and increased financial security is not the only source of emotional release. In some instances a change to poorer economic status may provide a relaxation in tension and be followed by pregnancy. Psychiatrists attribute this to the expiation of old guilt feelings through suffering and sacrifice.

The male who shows evidence of seminal deficiency due to mental fatigue is also prone to complain of lack of sex desire, impotence and premature ejaculation. The chances of successful pregnancy will be increased immeasurably by encouraging such a male to take a vacation and reorganize his existence to eliminate the stress factors. In the more extreme instances psychiatric help may be necessary.

What about Endocrine Factors in the Sterility Problem?

Direction of investigative studies in the problem of infertility toward the endocrine system usually takes place after an interrogation and complete physical examination of the patient have failed to unearth organic or other causes. Much information may be garnered through conversation with the patient which may arouse suspicion that the individual problem has an endocrine background.

The same questions asked to help the patient determine the approximate time of ovulation may indicate that the underlying defect is obviously in the field of faulty endocrine gland function. Since many endocrine defects manifest themselves at the time of puberty, one would like to know what the girl's developmental status was at that time. Had she developed a feminine figure at that time or was development delayed? Was she obese? Were there any signs or symptoms of thyroid deficiency, and have any of the symptoms persisted? Did she have hirsutism in adolescence? Did it have a male distribution, and has it persisted? From the point of view of function one would like to know the date of the menarche as well as the menstrual pattern at the onset and since that time. Were the periods delayed in onset for an appreciable time beyond the usual age of fourteen? Once established, what was the menstrual pattern, and was the interval constant? What was the nature and duration of the menstrual flow? Is there any suggestion of anovulatory bleeding? Has the patient ever had dysmenorrhea to suggest that ovulation has occurred? Has the dysmenorrhea increased in severity?

There can be little doubt that much sterility can be attributed to faulty endocrine equipment or function. It is not always easy to pinpoint the defect, particularly in the field of faulty function. As yet we have insufficient knowledge of (1) how the pituitary hormones act on the target end-organs; (2) how the pituitary gonadotropins reach the cells in the target organs; (3) how much the pituitary hormone production is modified by other endocrine glands or nervous reactions; (3) how the target organs respond selectively to the proper hormones; and (5) what determines or governs the response of a particular tissue to a particular hormone.

When the defect is a basic one, such as is found in pituitary infantilism, the lack of development in the uterus, ovary, penis or testis is evident. Lesser degrees of impairment may not be so obvious in an otherwise normally developed woman or man. In this group anovulatory bleeding may appear in the female and oligospermia in the male.

THE PITUITARY.   We have noted that testicular and ovarian atrophy occur in pituitary infantilism and that Froehlich's syndrome, as well as other lesions of the hypothalamus, is associated with incomplete development of the entire genital tract as well as the gonads. It is also true that pituitary tumors in both sexes will eventually result in sterility, just as Simmonds's disease does in the female. There can be no doubt that the pituitary hormones stimulate the gonad.

We recognize that there are at least two pituitary gonadotropic hormones, FSH and LH, each of which has its own physiologic action. FSH, for instance, stimulates the growth of ovarian follicles in the female and induces spermatogenesis in the male. The luteinizing hormone (LH), together with FSH, initiates ovulation and is responsible for the development of the corpus luteum in the female, as well as influencing the secretion of androgen in the male. Each is a separate or separable entity with individual properties clinically, but biologically the combined factors are needed to produce such phenomena as ovulation.

The successful use of the pituitary gonadotropins to initiate ovulation or increase spermatogenesis until 1961 has been most disappointing. Since they were foreign proteins usually derived from the pituitaries of sheep or hog, they were capable of producing hypersensitivity or anaphylactic shock and were therefore dangerous. To circumvent this disadvantage attempts have been made to induce ovulation and stimulate spermatogenesis by the use of chorionic gonadotropin derived from the urine of pregnant women and equine gonadotropins from the blood of pregnant mares. There is no doubt that they will stimulate follicular development and produce luteinization. They do not, however, induce ovulation or stimulate spermatogenesis. Moreover, they are thought to produce antihormones which neutralize the patient's own hormones. Newer preparations show greater promise of success.

THE THYROID. Thyroid function is directly concerned with fertility in both male and female. It is a well known observation that increased thyroid activity takes place at adolescence, during pregnancy and in the menopause. These are periods of changing sex function. In the male deficient spermatogenesis is seen in both hyperthyroidism and hypothyroidism. Fertility is most influenced by the deficient production and secretion of thyroid hormone in *hypothyroidism*. This is less apparent in *hyperthyroid* states. Between 20 and 25 per cent of childless couples will show evidence of hypothyroidism in one or both partners. The usefulness of thyroid extract therapy of the childless couple is well documented, with a figure in the neighborhood of 10 per cent success. Thyroid extract is given for the prevention of abortion on the basis that the rise in serum iodine seen in normal pregnancy is absent in the abnormal. The mechanism of action of thyroid hormone upon the gonad, however, is incompletely understood. We still are uncertain of how thyroid hormone acts on specific cells or what happens when it is through exerting its effect. The empirical use of thyroid hormone has been helpful in the female, but has had little influence in increasing spermatogenesis. Its use is still important in therapy of males who demonstrate a definite metabolic lack, for adequate thyroid function is essential to the promotion and maintenance of functioning gonadal cells.

THE ADRENAL. The exact role of the adrenal in infertility problems is also incompletely understood. We know that hyperfunction of the adrenal cortex is sometimes associated with amenorrhea. It has been shown that cortisone therapy may depress such adrenal hyperfunction with restoration of normal menstrual cycles and normal pregnancy. It is also true that severe degenerative adrenocortical disease is frequently associated with sterility. Nevertheless the part played by adrenal gland function is not clear, nor do we know whether the action of its hormones is directly on the gonad or mediated through the pituitary, if it does play a part.

What Information May Be Gained from Physical Examination?

The detailed history obtained from both female and male partners may suggest the presence of a constitutional disease or the possibility of organic disturbance in either ovary or testis.

COMPLETE PHYSICAL EXAMINATION. The physical examination must be complete and not confined to an evaluation of the pelvic organs. The primary aim in performing the general examination is to uncover evidence of any constitutional disease or organic abnormality that might prevent pregnancy or make it inadvisable from the point of view of the patient's health, either temporarily or permanently. Primarily, one would want to exclude the possibility of the presence of cardiac, renal, hypertensive, chronic infectious and anemic conditions, syphilis, tuberculosis or nephritis, as well as malignant tumors, particularly of breast or uterus. Any evidence of their presence should be further checked by appropriate laboratory and x-ray studies. In addition, by general examination one may discover evidence suggesting faulty function of the endocrine system. Scanty or abnormally distributed body hair,

together with other evidences of failure to develop the usual secondary sex characteristics of an adult woman's breasts or external genitalia, may indicate basic endocrine
defects, perhaps primary in the pituitary. Excessive body hair, particularly if it has
a male distribution, suggests a tumor or malfunction of either the adrenal or ovary,
or both. When hirsutism is combined with obesity, one may become suspicious of
ovarian dysfunction, such as is seen in the Stein-Leventhal syndrome. Or the obesity
may be present with a dry skin and coarse hair, suggesting thyroid hypofunction.
Conversely, other physical findings may raise a suspicion of hyperfunction of the
thyroid.

Obesity may be secondary to endocrine gland dysfunction or may be simply the
result of excess caloric intake over need. In some instances obesity may be traced to
psychogenic cause. Whatever the explanation, obesity is frequently associated with
relative infertility. If the obesity is secondary to endocrine abnormality, it usually
manifests itself in underdevelopment in the genital tract and usually in the gonad,
whether ovary or testis. This may be secondary to disturbances in the pituitary or
thyroid, or less commonly the hypothalamus. Froehlich's syndrome is an excellent
example. Here, as a result of pituitary failure, there is inadequate development of the
entire male genital tract, including the testis. Such defects are basic, and the likelihood of fertilization is naturally reduced. In the female the evidence would be confined
to an evaluation of the secondary sex characteristics, including the external genitalia.
When obesity is simply due to caloric excess coupled with a lack of exercise, or to
psychic unrest, much can be accomplished by an intelligent weight reduction program
and psychiatric therapy.

The Local Vaginal and Rectal Examinations

The pelvic examination is concerned with a search for and an evaluation of
lesions of the vulva, vagina, cervix, uterus, tubes and ovaries in relation to the likelihood of their influencing the initiation and maintenance of pregnancy (Figs. 28–1,
28–2).

On local examination of the vulva one can obtain considerable useful information
as to the state of the hymen, the size of the introitus and vaginal canal, the likelihood
or possible explanation of vaginismus, as well as the presence of any infection of the
vulva or vagina. It also helps to confirm other stigmata of underdevelopment secondary to endocrine cause.

VAGINAL INFECTION.   Although there is no direct evidence that vaginal
infections such as those due to *Trichomonas vaginalis* or Monilia actually cause sterility,
they do not make reproduction easy. Many women get pregnant despite obvious
vaginal infection, but others will not be successful until the infection has been cleared
up. The spermatozoa must be deposited in the vagina and enter the cervical canal
before pregnancy can occur. In subfertile patients or those who show suggestive
evidences of biological hostility to their husband's sperm it is clear that these infections
should be eliminated.

ANATOMY OF THE VAGINAL CANAL IN RELATION TO THE TECHNIQUE OF COITUS.
The female anatomy may also interfere with proper penetration and placement of
the ejaculate. It is not enough to ensure a successful pregnancy to have a male partner
capable of producing healthy, active sperm of good quality and adequate concentration. A highly fertile ejaculation does no good if it is not planted in the vaginal
canal in the neighborhood of the posterior fornix adjacent to the cervical os. A

narrow vagina, disproportion in the size of the organs, vaginismus or dyspareunia may obstruct the canal and interfere with the deposit of semen on the cervix. The magnitude of the problem is compounded if the male partner has a small penis deeply imbedded in fat and the cervix is placed high in the vagina. Contact with the penetrating phallus is absent, and the sperm are not deposited in the proper area. This may not be important in a highly fertile couple, but when one or both members are subfertile, it is of the utmost importance. Should the male partner be impotent, have hypospadias or suffer from premature ejaculation, the proper placement of the sperm is that much more essential. The position of the fundus of the uterus is also important. A retroverted uterus often obliterates the posterior vaginal fornix where the sperm normally form a pool, and the seminal discharge tends to escape.

CERVICAL ANATOMY AND PATHOLOGY. One of the most common organic causes of sterility is a lesion of the cervix which sets up a mechanical block to the passage of the spermatozoa, as in the case of a polyp. Or sperm transit is delayed by an overproduction of mucus as a part of cervical infection. The cervical infection may be superficial and external, as seen in cervical erosions which we recognize by the red, granulating, papillary, often ulcerated surface of the exposed cervical epithelium. On the other hand, the infection may be deep-seated in the endocervical glands. Infection here is apt to obstruct the passage of sperm in two ways. In the first place the endocervical canal is often so distorted as to become stenotic. In the second place the infection may produce a heavy, thick, tenacious, purulent discharge which enmeshes and destroys the spermatozoa. If the cervix is enlarged, fixed and boggy, the infection within the cervix is likely of long standing.

The appearance of the cervix may suggest inadequate development. This can be the explanation of an infertile state. An elongated, conical cervix with a pin-point os is usually the mark of an infantile uterus. In the mature, fully developed uterus the fundal measurements exceed those of the cervix. In the poorly developed uterus the cervix is relatively long in proportion to the size of the fundus.

THE UTERUS AND ADNEXA. Evaluation of the size, position, contour and mobility of the uterus should be carried out both by vaginal and rectal examinations. The same is true of estimation of the extent and nature of disease in the adnexa. The pelvic floor can best be palpated by rectal examination. For example, the diagnosis of endometriosis is commonly made by feeling nodular thickenings in the uterosacral ligaments and pelvic floor, together with a loss of mobility in both uterus and broad ligament. It is much easier to discover this on rectal examination.

Many pelvic tumors and malpositions of the uterus are compatible with fertility, but others either materially reduce the likelihood of pregnancy or make it next to impossible. Certain pelvic infections make pregnancy impossible or even dangerous. Other pelvic gynecologic conditions are associated with relative infertility. It has been said that in 5 per cent of the women who seek aid for sterility the pelvic disease requires more immediate attention than the fertility failure.

Malpositions of the Uterus. To the normally fertile couple a retroversion which can be replaced in normal position, though it may not stay there, is no deterrent to repeated pregnancies. If the couple is subfertile, a number of detrimental factors appear. The cervix points toward the anterior vaginal wall and never has an opportunity to bathe in the seminal pool of the posterior fornix. Moreover, the retroverted position tends to obliterate the posterior cul-de-sac and interferes with retention of semen in the vagina. If the uterus is fixed in retroversion or is deeply recessed in the vagina, the ease with which the patient becomes pregnant is reduced for both fertile

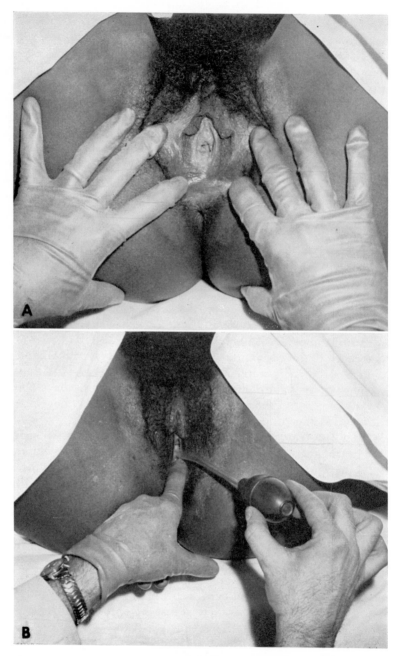

Fig. 28-1.   *A,* Inspection of the vulva and introitus is accomplished by spreading the labia. Good illumination is essential. *B,* The glass tube, with aspirator bulb, is next introduced to obtain material for a vaginal smear, before any lubricant is applied or digital examination is made. *C,* The labia are palpated for abnormalities, particularly enlarged Bartholin's glands. *D,* The vaginal speculum is next introduced, after proper lubrication, and guided by the fingers.

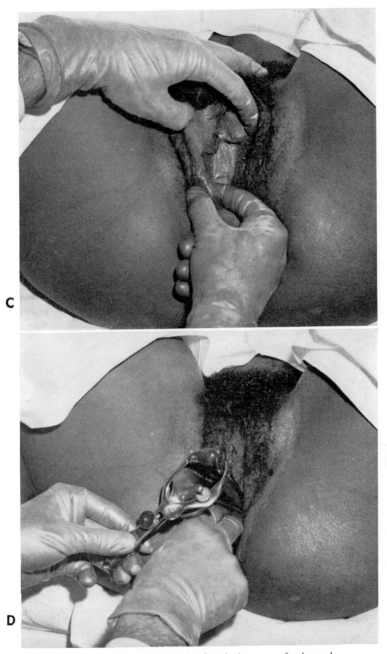

Fig. 28-1. *Continued.* See facing page for legend.

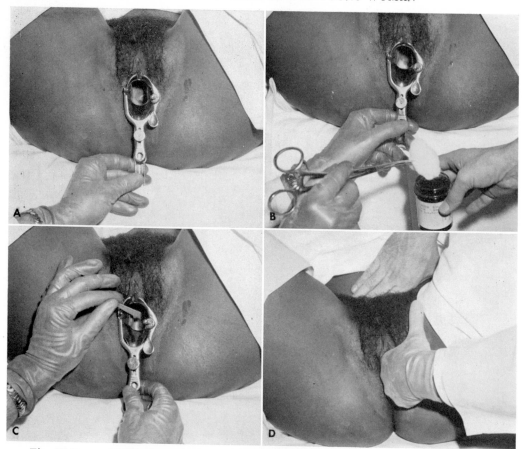

Fig. 28-2.　　*A*, With the vaginal speculum in place and with good illumination, the vagina and cervix are inspected. *B*, A Schiller iodine test is made by swabbing the cervix with Schiller's solution and then cleansing off the excess. *C*, If desired, a cervical and endocervical scraping may next be taken for cytologic study, with use of a wooden spatula. *D*, Finally, bimanual palpation identifies and localizes any abnormality of the uterus, tubes or ovaries.

and subfertile couples. Two factors are involved in the uterus fixed in retroversion that bear on fertility. One is the improper placement of semen, as already discussed, and the other is the element of chronic passive congestion, which interferes with normal tubal and uterine functions.

These factors are accentuated when the cervix is unhealthy because of chronic infection or the presence of an occluding polyp. They apply in the most exaggerated form when uterine prolapse or enterocele is present (Fig. 28–3). The seminal fluid can be neither collected nor retained under these conditions.

The Presence of Uterine Fibroids.　　Whether or not a fibroid tumor in the uterine wall influences fertility depends on its location. The subserous fibroid, for instance, may complicate an established pregnancy through torsion or degeneration, but it will not prevent the patient from becoming pregnant. In most instances an *intramural* fibroid is no barrier to conception. If, however, it is located at the cornual portion of the uterus, it may occlude the interstitial portion of the tube and either prevent the spermatozoa from getting into the tube or the impregnated ovum from getting out. An intramural fibroid located at the internal os may obstruct the cervical canal and deny entrance to the ascending spermatozoa or complicate a pregnancy at the time of delivery (Fig. 28–4, *A*). A large intramural fibroid tends to encroach on and distort the endometrial cavity and thus reduce the chance of conception. It may become so large that pregnancy would be considered inadvisable until it is removed. These patients are excellent *candidates* for *myomectomy*. Successful pregnancy may be expected to follow a properly performed myomectomy in approximately 40 per cent of patients so treated. Intramural fibroids may then be the sole factor in the sterility problem.

The greatest offenders are the *submucous fibroids,* which either originate close to and grow in the direction of the endometrial cavity or expand into it from an original source within the uterine wall (Fig. 28–4, *B*). The same may be said of large uterine polyps. Myomectomy for submucous fibroids is feasible, but it is more complicated, and there is less chance of a subsequent successful pregnancy. The uterine fibroid may thus be the source of the sterility because of its position or associated endocrine dysfunction. Such patients are prone to have a persistent proliferative or hyperplastic endometrium without progestational effect.

Ovarian Tumors.   Palpation of an ovarian cyst which persists for several months calls for surgical intervention before embarking on further study of a sterility problem. Such cysts are not physiologic and are potentially dangerous because of their possible malignant alteration, their tendency to consume increasing amounts of the normal ovarian tissue with continued growth and the likelihood of torsion once the pregnancy is established and progresses. The larger the cyst, the greater the urgency for surgery.

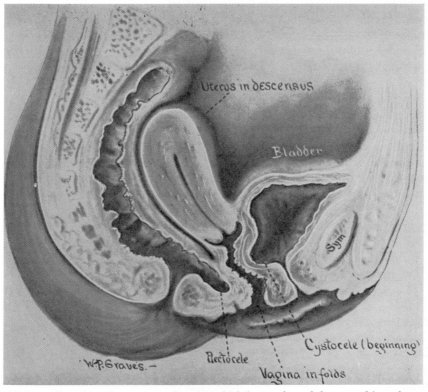

Fig. 28-3.   Drawing of a retroverted uterus which has prolapsed downward into the vagina. As a consequence the vaginal cavity is shortened and folded and may be compressed anteriorly by a cystocele and posteriorly by a rectocele. (From W. P. Graves: *Gynecology.*)

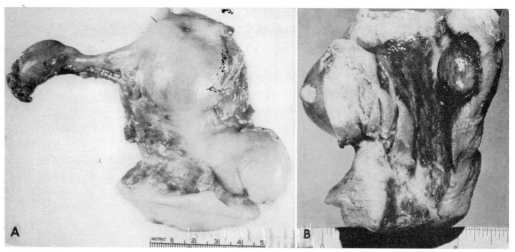

Fig. 28-4.   *A*, The nodule on the right side of the uterus just above the cervix is a fibroid tumor so located adjacent to the cervical canal as to interfere with impregnation or parturition, or both. *B*, A uterus opened to show a submucous fibroid bulging into the endometrial cavity on the right and an intramural fibroid on the left side of the illustration.

When operation is performed, the emphasis should be on excision of the cyst rather than oophorectomy. Conservation of as much ovarian tissue as possible is important, even though the opposite ovary appears completely normal, if the level of fertility is to be preserved.

CHRONIC PELVIC INFECTIONS.   By and large, pelvic infections interfere with or prevent conception through their effects upon the fallopian tubes. To a less extent chronic endocervicitis or endometritis may be implicated. The infection, whether it be caused by streptococcus secondary to abortion or sequelae of surgery to cervix or endometrium, gonoccoccus or tuberculosis, results in tubal damage, either intrinsic or extrinsic, and makes conception either impossible, more difficult or more dangerous. Tubal occlusion may follow any sort of pelvic peritonitis. Pelvic peritonitis after appendiceal rupture is a good example.

Streptococcal Infections.   Such infections produce a perisalpingitis and interfere with tubal function to greater or less degrees. Motility of the tube is impaired, and in extreme degree the tube becomes fixed. The fimbriated ends of the tubes are frequently occluded by the peritubal adhesions.

Gonococcal Infections.   Gonococcal exudations destroy the mucosa of the tube and create irregular occlusions of the tubal lumen. Admission to the tubal interior likely is denied to both the ova and spermatozoa.

Tuberculous Infection.   Such lesions are dangerous to the patient's general health. Pregnancy is contraindicated as long as active infection exists. Tuberculosis is usually discovered accidentally in the course of endometrial sampling in the sterility workup. The incidence of genital tuberculosis in the world population varies, depending on existing living conditions. It has been said to occur in 5 per cent of women under investigation for sterility. The primary source is usually tubal. The endometrium is involved in 50 per cent of cases. Unless the endometrium is infected and the biopsy is taken just before the onset of the menstrual period, tuberculosis localized in the tube may go unrecognized. In established cases its mucosa is destroyed, and the tube becomes irregular, fixed and stony hard. The tubes take on the shape of tobacco pouches and are occluded, and pregnancy is impossible (Fig. 28–5). In milder degrees of infection within the endometrium the secretory phase may be absent. The repeated reports of acute and chronic endometritis from endometrial biopsy specimens should arouse the suspicion of possible tuberculosis.

Whenever thickening, fixation and tenderness of the pelvic floor are noted on pelvic examination in association with palpable adnexal masses, chronic pelvic inflammatory disease should be suspected, and its treatment takes precedence over the investigation for sterility.

Endometriosis. Though the fimbriated ends of the fallopian tubes are almost invariably open in the patient who has endometriosis, sterility is commonly encountered. There seems to be a relative infertility factor even in patients with minimal evidence of endometriosis.

The reason why patients with endometriosis tend to have a sterility problem is complicated. Although the patient may have widespread dissemination of ectopic implants of endometrium throughout the peritoneum of the cul-de-sac and utero-sacral ligaments, nevertheless the fimbriated ends of the tubes are almost invariably

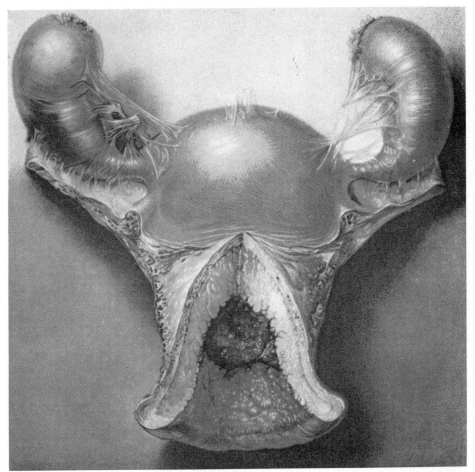

Fig. 28-5. Florid example of tuberculous salpingitis with peritubal adhesions and endometrial tuberculosis. (From a drawing by Max Brödel in T. S. Cullen; *Cancer of the Uterus.*)

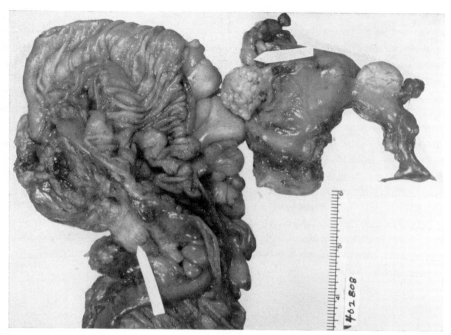

Fig. 28-6.   Endometriosis with adhesions between tubes, ovaries and sigmoid colon. The pointers indicate endometriotic foci in tubo-ovarian adhesions and in the colonic wall.

open. Rarely do we find involvement of the intramural portions of the tube at the cornual end. Usually the ovaries are involved, and ovarian "chocolate cysts" can often be felt on vaginal and rectal examinations. When the ovaries are involved, one can explain the lack of fertility on functional grounds. It is possible, however, to have widespread pelvic endometriosis without ovarian involvement, and this type invariably produces uterine and often tubal fixation (Fig. 28–6). It is not enough to have the fimbriated ends of the tubes patent unless there is also free mobility of both uterus and tubes. In many instances endometriosis is present without characteristic physical findings.

EVALUATION OF THE PHYSICAL EXAMINATION AND HISTORY.   When organic gynecologic or systemic diseases have been discovered in the course of either the history or physical examination, they should be evaluated in relation to their bearing on a pregnancy that may follow. (1) Is the disease process or local condition such that the pregnancy should be prevented rather than encouraged, because of danger to the patient's health? (2) Can the condition be corrected so that it is proper to consider the possibility of pregnancy at a later date? (3) Does the local disease in uterus or adnexa make pregnancy impossible, or can corrective therapy effect a situation favorable to pregnancy? (4) Should therapy be carried out immediately, or can it be postponed until other methods have been tried and failed? Will a program of delay jeopardize the chances of future success?

In many instances the nature of the abnormality, and to a certain degree its location, call for corrective therapy independent of its influence on the possibilities of subsequent pregnancy. In other situations corrective therapy needs to be undertaken only because of the chance that the initiation of pregnancy may become easier. If there are no symptoms and there is no danger inherent in the abnormality itself, good medical judgment would call for an examination of the husband before embarking on any extended medical or surgical corrective procedure. There would be little sense in performing an operation for an inconveniently placed fibroid, minimal endometriosis or obstruction of the fimbriated ends of the tubes if the husband had complete azospermia or suffered from a chronic debilitating illness.

If nothing abnormal is discovered on either the history or physical examination of the female partner, it is advisable at this stage of the investigation to examine the husband. Many special diagnostic tests used in the workup for sterility in the female are time-consuming and expensive, while some may be dangerous. The basic fault lies with the male approximately half the time. This fact should be communicated to the husband, who should also be advised that both spermatozoa and ova are needed to produce a pregnancy. After his wife has gone through the preliminary investigations and no obvious cause for reproductive failure has been discovered he may be less reluctant to submit to examination. By interrogation, physical examination and the performance of a few tests it should be a relatively simple matter to evaluate the role of the male partner. The diagnostic tests for male infertility are far less complicated and confining than those devised for the female. They are considered in the next chapter.

What Program Should Be Followed When Both Partners Appear Normal?

When the examination of both partners has failed to show any definite cause as to why conception should not take place, one can afford to wait six months or a year before carrying out further investigative studies in the female. The best results in most of the large series reporting experience with sterility problems seem to occur uniformly in the group in which both parties have been examined, instructed and assured that no obvious abnormalities are present. The emotional release from simple reassurance of normality may be all the patient needs to initiate a pregnancy in many instances. One cannot underestimate the value of the information imparted in the course of the interviews. The most important contribution made by the physician may concern the approximate timing of ovulation in relation to the frequency of intercourse. At best this is an estimate, but for the woman with a normal twenty-eight-day cycle ovulation probably does occur somewhere between the twelfth and fourteenth days. This important bit of advice coupled with general instruction on maintenance of normal health and nutrition may prove to be sufficient.

If no pregnancy is forthcoming after six months or a year on this regimen, further investigation of the female is warranted. Obviously, if a woman has married later and is trying to get pregnant in the middle or late thirties, one may choose to begin the additional investigations earlier.

What Special Diagnostic Procedures Are Available for More Detailed Investigation in the Female?

The investigations should be concentrated on the three most important factors in the physiology of conception. Since there is a limited time during which the spermatozoa may fertilize an ovum in the fallopian tube, we will want to know (1) whether ovulation has occurred and the closest possible estimate of when it took place; (2) whether there has been any obstacle in the transit of the spermatozoa from cervix to the outer portion of the tube where fertilization occurs; (3) whether there is any reason why the ovum is prevented from entering the tube at the fimbriated end.

What Methods Do We Have of Determining the Date of Ovulation?

ENDOMETRIAL BIOPSY.   Since we know that menstruation may occur in the absence of ovulation, it is of basic importance to know whether ovulation has taken place. We have shown that measurable changes are seen in the endometrium under the influence of progesterone. Progesterone can ordinarily only be produced if ovulation has occurred and a corpus luteum has developed. A sample of endometrium should be taken with a curet in the second half of the menstrual cycle. This is a simple office procedure which causes the patient minimal discomfort.

When Should the Biopsy Be Taken?   A regular sequence of events takes place in the endometrium which permits fairly accurate dating. If evidence of ovulation alone is sought, the sample should be taken on the first day of the next menstrual period. This obviates the danger of interrupting any pregnancy that may have started. If the object of the biopsy is to obtain data as to the exact date of ovulation, it should be taken around the twenty-second or twenty-third day, when the maximum amount of information can be obtained which will help to pinpoint the probable ovulation day. In either case the finding of a secretory endometrium is presumptive evidence that the patient has ovulated. If a proliferative type of endometrium is found at a phase in the cycle when one would normally expect to find progestational changes, then we may reasonably assume that ovulation has not occurred and that the bleeding is anovulatory.

If one is interested only in whether or not ovulation has taken place and is reluctant to take a biopsy specimen of the endometrium, either because of the fear of interrupting a pregnancy or the danger of infection, an ingenious spoon-shaped device may be inserted in the vagina just before the onset of the period. It is held in position beneath the cervix with a tampon (e.g. Tampax) for approximately twelve hours. This is a great convenience, for the menstrual period may begin at night, on a holiday or a weekend when patient and physician contact is more difficult. The menstrual discharges are collected during this time and then placed in a container filled with physiologic saline solution. After centrifuging, the tissue is fixed and stained, and a useful sample of the endometrium is obtained.

Sampling of the endometrium, whether by biopsy or other collecting device, is an excellent method of determining that ovulation has occurred. It gives only presumptive evidence of the date on which it happened.

WHAT TESTS ARE AVAILABLE TO TIME THE DAY OF OVULATION?   To date none of the tests designed to pinpoint the time of ovulation have received universal acceptance. Most of those in common usage give evidence of ovulation after the fact. This is true whether one measures vaginal acidity, changes in the vaginal epithelium, viscosity and acidity of the cervical mucus, basal body temperatures, endometrial biopsy or pregnanediol excretion on twenty-four-hour urine specimens. Other tests such as the rat ovarian hyperemia test and the measurement of changes in vaginal electropotential give promise of greater accuracy, but are still experimental and have not been generally adopted. Approximating the date of ovulation is important, since we are not yet in a position to determine it exactly. Therefore we must get the maximum amount of information out of the tools at hand.

The Basal Body Temperature.   Probably the most widely used method of determining ovulation is the recording of the body temperature the first thing on waking in the morning each day throughout the cycle. The temperature had best be taken by rectum and preferably at the same time every day. This test has the distinct advantage of convenience. It is performed by the patient and requires only that she (1) know how to read a thermometer, for the fluctuations are not great; (2) that she do it scrupulously and on a regular time schedule; and (3) that she record the temperature as she reads it.

There appears to be a definite relation between the fluctuation in the basal body temperature and ovarian function. Under the influence of estrin, in the early part of the cycle, the basal body temperature shows a steady drop day by day until a low point is reached just before ovulation. The drop is minimal and usually does not exceed half a degree, but it is definite. When ovulation is believed to occur, there is a further drop of five tenths of a degree followed by a similar rise on the following day and continuing each day, as the corpus luteum becomes more active and progestin is produced, until the basal temperature reaches a level approximately a full degree higher than the lowest recorded reading. As long as the corpus luteum is active the

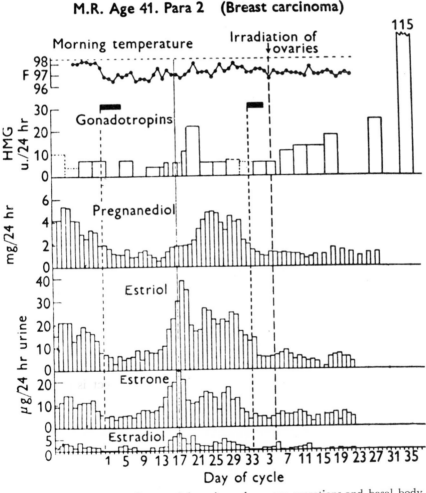

M.R. Age 41. Para 2   (Breast carcinoma)

Fig. 28-7.   Correlation by Brown of the urinary hormone excretions and basal body temperatures during an ovulatory cycle. Ovulation likely occurred on day 17, and morning temperatures thereafter were generally higher than in the proliferative phase. The patient had breast cancer, but her ovarian cyclic functions were not abnormal. (J. B. Brown: Urinary Excretion of Oestrogens during the Menstrual Cycle. *Lancet* Vol. 1, 1955.)

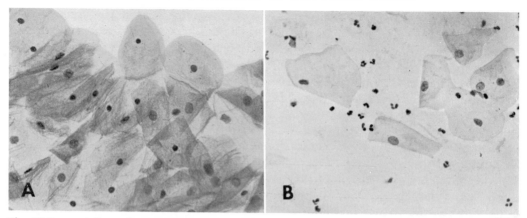

Fig. 28-8.   *A,* Preovulatory vaginal smears show a predominance of cornified cells with pyknotic nuclei. *B,* After ovulation more vaginal cornified cells are folded, and their nuclei are relatively vesicular.

temperature remains elevated. If pregnancy takes place, no drop in temperature occurs, but if it does not and the corpus luteum regresses, the temperature readings gradually recede (Fig. 28–7; see also Fig. 15–11).

To the person thoroughly versed in the interpretation of basal temperature charts it is possible to gain a good deal of presumptive evidence of fluctuations in ovarian activity. An irregular pattern may suggest, for example, failure of ovulation or poor and delayed corpus luteum function. To the general practitioner, who sees far more sterility problems than the specialist and has far less time to devote to the investigation of the cause, it is a most useful and practical test. With it he can get a pretty definite idea whether ovulation has taken place and a fair estimate of when.

WHAT INFORMATION CAN WE ACQUIRE FROM A VAGINAL SMEAR?   This is a simple test based on the cyclic variation that takes place in the epithelial cells of the vagina in response to ovarian hormone activity. Cornification takes place in the superficial layer under the influence of estrin stimulation. As the time of ovulation approaches an increasing degree of pyknosis is noted in the nuclei, which become gradually smaller, often fragmented and occasionally absent. Large cells with a minimum of granules are desquamated at the ovulatory point. After ovulation, under the influence of progesterone the cornification element disappears, and the epithelial cells in the vagina are relatively larger and now have large vesicular nuclei, while the cytoplasm becomes rich in granules (Fig. 28–8).

Though the changes do occur, it is not always easy to establish a sharp enough end-point to state that ovulation occurred at a specific time, and in sterility cases this test is useful mainly in establishing whether an estrogen effect is present or absent. Occasionally an unexpected diagnosis of cancer or pregnancy may result.

WHAT ABOUT THE CERVICAL AND VAGINAL SECRETIONS?   We have noted that a rapid change in the vaginal acidity to a pH of 7 or 8 takes place at the approximate time of ovulation. This can readily be tested by using indicator papers. Along with the change in acidity there are alterations in the physical characteristics of the cervical mucus which reflect the action of hormones on the endocervical glands. At ovulation the normally thick, heavy, gelatinous mucus becomes clean, thin and stringy. When placed on a glass slide, it crystallizes and forms a characteristic "fern" pattern. When one attempts to pick up the mucus with forceps, it tends to separate into thin threadlike strands as the jaws of the forceps separate. This is the so-called

Spinnbarkeit. At ovulation the tensile strength of these thin threads of mucus is much higher and a greater degree of stretching is possible than at any other phase of the cycle.

It is this change in the acidity and consistency of the cervical mucus that allows the spermatozoa to adapt to the vaginal secretion and pass into the endometrial cavity more readily. It is a good test and has many useful applications, but unfortunately it does not define the ovulatory date with any exactitude.

What Information Can Be Gained from Estimating Pregnanediol Excretion in the Urine? Since sodium pregnanediol glucuronide, or pregnanediol, is the metabolic end-product of progesterone, for all practical purposes the estimation of its excretion in the urine might seem to pinpoint the day of ovulation. Little is found in the early estrin phase of the menstrual cycle. The peak of its excretion is noted between the twenty-first and twenty-sixth days of the cycle (Fig. 28–9). The recovery of pregnanediol in the urine is simply *post hoc* confirmation that ovulation has occurred, but it does not help in specific dating. The method is expensive, time-consuming and not sufficiently informative, in its present method of assay, to be very useful.

Until recently it was generally believed that pregnanediol appeared only in the second half of the cycle, following ovulation and the development of a corpus luteum.

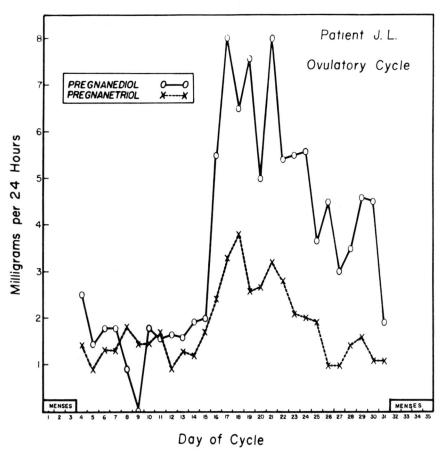

Fig. 28-9.   The rise in urinary excretion of pregnanediol from about 2 to 7 or 8 mg. per 24 hours occurred at midcycle after ovulation, as is usually the case.

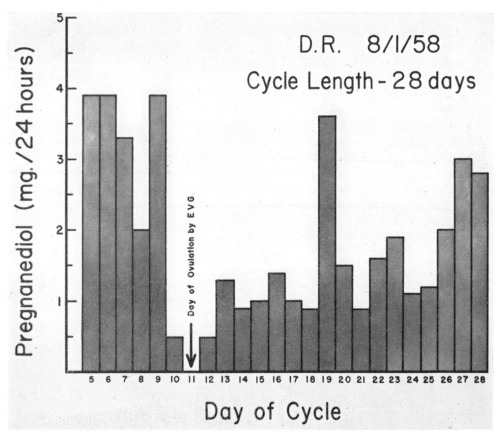

Fig. 28-10.   Example of a cycle during which the low point of pregnanediol excretion and the electrovaginal potential (EVG) both pointed to ovulation on the eleventh day of a 28-day intermenstrual period.

More refined analysis now indicates that small amounts of pregnanediol are present in the estrin phase. The significance of these findings is not immediately apparent, and for practical purposes we must rely on the recovery of significant amounts in the progestational phase.

ARE THERE ANY TESTS WHICH DO LOCALIZE THE OVULATORY DATE?   None of the methods in general usage have any great degree of accuracy, though there are two methods which have not been universally accepted, but do show promise of providing more precise information as to the actual date. Both tend to throw some doubt on the constancy of the duration of the postovulatory phase. Much of the present-day dating is based on the assumption that the menstrual period occurs fourteen plus or minus two days after theoretical ovulation has taken place. From the two experimental approaches to the problem there is a suggestion that ovulation occurs earlier in the cycle than we formerly supposed.

The Two-Hour Rat Test of Farris.   This test is based on the fact that the urine of women who are ovulating normally will produce hyperemia in the ovaries of Wistar rats in increasing degrees over a four- or five-day period preceding their ovulation. The end-point to one familiar with the technique is sharp, but unfortunately the procedure requires a specific strain of rat, and other observers have had less success with the interpretation of the color changes in the ovary that denote ovulation. The clinical results reported from the use of the test are provocative and impressive.

Determination of the Variation in Electropotential in the Vagina. The hope that it would be possible to determine the time of follicular rupture by electrical readings had until recently been unfulfilled. The changes observed were believed to be the result of the action of hormones upon the superficial vaginal capillaries, but not actually correlated with ovulation. Although there is as yet no conclusive proof that ovulation does take place at the time that the differences in electropotential occur, nevertheless there is recent indirect evidence that the two may be synchronous (Fig. 28–10). Patients who have a sterility problem have concentrated intercourse solely on the day selected by the electropotential machine as the day of ovulation and been rewarded by pregnancy in an impressive number of instances. This work and that of the appearance of hyperemia in the Wistar rat ovary need further confirmation.

What about the So-Called Huhner or Postcoital Test?

An ejaculate normal in volume, number and motility of sperm, and free of abnormal forms, will not produce a pregnancy if it cannot pass beyond the cervical barrier and enter the endometrial cavity. The failure may be due to obstructions to the passage of sperm within the cervical canal or to the hostility of the cervical secretions to the spermatozoa. Aspiration of cervical mucus after coitus is a most valuable and practical method of determining whether healthy viable sperm survive in the environment to which they will be exposed.

The maximal amount of information is acquired when the test is performed at the suspected time of ovulation so that the cervical mucus will be most receptive. If it is impossible to date ovulation, the specimen should be taken anywhere between the tenth and the fourteenth days of a regular twenty-eight-day cycle. The test should be performed within two hours after the time of intercourse and preferably after several days of abstinence.

The actual technique for carrying out the test is not complicated. The vaginal fornix is exposed with a nonlubricated speculum. The pooled secretions are aspirated with a dry pipet, placed on a glass slide and covered with a glass coverslip. When examined under the microscope, most of the spermatozoa will be inactive and may be presumed to be dead. The information obtained is valuable, however, for the sperm have at least been deposited in the vicinity of the cervix. After this the vagina is wiped clean of all contents, and the mucoid secretions are removed from the endocervical canal. This had best be done with an aspirating syringe, using suction rather than forceps. In this manner the full extent of the mucus plug is extracted, and some estimate of the degree to which the spermatozoa have penetrated can be made. The secretions are placed on a glass slide and examined under a microscope, using both high and low powers.

The interpretation of the test is most important. There is no general agreement as to the number of active, motile, migrating sperm that need be present to consider the test normal. Somewhere between twenty-five and fifty healthy sperm per high-power field may be regarded as essential to successful pregnancy. If only a single spermatozoon is observed, the test will indicate that intercourse has been satisfactorily performed and that the sperm at least have reached the proper destination. Total lack of spermatozoa in either the vaginal pool or cervix, on the other hand, would suggest faulty deposition, provided the sperm are normal. When no motile aggressive sperm are found in the cervical canal despite their known presence in the secretion of the vaginal fornix, then one may presume that it has been impossible for them to enter the canal. If, on the other hand, a few are active, while the rest are inactive or dead, one may rightfully assume that the cervical secretions are hostile to the spermatozoa.

The hostility of the cervical secretions to the penetrating sperm can be roughly assessed at this time by another simple test (Kurzrok-Miller). If one places a sample of cervical mucus, taken at the time of ovulation, immediately beside a sample of semen, penetration of the mucus by the sperm cells can be followed under the microscope, provided no incompatibility exists. This is not conclusive evidence, but it does provide a possible lead for further investigation.

It would be unwise to accept the observations of a single postcoital test as complete evidence. The Huhner test should be repeated under normal living conditions, after more prolonged periods of abstinence, and at varying intervals of time after intercourse before making final decisions. When apparent hostility of either vaginal or cervical secretions exists, one may wish to perform the test after giving a precoital douche of Ringer-Locke solution.

Normally we would expect to find from fifty to several hundred active progressive sperm per high-power field several hours after intercourse. If fewer than twenty-five are found within two hours after coitus, there is a definite barrier to successful conception.

What about the Inability of either Sperm or Ova to Enter the Fallopian Tube?

It is obvious that there must be a union of ovum and sperm before pregnancy can occur. If tubal occlusion or spasm prevents the sperm from entering the tube or a lack of normal tubal activity or adhesions of the fimbriated end deny entrance of the ovum, their union cannot be consummated. One may elect to acquire this basic information before doing the other diagnostic tests. In this discussion we have assumed that history and physical examination revealed no cause to suspect that tubal occlusion was present.

There are two methods of determining tubal patency.

TUBAL INSUFFLATION.   It is common practice to attempt to pass either carbon dioxide or air into the uterus and through the tubes before injecting any radiopaque material and securing x-ray evidence of tubal abnormality or lack of it. In the first instance one obtains information as to tubal motility, as well as patency, while hysterosalpingography pinpoints the actual site of obstruction in the tube (Fig. 28–11).

Carbon dioxide is the gas of choice. It is absorbed slowly and is less dangerous than air injection. Whatever vehicle is used, it is inadvisable to introduce the gas at pressures in excess of 200 mm. of mercury when one is using the test as a diagnostic tool. One may deliberately take a calculated risk and use higher pressures for therapeutic reasons. Fatal air emboli have been recorded when excessive pressures were used.

There are three ways of assessing the patency of the tubes: (1) The pressures recorded on the manometer are initially high, e.g. 200 mm. of mercury. If this pressure drops to a level of from 60 to 8 mm. of mercury, the tubes are patent and the gas has passed into the abdominal cavity. (2) The passage of gas through the tubes and into the abdomen is accompanied by a low-pitched sound, recurring intermittently and readily audible with a stethoscope placed on the lower part of the abdomen. If

Rubin Test - CO$_2$

the pitch is high and the pressure elevated, the tubes are probably stenotic. One with much experience may be able to determine whether one or both tubes are patent. (3) If the tubes are patent, the free gas escaping from the tube into the abdominal cavity accumulates beneath the diaphragm and produces pain on the top of the right shoulder when the patient assumes an upright position. This is a variable complaint, for some patients do not have it, but when it is present, it is an indication that at least there is a degree of patency. It is not evidence of a normal tube unless the symptom is produced with a normal amount of gas introduced at reasonable pressures.

Failure of carbon dioxide to pass through the tubes, as shown by failure of the pressure to fall from the initially high level of 200 mm. of mercury, even with the gas supply shut off, is a pretty good indication that both tubes are blocked. Before accepting this as complete evidence, repeated tests should be done, for it is possible that tubal spasm at the conical medial ends of the tubes will deny passage to the gas even when the pressures are high. To counteract this possibility it may be advisable to use an antispasmodic, such as an ampule of amyl nitrate, 1/100 grain of nitroglycerin or 50 gm. of Demerol.

By insufflation one may also get an idea of the motility of the tubes as well as their patency. A recording device (kymograph) normally registers minor fluctuations in pressure varying from 10 to 30 mm. of mercury every 5 to 10 seconds. These represent normal peristaltic activity in the tubes. Absence of these minor oscillations suggests that the tubes are fixed either by disease in the pelvis or peritubal adhesions when no obstruction is found within the tubes themselves.

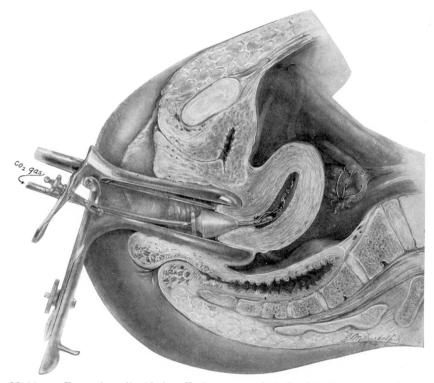

Fig. 28-11. For carbon dioxide insufflation a cannula is fixed in the cervix, and the gas under pressure is released into the uterus. Normally it passes out through the tubes. This examination is often called the Rubin test. (From Wharton: *Gynecology*.)

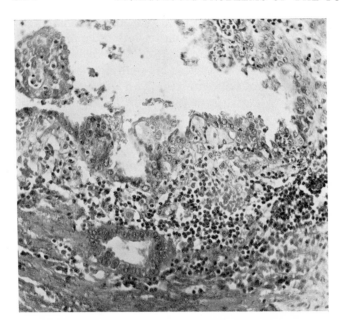

Fig. 28-12.   Tubal granulomatous inflammatory reaction to instillation of oil, as a complication of hysterosalpingograph. The large, pale macrophages contain the lipoid medium.

Tubal insufflation is an office procedure which under most circumstances produces a minimal amount of discomfort to the person with normal sensitivity. There is some pain when the cannula is introduced into the cervix and a moderate increase when the gas pressure is increased. A severe pain in the abdomen on one or both sides is an indication of obstruction to the tube, usually at the fimbriated end, and distention of the tubal wall. For this reason the test should never be done under anesthesia.

The chief contraindication concerns the likelihood of infection, either fresh or the lighting up of an old one. The test should not be done if there is any indication of an infection in either the tubes, cervix or vagina. A repeat test should be done only after a month has been allowed to elapse and not then if the previous examination has produced an inflammatory reaction in a pelvis previously felt to be normal. Some authorities believe this finding to be presumptive evidence of tuberculosis latent in the tubes or uterus.

The timing of the insufflation is most important. It should never be done in the presence of active uterine bleeding or impending menstruation. To get the maximal information with the least chance of danger it is best to perform the test in the latter part of the first week following the period. When performed at this time, it is late enough in the cycle to avoid (a) the risk of forcing desquamating epithelium back into the tubes, (b) gas embolus through the large uterine veins which may be open. It is early enough to avoid the interruption of pregnancy, since no ovulation has yet occurred. When it is done just before the menstrual period, the fully developed endometrium may occlude the cornual ends of the tubes and prevent the normal passage of gas. There is another reason for doing the test early in the cycle. Clinically, there is some circumstantial evidence that insufflation may induce ovulation and increase the chances of pregnancy. Insufflation therefore can be a therapeutic as well as a diagnostic maneuver.

HYSTEROSALPINGOGRAPHY.   The failure of gas to pass through the tubes is fairly good evidence of tubal occlusion, but the localization of the block is still uncertain. Such information can be obtained by injection of a radiopaque oil into the uterine cavity and tubes. If there is no obstruction to the introduction of the oil, x-ray study will show a well defined outline of both uterine cavity and tubes. The oil should be water-soluble and not irritating to the uterine and tubal epithelium. Some oils in the past stimulated a granulomatous foreign body reaction, remained in the tubes and produced chronic reactive inflammation (Fig. 28–12). In no instance should the radiopaque oil be introduced under pressure. One may force the dye into the general circulation through the uterine veins or produce a tubal rupture by over-distention of its walls. When aqueous iodine solution is used for tubal and uterine visualization, the examination should be carried out in the fluoroscopy room. In this manner the material can be seen escaping into the abdominal cavity through the open fimbriated ends.

In addition to information as to tubal function and disease the later review of the plates may show irregularities in the outline of the endometrial cavity. Congenital defects, polyps or submucous fibroids may be revealed for the first time.

How Do You Interpret Findings of the Hysterosalpingography?   If there is no obstruction to the flow of the radiopaque material, it escapes so rapidly into the peritoneal cavity that the tubal lumens are not distended. Any obstruction to the lumens due to internal disease or kinking due to peritubal adhesions will interrupt the continuity of flow and produce dilation of the tubes. When a tube is distended and isolated blotches of the contrast material are seen, one may reasonably suspect that the patient has a hydrosalpinx due to closure of the fimbriated end of the tube. If the passage is slow, if the tubes are moderately distended, but the oil finally enters the abdominal cavity as seen by fluoroscopy if the water-soluble oil is used, or if intraperitoneal droplets appear on a twenty-four-hour x-ray plate when Lipiodol is used, one may feel certain that partial obstruction is present.

The material may never enter the tubes. This may be due to lesions at the tubal ostia on the uterine side or, as in tubal insufflation by gas, the obstruction may be due to spasm. A spiked shadow at the cornual end, which is said to resemble a dog ear, seems to be indicative of tubal spasm rather than organic obstruction. It is therefore not advisable to conclude that the tubes are completely blocked on the basis of a single uterotubogram. The test should be repeated. The same timing factors as for tubal insufflation with gas are utilized when oil is used. The injection should be made between the fourth and the seventh days after the completion of the menstrual period, primarily to avoid the blocking effect of any menstrual debris at the cornual ends, with the added advantage of avoiding disturbance of any possible pregnancy.

What about Culdoscopy and Peritoneoscopy?

After a complete workup has been done one may wish to check the suggestions of intra-abdominal disease by direct inspection of the uterus and adnexa, by inserting either a culdoscope through the posterior fornix of the vagina or a peritoneoscope through the abdomen. Some additional information may be obtained, but the great majority of gynecologists prefer laparotomy. Definitive corrective measures can be carried out by abdominal exploration, while observation alone is possible either with culdoscopy or peritoneoscopy. The greatest usefulness might be in the patient who has a completely negative workup after both physical examination and tubal evaluation studies.

TREATMENT OF FEMALE STERILITY

A discussion of the treatment of sterility in the female becomes a summary of the efforts exerted to find the cause. How do we treat the woman when no cause for infertility is found? The greatest degree of success in treatment of sterility has followed the initial phases of the investigation, when a complete and exhaustive history has been taken and a physical examination has failed to disclose any systemic or local reason why pregnancy should not take place. When there are obvious nutritional deficiencies, the diet should be corrected to high protein intake supplemented with a liberal amount of vitamins and minerals. All the vitamins are essential, though there is less clinical evidence that vitamin E and wheat germ oil have all the value ascribed to them. If the patient is obese, she should be placed on a sensible weight reduction diet.

Though laboratory evidence of the usefulness of thyroid therapy is lacking, most gynecologists feel empirically that it has value. If there is a basal metabolic deficit, there is no question but that thyroid hormone should be given. One may choose to use L-triiodothyronine rather than thyroxin because of its alleged more specific effect on cell metabolism. When there has been an obvious overindulgence in the use of coffee, tobacco or alcohol, their use should be restricted. The elimination of stress in everyday living should be sought, and when possible, intelligent vacation planning should be emphasized.

Probably the greatest returns follow the instructions given to the patient, with particular concentration on the timing, frequency and technique of intercourse. The patient may now be reassured that nothing is basically wrong. The husband must thereafter be checked to be sure that he is a capable partner to the initiation of pregnancy. When both are normal, the reassurance of the fact brings such emotional release that pregnancy often results without any further corrective therapy.

What Do You Do about Any Organic Disease Discovered on Physical Examination?

Abnormalities uncovered in the course of the physical examination or laboratory workup may affect the production of ova. More likely the union of egg and sperm is prevented by organic lesions which interfere with transit of either one to the point of fertilization.

THE VAGINA AND CERVIX. Since the vaginal acidity may prove inimical to the existence of the sperm, all infections such as with *Trichomonas vaginalis* should be eradicated. To enhance the likelihood of cervical inseminations, at the approximate time of ovulation an alkalinizing precoital douche of Ringer-Locke solution should be used.

The cervix itself may harbor infection either in its superficial portion or deep in the canal in the endocervical glands. Erosions and endocervicitis should be eliminated by cervical cauterization. This treatment must be thorough, but care must be exercised to prevent the creation of cervical stenosis. When a cervical stenosis is found without infection, dilation should be done, and any polyps present should be excised. Cervical dilatation may be a useful device in therapy in the absence of any organic lesion. There is clinical evidence that any intracervical or intrauterine manipulation stimulates the uterus and adnexa either to ovulate or to function in a generally more normal fashion.

SURGERY FOR THE UTERUS.   The presence of tumors or malposition of the uterus may interfere with the initiation of pregnancy. Intrauterine polyps, submucous fibroids, retroversion, pelvic congestion or congenital anomalies may be the basic explanation of reproductive failure. Intrauterine polyps can be removed by curettage. Retroversion can be corrected by manual replacement of the uterus in normal position and maintained there by an intravaginal supportive pessary (Smith-Hodge). In rare instances an intra-abdominal surgical suspension may be indicated. Treatment of the other entities must be considered on their own merits, in relation to their likelihood of interfering with conception.

SURGERY FOR THE OVARY.   When there are cysts of the ovary which do not appear to be physiologic, surgical excision is indicated. Menstrual abnormalities combined with clinical suggestions of the Stein-Leventhal syndrome may warrant surgical exploration and wedge resections of the ovaries (see Fig. 18-6). The presence of chocolate cysts and evidence of widespread endometriosis of the pelvic peritoneum may call for abdominal exploration on their own right. Many gynecologists are skeptical of the value of conservative surgery for endometriosis when the prime reason for exploration is infertility. There appears to be an infertility element in all endometriosis cases, yet there are many reported series claiming success approaching 30 or 40 per cent after excision of endometrial implants from the ovary and peritoneum

SURGERY FOR THE TUBE.   Before one accepts as final a decision as to the patency of the uterine ends of the tubes, one may take a calculated risk and try to open up the ostia by increasing pressures during tubal insufflation to levels approaching 300 mm. of mercury. There are enthusiastic reports in the literature, with successful results recorded approaching 40 per cent for patency and 18 per cent for subsequent pregnancy. The risks are there, and the method should be used with caution. Since the results of surgery for correction of obstruction at the uterine ends of the tubes by resection of the offending areas and implantation of the remaining portions of the tubes into the endometrial cavity are obviously poor, one may choose to assume the risks. The successful results in the most favorable cases do not exceed 25 per cent and over-all are not much better than 5 per cent.

When obstruction of the tubes occurs at the fimbriated ends, as indicated by pain caused by insufflation or as seen following the uterotubogram, surgery may be indicated. The same may be said when investigative studies show disturbances in the motility of the tubes caused by peritubal adhesions. Improvements in techniques, with the use of polyethylene tubing to maintain the patency of the tubes and a plastic cap to cover the reconstructed fimbria and to prevent adhesions immediately postoperatively, have encouraged many gynecologists to resort to surgery more frequently than in the past. The results are still pretty discouraging. Since they are no better, one must be sure that all other factors in the sterility problem are essentially normal. If the patient understands that the likelihood of success is not great and she is willing to assume the risks, surgery is justifiable.

THE USE OF CHEMOTHERAPY COMBINED WITH HEAT.   In the presence of moderate degrees of pelvic inflammation the combination of heat and antibiotics may be worth trying. The heat may be applied daily in the form of intensive douches, either the Elliott treatment, which uses an intravaginal rubber bag through which hot water circulates, or pelvic diathermy. Some resolution of inflammation may be expected from the heat. The increased vascularity enhances the effectiveness of antibiotics, such as penicillin in doses varying from 600,000 to one million units daily. This regimen must be carried out for several months.

What Do You Do When the Investigations Point to Endocrine Cause?

Any disturbance in function of the endocrine system is bound to influence the initiation of pregnancy. In most instances there is a measurable indication of faulty function, but occasionally the only indication is a low fertility index. Approximately one third of the women who have a sterility problem can trace their difficulty to disturbed function of the endocrine system.

The chief manifestations, as previously noted, are (1) disturbances of the menstrual rhythm, even to the point of amenorrhea, (2) menstruation without ovulation, and (3) inadequate secretion of progesterone.

BASIC REQUIREMENTS IN ENDOCRINE THERAPY.   Since the proper function of the endocrine system depends on proper receptivity and utilization of the stimulating hormones at the cell level in the target organs, thyroid therapy is a useful adjunct. Faulty thyroid function may exist in the presence of a normal test for protein-bound iodine, basal metabolism or blood cholesterol determination. When this is suspected, it may be better to use L-triiodothyronine rather than Thyroid, USP.

We have previously commented on the role of nutrition, vitamin deficiency, obesity, intercurrent diseases and nervous tension in the proper functioning of the endocrine system. Before one embarks on a course of substitution endocrine therapy, the above-mentioned elements must be brought as near to normality as possible.

TREATMENT OF INADEQUATE OR ABSENT MENSTRUATION.   When the history indicates that the menstrual flow is scanty or absent, there is an obvious defect in the pituitary-ovarian-uterine axis. If the amenorrhea is primary, little can be done to correct it. The mechanism, diagnosis and treatment have been discussed (Chap. 21). If there is a suggestion of the Stein-Leventhal syndrome, one may advise abdominal exploration and wedge resections of the ovaries.

When amenorrhea appears after months or years of relatively normal menstruation, the defect likely is less basic. Secondary amenorrhea is most common in the Stein-Leventhal syndrome. If other stigmata are present, exploration is justifiable. In many instances hypoplasia of the uterus is present, owing to inadequate hormonal stimulation. Combined estrin and progestin therapy may build up the size of the uterus and render it more susceptible to hormonal stimulation from its own endocrine system. The effect of adrenal dysfunction may manifest itself by altering the menstrual cycle in the direction of amenorrhea. Cortisone suppression therapy then may restore the cycle and make pregnancy possible.

Until recently the *pituitary hormones*, singly or in combination, were not very effective and were even dangerous. Their value in re-establishing a regular menstrual pattern seemed to be negligible, and their influence on initiation of pregnancy nonexistent.

IRRADIATION OF THE PITUITARY OR THE OVARY with small doses has its enthusiastic advocates and violent opponents. Those who believe in it claim an extremely high percentage of success (80 per cent) when the main problem in infertility is amenorrhea or scanty menstruation. Those who believe that ionizing radiation in whatever dosage is basically destructive do not advise any irradiation. Those who advocate it point to a high percentage of delivery of normal infants at term and a persistence of a regular menstrual rhythm after that. If it is to be given, the radiation should precede the suspected ovulatory interval to avoid damaging any pregnancy that may have started.

What Can Be Done for the Patient with Anovulatory Bleeding?

A pattern of menstrual bleeding without ovulation is a serious problem to the girl who is trying to become pregnant. The diagnosis is made by the finding of a proliferative endometrium at any point in the second half of the menstrual cycle. This is presumptive evidence that ovulation and luteinization have not taken place. Once this type of bleeding becomes fixed, it is a hard job to reverse the process. Usually the endometrium proliferates abundantly, owing to the stimulation of estrin unbalanced by progestin, and the ovary is considered to be the source of the difficulty. The fault may lie within the endometrium, which may fail to respond properly to stimulation by the normal ovarian hormones. In such cases the endometrium will be atrophic, yet pregnanediol may be found in the urine.

COMBINED ESTRIN AND PROGESTIN THERAPY.   The most common method of correcting anovulatory bleeding is to place the patient on combined estrin and progestin therapy for several months. In this manner the ovary is placed at rest while the uterus continues to be stimulated, in the hope that it will rebound with added vigor when the substitution therapy is discontinued. The effect is on the ovary and not the pituitary. Newer combined preparations of estrin and progestin have become available which facilitate the management of this type of therapy. For intramuscular injection, preparations such as Delalutin and Delestrogen can be used. The physician may prefer to use progestin as an oral medication for the sake of convenience to both patient and himself. Enthusiastic reports are now appearing in the literature since the use of 10 mg. of Enovid or Provera.

THE PITUITARY HORMONES.   Since the primary defect is failure of ovulation, it would seem logical to give the pituitary hormones. As yet the pituitary hormones are imperfect, and their use is attended with some danger. There have been enthusiastic users of the gonadotropic substance found in pregnant mare's serum. It is claimed that not only has a progestational endometrium been produced, but also that pregnancies have occurred in women previously sterile because of anovulatory cycles. In view of the general disagreement as to their true value and the universal acceptance that severe anaphylactic reactions may follow the injection of the pituitary hormones to induce ovulation, this therapy must be regarded as experimental. We know too little of the dosage and timing to recommend their indiscriminate use. Moreover, there is the added objection that antihormones may develop which inhibit the hormones already being produced by the patient's own endocrine system.

The same objections are raised to the combined use of pregnant mare's serum and chorionic gonadotropin, which seem to have a synergistic action and thereby provide greater stimulation to the ovary which does not ovulate normally.

Purified extracts from the human pituitary gland combined with chorionic gonadotropin have recently been used clinically and have demonstrated some measure of capacity to induce ovulation. In a few instances pregnancies have resulted. The undesirable side effects appear to be minimal. The hormone is not yet available for general clinical use.

IRRADIATION OF THE OVARY AND PITUITARY.   Though small-dose irradiation of the ovary and pituitary seems to work successfully when the patient is amenorrheic, it apparently is less useful when menstrual bleeding occurs from an anovulatory endometrium.

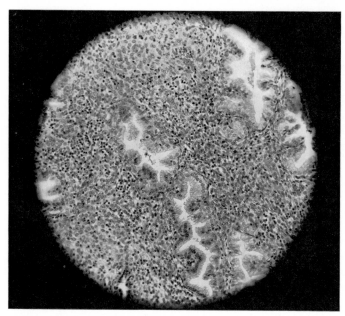

Fig. 28-13.   Example of a secretory endometrium deficient in predecidual stromal reaction. The glandular epithelium shows secretory exhaustion, and the stroma is infiltrated with lymphocytes, consistent with the appearance approximately 2 days before onset of menstruation. The stroma is compact, however, and without evidence of corpus luteum effect.

What Can Be Done for the Patient with a Deficient Progestational Phase?

It is not uncommon to receive a report from the pathologist of a poorly developed progestational endometrium when endometrial samples are taken in women with sterility problems (Fig. 28–13). An indication that this is true is seen on close scrutiny of the basal temperature charts and the electropotential readings. This progestational deficiency may be the sole cause for failure to initiate a pregnancy. If the endometrium is inadequately prepared to nourish an impregnated ovum, a conceptus never becomes properly implanted.

It is now possible to imitate a healthy appearance of a secretory endometrium by using the new oral progestational agents such as Enovid or Provera in 10-mg. doses from day 15 to day 25 for 3 consecutive months. As a supplement, thyroid extract and vitamin C may be given.

REFERENCES

General

Banks, A. L., Rutherford, R. N., and Coburn, W. A.: Fertility Following Adoption; Report of 31 Cases. *Fertil. & Steril.*, 12: 438, 1961.
Buxton, C. L , and Southam, A. L.: *Human Infertility*. New York, Paul B. Hoeber, Inc., 1958.
Farris, E. J.: *Human Ovulation and Fertility*. Philadelphia, J. B. Lippincott Company, 1956.
Gebhard, P. H., Pomeroy, W. B., Martin, C. E., and Christensen, C.V.: *Pregnancy, Birth and Abortion*. New York, Paul B. Hoeber, Inc., 1958.
Guttmacher, A. F.: Early Attitudes toward Infertility. *Fertil. & Steril.*, 4: 250, 1953.
Horne, H. W., Jr.: Coital Positioning in Infertility. *Fertil. & Steril.*, 12: 319, 1961.
Mazer, E., and Israel, S. H.: *Diagnosis and Treatment of Menstrual Disorders and Sterility*. 4th Ed., edited by S. L. Israel. New York, Paul B. Hoeber, Inc., 1959.

Newell, J. W., and Rock, J.: Upper Age Limit of Parturition; Review of Literature. *Am. J. Obst. & Gynec.*, 63: 875, 1952.

Penrose, L. S.: Mongolian Idiocy (Mongolism) and Maternal Age. *Ann. New York Acad. Sc.*, 57: 494, 1954.

Rubin, I. C.: *Uterotubal Insufflation.* St. Louis, C. V. Mosby Company, 1947.

Sawin, P. B.: The Influence of Age of Mother on Pattern of Reproduction. *Ann. New York Acad. Sc.*, 57: 564, 1954.

Stone, A., and Ward, M. E.: Factors Responsibile for Pregnancy in 500 Infertility Cases. *Fertil. & Steril.*, 7: 1, 1956.

Tietze, C.: Statistical Contributions to the Study of Human Fertility. *Fertil. & Steril.*, 7: 88, 1956.

Tietze, C., Guttmacher, A. F., and Rubin, S.: Time Required for Conception in 1727 Planned Pregnancies. *Fertil. & Steril.*, 1: 338, 1950.

Turner, V. H., Davis, C. D., and Carter, B.: Correlation of Estimated Prognosis with Some Findings and Results in 750 Sterile Couples. *Am. J. Obst. & Gynec.*, 70: 1189, 1955.

Tyler, E. T.: *Sterility: Office Management of the Infertile Couple.* New York, McGraw-Hill Book Company, Inc., 1961.

Villee, C. A.: *Control of Ovulation.* New York, Pergamon Press, 1961.

Weir, W. C., and Weir, D. R.: The Natural History of Infertility. *Fertil. & Steril.*, 12: 443, 1961.

Whitelaw, M. J.: What Is Normal Female Fertility? *Fertil. & Steril.*, 6: 103, 1955.

Witschi, E.: Overripeness of the Egg as a Cause of Twinning and Teratogenesis: A Review. *Cancer Res.*, 12: 763, 1952.

Young, W. C.: Gamete Age at the Time of Fertilization and the Course of Gestation in Mammals; in E. T. Engle, ed.: *Pregnancy Wastage.* Springfield, Ill., Charles C Thomas, 1953, p. 38.

The Pituitary

Bahn, R. C., Lorenz, N., Bennett, W. A., and Albert, A.: Gonadotropins of the Pituitary Gland and the Urine of the Adult Human Female. *Endocrinology*, 53: 455, 1953.

Buxton, C. L., and Herrmann, W.: Induction of Ovulation in the Human with Human Gonadotropins. *Am. J. Obst. & Gynec.*, 81: 584, 1961.

Noble, R. L., and Plunkett, E. R.: Biology of the Gonadotropins. *Brit. M. Bull.*, 11: 98, 1955.

Palmer, A.: Chorionic Gonadotropin—Its Place in the Treatment of Infertility. *Fertil. & Steril.*, 8: 220, 1957.

Simpson, M. E., and van Wagenen, G.: Experimental Induction of Ovulation in the Macaque Monkey. *Fertil. & Steril.*, 9: 386, 1958.

The Ovary

Day, L. A., and Smith, P. L.: The Reproductive Career of Women with Ovarian Dysfunction. *Am. J. Obst. & Gynec.*, 60: 93, 1950.

Hartman, C. G.: How Variable Is the Functional Life of the Human Corpus Luteum Menstrationis? *Obst. & Gynec.*, 7: 323, 1955.

Hertig, A. T., Rock, J., Adams, E. C., and Menkin, M. C.: Thirty-Four Fertilized Human Ova, Good, Bad and Indifferent, Recovered from 210 Women of Known Fertility. A Study of Biologic Wastage in Early Human Pregnancy. *Pediatrics*, 23: 202, 1959.

Hisaw, F. L.: Development of the Graafian Follicle and Ovulation. *Physiol. Rev.*, 27: 95, 1947.

Topkins, P.: Endometrial Biopsy Determination of Incidence of Ovulation in 402 Regularly Menstruating Women. *Fertil. & Steril.*, 4: 76, 1953.

The Adrenal

Herrmann, W., Buckner, F., and Morris, J. McL.: The Problem of "Mild" Adrenal Hyperplasia. *Fertil. & Steril.*, 11: 74, 1960.

Jones, H. W., Jr., and Jones, G. E. S.: The Gynecological Aspects of Adrenal Hyperplasia and Allied Disorders. *Am. J. Obst. & Gynec.*, 68: 1330, 1954.

West, C. D.: Evaluation of the Role of the Adrenal Cortex in Infertility. *Fertil. & Steril.*, 10: 102, 1959.

The Thyroid

Cominos, A. C.: Thyroid Function and Therapy in Reproductive Disturbances. *Obst. & Gynec.*, 7: 260, 1955.

Kurland, I. I., and Levine, W.: Hypothyroidism in Relation to Reproductive Disorders. *Fertil. & Steril.,* 10: 132, 1959.
Slater, S., Perlmutter, M., Solomons, E., and Numeroff, M.: Thyroid Function in Infertility and Habitual Abortion. *Fertil. & Steril.,* 11: 221, 1960.
Tyler, E. T.: The Thyroid Myth in Infertility. *Fertil. & Steril.,* 4: 218, 1953.

Diagnostic Evaluation of the Infertile Couple: General Discussion

Hartman, C. G.: A Half Century of Research in Reproductive Physiology. *Fertil. & Steril.,* 12: 1, 1961.
Simmons, F. A.: Diagnostic Techniques and Treatment of Sterile Couple; in J. V. Meigs and S. H. Sturgis, eds.: *Progress in Gynecology.* New York, Grune & Stratton, Inc., 1946, Vol. I, p. 246.
Southam, A. L.: What to Do with the "Normal" Infertile Couple. *Fertil. & Steril.,* 11: 543, 1960.

Endometrial Biopsy

Foss, B. A., Horne, H. W., Jr., and Hertig, A. T.: Endometrium and Sterility. *Fertil. & Steril.,* 9: 193, 1958.
Gillam, J. S.: Study of the Inadequate Secretion Phase Endometrium. *Fertil. & Steril.,* 6: 18, 1955.
Glass, S. J., Miller, W., and Rosenblum, G.: Secretory Hypoplasia of the Endometrium. *Fertil. & Steril.,* 6: 344, 1955.
Noyes, R. W.: Uniformity of Secretory Endometrium. *Obst. & Gynec.,* 7: 221, 1956.

Basal Body Temperature

Benjamin, F.: Basal Body Temperature Recordings in Gynaecology and Obstetrics. *J. Obst. & Gynaec. Brit. Emp.,* 67: 177, 1960.
Siegler, S. L., and Siegler, A. M.: Evaluation of Basal Body Temperature. An Analysis of 1012 Basal Body Temperature Recordings. *Fertil. & Steril.,* 2: 287, 1951.

Cervical and Vaginal Secretions

Cohen, M. R., Stein, I. F., Sr., and Kaye, B. M.: Spinnbarkeit, a Characteristic of Cervical Mucus. Significance at Ovulation Time. *Fertil. & Steril.,* 3: 201, 1952.
Roland, M.: A Simple Test for the Determination of Ovulation, Estrogen Activity, and Early Pregnancy Using Cervical Mucus Secretion. A Preliminary Report. *Am. J. Obst. & Gynec.,* 63: 81, 1955.
Zondek, B.: Arborization of Cervical and Nasal Mucus and Saliva. *Obst. & Gynec.,* 13: 477, 1959.

Pregnanediol

Ober, W. B., and Kaiser, G. A.: Pregnanediol. Methods, Limitations and Applications. *Am. J. Clin. Path.,* 35: 297, 1961.
Parsons, L., Whittaker, J. O., and Lemon, H. M.: Evaluation of Electrovaginal Potential Recordings as a Therapeutic Guide in Gynecological Problems. *Am. J. Obst. & Gynec.,* 79: 736, 1960.
Rogers, J.: Clinical Significance of Pregnanediol Excretion. *Fertil. & Steril.,* 6: 513, 1955.

Specific Tests to Date Ovulation

Behrman, S. J.: Detection of Ovulation. *Postgrad. Med.,* 27: 12, 1960.
Cohen, M. R., and Hankin, H.: Detecting Ovulation. *Fertil. & Steril.,* 11: 497, 1960.
Doyle, J. B., Ewers, F. J., Jr., and Sapit, D.: The New Fertility Testing Tape: A Predictive Test of the Fertile Period. *J.A.M.A.,* 172: 1744, 1960.
Farris, E. J.: Prediction of Day of Human Ovulation by Rat Test as Confirmed by 50 Conceptions. *Am. J. Obst. & Gynec.,* 56: 347, 1948.
Parsons, L., MacMillan, H. J., and Whittaker, J. O.: Abdominovaginal Electric Potential Differences, with Special Reference to the Ovulatory Phase of the Menstrual Cycle. *Am. J. Obst. & Gynec.,* 75: 121, 1958.

Sevag, M. G., and Colton, W. W.: Simple Chemical Method for the Determination of Ovulation Time in Women. *J.A.M.A.*, 170: 13, 1959.

Speck, G.: The Determination of the Time of Ovulation. *Obst. & Gynec. Surv.*, 14: 798, 1959.

Tietze, C.: Probability of Pregnancy Resulting from a Single Unprotected Coitus. *Fertil. & Steril.*, 11: 485, 1960.

Huhner or Postcoital Test

Gassner, F. X., Goldzieher, J. W., Masken, J. F., and Hopwood, M. L.: The Objective Measurement of Sperm Motility. *Fertil. & Steril.*, 10: 488, 1959.

Guard, H. R.: New Technic for Sperm Mucus Penetration Tests Using a Hemocytometer. *Fertil. & Steril.*, 11: 392, 1960.

Rubenstein, B. B., Strauss, H., Lazarus, M. L., and Hankin, H.: Sperm Survival in Women. Motile Sperm in the Fundus and Tubes of Surgical Cases. *Fertil. & Steril.*, 2: 15, 1951.

Tubal Insufflation, Hysterosalpingography and Culdoscopy

Goldberger, M. A., Marshak, R. H., and Davids, A.: Hysterography and Hysterosalpingography; Evaluation of 2500 Cases. *New York State J. Med.*, 50: 2697, 1950.

Kelly, J. V., and Rock, J.: Culdoscopy for Diagnosis in Infertility; Report of 492 Cases. *Am. J. Obst. & Gynec.*, 72: 523, 1956.

Measday, B.: An Analysis of the Complications of Hysterosalpingography. *J. Obst. & Gynaec. Brit. Emp.*, 67: 663, 1960.

Palmer, A.: Ethiodol Hysterosalpingography for the Treatment of Infertility. *Fertil. & Steril.*, 11: 311, 1960.

Riva, H. L., Hatch, R. P., and Breen, J. L.: Culdoscopy; An Analysis of 1500 Consecutive Cases. *Obst. & Gynec.*, 12: 610, 1958.

Rubin, I. C.: Uterotubal Insufflation. *Fertil. & Steril.*, 5: 311, 1954.

Youssef, A. F.: Colposcopy. The Results of Its Routine Employment in 1000 Gynaecological Patients. *J. Obst. & Gynaec. Brit. Emp*, 64: 801, 1957.

Hormone Therapy

Durham, W. C.: Progestational Steroid Requirements for Inducing and Maintaining Decidua in Women. *Fertil. & Steril.*, 12: 45, 1961.

Gemzell, C. A., Diczfalusy, E., and Tillinger, K.: Clinical Effect of Human Pituitary Follicle Stimulating Hormone (FSH). *J. Clin. Endocrinol. & Metab.*, 18: 1333, 1958.

Jones, G. S., Azez, Z., and Urbina, G.: Clinical Use of Gonadotropins in Conditions of Ovarian Insufficiency of Various Etiologies. *Fertil. & Steril.*, 12: 217, 1961.

Kotz, H. L., and Herrmann, W.: A Review of the Endocrine Induction of Human Ovulation. *Fertil. & Steril.*, 12: 96, 196, 299, 375, 493, 1961.

Tyler, E. T., and Olson, H. J.: Fertility Promoting and Inhibiting Effects of New Steroid Hormonal Substances. *J.A.M.A.*, 169: 1843, 1959.

Cortisone Therapy

Jeffries, W. McK.: Further Experience with Small Doses of Cortisone and Related Steroids in Infertility Associated with Ovarian Dysfunction. *Fertil. & Steril.*, 11: 100, 1960.

Jones, G. E. S., Howard, J. E., and Langford, H.: The Use of Cortisone in Follicular Phase Disturbances. *Fertil. & Steril.*, 4: 49, 1953.

Paldi, E., Fuchs, K., and Peretz, A.: Treatment of Sterility with Cortisone. *Fertil. & Steril.*, 11: 489, 1960.

West, C. D.: The Evaluation of the Role of the Adrenal Cortex in Infertility. *Fertil. & Steril.*, 10: 102, 1959.

Radiation Therapy

Israel, S. L.: Repudiation of Low-Dosage Irradiation of Ovaries. *Am. J. Obst. & Gynec.*, 76: 443, 1958.

Kaplan, I. I.: Treatment of Female Sterility with X-ray Therapy Directed to the Pituitary and Ovaries. *Am. J. Obst. & Gynec.*, 76: 447, 1958.

Muller, H. J.: Damage to Posterity Caused by Irradiation of the Gonads. *Am. J. Obst. & Gynec.*, 67: 467, 1954.

Neel, J. V.: Delayed Effects of Ionizing Radiation. *J.A.M.A.*, 166: 908, 1958.

Surgical Treatment

Allen, W. M., and Woolf, R. B.: Medullary Resection of Ovaries in Stein-Leventhal Syndrome. *Am. J. Obst. & Gynec.*, 77: 826, 1959.

Andrews, M. C., and Andrews, W. C.: Plastic Reconstruction of the Fallopian Tubes Using Polyethylene Catheters. *Am. J. Obst. & Gynec.*, 70: 1232, 1955.

Easterday, C. L., and Reid, D. E.: Incompetent Cervix in Repetitive Abortion and Premature Labor. *New England J. Med.*, 260: 687, 1959.

Evans, T. N., and Riley, G. M.: Polycystic Ovarian Disease (Stein-Leventhal Syndrome). Etiology and Rationale for Surgical Treatment. *Obst. & Gynec.*, 12: 168, 1958.

Green-Armytage, V. B.: Recent Advances in Surgery of Infertility. *J. Obst. & Gynaec. Brit. Emp.*, 66: 32, 1959.

Mutch, M. G., Jr.: Sterility and Tuboplasties; Critical Analysis of 42 Cases. *Fertil. & Steril.*, 10: 240, 1959.

Page, E. W.: Incompetent Internal Os of the Cervix Causing Late Abortion and Premature Labor. Technique for Surgical Repair. *Obst. & Gynec.*, 12: 509, 1958.

Steinberg, W.: Treatment of the Cervical Factor in Sterility. *Internat. J. Fertil.*, 2: 71, 1957.

Artificial Insemination

Behrman, S. J.: Artificial Insemination. *Fertil. & Steril.*, 10: 248, 1959.

Mastroianni, L., Jr., Laberge, J. L., and Rock, J.: Appraisal of the Efficacy of Artificial Insemination with Husband's Sperm and Evaluation of Insemination Technics. *Fertil. & Steril.*, 8: 260, 1957.

Pommerenke, W. T.: Artificial Insemination: Genetic and Legal Implications. *Obst. & Gynec.*, 9: 189, 1957.

Potter, R. G., Jr.: Artificial Insemination by Donor; Analysis of 7 Series. *Fertil. & Steril.*, 9: 37, 1958.

Chapter 29

Investigation and Treatment
of the Male Factor in Sterility

What Information Can Be Gathered from Interviewing and Examining the Male?

The pattern of history-taking closely follows that used in the woman. Age is less of a factor in male fertility. Many males maintain their ability to produce healthy, active sperm until they are well along in years.

THE PAST HISTORY is important in its relation to the patient's general health of the moment. Any severe constitutional disease, such as tuberculosis, cardiorenal disease, nephritis, gastric ulcer or hepatitis that was present in the past, may have a direct bearing on the male's present ability to produce healthy spermatozoa. Any acute infection in the past accompanied by a high fever may have damaged the testicular seminiferous tubules and permanently affected spermatogenesis. This is particularly true of mumps, gonorrhea, streptococcal infections, pneumonia and tuberculosis. The infection could have been either local or systemic. Local infections which produce suppuration will create a deficiency in the production of spermatozoa in proportion to their severity. Damage both to the testicular interstitial tissue and seminiferous tubules can also follow any trauma which injures the blood supply. If the hemorrhage is sufficiently severe, degenerative changes follow to the point of atrophy. The same atrophy can result from the pressure of a large hernia or varicocele. Similar testicular damage may occur from blood vessel trauma incidental to the repair of a hernia or varicocele.

Exposure to x-radiation given for skin disease in and around the scrotum can affect spermatogenesis adversely. High testicular temperature caused by congenital defects such as cryptorchidism, occupation or tight clothing tends to produce degeneration in the seminiferous tubules and defective spermatogenesis. A history of prostatitis, either specific or nonspecific, is extremely important, since the sperm, though produced normally, may not be properly conditioned because of disturbed prostatic or seminal vesicle secretions. It may be well to question the patient about neurologic symptoms such as headaches, nervous disorders or vertigo, particularly if there has been a history of severe head injury with loss of consciousness. Residual damage to the pituitary or hypothalamus could be present.

PRESENT STATUS.   Occupational hazards in the life of the male are many. Some affect spermatogenesis adversely. Any job held either now or in the past which exposed the patient to radiation effects, such as employment as an x-ray technician, electronic worker and radar operator, or exposure to inorganic forms of lead may interfere with the normal production of sperm. The same may be said of occupations that involve working in extremes of hot or cold, such as stokers, bakers, athletes and truck drivers. Many of these occupations directly affect spermatogenesis, but a greater deficiency will be noted in the group whose work calls for a considerable expenditure of nervous energy. Overwork can be a factor, but the effect is compounded by jobs associated with abnormal tension.

The present state of health is important. There can be little doubt that the ability to produce an adequate quantity of healthy sperm depends in part on a sound state of physical and mental health. Many men in a debilitated condition, if highly fertile from the beginning, can continue to produce normal sperm. Nevertheless some men are subfertile because of their basic equipment, and their deficiencies are accentuated by the habits which are a part of their daily existence.

HABITS.   When a couple has been unable to conceive, it may be well to look into their everyday living habits. Though there is no direct proof, the excessive use of *tobacco* can influence spermatogenesis. This may operate through its effect on general health, with less evidence that the gonad is influenced. Men, particularly those who have indoor jobs that create nervous tensions, have been restored to normal sperm production by restricting the use of cigarettes. This is less true for pipe and cigar smokers, but there can be no question that any male who is partner to a sterility problem will increase his contribution appreciably by practicing moderation in his use of tobacco.

Alcohol consumption plays an even larger role in influencing spermatogenesis, for there is ample evidence that both acutely and chronically alcoholic persons have a lower fertility index than abstainers. Again, this may not influence a male of high fertility, but it does operate when sperm production is borderline. The effect of alcohol is probably general, but there appears to be a local gonadal influence as well. Moderation in the use of alcohol should be practiced by the subfertile male. It may be wise to try to get some idea why the male drinks. If the reasons are psychogenic, a little alcohol may provide tension release and a more normal approach to the sexual act. The general state of health can be influenced by exercise, vacations and dietary habits.

EXERCISE.   Many men settle down into a sedentary existence after marriage, though they may have been very active before. Conversely, the athletically inclined male may throw himself violently into work and activities for which he is improperly conditioned and thereby overdo the exercise. A moderate amount of exercise should be encouraged in both partners.

VACATIONS.   These should provide an emotional release, if properly oriented. The more his work involves mental strain and fatigue, the longer a man's vacation should be. Under the stress of competition for the dollar which now motivates many people, it is not uncommon to find that the male has taken little or no vacation for years. When he has taken time off, he tends to spend the vacation doing the same things he does during his regular working days. Relaxation and a complete change of scene as well as type of activity should be sought.

DIET.   Many young men, particularly those who try to carry on extracurricular work while going to college, have a nutritional problem. Their infertility is compounded by nervous tension combined with an inadequate caloric and vitamin intake. The diet should be reasonably balanced with adequate protein content.

Under the stress of work many men will eat little breakfast or lunch and concentrate on the evening meal. It is far better to eat smaller amounts of food at regular intervals. The daily food intake should include a glass of milk, fresh fruit, vegetables, meat or fish, at least one egg, salad and cereal. Along with this there should be an adequate intake of vitamins, particularly A, B and E. If lacking in the diet, they should be supplied in supplemental forms. Vitamin therapy is simply one adjunct to dietary intake and affects spermatogenesis through the medium of nutrition.

OTHER FACTORS.   It may be well to question tactfully the proficiency of the male in the *technique of intercourse*. Some men, depleted by their occupation or manifesting psychogenic tendencies, suffer from impotence and premature ejaculation. Some will be taking hormones to correct their inadequacies. In most instances gland preparations or testosterone taken to increase the libido or sperm production either does nothing or actually depresses sperm production. Testosterone, if taken long enough, even in small quantities, will produce azospermia. Much can be accomplished through reassurance and instruction. If the psychogenic elements are deep-seated, a psychiatrist may be called in consultation. Instruction in the technique of intercourse may be rewarding, particularly if interrogation reveals that the male has little concept of what it is all about. His own clumsiness may account for dyspareunia in the female and unsatisfactory performance of the sex act. This may be of basic importance to the subfertile couple.

The frequency and timing of intercourse have been discussed for the female partner and need only be repeated for the instruction of the male.

PHYSICAL EXAMINATION.   *General physical examination* in the male is chiefly concerned with any evidence that may indicate an endocrine imbalance. Faulty spermatogenesis may be attributed directly to inadequate endocrine function. The majority of endocrine defects are congenital and should be evident in the adolescent growth period. If the disturbances are minimal in the adult, it may not be easy to recognize them from physical examination or laboratory study. It has been said that the time to diagnose and correct endocrine disturbances is in adolescence, for it may be too late to do much about it by the time the child becomes adult. The physician who unwisely counsels the family to let nature take its course in the hope that the defect will correct itself with time does the patient and family a disservice. Early diagnosis and treatment are important. The most dramatic example of need for early correction is seen in the problem of the undescended testicle, whether unilateral or bilateral.

What Is the Clinical Evidence for Endocrine Dysfunction?

Most severe endocrine disturbances present stigmata that can be recognized on general examination. There are all degrees of hypogonadism, for example. If the process begins before puberty, evidence of the defect is obvious. When it begins after puberty, the variations from the normal are less dramatic, and the only indication of endocrine failure may be deficient spermatogenesis. The male with basic hypogonadism sometimes will show, in addition to the lack of development in gonads and secondary sex characteristics, an overgrowth of the long bones and a fat distribution simulating that of the female, particularly in its concentration about the hips.

Another striking characteristic is a scanty growth of hair in the pubic, axillary and facial areas. One should ask when the patient first started to shave. This could be a lead in tracing the endocrine disturbance back to adolescence. It is interesting to note the extent of recession of hair in the temporal areas of the scalp. Though scanty hair distribution is noted in other areas, the hypogonad or eunuchoid patient does not show this bitemporal alopecia. Baldness may be an indication of virility.

Malfunctions of the thyroid gland, both in excess and in deficiency, are common in men with infertility problems. The clinical aspects of hyperthyroidism are clearly evident on physical examination. A more common defect is on the side of inadequate production of thyroid hormone. The male with well developed hypothyroidism may present the clinical picture of myxedema coupled with obesity, dry skin and coarse hair. There is usually a history of easy fatigue and intolerance to cold. Many males with a less well established hypothyroid state will have a depressed basal metabolism without much in the way of symptoms. Since adequate thyroxin or its end-product is essential to maximal cell function of the target organs, an evaluation of thyroid function is part of the investigation of the infertile male, regardless of symptoms. Replacement is indicated whenever the sperm count is reduced and thyroid function is low.

Examination of the External and Internal Genitals

This is the most important part of the examination. With the patient in the recumbent position the genitalia should be inspected and palpated. In examination of the penis one should observe the size, as well as any evidence of hypospadias or scars that would suggest previous venereal infection. Any urethral discharge should be noted and examined microscopically and bacteriologically. The size of the scrotum and the position of the testes within it should be recorded. One or both testicles may lie within the inguinal canal or high up in the scrotum. The size, consistency and proper rotation of the testes are also important to observe. If the testis is abnormally large, transillumination of the scrotum may reveal a hydrocele with a normal or small testis. Any tumor of the testis should be excised and examined pathologically. The epididymis must be palpated and evaluated for any induration or swelling that might suggest the presence of a spermatocele or a residuum of tuberculosis or gonorrhea. The vas deferens is best felt with the patient lying down. In some instances it is absent on one side or the other. Any beading felt along its course raises a suspicion of previous gonorrheal infection.

The accessory sex glands, chiefly the prostate and seminal vesicles, are palpated by rectal examination. This can best be done by having the patient lean forward over the table with the forearms resting on the table-top. The examination should be performed gently with a well lubricated gloved finger. The patient is provided with a glass slide to collect any discharge from the penis during the exploration of the seminal vesicle and prostate regions. After inspection of the anal opening for any hemorrhoids or fissures in ano the examining finger is inserted into the anal canal. Just within the anal sphincter one might palpate two firm nodules on either side. These are the so-called Cowper's glands. They are never palpable unless diseased. As the finger passes higher up along the anterior wall of the rectum the prostate is palpated. This should be gently examined for any areas of induration that would suggest prostatic infection. If the seminal vesicles, which are located in close proximity to either side of the prostate and just above it, are indurated, they are probably involved either in an interstitial vesiculitis or perivesiculitis. If they are distended, the seminal vesicles may be felt, but unless they are diseased they are usually not palpated as a distinct entity.

With the exploration completed the examination concludes by gently massaging the prostate and seminal vesicles and stripping the prostate from above, downward and inward. Any fluid escaping from the penis should be collected on a slide and examined microscopically for the presence of red or white blood cells, spermatozoa and other cells. It is difficult to distinguish between seminal vesicular secretion and that obtained from the prostate. Practically, it makes little difference, for infection in one will produce infection in the other. It is possible that no secretion will be obtained on the first examination, and the test should be repeated on subsequent visits. Usually a paucity of secretion is found in the subfertile patient, but definite conclusions cannot be made without repeated tests. After thorough microscopic examination of the wet slide it should be sent for gram stain and laboratory appraisal.

Routine Laboratory Examinations

These should be done for screening purposes. The minimal tests required are a blood serologic examination, a complete blood cell count and sedimentation rate, urinalysis, blood urea nitrogen, blood sugar and finally a basal metabolic rate or other test of thyroid function. If the examination discloses any evidence of faulty endocrine function, one may elect to do a urinary FSH, 17-ketosteroid examination or blood glucose tolerance test, together with x-ray studies of the sella turcica and a careful examination of the visual fields.

SEMEN ANALYSIS.   If no abnormalities are observed, the key test comes in obtaining semen for complete study. This specimen may be obtained by masturbation and collection of the ejaculate in a clean dry bottle with an adequate stopper. Care must be taken that none is spilled, for an estimate of the total volume is important. It must be examined within two hours of the time of collection. The bottled specimen is a far better method of collection than that with a condom, which is common practice. The material may be transported at normal temperature, and efforts to keep it at body temperature are cumbersome and unnecessary.

It is customary to have the male refrain from intercourse for five days before the specimen is collected. Some investigators prefer to examine the ejaculate without a preliminary period of abstinence, feeling that this most nearly approximates the regular demands placed on the functioning testes. If either no sperm or defective spermatozoa are found, the test is repeated after five days, during which the patient refrains from intercourse. The test performed in this manner will give effective evidence of the length of time required for the patient to restore the sperm to their most effective state.

The sperm are then analyzed to determine whether there is (1) adequate volume with normal viscosity. There should be at least 2.5 cc. total volume. The viscosity is checked with a bacteriologic loop. Any increase in viscosity should be considered abnormal. (2) A sufficient quantity of sperm per cubic centimeter of ejaculate. The minimal number of sperm required for initiation of pregnancy has not been established, but it is customary to accept the figure of 60 million per cubic centimeter. (3) Adequate motility and progression of the sperm. At least 40 to 50 per cent of the spermatozoa should be vigorous and active. (4) An overabundance of abnormal forms. It is possible for pregnancy to occur when there are as many as 30 or 40 per cent of abnormal forms, but the male would have to balance this by adequacy in other essential requirements. Usually normal males will have about 10 per cent of spermatozoa which do not have the proper conformation. By and large, the more abnormal forms present, the less the likelihood that pregnancy will follow.

A true estimate of testicular function should not be made on the basis of examination of a single specimen or upon finding a deficiency in one of the normal requirements listed above. Repeated examinations are needed at regular intervals. A final evaluation of the sperm will depend on a combination of factors. A diminished volume of sperm with a normal count and motility may be effective if there are not too many abnormal forms. On the other hand, a specimen with normal numbers of sperm should be regarded as unlikely to initiate a pregnancy if the motility is poor and the number of abnormal forms is high.

When Does One Do a Testicular Biopsy, and What Information Can Be Gathered?

Referring back to the physiology of conception, it is obvious that the male who has a complete absence of sperm has a defect either in the testes, where the spermatozoa are produced, or in the conducting system, namely, the epididymis or vas deferens. Bilateral testicular biopsies will pinpoint the source of the trouble. They also provide useful information in patients who have an inadequate number of sperm because of congenital defects, degenerative or inflammatory lesions. This is a simple procedure which may be carried out in the office or outpatient clinic under local anesthesia. The patient is immediately mobilized, and no time is lost from his work.

If the testicular biopsy specimens reveal microscopic evidence of normally functioning seminiferous tubules, the testes are obviously not at fault, and search for obstructive lesions must be made in the epididymis or vas deferens. As noted in the discussion on physical examination, such lesions can often be felt. In a certain number of cases the vas deferens may be congenitally absent. The obstructive lesion may be overcome in certain instances by anastomosing the duct above and below the obstruction.

When the biopsy specimens show a complete lack of testicular germinal epithelium, there is no form of therapy, hormonal or otherwise, that will overcome the sterility problem, which must be considered absolute. Three common types of defective spermatogenesis are observed in biopsy specimens: (1) In certain instances normal tubules lined by the supporting Sertoli cells are present, but there is a complete absence of spermatogenic cells. (2) In others spermatogonia, primary and secondary spermatocytes appear normal, but the final stages of development to spermatids and spermatozoa do not take place (Fig. 29–1, *A*). (3) Finally, in the so-called Klinefelter syndrome the tubules are completely atrophic and hyalinized, with absent spermatogenic activity. Compensatory or idiopathic apparent hyperplasia of the Leydig cells is common in this syndrome, and the patient frequently has gynecomastia (Fig. 29–1, *B*). Usually the testes are small, but an identical biopsy appearance may be found in patients who have normal-sized testicles and no gynecomastia.

Degenerative lesions of the testicle are usually caused by circulatory damage, toxic effects of acute infection, wasting diseases, nutritional deficiency and endocrine defects that have appeared after the testicle developed beyond the stage of puberty. The degree of damage varies widely and is proportional to the severity of the exciting cause. All active seminiferous tubules may have become entirely hyalinized, or the degeneration may appear only in patches. The latter is claimed to be common after mumps. It may be possible in certain instances to correct the factor producing the

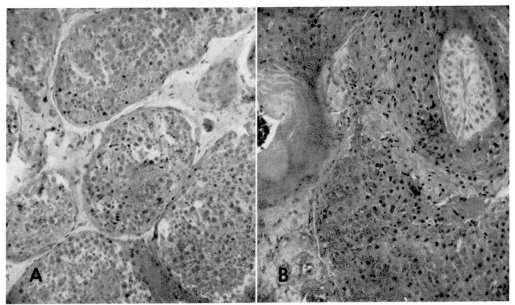

Fig. 29-1. *A*, Abnormal testicular tubules with so-called maturation arrest of spermatogenesis. The prespermatogonia and spermatogonia divide normally, but many miotic divisions result in cells that degenerate and provide the small dark masses of nuclear debris. Mature spermatozoa are rare. *B*, The testicular tubules in Klinefelter's syndrome are either completely hyalinized or lined only by Sertoli cells. The sheets of interstitial cells of Leydig shown may be obvious because of the atrophy of tubules rather than true hyperplasia.

degeneration and bring about a certain degree of restoration of tubular activity, provided the cause is recognized sufficiently early. An example of this would be the repair of a large hernia or varicocele that caused pressure on the blood supply to the testis. Degenerative changes in the testis are not as basic or irreversible as those caused by developmental failure.

Inflammatory lesions also appear after the testicle has fully matured. Rarely is the testicle damaged by infection in infancy or childhood. The worst damage is produced by fibrosis that follows cellular infiltration and edema as a normal histologic sequence. All degrees to the point of total atrophy are seen.

It is at once apparent that the simple performance of testicular biopsies gives the maximal amount of information, with the least expenditure of time and money, in attempting to evaluate the male factor in sterility. Either the sterility is absolute and no further investigation of either male or female need be done, or the direction the therapy should take is made clearer. Artificial insemination may provide an answer if the male partner is incurably sterile.

TREATMENT OF MALE INFERTILITY

The same general factors that apply in the female are operative in the male. The basic fault in the male lies either in inadequate production of sperm or in their transmission. The testicular biopsy will differentiate between the two.

DEFICIENT SPERMATOGENESIS. Instruction in the frequency and timing of intercourse is essential and often rewarding. Correction of abnormal living habits, occupations which may contribute to the sterility problem, or dietary inadequacies are all of basic importance if spermatogenesis is to improve in any given individual. If any latent source of infection is present, it should be eradicated. Chronic disorders such as anemia, diabetes mellitus, disturbed liver function or kidney infection may influence spermatogenesis. Whenever possible, the patient should be brought into the best possible health.

Improvement in any deficiency of sperm production will be more profoundly influenced by these measures than by the use of endocrine therapy. Except for the use of thyroid extract, there is little evidence that spermatogenesis is influenced to any great extent. It has been suggested that those who theoretically were improved by hormone therapy were either undergoing spontaneous regeneration or varied in their sperm production normally. The use of the pituitary hormones, pregnant mare's serum or chorionic gonadotropin alone or in combination should be reserved for the male who is obviously either eunuchoid or hypogonadal.

The use of testosterone in the patient who is found to have an inadequate number of spermatozoa has been advocated and has received some enthusiastic support in recent years. By design testosterone propionate (75 mg.) is injected 3 times a week in doses of 25 mg. each until the spermatozoa disappear entirely from the specimen of semen. The testosterone is then discontinued in the hope that a rebound phenomenon will occur. This is the equivalent of putting the ovary to rest by substituting estrin and progestin therapy. The increased production of sperm by the testes when the testosterone is omitted is more readily measured in the male than ovarian rebound in the female. The beneficial effects, if any, must be on the basis of the rebound, for there is little evidence that testosterone does anything but depress spermatogenesis.

What Treatment Can Be Offered When Sperm Transmission Is Inhibited?

SURGERY.   Earlier in the discussion of the various factors which might influence the transmission of sperm we noted that such pathologic conditions as spermatocele, hydrocele, varicocele or the presence of a large hernia were frequently implicated. Surgical removal or correction of these entities is obviously indicated.

When there has been a past history of gonorrhea, and physical examination reveals an indurated epididymis on both sides, the cause of the azospermia may be due to obstruction at these points. If testicular biopsy shows normal sperm production, one may elect to perform a short-circuiting operation (epididyvasotomy) around the obstruction, particularly when it is found at the lower epididymal pole. Approximately one third of such operations at present may be considered successful. The group that failed at least had the satisfaction of knowing that everything possible has been done to remedy a situation which otherwise could only be regarded as hopeless.

Local abnormalities of the penis such as hypospadias, epispadias and stricture of the urethra can be corrected by either surgery or dilatation. Attempts to wash out the seminal vesicles by scrotal vasotomy or catheterization of the ejaculatory ducts by endoscopy have not been very successful.

NONOPERATIVE TREATMENT.   One of the most satisfactory and rewarding methods of therapy for azospermia or oligospermia due to obstruction is simply a properly performed periodic prostatic massage. The massage should be done twice weekly for several months. The duration will depend on how long it takes to reduce the number of white cells to about ten to fifteen per high-power field, or until the urine specimen after massage is free of shreds of mucus. The results are better when the obstruction is due to mucus rather than infection. The massage is best carried out when the bladder is full. For the first few times the massage may be painful.

REFERENCES

Charney, C. W.: Treatment of Male Infertility with Large Doses of Testosterone. *J.A.M.A.*, 160: 98, 1956.

Cohen, M. R., and Stein, I. F.: Sperm Survival at Estimated Ovulation Time; Comparative Morphology and Relative Male Fertility. *Fertil. & Steril.*, 2: 20, 1951.

Farris, E. J.: The Number of Motile Spermatozoa as an Index of Fertility in Man. A Study of 406 Semen Specimens. *J. Urol.*, 61: 1099, 1949.

Farris, E. J., and Colton, S. W.: Effects of L-Thyroxine and Liothyronine on Spermatogenesis. *J. Urol.*, 79: 863, 1958.

Harrison, G. A., and Harris, R.: Thermoregulation of the Testis at High Temperature. Studies on Fertility. *Proc. Soc. Study of Fertility* (Oxford), 8: 76, 1956.

Heckel, N. J.: Production of Oligospermia in Man by Use of Testosterone Propionate. *Proc. Soc. Exper. Biol. & Med.*, 40: 658, 1939.

Heller, C. G., and Maddock, W. O.: Use of Androgens in Men. *Bull. New York Acad. Med.*, 24: 179, 1948.

Horrax, T. M.: Liothyronine in the Treatment of Male Infertility. *J. Urol.*, 80: 49, 1958.

Howard, R. P., Sniffen, R. C., Simmons, F. A., and Albright, F.: Testicular Deficiency. A Clinical and Pathologic Study. *J. Clin. Endocrinol.*, 10: 121, 1950.

MacLeod, J., and Gold, R. Z.: The Male Factor in Fertility and Infertility. II. Spermatozoon Counts in 1000 Men of Known Fertility and in 1000 Cases of Infertile Marriage. *J. Urol.*, 66: 436, 1951.

Idem: The Male Factor in Fertility and Infertility. Effect of Continence on Semen Quality. *Fertil. & Steril.*, 3: 297, 1952.

Miller, D.: The Importance of Simultaneous Evaluation of the Husband and Wife in Sterile Marriage. *Am. J. Obst. & Gynec.*, Supp., 61A: 711, 1951.

Shettles, L. B.: The Relation of Nutrition to Spermatogenesis. Proceedings of 3rd Annual Conference on Sperm. Biol. *J. Nat. Conf. Maternal Health*, 1942, p. 28.

Idem: Observations on Human Spermatozoa. *Bull. Sloane Hosp. for Women*, 6: 48, 1960.

Simmons, F. A.: Diagnosis and Treatment of Infertile Male. Nelson Monographs, Arch. Surg. New York, Nelson & Sons, 1951.

Sohval, A. R.: Anatomy and Endocrine Physiology of the Male Reproductive System; in J. T. Velardo, ed.: *Endocrinology of Reproduction*. New York, Oxford University Press, 1959, p. 243.

Swyer, G. I. M., Tulloch, W. S., and Boyd, R. H.: Discussion on Male Infertility. *Proc. Roy. Soc. Med.*, 46: 835, 1953.

Teitelbaum, H. A., and Gantt, W. H.: Effect of Starvation on Sperm Count and Sexual Reflexes. *Science*, 124: 363, 1956.

Williams, W. W.: *Sterility: The Diagnostic Survey of the Infertile Couple*. Springfield, Mass., the author, 1953.

Zanartu, J., and Hamblen, E. C.: Effect of Oligospermia in Insemination and Fecundation in Fertile Women. *Fertil. & Steril.*, 11: 248, 1960.

Chapter 30

Habitual Abortion

THE NEXT main problem germane to the discussion of sterility is concerned with inability to maintain a pregnancy once it is initiated. This may be due to (1) faulty germ plasm of either the sperm or ovum, or perhaps both; (2) a faulty environment within the uterus which prevents proper implantation of the fertilized ovum; or (3) finally, biochemical alterations within the endometrium that interfere with adequate nourishment of the implanted conceptus. This sterility is relative, for the beginning of pregnancy has been achieved, but the pregnancy terminates in a spontaneous abortion either early or later in its course. The patient never is able to deliver a normal viable infant.

Pregnancy may cease after the premature delivery of an infant that never became viable at any point, or go through to term only to produce a stillbirth. These two problems fall within the scope of the discussion of sterility, since the basic factors are somewhat akin to the elements that produce early abortion. Nevertheless, they more rightfully belong in the field of obstetrics and will not be discussed here.

Within the province of the gynecologist we find the following entities: (*a*) habitual abortion, (*b*) threatened abortion, (*c*) incomplete abortion, (*d*) inevitable abortion, (*e*) missed abortion, and (*f*) ectopic pregnancy. All usually terminate pregnancy early from the three basic causes mentioned above.

It has been said that the incidence of spontaneous abortions among all pregnancies rests somewhere in the neighborhood of 10 per cent. The majority among these will undoubtedly be due to random factors which are not necessarily repetitive in subsequent pregnancies. A pessimistic attitude toward the likelihood of abnormal gestation in a succeeding pregnancy is therefore unjustified. Normal delivery of a live healthy infant may be expected in 85 per cent of cases after one spontaneous miscarriage and roughly in 60 per cent after a second repeated similar incident. One may be reasonably accurate in assuming that a great part of the failure is due to chance. Recurrent elements begin to appear when three or more successive pregnancies terminate in spontaneous abortions. In this group one should seek a basic defect, for if this is uncorrected, less than 25 per cent of the women with this kind of obstetrical history can be expected to deliver a normal child in the next pregnancy. Such a patient would be regarded as suffering from *habitual abortion*. It is in this group that one should be energetic in seeking the cause and instituting treatment.

What Part Do Defects of Germ Plasm Play?

The likelihood of initiation and maintenance of a pregnancy increases when both ovum and spermatozoa are relatively healthy. Fortunately nature is very selective about the fitness of the embryo and apparently tends to discard undesirable fertilized ova. When the products of abortion are studied pathologically, 90 per cent will show defects of sufficient magnitude to make continued viability of the embryo impossible. Those not eliminated early frequently continue to grow for a time, but the pregnancy usually terminates before the fetus becomes clinically viable, owing to its gross developmental abnormalities.

In the male the defect in the germ plasm may be forecast by observing a number of abnormal forms present on examination of the semen. If the ejaculate contains more than 40 to 50 per cent of abnormal sperm heads, the pregnancy usually ends in spontaneous abortion. The factors which bear on faulty spermatogenesis in the male have been discussed previously. In addition to the local and systemic factors that influence the production of healthy sperm, one should pay particular attention to thyroid function. There is little question that hypothyroidism even in mild degree does influence spermatogenesis adversely.

It is not quite as easy to detect defective ova in the female, for those that are not fertilized cannot ordinarily be recovered. We have no way of knowing which are bad and which are good. Earlier we noted that a higher percentage of abnormal pregnancies appears in adolescence when the ovaries are immature and in the forties when the influence of the endocrines is on the wane. In either case the fault may be ascribable to faulty ovogenesis. The incidence of spontaneous abortions due to defective germ plasm in the ova may be much higher than the usual estimate of

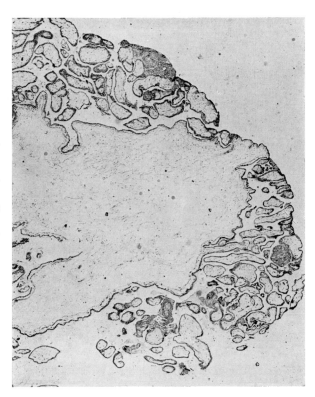

Fig. 30-1. A blighted ovum that was aborted and studied pathologically. The ovisac is empty except for proteinaceous fluid, and the embryo, if it ever existed, has been completely resorbed. The chorionic villi around the outside are avascular and partially degenerated. These are common findings in spontaneous abortion.

10 per cent, for undoubtedly many women abort without knowing it. Fertilized ova presenting pathologic evidence of germ plasm defects have been recovered from hysterectomy specimens in women who have not missed a period. The defect would seem to be in the ova rather than unsuitable environmental conditions within the uterus. Approximately half of all abortions are due to so-called blighted ova (Fig. 30–1).

Some part of the developmental defect in sperm or ova may be traced to genetic cause, but the greater portion may be due to faulty function of the endocrine system. The effect is chiefly noted in the endometrium, where deficient gonadal stimulation has prepared an inadequate bed for implantation of the conceptus, but ovogenesis is also profoundly influenced. One notes a high incidence of menstrual irregularity in the history of women subject to recurring abortion.

What Part Do Abnormal Uterine Conditions Play in Habitual Abortions?

In addition to union of healthy sperm and ovum the uterine environment must be favorable if the pregnancy is to survive the phase of implantation. Congenital or acquired deformities within the uterus are not conducive to the development of a normal pregnancy. We have discussed the relations of fibroids and polyps, particularly the submucous fibroid, to the problem of sterility. Though hidden, its presence may be suspected by the history of heavy menstrual bleeding and is confirmed by curettage or hysterosalpingography. Congenital defects such as bicornuate uterus or one presenting either partial or complete septation are discovered in the same way (Figs. 30–2, 30–3). The retroverted uterus is usually not a deterrent to pregnancy, but when repeated abortions occur in a patient who shows evidence of pelvic congestion from malposition of the uterus, it would be well to replace it in normal position and hold it there, as with a pessary.

In many instances the only sign that the uterine environment is unsuitable is the presence of clinical stigmata that suggest hypoplasia or underdevelopment in the uterus itself. Such a uterus may menstruate normally, but be poor soil for the maintenance of a pregnancy. Invariably there will be other evidence pointing to general lack of genital development. The cervix is usually long and conical and out of proportion to the size of the fundus, while the endometrial cavity and vagina are shallow. The underdevelopment reflects insufficient estrin stimulation. Pregnancy is unlikely in such a uterus unless exogenous estrin is supplied to supplement the amount pro-

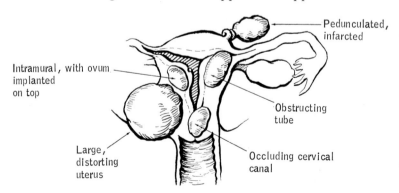

Fig. 30-2.   Five ways in which uterine fibroid tumors can interfere with pregnancy or contribute to abortion.

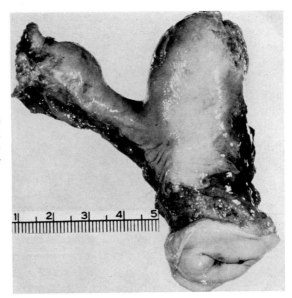

Fig. 30-3. A partially bicornuate uterus, congenitally malformed and often unable to support the development of a pregnancy to the stage of fetal viability, after premature delivery.

duced normally. The so-called infantile uterus can be made to hypertrophy and approach normal adult size on such a regimen. To maintain the pregnancy it may be necessary to continue with small doses of estrin when the uterus has previously shown signs of underdevelopment.

What Biochemical Factors Influence Implantation and Subsequent Nutrition of the Embryo?

In the earlier discussion on the physiology of menstruation we noted the histologic changes that occurred in the endometrium under the influence of the ovarian hormones in anticipation of the receipt of the impregnated ovum. The intrinsic metabolism of the endometrium is concerned with the preparation of a proper site for implantation of the ovum, and also with its nourishment once the trophoblastic cells invade its substance.

Continued proliferation of the trophoblastic cells which will eventually form the placenta and membranes depends on an adequate supply of carbohydrate in a form that can be readily assimilated. The demand is immediate after implantation, and the need continues through the early weeks of pregnancy. Proteins, fats, vitamins and inorganic materials are present in large quantities and are also essential, but the basic need is carbohydrate for glycolysis.

We have noted the preparation of the endometrium in anticipation of possible pregnancy early in the estrin phase of the menstrual cycle. By histochemical methods alkaline phosphatase can be found in the cells of the endometrial glands and the endothelial cells of the arterioles supplying the endometrium before one detects any glycogen in the cells. This is the enzyme previously concerned with breaking down the glycogen into the more readily utilizable glucose and fructose which the trophoblasts need in large quantities in the early phases of implantation. The concentration of alkaline phosphatase increases as the ovulation date approaches and pregnancy becomes imminent.

After ovulation and preceding implantation glycogen is mobilized from its position at the base of the endometrial cells lining the glands and is released into the lumens of the glands where the alkaline phosphatase by enzymatic action converts it into glucose and fructose. It is interesting to note that though alkaline phosphatase is found in abundance, glycogen is absent in the patient who has anovulatory cycles or microscopic evidence of hyperplasia. These findings are also common to the girl with a sterility problem. In some instances the histologic pattern approaches the normal, but the quantities of glycogen secreted and the amount of alkaline phosphatase are subnormal. In others, particularly those with histologic evidence of imperfect arteriolar development, adequate amounts of glycogen are found, but alkaline phosphatase is lacking.

When the intrinsic metabolism is adequate and sufficient nourishment is supplied, the embryo will continue to grow. Any factor that adversely influences the preparation of the endometrial bed or interferes with normal nutrition will create a barrier to subsequent pregnancy. We have noted that anemia, constitutional disease, acute or chronic illness and psychogenic factors, among others, may be responsible for repeated abortions in some or occasional abortions in others. It is not easy to decide in such cases whether sterility or abortion is due to germ plasm defect or improper environment. Approximately 70 per cent of patients who abort are said to show deficient endometrial carbohydrate metabolism. The most likely cause of repeated abortions can be traced to faulty function in the endocrine system. There appears to be an intimate correlation, for example, between a healthy endometrium and normal glycogenesis. Not only do insufficient pituitary stimulation and ovarian response produce an abnormal endometrial pattern, but also profound disturbances occur in carbohydrate metabolism.

Functional inadequacy of the endometrium may affect the development of the chorion or other parts of an immature placenta. One may find avascular and edematous young chorionic villi, together with lack of development and even degeneration of their trophoblastic cells. This in turn may result in the production of insufficient amounts of chorionic gonadotropin upon which the continued life of the corpus luteum depends. In most instances the growing embryo depends upon the proper function of the corpus luteum for at least ten weeks immediately after implantation. Despite the fact that pregnancy has occasionally continued when the corpus luteum has been removed surgically in the first two months after conception, nevertheless many more pregnancies have been interrupted by this maneuver. Eventually the growing placenta takes over the functions of the corpus luteum by secreting increasing amounts of estrins and progestins. The complete transfer of responsibility for the maintenance of pregnancy from the corpus luteum to the placenta usually takes place about the fourteenth week after fertilization. In certain women this transfer may occur earlier, as shown by failure of the patient to abort when the corpus luteum is removed.

As a result of endocrine malfunction and interference with the normal development of the placenta a vicious circle may develop. The failing chorionic gonadotropin is inadequate in quantity to sustain the corpus luteum upon which it temporarily depends for existence. The interplay of hormones in the maintenance of pregnancy is evident. The corpus luteum of pregnancy is responsible for the secretion of (1) estrin, which is responsible for the production and continued maintenance of an endometrium suitable for implantation of the impregnated ovum; (2) progestin, which creates within the endometrium a sufficient store of nourishment in a form that the growing embryo can use. Success in furthering growth of the young placenta also will depend in part on how well the thyroid has prepared the cells of the endometrial glands to carry out the intricate metabolic processes required to encourage embryonic implantation and growth. Adequate supply of a variety of hormones is necessary for the successful initiation and continuance of a pregnancy. It is not always easy to locate the fault when abortion occurs repeatedly.

Clinically, one gets some indication that abortion is imminent when the level of excretion of chorionic gonadotropin falls sharply. Temporary reductions may be compatible with continued growth of the embryo, but a progressive decline certainly indicates trouble which will probably lead to abortion. It is difficult to decide at times as to which is the cart and which the horse, for the decline in hormonal excretion may be due to a failure of corpus luteum function from other causes, rather than to the intrinsic metabolic defects of trophoblasts. The level of chorionic gonadotropin is assayed by injecting into a rabbit 5 cc. of the first morning specimen of urine. This is the Friedman test. Recordings are made upon the reaction of the rabbit ovary to the injected material. If the urine is of proper specific gravity, usually 1.020, a negative test would suggest death of the embryo, and a forecast of abortion can be made. A weakly positive reaction indicates trouble, for the amount of chorionic gonadotropin secretion is less than adequate, but it may still be possible to salvage the pregnancy by proper substitution therapy, in the form of either progestin or chorionic gonadotropin. Serum injection may provide a more accurate test.

Just as deficiency in chorionic gonadotropin indicates a pathologic implanted conceptus, so a drop or progressive decline in the level of sodium pregnanediol excretion suggests failure of corpus luteal function. The decline in the level of this metabolite of progestin often antedates the appearance of uterine bleeding and may be the first harbinger of impending abortion. The decline cannot be demonstrated in all patients who are about to abort, but a negative pregnanediol determination may be regarded as a pretty fair indicator that abortion is imminent.

The association of inadequate thyroid function with habitual abortion has been well documented. Approximately three quarters of patients so harassed will demonstrate thyroid deficiency. When thyroid function is measured by basal metabolic rate determinations, levels in the range of -10 to -20 are commonly found. Perhaps an estimation of the protein-bound iodine level in the serum may be a better index of thyroid gland function. Normally the level in pregnant women becomes elevated at the beginning of pregnancy, reaching levels in excess of 8 gammas, where it remains until pregnancy terminates. If there is no abrupt rise with the onset of conception, one may anticipate an early extrusion of the products of gestation.

TREATMENT OF HABITUAL ABORTION

The patient who has aborted more than once in successive pregnancies may be expected to do it again. The likelihood of successful pregnancy decreases sharply when the incident is repeated on three successive tries. Success in preventing further recurring episodes will depend in large part upon the seriousness of the underlying defects which may cause it and our ability to correct them. The contributing factors have been outlined in the preceding discussion.

The next concern is how to help the patient retain a pregnancy once conception has started. Measures that can be taken will be discussed in the order of their most practical application.

DIETARY DEFICIENCY.   There can be little doubt that the chances of successful pregnancy will be materially increased if the diet is adequate in proteins, carbo-hydrates, minerals and vitamins. Of the last, the two most important are vitamins C and E. There is experimental evidence that (1) vitamin C is important in enhancing the effect of progesterone upon the endometrium, and (2) levels of ascorbic acid in the pregnant woman reflect the voracious requirements of the growing embryo, particularly in the first eight weeks, for they are only slightly above the lower limits of normal during this period. No one seems to be very certain of the mechanism by which vitamin E influences threatened abortion. The rationale for its use is closely akin to the empirical use of thyroid in the absence of laboratory confirmation of any deficiency. Actually, our normal diets are rarely lacking in vitamin E, and no ap-preciable diminution is noted in pregnancy. Despite these observations, therapy for habitual abortion would be incomplete without vitamin E supplements. There is ample evidence from clinical experience that the use of alpha tocopherol acetate will raise the level of vitamin E in doses of 300 mg. daily and that vitamin E is important in maintaining a pregnancy in patients who give a history of habitual abortion.

THYROID SUPPLEMENT. Since nearly three quarters of the patients who suffer a repeated loss of early pregnancies show laboratory evidence of thyroid inadequacy, substitution therapy is of the utmost importance in prophylaxis. We have noted that adequate sensitization of the target organ cells by thyroxin is basic for the proper response to and utilization of gonadal hormones. It is thought to affect both the quality of the germ plasm and the intrinsic metabolism of the endometrium.

REGULATION OF LIVING HABITS. It is axiomatic that the patient who has repeated abortions must restrict some of her activities. Household duties are not contraindicated, but strenuous exercise and prolonged automobile trips should be outlawed. A moderate amount of activity within the realm of reason is far better than confinement to bed, unless pain or vaginal bleeding makes it advisable. For the same reason that strenuous exercise is contraindicated, sexual intercourse should be pro-hibited until the pregnancy is well established. In recent years much has been written on the psychosomatic aspects of repeated abortion. Retiring to bed without adequate reason can only accentuate the sense of apprehension which already is a part of the psychic background of habitual abortion.

HORMONAL SUBSTITUTION. Though much of the basic cause for habitual abortion can be traced to faulty endocrine function, the use of hormones to maintain pregnancy has not been very rewarding, unless a definite deficiency can be demon-strated. Whether the hormone is given in the form of estrin, chorionic gonadotropin or progesterone, the main consideration is to bolster a failing corpus luteum and aid progesterone production. To this end a regimen of *synthetic estrin* has been used with enthusiasm by some and reservation by others. Increasing doses of oral diethyl-stilbestrol are given, beginning in the sixth week of pregnancy. The initial dose of 5 mg. daily is increased by 5 mg. each 2 weeks until the patient is receiving 25 mg. daily. Thereafter doses are increased at a rate of 5 mg. each week until the thirty-fifth week, when the regimen terminates.

Progesterone substitution as a direct supplement seems most logical. It is effective as an intramuscular injection whenever a deficiency of progesterone, as measured by sodium pregnanediol excretion, can be established. One may choose to use progester-one substitution empirically. Theoretically, the endocrine defect is in progesterone production or utilization. Since the progesterone is usually given by injection every other day for four to five months, the therapy becomes tiresome as well as expensive. Oral preparations of progesterone to date have not been as dependable. Longer-acting synthetic progesterone-type preparations which are effective by the oral route are now available for clinical use.

Though the value of the supportive regimen may be challenged, it is logical and certainly does not cause harm. Actually, it is difficult to prove that progesterone substitution does any good. Most of the enthusiastic reports of successful progesterone therapy have come in patients who have had two successive spontaneous abortions, when the chance of a normal pregnancy later is still in the neighborhood of 60 per cent. With combinations of estrin and progesterone salvage of pregnancies in excess of 60 per cent has been reported. By and large, the other methods mentioned are more likely to produce fetal salvage than hormonal substitution.

REFERENCES

Etiology and Diagnosis

Benson, R. C., and Traut, H. F.: The Vaginal Smear as a Diagnostic and Prognostic Aid in Abortion. *J. Clin. Endocrinol.*, 10: 675, 1950.

Berle, B. B., and Javert, C. T.: Stress and Habitual Abortion. Their Relationship and the Effect of Therapy. *Obst. & Gynec.*, 3: 298, 1954.

Calderone, M. S.: *Abortion in the United States.* New York, Paul B. Hoeber, Inc., 1958.

Corner, G. W., and Bartelmez, G. W.: Early Abnormal Embryos of the Rhesus Monkey; in E. T. Engle, ed.: *Pregnancy Wastage.* Springfield, Ill., Charles C Thomas, 1953, p. 3.

Cross, R. G.: Repeated Abortions, Miscarriages, and Stillbirths. Value of Antisyphilitic Treatment. *Lancet*, 2: 754, 1946.

Davis, A.: 2665 Cases of Abortion. A Clinical Survey. *Brit. M.J.*, 2: 123, 1950.

Eastman, N. J.: *Williams Obstetrics.* 10th Ed. New York, Appleton, 1950.

Falls, F. H.: Pregnancy in the Bicornuate Uterus. *Am. J. Obst. & Gynec.*, 72: 1243, 1956.

Glass, B.: The Relation of Rh Incompatibility to Abortion. *Am. J. Obst. & Gynec.*, 57: 323, 1949.

Gutterman, H. S.: Progesterone Metabolism in the Human Female, Its Significance in Relation to Reproduction. *Rec. Progress Hormone Res.*, 8: 293, 1953.

Hertig, A. T., and Livingstone, R. G.: Spontaneous, Threatened and Habitual Abortion; Their Pathogenesis and Treatment. *New England J. Med.*, 230: 797, 1944.

Hertig, A. T., and Rock, J.: A Series of Potentially Abortive Ova Recovered from Fertile Woman Prior to the First Missed Menstrual Period. *Am. J. Obst. & Gynec.*, 58: 968, 1949.

Idem: Abortive Human Ova and Associated Endometria; in E. T. Engle, ed.: *Menstruation and Its Disorders.* Springfield, Ill., Charles C Thomas, 1950, p. 96.

Hon, E. H., and Morris, J. McL.: Gonadotrophin Titers in Disturbed Pregnancies. *Surg., Gynec. & Obst.* 101: 59, 1955.

Huber, C. P., Melin, J. R., and Vellios, F.: Changes in Chorionic Tissue of Aborted Pregnancy. *Am. J. Obst. & Gynec.*, 73: 569, 1957.

Hughes, E. C., Lloyd, C. W., Van Ness, A. W., and Ellis, W. T.: The Role of Endometrium in Implantation and Fetal Growth; in E. T. Engle, ed.: *Pregnancy Wastage.* Springfield, Ill., Charles C Thomas, 1953, p. 51.

ailer, J. W., and Longson, D.: Hormonal Changes during Pregnancy. *S. Clin. N. Amer.*, 37: 341, 1957.

Javert, C. T.: Repeated Abortion. Results of Treatment in 100 Patients. *Obst. & Gynec.*, 3: 420, 1954.

Idem: Stress and Habitual Abortion. *Obst. & Gynec.*, 32: 98, 1954.

Idem: *Spontaneous and Habitual Abortion.* New York, McGraw-Hill Book Company, Inc., 1957.

Jöel, C. A.: The Role of Spermatozoa in Habitual Abortion. *Fertil. & Steril.*, 6: 459, 1955.

Jones, H. W., Jr., Delfs, E., and Jones, G. E. S.: Reproductive Difficulties in Double Uterus. The Place of Plastic Reconstruction. *Am. J. Obst. & Gynec.*, 72: 865, 1956.

Kistner, R. W.: Habitual Abortion, General Consideration and Management. *Medical Sc.*, June 10, 1959, p. 782.

Mann, E. C.: Psychiatric Investigation of Habitual Abortion. Preliminary Report. *Obst. & Gynec.*, 7: 589, 1956.

Idem: The Role of Emotional Determinants in Habitual Abortion. *S. Clin. N. Amer.*, 37: 447, 1957.

Idem: Habitual Abortion, a Report in Two Parts on 160 Patients. *Am. J. Obst. & Gynec.*, 77: 706, 1959.

Masters, W. H., Maze, L. W., and Gilpatrick, T. W.: Etiological Approach to Habitual Abortion. *Am. J. Obst. & Gynec.*, 73: 1022, 1957.

Melinkoff, E.: Questionable Necessity of Corpus Luteum. *Am. J. Obst. & Gynec.*, 60: 437, 1950.

Randall, C. L., Baetz, R. W., Hall, D. W., and Birtch, P. K.: Pregnancies Observed in the Likely-to-Abort Patient with or without Hormone Therapy before or after Conception. *Am. J. Obst. & Gynec.*, 69: 643, 1955.

Shettles, L. B.: The Living Human Ovum. *Am. J. Obst. & Gynec.*, 76: 398, 1958.

Speert, H., and Guttmacher, A. F.: Frequency and Significance of Bleeding in Early Pregnancy. *J.A.M.A.*, 155, 712, 1954.

Tietze, C., Guttmacher, A. F., and Rubin, S.: Unintentional Abortion in 1479 Planned Pregnancies. *J.A.M.A.*, 142: 1348, 1950.

Tompkins, W. T.: Nutrition and Nutritional Deficiencies in Pregnancy; in C. B. Lull and R. A. Kimbrough, eds.: *Clinical Obstetrics.* Philadelphia, J. B. Lippincott Company. 1953, p. 163.

Venning, E. H.: Clinical Value of Hormone Estimations. *Brit. M. Bull.*, 11: 140, 1955.

Wall, R. L., Jr., and Hertig, A. T.: Habitual Abortion, a Pathologic Analysis of 100 Cases. *Am. J. Obst. & Gynec.*, 56: 1127, 1948.

Weil, R. J., and Stewart, L. C.: The Problem of Spontaneous Abortion. III. Psychosomatic and Interpersonal Aspects of Habitual Abortion. *Am. J. Obst. & Gynec.*, 73: 322, 1957.

Wengraf, F.: *Psychosomatic Approach to Gynecology and Obstetrics.* Springfield, Ill., Charles C Thomas, 1953.

Wislocki, G. B., Dempsey, E. W., and Fawcett, D. W.: Some Functional Activities of the Placental Trophoblast. *Obst. & Gynec. Surv.*, 3: 604, 1948.

Youssef, A. F.: The Uterine Isthmus and Its Sphincter Mechanism, a Radiographic Study. *Am. J. Obst. & Gynec.*, 75: 1320, 1958.

Zondek, B., and Goldberg, S.: Placental Function and Foetal Death. (1) Urinary Gonadotrophin Titration Test in Early Pregnancy. (2) Urinary Oestriol Excretion Test in Advanced Pregnancy. *J. Obst. & Gynaec. Brit. Emp.*, 64: 1, 1957.

Treatment

Baird, D.: Preventive Medicine in Obstetrics. *New England J. Med.*, 246: 561, 1952.

Barter, R. H., Dusabek, J. A., Riva, H. L., and Parks, J.: Surgical Closure of the Incompetent Cervix during Pregnancy. *Am. J. Obst. & Gynec.*, 75: 511, 1958.

Bos, C., and Cleghorn, R. A.: Psychogenic Sterility. *Fertil. & Steril.*, 9: 84, 1958.

Davis, M. E., and Plotz, E. J.: The Metabolism of Progesterone and Its Clinical Use in Pregnancy. *Rec. Progress Hormone Res.*, 13: 347, 1957.

Dieckmann, W. J., Davis, M. E., Rynkiewicz, L. M., and Pottinger, R. E.: Does the Administration of Diethylstilbestrol during Pregnancy Have Therapeutic Value? *Am. J. Obst. & Gynec.*, 66: 1062, 1953.

Easterday, C. L., and Reid, D. E.: The Incompetent Cervix in Repetitive Abortion and Premature Labor. *New England J. Med.*, 260: 687, 1959.

Fisher, J. J.: The Effect of Amputation of the Cervix Uteri upon Subsequent Parturition. A Preliminary Report of 7 Cases. *Am. F. Obst. & Gynec.*, 62: 644, 1951.

Goldzieher, J. W., and Benigno, B. B.: The Treatment of Threatened Recurrent Abortion. *Am. J. Obst. & Gynec.*, 75: 1202, 1958.

Jones, G. S.: Abortion and Corpus Luteum Deficiency. *Obst. & Gynec. Survey*, April, 1959.

Lash, A. F.: The Incompetent Internal Os of the Cervix; Diagnosis and Treatment. *Am. J. Obst. & Gynec.*, 79: 552, 1960.

Morgan, J., Hackett, W. R., and Hunt, T.: The Place of Progesterone in the Treatment of Abortion. *J. Obst. & Gynaec. Brit. Emp.*, 67: 323, 1960.

Rawlings, W. J., and Krieger, V. I.: Studies in the Prevention of Abortion Due to Corpus Luteum Deficiency. *M. J. Australia*, 2: 561, 567, 1958; in *Obst. & Gynec. Surv.*, 14: 240, 242, 1959.

Russell, K. P.: Thyroid Disease in Pregnancy, Its Detection and Management. *Obst. & Gynec.*, 8: 207, 1956.

Smith, O. W.: Diethylstilbestrol in the Prevention and Treatment of Complications of Pregnancy. *Am. J. Obst. & Gynec.*, 56: 821, 1948.

Smith, O. W., and Smith, G. Van S.: Use of Diethylstilbestrol to Prevent Fetal Loss from Complications of Late Pregnancy. *New England J. Med.*, 241: 562, 1949.

Speert, H.: Pregnancy Prognosis Following Repeated Abortion. *Am. J. Obst. & Gynec.*, 68: 665, 1954.

Starr, P.: Diagnosis and Treatment of Hypothyroidism. *Postgrad. Med.*, 17: 73, 1955.

Chapter 31

Threatened and Inevitable Abortion

THOUGH a defective pregnancy may be forecast by (1) a failure to maintain the morning body temperature, (2) decline in urinary sodium pregnanediol excretion, (3) an abrupt drop in the excretion of chorionic gonadotropin in advance of any clinical sign, the chief indication that abortion is imminent comes with the appearance of vaginal bleeding. It may appear for only a day as profuse bleeding or continue for weeks as vaginal spotting. The more persistent and profuse the vaginal bleeding, the greater the chance of abortion. At times the blood is bright and fresh, while at others dark brown blood is passed, suggesting that the process is of long duration and perhaps in relative abeyance at the moment. If the spotting persists for several weeks, the chances of saving the pregnancy decline rapidly.

Bleeding from the vagina usually precedes the onset of pain, particularly if the pregnancy is to terminate early. Occasionally they occur together. When pain is the first presenting symptom, late abortion is the rule. The combination of bleeding, during an established pregnancy, with cramplike pain suggests that the uterus is trying to extrude a defective gestation.

A distinction must be made, however, between a threatened and an inevitable abortion, in order that proper therapy be instituted early enough to do any good. We recognize that many abortions are due to a so-called blighted ovum, but not all are defective, and the early appearance of bleeding simply means that the pregnancy is threatened. Even though we know that a single episode involving loss of an increasing amount of bright blood is associated with abortion due to blighted ovum in over 90 per cent of cases, one can afford to temporize with therapy for a short time or until the hand is forced by excessive bleeding.

The distinction between a *threatened abortion* and an inevitable abortion is usually made by evaluation of the amount of blood loss in relation to the duration of the vaginal bleeding. If bleeding has been profuse or prolonged, in all probability the pregnancy is undesirable, and no effort should be made to save it. This is particularly true if speculum examination shows that the cervix has become either dilated or effaced. Abortion in such a patient is *inevitable* (Fig. 31–1).

One may wish to confirm the clinical impression by objective data. The simplest means of doing this is to check the morning body temperature. Failure to maintain the previously high level may suggest that all is not well with the embryo. The Aschheim-Zondek test on mice, the Friedman test on a rabbit or a frog test of the patient's urine may be helpful if the results are either negative or weakly positive. In this instance an insufficient amount of chorionic gonadotropin is being produced,

383

STAGES OF ABORTION

SYMPTOMS

TREATMENT

THREATENED ABORTION

Hemorrhage
  moderate,
  increasing
Cervix closed

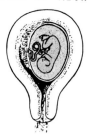

THREATENED ABORTION

Two days' bed rest

INEVITABLE ABORTION

Hemorrhage
  increasing
Uterus contracting
Cervix dilating
Placenta detaching

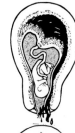

INEVITABLE ABORTION

Endocrine therapy
  useless
Replace blood
  as necessary

INCOMPLETE ABORTION

Hemorrhage
  increasing
Uterus contracting
Cervix dilated
Placenta
  detached,
  partially expelled,
  fragments remain.

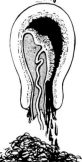

INCOMPLETE ABORTION

Pentothal sodium i.v.
Curettage with large,
  sharp curette
Ovum forceps
Pitocin drip i.v.
Send tissue for pathological
  examination for hydatid
  tissue, adenocarcinoma,
  sarcoma, polyps.

COMPLETE ABORTION

Hemorrhage
  may continue
Active labor
Cervix dilated
Fetus and placenta
  delivered
Fragments remain

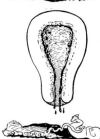

COMPLETE ABORTION

No packing needed
Curettage may be
  necessary

MISSED ABORTION

Decidual bleeding trapped
Uterus shrinks in size
Minor cramps
Placenta and fetus necrotic
Cervix not dilated
Poor response to oxytocics

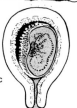

MISSED ABORTION

Wait for bleeding;
  then curettage
  or abdominal
  hysterotomy

Fig. 31-1.   Diagrammatic summary of various types of abortion and their treatment. Note that the cervix is not dilated in threatened or missed abortion, and the therapy is expectant. (Courtesy of Tenney and Little: *Clinical Obstetrics.*)

and abortion is inevitable. A decline in the excretion of sodium pregnanediol suggests progesterone deficiency, but does not differentiate threatened from inevitable abortion.

When the vaginal spotting or appearance of fresh bleeding is of recent date, short duration and moderate quantity, the growth pattern of the developing embryo has been compromised, and an abortion is threatened. It is still possible to salvage the fetus if active supportive measures are instituted promptly. This is particularly true if the cervix remains closed. The appearance of bleeding and colicky pain is a warning signal to a patient who has had repeated difficulty previously in trying to keep a pregnancy going.

To the patient who is having her first episode of vaginal bleeding in the early weeks of pregnancy, other factors than threatened abortion must be ruled out. A patient with localized abdominal cramps and bleeding could have an ectopic pregnancy. The bleeding may be coming from a cervical polyp or less commonly a cancer of the cervix. Inspection of the cervix and palpation of the uterus for size, contour, mobility and tenderness may give the clue to the proper diagnosis. Usually the size of the uterus will be compatible with the duration of pregnancy. The presence of a mass behind the cervix, which produces pain on motion, and a uterus smaller than one would expect for the duration of the pregnancy may make one suspicious of a possible ectopic gestation. An asymmetrical uterus could be a pregnancy in either a bicornuate or fibroid uterus.

How Do We Treat a Threatened Abortion?

When the decision has been made that the pregnancy can still be salvaged, immediate steps should be taken to support it in every possible way. The patient should be put to bed at once and kept there as long as the vaginal bleeding continues and for a short period after the bleeding has stopped. Since the patient is unquestionably apprehensive about her condition, she should be given mild sedatives. The cramps are usually not severe enough to require narcotics. Since the differential diagnosis between threatened abortion and ectopic pregnancy is a difficult one to make, heavy medication for pain is contraindicated. If the patient has obvious symptoms or a history suggesting thyroid deficiency, one may give thyroid extract substitution in 2-grain doses daily. In patients with threatened abortion estrin therapy has given satisfactory results, according to the reports of many gynecologists. The plan of therapy has been previously outlined (Chap. 30). Progesterone replacement in 25-mg. doses daily by injection may be used until the bleeding ceases. Thereafter it should be given three times weekly until the placenta has taken over hormonal control, usually about the fourth month of pregnancy. Of all the methods of therapy, bed rest, restricted activity and thyroid substitution seem to be as efficacious as any.

How Do We Treat Inevitable Abortion?

When the physician has decided that abortion is inevitable, and the pregnancy is sufficiently jeopardized to make any attempts to prolong it inadvisable, one may proceed conservatively and pursue a policy of watchful waiting. During the active bleeding phases the patient should be put to bed. Usually she will pass the products of conception without complication. If the bleeding is excessive, the patient should be hospitalized, and the uterus curetted. Many gynecologists prefer this method of handling inevitable abortion, feeling that an early and complete removal of the degenerating placental products results in fewer complications and a shorter recovery period.

What Is the Treatment of an Incomplete Abortion?

When the patient actually passes recognizable fetal tissue in the course of her episodes of cramps and uterine bleeding, she has an incomplete abortion. The cervix is dilated and usually effaced. Normally one expects that the patient who has completely extruded the products of her defective pregnancy will stop bleeding after two or three days. Incomplete evacuation of the uterus leads to profuse vaginal bleeding accompanied by gushing spells in recurring episodes for several weeks. Though the bleeding approaches the magnitude of vaginal hemorrhage at periodic intervals, it is rarely severe enough at any time to cause the patient to faint or to present a clinical picture of acute blood loss. The pregnant woman can withstand an astonishingly large loss of blood. Fatal hemorrhage is almost unknown. Replacement of lost blood, however, is a major factor in the treatment of incomplete abortion.

The other important factor is infection. Since the cervix is open, the mucus plug gone, and tissue has been extruded, the normal protection to bacterial invasion of the endometrial cavity has been lost, and the uterus should be regarded as potentially infected. The degree of infection will depend on local conditions plus the virulence of the invading organism, which is usually a streptococcus. When bacterial invasion is extreme, the patient will present all the symptoms of spreading uterine sepsis, such as prostration, local tenderness in the vaginal vaults, fixation of the uterus, nausea, vomiting and even chills and fever. This is the picture of a septic abortion with septicemia and will be discussed under pelvic inflammation (see Chap. 41).

At the other end of the spectrum the patient may have a mild degree of infection confined to the uterus as the result of invasion of the uterine cavity by saprophytic organisms which normally inhabit the vagina. Since the pregnancy has died, saprophytes attack the degenerating placenta and contribute to the dissolution of the remaining products of conception. Putrefaction sets in within the mass of tissue, which in a sense represents an intrauterine foreign body. Actually, the infection is localized in the degenerating placental remnants and is not therefore a true infection of the uterus itself. The patient may have a low-grade fever and even elevation of the pulse rate, but they are due to absorption of toxic substances from the putrefying uterine contents and not from true infection of the uterus.

The proper management of incomplete miscarriage depends on how extensive and prolonged the blood loss may be and the extent of the sepsis within or of the uterus.

1. If there is no fever and the blood loss is sporadic or minimal, the patient should be sent to bed and given a sedative. The most reassuring thing the physician can do to put the patient's mind at ease is to convince her that the present episode is pure accident and need not be repeated in her subsequent obstetrical life. Blood should be replaced by transfusion, according to need, as measured by hemoglobin and hematocrit determinations. Any obvious tissue protruding from the cervix should be removed. The majority of patients with uncomplicated incomplete miscarriage will pass the residual products of the degenerated placenta after a few days on this sort of regimen.

2. Should the process be prolonged or the vaginal bleeding assume dangerous proportions, it will be safer to empty the uterus by curettage, provided the evidence

of infection is minimal. It is of the utmost importance for the uterus to be emptied completely of its contents, for it is dangerous to re-enter the endometrial cavity after the initial curettage. To avoid the likelihood of stirring up infection within the uterus as a result of the manipulation, streptomycin and penicillin should be given both before and after the curettage. Bleeding may be heavy at the time the uterus is being emptied and may lead the surgeon into the trap of packing the uterus and vagina. This practice should be avoided. The best method of reducing the bleeding is complete evacuation of the uterus.

3. In the presence of fever, the treatment of incomplete abortion becomes confused. Some gynecologists and obstetricians prefer the conservative approach of bed rest and supportive therapy, while others advocate prompt surgical evacuation of the uterine contents. Following the conservative method of therapy, the patient is placed on bed rest and given antibiotic chemotherapy along with blood replacement. The treatment continues until either the patient completes the abortion or the temperature returns to normal and stays there for one to two weeks. Attempts are made to assist the uterus in getting rid of the products of conception by giving parenteral estrin, with the idea of sensitizing the uterus to contractions set up by the administration of quinine and ergotrate. In our opinion a medical regimen of this sort is unlikely to produce results, for the uterus has demonstrated no response to endogenous hormones. If the fetus has not been expelled after two weeks of bed rest without fever, the exponents of conservative management feel that the uterus can now be curetted with far less risk.

4. If there are no outward indications of a spread of infection beyond the confines of the uterus, the proponents of immediate active intervention believe that curettage can be performed with minimal morbidity and an infinitesimal mortality risk. This is based on the feeling that the fever is due to a saphrophytic infection of the retained products of conception and represents toxic absorption rather than true uterine infection. Chemotherapy with antibiotics is given both before and after evacuation. This method of handling the problem has become increasingly popular. It has the distinct advantage of ridding the uterus of its noxious contents early, before secondary infection can set in, and it does materially reduce the economic loss that must follow a prolonged bed rest and subsequent convalescence.

What Is the Management of Missed Abortion?

Occasionally after an initial episode of vaginal bleeding and lower abdominal cramps the symptoms subside and the threat of abortion seems to have passed. Unfortunately this may not be true, for sometimes the uterus does not continue to increase in size, as one would expect with a young viable embryo. In all probability the fetus has died. A drop in the basal body temperature or a negative pregnancy frog test of the urine will confirm the clinical impression. In most cases one can afford to let the uterus expel its contents when it will, provided the patient can adjust to the emotional strain of continuing to carry a dead fetus. If not, it will be better to empty the uterus by curettage.

There is another vital reason for considering emptying the uterus. The symptoms of missed abortion are identical with those of chorionepithelioma. One can afford to delay curettage only if the diagnosis of missed abortion is certain. Again, a pregnancy test of the urine repeated every two weeks will be helpful in making the differential diagnosis. The Friedman or frog test depends on the amount of chorionic gonadotropin produced by the trophoblast of the growing placenta. Recently quantitative studies to measure the excretion of chorionic gonadotropin have been carried out on male frogs and toads. The frog determinations are less accurate because of seasonal changes in sensitivity. The male toad of the variety Bufo marinus, on the other hand, shows a constant response throughout the year. When the values are high, the chances of the patient having a hydatidiform mole or choriocarcinoma are excellent, while low values indicate either abortion or ectopic pregnancy. In missed abortion there would be no gonadotropic activity. The problem of chorionepithelioma will be discussed later (see Chap. 33).

Testing for chorionic gonadotropin by means of newly available commercial antiserum may eventually supplant the pregnancy tests that utilize animals. The method is still too new to be certain of its accuracy and scope.

REFERENCES

Ainslie, W. H.: Treatment of Threatened Abortion. *Obst. & Gynec.,* 13: 185, 1959.

Baden, W. F., and Baden, E. E.: Cervical Incompetence: Repair during Pregnancy. *Am. J. Obst. & Gynec.,* 74: 241, 1957.

Barnes. L. W.: Urinary Excretion of Pregnanediol after Intravenous Administration of Progesterone in Threatened Abortion. *Am. J. Obst. & Gynec.,* 75: 53, 1958.

Bobrow, M. L., and Friedman, S.: Incomplete Abortion. A Twenty-Five Year Review of Cases Seen at a Large Municipal Hospital. *Am. J. Surg.,* 95: 938, 1958.

Borglin, N. E.: Missed Abortion. An Analysis of a 10 Year Series. *Acta Obst. et Gynec. Scandinav.,* 36: 512, 1957.

Diddle, A. W., O'Connor, K. A., Jack, R., and Pearse, R. L.: Evaluation of Bed Rest in Threatened Abortion. *Obst. & Gynec.,* 2: 63, 1953.

Eastman, N. J.: Therapeutic Abortion. *Obst. & Gynec. Survey,* August, 1958.

Gray, J. D., Tupper, C., and Rowse, J. A.: The Problem of Spontaneous Abortion. VII. Prematurity and Spontaneous Abortion. *Am. J. Obst. & Gynec.,* 78: 325, 1959.

Guterman, H. S., and Tulsky, A. S.: Observations on the Use of Progesterone in Threatened Abortion, with Special Reference to Pregnandiol Excretion as a Guide to Therapy. *Am. J. Obst. & Gynec.,* 58: 495, 1949.

Henry, J. S.: Some Biological Aspects of Spontaneous Abortion. *Am. J. Obst. & Gynec.,* 73: 1229, 1957.

King, A. G.: Threatened and Repeated Abortion. Present Status of Therapy. *Obst. & Gynec.,* 1: 104, 1953.

Singh, B. P., and Morton, D. G.: Blood Protein-Bound Iodine Determinations as a Measure of Thyroid Function in Normal Pregnancy and Threatened Abortion. *Am. J. Obst. & Gynec.,* 72: 607, 1956.

Wide, L., and Gemzell, C. A.: An Immunological Pregnancy Test. *Ann. Endocrinol.,* 35: 261, 1960.

Chapter 32

Ectopic Pregnancy

PURSUING the discussion of faulty implantation of the embryo, one automatically next considers other sites outside the endometrial cavity where the fertilized ovum may elect to rest and grow. Such a pregnancy is called *ectopic* or *extrauterine*. Though the terms are used synonymously, the designation "ectopic" is more nearly accurate, for pregnancy may grow in the interstitial portion of the uterine wall or at the cornual end of the tube. Actually, these are abnormal implantations, but still may not be extrauterine. When implanted outside the endometrial cavity, a beginning pregnancy may be found in any portion of the fallopian tube, in the ovary or on the peritoneal surface within the abdomen. Descriptive terms such as "interstitial," "isthmic," "abdominal" and "ovarian" are often used, depending on the primary location (Figs. 32–1, 32–2). In most instances a single ectopic gestation is found in the outer or "ampullary" portion of the fallopian tube. Rarely, a normally implanted pregnancy is noted within the uterus, while another, ectopic pregnancy exists in the tube. Bilateral tubal pregnancies have been reported.

How Common Is Ectopic Pregnancy?

The actual incidence of ectopic pregnancy is hard to determine. It is said to be in the region of 10 per cent. The symptoms of unruptured ectopic pregnancies are so vague and minimal, however, that many cases go undiagnosed. Not all ectopic pregnancies progress to the point of tubal rupture. The vaginal bleeding may be no more than one anticipates from a normal period. Moreover, the differential diagnosis between ectopic pregnancy and abortion is not always clear-cut. An identical clinical picture can be produced by a ruptured ovarian follicle, mild appendicitis or torsion of the pedicle of an ovarian cyst.

Why Does the Ectopic Implantation Occur in the Tube?

Fertilization of the ovum normally takes place in the outer or ampullary portion of the fallopian tube. From this position it gradually descends, over a period of three to four days, into the uterus. The rate of passage becomes slower as the impregnated ovum approaches the narrow uterine end of the tube. The slowness of transit may be by design: (1) to give progestin more time to prepare the endometrium, or perhaps (2) to allow the tubal fluid to condition the embryo for implantation.

Obviously there are a number of factors that may either delay fertilization, interfere with normal development of the ovum or obstruct passage of the impregnated

389

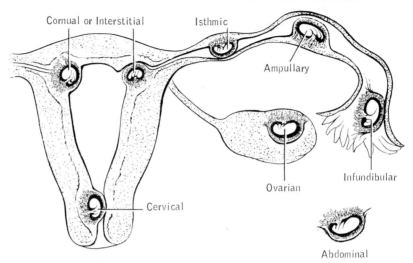

Fig. 32-1.   Various ectopic implantation sites of pregnancy in the uterus, tube, ovary and peritoneal cavity.

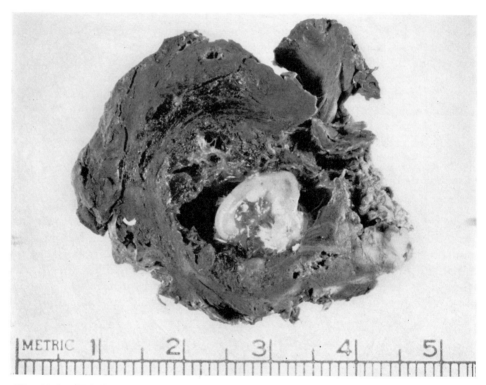

Fig. 32-2.   Tubal ectopic pregnancy with the embryo in place, surrounded by a blood clot.

ovum into the uterus. All may lead to an ectopic pregnancy implanted within the tube. Of them all, established chronic salpingitis is considered most often responsible.

How Does Delay in Fertilization Affect the Etiology?

Normally the sperm anticipate the appearance of the ovum in the fallopian tube. Time is apparently needed (1) to permit the accumulation of a sufficient number of spermatozoa and (2) to allow the tubal fluid an opportunity to condition the spermatozoa so that one sperm may penetrate the ovum. Anything that will delay either the sperm or ovum from reaching the point of impregnation will interfere with normal fertilization. In most instances the aging sperm can no longer penetrate the egg. When penetration does occur, developmental abnormalities appear which are incompatible with continued growth of the ovum. Perhaps after ovulation the ovum may float aimlessly about in the peritoneal cavity, owing to mischance or inefficient ciliary action of the tubal fimbriae.

What Factors Interfere with the Normal Development of the Ovum in the Tube?

In most instances the etiology of ectopic tubal pregnancy is linked to mechanical interference with the passage of the fertilized ovum. Not infrequently in the woman having her first pregnancy the tube that contains an ectopic gestation appears otherwise normal, and no obstructive element is found. It is possible that abnormal physiology and intrinsic metabolism of the tubal epithelium may be fully as important in ectopic pregnancy as the impatency of the tubal lumen. We know little about the histology or histochemistry of the tubal epithelium. Is the chemical environment of the tube a necessary prerequisite to impregnation? Can an ovum be fertilized in a patient who has had both tubes removed? The tubal fluid may have a more useful function than that of a simple transport medium. It is thought to play a role in conditioning the spermatozoa, augmenting their power to penetrate the ovum, but it may also prove important in guaranteeing the survival and safe transport of the impregnated ovum into the uterus.

One may postulate that a normal metabolic environment within the fallopian tube preserves the zona pellucida of the impregnated ovum and prevents ectopic implantation during its passage through the tube. Should abnormal metabolic con-

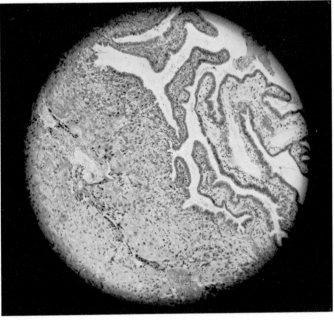

Fig. 32-3. Scanty stromal decidual reaction typical of the inadequate nidation site for implantation found in tubal ectopic pregnancy.

ditions be present, the histolytic process responsible for its dissolution might begin while the fertilized ovum is still within the tube. Unless implanted promptly, it will die. Seeking the most favorable environment, the blastocyst implants in the tubal epithelium. Some believe that the embryo is attracted to aberrant islands of endometrial epithelium which are occasionally noted in histologic review of tubal epithelium. There is considerable controversy as to whether such epithelial nests occur with sufficient frequency to explain implantation on the tubal mucosa. Certainly the same events may occur in a patient who has a normal, well differentiated tubal epithelium, as shown by study of large groups of tubal pregnancies. If endometrial islands are present, the likelihood of implantations on such sites would increase materially.

The extent to which an ectopic gestation will progress within the tube depends in part on the location and the ability of the tubal epithelium to sustain the pregnancy. The extent of the decidual reaction in the tubal stromal cells varies, but it is often completely absent and is never adequate to supply the voracious invasive appetite of the growing trophoblast (Fig. 32–3).

What Elements Impair the Normal Transport of the Ovum within the Tube?

These are chiefly three in number. In the vast majority of instances the source of the difficulty may be traced to some old inflammatory process either in or around the fallopian tube. Less commonly the explanation may be found in congenital maldevelopment.

INFLAMMATORY CHANGES WITHIN THE TUBE.   Certain disease entities such as gonorrhea primarily attack the tubal epithelium and create an endosalpingitis. When the infection is extensive, sufficient epithelial destruction will have taken place to obstruct completely the tubal lumen at the uterine end and deny admission of the spermatozoa. In milder degrees of infection, however, the obstructive process is not enough to prevent the entrance of the sperm, but it is sufficiently well developed to interfere with the passage of the fertilized ovum, which is naturally larger than a spermatozoon. That factors other than mechanical obstruction are operative is indicated by the fact that ectopic pregnancy is rare in patients with tuberculous salpingitis, yet this disease also primarily attacks the tubal epithelium. In mild and moderate endosalpingitis two things usually happen: (a) The tubal epithelium covering the plicae is destroyed, the cilia of the tubal cells disappear, and mechanical obstructions appear within the lumen, due to the formation of crypts, blind passages or follicles formed by adhesions of the tubal plicae. The tubal muscle may have been involved in the original inflammatory process, and the normal peristaltic action of the tube becomes impaired by fibrosis. This factor, coupled with the loss of cilia, destroys the normal mechanism by which the fertilized ovum is transported to the uterus.

The pathologic changes occurring in the fallopian tube as a result of infection will be discussed in greater detail under pelvic inflammation (see Chap. 44).

INFLAMMATORY CHANGES OUTSIDE THE TUBE.   Perhaps the most important factor in the etiology of ectopic pregnancy is that of a previous pelvic infection which results in the formation of adhesions both in and around the tubes. The infection may be due to a variety of causes, most commonly venereal, postabortional or puerperal. Extensive pelvic adhesions often occur after ruptured appendicitis and subsequent pelvic peritonitis. Widespread adhesions in the pelvis can follow a previous pelvic laparotomy in the absence of any known infection.

Whatever the explanation, as a result of the pelvic inflammatory process, adhesions and fibrous bands form around the tube which tend to interfere with its normal motility and in addition produce mechanical kinking and pressure on the tubal lumen.

CONGENITAL FACTORS OR ABNORMALLY PLACED TUMORS. Certainly some bizarre types of tubal pregnancy are traceable to maldevelopments, but less obvious congenital factors may also explain some ectopic pregnancies. It is difficult to assess correctly the importance of the small tubal diverticula, accessory ostia and occasional twists that one sees in the otherwise normal, uninfected fallopian tube. Possibly the tubal diverticula may serve to trap the fertilized ovum and delay its migration into the uterus.

There are recorded cases in which pregnancy has developed in a rudimentary uterine horn or fallopian tube that has no connection with the endometrial cavity. The only possible way for the spermatozoa to get into such a rudimentary tube is by migration across the peritoneal cavity from the opposite normal tube. Either the ovum was evidently extruded from the ovary on the side of the imperfect tube, or one can postulate migration of the ovum across from the opposite ovary.

In addition to inflammatory and fibrotic obstructions to the passage of the fertilized ovum one may occasionally encounter a tubal fibroma, polyp or endometriosis that partially occludes the lumen. Abnormally situated uterine fibroids or adherent ovarian cysts also can distort or obstruct the lumen of the fallopian tube.

How Does the Ectopic Embryo Grow?

The impregnated ovum may implant anywhere along the course of the tube, but primarily one finds the ectopic pregnancy in the outer two thirds or ampullary portion of the tube, just lateral to the narrow isthmic section. The embryo implants and tries to grow in the same manner as in the endometrial cavity, but it has a far less favorable soil to deal with. Some decidual reaction occasionally may take place within the stromal cells under the tubal epithelium, but there is usually too little of it to form much of a bed. It is the nature of the trophoblast to invade the surrounding tissue in search of sustenance. Since there is little in the way of decidual bed, the voracious trophoblasts invade the muscle wall directly. The degree of this invasion is determined by the thickness of the decidual bed. The extent of such muscle wall invasion may explain the duration of viability of the ectopic implant. Sometimes the implantation is sufficiently well developed so that even though the tube is distended until it ruptures, the pregnancy may survive for months, or even to term. But in the vast majority of cases the pregnancy terminates in the second or third month by tubal abortion or rupture, or both.

In response to the demands of the growing ectopic pregnancy the tube tries to respond by dilatation and increase of the blood supply to the area of the implant, just as it does in the endometrium. The tubal mucosa lacks the elements necessary to nourish and sustain the fetus, for it was never designed to do so and cannot readily adapt to the increased demand. The trophoblasts continue to burrow into the wall of the tube, which eventually becomes abnormally stretched and thinned out to form a fragile sac containing the chorionic vesicle and the embryo. The eroding chorionic villi progressively weaken the tubal wall and erode the underlying blood vessels. As a result of the mechanical stretching and blood vessel invasion extensive hemorrhage takes place both within the embryonic sac and between it and the tubal wall. In this manner the tubal pregnancy is destroyed and separated from the original site of implantation.

Once it has separated, several things may happen to the dying embryo: (1) As blood floods into the chorionic sac the sac becomes so overdistended that it ruptures into the lumen of the tube. There it forms a so-called tubal blood mole, which is not unlike the hemorrhagic tissue (Breus's mole) recovered in a true uterine abortion.

2. If the separation occurs early enough or the tubal bleeding is not too extensive, the conceptus may absorb either entirely or in part without producing anything more than moderate lower abdominal pain for a few days and practically no vaginal bleeding. Rarely does suppuration occur. If absorption is incomplete, evidence of its previous existence can sometimes be found within the tube several years later when laparotomy is performed for another cause. On microscopic section one may see remnants of hyalinized villi.

3. In a so-called *tubal abortion* the patient may extrude the tubal blood mole out through the fimbriated end of the tube, either completely or incompletely, provided the life span of the ectopic pregnancy was not prolonged beyond a two- or three-months' period, after which it is too large to pass, and the fimbriated end tends to close. The factor that caused the expulsion of the dying ovum was probably reversed peristaltic muscular contractions of the tube, initiated by irritation from bleeding within the lumen. The force of the contraction may be sufficient to eject the entire unwanted pregnancy out the tubal ostium into the abdominal cavity. Thus the tubal abortion is said to be *complete*. On the other hand, the abortion may be *incomplete* when it is not entirely expelled from the tube or some connection with the original implantation site remains. The severity of the symptomatology produced will vary, depending on the amount of hemorrhage and the duration and extent of the process of tubal extrusion.

4. The fallopian tube itself may rupture directly into the abdominal cavity or develop a slow hemorrhagic leak rather than extrude blood into the tubal lumen. The main precipitating factors that cause a tube to rupture are (*a*) the extent of erosion by the chorionic villi, (*b*) the capacity of the tubal lumen to distend.

Abrupt changes in intraluminal pressure such as are due to hemorrhage may be enough to precipitate a *spontaneous rupture*. Sudden muscular effort on the part of the patient may be all that is needed to trigger a tubal rupture. For example, rupture of an ectopic pregnancy often follows sexual intercourse. Tubal rupture may be expected to occur if the ectopic implant occurs in the interstitial isthmic portion of the tube. Because of its location and structure there is less opportunity for the tube to distend. The eroding chorionic villi directly invade the musculature and blood vessels. Rupture occurs despite the fact that the fimbriated ends of the tubes usually remain open. Rupture also occurs frequently in the outer portion of the tube, regardless of whether the fimbriated end is open or closed. This is considered due to the direct eroding action of the trophoblast and subsequent thinning of the muscular wall.

What Is the Fate of the Embryo after It Leaves the Tube, either by Rupture or Abortion?

AFTER TUBAL ABORTION.　　　If the hemorrhage is sudden and severe, the tubal contraction is usually sufficient to force the abortus completely out through the open end of the tube into the abdominal cavity. The symptoms are usually extreme and are chiefly those of intraperitoneal hemorrhage. It is impossible clinically to distinguish a tubal rupture from tubal abortion when this train of events has occurred. When abdominal exploration is done, the tube itself will be greatly distended with blood, and a large clot containing the remains of the pregnancy is found in the cul-de-sac. Often this is covered by a sort of pseudomembrane that walls it off from the overlying intestine. If there have been repeated minor episodes of bleeding from the open end of the tube preceding the acute hemorrhagic phase, this protective membrane composed of organized hemorrhage may be fairly thick (Fig. 32–4).

In the great majority of cases repeated incidents of minor bleeding have taken place over a period of several days. If no sudden increase in tubal contraction occurs, the continued loss of blood permits considerable coagulation, and an organizing clot is found, complete with fibrous cover, around the end of the tubal ostium. The process is a gradual one with mild symptomatology. It may go unrecognized until it is large enough to be palpated as adnexal tumor or give symptoms suggesting pelvic inflammatory disease. When the bleeding is more pronounced, the blood continues to escape into the peritoneal cavity, but it does not reach the proportions of a true intraperitoneal hemorrhage. The symptoms are usually sufficiently pronounced to make abdominal exploration advisable. The aborting embryonic sac can frequently be found protruding from the open ostium with a flimsy attachment to the original implantation site. Evidence of recent and old bleeding can be seen in and around the open end of the tube and in the pouch of Douglas. The operator usually completes the abortion by milking the remaining contents out through the open end of the tube. The distention of the tubal lumen with blood does not persist, and at subsequent abdominal exploration no evidence of a previous tubal abortion can be detected.

AFTER TUBAL RUPTURE.   The extent of rupture of the fallopian tube depends on the distensibility of the tube and the degree of trophoblastic erosion. Gradually, as the tubal musculature thins out, either a sudden spontaneous rupture occurs into the abdominal cavity or the broad ligament is invaded. The latter pathway, though uncommon, is taken chiefly when the implantation site is in the region of the isthmus, since no other place exists for it to go, particularly if the pregnancy is implanted on

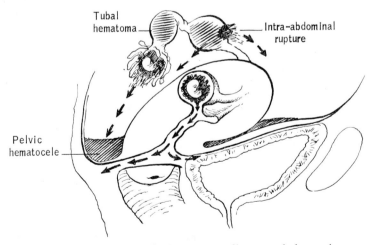

Fig. 32-4.   Four varieties of hemorrhage may complicate a tubal ectopic pregnancy: (*a*) tubal abortion with intraperitoneal bleeding produces a pelvic hematocele; (*b*) localized bleeding leads to a tubal hematoma around the implantation site; (*c*) the tube ruptures intraperitoneally; and (*d*) hemorrhage dissects along intraligamentous routes to reach the vaginal or bladder walls.

the floor of the tube rather than the top or sides. This can also occur when the ectopic implant is similarly placed in the outer portions of the tube. It is known as an "intra-ligamentous rupture" in contradistinction to that of the "intraperitoneal rupture," which takes place when the break in the tubal musculature occurs on the roof or sides of the fallopian tube.

The invasion of the tubal musculature by the chorionic villi and trophoblast may take place at spaced intervals, so that no one spot takes the full brunt of the destructive process. In this case the tube leaks rather than ruptures, and an encapsulated hemorrhagic mass surrounding the tube prevents sudden rupture into the abdominal cavity. This is called a "tubal hematocele." Given enough strain or increased intracapsular tension from hemorrhage, a secondary rupture into the abdomen may follow. In most instances no further growth can be expected from the embryo which has been expelled violently into the peritoneal cavity or through the base of the tube into the broad ligament, for it has been destroyed either by the original hemorrhage into the sac or by separation of the placenta from the implantation site. Rarely the placental villi emerge through minor rents in the tubal musculature and gradually come to occupy a position outside the tube, either in the abdominal cavity or broad ligaments. These conditions will be discussed later.

How Is the Uterus Affected by a Developing Ectopic Pregnancy?

While all this is going on in the tube some changes are noted in both the uterine musculature and endometrium. The more pronounced effect is observed in the endometrium.

The uterus does enlarge and in many instances becomes soft, but it is not always easy to detect the enlargement, particularly if the symptoms of ectopic pregnancy appear as early as six weeks after the last menstrual period. Should the pregnancy in the tube remain viable beyond the third or fourth month, a definite increase in uterine size is noted. Neither does it reach the proportions of an intrauterine pregnancy of the same duration, nor is softening of the cervix apparent.

The endometrium temporarily responds to the hormonal stimulation of the developing ectopic pregnancy. It may be expected to continue to show decidual changes consistent with pregnancy only as long as it receives proper hormonal stimulation. Often this stimulation disappears several weeks before symptoms related to ectopic pregnancy develop. Consequently no assistance in the diagnosis of tubal ectopic pregnancy can be expected from uterine curettings. Usually an ordinary proliferative, secretory or menstrual endometrium will be present, without evidence of a decidual reaction of pregnancy. Once the fetus has died, hormonal stimulation from the immature chorionic villi and the corpus luteum rapidly decreases. Since the uterine decidua depended upon the progesterone which has now been withdrawn, it too degenerates.

If the hormonal withdrawal is rapid, the patient may have sudden vaginal bleeding and present the clinical picture of a miscarriage. Examination of the blood clot expelled may show microscopic evidence of a complete decidual cast. The actual changes taking place in the endometrium are similar to those that occur during normal menstruation. One cannot correlate the death of an ectopically implanted embryo with the date of the expulsion of the decidual cast. The embryo may have died several days or even weeks before.

If the life of the tubal embryo is in jeopardy, the level of the circulating gonadotropins may fall to the point at which some vaginal bleeding occurs. Usually uterine curettage is not performed, for the differential diagnosis between threatened uterine abortion and ectopic pregnancy cannot be made with accuracy. If for good reason curettage is done, the endometrium may or may not show decidua without villi, but this cannot be counted on to make a correct diagnosis of ectopic pregnancy.

When progesterone stimulation is gradually withdrawn over a protracted period of several weeks, the endometrium is thrown off in patches and the vaginal bleeding may be very scanty. Actually, as already mentioned, the endometrium may have undergone complete regeneration, and curettage shows only a normal cyclical endometrial phase. This fact should be noted again, for one may miss the diagnosis of ectopic pregnancy if too great reliance is placed on the interpretation of the endometrium obtained by endometrial biopsy or curettage. It has been said that the longer the symptoms of external bleeding have been present, the less likely one is to find decidua in endometrium obtained by these methods.

The vaginal bleeding in patients with an ectopic pregnancy comes largely from changes within the endometrium rather than bleeding from the implantation site within the tube. An occasional viable embryo in the tube will be found in the presence of vaginal bleeding, but such cases are the exception, not the rule. Bleeding in this instance is probably due to a local condition at the site of tubal implantation.

How Useful Are Hormonal Tests in the Diagnosis of Ectopic Pregnancy?

The interpretation of the Aschheim-Zondek, Friedman or frog test of urine in ectopic pregnancy can be most misleading. As long as the embryo lives, assay of the urine for circulating gonadotropins will be positive. It becomes negative when the trophoblast is no longer functional. Unfortunately the tests are unreliable at a time when you need them most, namely, before tubal rupture or abortion has taken place. If the symptoms are mild and abnormal vaginal bleeding has been present for only a short period, the pregnancy tests may vary from strongly to weakly positive. Thus in an early gestation the tests do not differ materially from those found in threatened abortion. When the internal bleeding and pain are of longer duration, the tests are usually negative even though the trophoblasts continue to digest the tubal musculature and produce intraperitoneal bleeding. It is obvious that one may have either a positive or a negative pregnancy test and still have a tubal pregnancy. The danger lies in the false sense of security engendered when the urine test is reported as negative. If one can be sure of what is actually going on in the uterus or tube, the tests may be helpful, but one should not rely on them completely.

How Do We Make a Diagnosis of Pregnancy?

The diagnosis of early unruptured ectopic pregnancy is made largely on suspicion. The symptoms and signs are so minimal that they are often indistinguishable from a slightly abnormal menstrual period or at the most from those which customarily accompany a threatened uterine abortion. Unless the clinical suspicion of ectopic pregnancy is aroused, the patient may well go on to tubal or cornual rupture. When tubal abortion or rupture occurs, the symptoms are usually violent and call for immediate surgical action. The symptoms then are not pathognomonic of ectopic pregnancy, but of intraperitoneal hemorrhage, which may be due to a tubal pregnancy or to any one of a number of other pathologic conditions in the pelvis.

TUBAL PREGNANCY BEFORE ABORTION OR PERFORATION AND THE OCCURRENCE OF INTRAPERITONEAL HEMORRHAGE. In its incipient stage an ectopic pregnancy does little to disturb the health of the woman or do more than raise a question of pregnancy. No indication will be given that the pregnancy is abnormally located. One normally associates morning nausea and breast enlargement with a developing pregnancy, but in most instances the tubal pregnancy terminates too early for these symptoms to develop. About all the healthy young woman with a normally regular menstrual pattern observes is that there is some delay in the appearance of menstruation, which is then followed by a spotting type of vaginal bleeding several days or weeks later. Even this may be lacking. Approximately one third of women who subsequently turn out to have an ectopic pregnancy had no interruption in their periods at all. In this case the period was not quite normal or perhaps appeared two or three days before the expected time.

In many instances there is no great departure from the normal either in the amount or the nature of the menstrual flow. Most frequently the menstrual bleeding will be spotty with a tendency to appear intermittently, leaving only regional soreness in the abdomen. Approximately one fifth will describe a moderate bloody discharge not much removed from normal. By and large most patients are ambulatory, but 10 per cent will have a sudden gush of heavy vaginal bleeding and require bed rest or hospitalization. In whatever form it appears vaginal bleeding usually heralds the death of the ovum in the tube, either because of hemorrhage into the sac or separation of the placenta from the implantation site.

Pain is a significant symptom and certainly the most common of all in patients who have ectopic pregnancy. When the tubal pregnancy continues to grow, the duration of amenorrhea increases, and vaginal bleeding does not appear as an early symptom. Not infrequently, however, such a patient will have recurring attacks of lower abdominal pain, usually localized to one side or the other, as the tube distends to accommodate the growing embryo. Pain may be so minimal that the patient completely disregards it. Whenever sharp, colicky, spasmodic pain appears in a healthy girl with a pregnancy, one should immediately become suspicious of the possibility that it is ectopic.

PELVIC EXAMINATION. Once the diagnosis of ectopic pregnancy has been raised, every effort must be made to confirm it or rule it out. A general physical examination should be performed, but rarely does it help in the differential diagnosis. Breast changes, particularly enlargement in the upper outer quadrants, suggest pregnancy, but they may be absent and do not help in the localization. Chief reliance must be placed on the vaginal examination. In this examination we are more interested in the findings in the adnexa than in the uterus. At this stage of development of normal pregnancy the uterus may be enlarged and the cervix soft, but it is so early that these signs may be absent. If present, they do not help us in locating the pregnancy.

A movable tender mass lying lateral to the uterus, on one side only, is a significant finding. Since the tube is as yet unruptured, the size of the mass may vary and with it the degree of tenderness. If small, it may feel smooth, ovoid, elastic and not particularly tender. When large and unruptured, it is often felt as a sausage-shaped mass separate from the uterus, while the opposite adnexal region seems essentially normal. The mass is usually tender, for the tube is overdistended. *Pain and tenderness may be accentuated when the cervix is moved with the examining finger.* If one can feel pulsating vessels on the under side of the palpable adnexal mass, further suspicion of an ectopic pregnancy is aroused. Rarely can this be felt when the conceptus in the tube is still small.

In summary, one may state that ectopic pregnancy must be ruled out before considering any other diagnosis when a healthy young woman consults you because of (1) a history of slight vaginal spotting or bleeding several days or weeks after a missed period, (2) unilateral abdominal pain which you associate with the presence of a palpable, tender mass.

What Is the Differential Diagnosis of Unruptured Tubal Pregnancy?

The possibility of the presence of an ectopic pregnancy has been considered, but other pathologic entities may simulate an eccentrically placed pregnancy. For example, a persistent corpus luteum cyst can delay menstruation for a time and be followed by vaginal spotting. On examination one feels the same ovoid, tender unilateral mass. Other signs of pregnancy of course are lacking. It may be necessary to use hormonal pregnancy tests or even curettage to aid in establishing the diagnosis. One can normally expect the frog test to be negative, but occasionally a positive test will be reported.

The pathologic condition most commonly found that adds confusion to the diagnosis of ectopic pregnancy is the *threatened abortion*. The symptoms and physical findings are similar in both ectopic pregnancy and threatened abortion. There are a few distinguishing factors which may be helpful in the differentiation when considered together, for no single one can be considered pathognomonic. (1) The symptoms of ectopic pregnancy manifest themselves earlier in relation to the last menstrual period than do those of threatened abortion. (2) The uterus tends to be larger and the cervix softer in threatened uterine miscarriage. (3) In ruptured ectopic pregnancy the pain is characteristically localized to one side or the other of the midline and may be sharp and cramplike. The pain of threatened uterine abortion is less severe, in its early phases, with a tendency to center over the suprapubic area. (4) A unilateral adnexal swelling may be felt in both conditions in approximately the same location. In threatened uterine miscarriage this is the corpus luteum of pregnancy. In the early unruptured phase of tubal pregnancy there is little to differentiate the two situations unless one can happen to feel pulsating vessels on the under side of the adnexal mass. (5) The vaginal bleeding pattern after delayed menstruation is not dissimilar, though it does appear earlier in tubal pregnancy than one would expect in a uterine abortion. When placental fragments are recovered in the vaginal discharge, a diagnosis of incomplete rather than threatened uterine abortion can be made.

Other entities which may confuse the clinician in making a diagnosis of unruptured ectopic pregnancy are (*a*) salpingitis, (*b*) appendicitis, (*c*) rupture of an ovarian follicle or corpus luteum cyst, (*d*) an ovarian cyst with a twisted pedicle. Each condition carries some distinguishing factor that helps in differentiation. For example, salpingitis is apt to be bilateral and associated with fever and leukocytosis. In appendicitis there will be no delay in menstruation. An ovarian cyst may have been noted on examination previously. No palpable adnexal tumor will be felt when the vaginal bleeding and pain are due to unruptured follicle cysts. The factor common to all four lesions is the lack of delay in menstruation.

When Do We Do a Curettage, and How Much Information Can Be Gained?

Naturally one would not elect to do a curettage for diagnosis if there were any chance that the pregnancy was still viable within the uterus. If, however, the patient has been having bleeding for several days or weeks, and the diagnosis is still in doubt, curettage may be helpful. For example, if the curetted material reveals decidua without villi, one may reasonably assume either that there is an ectopic pregnancy or that an intrauterine abortion has already occurred. Although this is a good working rule, it cannot be relied upon completely.

Absence of decidual change in the endometrium unfortunately does not mean that a pregnancy may not exist in the tube. The curettage has usually been postponed until we are certain that no viable pregnancy exists in the uterus, or the patient has had symptoms of vaginal spotting, and the ovum has been dead for some time before she consults the physician. During this period the endometrium may well have regenerated, and one may recover a normal secretory phase while living trophoblast remains in the tube. One should be on guard, for the findings of a normal secretory endometrium on endometrial biopsy or curettage otherwise may lull you into a false sense of security. The longer the symptoms have persisted, the greater the likelihood that the endometrium will fail to demonstate any decidual change.

What Other Methods Are Available to Establish a Diagnosis?

The value of the pregnancy tests of urine has been discussed already. They are useful in establishing the diagnosis of pregnancy and help to rule out salpingitis, appendicitis and ovarian follicle rupture, but they are not of much use in localizing the pregnancy.

Posterior colpotomy, culdoscopy and needle puncture of the cul-de-sac are helpful only if positive evidence is obtained. When the pregnancy is still in the fallopian tube, one would not expect to find blood in the cul-de-sac if an exploring needle is introduced. Likewise visualization of the tubes by culdoscopy or posterior colpotomy is often unsatisfactory, unless the tubal mass is of appreciable size or the entire length of both tubes can be thoroughly inspected. The disadvantages of curettage, culdoscopy, needle puncture of the cul-de-sac or posterior colpotomy all point up the fact that the diagnosis of unruptured ectopic pregnancy is made mainly on suspicion aroused by observing a combination of circumstances rather than the pathognomonic features of any one observation. When an unruptured tubal pregnancy is suspected, the patient should be hospitalized.

How Do We Treat an Unruptured Ectopic Pregnancy?

The most important factor in treatment is prompt diagnosis, for the stretching and eroding processes in the tube may accelerate rapidly and the symptoms reach catastrophic proportions suddenly. All too frequently patients are discharged from the hospital after a period of observation only to sustain tubal rupture shortly after returning home. In some instances the tube may rupture on the ward while under observation. If the adnexal mass shows any enlargement, immediate intervention is imperative. The patient should preferably be explored surgically if the symptoms continue after reasonable attempts to make a diagnosis.

The established surgical procedure has always been removal of the involved tube in its entirety. Since there is no reason to implicate the ovary on the affected side, it is usually left undisturbed. Recently there has been some agitation to remove this ovary, on the theory that the opposite ovary would then be the sole source of ovum production, and because of its intimate anatomic relation with the remaining tube, the chances of pregnancy would be augmented. This line of reasoning is highly debatable. Again, there has been some departure in therapy from the old established axiom that the tube must be removed under any conditions. The time-honored concept was based on the belief that the tube was basically defective, either because of salpingitis or congenital malformation. Yet we know that many girls with normal genital development and no past history of tubal infection have had their first pregnancy in the tube.

There is logic, then, in suggesting that, after due consideration of the extent of damage created by the pregnancy in the tube, as well as the condition of the opposite tube and ovary, salpingostomy may be the treatment of choice. On several occasions the tube has been opened, the pregnancy extruded and the defect closed with gratifying results. One girl who had only one intact tube has delivered two children after removal of an unruptured pregnancy from the tubal lumen. It is a matter of surgical judgment based on a critical review of the existing situation whether the entire tube should be removed or whether one can afford to remove the pregnancy and leave the tube.

TUBAL ABORTION OR RUPTURE.   The clinical phenomena associated with tubal abortion or rupture are directly referable to the extent of the hemorrhage and the speed with which it occurs. The symptoms actually are those of intraperitoneal hemorrhage and vary, depending on how badly the peritoneum has been insulted.

THE EXTENT OF VAGINAL BLEEDING IN RUPTURE OR ABORTION OF THE TUBE. By and large the symptoms of tubal rupture or abortion are centered in the abdomen, but the uterus does take part to a greater extent than is evident when the tubal gestation remains unruptured. The amount of vaginal bleeding increases and becomes less sporadic and darker in color. As long as the vaginal bleeding is moderate in amount there may be no great variation from that seen in a normal menstrual period, which the patient frequently believes it to be, though she is often concerned that it does not stop at the expected time. Decidua may be expelled in patches, and the possibility of ectopic pregnancy may never be considered, but more frequently a complete uterine cast of decidua is passed. When this occurs, one should immediately suspect the diagnosis of gestation within the tube.

What Symptoms and Physical Findings Are Associated with Severe Intraperitoneal Hemorrhage?

There is little doubt about the diagnosis and the course of action when sudden intraperitoneal hemorrhage of major proportions occurs either from tubal rupture or complete tubal abortion. The insult to the peritoneum is immediate and massive. The symptoms of shock that follow are partly due to the peritoneal damage, but more to the actual amount of blood lost.

The extent of total blood loss varies both in amount and timing. Usually there is a history of mild, intermittent, cramplike pain occurring on one side of the abdomen associated with vaginal spotting or moderate flow from the vagina several days or weeks after a missed menstrual period. The patient may be shopping or carrying on her household duties with minimal discomfort when suddenly without other warning she is seized with a sharp overwhelming pain which may produce fainting or force her to lie down. The initial attack can be, but rarely is, fatal. One patient went into shock, lay down and died in a few hours before anything could be done for her. A fatal termination is extremely rare. Usually the patient recovers and may even carry on her work after a few hours with only mild faintness and weakness as a residual. In this case the hemorrhage which began briskly had gradually subsided, permitting temporary recovery. Not infrequently a second hemorrhage provides a repetition of the initial episode. Any sudden exertion such as straining at stool, lifting heavy objects, doing her housework or sexual intercourse may be the precipitating cause. Blood in the cul-de-sac from the original hemorrhage which subsided may produce an urge to defecate and produce a repetition of the primary incident.

When the patient collapses, all the symptoms of shock from intraperitoneal hemorrhage are present. A severe agonizing pain in the lower abdomen occurs, and pain may be referred to the upper part of the abdomen or supraclavicular area. The patient has a cold, clammy, colorless skin, a rapid thready pulse and a falling blood pressure. If the hemorrhage is extreme or continues, the patient becomes restless and exhibits the labored respiration characteristic of air hunger, while the temperature falls to subnormal. The extent to which the classic picture of shock is present will depend on how rapidly a large amount of blood is lost. It is the rapidity rather than the total amount of blood lost that is important. For example, if the hemorrhage occurs intermittently over a period of days, the blood lost may be equal in all to that of an original sudden hemorrhage, but the only indication of it may be an elevated pulse and other symptoms suggesting anemia.

Physical examination in the acute phase will reveal a distended, tender abdomen, often with dullness to percussion in the flanks. The abdominal wall feels doughy, and the same sensation is noted on palpation of the vaginal fornices. Except for local tenderness, made worse by moving the cervix, the only thing felt by vaginal examination is a fullness in the cul-de-sac with the doughy sensation. On rectal examination the cul-de-sac can be found bulging into the anterior rectal wall. It has no outline and is not under tension. The tenderness is definite, but it is not as acute as that found in pelvic inflammation. There is seldom any doubt that the pelvis is full of blood and nothing else. Occasionally one may outline, in addition, a tender sausage-shaped mass on one side of the uterus, but usually the pelvic mass has no outline.

In the face of the acute symptoms and physical findings suggesting intraperitoneal hemorrhage there is no reason to refine the diagnostic examination. The most likely cause in a woman of this age is tubal rupture or abortion.

TREATMENT OF PATIENTS WITH ACUTE INTRA-ABDOMINAL HEMORRHAGE

Again the important element in therapy is prompt diagnosis and even more rapid abdominal exploration. The degree of shock varies and must be combated by saline solution, glucose infusions and blood replacement. It is a basic surgical principle that the patient's condition should be stable before attempting operation. With a patient bleeding massively into the peritoneal cavity there may be no time to do more than to transfuse the patient with blood injected into a major artery such as the femoral and follow it with intravenous blood replacement as the operation proceeds. Speed is of the greatest importance.

Once the bleeding is controlled the emergency passes, but the operative procedures should not be prolonged. The damaged fallopian tube should be removed as expeditiously as possible. If the patient is in reasonable condition, one may also excise the cornual portion of the tube to prevent the subsequent development of salpingitis in the stump. If haste is essential, simply the damaged portion of the tube should be removed. If possible, the ovary on the damaged side should be left, but if it is intimately matted together, it may be easier and far quicker to take out both the tube and ovary. Any obvious clots should be wiped out, but with the patient in poor shape the surgeon should not waste time in needless peritoneal toilet. With the bulk of the clot removed the rest will absorb. If a blood bank is available, replacement of blood should continue up to the estimated amount of loss as the operation proceeds and thereafter. When no blood is available, one may safely transfuse the patient from her own blood recovered from the pelvis, provided it appears normal and the history of sudden rupture dates back no longer than thirty-six hours. It must first be strained through gauze to remove the clots and then be citrated. Obviously, the patient's appendix should not be removed if she is in poor general condition.

What Are the Symptoms of Moderate Intraperitoneal Bleeding from Tubal Rupture or Abortion?

The dramatic course of events that follows acute and repeated intra-abdominal hemorrhage leaves little question about the diagnosis, and there is no occasion to delay the obvious therapy. The majority of patients who have had one severe hemorrhagic incident or who bleed moderately but continuously from the tube into the abdominal cavity or broad ligament recover from their shock and enter the hospital in less of an emergency. The patient may complain of abdominal discomfort, pressure on the rectum, and diarrhea and have a slight fever and leukocytosis, but the acute phases have passed. A sudden transition to an emergency status may take place, but for the moment the process is in abeyance. On vaginal examination one again feels the same doughy fullness in the cul-de-sac characteristic of the presence of blood. If there has been recovery after a major episode, the same consistency is felt in both vaults. When the bleeding episodes have recurred repeatedly, there may be an accumulation of a fair amount of blood in the cul-de-sac, but there is a greater tendency for the fullness to localize on the affected side. This is usually the situation when intermittent bleeding follows partial extrusion of a tubal mole, as in tubal abortion, or when partial leakage from the wall of the tube has caused a peritubal hematocele.

There is no occasion to rush such a patient to the operating room for emergency surgery. Frequently the slight temperature elevation, local tenderness and the presence of adnexal masses raise the question of the differential diagnosis between tubal abortion and pelvic inflammation. One can afford to take time to establish a diagnosis.

In such a case needle puncture of the cul-de-sac may help. If old blood is recovered, ectopic pregnancy is suspected. The urine test for pregnancy and endometrial sampling may be helpful in making the diagnosis, provided too much reliance is not placed on negative reports.

While under observation the local conditions in the pelvis should be re-evaluated. The pelvis should improve under a supportive and antibiotic chemotherapy regimen if the underlying disease is not an ectopic pregnancy. If it does not improve or if the situation gets worse, surgical exploration is indicated.

TREATMENT OF THE PATIENT WITH MODERATE INTRAPERITONEAL BLEEDING FROM TUBAL RUPTURE OR ABORTION

Since there has been no indication for emergency surgery, the physician has had plenty of time to get the patient in the best possible condition for operation. The operation is being done at the time of election. The surgeon then can well afford to take the time to appraise fully the entire situation in the pelvis.

Recurrent bleeding, never massive enough to precipitate an immediate operation, but enough to cause a pelvic mass, is frequently the result of an incomplete attempt to extrude a blood mole from the tube. It continues to bleed in varying amounts. In many instances it is possible to milk the rest of the tubal abortion out through the open fimbriated end without sacrificing the fallopian tube. The operator takes a calculated risk that the tube was not irreparably damaged by the ectopic pregnancy, nor was chronic disease the reason for the present occurrence. This may be important to the girl who has only one tube, either because the other one has been removed or is now seriously impaired. On the other hand, if the patient's family is complete, it may be wise to remove not only the fallopian tube on the affected side, but the other one as well, should it be grossly damaged. One should not be confused by the chemical reaction to old blood sometimes seen on the surface of either tube. Frequently this will produce a subacute inflammatory reaction on the peritoneal surface. It is a good and sufficient reason for removing the old blood, but an inadequate cause for removal of the tube. If the decision is made to remove both tubes, hysterectomy should be done, leaving both ovaries *in situ*.

All the old blood should be removed from within the pelvis and around the tube. It is possible that it may all absorb even when large amounts are left, but it is more likely to fibrose and cause a low-grade pelvic peritonitis.

There is no reason why the appendix should not be removed, since time is not a factor. Though old blood is theoretically a good bacterial culture medium, there is little likelihood of peritonitis, particularly when the patient's resistance is supported by antibiotic drugs.

What Happens if Abdominal Exploration Is Not Done?

The diagnosis of ectopic pregnancy may be missed because the diagnosis was not considered, and the patient can recover completely. Whenever the question has been raised, however, the patient probably should be subjected to exploration, even after the danger of further bleeding has passed. It is amazing how much old blood can be tolerated in the pelvis without producing much in the way of pain or discomfort, once the acute insult to the peritoneum has been overcome. Except for a low-grade fever which is probably secondary to absorption of the old blood, the only symptoms are those of pressure on the rectum or bladder.

When there has been a profuse intraperitoneal hemorrhage with recovery or there have been repeated episodes of bleeding of lesser magnitude, the old blood in the pelvis gradually walls itself off from the intestine and omentum by forming a pseudomembrane or fibrous capsule. This is of varying thickness, depending on how long the process has been going on. The pelvic blood simply organizes to form a localized pelvic hematoma. This may fill the entire pelvis or localize around the tubal ostium.

If the mass is small, it can be felt only on vaginal or rectal examination, but if large, it may be palpated above the level of the symphysis, usually more on one side than the other. As one might expect, the percussion note is flat over the lower abdomen, while tympany is noted over the intestines that have been pushed into the upper abdomen by the underlying mass. The findings are not unlike those accompanying a twisted ovarian cyst with hemorrhage into its interior or infarction of a large pedunculated fibroid.

On vaginal examination a diffuse mass of varying size can be felt merging into the abdominal mass and lying behind the uterus, partly or completely filling the pelvis, jutting into the rectum or vagina and forcing the uterus anteriorly against the pubic symphysis. If the mass is more noticeable on one side, it may push the uterus to the opposite side. Soft spots may appear in the otherwise doughy, elastic mass which reflect the normal process of blood clot liquefaction and absorption. When firm hard areas are felt with adjoining soft areas, differentiation from a semisolid and semicystic ovarian tumor may be difficult.

TREATMENT OF LATE SEQUELAE OF INTRAPERITONEAL BLEEDING FROM TUBAL RUPTURE OR ABORTION

It is entirely possible, though it is difficult to prove, that many tubal ruptures pass through an acute phase incident to extravasation of blood from the tube into the peritoneal cavity and stabilize without appreciable subsequent discomfort. Blood accumulates as the result of gradual but continued leakage from either a rupture or tubal abortion. There is never enough blood loss at any one time to cause a peritoneal insult sufficient to require an immediate surgical intervention. The only indications of blood loss may be simply tachycardia and anemia.

As the blood collects in the pelvis after extensive bleeding or around the end of the tube if lesser amounts have occurred, it tends to fibrose and organize. Along with the organization of the clot and formation of the protective fibrous membrane that partially walls it off from the intestine, multiple adhesions form in the lower pelvis, involving the tube and adjacent organs.

The treatment will depend largely on the extent of hemorrhage and its location. It may be felt rising out of the pelvis and filling the lower part of the abdomen on one or both sides. If localized around the tubal ostia, it can be felt vaginally or by rectum as a tubo-ovarian mass. Although it may be possible to drain a collection of old blood which has undergone liquefaction through the vagina adequately in most instances, it is far better to explore the abdomen surgically in order that a more complete pelvic toilet may be done. This is especially necessary if preservation of the patient's reproductive function is of the utmost importance. Peritubal adhesions due to organizing blood clot do nothing to preserve the normal motility of the remaining otherwise unaltered tube.

What Happens When Viable Placental Tissue Is Extruded into the Peritoneal Cavity or Broad Ligament?

In most instances the conceptus extruded through the open end of the tube or through a rent in its side has already been destroyed by the hemorrhage associated with the dislodgment of the placenta in the first place. In rare instances, said to be about once in 15,000 deliveries, the embryo continues to survive within the peritoneal cavity or broad ligament. The great majority of these die in the early months of pregnancy, but a few continue to term only to die or be found malformed at the time of delivery. It is possible for the embryo to die without the patient's being aware of it. One would expect that such a course of events would precipitate an early pelvic infection and intestinal obstruction as the fetus underwent decomposition. It is rather amazing that it does not always do so, for one might anticipate that intestine would become adherent to the necrotic mass. Yet there are recorded instances in which the organization of the dead fetus progressed without incident, became coated with lime salts and formed an abdominal lithopedion. Some of these are known to have been present for years, to be recognized only when the patient has come to autopsy or undergone abdominal exploration for what was believed to be an ovarian cyst.

It may be possible for the impregnated ovum to implant directly on the peritoneal surface of the lower abdominal cavity. The great majority of intra-abdominal or intraligamentary pregnancies are secondary. The point of implantation was primarily in the tube, but migration has taken place either because the viable ovum has been extruded from the tubal ostium and eventually lost its placental attachment to the original implantation site, or it has grown out through a rent in the wall.

In the early growth phase the symptoms are identical with those of an unruptured tubal pregnancy or, at the most, tubal abortion. The intermittent attacks of pain in the lower part of the abdomen of a patient known to be pregnant suggest either that the tube is being distended or that some hemorrhage is taking place into the abdominal cavity. At the time of tubal abortion or when a breakthrough occurs in the tubal wall, there may be some vaginal bleeding. The bleeding, either vaginal or rectal, promptly subsides if the fetus retains its viability. The symptoms then are minimal and consist chiefly of lower abdominal discomfort or mild pain.

It may be impossible in summarizing the evidence gathered from the history and physical examination to say whether the patient has had a threatened abortion and recovered or whether the pregnancy is a normal intrauterine pregnancy once the acute phases have passed. The close proximity of an enlarging adnexal mass to the uterus often gives a false impression that the enlargement is due to uterine pregnancy. As the pregnancy enlarges, however, one may become suspicious of the cervix, which should become increasingly soft if a viable pregnancy is within the uterus. If the pregnancy is ectopically placed, the cervix will be unchanged. This does not help to localize the pregnancy outside the uterus, for it could still be within an expanding tube or lie in either the abdominal cavity or broad ligament. It is practically impossible to distinguish between an intraligamentary and an abdominal pregnancy.

Since most of these ectopic pregnancies die in the early months, the symptoms of lower abdominal discomfort and pain increase until laparotomy is done with a diagnosis of extrauterine pregnancy. An acute episode of pain is usually synchronous with the death of the fetus. The management of an abdominal pregnancy which goes through to term involves many problems. These fall within the province of the obstetrician and will not be discussed in this volume.

REFERENCES

Development of Ectopic Pregnancy

Anderson, G. W.: Racial Incidence and Mortality of Ectopic Pregnancy. *Am. J. Obst. & Gynec.*, 61: 312, 1951.

Beacham, W. D., Webster, H. D., and Beacham, D. W.: Ectopic Pregnancy at New Orleans Charity Hospital. *Am. J. Obst. & Gynec.*, 72: 830, 1956.

Bercovici, B., Pfau, A., and Liban, E.: Primary Ovarian Pregnancy. Report of 3 Cases, One with Implantation in an Endometrial Cyst of Ovary. *Obst. & Gynec.*, 12: 596, 1958.

Berlind, M.: The Contralateral Corpus Luteum; An Important Factor in Ectopic Pregnancies. *Obst. & Gynec.*, 16: 51, 1960.

Bobrow, M. L., and Winkelstein, L. B.: Intrafollicular Ovarian Pregnancy. *Am. J. Surg.*, 91: 991, 1956.

Bossart, L. J., and others: Unruptured Primary Ovarian Pregnancy. *Am. J. Obst. & Gynec.*, 69: 1366, 1955.

Crawford, E., and Hutchinson, H.: A Decade of Reports on Tubal Pregnancies Condensed from Literature, Plus 300 Consecutive Cases without a Death. *Am. J. Obst. & Gynec.*, 67: 568, 1954.

Ellis, R. W.: Ovarian Pregnancy. *Obst. & Gynec.*, 14: 54, 1959.

Fulsher, R. W.: Tubal Pregnancy Following Homolateral Salpingectomy. A Review of 67 Cases Described in Literature and Report of 4 New Ones. *Am. J. Obst. & Gynec.*, 78: 355, 1959.

Goodman, D., Elia, A. D., and Friedell, G. H.: Simultaneously Aborted Intrauterine and Tubal Pregnancies. Report of a Case. *Obst. & Gynec.*, 16: 53, 1960.

Jarcho, J.: Ectopic Pregnancy, with Special Reference to Abdominal Pregnancy. *Am. J. Surg.*, 77: 273, 1949.

McKenzie, C. H.: Ovarian Pregnancy Associated with Endometriosis in Same Organ. *Am. J. Obst. & Gynec.*, 45: 126, 1943.

Nelson, H. M., and Guindi, S.: Ectopic Pregnancy. *Postgrad. Med.*, 28: 343, 1960.

Roth, D. B.: Ectopic Pregnancy. Is It Increasing? *Obst. & Gynec.*, 13: 544, 1959.

Speert, H., Nash, W., and Kaplan, A. L.: Tubal Pregnancy: Some Observations on External Migration of Ovum and Compensatory Hypertrophy of the Residual Ovary. *Obst. & Gynec.*, 7: 322, 1956.

Diagnosis and Treatment

Bobrow, M. L., and Winkelstein, L. B.: The Value of Centesis as a Diagnostic Procedure in Ruptured Ectopic Gestation. *Am. J. Obst. & Gynec.*, 69: 101, 1955.

Bradbury, W. C.: Technic of Posterior Colpotomy. *West. J. Surg.*, 60: 377, 1952.

Decker, A.: Culdoscopy. *Am. J. Obst. & Gynec.*, 63: 654, 1952.

Durfee, R. B.: Posterior Colpotomy Incisions in Gynecologic Disease. *J.A.M.A.*, 169: 1594, 1959.

Rosenblum, J. M., Dowling, R. W., and Barnes, A. C.: Treatment of Tubal Pregnancy. *Am. J. Obst. & Gynec.*, 80: 274, 1960.

Rosenthal, A. H.: Rupture of the Corpus Luteum, Including Four Cases of Massive Intraperitoneal Hemorrhage. *Am. J. Obst. & Gynec.*, 79: 1008, 1960.

Skulj, V.: Significance of Tubal Pregnancy in the Reproductive Life of Women. *Am. J. Obst. & Gynec.*, 80: 278, 1960.

Williams, P. C., and Enriquez, R. V.: Ectopic Pregnancy. *M. Clin. N. Amer.*, 45: 115, 1961.

Wooten, E. L.: Use of Posterior Colpotomy in the Diagnosis and Treatment of Ectopic Pregnancy and Other Lesions of the Pelvis. *Am. J. Obst. & Gynec.*, 80: 727, 1960.

Chapter 33

Hydatidiform Mole

and Chorionepithelioma

THE TWO entities hydatidiform mole and chorionepithelioma represent further byproducts of the problems of reproduction. Though they have a different clinical course and the pathologic patterns are dissimilar, they are commonly discussed together, for chorionepithelioma may appear in a patient who has previously extruded a mole. This is not an invariable association, for chorionepithelioma can follow an abortion, ectopic pregnancy or even a normal full-term gestation (Fig. 33–1). The hydatidiform mole is not infrequent and usually runs a completely benign course, with many patients capable of becoming pregnant and delivering normal healthy infants after its extrusion. Chorionepithelioma or choriocarcinoma, on the other hand, is an uncommon but highly lethal tumor, nearly unique in that it is the outstanding example of the rare instance in which a malignant tumor of one individual, the fetus, kills another, the mother.

HYDATIDIFORM MOLE

Definition of a Hydatidiform Mole

A hydatidiform mole, which in general gynecologic parlance is loosely called a mole, and occasionally a vesicular mole, is a benign but abnormal product of pregnancy which has remained too long in the uterus. The word "mole" means "mass" and of course has several other meanings. For example, an ordinary abortion with tuberous (lumpy) subchorionic hematomas is classified as a Breus mole. The fetus of a hydatidiform molar pregnancy is either stunted, necrotic or entirely absent. Under normal conditions the uterus expels the abnormal gestational products when the patient aborts approximately six weeks after the missed menstrual period, or eight weeks after conception. If the trophoblast maintains its viability beyond this time and the products are not extruded, a "missed abortion" results.

A completely developed hydatidiform mole exhibits characteristic pathologic changes in the chorionic layers of the gestation sac. There are three basic histologic findings located chiefly in the chorionic villi. (1) Cystic degeneration appears in the villi with hydropic swelling in the main portions. (2) There is notable lack of vascularization within the villi. This lack almost inevitably is associated with the death of the embryo. (3) Despite the lack of vascularization, the villi remain viable, and mild

408

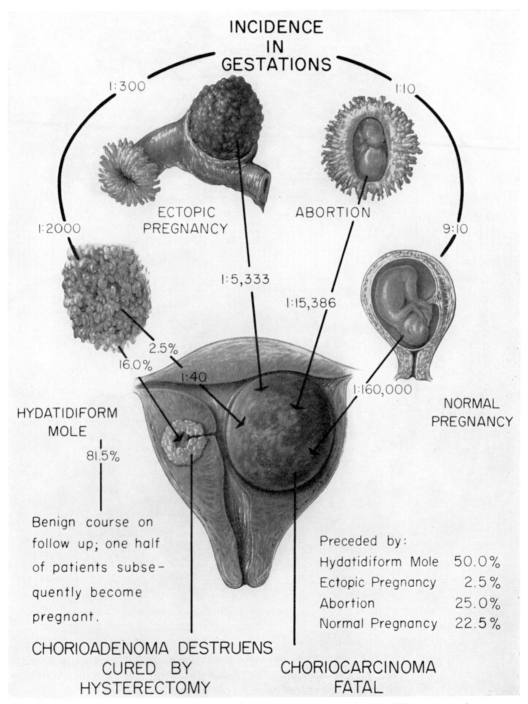

Fig. 33-1.   The relative frequency of choriocarcinoma complicating different sorts of pregnancy is indicated. The hydatidiform mole may develop into either chorioadenoma destruens or choriocarcinoma. (From A. T. Hertig and H. Mansell: Hydatidiform Mole and Choriocarcinoma. Fascicle, Armed Forces Institute of Pathology.)

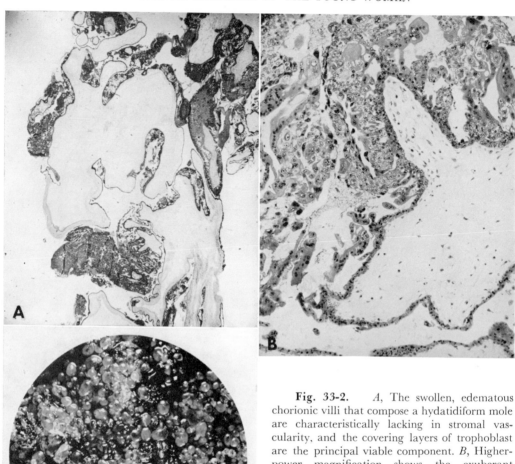

Fig. 33-2. *A,* The swollen, edematous chorionic villi that compose a hydatidiform mole are characteristically lacking in stromal vascularity, and the covering layers of trophoblast are the principal viable component. *B,* Higher-power magnification shows the exuberant growth of both cytotrophoblast and syncytial trophoblastic layers in the maternal vascular sinusoids. *C,* The pale, grapelike clusters of edematous chorionic villi are characteristic of hydatidiform mole.

or notable proliferation of the covering of the trophoblastic tissue is noted (Fig. 33–2, *A, B*). The fetus dies, but the chorionic tissue is retained within the uterus and continues to live and temporarily to grow.

The functioning trophoblastic tissue produces the chorionic gonadotropin in sufficient quantity to create a positive urine test for pregnancy, though the fetus is dead. It is characteristic of the mole that excessive quantities of gonadotropin are manufactured. Since there is a total loss of any connection between the original fetal circulation and that of the villi, the villi begin to degenerate, pull apart easily and become distended with fluid, which under normal conditions would be absorbed or utilized. Progressive swelling of the villi follows, and eventually grapelike masses are formed which we recognize grossly and are characteristic clinically (Fig. 33–2, *C*).

This train of events begins to appear when the abnormal products of the pregnancy are retained longer than ten weeks. Examination of the placental villi passed or curetted from the uterus at this time will show some of the villi to be swollen and edematous (Fig. 33–3). If the placenta survives beyond the twelfth week, in the absence of a viable embryo, fully half or more of the villi will appear microscopically swollen and edematous. This is termed a "transitional" hydatidiform mole (Fig. 33–4). Beyond the fourteenth week the mole has fully matured and presents a typical

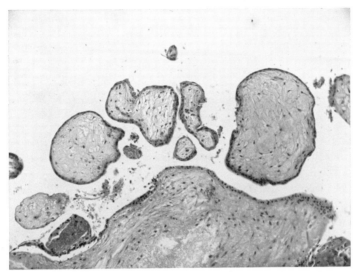

Fig. 33-3.   The chorionic villi of a missed abortion are avascular, and begin to show focal degeneration and stromal edema about the tenth week after conception.

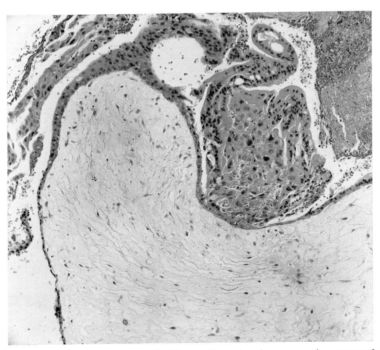

Fig. 33-4.   In a missed abortion retained over 12 weeks after conception, most of the chorionic villi have degenerated stroma, and at least half are edematous, with viable trophoblast proliferating on the surface. This constitutes a "transitional mole."

picture both grossly and microscopically. Grossly, one finds the uterus enlarged and distended by thousands of watery, pale, smooth, grapelike clusters of translucent villi. As the patient goes into labor and spontaneously tries to abort the mole, these grapelike masses are passed into the vagina. Almost invariably this is accompanied by bleeding of some magnitude.

It is obvious that many of the pathologic characteristics of the mole are similar to those found in a few chorionic villi from a patient who has had a retained blighted ovum or missed spontaneous abortion. Usually the uterus expels the blighted ovum early, at least by the ninth or tenth week after fertilization, while the vast majority of moles are discovered around the nineteenth week.

What Is the Explanation of the Development of a Mole?

Much thorough investigative effort has been expended in search for the cause of the recognizable changes within the hydatidiform mole, but the real explanation is still incompletely known. Obviously, the mechanisms are closely linked to the cause of the abortion, with many of the same factors at work. For example, one cannot disregard the environmental factors within the endometrium or even tube, where moles have occasionally been found after an ectopic pregnancy. External factors bearing on both ovogenesis and spermatogenesis apply equally well to abortions or to moles. We know that both the ova and the spermatozoa are sensitive to the effects of toxic agents, vitamin deficiency, temperature changes and hormonal imbalance. Age is definitely a factor, for moles tend to occur at both ends of the menstrual spectrum. There is a striking tendency for a molar pregnancy to appear in the juvenile phase of reproductive life and again after the age of forty. It is said to be twenty times more likely for a woman to have a mole when pregnancy takes place after the age of forty. This is particularly true if it is the first pregnancy. The development of a mole in the adolescent period may be related to the immaturity of the ovary, with some evidence that it may not yet be ready to sustain a normal pregnancy. In the older age group, on the other hand, there appears to be a background of inadequate hormones.

Both the male and the female are implicated in the etiology of the hydatidiform mole. A number of theories localize the defect to the ovary, and particularly to the follicle. Another school believes the male to be the source of the maldevelopment, suggesting that chorionic tissue may emanate exclusively from the male. Supporting arguments are advanced for both points of view, but the fact remains that the true cause is really not known.

How Common Is the Hydatidiform Mole?

The actual incidence of hydatidiform mole is difficult to determine. As we have noted, many abortions, if retained, would likely have developed into moles. Ten per cent of all pregnancies are said to terminate in abortion, but the frequency of the mole is not much greater than one in 1500 to 2000 pregnancies. Geography makes some difference. For example, the incidence is definitely higher in some Far Eastern countries (Philippines, China), where mole formation occurs approximately once in every 500 pregnancies. This may be due to the fact that early marriage is common in these countries, and the age factor comes into play. Moles also tend to appear in women of high fertility. This factor is also operative in the increased incidence in these geographical locations.

The fact that there appears to be some tendency for hydatidiform mole to occur at both ends of the reproductive period does not mean that it cannot occur in other age groups. The majority will appear during the phases of greatest reproductivity, namely, the age groups between twenty-five and thirty-five.

Diagnosis of Hydatidiform Mole

What Is the Most Important Symptom?   The pathologic changes begin early, but rarely produce symptoms until *vaginal bleeding* appears after ten or more weeks of amenorrhea. The bleeding varies widely in nature as well as in the manner and amount of blood lost. When intermittent spotting occurs, the bloody discharge is usually blackish in color, grading off to brown, red or pink, depending on the amount being lost. Bleeding may be profuse, in which case the color is apt to be red. Whatever the color or however it occurs, the patient with a hydatidiform mole almost invariably bleeds. Certainly this is the most important single symptom, but there is little to distinguish it from an early abortion, except that the mole is apt to occur later in the pregnancy, beyond the tenth week. The bleeding occurs without pain, and uterine cramps are usually absent.

Is the Uterus Always Enlarged?   The size of the uterus may prove helpful, for approximately 40 per cent will show a uterine enlargement greater than one might expect from the duration of the pregnancy. On the other hand, the patient can have a hydatidiform mole when the uterus is of normal size, and approximately one third will have a uterus smaller than one would anticipate from the date of conception. In all probability the size of the uterus reflects the viability of the mole. When uterine enlargement is present, it may be considered pathognomonic of a mole, provided twin pregnancy, hydramnios or pregnancy within a fibroid uterus can be ruled out. The presence of a mole cannot be ruled out when the uterus is either normal or small in size.

The diagnosis is obvious when the patient passes a placental mass, which grossly resembles a cluster of white grapes, from the dilated cervical os of an overenlarged uterus. The placenta may be completely replaced by the edematous mass of dilated vesicles, or the involvement may be spotty. Though the early bleeding occurs without pain, expulsion of the mole is usually accompanied by uterine cramps.

What Can We Learn from X-ray, Palpation and Auscultation?   The uterus may simply have enlarged at an accelerated pace to a size out of proportion to that expected of a normal pregnancy when the size is compared to the date of conception. For example, with the presence of a mole in a pregnancy calculated by dates to be of three months' duration, the uterus may feel the size of a five months' pregnancy. One might expect at this time to be able to palpate fetal bone structure, see it by x-ray or detect a fetal heart beat. If, on the other hand, the uterus has not enlarged, little can be gained by x-ray scout films, for fetal bones are usually not seen until after the third or fourth month.

How Long Does a Mole Persist?   The duration of life of the mole varies and is in part dependent on the vitality of the trophoblasts which produce the chorionic gonadotropin. If the trophoblastic activity is high and the uterine musculature sluggish, the life of the mole may be extended beyond the nineteenth week, the time when most of them are expelled. Those moles with less vitality are probably extruded early and become confused with abortions, but the more vital may deliver much later. Some have been reported as late as two years after the start of pregnancy.

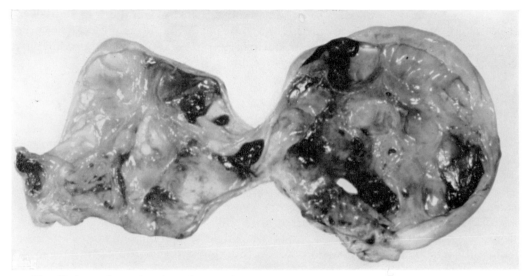

Fig. 33-5.   A grossly enlarged ovary that measured approximately 10 cm. in diameter contained multiple theca lutein cysts, microscopically. This finding on both sides at operation suggested the presence of an intrauterine hydatidiform mole, which was confirmed by curettage.

WHAT OTHER SIGNS AND SYMPTOMS OF ABNORMAL PREGNANCY MAY OCCUR? When the life of the mole has been prolonged beyond the ten-week period, signs of *early toxemia* may present themselves. Approximately half of the patients with a hydatidiform mole will experience intractable vomiting, and more than a third will demonstrate *hypertension* and *albuminuria* and experience *headaches*. Some or all of these symptoms are frequently present, but not always at the same time. Symptoms of this sort which suggest eclampsia are significant when they occur so early in pregnancy, for they are rarely early findings when a pregnancy is developing normally. The explanation can probably be traced to the high level of circulating chorionic gonadotropin, for the symptoms usually appear in the patient who has a rapidly enlarging uterus indicative of increased vitality of the molar tissue.

HOW SIGNIFICANT IS OVARIAN ENLARGEMENT DUE TO THECA LUTEIN CYSTS? Under the stimulation of the luteinizing component (LH) of chorionic gonadotropin the ovaries of the patient with a mole tend to undergo widespread luteinization of the follicles and to develop theca lutein cysts. These cysts vary in size from 1.5 to 15 cm. The majority are small, but in many instances they are large enough to be palpable on examination (Fig. 33–5). Nevertheless the fact that enlarged ovaries are not felt does not eliminate the possibility that the patient may have a mole.

Though bilaterally enlarged ovaries contribute to the diagnosis of hydatidiform mole, they should not influence the subsequent treatment. It is a curious fact that the lutein cysts seem to grow rapidly after the mole has delivered and equally fascinating that they disappear spontaneously. Within two or three months the ovaries are back to normal size. Since these cysts are benign and do regress, one should not be tempted into surgical moves to correct them. In fact, you do the patient a good turn by leaving them alone.

It has been suggested that their presence provides protection against subsequent development of chorionepithelioma. Although cystic enlargement of the ovary is sometimes present with chorionepithelioma, more often it is not. Estrin seems to provide a brake against excessive activity of trophoblastic growth. The enlarged cystic ovaries should then be an excellent defense. The patient without ovarian enlargement may be a more likely candidate for malignant changes in the mole.

The arguments for and against removal of the ovaries, when the patient has chorionepithelioma, will be discussed later. Theca lutein cysts in the presence of a benign mole should be left alone.

WHAT DO LUTEIN CYSTS LOOK LIKE MICROSCOPICALLY?   Characteristically, these theca lutein cysts imitate corpora lutea. The cysts are lined by readily recognizable bright yellow tissue, grossly. Under the microscope the cyst wall is composed of enlarged, polygonal, luteinized theca interna cells arranged in two or three layers (Fig. 33–6). Except for the different architecture and smaller cell size, their appearance is not unlike adrenal cortical cells.

WHAT LABORATORY TESTS ARE HELPFUL?   Laboratory tests are useful in making the diagnosis of a hydatidiform mole and in evaluating the malignant potential both in the initial phases and in subsequent follow-up. They must be interpreted intelligently and with proper regard to the clinical history and findings. None are infallible. The two tests most commonly done are (*a*) quantitative determinations of chorionic gonadotropin and (*b*) histologic interpretation of the curetted endometrial lining and the entire mole. Occasionally the *vaginal smear* will reveal odd multinucleated cells which resemble trophoblasts and are not usually seen in the smears of a pregnant patient. This may suggest that a mole is present.

What Information Do We Get from the Aschheim-Zondek Type of Test?   Quantitative determinations of the amount of circulating chorionic gonadotropin have received widespread acceptance as a method of establishing the diagnosis of hydatidiform mole. Actually, such tests are of limited practical value when used as the only criterion for an accurate diagnosis. There is too much individual variation in these tumors to rely on such information completely. The amount of chorionic gonadotropin recovered depends upon how much trophoblastic tissue is present and how active it is. There seems to be a relation between the amount of hormone and the vitality of the mole. Since some moles may be inactive or incapable of producing large amounts of hormone, it is possible for a patient to have a hydatidiform mole though the quantitative tests show less than the normal amount. If one is to place much faith in the tests, one must correlate the age of the pregnancy with the size of the mole. Some normal pregnancies at ten weeks produce levels of chorionic gonadotropin in excess of those

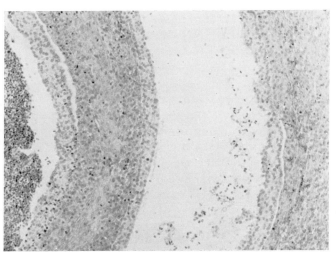

Fig. 33-6.   Theca lutein cysts are lined by partially luteinized granulosa cells, beneath which are several layers of darker-staining, luteinized theca interna cells.

found in a mole. Moreover, other complications of a normal pregnancy such as pernicious vomiting often are associated with high levels.

It is obvious that the mere presence of a high level of chorionic gonadotropin neither makes nor rules out a diagnosis of hydatidiform mole. If one places too much stress on such findings, there is grave danger that a normal pregnancy may be interrupted or the uterus be sacrificed.

Chorionic gonadotropin recovered from the spinal fluid has greater significance, for it is most unlikely that a single normal pregnancy will produce it. Normal twin pregnancies, however, do so. Therefore the test is not infallible in any situation, but is useful when interpreted intelligently in connection with other clinical findings. As a final word of caution the quantitative tests, to have any significance, must be based on determinations from a series of specimens rather than a single 24-hour urine specimen.

How Helpful Are Other Hormonal Studies in Establishing a Diagnosis?   The same conclusions that apply to the excretion of chorionic gonadotropin are operative when one attempts to measure the excretion of other hormones in the presence of a mole. In a normal pregnancy which progresses beyond the third month one expects to find a rising titer of both estrin and pregnanediol. The reverse is true in the patient with a hydatidiform mole. The trophoblasts continue to put out increasingly large quantities of chorionic gonadotropin, but they seem to lose their power to produce either estrin or progestin. The findings, however, are relative, and in general we must conclude that quantitative serial determinations of the urinary secretion of estrin, pregnanediol and 17-ketosteroids have little practical value in establishing the diagnosis of a mole.

Treatment

We have noted that the malignant chorionepithelioma may occur after a normal or ectopically placed pregnancy, but it frequently does follow a mole. Because of this the treatment of the mole automatically falls into two phases. In the first place, we are concerned with the best method of evacuating the uterus according to the individual conditions which prevail, and whether or not there is any indication that malignant degeneration has occurred. In the second place, we should consider the best plan for carrying out a clinical follow-up which must go on for at least five years after delivery of a hydatidiform mole.

WHAT METHODS ARE USED TO EVACUATE THE MOLE?   The great majority of gynecologists prefer to empty the uterus promptly once the diagnosis of a mole has been made beyond a shadow of a doubt. A few feel that the danger of malignancy has been overemphasized, since most moles run a benign course. They prefer to allow the patient to abort the mole spontaneously, provided the bleeding is not excessive.

Obviously, if the patient has gone into labor and is passing grapelike clusters of tissue through a dilated cervical os, she should be allowed to continue. The spontaneous expulsion of the mole may be complete, as shown by a reduction in the size of the uterus and the cessation of bleeding. If bleeding continues, however, one must assume that gestational products remain. These must be eliminated by curettage under anesthesia with either blunt curet or ovum forceps. It is possible to do this with finger dissection if the os is sufficiently dilated, but the blunt curet is the instrument of choice. Astonishing amounts of hydatidiform villi are curetted, frequently enough to fill a large pan (Fig. 33–2, *C*). There are dangers in curettage, for the uterus containing a mole is definitely softer than in a normal pregnancy. It is, therefore, all too easy either to tear the cervix or to perforate the fundus. The uterus must be completely emptied, for the bleeding is often excessive and will not cease until all the products are removed. The molar products should be thoroughly examined microscopically for possible malignant change. Particularly important are the curettements from the uterine wall.

The majority of patients will extrude the mole spontaneously, but not infrequently the patient fails to pass the typical grapelike bodies, does not go into spontaneous labor, yet bleeds persistently and often profusely through a cervix which has not dilated. The uterus must be evacuated to control the bleeding. There are two main schools of thought as to how this may best be accomplished.

1. Most gynecologists seem to favor the vaginal approach to uterine evacuation of the mole, feeling that the uterus can be satisfactorily emptied either by curettage or vaginal hysterotomy. There appears to be little danger of disseminating chorionic implants by this method, for unquestionably any dissemination will already have occurred, before the symptoms call for operative intervention. In general, curettage is preferred to hysterotomy. The only excuse for doing a vaginal hysterotomy would be uncertainty of the operator's ability to remove all the contents. If this is true, the explanation should be sought by thoroughly exposing the uterine cavity to rule out possible invasion of the muscle wall. If hysterotomy seems indicated, it is probably better to do this by the abdominal approach. It is not always easy to determine whether a mole is actually penetrating the uterine wall or whether the area under suspicion simply represents necrotic tissue and old blood. The mere suspicion of invasion may lead to an unnecessary hysterectomy because of fear of malignant degeneration in the mole. This is the reason why the majority of obstetrician-gynecologists prefer curettage to abdominal hysterotomy.

2. The proponents of abdominal hysterotomy present a good case, pointing out that simple emptying of the uterus may be unsatisfactory and frequently is dangerous when the patient bleeds excessively from a uterus with an undilated cervix. The softer uterine consistency in the presence of a mole increases the chance of cervical tear and fundal perforation. They believe that the uterus can be more completely emptied and the bleeding better controlled when abdominal hysterotomy is performed. Moreover, direct inspection of the uterine cavity allows the surgeon to determine whether or not there is any gross invasion of the wall. It is easy to be in error in this evaluation, but one might well question whether any more uteri are sacrificed unnecessarily because of this than are lost by the uncertainty that follows bleeding after an incomplete evacuation by curettage. If gross invasion is present at the time of abdominal hysterotomy, a total hysterectomy with preservation of the ovaries may save the patient's life. Since it is common practice to follow up patients for at least five years after expulsion of a hydatidiform mole, one may be on safer ground in evaluating the prognosis if one has looked at the implantation site directly.

How Valuable Is the Pregnancy Test in the Follow-up Period?   It is of prime importance that the patient have periodic examinations after spontaneous extrusion of a mole or curettage for retention of molar products, whether she has symptoms or not. Usually any tendency for a malignant chorionepithelioma to develop will manifest itself within a matter of a few weeks or months after the expulsion of a mole. This is the period of greatest danger and the one requiring the closest supervision. Nevertheless a choriocarcinoma (chorionepithelioma) may appear several years after a mole has been passed. One cannot relax completely until many years have passed. Quantitative determinations of chorionic gonadotropin on 24-hour urine specimens provide the easiest means of carrying out a follow-up program. Though it takes longer to do (five days) and is more expensive, the Aschheim-Zondek test performed on immature mice is more accurate than the other biological tests, including the Friedman and frog tests.

After the delivery of a normal child the pregnancy test becomes negative within a week or ten days. After expulsion of a mole it may remain positive for a month or more. Approximately 70 per cent will be negative at the end of a month. By the end of 3 months close to 95 per cent will be found to have a negative pregnancy test.

The follow-up program, utilizing repeated determinations of chorionic gonadotropin, should begin approximately two months after the mole has been passed, unless the patient has recurrence of vaginal bleeding. In this case the possibility of malignant change should be considered at once. Before two months the pregnancy test does not help much, for the values continue to remain high even though no molar fragments are present.

The chief reliance before two months have passed must be placed on an evaluation of the size of the uterus. If the uterus does not involute properly or increases in size, and bleeding from it reappears, curettage is indicated, provided the patient has made an all-out effort to keep from getting pregnant again. Microscopic interpretation of the curetted material will in most instances give a pretty clear picture of the nature of the molar fragments and the likelihood of malignant change. This is not 100 per cent true, for the malignancy may lay hidden in one cornu of the endometrial cavity and be missed on curettage, or it may be buried in the uterine musculature. By and large, however, the curetted material will give accurate information as to conditions within the uterus.

If the titer of the gonadotropins remains high or shows a sudden increase after the curettage, one should suspect occult malignancy despite the evidence of curettage. If the patient also bleeds from a uterus that fails to revert to normal size, hysterectomy is indicated.

One of the most difficult differential diagnoses to make immediately after extrusion of a mole is whether the failure of the uterus to involute and the chorionic gonadotropin level to fall really represent persistence of molar fragments or malignant change within them or whether the patient is simply pregnant again. One does not like to interrupt a normal pregnancy under the mistaken impression that the signs and symptoms are due to a mole. For this reason patients who have passed a hydatidiform mole should be advised to keep from getting pregnant for at least one year thereafter.

After the two-month period the pregnancy test is performed twice a month, if the initial test is negative, until one year has elapsed. A single negative Aschheim-Zondek test does not exclude the possibility of chorionepithelioma. One should not become panicky, on the other hand, if the test is positive. The mere persistence of a positive test does not mean that the patient necessarily has malignant disease. There is no need to rush into immediate hysterectomy. Much of the malignant potential of the mole is of low grade. Those of higher grade usually disseminate so widely early in their course of development that hysterectomy will not cure them. One can therefore afford to take the time to be sure of the diagnosis before carrying out definitive therapy. Certainly no overt act should follow the findings of a single positive pregnancy test. The important thing is to know whether the titer is rising or falling. The test should be repeated twice a week as long as it is positive. Any sudden increase in the titer should be looked upon with alarm, provided that several tests continue to show a rise. Hysterectomy, leaving the ovaries and tubes, is then indicated and should be performed promptly.

After hysterectomy the biologic test should be repeated every two weeks for at least six months after the first negative report. After this, if the reaction continues to be negative, the interval can be stretched to three months, but tests should be carried out for at least three years.

WHY IS PATHOLOGIC EXAMINATION OF MOLAR PRODUCTS IMPORTANT? By evacuating the uterus of all molar products the surgeon has completed the first phase of the treatment of the hydatidiform mole. Such a patient, however, must be closely followed up for several years after the mole has been passed. We recognize that most moles have a benign course, for the majority of patients recover and go on to deliver normal babies. Nevertheless most chorionepitheliomas, though they are rare entities, give an antecedent history of a mole. These tumors do have some variations in their lethal potential, but only approximately one sixth of all malignant moles are fatal. We are primarily concerned, then, with the question of whether the initial mole was entirely benign or whether any part of the curettings or portion of the mole showed any suspicion of malignant change. The problems of accurate classification and evaluation of the prognosis in hydatidiform moles have plagued the gynecologist and the pathologist for years. More elaborate classifications have been evolved, but for practical purposes it seems expedient simply to classify hydatidiform moles as benign, suspicious or malignant.

Regardless of the method by which the surgeon elects to empty the uterus, all products of the molar gestation must be submitted and undergo thorough microscopic study. All too frequently the pathologist receives the mole, but not the curettings, and the best indication of any invasive process will be found in the curetted material. Accurate morphologic diagnosis is important in order that the chorionepithelioma (fully developed malignancy in a mole) be distinguished from (1) an early or abnormal previllous pregnancy. Such a pregnancy may have an ovisac and perhaps an embryonic disk, but no genuine trophoblastic anaplasia (Fig. 33–7, *A*). (2) Syncytial endometritis. This is a physiologic situation in all pregnancies, with infiltration of maternal decidual tissue by individual microscopic trophoblastic syncytial cells, but no sheets of trophoblasts. Anaplasia or obvious cancer invasion is lacking (Fig. 33–7, *B*). (3) Placental polyp, when a portion of the cotyledon has been left behind in a superficial vascular sinusoid. The retained villus is composed of placental connective tissue covered with senile trophoblast that shows no anaplasia. (4) Benign or borderline malignant hydatidiform mole, which includes recognizable chorionic villi without definite evidence of myometrial invasion. (5) Chorioadenoma destruens. This is a circumscribed intramyometrial tumor which contains recognizable chorionic villi as well as anaplastic cytotrophoblasts and syncytial trophoblasts. It is locally invasive, but usually does not metastasize.

WHAT DOES A BENIGN MOLE LOOK LIKE MICROSCOPICALLY? A benign mole is composed of edematous avascular chorionic villi covered by the two conventional layers: (*a*) the inner cuboidal layer of cytotrophoblast (Langhans layer) and (*b*) the outer syncytial trophoblast. Pyknotic nuclei and degenerating cells are present, as well as mild local thickening of the trophoblastic layer (Fig. 33–7, *C*).

No untoward complications are anticipated from this type of mole, provided it has been completely removed from the uterus. If bleeding continues after evacuation,

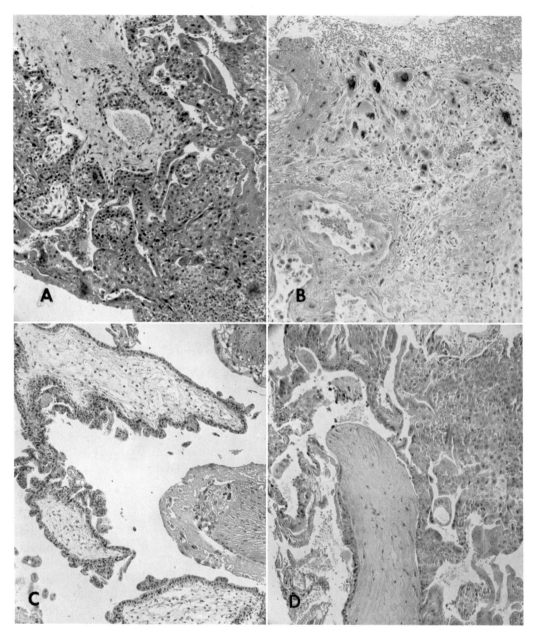

Fig. 33-7.   *A*, Embryo surrounded by previllous and early villous trophoblast, which was unexpectedly found in curettings. The normally exuberant young trophoblast should not be confused with
choriocarcinoma. *B*, Syncytial trophoblastic giant cells normally infiltrate the decidual uterine lining
in every pregnancy. Syncytial endometritis is thus a physiologic condition accompanying intrauterine
placentation. *C*, In benign hydatidiform mole the villi are covered by 2 layers of fairly regularly arranged
trophoblastic cells. *D*, In a suspicious mole sheetlike growths of cytotrophoblastic cells may occur, and
the syncytial cells are variable in size and staining qualities. No invasion is found, however.

if the uterus fails to involute and the pregnancy test remains positive, in all probability molar products have been left behind. There is lesser concern that a malignant change may have occurred.

What Constitutes a Suspicion of Malignancy within a Mole? This is the group that provides the greatest controversy and the most uncertainty as to proper treatment. Approximately half the moles which appear to be histologically malignant never exhibit any clinical signs of cancer. This is why it is important for the pathologist to receive and examine by multiple section technique samples from both the mole and the curetted endometrium. It is axiomatic that abnormal trophoblastic activity in the endometrial lining will give a poorer prognosis than an isolated area in a villus on the periphery of a mole. The most dangerous parts are obviously in and beneath the region of the placental implantation site.

The most important factor to determine is the extent of the invasive behavior of the trophoblastic cells (Fig. 33–7, *D*). This is not easy, for the trophoblast is normally aggressive from the time the fertilized ovum first implants on the endometrial surface. Syncytial trophoblasts actually habitually erode into blood vessels even before recognizable villi are formed. Individual syncytial trophoblastic cells regularly infiltrate the underlying endometrium, where they locally replace the endothelial cells in the blood vessel walls. They also circulate in the blood stream, and even under normal conditions they are found in pulmonary capillaries of all pregnant women. The endometrial infiltration, as mentioned, is called syncytial endometritis.

Another misleading aspect is the fact that trophoblastic cells remain undifferentiated or immature in appearance. They often have cytoplasmic basophilia and abundant nuclear chromatin, befitting cells with active metabolic and hormonal functions. Thus they normally have some of the characteristics of neoplastic growth. If these cells ordinarily exhibit some immaturity and have the property of invasion, the pathologist is bound to have considerable difficulty in trying to determine whether the growth pattern is normal, premalignant or that of established invasive cancer.

A truly malignant tumor of the chorion is made up of cytotrophoblasts and syncytial trophoblasts. The tumor has almost no stroma and has no blood supply. It exists as a parasitic growth in the blood stream, acquiring sustenance for continued growth through the propensity of the trophoblasts to invade the blood vessels of the uterine musculature. This invasive characteristic can best be evaluated by a study of the curetted endometrium. There will always be a few cases in which enough uncertainty exists to warrant hysterectomy.

Do All Malignant Moles Have the Same Lethal Potential? The two forms of malignancy that occur in the uterus after delivery of a mole are chorioadenoma destruens (invasive mole) and chorionepithelioma (choriocarcinoma). The former appears only after malignant transformation has occurred in a hydatidiform mole, while the latter may follow pregnancy anywhere, whether normal or abnormal. The more abnormal the pregnancy, the greater the likelihood of cancer. By far the greatest number follow the delivery of a mole. Less frequently they are seen after ectopic pregnancy or abortion.

Chorioadenoma destruens and chorionepithelioma vary in their lethal potential. The invasive mole is just that, for it is locally malignant only. It may perforate the uterus and kill the patient from hemorrhage or sepsis, but it does not do so by metastases. This is curious, for there is ample evidence that chorionic tissue is normally disseminated widely to the lung and other remote areas. Chorioadenoma destruens can be cured by hysterectomy, in contrast to chorionepithelioma, which is almost invariably fatal when it develops after a molar pregnancy.

CHORIOADENOMA DESTRUENS (INVASIVE MOLE)

The diagnosis is made, when the uterus has been opened, from tissue specimens taken from the implantation site of the mole, at the time of either abdominal hysterotomy or hysterectomy. Surgical intervention was necessary because of the persistence of bleeding after expulsion of the mole and subsequent curettage, together with the finding of an enlarging uterus and a rising titer of chorionic gonadotropin.

On gross examination the interior of the uterus shows a typical hemorrhagic mass, spherical in shape, buried in the myometrium (Fig. 33–8, *A*). This could be simply necrotic tissue or old blood, but it is important that this blood clot be examined, since approximately 16 per cent of all moles will show evidence of invasion of the uterine musculature.

Microscopic study usually reveals the presence of invasive molar tissue within the muscle wall. The chorionic villi are often still discernible superficially. From the chorionic villi sheets and free "tissue-culture-like growths" of syncytial trophoblasts and cytotrophoblasts have invaded the myometrium. Anaplasia is present, but the neoplasm is not wildly undifferentiated, and it is still possible to recognize the villous placental tissue of origin (Fig. 33–8, *B*). The combined gross and microscopic findings define chorioadenoma destruens.

Total hysterectomy, leaving the ovaries, is the obvious treatment, for though the degree of malignancy *may be low*, the trophoblasts have demonstrated their power to invade. The variations in the rate of growth and the ability to metastasize could be due to natural protective factors rather than any loss in malignant potential. There seems to be some evidence that the same factors which absorb or destroy the chorionic villi in the implantation site of a normal pregnancy also operate to restrict the pattern and rate of growth when anaplasia is present in a mole.

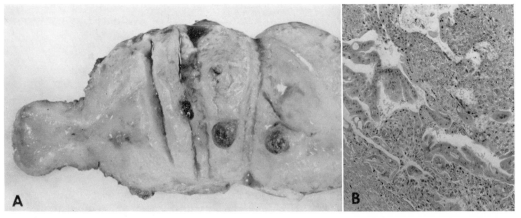

Fig. 33-8.   *A*, Nodules of chorioadenoma destruens in the myometrium are characteristically spheroid, red and friable. They are smaller and better demarcated than uterine choriocarcinoma. *B*, Microscopically, chorioadenoma destruens shows trophoblastic growth within the myometrium, obviously invasive, but relatively well differentiated. In places actual villi with stroma are found in the myometrium, something that does not occur in choriocarcinoma.

CHORIONEPITHELIOMA (CHORIOCARCINOMA)

How Do the Gross and Microscopic Pictures of Chorionepithelioma in the Uterus Differ from Those of Chorioadenoma Destruens?

The same clinical findings, laboratory studies and symptoms have provided indications for surgical intervention in both entities. It is important to differentiate the two, both grossly and microscopically, because of the highly lethal nature of chorionepithelioma. Since chorionepithelioma may follow a normal delivery, ectopic pregnancy or abortion, it is important that all abnormal placentas and gestational products be examined pathologically for possible trophoblastic malignancy.

THE GROSS PICTURE. Grossly, a choriocarcinoma will show multiple, firm, purple, typically hemorrhagic nodules of tumor tissue when the uterine cavity is opened at the time of hysterotomy or after hysterectomy (Fig. 33–9). No hydropic villi are evident. The tumor masses, which are made up of wildly growing trophoblasts, may extend through the uterus and involve the adjacent lymphatics and veins in the parametrium (Fig. 33–10). Rarely are the margins discrete, for they tend to merge into the surrounding muscle. The pure trophoblast has extensively invaded the blood vessels, and widespread metastases occur early.

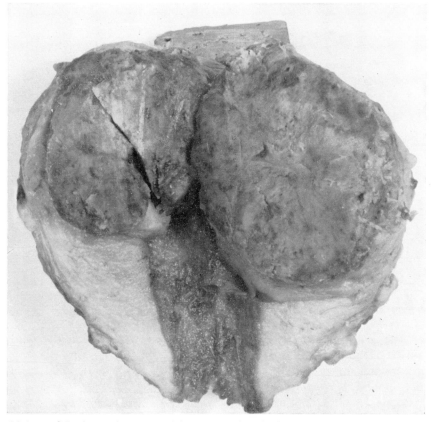

Fig. 33-9. Massive replacement of the myometrium by hemorrhagic, friable and poorly demarcated choriocarcinoma. This tumor developed after a normal pregnancy at Massachusetts Memorial Hospitals, and the patient died 10 months after hysterectomy with lung metastases.

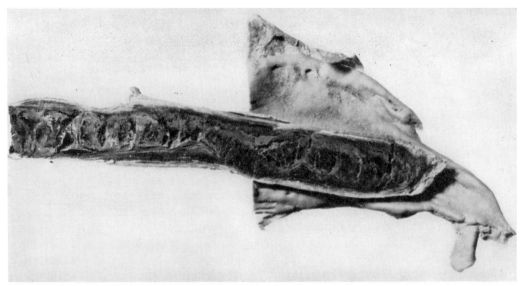

Fig. 33-10.   Choriocarcinoma may grow in the parametrial veins as a solid cord of tumor mixed with blood clot.

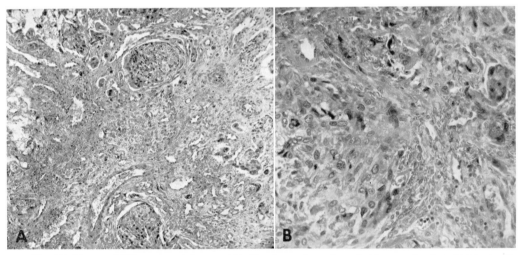

Fig. 33-11.   *A,* The myometrium and its blood vessels are invaded by anaplastic individual cells and masses of malignant trophoblastic tissue in choriocarcinoma. In places there are the characteristic hemorrhages which give the tumors a typical red color grossly. *B,* Cytotrophoblastic cells growing in sheets show abnormal variations in their size, shape and staining in choriocarcinoma, and the intermingled multinucleated syncytial trophoblastic cells are equally anaplastic.

THE MICROSCOPIC PICTURE.   On microscopic examination the wild uncontrolled growth of the trophoblast is immediately apparent. The tumor is composed of tangled masses and sheets of anaplastic cells, both large and small, which resemble the previllous trophoblast. No actual chorionic villi are seen, however. Varying quantities of cyto- and syncytio-trophoblasts are found in different parts of the tumor in the same patient. There is some suggestion that the vitality of the lesion may be somewhat less when the preponderance favors the syncytial trophoblast. The tumor of greatest activity and lethal potential is associated with more cytotrophoblastic cells, showing many mitotic figures and much immaturity of trophoblasts. Typically, these malignant trophoblasts erode small vessels and lie in pools and sinusoids of unclotted blood, usually in the border zone between active trophoblastic tissue and the areas of necrosis which are common in these tumors (Fig. 33–11). It is the propensity of the neoplastic trophoblast to invade blood vessels that makes early tumor embolism and multiple metastases to the lung and other areas such common occurrences.

WHAT ARE THE VARIATIONS FROM THE GROSS AND MICROSCOPIC PICTURES OF CHORIONEPITHELIOMA? It is an interesting and not too uncommon observation to find metastases from chorionepithelioma, without any gross or microscopic evidence of disease in either the endometrium or myometrium. It would seem that regression takes place at the point of origin as the secondary deposits take root and grow. When the malignant process is buried in the uterine wall, curettage of the endometrium or direct inspection of the uterine cavity also may fail to demonstrate any lesion within the uterus.

On What Does the Final Diagnosis of Chorionepithelioma Rest?

The final diagnosis of chorionepithelioma must rest on the microscopic interpretation of the material presented, coupled with the clinical findings. The biologic tests for chorionic gonadotropin offer too many variables. For example, though they may represent exceptions rather than the rule, it is possible to have a chorionepithelioma with a negative test for gonadotropin and, conversely, a positive test with no demonstrable chorionic tissue. It is fair to say that not all pathologists agree on all histologic interpretations, but by and large it is safer to rely on the tissue pathology than on laboratory determinations of the amount of chorionic gonadotropin. The difficulty in establishing a histologic diagnosis is greater when a uterine lesion convenient to biopsy is being examined than is true of a metastatic site, for example in lung.

WHAT SYMPTOMS AND SIGNS ARE PRODUCED WHEN THE CHORIONEPITHELIOMA IS PRESENT WITHIN THE UTERUS? There are no pathognomonic symptoms of chorionepithelioma of the uterus per se. We suspect the diagnosis when *uterine hemorrhage* occurs or excessive bleeding persists from a uterus that fails to involute or increases in size. The suspicion is strengthened when the titer of urinary chorionic gonadotropin reappears and continues to rise several months or even years after the termination of a normal pregnancy, hydatidiform mole or an abortion. The bleeding could be due to retained products of an old pregnancy or an accident to a new one. It is possible that molar fragments are retained. The most important thing to rule out, though its occurrence may be rare, is a true chorionepithelioma.

It is possible for a chorionepithelioma to be hidden in the wall of the uterus without involving the endometrium. In this case bleeding will not occur. The only suggestion other than the rising titer of chorionic gonadotropin will be the size of the uterus, which either fails to involute or increases in dimension. Rarely does it get beyond the size expected of a two months' gestation, but the contour is often irregular and indistinguishable from a fibroid uterus. The tumor in the uterus does not have to be very large to produce widespread distant metastases; in fact the secondary extension of the disease, whether it occurs in lung, liver or brain, may be larger than the primary tumor at the time it is discovered.

It is a well documented observation that not infrequently distant metastases

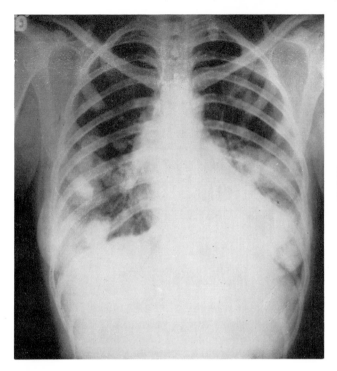

Fig. 33-12. Multiple nodular pulmonary metastases from a uterine choriocarcinoma are a common finding in this condition.

appear with only a scar to mark the original site of origin within the uterus. This is a quality peculiar to chorionepithelioma and has no counterpart in tumor growth anywhere else in the body. The same peculiar situation occurs in some testicular choriocarcinomas which show abundant metastases, yet with no primary tumor that can be recognized as such. The mechanism of this phenomenon is not known. It may be that the free trophoblastic cells, which we know appear in the lung during a normal pregnancy, and are frequently found after moles, actually undergo a malignant transformation in some chorionepitheliomas. The trophoblasts at the implantation site could enter the blood stream by direct penetration without any appreciable invasion of the myometrial wall. It is possible that the same functions are at work in tumor regression that cause the normal placental site to disappear and the syncytial emboli to disappear from the lung.

What Symptoms Are Produced by the Metastases? We have noted that the primary site within the uterus often disappears once the metastasis is firmly established. In instances of this sort the customary bleeding will be absent, and the first indication of any trouble is often produced by the metastases. The metastases are widespread and frequently multiple. They are found in nearly every organ of the body. Lung, liver, brain, kidney, spleen, bowel and ovary are involved in approximately the order named. Purplish nodules can often be seen in the vagina, vulva and cervix. These metastatic lesions may arrive there by lymphatic spread, but by and large the dissemination is by the hematogenous route. By far the greatest number (60 to 80 per cent) occur in the lung.

The first indication of trouble is often the appearance of a persistent cough, hemoptysis or simply shortness of breath. The x-ray film will usually confirm the presence of a solitary nodule or widespread metastases in the lung fields (Fig. 33–12). Sometime x-ray examination reveals extensive lung involvement in the patient who has no symptoms at all. One should be suspicious of a negative report in the presence of clinical symptoms, for tumor has been found in the lung postmortem when none showed by x-ray examination. If there is doubt, laminograms of the chest should be taken.

Usually the metastases manifest themselves within the first year, but occasionally years may elapse from the time of the delivery of a mole, abortion, ectopic or normal pregnancy before the first symptoms appear. In all probability, during this long latent period, the metastases simply remained in a quiescent state. On the other hand, one cannot completely rule out the possibility that the tumor originated in a teratoma located in the lung rather than in the placental trophoblast. Such tumors have been known to appear in nulliparous and virginal women in the absence of any pregnancy.

There is another fascinating thing about metastases from chorionepithelioma, namely, their tendency to spontaneous regression. This is particularly true of lung metastases, though it may occur in other areas. Usually the phenomenon is observed after the primary site has been removed by hysterectomy, but it has followed excision of vaginal metastases and in a few instances has occurred spontaneously without any therapy.

Because the tumor invades blood vessels and has a tendency to necrosis, the predominant symptom will be hemorrhage. When it occurs in an area that has an outlet, the symptoms will be obvious bleeding. For example, tumor in the vagina will produce bleeding and a foul discharge. Tumor in the intestinal tract will cause abdominal pain and bloody stools. Hematuria and dysuria will be present if the tumor is in the kidney or bladder. Hemoptysis, coughing and chest pain are usually present if the lung is involved.

When the metastasis occurs in a nonexpansile area, the chief symptoms are usually those of pressure produced by the hemorrhage and necrosis. Hence headaches, loss of consciousness or speech, blurring of vision, convulsions and paralysis are frequent symptoms in the patient who has cerebral metastases. When the liver is involved, one can expect jaundice and bilirubinuria. Again the symptoms may vary according to the activity of the tumor, and spontaneous regression has been noted to follow hysterectomy, in these regions as well as the lung. These observations often go hand in hand with a reduction in the titer of the chorionic gonadotropins. One should not get the idea that spontaneous regression is common, for chorionepithelioma is a rapidly fatal disease, and in most instances death follows within six months of the time the diagnosis is made.

SUMMARY OF THE DIAGNOSTIC CRITERIA.   It is obvious from the preceding discussion that none of the tests themselves are foolproof in establishing a diagnosis of chorionepithelioma. The vaginal smear as a diagnostic implement has not been mentioned, but it too is useful only if it is positive. A negative smear means nothing. To be accurate in all cases it is necessary to pool the data and observations from the clinical history, the hormonal assays and the histologic review of the sections of the tumor specimen. The great majority (75 per cent) can be diagnosed on the basis of the following criteria: (1) A history of previous pregnancy terminating either normally or pathologically as a mole, ectopic pregnancy or abortion; (2) the appearance of vaginal bleeding from a uterus that is larger than one would anticipate in a normal pregnancy. These are important observations, but they should be confirmed by quantitative hormonal studies and pathologic review of the tumor from the material obtained at either curettage or hysterotomy. The chances are that the patient has a serious tumor if the histologic findings are suspicious or definitely malignant, and the patient has a rising titer of chorionic gonadotropins.

Treatment

The treatment of choice in chorionepithelioma is primarily surgical, whether the process seems to be confined to the uterus or whether metastases have been demonstrated elsewhere. Before discussing surgical removal of the uterus it will be well to consider briefly other forms of therapy.

A conservative school feels that a true chorionepithelioma cannot be cured by surgical or any other means. Rather than submit the patients to the rigors of surgery which is destined to be nonproductive, they prefer to rely on supportive therapy only. Treatment is entirely palliative, with transfusions of blood as the chief instrument. This is designed to combat the anemia and increase the patient's general resistance with the hope that specific antibodies against the growth of chorionic cells may develop. This is the basis for giving transfusions of blood taken from pregnant women donors.

The conservative attitude toward therapy is entirely defeatist and has little to recommend it.

The *use of hormone therapy* has had many advocates. Estrin in daily dosage up to 1000 mg. (1 gm.) has been given on the theory that it will supplement the low estrin levels commonly encountered in chorionepithelioma and thereby introduce a braking effect on the proliferation and activity of the trophoblastic cells which are responsible for the production of chorionic gonadotropins. Well documented cases occur in the literature which support the contention that the titer of chorionic gonadotropin falls and lung metastases diminish as seen by x-ray film after the administration of large doses of oral estrogen. It has been suggested that better results might be obtained if it were to be given intramuscularly.

Though testosterone has been used, largely on the same basis that estrin has been given, the results are not very favorable. The same thing may be said of any of the hormones designed to suppress the activity of the pituitary. Since surgical hypophysectomy fails to have any influence on this kind of tumor growth, it is hard to see how we can expect much from hormonal depression of pituitary function.

Antifolic acid derivatives such as Methotrexate have helped some women who have had inoperable lung metastases. The effects in most cases and in whatever manner given are largely palliative. The disease process is temporarily arrested, and the symptoms abate for a limited time only.

SURGICAL TREATMENT OF THE PRIMARY TUMOR IN THE UTERUS.   With the diagnosis of chorionepithelioma firmly established, the treatment of choice is total removal of the uterus, regardless of whether remote metastases are present or not. The removal of the primary source of the tumor appears to have a favorable influence on the distant extensions of the disease (Fig. 33–13).

There is considerable basis for argument as to how much tissue should be removed. Unless there is obvious involvement of the paracervical and paravaginal lymphatics or veins as well as the regional nodes, there is no occasion to do a Wertheim hysterectomy and pelvic node dissection. Since we know that chorionic tissue is recoverable in remote areas even with a normal pregnancy, it is unlikely that wholesale removal of all the pelvic contents will improve the prognosis.

On the other hand, all obviously involved tissue should be removed within the limits of surgical judgment.

Should the Ovaries Be Removed?   One can debate whether the ovaries should be removed. For years it has been standard procedure to do a total hysterectomy and bilateral salpingo-oophorectomy for chorionepithelioma. There is a great temptation to remove them, because (1) it is a malignant process; (2) the ovaries do present cystic enlargement. Since we know that the ovarian enlargement regresses after hysterectomy with removal of the primary tumor, and there is some evidence that the ovary exerts a protective action through estrin on the growth of chorionic hormone-producing cells, it would seem wise to leave the ovaries, provided they are not implicated in the primary disease process. This would be true particularly if remote metastases were present. The burden of proof, however, is on the surgeon who says that the ovaries are not involved.

The follow-up program after hysterectomy, using biologic tests for chorionic gonadotropin and scanning x-ray films of the chest, has been outlined previously.

SURGICAL TREATMENT OF THE METASTASES. It is within the realm of good surgical judgment and in keeping with full consideration of the natural history of chorionepithelioma to remove isolated metastases in accessible areas, whether local or distant. In many instances it is possible to excise local lesions on the vulva and vagina without being too destructive. If preliminary investigation seems to indicate that solitary metastases are present in lung or kidney, they may be successfully removed by lobectomy, pneumonectomy or nephrectomy. There are reports of successful excision of solitary metastases to brain and spinal canal. The chances of success are increased if the preliminary workup gives evidence that the tumor is rather slowly growing and has only recently shown signs of increased activity.

WHAT OTHER FORMS OF TREATMENT ARE AVAILABLE FOR THE TREATMENT OF METASTASES? *Irradiation.* One might expect that some form of irradiation treatment would be effective, since the primary tumor arises from embryonic tissue that should be sensitive to radiation. It is surprising that none of the radiation media, such as x-ray, radium or radioactive substances, have had any consistently beneficial

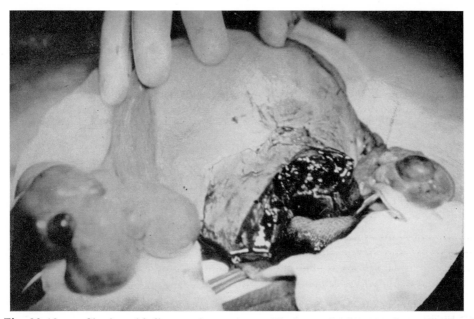

Fig. 33-13. Chorionepithelioma at hysterectomy. The hemorrhagic tumor is seen bulging from the cut surface of the incised uterus. The grossly enlarged ovaries filled with theca lutein cysts are demonstrated. Hysterectomy is the treatment of choice once a diagnosis of choriocarcinoma is established.

effect upon chorionepithelioma, either locally or in the metastases. The fact that they have not may be due to the destructive effect of irradiation on ovarian function. This may upset the natural defense factor which seems to operate through the ovary and be concerned with the production of estrin. We have noted that estrin seems to have an inhibiting effect on the growth of chorionic tissue. The general impression is that irradiation alone has little beneficial effect, at least on the primary tumor. Occasionally a favorable response of an isolated metastasis in lung or kidney is reported. There is, therefore, no reason to withhold x-ray treatment if the ovaries have already been removed. X-ray treatment has been given in combination with other forms of therapy, with the results reportedly successful.

Chemotherapy. Recently nitrogen mustard has been used in combination with x-ray treatment on the theory that one would supplement the other and enhance the destructive effects upon the trophoblast. The patient seems to feel better and gain weight and appetite after the use of intravenous nitrogen mustard, but a sufficient number of cases showing a continued favorable response is not yet available. Nitrogen mustard has been used after total hysterectomy and without x-ray, but again too infrequently to evaluate it. The same may be said for radioactive phosphorus.

Methotrexate and related chemotherapeutic agents, in use at the National Institutes of Health, have recently produced some astonishing remissions and apparent cures in chorionepithelioma. This is one of the outstanding instances of success in control of a disseminated cancer after drug therapy, if these agents continue to prove effective in more cases over a longer period of time. Amethopterin (Methotrexate) has been called the first chemotherapeutic agent to cure a cancer.

REFERENCES

Hydatidiform Mole

Bardawil, W. A., Hertig, A. T., and Velardo, J. T.: Regression of Trophoblast. Hydaditiform Mole. A Case of Unusual Features, Possibly Metastases and Regression. Review of the Literature. *Obst. & Gynec.*, 10: 614, 1957.

Bressler, R., and Forsyth, B. R.: Serum Leucine Aminopeptidase Activity in Normal Pregnancy and in Patients with Hydatidiform Mole. *New England J. Med.*, 261: 746, 1959.

Corscaden, J. A., and Shettles, L. B.: Hydatidiform Mole and Choriocarcinoma. *Bull. Sloane Hosp. for Women*, 5: 41, 1959.

Crisp, W. E.: Hysterectomy Is the Treatment for Hydatidiform Mole. *West. J. Surg., Obst. & Gynec.*, 65: 53, 1957.

Delfs, E.: Quantitative Chorionic Gonadotrophin (Prognostic Value in Hydatidiform Mole and Chorionepithelioma). *Obst. & Gynec.*, 9: 1, 1957.

Douglas, G. W.: The Diagnosis and Management of Hydatidiform Mole. *S. Clin. N. Amer.*, 37: 379, 1957.

Grady, H. G.: Hydatidiform Mole and Choriocarcinoma. *Ann. New York Acad. Sc.*, 75: 565, 1959.

Hertig, A. T., and Sheldon, W. H.: Hydatidiform Mole—A Pathologicoclinical Correlation of 200 Cases. *Am. J. Obst. & Gynec.*, 53: 1, 1947.

Hunt, W., Dockerty, M. B., and Randall, L. M.: Hydatidiform Mole. A Clinicopathologic Study Involving "Grading" as a Measure of Possible Malignant Change. *Obst. & Gynec.*, 1: 593, 1953.

Logan, B. J., and Motyloff, L.: Hydatidiform Mole. A Clinical and Pathological Study of 72 Cases with Reference to Their Malignant Tendency. *Am. J. Obst. & Gynec.*, 75: 1134, 1958.

McCormick, J. B.: Gonadotrophin in Urine and Spinal Fluid. Quantitative Studies for Chorionic Moles and Choriocarcinomas. *Obst. & Gynec.*, 3: 58, 1954.

Novak, E.: Pathological Aspects of Hydatidiform Mole and Choriocarcinoma. *Am. J. Obst. & Gynec.*, 59: 1355, 1950.

Page, E. W.: Relation between Hydatid Moles, Relative Ischemia of Gravid Uterus, and Placental Origin of Eclampsia. *Am. J. Obst. & Gynec.*, 37: 291, 1939.

Reed, S., Coe, J. I., and Berquist, J.: Invasive Hydatidiform Mole Metastatic to the Lungs. Report of a Case. *Obst. & Gynec.*, 13: 749, 1959.

Savage, M. B.: Trophoblastic Lesions of the Lungs Following Benign Hydatid Mole. *Am. J. Obst. & Gynec.*, 62: 346, 1951.

Shiffer, M. A., Pomerance, W., and Mackles, A.: Hydatidiform Mole in Relation to Malignant Disease of the Trophoblast. *Am. J. Obst. & Gynec.*, 80: 516, 1960.

Smalbraak. J.: *Trophoblastic Growths. A Clinical, Hormonal and Histopathologic Study of Hydatidiform Mole and Chorioepithelioma.* Amsterdam, Elsevier Publ. Co., 1957.

Stanton, E. F.: Pregnancy after Forty-Four. *Am. J. Obst. & Gynec.*, 71: 270, 1956.

Chorionepithelioma

Arias, R. E., and Bertoli, F.: Metastatic Choriocarcinoma without Primary Lesion. (Report of a Case). *Obst. & Gynec.*, 13: 737, 1959.

Buckle, A. E.: Further Experience with Methotrexate in Choriocarcinoma. *Brit. M.J.*, 1: 173, 1961.

Editorial: Chemotherapy of Choriocarcinoma and Related Trophoblastic Tumors in Women. *J.A.M.A.*, 168: 894, 1958.

Hertz, R., Bergenstal, D. M., Lipsett, M. B., Price, E. B., and Hilbish, T. F.: Chemotherapy of Choriocarcinoma and Related Trophoblastic Tumors in Women. *J.A.M.A.*, 168: 845, 1958.

Jackson, R. L.: Pure Malignancy of the Trophoblast Following Primary Abdominal Pregnancy. *Am. J. Obst. & Gynec.*, 79: 1085, 1960.

Kistner, R. W.: Malignant Syncytioma Following Benign Hydatidiform Mole. *Am. J. Obst. & Gynec.*, 63: 888, 1952.

Li, M. C., Hertz, R., and Bergenstal, D. M.: Therapy of Choriocarcinoma and Related Trophoblastic Tumors with Folic Acid and Purine Antagonists. *New England J. Med.*, 259: 66, 1958.

Maier, H. C., and Taylor, H. C., Jr.: Metastatic Chorionepithelioma of the Lung Treated by Lobectomy. *Am. J. Obst. & Gynec.*, 53: 674, 1947.

Novak, E., and Seah, C. S.: Choriocarcinoma of the Uterus (a Study of 74 Cases from the Mathieu Memorial Chorionepithelioma Registry). *Am. J. Obst. & Gynec.*, 67: 933, 1954.

Park, W. W., and Lees, J. C.: Choriocarcinoma: General Review, with Analysis of 516 Cases. *Arch. Path.*, 49: 73, 205, 1950.

Stahmann, F. S.: Choriocarcinoma Associated with Normal Pregnancy. *Obst. & Gynec.*, 10: 689, 1957.

Chapter 34

Congenital Abnormalities
in Relation to Sterility

THE VARIOUS forms of uterine maldevelopment are usually discovered in the twenty- to thirty-year age group, largely because they are implicated in the problems of fertility or the maintenance of pregnancy. It is important that the anatomic variations be recognized as early as possible, before they take on pathologic significance through complications that may arise in pregnancy. The majority of cases come to light in investigations of the reasons for infertility, for the most common anomalies of the uterus are frequently not detectable on routine physical examination. Although there seems to be no reason to believe that patients with uterine maldevelopment are infertile because of the variation from the anatomic normal, nevertheless many of these patients do have trouble in conceiving because of associated pathologic conditions The problem for the pregnant patient lies in the difficulties encountered in delivering a live full-term infant.

What Is the Embryonic Explanation for the Maldevelopments?

In order to understand fully the various types of congenital abnormality found within the uterus, it is necessary again to consider briefly the embryology of the genital tract.

In the earliest phase of development the mesonephric tubercle and the gonad are intimately in contact. As yet there has been no indication whether the embryo will develop as a male or female. If it is to be a female, the müllerian duct system predominates, and from the ducts spring the uterus, tubes and vagina, while the male duct system (wolffian ducts) is rudimentary (Fig. 34–1). This change begins toward the end of the second month and proceeds slowly. As in other higher mammals, fusion of the two müllerian ducts takes place in the lower portion of the uterus, so that it opens into the vagina as a single structure, the cervix. As yet there is no definite point of differentiation between the fused or cervical portion of the uterus and the vagina. Gradually, beginning in the third month, the demarcation becomes apparent as the vagina acquires patency. Fusion of the two müllerian ducts and the establishment of the vaginal canal are usually complete by the fifth month. Under the influence of the natural hormones the genital apparatus develops rapidly in the last trimester of pregnancy.

432

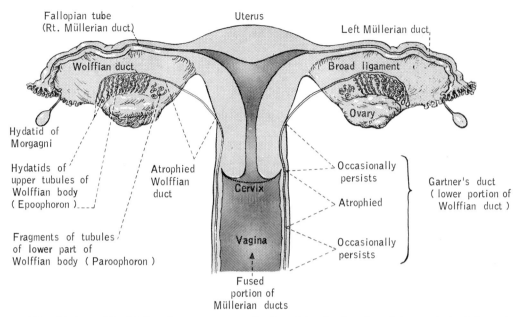

Fig. 34-1. Vestigial male organs normally found in the female pelvis are derived from the wolffian body and the wolffian duct. They are situated in the broad ligament, the uterine wall and the vaginal wall and may give rise to parovarian cysts or cysts and tumors in the broad ligaments or vaginal walls.

It is obvious from this brief recording that (*a*) a variety of forms of maldevelopment may appear, either because the müllerian ducts fail to fuse properly or because some portion of the system develops imperfectly or not at all; (*b*) because of the close proximity of urinary and genital primordia in early embryonic life, many uterine maldevelopments are accompanied by defects in the urinary system.

What Types of Malformation Are Found?

All degrees of duplication and partitioning of the uterus are possible, ranging from a complete duplication of the uterus, tubes and vaginal canal, such as one sees in the so-called double uterus with a septate vagina, to the simple uterus arcuatus, which has nothing more abnormal than an indentation in the fundal portion. The uterus didelphys is a comparatively rare finding, but is well known, for the picture is so striking that its occurrence is frequently reported in the literature (Figs. 34–2, 34–3). The arcuate or heart-shaped uterus is by all odds the most frequent of all the anomalies. The fusion is nearly complete, and the appearance is so nearly normal that it may pass unnoticed.

Both the arcuate and didelphic types of uterus, with all the variants in between, are obvious examples of either complete or partial failure of union of the two müllerian ducts. The finding of a single cavity and one tube and ovary (uterus unicornis) is an example of unilateral failure in development. This usually takes place within the first month of fetal life. Because it is a fundamental developmental defect, there are apt to be other anomalies in the genitourinary tract, such as absence of a kidney and ureter on the same side as the uterine defect. A combination of failure of fusion of the müllerian ducts, coupled with maldevelopment, is apparent in the occurrence of a double uterus with one normal and one rudimentary horn, which may or may

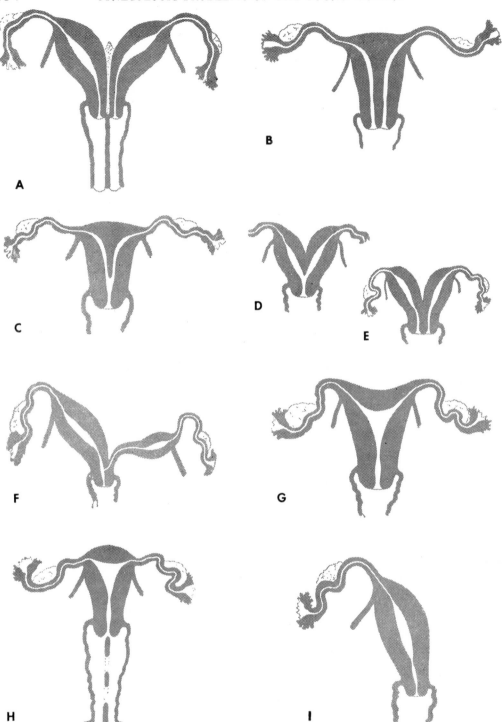

Fig. 34-2. Uterine anomalies. *A,* Uterus didelphys with double vagina; *B,* uterus septus duplex with single vagina; *C,* uterus subseptus unicollis; *D,* uterus bicornis unicollis, a variant of so-called bipartite uterus; *E,* uterus duplex; *F,* uterus bicornis unicollis with one connected rudimentary horn. In a related anomaly the smaller horn is unconnected. *G,* Uterus arcuatus; *H,* septations of vagina; *I,* uterus unicornis.

not connect with the vagina. Eighty per cent of the time it does not. This is the so-called uterus bicornis unicollis with a rudimentary horn. Jarchos's classification of uterine malformation lists the anomalies in the following order (see also Fig. 34-2):

1. Uterus didelphys (double uterus, cervix and vagina)
2. Uterus duplex bicornis bicollis (double uterus with two horns, two bodies, two cervices and a normal vagina)
3. Uterus bicornis unicollis (a single endometrial cavity with two horns, a single cervix and a normal vagina)
4. Uterus, septate (a complete longitudinal partition from fundus through the cervix)
5. Uterus, subseptate (a partial partition of the endometrial cavity)
6. Uterus arcuatus (a depression in fundus)
7. Uterus unicornis (a single cavity with one tube and ovary)
8. Uterus bicornis unicollis with a rudimentary horn.

The other forms of genital maldevelopment, such as congenital absence of the uterus or vagina, as well as congenital atresias and partitions blocking the vagina and cervix, are usually discovered at puberty or during infancy and were discussed in the appropriate age groups.

Why and When Do the Uterine Anomalies Occur?

The actual reason for the maldevelopment is not clear. It may be faulty germ plasm, hormonal failure during intrauterine life or simply inadequate or arrested embryonic fusion. Complete failure in development usually occurs early in the first month of embryonic life. Complete duplication, as in uterus didelphys, probably occurs during the second month from faulty fusion of the two müllerian ducts. Should there be a rudimentary horn, the defect is due either to faulty development or to partial tissue suppression that occurs at approximately the same period of fetal growth.

The less severe examples of uterine anomalies occur after the third or fourth month, because of incomplete fusion. Thus we have the various forms of bicornuate uterus, double cervices or varying kinds of uterine partition.

The arcuate or heart-shaped uterus appears after the fifth month.

How Common Are Congenital Anomalies of the Uterus and Vagina?

The actual incidence is difficult to determine. Many of the abnormalities produce no symptoms, interfere in no way with fertility or subsequent pregnancy and consequently are never discovered. Many that are found at autopsy or in the course of operation for other cause are never reported. The incidence is said to range between 0.004 and 3.8 per cent. Expressed in another way, 1 in 1500 obstetrical cases and 1 in 2000 gynecologic cases will prove to have some variation from the normal.

Do Anomalies Influence the Likelihood of Conception?

The consensus is that the malformations are not per se the cause of infertility. Usually there are other developmental factors as well, for conception readily takes place when the ovary and endometrium mature. On the other hand, if the entire process is a developmental failure associated with atresia, it is hard to believe that malformation does not have some influence in causing infertility, particularly since many cases are discovered as part of fertility investigations. The presence of uterine malformations does not preclude the chance of pregnancy, though it certainly does not increase the possibilities.

What Happens to the Patient Who Does Conceive?

Congenital anomalies have clinical importance because of the many obstetrical complications that can take place in the patient who is pregnant with a malformed uterus. Unfortunately the failure of the uterus to develop normally may go entirely unrecognized until pregnancy occurs, or a failure to conceive prompts investigation as to the cause. A woman may go through life without the knowledge that there is a double uterus or vagina. Fertility is unimpaired, and some pregnancies, even twin infants, have been delivered from a uterus didelphys. One may fail to recognize an arcuate uterus or to suspect the presence of a septum in association when the diagnosis is made.

Though the delivery of a normal infant and rarely twins is possible in a patient with uterus didelphys, the usual history is one of abortion or premature labor. When the pregnancy continues to term, the labor is usually prolonged, probably because of inadequate muscular development in the uterine wall coupled with a rigid, fibrous cervix.

There is a tendency on the part of all pregnant malformed uteri to abort spontaneously. A little over 50 per cent go to term as against a normal rate of 85 per cent. Abortion is particularly likely to occur when the pregnancy takes place in a septate uterus, whether partial or complete. Approximately one third of all pregnancies occurring in a uterus with a bicornis unicollis, complete or subseptate defect will abort in the second trimester of pregnancy. The explanation probably rests upon the lack of a proper implantation site that will supply sufficient space to permit normal expansion with the growing fetus. Approximately one third to one half of patients who have uterus didelphys or uterus bicornis bicollis will also abort (Fig. 34–3).

Pregnancy in one horn of a double uterus may proceed to term, when it produces its own peculiar complications, but abortion is also frequent. This may be anticipated if the patient continues to bleed from the nonpregnant horn. It may be bleeding from a decidual cast, for the endometrium in the nongravid side is being stimulated by the same hormones that influence the normal pregnancy, but it is far more likely to herald an impending abortion.

Pregnancy may take place in the rudimentary horn of a bicornuate uterus and lead to dramatic complications. It is not easily recognized, and the enlarging mass, seemingly adnexal, may be considered a growing fibroid. Since the musculature is incompletely developed and there is no communication with the vagina at least 80 per cent of the time, any pregnancy in the rudimentary horn carries all the dangers present in an interstitial or ectopic pregnancy. Intra-abdominal rupture usually takes place somewhat later than in an ectopic tubal pregnancy, about the tenth week, and can result in a fatal hemorrhage, if not recognized.

What Happens if the Patient Does Not Abort Spontaneously?   A variety of complications occur in the patient with a malformed uterus who carries the pregnancy to term. Although normal pregnancy is possible and even likely, if the patient has a single uterine cavity, tube and ovary (uterus unicollis), the majority of uterine anomalies produce a considerably lowered percentage of viable babies. The viable birth rate has been reported to be 64 per cent as compared to 93 per cent in women without malformations.

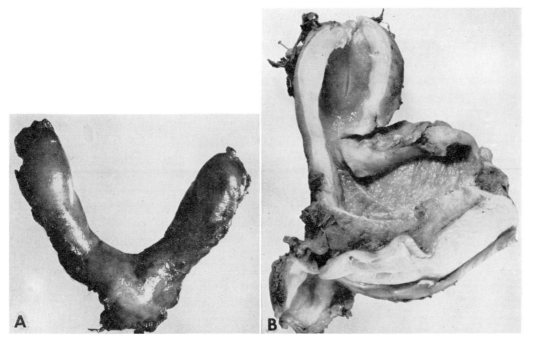

Fig. 34-3.   *A*, Uterus didelphys, similar to that in Figure 34–2, *A*, but with a single vagina. Maintenance of a pregnancy in such a situation is rather unlikely. *B*, Uterus similar to that in Figure 34–2, *F*, a uterus bicornis unicollis with a rudimentary horn. Reproductive failures may lead to discovery of this type of anomaly.

It depends somewhat on the extent of the malformation, but even the arcuate uterus provides a high percentage of complications which are chiefly fetal prematurity, postmaturity, prolonged labor, sudden intrauterine fetal deaths, and breech and transverse presentations, as well as retained placenta. Bleeding during the third stage of labor and in the immediate postpartum period is much more pronounced. Dystocia and obstruction to the normal passage of the infant by the enlarged nonpregnant horn create other problems at the time of delivery. Perhaps because of malformation of the placenta due to defective implantation, a high percentage of fetal abnormalities such as polydactylism and intrauterine amputations is observed in pregnancy within the malformed uterus. Because of the prolonged difficult labor the cesarean section rate is usually much higher than normal. This is probably based on the unsupported fear of uterine rupture, which actually occurs infrequently. Hemorrhage, pain simulating a clinical history of acute surgical condition of the abdomen and malpresentations are the chief antepartum complications. Toxemia and other medical complications at term are no higher than one finds in normal pregnancy.

How Is the Diagnosis of Uterine Anomaly Made before the Appearance of Pregnancy?

In many instances the existence of uterine anomalies is totally unsuspected until (*a*) the patient is investigated for the cause of infertility, or (*b*) the patient is examined for symptoms related to the uterus or adnexa.

The history is sometimes helpful, with *pain* the most consistent symptom. Patients who have a bicornuate uterus frequently have severe *dysmenorrhea*. The menstrual bleeding pattern is deranged in two ways: (1) the bleeding is apt to be both profuse and delayed; (2) the two uterine horns may respond independently to hormonal stimulation, so that the patient has bimonthly periods, each lasting two or three days. Severe menorrhagia is common and may require curettage for relief. The presence of a double uterus is frequently discovered at this time. Unless there is partitioning of the vagina or malposition of one horn of a bicornuate uterus, dyspareunia and other difficulties encountered in coitus are more uncommon than one might expect. The most helpful factor in the history is the story of repeated miscarriages seemingly without cause.

The history of pain or menstrual functional irregularity and the desire for pregnancy bring the patient to the physician for examination. If aware of the possibility, the examiner is unlikely to miss a uterus didelphys or a uterus duplex, provided he does a careful vaginal speculum examination. The other malformations, particularly the septate, subseptate and arcuate types of uterus, are less readily diagnosed on physical examination. If the depression on the fundus of the uterus is pronounced, it may be possible to feel it, but frequently it does not become evident until pregnancy occurs and the uterus enlarges. As pregnancy advances, one side of the uterus appears to grow at the expense of the other, and suspicion is aroused.

The one uterine abnormality that gives rise to the most serious complication of the many that may occur in pregnancy is the rudimentary horn. A growing fetus expanding in the environment of a rudimentary horn that is deficient in normal muscular development is certain to exert more pressure than the walls can stand, and intra-abdominal rupture is more than likely. The resulting hemorrhage is brisk, profuse and often fatal.

The differential diagnosis between an ectopic pregnancy and one in a rudimentary uterine horn is often difficult, but must be established. The following observations based on history and physical findings may be important:

(*a*) On physical examination the adnexal mass seems to be more firmly attached to the main body of the uterus, and over a wider area.

(*b*) The entire uterus seems to be larger and the cavity more irregular than one would expect in an ectopic pregnancy. The differentiation from a pedunculated fibroid may be difficult.

(*c*) Abnormal vaginal bleeding, which is usually the first indication of death of the embryo within the tube, usually occurs somewhat later, after the tenth week, when the pregnancy exists in the rudimentary uterine horn.

(*d*) The adnexal mass is usually much larger than one would expect of an ectopic tubal pregnancy.

Uterosalpingography unearths more anomalies of the uterus and genital tract than any other single diagnostic procedure. Photographic evidence is essential, for gas insufflation gives no indication of any defect.

The discovery of a maldevelopment in the genital tract makes an investigation of the urological system imperative. The related suppression in development or the absence of guiding wolffian duct factors, such as a kidney or a ureter on one side, may result in a unicornuate uterus, tube and ovary (uterus unicollis). This is not an uncommon finding. It may occur with any of the many types of uterine anomaly.

What Nonpregnant Complications May Appear?

An early diagnosis is important, for many obstetrical complications can be dealt with more effectively if the uterine defect is recognized before the pregnancy takes place.

The nonpregnant complications, in addition to the tendency of the abnormally developed uterus to produce excessively heavy menstruation and occasionally twice monthly periods, are (*a*) the likelihood of developing a huge hematometra when there is no communication of a rudimentary horn with the vagina or main body of the uterus (Fig. 34–2, *F*) and (*b*) the possibility of malignant disease developing in one endometrial cavity of a double uterus. The sole presenting sign in association with vaginal bleeding may be the presence of a polyp. This may be visible, while the cancer lies hidden in the other cavity. Both such types of hematometra and adeno-carcinoma have been noted in our personal experience.

What Kind of Corrective Treatment May Be Given?

It is a good general principle not to operate for the sole purpose of correcting an abnormality, unless the patient has had a history of repeated abortions, many protracted, complicated labors or other difficulties unconnected with pregnancy. If there has been a history of repeated pregnancy in a septate, subseptate or arcuate uterus, one may legitimately operate to remove the septum by longitudinal section of the uterine body and reconstruction of the uterus, so that a single endometrial cavity results. When a rudimentary horn is found at exploration because of the symptoms it produces or as an incidental discovery, the abnormal portion of the uterus should be excised.

There is no reason to perform surgical excision or reconstructive procedures in a patient with a double uterus as long as there is no vaginal partition to interfere with intercourse. It is important in the face of abnormal vaginal bleeding requiring curet-tage that both cavities be thoroughly curetted. Occasionally the longitudinal partition may lie in close approximation to the side wall of the vagina, and the presence of a double uterus may not be suspected. Vaginal septa may require excision because of dyspareunia created by the obstructing bands or partitions.

Although fertility is unimpaired, obstetrical complications may be frequent and the percentage of viable babies materially lower than the normal expectancy in the malformed uterus. There is no indication for sterilization unless the episodes at delivery have been repeatedly exacting or dangerous. Though the fetal mortality rate is nearly 10 times higher in the malformed uterus, the maternal mortality rate ranges from zero to 1.5 per cent.

REFERENCES

Bergman, P.: Treatment of Sterility of Intra-uterine Origin. *Clin. Obst. & Gynec.*, 2: 852, 1959.

Gillespie, E. C.: Principles of Uterine Growth in Pregnancy. *Am. J. Obst. & Gynec.*, 59: 949, 1950.

Hervet, E.: Uterine Malformation. New Observations of Reparative Surgery. *Gyn. Obst. Paris*, 9: 504, 1957; *Internat. Abst. Surg.*, Feb., 1959, p. 163.

Jarcho, J.: Malformations of the Uterus. Review of the Subject, Including Embryology, Comparative Anatomy, Diagnosis and Report of Cases. *Am. J. Surg.*, 71: 106, 1946.

Jones, H. W., Jr., Delfs, E., and Jones, G. E. S.: The Reproductive Difficulties in Double Uterus. The Place of Plastic Reconstruction. *Am. J. Obst. & Gynec.*, 72: 865, 1956.

Kern, W. H., and Henriksen, E.: Chorioadenoma Destruens in a Uterus Duplex Bicornis. Report of a Case. *Am. J. Obst. & Gynec.*, 80: 532, 1960.

Strassmann, E. O.: The Strassmann Operation for Double Uterus; A Fifty Year Experience. *Obst. & Gynec.*, 10: 701, 1957.

Williams, W. W.: Spermatic Abnormalities. *New England J. Med.*, 217: 946, 1937.

Chapter 35

Secondary Amenorrhea:
Diagnosis and Treatment

FAILURE of menses to appear in a woman who has previously had periods that occurred rhythmically is called secondary amenorrhea. The basic defect in the pituitary-ovarian-uterine axis obviously cannot be as severe as that encountered in a girl who has never had menstrual periods. The secondary amenorrhea may last for months or years, and the causes may range from psychiatric ones to poverty. The reason for the lack of menstrual flow may be (1) organic, due to pathologic changes in the uterus, ovary or pituitary; (2) due to overactivity or inadequate function of other endocrine glands such as the thyroid, adrenal or pancreas; or (3) attributed to abnormal psychogenic states.

What Pathologic Changes Appear in the Pituitary-Ovarian-Uterine Axis Which Might Account for Secondary Amenorrhea?

THE UTERUS.   It is obvious that menstruation can occur only if the endometrium lining the uterine cavity is present and is properly receptive to the stimulating action of the ovarian hormones. In secondary amenorrhea the endometrium, by history, has evidently been responsive in the past. For a variety of reasons the response is now lacking.

The most likely cause of endometrial atrophy in this age group is infection within the uterus of such severity that the endometrium is damaged and rendered unresponsive to hormonal stimulation. Tuberculous endometritis is apt to result in amenorrhea, although profuse and irregular menstruation is common during the early active stages of the disease. Ill-advised attempts at abortion, such as instillation of cauterizing substances into the endometrial cavity, can produce permanent endometrial atrophy. After overenthusiastic curettage the endometrium may not regenerate adequately. Should one use intrauterine radium for purposes of controlling excessive menstrual bleeding, one runs the risk of doing permanent damage to the endometrium. In modern gynecologic therapy radium would not be used in this age group.

Whether the amenorrhea is due to intrinsic deficiencies in the endometrium itself or is secondary to a lack of proper hormonal stimulation can readily be tested by giving estrin orally in the form of diethylstilbestrol, 2 mg.; Premarin, 1.25 mg.; or Estinyl, 0.5 mg. daily for a 3-week period. Bleeding from estrogen withdrawal should

440

follow within a week or ten days after cessation of therapy if the endometrium is present and capable of responding to the hormones.

THE OVARY.   The basic cause for the amenorrhea may rest in the ovary itself. The patient can menstruate only if the ovary is capable of receiving stimulation from the pituitary gonadotropins and in turn produces its own hormones. If the patient does not bleed and the endometrium is evidently intact, the defect is likely primarily an estrogen lack. When ovarian failure is complete, no estrin is produced, and the endometrium becomes quiescent and tends to atrophy, although it retains its power to respond to the administration of exogenous estrin.

The most likely causes of amenorrhea due to ovarian failure in this age group are pituitary hypergonadotrophic activities which may result in the creation of the polycystic ovary syndrome, ovarian hyperthecosis or pituitary failure with induction of a premature menopause.

The Polycystic Ovary, Stein-Leventhal Syndrome and Hyperthecosis

The pathologic findings to be described are typical of the polycystic ovary and often occur as part of a more advanced clinical representation, the Stein-Leventhal syndrome.

POLYCYSTIC OVARY.   Here the multiple, immature unruptured follicles appear crowded directly beneath a thickened ovarian capsule. The ovarian capsule is smooth, shining and gray-white, like the testicular tunica vaginalis (Fig. 35–1). Because of the restrictive barrier presented by the thick capsule surrounding the ovary, the follicle apparently cannot come to full maturation, and the ovum thus cannot escape to complete ovulation. Increased pressure within the follicle which has been stimulated but cannot expand may lead secondarily to pressure atrophy of the hormone-producing ovarian stroma and to amenorrhea, which may be either partial or complete, depending on the degree of ovarian failure.

A low level of urinary estrogenic activity can usually be demonstrated in these

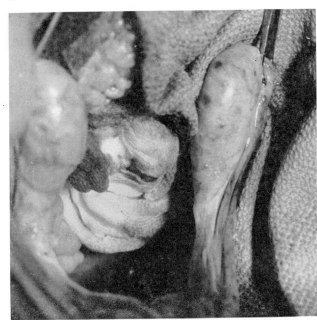

Fig. 35-1.   Polycystic ovaries at operation appear enlarged, smooth and pearly gray. Small translucent cysts are evident, but the normal gyri and signs of corpus luteum formation are absent.

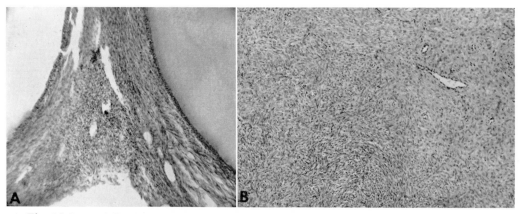

Fig. 35-2.   *A*, Portion of a polycystic ovary to demonstrate that these cysts are of follicular type, lined by granulosa cells and without a notably luteinized theca interna. *B*, Excessive ovarian luteinization, as shown in the right half of the figure, is associated with the Stein-Leventhal syndrome and less specific types of secondary amenorrhea.

cases, despite the amenorrhea, but the FSH is rarely elevated, since some estrin is being produced. If the ovarian atrophy progresses, the amounts of the follicle-stimulating hormone recovered in the urine will increase.

STEIN-LEVENTHAL SYNDROME.   At times the gonadotropic activity involves a relatively greater release of LH than FSH. In such instances the multiple follicular cysts become large, and elements of luteinization are seen more often on pathologic study (Fig. 35–2, *A*). This may be associated with the so-called Stein-Leventhal syndrome. Characteristically, it appears in the woman who is obese with a touch of hirsutism to go along with the amenorrhea and infertile state. We now recognize that the same pathologic condition can be found in women who are outwardly normal in their appearance and are neither fat nor hirsute. We noted the appearance of this syndrome in the adolescent girl and described many of its manifestations at that time, but the process varies in degree and rate of progression, so that it may manifest itself for the first time in the twenties as one of the problems causing infertility.

HYPERTHECOSIS.   The excess stimulation provided by the gonadotropic hormones in certain instances may produce extreme degrees of luteinization of the ovarian stroma, due to LH activity, with or without any increased follicle stimulation by the FSH element. Evidence for overactivity of the pituitary gonadotropic LH can be seen in the form of luteinized theca cells beneath the walls of follicle cysts as well as in the solid, luteinized ovarian stroma (Fig. 35–2, *B*). This ovarian hyperthecosis also interferes with ovulation and tends to create varying degrees of amenorrhea and masculinization. It may be permanent, but like the polycystic ovary syndrome, the defect is frequently less than complete, and normal ovulatory bleeding may occur once or twice a year.

PREMATURE SENILITY (PRECOCIOUS MENOPAUSE).   It is generally agreed that the female child is born with a variable complement of ovarian follicles. Exhaustion of the follicles may follow prolonged overstimulation by the pituitary hormones. There are many well documented cases of persistent amenorrhea dating from the late twenties and early thirties. In some instances a familial tendency is noted. One must postulate that either such patients have fewer ovarian follicles for genetic reasons, or the normal complement has been used up through excessive pituitary gonadotropic activity or for other reasons.

As a result of the overproduction of gonadotropins by the basophilic cells of the pituitary, multiple immature follicles become cystic and a smooth enlargement of the ovary develops, as mentioned above. This polycystic condition is frequent in women and can be created in animals by injecting gonadotropic hormones. Despite increased amounts of follicle-stimulating hormones, ovulation does not occur. Instead, the intact cystic follicles line up beneath a thickened, superficial ovarian stroma. If the quantity of the follicles is limited and the stimulation overactive, the follicles may eventually become exhausted, and a premature menopause appears.

How Do You Test for Primary Ovarian Failure?

Fundamentally, the evidence for the failure of the ovary to produce estrin should be substantiated by obtaining (1) vaginal smears. (2) endometrial biopsies, and (3) urinary assays for estrogen and follicle-stimulating hormone.

If adequate laboratory facilities and trained personnel are available, the diagnosis should be made in this way. One should keep in mind, however, that (1) the response of the vaginal epithelium does not always reflect the degree of biological activity of the ovarian hormones, nor localize the source of its production; (2) the endometrial biopsies do not always permit one to distinguish between minimal amounts of estrogen activity and none at all; and (3) the same criticism may be leveled at the laboratory determination of estrogen and FSH. Moreover, all three are costly and take time to perform.

PROGESTERONE WITHDRAWAL TEST. There is a simple test available which gives the maximum amount of information with the minimal expenditure of time and money. It is useful in differentiating between relative and absolute failure of ovarian activity. If the endometrium is capable of responding, an injection of 10 mg. of progesterone given intramuscularly every day for 5 days will produce uterine bleeding within 72 hours thereafter, provided the ovary is secreting estrin. If the ovary is totally inactive, there will be no vaginal bleeding. When there is any doubt about the responsiveness of the endometrium, this can be checked easily by administering estrin and awaiting the appearance of estrogen withdrawal bleeding. The ovary is producing at least some estrin when bleeding occurs, and we know that the defect is relative and not absolute. The new, longer-acting progesterone preparations should not be used in this test for the reasons advanced on page 452.

If no bleeding occurs after progesterone withdrawal and the endometrium is responsive, then the source of the ovarian failure must be sought elsewhere. It still may be primary in the ovary, but it could be the result of inadequate stimulation by the pituitary gonadotropins. Urinary assays for follicle-stimulating hormone should then be done. An elevated urinary FSH in the presence of a progesterone test which fails to produce uterine bleeding is definite proof that the basic defect lies in the ovary.

Metropathia Hemorrhagica

In the condition known as metropathia hemorrhagica the patient may have persistent periods of amenorrhea of up to eight or twelve months, followed by an excessive and prolonged menstrual flow. The ovarian defect in this instance is a relative one, due to failure of ovulation to occur.

After months of amenorrhea, during which time the uterus has built up an abundance of hyperplastic endometrium, the patient either bleeds spontaneously or does so after the administration of progesterone. This latter bleeding is known as a "medical curettage." After this the patient may either resume a normal cyclic bleeding pattern or go back into an amenorrheic phase. If she does the latter, it may be impossible to reproduce bleeding after the progesterone withdrawal test. This would suggest that there may be differences in individual requirements for estrin priming of the endometrium. No two persons are the same in this respect, and the output of the ovarian hormones may vary in the same woman from month to month.

Prolongation of the Corpus Luteum Effect

The duration of activity of the corpora lutea has not been completely established. It is said normally to be in the range of ten to twelve days. When the effect is prolonged beyond that time, the patient in most instances is pregnant. Although the most likely source of the luteotropin then is the placenta, where it is produced as chorionic gonadotropin, there is still a possibility that the pituitary may put out a similar hormone in excess.

This may be related to the mechanism by which the adrenal cortex is stimulated and acts sometimes to suppress menstruation. Amenorrhea might then result from the action of adrenal androgen in inhibiting either corpus luteal function or the normal cyclic secretion of luteotropin by the pituitary.

The menstrual cycle may be delayed by the persistence of a corpus luteum cyst to the point at which the patient may miss one or two periods. Occasionally there is a minor degree of spotting, and less often chronic menstruation lasting up to forty days. If the patient suddenly bleeds into the peritoneal cavity from a minor laceration in the wall of a persistent corpus luteum cyst, the history of amenorrhea, spotting, pain and the palpation of an adnexal mass may lead to confusion in differentiating it from an early, ruptured tubal ectopic pregnancy. If one can be sure that the patient is not pregnant and that the adnexal mass is truly a corpus luteum cyst, operation is not indicated. When there is no such assurance, abdominal exploration is essential.

ALTERED FUNCTION OF OTHER ENDOCRINE GLANDS AND THEIR RELATION TO AMENORRHEA

It is a well known observation that disturbed function in either the adrenal or thyroid gland may lead to amenorrhea. Other factors such as malnutrition may be present which make the relation between endocrine dysfunction in these glands and the appearance of secondary amenorrhea somewhat obscure.

The Adrenal Gland

The relation between adrenal cortical function and ovarian activity has been studied extensively both in laboratory animals and in human subjects. It has been shown in animal experiments, for example, that amenorrhea appears in the presence of adrenal insufficiency. The same observations can be made in the human patient with Addison's disease. The effect does not seem to be a direct one, however, for it is intimately related to other factors concerned with body economy. When adrenal cortical insufficiency develops, not only are the gonadotropic stimuli depleted, but profound changes also occur in electrolyte balance, particularly in sodium and chloride metabolism and water retention. In fact, the menstrual function can be maintained so that even the addisonian patient can become pregnant if adequate replacement of sodium, chloride and water is provided.

At the opposite end of the spectrum there has been general agreement that hyperactivity of the adrenal cortex will often suppress ovarian function and lead to genital atrophy. The effect, as in Cushing's syndrome, is variable. It may be produced indirectly through the action of the adrenal cortical steroids upon the cells of the anterior pituitary which are concerned with gonadotropin production. It is also possible, however, that the effect may be a direct one upon the ovary, with resulting secondary disturbance in pituitary gonadotropic function.

WHAT ARE THE MANIFESTATIONS OF HYPERACTIVITY OF THE ADRENAL CORTEX IN THE ADULT FEMALE?   The two most common clinical entities associated with hyperactivity of the adrenal cortex are (1) Cushing's syndrome, in which there is a profound metabolic disturbance associated with overactivity in the mechanism of converting protein into carbohydrate, and (2) the adrenogenital syndrome.

Cushing's syndrome appears in adolescence and early adult life and has been described in detail elsewhere (p. 241). The adrenogenital syndrome may be congenital. This form of disturbed adrenal function has been discussed in the section on the problems of infancy and early childhood (p. 59).

The adrenogenital syndrome may manifest itself after the onset of puberty. Then it is an acquired rather than a congenital form of the syndrome. The symptoms vary widely, and there may be no obvious abnormality present on physical examination except hirsutism. This is heaviest on the face as whiskers and on the body as hair on the chest and abdomen (Fig. 35–3). With more extreme degrees of increased androgen production the physical signs of genital dysfunction and atrophy begin to appear. The

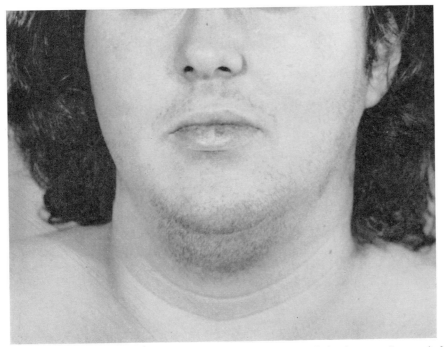

Fig. 35-3.   Facial hirsutism without other evidence of masculinization may be one indication of the adrenogenital syndrome. Some cases are of unknown, possibly genetic, origin, without evidence of any adrenogenital dysfunction.

breasts become flat, the clitoris enlarged, the patient becomes more muscular and develops a male type of baldness, acne appears, the voice deepens, libido is diminished or lost, and the patient becomes amenorrheic.

These are serious danger signs in the adolescent child or young woman, for they are apt to be due to adrenal neoplasm rather than adrenal hyperplasia. In earlier discussion it was pointed out that the 17-ketosteroid excretion may be as much as ten times normal. Several urinary determinations should be done, for one may get a false impression of the state of adrenocortical activity from a single specimen. When cortisone is given, the 17-ketosteroid level supposedly drops promptly to the normal range if the underlying metabolic disturbance is due to adrenal cortical hyperplasia. It remains elevated when adrenocortical adenoma or carcinoma is present.

Further help can be obtained from the laboratory in making the differential diagnosis between the two. The 11-oxygenated-17-ketosteroid level is elevated in adrenal hyperplasia, while urinary dehydroisoandrosterone appears in large amounts in the presence of tumor. It is interesting to note that in both hyperplasia and tumor the level of urinary estrogens is increased, yet the patient has signs of external genital atrophy. It is possible that the source of the excessive urinary estrin may stem from the breakdown of androgen into estrin. One may also postulate that the excessive amount of androgen prevents the utilization of estrin at the cell level, resulting in an increase in the amount excreted.

One should be suspicious of a young girl who exhibits amenorrhea or increasing hirsutism and shows a high level of urinary estrin, together with a continued elevation in 17-ketosteroids after cortisone. Such patients are apt to have adrenocortical neoplasms. When this is suspected, the patient should promptly be explored surgically, and the tumor removed. Some are benign, while others are malignant. X-ray treatment has been ineffective in the treatment of both adrenal hyperplasia and tumors.

WHAT OTHER FACTORS HAVE A BEARING ON ADRENAL FUNCTION AND LEAD TO SECONDARY AMENORRHEA? Disturbances in adrenocortical function may be due to metabolic alterations, as noted in Cushing's or the adrenogenital syndrome, or caused by actual destruction of adrenal tissue by pathologic processes such as cancer or tuberculosis. When normal adrenal cortex is destroyed, the clinical manifestations may not be immediately apparent and may occur only when enough of the normal tissue is replaced or when debilitating complications arise.

Chronic Illness and Malnutrition. In Addison's disease, by definition the adrenal cortex is damaged to varying but significant degrees. The hormone production is materially reduced to the point at which the urinary 17-ketosteroids may be absent. Nevertheless ovarian function may continue undisturbed until the patient becomes so depleted in her nutritional state that the pituitary stimulus no longer is adequate. Apparently the anterior lobe of the pituitary will not produce follicle-stimulating hormone unless there is an adequate intake of protein and vitamin B. Essential amino acids are requisite to the formation of FSH. Any chronic illness or condition which is associated with malnutrition may then be the cause of secondary amenorrhea, and this may occur in the absence of any noticeable drop in urinary 17-ketosteroid excretion.

What Effect Does the Thyroid Have in the Production of Secondary Amenorrhea?

An interrelation between thyroid and ovarian function is well substantiated. One has only to note the clinical observation that the thyroid enlarges at puberty, during pregnancy and at the time of the menopause. The mechanism by which the thyroid exerts its effect on ovarian function is not clear. It may do this directly or through the mechanism of the pituitary. The relation may also be reciprocal. There is some evidence that large doses of estrin depress both gonadotropic and thyroid-stimulating hormone production by the pituitary. Clinically, however, there is a suggestion that estrin stimulates the thyroid to greater activity, while estrogen withdrawal decreases thyroid function. Just what the mechanism may be obviously is in doubt, but that there is such a relation is abundantly clear.

It may be that the level of thyroid function affects the menstrual cycle through its action on the gonadotropic cells of the anterior pituitary. We know, however, that the fundamental purpose of the thyroid hormone is to stimulate the metabolic activity of all living cells. It is far more likely, then, that the cause of the amenorrhea accompanying myxedema lies in a disturbance in this basic thyroid function. The receptiveness of the ovarian follicular cell to stimuli from pituitary gonadotropin and the ability of the ovary to respond by putting out its own hormones will depend both on the general state of nutrition and on the conditioning of the cells in the ovarian follicle by the thyroid hormones.

Confusion as to the role of the thyroid hormone in regulating the menstrual cycle comes about when we observe clinically that the hypothyroid state may be associated with either profuse menstruation or amenorrhea.

THE HYPOTHYROID PATIENT.   The theory that amenorrhea results from depressed thyroid function, which interferes with normal cellular activity in the ovarian follicle, gains some support from the clinical observation that simple replacement of thyroid extract will often restore normal ovulatory menstrual cycles. We further note that any condition or state which leads to malnutrition or faulty intake of food will tend to depress ovarian activity and result in amenorrhea. Obesity and the hypothyroid state go hand in hand. In some instances the menstrual bleeding pattern can be returned to normal by a simple weight reduction regimen, but in others thyroid replacement therapy will be necessary to bring it about.

It is an interesting clinical observation that the patient with true adult myxedema usually has secondary amenorrhea, while the girl with moderate depression of thyroid function bleeds excessively. After surgical removal of the thyroid gland myxedema may result, but rarely do these patients have amenorrhea. Nearly all of them bleed excessively.

Whether the hypothyroid patient has secondary amenorrhea or bleeds too much, it seems paradoxical that the menstrual flow will generally return to a normal pattern, in both duration and amount, when thyroid extract is given. This is not invariably true of the patient who has myxedema. Sometimes the basal metabolic rate may be elevated to normal, but the menses do not reappear. One wonders whether such patients may also have some degree of pituitary failure. Occasionally one observes that myxedema seems to follow upon an excessively heavy menstrual period or acute blood loss and shock at the time of delivery. The etiology could be akin to that advanced to explain Sheehan's disease, namely, some degree of ischemic necrosis in the anterior lobe of the pituitary.

Although many theories have been suggested to explain why one patient with hypothyroidism bleeds heavily with her periods and another does not bleed at all, no satisfactory explanation is yet forthcoming. It is possible that the myxedema patient who does not resume a normal cycle after thyroid therapy may have some pituitary defect, like a variant of panhypopituitarism.

THE HYPERTHYROID PATIENT.   In general, patients who have overactive thyroid function and are truly hyperthyroid have irregular, scanty menstrual flow, and frequently are amenorrheic. This is in all probability due to a decreased production of pituitary gonadotropin, secondary to effects of the excessive thyroxin liberated from a hyperplastic thyroid gland. Restoration of normal menstrual function takes place when the basal metabolism, after therapy, returns to normal levels.

THE PSYCHOGENIC FACTORS IN SECONDARY AMENORRHEA

It is a well known fact that women exposed to emotional shock, marital maladjustments, changes in their environment or any other state that produces stress may not menstruate for one or more months thereafter. The assumption is made that functional changes in the central nervous system are responsible. This theory is based largely on animal experiments, wherein bilateral damage to certain parts of the hypothalamus is produced surgically. After such trauma, changes or interruptions in the estrous cycle appear. One postulates in stress phenomena that a block is set up in the hypothalamus which interferes with the production or release of the pituitary gonadotropins. This has been called hypothalamic amenorrhea. In all probability the term is poorly chosen, for it is impossible to carry over experimental animal experience and apply it to human beings in this situation.

There can be no doubt, however, that women have secondary amenorrhea following psychogenic trauma. The basic functional disturbance would also appear to be central in origin, for the ovarian follicle does not produce enough estrogen, nor the adrenal an adequate amount of 17-ketosteroids. Despite the apparent deficiency of estrogen, the follicle-stimulating hormone level is not elevated. It is interesting to note that almost invariably patients who have a psychogenic component to their amenorrhea fail to respond to progesterone withdrawal tests, thereby suggesting that estrin production is in abeyance. It would appear that pituitary gonadotropic cells are functioning at a low level.

What Is the Psychiatric Explanation of Secondary Amenorrhea?

Psychiatrists feel that many kinds of endocrine dysfunction in the female, which appear in the realm of gynecology, are conditioned or modified by emotional factors that may be either exciting or depressing. The emotional stimuli act centrally through the pituitary or hypothalamus to prevent the production or liberation of the pituitary gonadotropins. Failure to menstruate is believed to be due to the inability of the pituitary to produce or release the luteinizing hormone, since ovulation is also inhibited. Many investigators are well aware of the inadequacies of this theory and are ready to admit that they are not certain whether the hormonal imbalance predisposes the patient to psychic conflict or whether the mental unrest precipitates the hormonal disturbance.

Whatever the mechanism, one can hardly deny that gynecologists see many women who have no organic disease, show no suggestion of adrenal or thyroid dysfunction, appear adequately nourished and well, and yet may have amenorrhea. Frequently one can obtain a history of severe emotional shock, grief, profound unhappiness in a new environment, fear of pregnancy or the obligations of marital life, or sexual maladjustment.

Obviously there are all manner of psychologic disturbances, some of them relatively superficial, while others involve fundamental personality changes. Their impact on endocrine function varies with the degree of psychiatric disturbance.

MINOR PSYCHIC EMOTIONAL PROBLEMS.   In most instances the simpler forms of emotional conflict are concerned with rejection of the feminine role. In all other respects the patient is in tune with her environment and life's problems. She simply does not want to be a female. This reaction may not be constant, so that at times the two sexual elements may be in conflict with each other, and the patient has some difficulty in deciding just what she wants to be. Guilt feelings may appear if she has reacted strongly against being a female in the past, when that part of her psyche that wants to be a complete woman is in the ascendency. The underlying psychiatric defect is not great, and the patient will usually resume normal menstrual periods with moderate psychiatric assistance.

MAJOR PSYCHIATRIC PROBLEMS.   The psychiatric disturbance may run much deeper in some patients who have secondary amenorrhea. In general, this group of patients tends to be very immature, and they reflect their inability to cope with the problems of everyday living in a variety of ways. These women are apt to be unstable emotionally and may flare up and react violently if one of their demands, which are often childish, is not satisfied at once. Though they apparently need to be dependent on someone, as an emotional crutch or for guidance, they are quick to take offense at criticism, whether real or implied, and may become angry for little cause.

Fundamentally, they are afraid of everything and go to great lengths to avoid anything that would likely develop into a fear situation. Thus they tend to avoid marriage, or if they find themselves trapped in it, they will try to get out of any marital relation that might lead to pregnancy. These patients also reject the feminine role and would prefer to be boys. If the menstrual periods stop, they are delighted and prefer that they remain suppressed. Some profoundly disturbed patients go to bizarre extremes such as standing upright to urinate, in order to prove to themselves that they are really males whose male attributes are simply hidden.

What Are the Hormonal Relations in Secondary Amenorrhea of Psychogenic Origin?

When one tries to work out a pattern of what to expect in the way of hormone excretion in relation to a given psychiatric state, one is obviously in an ambiguous situation. There is too much that we do not know in both endocrinology and psychiatry.

Interesting observations have been made on hormonal excretion in psychogenic amenorrhea. There appears to be some correlation between the degree of psychic unrest and variations in the urinary excretion of 17-ketosteroids and hydroxycorticoids. Investigators have noted a definite relation between the immaturity of the individual personality and adrenocortical functional instability.

In the woman who has a relatively minor psychiatric problem, which deals largely with rejection of the feminine role, the sole endocrine imbalance lies in the ovary. The adrenal element is lacking, for no variation is noted in the levels of either the 17-ketosteroids or the hydroxycorticoids. In the girl who has a fundamental psychiatric problem the adrenal gland is implicated, as well as the pituitary-ovarian axis. The psychic disturbance is much more profound when both are involved. In these patients the 17-ketosteroids show peak excretion during periods of stress, while the hydroxycorticoids remain at a subnormal level. One can hardly reason from these observations, but the findings are important and deserve further explanation. The psychiatrist and the gynecologist can learn much from combined investigative work.

TREATMENT OF SECONDARY AMENORRHEA

The problem in therapy of the patient with secondary amenorrhea differs materially from that in primary amenorrhea. Obviously the defect in the pituitary-ovarian-uterine axis is not so basic, since the patient did menstruate at one time. If one can identify the source of the difficulty, treatment has a far greater chance of success than in primary amenorrhea. The degree of success will depend upon the duration of the amenorrhea and the nature of the deficiency or blocking agent. The longer the amenorrhea has persisted, the more refractory the uterus becomes and the harder it is to bring about a restoration in the menstrual flow.

The fundamental cause of the amenorrhea, as already discussed, may be dysfunction in any one of the elements that make up the axis, but more often the source of the disturbance will be found in some factor that either has interfered with normal good health or has upset mental equilibrium. The menstrual cycle is a sensitive indicator of the general state of health and may give the first indication that the patient's well-being is in jeopardy.

The possible causes of secondary amenorrhea are many and varied, as we have seen. Amenorrhea may be due to systemic or organic disease, endocrinopathy or psychic unrest. The primary source for the difficulty may rest in the ovary, thyroid, adrenal or central nervous system. The kind of treatment and the prognosis expected from it depend on the cause. The earlier the diagnosis is made and the younger the patient, the greater the chance of success. The history and physical examination are therefore of prime importance. Secondary amenorrhea is a symptom, not a disease.

With the Diagnosis Established, What Forms of Therapy Are Available for the Treatment of Secondary Amenorrhea?

When it has finally been established that the secondary amenorrhea is truly functional and not due to systemic organic disease or tumor, one may then concentrate upon the malfunctions of the endocrine system which are due to malnutrition, psychic cause or intrinsic defects within the endocrine glands themselves.

Our primary concern in therapy is to restore a normal menstrual cycle with the hope that future pregnancies will be possible. The patient may want a normal cycle and care less for pregnancy, but the re-establishment of a fully functioning reproductive system should be the physician's aim. Time is a factor only because the sooner the underlying difficulties are overcome, the better the chance that success will follow. Actually, the patient's health will not be damaged if menstruation is not restored, provided (1) any serious systemic disease has been ruled out, (2) the patient is unconcerned about the fact that she does not have her periods, and (3) she does not complain of the train of menopausal symptoms that sometimes accompany the cessation of menstruation.

CORRECTION OF THE NUTRITIONAL STATE. If the hormones are to act normally, the patient must be in a sound state of general physical and mental health. In many instances hormonal malfunction may be traced to faulty nutrition. We have noted the effect of inadequate food intake in patients who have amenorrhea with anorexia nervosa. The modern woman is very susceptible to the advertising blandishments which guarantee substantial loss of weight in amazingly short periods of time. Many diets are substantially lacking in the proper amounts of minerals and vitamins which are essential to adequate hormone production and utilization.

If the patient dates her failing menstrual function to the time when she went on such a diet or there is obvious suggestion from the history and physical examination of improper intake of foods or vitamins, much can be accomplished by prescribing a high caloric diet adequate in proteins and vitamin B. The essential elements are meat, milk, fruit and vegetables. A normal regimen of living must be established which will ensure plenty of sleep and exercise, combined with emotional stability in both work and play. Stability is very important, for many cases of secondary amenorrhea are obviously due to disturbed emotional balance. During the adjustment period sedatives or tranquilizing drugs are justified, provided one keeps in mind that drug addiction may itself contribute to amenorrhea.

WEIGHT REDUCTION. When amenorrhea is accompanied by obesity, a great deal can be accomplished by a weight-reduction diet. Not infrequently such a regimen will be rewarded by restoration of menstruation without any other form of therapy. It is a hard thing for a woman to go on a diet and stay on it, but if she has the added incentive of reclaiming her lost periods, she may gain sufficient character to accept the hardship such a diet entails. Actually, she will learn to keep it up if you can once get her to try it for a month. To assist her it is perfectly reasonable medicine to give her one of the drugs designed to suppress appetite, such as d-amphetamine in 5-mg. doses one hour before each meal, provided she has a normal blood pressure.

The Psyche and Obesity. Since compulsive eating is one manifestation of psychic unrest, an effort should be made to bring out any psychic conflict the patient may have. Many are fairly superficial, and the fact that the patient has had an opportunity to discuss her problems may actually be as much responsible for restoring a normal menstrual pattern as the actual loss of weight. In all probability it will do little good to put the patient on a weight-reduction diet if psychic factors are the basis for her obesity.

Thyroid Therapy and Obesity. As further support to the patient trying to lose weight to correct her amenorrhea, it has been customary to give these patients thyroid extract in daily doses of ½ to 1 grain. Many women in the reproductive age group, as well as those of adolescent or premenopausal age, have borderline hypothyroidism. Not all are obese, for many thin women have abnormal sensitivity to cold, do not perspire in warm weather and complain of fatigue without adequate cause. Frequently these patients are found to have basal metabolic rates of -10 to -20, or low values of protein-bound iodine in the serum to go with their amenorrhea. On physical examination they are prone to have a slow pulse, low blood pressure, dry skin and coarse hair. Many complain that they are losing their hair.

When the obese amenorrheic patient presents such an array of symptoms on taking her history, and the physical examination and laboratory tests are in support, the substitution of thyroid extract is a reasonable therapeutic adjunct to a weight-reduction regimen. There is less logic in its empiric use. The internist interested in thyroid disease will frequently insist that you accomplish nothing by substitution of thyroid in a euthyroid patient and that you may actually be doing harm. He feels that the use of thyroid in a patient whose gland functions normally simply discourages the thyroid from producing its own hormones. For the thyroid to be effective there should be evidence of thyroid deficiency.

PSYCHOTHERAPY. Previously we have discussed the role of the psyche in the production of amenorrhea. Some of the problems are deep-seated, but the majority can be traced to marital discontent, improper sex instruction, fear or plain inability to cope with the everyday problems of life. The psychic factor may be the activating cause or work indirectly, as we have seen in the obese patient with amenorrhea. It may be a contributing factor to other causes. Thus the patient who finds herself amenorrheic may become abnormally fearful that she is going through an early menopause and will never be able to have children. Fear then acts as a suppressive factor in normal hormonal function. In many instances the patient may resume her periods after simple frank discussions unencumbered with psychiatric verbiage. If there is no proof to the contrary, the physician will be wise to reassure the patient that not all chance of future pregnancy is lost if the periods can be restored to normal, but that if they cannot, her health is in no way endangered.

WHAT CAN BE ACCOMPLISHED WITH HORMONES IN THE TREATMENT OF SECONDARY AMENORRHEA? The greatest chance of success in the treatment of secondary amenorrhea lies in hormone therapy. The success of such therapy will depend upon how long the amenorrhea has been present.

If it has been present for less than two years, there is an excellent chance that progesterone therapy alone may restore menstrual function. If the patient responds to a test dose of 25 mg. of progesterone given intramuscularly for 4 days by having withdrawal bleeding within 72 to 96 hours, we have established the fact that (*a*) there is estrin present and that the pituitary and ovary are functioning, albeit inadequately; (*b*) the endometrial lining of the uterus is capable of responding to stimulation by the ovarian hormones.

It would be much more convenient if the test could be carried out with a single intramuscular injection, and recently a long-acting progesterone, 17-alphahydroxyprogesterone caproate, has become available in doses of 250 mg. per cubic centimeter. Unfortunately, the progesterone withdrawal test is inconclusive when given in this way, for progesterone is eliminated rather rapidly and its effect is over within forty-eight hours. For this reason we continue to rely on the intramuscular injection of 25 to 50 mg. of progesterone in oil for a period of either 2 or 4 days when we are testing the integrity of the pituitary-ovarian-uterine axis and particularly uterine sensitivity. The newer, longer-acting progesterones given orally, such as Norlutin, Enovid and Provera, and the intramuscular agent, 17-alphahydroxyprogesterone caproate (Delalutin), are reserved for replacement therapy over a longer period of time. When bleeding does follow the withdrawal of progesterone, the patient should be treated by intramuscular progesterone beginning on the eighteenth day after the onset of bleeding, for the next three or four months. For this purpose one may give the single injection of Delalutin (500 mg.) or spread the injection of Proluton over a 4-day interval, giving 25 mg. per day.

Amenorrhea of Longer Duration. If the amenorrhea has been present for longer than two years, the uterus may have become refractory to estrin stimulation. Lacking the rhythmic hormonal stimulation of estrin, the uterine musculature and endometrium become hypoplastic. Progesterone withdrawal bleeding, therefore, does not occur. In order to obtain the progesterone effect it will be necessary to prime the uterus with oral estrogen over a period of months. Large doses of oral estrin, such as 0.5 mg. of Estinyl, 2 mg. of diethylstilbestrol, or 5.0 mg. of the conjugated estrogen (Premarin) are necessary in daily doses for 3 weeks out of each month in order that the uterus be resensitized to estrogen stimulation. If the progesterone test has failed to produce withdrawal bleeding on the initial test, it usually takes three to six months of such estrogen priming before progesterone produces the desired effect. Only then can estrogen therapy be combined with progesterone in cyclic fashion to simulate the hormonal production by the ovary in a normal menstrual cycle. Therapy should then proceed according to a regular plan, giving any one of the estrogens in the dosage mentioned for twenty-one days. A single injection of 17-alphahydroxyprogesterone caproate (500 mg.) or 20 mg. of progesterone daily for 5 days should be given on the eighteenth day. This type of cyclic estrogen and progesterone therapy should be continued for several months.

What about the Use of Estrogen Alone? For the patient who wishes to restore normal menstrual cycles with the possibility of pregnancy in mind, estrogen has little to offer that cannot be produced better by progesterone. It is useful, however, in the patient who is unable to have periods produced by her own hormones, yet wishes to have bleeding which simulates menstruation for psychic reasons. It is also of value for its effect on other target organs that have become atrophic because of estrogen lack. As the result of oral estrogen replacement therapy the patient maintains or restores her feminine figure and has regular instances of monthly bleeding, though she has no chance of achieving pregnancy.

The other main use of estrogen is to test the sensitivity of the uterine epithelium to hormonal action. If bleeding does not follow progesterone withdrawal on the initial test, the physician may elect to give an intramuscular injection of 1 cc. of estradiol benzoate every other day for 10 days. If the uterine epithelium is properly sensitized, estrogen withdrawal bleeding will take place a few days after the last injection. We now know that the uterus is responsive, but this test does not tell us what we learn from the progesterone test. Progesterone withdrawal bleeding means that the patient is producing her own estrogens, but the uterus may still be refractory to the patient's own endogenous estrogen. This is why it may be necessary to prime the uterus with estrogen. The more concentrated intramuscular injection of estrogen, when used as a test, simply indicates the uterine responsiveness.

Pituitary Gonadotropins. When the ovary is in partial failure due to inadequate pituitary stimulation, the logical substitute in hormone therapy should be a gonadotropin of the pituitary. In fact there have been some enthusiastic reports in the Scandinavian literature of the successful use of pregnant mare's serum, 1500 International units, injected intramuscularly for 5 days, followed by 1500 units of chorionic gonadotropin given intramuscularly for 3 days. Normal cycles are said to have been restored to 40 per cent of women who had previously been amenorrheic for as long as 3 years.

Until recently investigators in the United States have not been favorably impressed with the combined use of chorionic gonadotropin and extracts of the pituitary. All agree that stimulation is possible, for these substances are known to produce ovarian cysts, but in general they seemed to do little to correct the fundamental defect. When they have been said to produce ovulation, the observations are open to question, for spontaneous ovulation has been known to occur without hormone therapy of any sort. Most observers held little brief for the use of chorionic gonadotropin alone, for it seemed to have no effect on the pituitary and stimulated the ovary only when a corpus luteum was already present.

The pituitary gonadotropins in use until recently have usually been extracts of sheep pituitary or preparations made from pregnant mare's serum. Since they were of animal origin, the problem of species specificity was all too obvious. The chief objection to their use was directed toward the severe anaphylactic reactions that were prone to occur. It was always dangerous to give them without preliminary desensitization tests. Moreover, some observers believed that they produced antihormones if they were injected over any length of time. In general, the use of such gonadotropins seemed to offer little in the treatment of secondary amenorrhea.

In the recent literature, however, reports have begun to appear which hold promise for the future. Multiple ovulation, as measured by basal body temperature, endometrial biopsy, vaginal smear, culdoscopy and laparotomy has been reported in the monkey and human being after the injection of purified extracts made from the pituitaries of these two species. Interestingly enough, the extracts of the human pituitary, obtained from autopsy subjects, were made without regard to sex or age of the subject. Buxton's experience with the human pituitary material in women amenorrheic from three to six years repeats that of Gemzell and closely parallels that of Van Wagenen and Simpson in monkeys, utilizing monkey pituitary.

In general, after this treatment the ovaries, as seen on direct observation, are enlarged with their surfaces studded with dark purplish-blue hemorrhagic areas, approximately 1 cm. in diameter, and presenting all the characteristics attributed to ovulation. In at least one instance microscopic study of these areas revealed fresh corpora lutea in different stages of development. The effect of the combined use of human chorionic gonadotropin followed by the injection of human pituitary gonadotropin appeared to be one of creating multiple points of ovulation; in one reported instance a patient gave birth after a twin pregnancy. In most of the cases in which menstruation was restored the endometrium was secretory with rather more than the normal amount of decidual reaction in the stoma. This form of therapy can scarcely be regarded as practical for the patients who after such treatment reacted favorably each time by ovulating and then menstruating once, but failed to continue to do so on their own when the therapy was withdrawn. It is significant, however, that human pituitary extracts can produce ovulation in the human ovary by the action of the gonadotropin.

X-ray Treatment.   Treatment of the ovary and pituitary, either alone or in combination, using small doses of irradiation, has been advocated for the restoration of the menstrual cycle in secondary amenorrhea, and several large series of successfully treated cases have been reported in the literature.

Theoretically, small doses of radiation are supposed to be stimulating without causing any recognizable histologic change in the cells of the ovary. The primary or developing follicles appear to be less affected than the granulosa cells of the larger, more mature follicles, while the corpora lutea and the interstitial tissues offer the greatest resistance to radiation effects. It is thus possible that newer follicles with a higher functional capacity may arise from the unchanged primordial follicles in the regenerative period following radiation.

Since the principal effect of irradiation is destruction of tissue, it is hard to understand how roentgen rays can be selective and attack the cells in any gland that are primarily responsible for dysfunction without damaging others that are entirely normal. Not only are there differences in the response of the individual ovary to irradiation, but also there must be a thin line of demarcation between a dose that is stimulating (if it exists) and one that is destructive.

In recent literature, as an aftermath to our fears of atomic radiation, there has been an increasing interest in the possibilities of the damaging effects of radiation upon embryonic cells. When x-ray treatment is given to the ovaries during the reproductive years, particularly between twenty and thirty, there is grave danger to the germ plasm. The production of mutations may result, however small the radiation dose. Warnings have been issued by radiologists as well as geneticists that x-ray treatment is not without its hazards. It is suggested that the total gonadal exposure should not exceed 50 roentgens during the female reproductive period.

Enthusiastic supporters of low dosage radiation therapy to the ovaries in amenorrheic cases, after an experience going back over thirty years, fail to note any deleterious effect from such radiation in patients, their offspring or subsequent pregnancies. They believe that the hazards are more theoretical than real and that mutations are unlikely to appear in sufficient frequency even in later generations for one to withhold radiation therapy from a patient who is amenorrheic and wishes to become fertile. Animal experiments, however, not only on fruit flies, but also on guinea pigs, rabbits and mice tend to support the geneticists, in that mutations are possible even when small doses of irradiation are given. It would appear that, although the hazards of radiation to the ovary are not fully understood, nor are the number and time of the appearance of mutations known, the dangers inherent in this form of therapy are greater than the benefits that may possibly follow.

What Are the Chances of Re-establishing a Menstrual Cycle and the Likelihood of Subsequent Pregnancy in Secondary Amenorrhea after Irradiation of the Ovaries?   It is a difficult undertaking to estimate the degree of success in the restoration of regular menstrual cycles by irradiating the ovaries or pituitary in a patient with secondary amenorrhea for the simple reason that spontaneous resumption of menstruation is known to occur in this group, in which the psyche plays such an important role. The published figures range from 35 to 70 per cent. After the restoration of the menstrual period approximately half of the patients become pregnant, but not all carry through to the delivery of a normal infant. The number of subsequent abortions has been estimated as about 25 per cent.

The degree of success, as in all therapy of secondary amenorrhea, will depend in part upon the length of time the patient has had her amenorrhea.

What about the Use of Low Dosage Irradiation to the Pituitary?   Theoretically, if small doses of irradiation will stimulate cells to increased production of hormones, the direction of treatment toward the pituitary should be ideal, in view of the dominant role that the anterior pituitary lobe plays in the initiation of menstrual function. Many advocates of the use of irradiation for secondary amenorrhea like to combine radiation of both the pituitary and genital regions. In all probability, any effect observed can be traced to the effect of irradiation upon the ovary rather than the pituitary. There is general agreement that small doses of irradiation to the anterior pituitary do not produce any notable alteration in hormonal production. Radiation has proved effective in cases of acromegaly and pituitary tumors when large destructive doses have been given.

Should Irradiation of the Ovaries Ever Be Done for the Restoration of the Menstrual Cycle in Secondary Amenorrhea?   There seems to be pretty general agreement that the use of irradiation to the ovaries and pituitary should be avoided. If it is used at all, it should be reserved for a patient who has exhausted all other kinds of therapy, but still wants desperately to have her menstrual periods. If she has never had menstrual periods (primary amenorrhea), or if there is a past history of partial oophorectomy, irradiation therapy should not be given. It will do no good in the first instance and may effect a permanent menopause in the second. If the patient does not care whether she menstruates or not, nothing need be done, for general well-being is not dependent upon cyclic menstruation. Many women lead satisfactory lives who have never menstruated.

SURGERY.   There is a place for surgery in the treatment of secondary amenorrhea. Some benign tumors of the adrenal and pituitary may be removed by surgical intervention, and menstrual function is then restored.

The most satisfactory results after surgical therapy come in the patients who have the Stein-Leventhal syndrome. Why this simplest of all operations, the removal of a wedge-shaped section of tissue from both ovaries, should prove so effective is not known. Those who have followed up these patients claim that no recurrence of the original underlying abnormality follows operation. This is important, for many of these patients have normal ovulatory cycles and become pregnant later. Early recognition and operation are important, for if left unoperated, many of these girls become sterility problems. The process eventually becomes irreversible as uterine atrophy continues and the uterus becomes more refractory to ovarian stimulation.

One may be reluctant to operate on a young girl, but if she has not menstruated by the time she is of college age or has periods every six months to a year, exploration is indicated, provided there is no other obvious explanation of her amenorrhea and all other methods of therapy have been tried and failed. It is reason enough to explore the abdomen to know exactly the state of genital development. If a young woman has never menstruated, she has the right to know whether she can ever menstruate and have children. Since there is a reasonable chance that she may have the Stein-Leventhal syndrome, for which there is a simple, dramatic cure, there is no excuse for not advising abdominal exploration. The operation is comparable in the risk and time spent in convalescence to that of appendectomy, which may usually be performed incidentally. There is another element to consider, namely, that the underlying pathologic picture of polycystic ovaries is not unlike that of the stromal hyperplasia commonly associated in later life with carcinoma of the endometrium and the breast. Since the process does not recur after operation, the operator may be providing cancer prophylaxis at an early age.

REFERENCES

General Observations

Bauer, H. G.: Endocrine and Other Clinical Manifestations of Hypothalamic Disease. A Survey of 60 Cases with Autopsies. *J. Clin. Endocrinol.*, 14: 13, 1954.
Bishop, P. M. F.: *Recent Advances in Endocrinology*. 7th Ed. New York, Blakiston Co., 1954.
Fluhmann, C. F.: *The Management of Menstrual Disorders*. Philadelphia, W. B. Saunders Company, 1956.
Hamblen, E. C., Esselbourn, V. M., and Swatelle, W. E.: Amenorrhea: Some Clinical Notes on Its Etiology, Diagnostic Evaluation and Therapy. *M. Clin. N. Amer.*, 37: 1077, 1953.
Jones, G. S.: *The Management of Endocrine Disorders of Menstruation and Fertility*. Springfield, Ill., Charles C Thomas, 1954.
Li, C. H.: Pituitary Growth Hormone as a Metabolic Hormone. *Science*, 123: 617, 1956.
Mazer, C., and Israel, S. L.: *Diagnosis and Treatment of Menstrual Disorders and Sterility*. 4th Ed., edited by S. L. Israel. New York, Paul B. Hoeber, Inc., 1959.

Pituitary-Ovarian-Uterine Axis

Rogers, J.: Disorders of Menstruation; in *Disease a Month* Series. Chicago, Year Book Publishers, Inc., April, 1957.

Scott, R. B.: Thickening of the Ovarian Tunica. Effect of Its Production Artificially upon Ovulation in Monkeys. *Fertil. & Steril.*, 7: 44, 1956.

Stein, I. F., and Leventhal, M. L.: Amenorrhea Associated with Bilateral Polycystic Ovaries. *Am. J. Obst. & Gynec.*, 29: 181. 1935.

Sternberg, W. H.: The Morphology, Androgenic Function, Hyperplasia and Tumors of the Human Ovarian Hilus Cells. *Am. J. Path.*, 25: 493, 1949.

Whittaker, S. R. F., and Whitehead, T. P.: The Diagnosis and Treatment of Hypopituitarism. *Brit. M.J.*, 2: 265, 1954.

Other Endocrine Factors

Bongiovanni, A. M.: Detection of Pregnanediol and Pregnantriol in Urine of Patients with Adrenal Hyperplasia. Suppression with Cortisone. A Preliminary Report. *Bull. Johns Hopkins Hosp.*, 92: 244, 1953.

Jailer, J. W.: Virilism. *Bull. New York Acad. Med.*, 29: 377, 1953.

Sikkema, S. H.: Triiodothyronine in the Diagnosis and Treatment of Hypothyroidism; Failure to Demonstrate the Metabolic Insufficiency Syndrome (Controlled Study). *J. Clin. Endocrinol.*, 20: 546, 1960.

Psychogenic Factors

Benedek, T.: Infertility as a Psychosomatic Defense. *Fertil. & Steril.*, 3: 527, 1952.

Rubenstein, B. B.: An Emotional Factor in Infertility; A Psychosomatic Approach. *Fertil. & Steril.*, 2: 80, 1951.

General Therapy

Krogan, W S., and Freed, S. C.: *Psychosomatic Gynecology.* Philadelphia. W. B. Saunders Company, 1951.

Rogers, J. and Mitchell, G. W., Jr.: The Relation of Obesity to Menstrual Disturbances. *New England J. Med.*, 247: 53, 1952.

Endocrine Therapy

Bickers, W.: Progesterone and Anhydrohydroxyprogesterone: A Comparative Study of Oral Administration. *J. Lab. & Clin. Med.*, 35: 265, 1950.

Birnberg, C. H., Livingston, S., and Davis, J. G.: Large-Dose Oral Progesterone Therapy in Menstrual Disorders. *Obst. & Gynec.*, 11: 115, 1958.

Buxton, C. L., and Herrmann, W. L.: Effect of Thyroid Therapy on Menstrual Disorders and Sterility. *J.A.M.A.*, 155: 1035, 1954.

Idem: Induction of Ovulation in the Human with Human Pituitary Gonadotrophins. A Preliminary Report. *Am. J. Obst. & Gynec.*, 81: 584, 1961.

Comninos, A. C.: Thyroid Function and Therapy in Reproductive Disturbances. *Obst. & Gynec.*, 7: 260, 1956.

Frank, R., and Guterman, H. S.: Comparison of Progesterone Preparations in Secondary Amenorrhea. *Fertil. & Steril.*, 5: 374, 1954.

Gemzell, C. A.: *Colloquia on Endocrinology.* Ciba Foundation. London, J. & A. Churchill, Ltd., 1960, Vol. XIII, p. 191.

Greenblatt, R. B.: Physiologic Effectiveness of Progesterone Vaginal Suppositories. *J. Clin. Endocrinol.*, 14: 1564, 1954.

Hammond, J.: Hormones in Relation to Fertility in Farm Animals. *Brit. M. Bull.*, 11: 165, 1955.

Haskins, A. L.: Adjunctive Estrogen Therapy. *Obst. & Gynec.*, 11: 49, 1958.

Jones, G. S.: *The Management of Endocrine Disorders of Menstruation and Fertility.* Springfield, Ill., Charles C Thomas, 1954.

Kotz, H. L., and Herrmann, W.: A Review of the Endocrine Induction of Human Ovulation. VI. The Gonadotropins. *Fertil. & Steril.*, 12: 375, 1961.

Parsons, L.: The Causes and Management of Uterine Hemorrhage. *M. Clin. N. Amer.*, 37: 1497, 1953.

Parsons, L., and Tenney, B.: Endocrine Therapy in Menstrual Disorders. *M. Clin. N. Amer.*, 34: 1537, 1950.

Umbaugh, R. E.: Superovulation and Ovum Transfer in Cattle. *Fertil. & Steril.*, 2: 243, 1951.

Van Wagenen, G., and Simpson, M. E.: Induction of Multiple Ovulation in the Rhesus Monkey (Macaca Mulatta). *Endocrinology*, 61: 316, 1957.

Radiation

Clemedson, C.-J., and Nelson, A.: General Biology; The Adult Organism; in M. Errera and A. Forssberg, eds.: *Mechanisms in Radiobiology*. New York, Academic Press, 1960, Vol. 2, p. 95.

Drips, D. G.: Ovarian Dysfunction in Young Women Treated with Low-Dosage Irradiation. *Am. J. Obst. & Gynec.*, 55: 789, 1948.

Haman, J. O.: X-ray Irradiation to Promote Ovulation. *West. J. Surg., Obst. & Gynec.*, 55: 107, 1947.

Israel, S. L.: The Repudiation of Low-Dosage Irradiation of the Ovaries. *Am. J. Obst. & Gynec.*, 76: 443, 1958.

Kaplan, I. I.: Third Generation Followup of Women Treated by X-ray Therapy for Menstrual Dysfunction and Sterility Twenty-Eight Years Ago, with Detailed Histories of the Grandchildren Born to These Women. *Am. J. Obst. & Gynec.*, 67: 484, 1954.

Idem: The Treatment of Female Sterility with X-ray Therapy Directed to the Pituitary and Ovaries. *Am. J. Obst. & Gynec.*, 76: 447, 1958.

Muller, H. J.: Damage to Posterity Caused by Irradiation of the Gonads. *Am. J. Obst. & Gynec.*, 67: 467, 1954.

Chapter 36

Amenorrhea Following Childbirth

THERE are three rather well known, but still rare, entities that result in the dramatic disappearance of the menstrual periods following pregnancy in a girl who previously had been completely normal. They are (1) Simmonds's disease, (2) Sheehan's syndrome, and (3) Chiari-Frommel syndrome. The actual mechanism to blame for the amenorrhea is not clear, but the relation to childbirth is definite. All three entities eventuate in varying degrees of panhypopituitarism. The production of the gonadotropins diminishes, and the function of the other endocrine glands is disturbed in proportion to the degree of damage to the anterior pituitary lobe. In nearly every instance both Simmonds's disease and the Sheehan syndrome have appeared after a traumatic or septic delivery associated with hemorrhage and shock, either during or immediately after childbirth. If the shock and hemorrhage are severe enough, the patient may die in the immediate postpartum period. When the hemorrhage is extensive enough to produce shock, but not enough to be lethal, it may result in an arterial thrombosis in the anterior portion of the pituitary gland, as in Simmonds's disease, or hemorrhagic necrosis brought on by prolonged ischemia, as noted in Sheehan's syndrome. The patient does not die, but exhibits the symptoms of panhypopituitarism in varying degrees either months or, as in Sheehan's syndrome, years after the initial damage.

SIMMONDS'S DISEASE

What Are the Signs and Symptoms of Simmonds's Disease?

One should suspect Simmonds's disease when a patient who was normal before the traumatic or septic birth of a child begins to complain of weakness and fatigue and shows a complete disinterest in sexual activity. Simmonds's original patient had puerperal sepsis eleven years previously, followed by amenorrhea, asthenia, vertigo, spells of unconsciousness, emaciation, anemia and premature senility. There may be only few symptoms and variable physical findings.

Experimentally, in animals large portions of the anterior pituitary lobe can be destroyed and replaced by scar tissue without producing any obvious alteration in endocrine function. Gonadotropic secretion and target-organ response may therefore vary, depending on the extent of damage to the anterior pituitary. Decrease in the output of the thyrotropic hormone produces the train of symptoms and physical

459

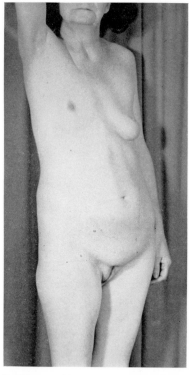

Fig. 36-1.   Appearance of premature senility in a woman of childbearing age with Simmonds's pituitary cachexia. The breasts are atrophic, the skin is thin and pale, and the body hair absent.

findings of hypothyroidism, which are the most easily recognized. They vary all the way from increasing cold sensitivity to an outright myxedema. In the majority the skin will be cool, dry, pale, thin and atrophic, and the eyebrows sparse.

The other endocrine glands are also affected. Lack of stimulation by FSH and decreased end-organ response will produce amenorrhea. Lack of the adrenocortico-tropic hormone encourages wasting of both tissues and muscle. The patient has a slow pulse and a low blood pressure and appears apathetic and listless. As androgen production declines, hair begins to fall out, first in the axillae and later from the scalp and pubic regions. The atrophic changes in the underlying connective tissue and skin and the loss of hair give the patient the appearance of being prematurely aged (Fig. 36–1). When damage to the pituitary is severe enough, the somatotropic hormone is produced in inadequate quantity. As a result the patient may lose her appetite, have spells of vomiting and may experience attacks of faintness or weakness due to hypo-glycemia.

What Other Entities May Simulate Simmonds's Disease?

Since the symptoms and physical findings are directly related to the extent of damage to the anterior pituitary, other pathologic entities can present the same picture. This is particularly true of chromophobe adenomas of the pituitary and other suprasellar tumors that either replace normal pituitary by overgrowing the function-ing cells or compress pituitary tissue by growth from outside the gland capsule. Sheehan's syndrome closely parallels the presenting picture of Simmonds's disease, for in this condition the pituitary is damaged by ischemic necrosis and hemorrhage secondary to severe shock from uterine hemorrhage suffered in the process of delivery.

The differentiation between pituitary or hypothalamic tumors and Simmonds's disease can be made by uncovering a history indicating a close relation to traumatic childbirth in the latter, and by the x-ray and neurologic findings. The patient with tumor should show x-ray evidence of enlargement or damage of the sella turcica, destruction of the clinoid processes, or disturbances in the neurologic pattern of the visual fields and appearance of the eyegrounds. The difference between Simmonds's disease and Sheehan's syndrome is largely one of degree and is directly dependent on the extent of destruction in the anterior pituitary lobe. By and large the damage in Simmonds's disease is more extensive.

How Does One Differentiate between Anorexia Nervosa and Simmonds's Disease?

The signs and symptoms of Simmonds's disease are not unlike those seen in anorexia nervosa, except that the defect is far more basic and the history entirely different.

The adolescent or young adult with anorexia nervosa has usually suffered a traumatic emotional experience. It may be due to a change in environment, a downgrading of her ego, or an unfortunate experience with men. As a result she loses all interest in food and begins to lose weight, as malnutrition takes its toll. The characteristic appearance of the patient with anorexia nervosa is one of profound emaciation and weight loss. Despite the wasting she continues to lead an active, vigorous life, with particular emphasis on "good causes." Moderately depressed, her thoughts are concentrated on (a) her aversion to food and (b) her distaste for the world and its evil ways. As a result of the malnutrition the pituitary fails to function normally. This is reflected in diminished thyroid and ovarian function. The patient not only loses weight rapidly, but also has a slow pulse and low blood pressure. Her basal metabolic rate drops, and signs of estrogen lack are obvious before she becomes amenorrheic.

The distinction between the two entities, which have many characteristics in common, is made fairly easily. In anorexia nervosa (1) the girl has a history of some element of emotional unrest; (2) she continues to be active while wasting away through malnutrition; (3) she does not lose her axillary and pubic hair, except when the condition is prolonged.

The patient with Simmonds's disease, on the other hand, may appear to be pudgy and fat rather than thin and emaciated. Actually, she has lost a considerable amount of tissue and muscle substance, but this is masked by the myxedema that comes from decreased thyroid function as the pituitary thyrotropic stimulus diminishes. With decreasing thyroid function the patient becomes apathetic and sluggish rather than hyperactive as in anorexia nervosa. The patient with Simmonds's disease shows circulatory changes in the skin, which becomes pale, thin and dry and provides little protection from the cold. The axillary and later the pubic hairs disappear. This is not true of anorexia nervosa. Finally the related condition, Sheehan's syndrome, can often be traced to a fairly recent traumatic birth.

It is important to remember that the patients with Sheehan's syndrome are not necessarily thin and emaciated despite the loss of tissue and muscle. This widespread impression is in error.

What Is the Clinical Picture in Sheehan's Syndrome?

Since the underlying pathology in both Simmonds's disease and Sheehan's syndrome is basically the same, though their etiology differs slightly, the discussion

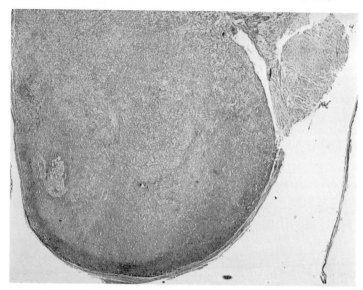

Fig. 36-2.   Pituitary necrosis has destroyed all the anterior lobe tissue shown except for the narrow, dark-stained rim just beneath the capsule. Even this degree of destruction is not always accompanied by clinicopathologic evidence of hypopituitarism.

of the laboratory findings and treatment will be deferred until the description of the clinical picture of Sheehan's syndrome.

The difference between Simmonds's disease and the Sheehan syndrome seems to be largely a question of the extent of anterior pituitary damage. Since Simmonds's disease is believed to be due to a thrombotic or embolic infarct, the chances of extensive tissue necrosis would appear to be greater than in Sheehan's syndrome, in which the cause is believed to be tissue anoxia secondary to severe uterine hemorrhage and shock incident to delivery. As a result there appear to be many more cases of unsuspected, or subclinical, Sheehan's syndrome than we would expect in Simmonds's disease.

When symptoms appear, their severity will depend on the extent of tissue necrosis within the anterior pituitary and the amount of scar tissue replacement. For example, the symptoms of Sheehan's syndrome may not become evident for months or years after the delivery. They may not manifest themselves until a subsequent childbirth or severe infection brings on an additional stress factor.

Sheehan has shown, through review of human patients post partum, and animal experiments tend to confirm, that the anterior lobe of the pituitary can suffer better than a 50 per cent degree of tissue damage without any reflection in altered function of the endocrine glands. Some damage is noted when 60 per cent of this portion of the gland is destroyed, and the symptoms become progressively more obvious as the pathologic damage becomes greater. Some symptoms do not appear until approximately 95 per cent of the anterior pituitary is destroyed. It is thus obvious that the pituitary can be severely damaged without causing any noticeable disturbance in the production of the pituitary gonadotropins (Fig. 36–2).

In the great majority of instances Sheehan's syndrome follows massive intra-partum or postpartum hemorrhage accompanied by shock. This need not be the sole etiologic explanation, however, for pituitary necrosis has been reported in the presence of severe postpartum infection or diabetes mellitus. Varying degrees of panhypopituitarism have been observed in previously normal patients after a delivery uncomplicated by hemorrhage or shock. For all practical purposes, however, hemorrhage, shock and pituitary necrosis are linked together.

There appears to be little relation between the extent of hemorrhage and shock and the extent of pituitary damage. One may have small, medium or large areas of necrosis. The symptoms, therefore, may show up in only one rather than all target organs. One may then lose the gonadotropic and thyrotropic hormones without the adrenocorticotropic function. These patients survive stresses placed upon them, but become amenorrheic and exhibit all the symptoms of thyroid deficiency. It is not uncommon to observe that patients who have had a severe hemorrhage with shock during pregnancy are apt to have diminished menstrual activity and sterility problems.

SHEEHAN'S DISEASE

What Is the Incidence of Sheehan's Syndrome?

The true incidence of Sheehan's syndrome is hard to come by. Sheehan feels that severe hemorrhage and shock will result in pituitary necrosis in over half of the patients so traumatized. Since the degree of necrosis varies in extent, and symptoms appear only when there has been considerable damage, it is obvious that pituitary necrosis following postpartum hemorrhage occurs more frequently than is generally recognized. Approximately 40 per cent of Sheehan's series of live patients followed up for some time after severe traumatic childbirth had partial or severe symptoms of hypothyroidism.

Israel and Schneeberg and their co-workers also believe that anterior pituitary necrosis is far from a rare sequel to postpartum hemorrhage. In their opinion minor changes frequently go unrecognized clinically. The patient may have moderate symptoms referable to faulty thyroid function and show nothing abnormal on physical examination. Any patient, then, who has experienced severe hemorrhage in the course of delivery should be kept under observation for years. One of Schneeberg's patients had pituitary damage of lethal amount, yet exhibited little in the way of symptoms until she died during an uncomplicated subsequent pregnancy. In the interest of preventive medicine it would be well to regard any patient who had a severe bleeding episode during pregnancy as a potential candidate for pituitary necrosis and to support her with ACTH and cortisone during times of stress.

What Are the Symptoms of Sheehan's Syndrome?

The classic symptoms are those of panhypopituitarism. Thus we may expect to find, in a well established case, (1) absence of lactation, (2) amenorrhea, (3) atrophy of the uterus and cervix as well as senile changes in the vaginal epithelium, (4) loss of axillary and pubic hair and gradual thinning of the eyebrows, (5) a dry, thin, pale skin which is sensitive to cold and does not perspire, (6) loss of appetite, vomiting and a tendency to spells of fainting and weakness because of the accompanying hypoglycemia, (7) a disturbance in the water and electrolyte balance, (8) an increasing disinterest in her home and family, as the patient becomes placidly inactive (Fig. 36–3).

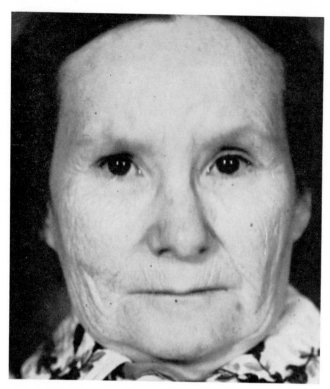

Fig. 36-3. The facial appearance of Sheehan's syndrome includes a sagging of the soft tissues, mild alterations of myxedematous type, and pallor.

It is evident from the foregoing discussion that only a few of this train of symptoms may be present. If only the gonadotropin or other single pituitary hormone is involved, the disturbance will be concentrated on its target organ. The symptoms may be minimal in amount.

What Are the Laboratory Findings in Simmonds's Disease and Sheehan's Syndrome?

The search for evidence to confirm pituitary insufficiency concentrates on target organ function.

Diminished gonadotropic function is suspected if the vaginal smear is atrophic and the endometrial biopsy reveals scanty material with a few atrophic glands. It is confirmed when the patient is amenorrheic, the uterus, external genitalia and breasts are atrophied, and the urinary assays for FSH are diminished or absent.

Inadequate thyroid function is suspected when the protein-bound iodine in the serum, basal metabolism or radio-iodine uptake are at low levels. The serum cholesterol level will be elevated. From combination with the physical findings mentioned, one may suspect that the thyrotropic hormone is inadequate or lacking.

The adrenal cortical function is measured by (*a*) urinary 17-ketosteroid excretion, (*b*) oral glucose tolerance test, (*c*) insulin tolerance test, (*d*) eosinophil response to ACTH, (*e*) serum sodium, potassium and chloride levels, as well as the carbon dioxide-combining power, (*f*) water excretion tests. The absence of diabetogenic effects of growth hormone can best be evaluated by the responses to the insulin tolerance and oral glucose tolerance tests.

In the laboratory evaluation all or only a few elements may be abnormal, in keeping with the clinical response to variable degrees of necrosis in the pituitary. Such tests are useful, however, in pinpointing the area of deficient target organ response.

What Treatment Can Be Offered the Patient with Simmonds's Disease or Sheehan's Syndrome?

Since considerable damage may be present in the pituitary in the absence of clinical manifestations, one of the most important elements in therapy is the recognition, or suspicion, of the presence of lesions in the pituitary. Of the two, Simmonds's disease is far more likely to manifest itself than Sheehan's syndrome, for the fundamental defect is more widespread.

Practically, one should become suspicious of a patient who either did not lactate after delivery or failed to regrow the hair shaved from the pubic area in anticipation of the delivery. It would also be good prophylactic medicine to keep under observation any patient who has had a severe uterine hemorrhage, complicated by shock, whether suggestive symptoms are present or not. The symptoms of Sheehan's syndrome may not appear for months or years.

The treatment, then, falls into three spheres of activity: (1) prompt treatment of shock and hemorrhage at the time of delivery, (2) prolonged observation of the patient who has had such an experience, (3) the treatment of symptoms when they appear.

It is obvious that the intensity of therapy will depend on the degree of damage, as manifested by the target organ response. If all the endocrine glands are involved, the anterior pituitary is too severely damaged for one to expect to accomplish anything except by total replacement therapy, which is not yet possible. About all the physician can do otherwise is to outline general supportive measures designed to improve hygiene and nutrition.

ACTH is the most practical of the hormones to replace. By and large the patient has no great difficulty in surviving stress periods caused by illness, severe infection or pregnancy when gonadotropic or thyrotropic function is lost or in abeyance. But the patient with adrenocortical insufficiency due to lack of pituitary stimulation must have substitution therapy with ACTH or corticosteroids before, during and after stress, or run the risk of fatal consequences.

If the pituitary damage is extensive, it is unwise to give thyroid extract to stimulate a sluggish metabolism. The endocrine glands have no need for increased oxygen consumption, since the body metabolism is totally depressed. Actually, the lowered metabolism may be a kind of protective mechanism.

When the damage is less severe, the emphasis in treatment should be directed toward the target organ that lacks adequate stimulation from the pituitary hormones. The usual case of Sheehan's syndrome lacks adequate gonadotropic and thyrotropic stimulation. Unfortunately, we do not have any dependable hormone that we can use to force the pituitary to put out more of the deficient hormones. All that can be done is to replace estrin and thyroid on a permanent schedule. The defect in the pituitary remains unchanged. As with all hormone substitution therapy, one can hope that the pituitary may be placed at rest long enough to have the gland recover spontaneously. If the adrenocorticotropic hormone is deficient, one can improve adrenal insufficiency by giving ACTH, but this is the only hormone that can be used for anything other than pure substitution.

THE CHIARI-FROMMEL SYNDROME

There are a few rare gynecologic entities that produce a dramatic combination of amenorrhea, persistent galactorrhea, a low production of pituitary FSH and atrophy of the uterus, ovaries and the vaginal tract. Perhaps the most dramatic is the so-called Chiari-Frommel syndrome, first described by Chiari in 1855 and later elaborated upon by Frommel in 1882. In this syndrome this chain of events invariably followed a normal pregnancy, although some element of faulty nutrition appeared as well.

What Are the Symptoms and Clinical Findings?

Although the patient becomes amenorrheic after the birth of the child, this often does not seem to concern her, despite the fact that the menstrual history had previously been normal. These patients are concerned about the persistent discharge of milk from the nipples. The quantity varies in amount, but may appear sufficiently abundant to prove troublesome. The discharge may continue for months or years (Fig. 36-4). There is one case reported in which it lasted for more than fifteen years. In most instances the amenorrhea is as permanent as the galactorrhea is persistent, although there are a few cases on record in which the menses resumed and subsequently pregnancy followed. The other symptoms, which may or may not appear, such as abdominal pain, backache, mental depression and hysterical outbursts, are nonspecific.

The factor of ovarian and uterine atrophy suggests that a pituitary stimulus is lacking. The ovaries are almost invariably small and atrophic, while the uterus in most instances is small. Endometrial biopsies show an atrophic endometrium, when any tissue can be curetted, and the urinary FSH is recovered in only small amounts. The breasts, however, despite the diminished or absent stimulation of estrin, remain large or even appear voluminous.

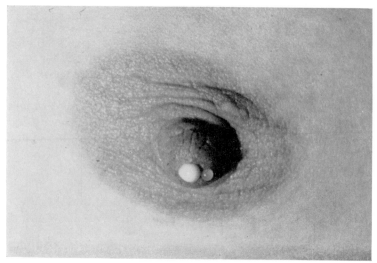

Fig. 36-4.   Persistent postpartum lactation produces the salient symptom in the Chiari-Frommel syndrome.

What Other Entities Simulate the Chiari-Frommel Syndrome?

The chief factor which distinguishes the Chiari-Frommel syndrome from other entities that produce the same train of events is its association with pregnancy. Persistent lactation has also been associated with acromegaly and chromophobe adenomas of the pituitary. Forbes and Albright reported a series of patients with galactorrhea, amenorrhea, uterine atrophy and low FSH, the great majority of whom had neither pituitary tumor nor any previous pregnancy. In all, however, there has been obvious evidence of pituitary deficiency as evidenced by the low FSH and the absence of estrogen effect on the target organs.

Why Do These Patients Have Persistent Galactorrhea?

The mechanism for the persistence of lactation is not entirely clear. As Forbes suggests, it is not due to the lack of FSH, for the hormone is produced in larger quantity in normal nursing mothers who have amenorrhea than in nonlactating mothers. Nor is it due to inadequate amounts of estrin, since (*a*) no lactation occurs after castration or in the menopausal state, and (*b*) some nursing mothers become pregnant.

The pituitary seems to be implicated in some way, though the defect appears to be selective. The only evidence for pituitary failure is the low FSH and deficient production of estrin. All the other factors are apparently normal. Albright has postulated that the pituitary is producing specific hormones in excess. There is some evidence that the source in the pituitary for this overproduction of hormone lies in the acidophilic cells. This is true in acromegaly, in which there is known hormonal overproduction by these cells. Cushing also considered that cells in chromophobe adenomas were often preacidophilic. It is thought that chromophobe adenomas cause lactation either because they produce a lactogenic hormone (prolactin) in excess, or because they interfere with the production of the pituitary hormones that normally inhibit lactation.

What Can Be Done for the Patient with the Chiari-Frommel Syndrome?

These patients are notoriously resistant to therapy. A few recover spontaneously and resume normal menstrual periods without medical aid. In the great majority this condition appears to be permanent. In some patients there appears to be enough of an element of malnutrition to warrant outlining a course of therapy designed to improve the general condition and the accompanying anemia. Hormone therapy has proved to be unproductive. Any suggestion of pituitary tumor should be thoroughly investigated.

REFERENCES

Chiari-Frommel Syndrome

Argonz, J., and Del Castillo, E. B.: A Syndrome Characterized by Estrogenic Insufficiency, Galactorrhea and Decreased Urinary Gonadotropin. *J. Clin. Endocrinol.*, 13: 79, 1953.

Ashkar, P. A.: Chiari's Syndrome; Report of a Case. *J. Obst. & Gynaec. Brit. Emp.*, 57: 78, 1950.

Christiansen, E. G.: Case of Chiari-Frommel Syndrome. *Acta Endocrinol.*, 24: 407, 1957.

Cohen, A.: Amenorrhoea and Prolonged Lactation, Including a Further Report on the Chiari-Frommel Syndrome. *Australasian Ann. Med.*, 8: 77, 1959.

Forbes, A. P., Henneman, P. H., Griswold, G. C., and Albright, F.: A Syndrome Distinct from Acromegaly, Characterized by Spontaneous Lactation, Amenorrhea and Low FSH Excretion. *J. Clin. Endocrinol.*, 11: 749, 1951.

Idem: Syndrome Characterized by Galactorrhea, Amenorrhea and Low Urinary FSH: Comparison with Acromegaly and Normal Lactation. *J. Clin. Endocrinol.*, 14: 265, 1954.

Greenblatt, R. B., Carmona, N., and Hagler, W. S.: Chiari-Frommel Syndrome: Syndrome Characterized by Galactorrhea, Amenorrhea, and Pituitary Dysfunction. Report of Two Cases. *Obst. & Gynec.*, 7: 165, 1956.

Krestin, D.: Spontaneous Lactation Associated with Enlargement of Pituitary, with Report of 2 Cases. *Lancet*, 1: 928, 1932.

Mendel, E. B.: Chiari-Frommel Syndrome. An Historical Review with Case Report. *Am. J. Obst. & Gynec.*, 51: 889, 1946.

Rolland, C. F., Matthew, J. D., and Matthew, G. D.: Pregnancy in Addison's Disease. *J. Obst. & Gynaec. Brit. Emp.*, 60: 57, 1953.

Russfield, A. B., Reiner, L., and Klaus, H.: The Endocrine Significance of Hypophyseal Tumors in Man. *Am. J. Path.*, 32: 1055, 1956.

Sharp, E. A.: Historical Review of Syndrome Embracing Uteroovarian Atrophy with Persistent Lactation (Frommel's Disease). *Am. J. Obst. & Gynec.*, 30: 411, 1935.

Sheehan's Syndrome

Brennan, C. F., Malone, R. G. S., and Weaver, J. A.: Pituitary Necrosis in Diabetes Mellitus. *Lancet*, 2: 12, 1956.

Cook, J. E., Bean, W. B., Franklin, M., and Embick, J. F.: Postpartum Necrosis of the Anterior Lobe of the Pituitary Gland: Sheehan's Disease. *A.M.A. Arch. Int. Med.*, 87: 517, 1951.

Gottshalk, H. C., and Tilden, I. L.: Necrosis of Anterior Pituitary Following Parturition. *J.A.M.A.*, 114: 33, 1940.

Hornabrook, R. W., and Caughey, J. E.: Hypopituitarism Following Postpartum Necrosis of Anterior Pituitary. *New Zealand M.J.*, 53: 210, 1954.

Israel, S. L., and Conston, A. S.: Unrecognized Pituitary Necrosis (Sheehan's Syndrome); Cause of Sudden Death. *J.A.M.A.*, 148: 189, 1952.

Schneeberg, N. G., Perloff, W. H., and Israel, S. L.: Incidence of Unsuspected "Sheehan's Syndrome" (Hypopituitarism after Postpartum Hemorrhage and/or Shock). Clinical and Laboratory Study. *J.A.M.A.*, 172: 20, 1960.

Sheehan, H. L.: Postpartum Necrosis of Anterior Lobe of the Pituitary. *Lancet*, 2: 321, 1940.

Idem: Incidence of Postpartum Hypopituitarism. *Am. J. Obst. & Gynec.*, 68: 202, 1954.

Simmonds's Disease and Anorexia Nervosa

Bliss, E. L., and Migeon, C. J.: Endocrinology of Anorexia Nervosa. *J. Clin. Endocrinol.*, 17: 766, 1957.

Cushing, H.: Basophil Adenomas of Pituitary Body and Their Clinical Manifestations (Pituitary Basophilism). *Bull. Johns Hopkins Hosp.*, 50: 137, 1932.

Dally, P. J., and Sargant, W.: A New Treatment of Anorexia Nervosa. *Brit. M.J.*, 1: 1770, 1960.

Du Bois, F. S.: Compulsion Neurosis with Cachexia (Anorexia Nervosa). *Am. J. Psychiat.*, 106: 107, 1949.

Farquharson, R. F., and Hyland, H. H.: Anorexia Nervosa; Metabolic Disorder of Psychologic Origin. *J.A.M.A.*, 111: 1085, 1938.

Ganong, W. F., and Hume, D. M.: Effect of Graded Hypophysectomy on Thyroid, Gonadal and Adrenocortical Function in Dog. *Endocrinology*, 59: 293, 1956.

Moulton, R.: A Psychosomatic Study of Anorexia Nervosa, Including the Use of Vaginal Smears. *Psychosom. Med.*, 4: 62, 1942.

Murdoch, R., and Govan, A. D. T.: Therapeutic Effect of Subsequent Pregnancy in Simmonds' Disease. Case Report. *J. Obst. & Gynaec. Brit. Emp.*, 58: 18, 1951.

Nemiah, J. C.: Anorexia Nervosa; Clinical Psychiatric Study. *Medicine*, 29: 225, 1950.

Perkins, R. F., and Rynearson, E. H.: Practical Aspects of Insufficiency of the Anterior Pituitary Gland in the Adult. *J. Clin. Endocrinol.*, 12: 574, 1952.

Plaut, A.: Pituitary Necrosis in Routine Necropsies. *Am. J. Path.*, 28: 883, 1952.

Chapter 37

Tumors Complicating Pregnancy

CARCINOMA OF THE CERVIX ASSOCIATED WITH PREGNANCY

CANCER of the cervix is primarily a neoplastic growth encountered in the woman in her mid-forties. The peak incidence is around forty-five years of age. Since cancer of the cervix produces few symptoms and tends to occur late in the menstrual span, the physician and the patient may give little thought to intermenstrual bleeding or spotting that occurs in the twenties or thirties, and certainly they rarely associate the symptom with a possible cancer. Cervical cancer, however, has been reported in infancy and in teen-age girls but usually as an adeno- rather than a squamous carcinoma. Unlike the prepuberal child, in whom the cervical cancer is apt to be an adenocarcinoma, the menstruating young girl—like the premenopausal woman—will show only 5 per cent adenocarcinomas, the remainder being epidermoid carcinomas. Approximately 7 per cent of all cervical cancers occur in women under the age of thirty.

It is not surprising, then, that cancer of the cervix may be present in the pregnant woman. The prognosis is uniformly poor. The reason why this is so is not altogether clear. It has been suggested that cancer of the cervix in the young woman, like malignancy in the breast, responds less well to standard forms of therapy. There is also a temptation to explain the poor results by a tumor-stimulating factor produced by the pregnancy itself, although there is no reliable evidence that pregnancy alters the rate of growth of a cervical cancer.

It is far more likely that the poor results reported in the treatment of cancer of the cervix associated with pregnancy are due to the fact that the telltale symptoms of bleeding or discharge were attributed to a benign cause and the true explanation never suspected until too late. We shall show in the more detailed discussion of carcinoma of the cervix in later chapters that the extent of the disease is the most important single factor in estimating the prognosis. The patient with cancer of the cervix and a concomitant pregnancy, just as in breast cancer, often has more extensive disease.

What Is the Incidence of Carcinoma of the Cervix Coexisting with Pregnancy?

The true incidence of the coexistence of cervical cancer and pregnancy is hard to come by, largely because (*a*) in the statistical reports of yesteryear, obstetrical practice discouraged vaginal examinations, so that undoubtedly some cases were overlooked; (*b*) the series now being presented include many carcinomas in situ that either might not be recognized or might not progress to the invasive stage until several years after delivery. This is due to the present widespread use of the vaginal Papanicolaou smear.

Reports of cervical cancer with pregnancy from individual institutions, even in the same geographic area, vary from 0.05 to 0.5 per cent of all pregnant women. A compilation of several large series from institutions throughout the world reveals 446 cervical carcinomas in a grand total of 1,108,352 pregnancies. The incidence, then, is approximately 0.045 per cent, or about one in every 2500 pregnancies. Roughly, 1.5 per cent of all cervical cancers will be associated with pregnancy.

How Is the Diagnosis Made?

The diagnosis of cancer of the cervix in a pregnant uterus is made when the physician is alert to the fact that any vaginal bleeding or discharge may herald the existence of a malignant growth. A variety of benign explanations, such as persistence of menstruation, threatened abortion, cervical erosion or cervicitis in early pregnancy and premature labor in the later phases, act as decoys to keep the physician's index of suspicion low.

It is particularly important to rule out the possibility of malignant disease rather than to attribute bleeding to a benign cause in a woman who has even a small amount of vaginal bleeding, whatever the stage of pregnancy. The nature, amount and duration are of no importance. Unlike cancer of the cervix in the nonpregnant woman, the lesion is apt to have an endocervical location which is far less likely to bleed than the exophytic kind of lesion. Approximately one third of the cases will have extensive disease without any bleeding at all.

What Steps Should Be Taken to Pinpoint the Cause of Bleeding?

1. The most important step in investigating the cause of any vaginal staining in a pregnant woman is to take a Papanicolaou smear. It will be unnecessary if physical examination reveals an exophytic kind of growth or an ulceration with firm hard borders, but it will be invaluable if the examiner encounters, as he so often does, simply an erosion or cervicitis in an edematous congested cervix.

2. The next step is to examine the patient with a vaginal speculum. We now know that no harm will come to the pregnancy, for it has been amply demonstrated that even repeated biopsies or actual cold-knife conization will not influence its course.

Cancer of the cervix has the same gross characteristics in the pregnant as in the nonpregnant state, but in its early stages the diagnosis is complicated by the edema, congestion and the other physiologic changes that occur in the epithelium incident to the pregnancy. Approximately one third of the patients will present no obvious alteration in the gross appearance of the cervical epithelium. In this instance a growth in the endocervical canal should be suspected. The remainder will have some sort of erosion, either simple or papillary. Papillary erosions are reasonably common, and since they are very friable and bleed easily, the gross appearance may be that of an exophytic carcinoma. The largest benign exophytic growths of the cervix in pregnancy are papillomas, often called cockscomb papillomas. They may be difficult to distinguish from carcinoma both clinically and pathologically, except by expert specialists.

Any ulceration should be regarded with grave suspicion. This is heightened when bleeding occurs with minimal trauma to an ulcerating lesion which has a hard, red, granular base and overhanging, irregular, firm edges.

3. Since therapy cannot be carried out without pathologic confirmation, a biopsy of any suspicious area must be taken. The changes in the cervical epithelium incident to pregnancy make choice of the proper area more difficult than in the nonpregnant cervix. Schiller's solution will be useful in selecting the area from which the biopsy should be taken. Due to the confusion offered by physiologic changes in pregnancy, cervical biopsies from a number of widely dispersed areas, including the endocervix, should be taken. This can be done with impunity, just as one would do in a nonpregnant cervix.

There is a lamentable tendency to take too few biopsies, which are altogether too small for the pathologist to make an adequate interpretation. The physician need not hesitate to take an adequate amount of tissue from a number of areas for fear that he will cause troublesome bleeding or induce abortion or premature labor. The pathologist has his own problems in interpreting the tissue presented to him because of the proliferative epithelial changes that occur normally in pregnancy. He has little chance in a problem case if he does not have enough tissue to work on. It is far better to lose the baby, which is not likely, through adequate biopsy procedures than possibly to lose both mother and baby by falsely interpreting the basic condition because the specimen was either insufficient in amount, or taken from the wrong place.

4. The next step in orderly sequence is to evaluate the extent of the cancer. This is not easy under the best of circumstances and is complicated in the pregnant cervix by pelvic congestion and edema. Unfortunately, the great majority of cases of cervical cancer in pregnancy are discovered in the last trimester when the disease is relatively far advanced. Occasionally, when the importance of the symptom of bleeding has been recognized and smears and a vaginal examination have been performed, carcinoma in the early stages of growth (League of Nations Stages I and IIa) may be encountered. In all probability the cancer did not develop under the influence of pregnancy, but was present before it began and was previously unrecognized. This points up to the necessity of early vaginal examination in the face of bleeding of any magnitude.

The extent of the growth has a direct bearing on the choice of therapy and is intimately linked to the prognosis. It is important, therefore, to form an estimate of the amount of cancer the patient has and the direction of its spread.

What about Interpretation of the Vaginal Smears?

When histologic review of biopsy specimens confirms the clinical impression that cancer is present, there is no problem except the choice and timing of therapy. When the smears are suggestive and the pathologic findings from the biopsy are inconclusive or negative, there is a real problem.

Because hormonal stimulation is at its height and fungus infection is common in the pregnant state, a number of variable cytologic elements appear in the vaginal smear of a pregnant woman. Because of the altered hormonal activity such smears are apt to contain an unusual number of basal cells, which vary in size and shape and often have hyperchromatic nuclei. Actually, there is no difference in the positive cancer smear in the pregnant and nonpregnant, except for the fact that basal cells, as noted above, often seen in the premenstrual phase of a normal cycle are present in greater numbers and are out of proportion to the number of cancer cells. The problem is

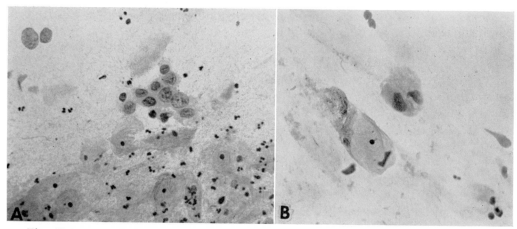

Fig. 37-1.   *A,* Malignant cells from the vaginal smear of a pregnant patient. The large, pale nuclei suggest cervical carcinoma in situ, as later proved by biopsy. *B,* Atypical benign cells in pregnancy, shown around one normal cornified cell.

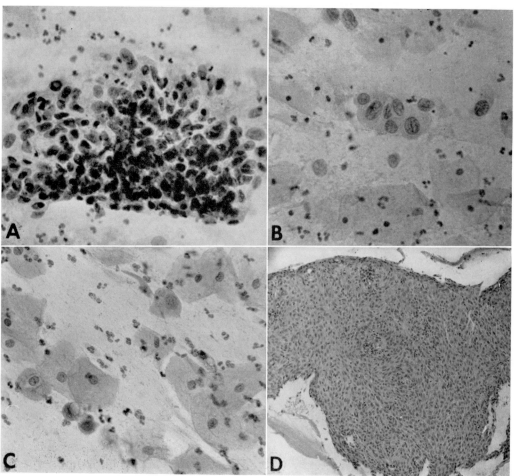

Fig. 37-2.   *A,* Obvious malignant tumor cells in a Class V Papanicolaou smear taken during pregnancy. *B,* Class IV or suspicious cells, not obviously cancerous, from the same patient as shown in *A. C,* Class III or suspicious smear from another pregnant patient. *D,* Biopsy with carcinoma in situ during pregnancy. The cervical carcinoma cells are often less hyperchromatic than they appear in nonpregnant women.

further compounded by the variety of leukocytic elements present, which may arise because of inflammatory conditions within the cervix such as erosions or the possible presence of trichomonads or monilia. As a result there is an increased amount of exfoliation of the cornified cells (Fig. 37–1).

These factors complicate proper classification of vaginal smears taken during the course of pregnancy. We are most concerned with the diagnosis of early lesions, for the more advanced lesions are clinically obvious or can be readily detected by biopsy. The very suspicious, so-called Class IV, or positive, Class V smears, will show probable or actual tumor cells, respectively, while Class III is in the suspicious class. Obviously, tissue diagnostic confirmation by biopsy is essential before definitive therapy is outlined. A reasonably high percentage will prove to have cancer of the cervix when a Class IV smear is reported, but the lesion may be in situ and not invasive. If the former, one can afford to temporize, while in the latter, immediate therapy is mandatory. Class III smears are simply suspicious, and a program of repeated checking by smears at regular intervals will suffice. (Fig. 37–2, *A, B, C*).

What about Interpretation of the Biopsy Specimen?

The problems encountered in interpreting vaginal smears from a pregnant patient are magnified when histologic evaluation is undertaken. The same complicating factors are present: (*a*) increased hormonal stimulation of the cervical epithelium and (*b*) the epithelial reaction to infection. The pathologist must also decide whether there is or is not invasion.

The trained pathologist will have little difficulty in the diagnosis of a frankly invasive cervical cancer. This comprises the largest group, for most of them are well established when the first biopsy is taken, but the problem arises in the early case in differentiating between hyperactivity of the basal layer and carcinoma in situ on the one hand, and carcinoma in situ with invasion on the other (Fig. 37–2, *D*).

Pregnancy produces characteristic changes in the cervical epithelium and the surrounding stroma. Actually, such changes represent simple magnification of the hormonal cycles normally present in the nonpregnant woman. Thus we have increased vascularity and edema of the stroma as well as stromal decidual reaction

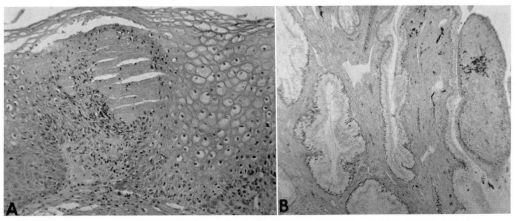

Fig. 37-3. *A,* Benign epithelial hyperplasia and stromal hyperemia normally found in the pregnant exocervix. *B,* Physiologic hyperplasia of endocervical glands in pregnancy results in formation of the mucous plug.

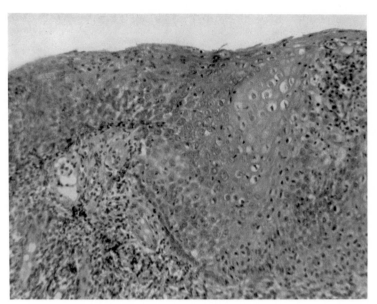

Fig. 37-4.   Cervical biopsy in pregnancy that presented a difficult differential diagnosis between epithelial hyperplasia and carcinoma in situ. After examination of multiple sections and pathologic consultations a final diagnosis of carcinoma in situ was rendered.

and signs of inflammation. The endocervical glands undergo hyperplasia of their epithelium, and many of them may show evidence of epidermidization. The squamous cervical epithelium itself shows proliferation in all its layers, but particularly in the basal cell layer. The individual cells occasionally exhibit varying degrees of anaplasia in both the basal and other layers. Characteristically, the nuclei increase in number and in mitotic activity, which is said to be five times greater in the pregnant cervix. Nuclei also tend to vary in size and shape, and occasionally have multiple nucleoli (Fig. 37–3).

Since these changes may be encountered in the epithelium of a normal pregnant woman, it is evident that the pathologist may have considerable difficulty in deciding whether the alterations in the epithelial pattern truly indicate neoplastic change. This is why it is important that adequate tissue material be presented to him. If the pathologic interpretation raises suspicion, but a firm diagnosis cannot be made from the tissue at hand, the surgeon should do a cold-knife conization of the cervix, under anesthesia, which will include not only the exocervix, but a segment of the endocervix as well. This can be done without endangering the pregnancy. Even with adequate tissue available, in the most difficult cases, it may be largely a question of the degree of atypism or altered polarity of the cells that allows the pathologist to make the distinction between benign pregnant epithelium and carcinoma, either in situ or invasive (Fig. 37–4).

What about Carcinoma in Situ in the Pregnant Cervix?

If the biopsy specimen is truly neoplastic and invasion has been ruled out, the physician is faced with only a minor problem in therapy. The real questions are whether the patient has any suggestive point of invasion of the basement membrane in the tissue examined or whether the specimen was taken from the area adjacent to

University, have attempted to replace fictional knowledge with fact. Their findings add information as well as dispel certain preconceived notions.

It is apparent from these studies that the sexual response of women may be divided into four distinct phases: (1) the excitement phase, (2) the plateau phase, (3) the orgasmic phase, and finally (4) the resolution phase.

What Happens during the Excitement Phase?

A woman may enter the excitement phase through a variety of media that stimulate her sexual interest. For the most part the emotional response will be initiated when any one or all of the known erogenous zones such as lips, breast, neck, inner thighs or clitoris are stimulated, either through the act of kissing or through manual manipulation. Sexual desire may also arise, however, as the result of viewing a suggestive movie or reading pornographic literature.

The initial response is often noted in the breasts, which respond to sexual excitement by (a) erection of the nipples, (b) vasocongestion. During this phase the nipple actually increases in length and broadens in base as the elastic and muscular fibers contract. The distended venous channels can be seen beginning on the chest wall and extending over the upper surface of the breast in the direction of, but never quite reaching, the areola, largely because of the rapid emptying of these veins into the deeper main channels. As the result of the venous engorgement, the breasts actually increase in size.

The external genitalia, as well as the vagina, respond to sexual excitation in a variety of ways. One of the first and most immediate indications of mounting sexual excitement is an increase in the amount of vaginal secretory lubrication. In the past the source of the vaginal fluid was attributed to the secretory activity of both Bartholin's gland and the cervix. Secretion of Bartholin's glands, for example, supposedly reduced the vaginal acidity and provided a more favorable environment for sperm survival. Actually, the production of secretion is so minimal that it could hardly influence the acidity to any appreciable extent. It is now also reasonably well established that there is no secretory activity on the part of the glands of a healthy cervix during sexual excitement.

Vaginal lubrication is an important response to rising sexual tension. Although there are no major glands in the vaginal epithelium, Masters observes a "sweating phenomenon" manifested by the appearance within ten to thirty seconds after stimulation of multiple and individual droplets that closely resemble ordinary perspiration, such as one sees on the skin. It is this sweating phenomenon on the part of the entire vaginal epithelium that provides the main lubrication and lowers the vaginal acidity.

The vasocongestive phenomenon is apparent in the external genitalia as sexual tension mounts during the excitement phase. This is most apparent in the clitoris and labia minora. The clitoris nearly doubles in size. The alterations in the color of the labia minora give a fair indication of the degree of sexual stimulation. As venous engorgement increases, the sexual skin changes from a pink to deep wine-red color, and the labia minora likewise double in size.

With continuation of the excitement phase the upper and inner portions of the vagina distend, and the cervix and body of the uterus, if not held down by disease, will retract into the upper pelvis. Thus the upper portion of the vagina tends to increase in both length and laterally.

The excitement phase will vary in length, depending upon the woman and her response to the technique of stimulation. If the reaction is favorable, the excitement phase may be relatively short, or it may abate if the stimulating force is applied forcefully or in a manner which disturbs the patient's psyche.

What Happens in the Plateau Phase?

The normal woman moves easily and readily into the plateau phase if the stimulation is pleasurable and is constantly maintained. The engorgement is generalized in the breasts, perineum and vagina. In the breast this is manifest in two ways: (1) the areolae become engorged so that they tend to engulf the nipple to such an extent that the nipple seems less erect, though it is actually unchanged; and (2) the breast itself increases in size and may be as much as a quarter larger than usual. The extent of response in the breast will depend in part upon the degree of alteration effected by previous pregnancies and lactation.

The outer third of the vagina with its bulbocavernosus muscle also becomes distended with venous blood and undergoes a moderate dilation. As a result of this physical alteration, which is peculiar to the plateau phase, the central portion of the vaginal lumen above it tends to narrow. This explains the gripping sensation experienced by men during intercourse, as the vaginal wall tightens around the shaft of the penis.

The woman is now fully prepared for the orgasmic phase. Vaginal lubrication is at its height, full engorgement has taken place, and the vaginal canal has widened and deepened to full extent. Whether or not the woman actually achieves an orgasm depends on a variety of factors. The length of the plateau phase is never the same for everyone, and is rarely predictable in the same woman. For example, she may progress rapidly into a sudden explosive orgasm or she may never achieve it despite the best efforts of both partners.

What Is an Orgasm?

Attempting to describe the sensations involved in the emotional climax (orgasm) is like trying to describe a headache to a woman who has never had one. A surprising number of women, however, have never had an orgasm and are extremely interested in knowing what it is like, in order that they may experience the sensation. It is a safe assumption that if the patient has had the experience, she will recognize it.

An orgasm usually begins as a tickling or tingling sensation, starting in the region of the clitoris, mounting in intensity until it spreads to both the internal portions of the vagina and the external genitalia. It is sharply localized to the genital area. The sensation is overpowering and uncontrollable, culminating in a sudden burst of ecstasy. Some women faint or burst into tears, while others cry out with expressions of love; some become violent and bite and scratch. These methods of expression are normal and simply reflect a sense of passion strong enough to do away with inhibitions. The degree of emotion varies with the individual partner. The more pronounced reactions should not be regarded as manifestations of an oversexed woman. Such women are highly emotional and passionate by nature, while others are less responsive. The great majority of women will each have a recognizable level of emotional response which is her own. The marriage will be happier if the husband is cognizant of his wife's particular pattern of expression.

In general there are two types of orgasm. (1) By far the largest number of women reach a peak of excitement only after a relatively long period of preliminary love-making, which may last up to fifteen minutes or more. The climactic sensation, however, is not maintained, and the intensity declines promptly. It is possible for such a woman to repeat the orgasm more than once. If the husband is aware of this, he may adjust his coital technique so that his wife derives more pleasure from their sex relations. (2) The woman of highly passionate nature is quick to arouse and reaches the height of her sensation within the first minute or so of the act of intercourse. Instead of subsiding promptly, the emotional pitch is maintained over a prolonged period of time. This sort of woman is capable of continuing intercourse for some time. If the man is concerned only with his own pleasure and is not aware of his wife's emotional pattern, he may leave her entirely unsatisfied.

SIMULTANEOUS CLIMAX.   There is a misconception about the emotional value of a climax which both partners arrive at simultaneously. This is said to be the ultimate in achievement, and many women are concerned because such experiences are foreign to them. There is no question that the excitement of the woman is increased when she can feel at the height of her own pleasure that she is giving happiness to the man she loves. But this is a difficult thing to achieve as a regular pattern. Too frequently the partners are so concerned with the thought that one may arrive at a climax before the other that all spontaneity is lost through the mental effort involved.

The Resolution Phase

If the patient fails to achieve a climax, it becomes a frustrating and trying experience that often may last for hours. Repeated performances of this sort without any relief tend to make a woman constantly unhappy, extremely nervous and thoroughly frustrated. The physiologic preparation, achieved during the excitement phase, subsides slowly and then only when all forms of sexual stimulation have ceased. On the other hand, if the patient does achieve an orgasm, she may go through a rapid resolution phase as sexual tension is released. This is the ultimate goal.

Are All Women Capable of Experiencing a Climax, and Is It Essential to Marital Happiness that They Should?

Although there are wide variations in the degree of sexual anesthesia, the great majority of women are fully capable of reaching a climax during sexual intercourse. In the past it was always assumed that the woman must have an orgasm to be completely happy in her marital existence. Not to do so was to incur the risk of causing a high degree of emotional tension, unrest and dissatisfaction with all the other factors inherent in the marital adjustment. Although this may still be true in individual instances, wider experience now suggests that many women find intercourse to be enjoyable and profitable, despite the fact that they may never have had an orgasm or any sensation comparable to it. After intercourse such a woman may experience a sense of relaxation and satisfaction, with the gradual subsidence of emotional tension. Intercourse then may be meaningful and entirely natural for the couple involved, and the physician should make no attempt to alter the pattern. The wife need not achieve a climax to receive pleasure from intercourse, nor does pleasure have any bearing on whether she can conceive and raise a family.

Some women are truly frigid, and though they love their husbands deeply, they are totally unable to acquire sexual satisfaction. In rare instances there may be anatomic deficiencies, such as insufficient nerve endings in the clitoris or posterior vaginal fornix or possibly some block in the transmission or receipt of nerve impulses in the reflex arc that leads from these areas to the genital reflex center in the spinal cord. More often, however, psychic factors operating at the level of the cerebral cortex inhibit the translation of sexual stimuli into a pleasurable response. Unless there is a true aversion to sex, the marital relation may proceed without disturbing either partner.

WHAT ARE SOME OF THE COMMON FACTORS WHICH APPEAR IN THE WOMAN WITH SEXUAL ANESTHESIA?

In many instances the marital problems, as they concern sex, stem from sheer ignorance or an assimilation of the person's mother's attitude toward sex. If this be the case, much can be accomplished by marital counseling and sex education before marriage takes place. A great majority of the psychosexual problems that become important enough to require the services of a psychiatrist in the years after marriage are actually preventable. If maladjustments exist at the start of the marriage, they will in most instances increase with the passage of the years unless something is done to prevent them. The time to do this is before the marriage occurs.

WHAT CAN THE PHYSICIAN DO BY WAY OF SEX EDUCATION IN PREMARITAL COUNSELING?

Most young girls who consult a physician for premarital advice appear to be primarily interested in preventing pregnancy for "a couple of years at least." The physician will be well advised to tell the prospective bride that no one has yet discovered a convenient time to have a baby.

Whenever possible, the physician should try to determine by careful sympathetic questioning how much the girl actually knows about sexual intercourse. The physician is likely to assume that the modern girl, through school instruction or vicarious premarital experience, is well versed in genital anatomy and physiology and the technique of the sex act. Such an assumption is in error. It may not be possible to pursue this line of questioning at the first visit, but an effort should be made if there is an opportunity to see the girl again before her marriage. Too many girls know too little, and though they have doubts, they are unwilling to express them for fear of being considered ignorant. In most instances the girl will welcome an opportunity to discuss her physical equipment, physiologic facts and a few technical details of the sex act. The physical examination that follows will assure her of the possibilities of her being able to produce a child.

Attitude toward Marriage

In far too many instances the girl's attitude toward marriage has been conditioned by the experience of her mother. This may be favorable or unfavorable. Some mothers will have imbued their daughters with the impression that sex is overrated, disgusting and unpleasant, but it must be tolerated by the young wife as part of her duty. This is particularly true if the girl is a child of a broken marriage or one in which marital maladjustments have been all too obvious. This is hardly the climate for forecasting the achievement of satisfaction from sexual intercourse. The physician can do much to allay the girl's fears and misconceptions if these factors become apparent in the course of his discussion of marital problems.

Fear of Genital Injury and Pain on Rupture of the Hymen

There are many preconceived notions about the pain and discomfort suffered by the girl in her first sexual experience. The fear of genital injury often persists into the adult state and so conditions the wife that she never has a chance to achieve satisfaction from intercourse. The girl is eager to follow the pattern set by her husband, but if his overenthusiastic efforts to be a man of the world offend the girl's modesty and are contrary to her premarital concepts, she may develop a dislike for sexual intimacies which persists.

There is no set pattern that must be followed on the first night of the honeymoon. The process is not a complicated one and should proceed without unpleasant incidents unless the male is abnormally ignorant or the girl overmodest. Both should understand that the initial penetration by the male organ results in stretching of the hymen to the extent that tearing occurs and may be accompanied by pain mixed with pleasure. The girl should be told to expect this, just as she may expect labor to be painful. Actually, she has nothing to dread from the so-called rupture of the hymen, for it need not be a painful experience. Particularly in this day and age when feminine hygiene during menstruation is accomplished by use of the intravaginal tampon, she may have no pain at all. Some pain may be expected, but the girl gradually learns to accept it as a necessary prerequisite to the pleasure she knows will follow.

Hemorrhage and the Resistant Hymen

One of the important parts of the premarital physical examination is the evaluation of the distensibility of the hymen. The gynecologist may recommend manual distention by graduated dilators or excision of the hymen under anesthesia as a premarital step.

Thoughtless application of force to a hymen that does not yield readily to reasonable pressure may produce excruciating pain and frightening blood loss. Such an experience can create sexual frigidity in a woman by adding traumatic support to the idea, which may already have been implanted in her mind by a frigid mother, that intercourse is a sacrifice that must be made to the lust of men. The understanding husband, faced with this situation, will desist from any further advances. It is far better to wait until his bride has recovered from the physical and emotional rigors of the wedding and is more relaxed.

In some instances the vagina may not be anatomically constructed to accept the full male organ during the first attempt at intercourse. If the rupture of a tough hymen has produced hemorrhage, the husband in his next attempt should take care to insert the organ gradually and not try to penetrate the vagina to the fullest extent until it can be done easily. The complaint of disproportion in size between the two organs is often offered by women who have developed a distaste for intercourse, as an excuse to avoid it. Too many cases of sexual frigidity date from a painful honeymoon experience springing from overenthusiastic attempts of an immature husband to prove his masculinity.

False Modesty

Based largely on childhood impressions and an immature knowledge of sexual problems, false modesty possesses many husbands and wives to a greater or lesser degree. Women have it more than men, and it is a common cause of marital unhappiness. When carried too far, it can defeat the whole purpose of achieving the ultimate in sexual satisfaction because it prevents the wife from abandoning herself to her natural emotions. For example, the young wife is apt to develop a pattern of behavior during intercourse based upon what she has been taught by her husband, to whom she looked for instruction. He may be entirely satisfied with her response. As she becomes more familiar with intercourse she may experience sensations that are more powerful than anything she has felt before. Because of her modesty she feels that she is wrong in having such feelings, but the conventional sex habits they have previously developed no longer completely satisfy her. She is reluctant to make any passionate advances for fear of shocking her husband, but she expects him to be aware of her heightened desire and to respond in kind. If he is not alert to her increasing passion and does nothing to satisfy her, because he is too preoccupied with his own pleasure, she becomes resentful and begins to lose her interest in intercourse. Her responses become more and more passive and unenthusiastic.

Her husband may be entirely unaware of this and believe his wife to be happy with their habitual pattern of intercourse. If he continues to be ignorant and never makes any effort to take the initiative, she had best forget her maidenly modesty and the fear that she may shock him and tell him of her unsatisfied desires. Not infrequently she will find that he too may have had similar ideas, but has been afraid to make them known to her. Variety in the sex act will add vitally to their marital happiness. Both should be assured that the desires they wish to express and their thoughts about satisfying them are entirely normal and in keeping with the common experience of other couples throughout the world.

Coital Technique

The girl approaching marriage should be told what anatomic areas produce the stimuli responsible for the orgasm. The woman differs from the man in that pleasurable genital stimuli are derived from two areas, the clitoris and the vagina, while the man has only the penis. It is also true that a woman is slower to arouse to the point at which she is ready for intercourse. A woman yearns to be loved and possessed, but she is resentful of being used simply as an instrument of man's pleasure, and in many instances she may appear to care as much for the preliminary love making leading up to intercourse as she does for the act itself. It is normal and natural for her to want to be prepared for intercourse by caresses and genital stimulation.

The Role of the Male

Much of the marital unhappiness traceable to the wife's relative indifference to intercourse can be attributed to ignorance on the part of the man. The husband should know which of the erogenous areas that she has seems to bring out the greatest emotional response. By experience he will learn to vary his attention from one area to another and to discover which of the many combinations seems to give his wife the greatest pleasure. He will come to recognize when his wife has been adequately prepared for intercourse by the nature of her response and the increase in the amount of vaginal secretion. If the husband does not attempt by romantic advances and preliminary love play to put his wife in a more receptive attitude, she may gradually develop disinterest in and distaste for intercourse.

Normal women, even when they are very passionate, can usually be satisfied by a single relationship when it is properly performed. After complete satisfaction she is not concerned with the urge to repeat the intimacies at too frequent intervals. Actually, after the honeymoon is over so many other factors appear in the routine of daily living that intercourse two or three times a week may be considered normal.

If the man is not sufficiently well versed in these basic facts, the gynecologist can do much to prevent future marital unhappiness by instruction during their premarital consultation. At that time it will also be advisable to inform the prospective husband about the bride's virginity. So many races and religious sects place such importance on the intact hymen as evidence of chastity that it is important that no false impressions should arise from inadequate evidence. If the husband finds that his wife experiences no pain or does not bleed with the first attempt at intercourse, he may not believe in her virginity despite her assurances. This can affect their subsequent marital happiness. Actually, the hymen varies in the ease with which it may be distended. If the wife has had previous sexual experience, she can readily deceive her husband by simulating pain. There are also many ways in which a hymen can be stretched, short of intercourse. The husband, therefore, before he becomes emotionally disturbed about his wife's virginity, should remember that chastity is concerned with thought as well as deed. Even the girl with an intact hymen may have experienced a wide variety of intimacies without submitting to the final act of penile penetration. If so, she can hardly be considered chaste in her attitude.

The Role of the Modern Gynecologist in Marital Counseling

In the past the gynecologist or other physician underestimated the value of his counsel when young women consulted him for marital advice. Being uncertain as to the direction such consultations should take and ill informed as to psychosexual details, the physician was prone to gloss over the problems in a manner which could only increase the patient's fears and apprehensions. Premarital counseling has largely taken the form of a few casual philosophical observations coupled with a general physical examination. The physician allots little time to permit a discussion of the fundamental questions about and attitudes toward the sexual act.

In the present age when the young girl has been exposed to much free interchange of information, supported in part by school instruction, the physician can hardly afford to be ill informed and to cut the interview short because he does not know how to conduct it.

Much can be accomplished through a sympathetic understanding and the review of simple facts. Some problems will be difficult or impossible to solve, but this should not deter the gynecologist from discussing these problems. With a little experience he can soon discover whether he should continue with the discussion or refer the patient to some other physician more competent to deal with the problem than he is.

Attitude of the Physician in Marital Counseling

Whether or not the discussion of maladjustments after marriage will be successful depends in a large part on the attitude of the physician during the interview. The most important requisite is that of a sympathetic listener. The majority of problems have no great depth and can readily be resolved by the simple process of listening and questioning until the patient eventually comes to understand the problem herself. To help the patient to see what is wrong, the gynecologist must be sympathetic but determined in his attitude. He must convince the patient of his profound interest in her problem without becoming too closely allied to it. It is easy to become over-sympathetic to the wife's recounting of her difficulties, particularly if the position of the husband is unknown. As a practical measure it is far better to take the side of the undeclared partner in order that the wife recognize her own defects. She will be anxious to have her physician believe that her husband is totally at fault, as well he may be, but in general both parties are culpable. A sympathetic attitude should not be construed as meaning total agreement with the patient's statement of the situation, whether real or fanciful.

WHAT ARE SOME OF THE FACTORS THAT CONTRIBUTE TO MARITAL UNHAPPINESS?

It has been said that the attitude of the partners toward sex is the basic cause of marital unhappiness. Add to this ignorance of the technique of intercourse, and most of the problems that are amenable to correction can be placed in one category or the other. The remainder have deep-seated psychiatric implications which are beyond the scope of the gynecologist.

Immaturity

One of the common explanations of marital maladjustment springs from the immaturity of one or both partners.

The wife may become increasingly perturbed because her husband seems incapable of accepting the responsibilities that go with being either a husband or parent. Though he receives physical relief and enjoyment from intercourse, he seems totally oblivious of the fact that he should contribute to his wife's happiness. She, therefore, tends to respond to his advances with increasing disinterest. This is likely to send the husband in search of pleasure elsewhere, particularly if it carries no obligation with it. If the couple has a child, he may become jealous of her attention to the infant and her seeming indifference to his needs. His grievance may or may not be real, but he often reacts by paying little or no attention to the child or to his wife's problems in trying to rear it. She usually fails to understand and reacts to his sexual demands with a minimal response.

The wife can also be immature in her acceptance of the responsibilities of marriage. She may cling to the thought of her carefree days when she was belle of the ball. Frequently she is too insistent in her demands for her husband's attention and inordinately jealous of his attention to other women, no matter how innocent. A vicious circle develops when the husband rebels.

The wife's immaturity may also appear in another guise with regard to child-birth. If she is reluctant to ruin her figure or share the complete domination of her husband with the child, she may remain entirely passive during intercourse, under the mistaken impression that if she does not become emotional she will not have a child.

The Urge to Reproduce and the Fear of Pregnancy

Both the urge to reproduce and the fear of pregnancy contribute to psychosexual maladjustment in marriage.

The primary aims in intercourse are (*a*) reproduction and (*b*) satisfaction. The man combines both factors in a single act. He receives his pleasure, feels physically relieved because of the semen discharged and fulfills his duty to posterity all at the same time. The woman discharges nothing and serves the species only after nine months have passed. Her sexual urge comes from her desire to be loved, and her basic instinct is to reproduce.

This has a direct bearing on achieving an orgasm. Many women apparently cannot have an orgasm without conscious or unconscious ideas about childbirth. If this thought is constantly present in the woman's mind, and another child is not wanted, this alone may be enough to prevent her from reaching a climax. On the other hand, the intense desire to have a child may be enough to prevent an orgasm. It is still possible for her to have a child, but the pleasurable elements in the union are lost in the intensity of the urge to reproduce. Occasionally one finds a woman who derives pleasure from intercourse and has a satisfactory orgasm, yet intercourse is followed by fits of depression. The emotional response may be violent during the act, perhaps because of the intensity of her desire to have a child. When she does have one, the relation becomes calmer and more normal.

Environmental Factors

There can be little doubt that the ordinary mechanics of living profoundly influence the woman's response to intercourse. If she is worn out by her household duties or the responsibilities involved in trying to be mistress of the home and carrying on a regular job at the same time, she is apt to have less enthusiasm for intercourse. This is particularly true if she does not receive as much pleasure as she would like, and it will not be long before she thinks that intercourse is highly overrated. Economic pressures and financial embarrassment precipitate worries that defeat the achievement of a relaxed mood conducive to successful coitus. In too many couples the fear of having a child that will wreck their economic status approaches the panic stage. This is hardly the atmosphere for acquiring complete sexual satisfaction.

Poor health on the part of either one may contribute to the problem, particularly when it is combined with fatigue.

The actual living conditions may play a role, especially among the newly married or those in straitened financial circumstances. Early in marriage the couple may be forced to live with one or the other's parents or in such crowded quarters that they are afraid to express themselves naturally. If a young child has to share the parent's bedroom, its presence may be enough to interfere with complete abandon in intercourse.

Some Psychologic Factors

Some of the frigidity is purely malicious. The desire to deprive the husband of pleasure because of the wish to get even with him is one manifestation. This is a simple question of maladjustment capable of correction, but other psychologic factors are far more deep-seated.

The more vicious form stems from faulty education in matters pertaining to sex. A puritanical background or mother's instructions may have implanted the thought in a woman's mind that intercourse is a sacrifice she must make. Since intercourse is not so painful as it is revolting, she makes no effort to respond. The home situation becomes complicated, and marital unhappiness is inevitable.

The reverse of this situation occurs in what is called benevolent frigidity. In this instance the woman is overcome with her motherly attitude toward her husband. She becomes too tender and is so occupied with pleasing him that she fails to derive any pleasure herself. The fact that she will afford him more satisfaction if she too obtains pleasure is lost in the intensity of her passive response.

The aggressive woman, on the other hand, who wishes to overpower her husband and to dominate him even in the act of intercourse will attempt to pursue her own rhythm, independent of her husband. Intercourse becomes a contest to see which of the two can achieve a climax first, or who can keep it up the longest. There are some homosexual attributes here that may so frighten the husband that he can no longer satisfy his wife.

The problems of sexual adjustment in the postmarital period are many and varied. Many will take origin from personality problems inherent in one or both partners, and the marital maladjustment simply reflects this long-standing personality defect. The gynecologist will rapidly become aware of the fact that the problems involved fall in the province of a psychiatric approach rather than simple reassurance and instruction.

WHY DO SOME WOMEN DEVELOP AN AVERSION TO SEXUAL INTIMACY?

We have noted previously that ignorance of technical details of the sex act is as much responsible for sexual maladjustment as the attitude toward sex.

If most women are capable of responding emotionally, why do some women begin to show reluctance in consummating sexual union? If the couple is otherwise compatible and still in love, the fault must lie in intercourse itself. It must be true that one of several things is happening: (1) coitus is painful; (2) the wife is not experiencing any pleasure from the act or is incompletely satisfied; (3) she is motivated by some premarital concept which controls her actions to a greater degree than she realizes; (4) she has developed a marital attitude which prevents a normal expression of her feelings.

In most instances the husband will not recognize the fact that intercourse has become distasteful to his wife, for she will rarely raise the issue for fear of hurting his feelings. She will complain bitterly about his conduct about the house, his disposition, the clothes he wears, his habit of reading when she wants to talk, but she will never tell him that he fails to satisfy her sexual needs.

It is at this point that the patient consults her gynecologist for some vague pelvic complaint totally unrelated to her underlying difficulty. Under careful questioning the patient may then admit that she is troubled by the fact that sexual intercourse is no longer satisfactory. Under sympathetic probing she may suggest that her husband does not spend enough time in preliminary love making and is far too concerned with his own pleasures, giving little thought to her needs. She may complain that he wants her to indulge in intercourse too frequently. Perhaps she feels that their intimacies tend to follow a monotonous, deadly routine of sameness in everything connected with sexual intercourse. She may wish to vary the pattern of coitus that is always performed in the same old manner, in the same bed and at the same time. These factors disturb her, but she is unwilling to discuss them with her husband and turns to the gynecologist for help. Unfortunately she does not make his role any easier by her reluctance to reveal the true nature of her concern.

There may be other factors that disturb her psyche and prevent her from deriving pleasure from their intimacy. She may, for example, resent her husband's spending so much of his energy on his work or recreation. She may feel that he does not pay enough attention to the children and does not help her in trying to solve their problems. Certain sexual practices that he regards as normal may offend her modesty and add a sordid note to their relations. Unless the patient has complete confidence in her husband, it will avail him little to assure his wife that certain forms of sexual indulgence are perfectly proper and normal. If these suggestions are contrary to her preconceived notions, she may regard his desires as peculiar to him and tailored to suit his own pleasure. It takes time and patience to overcome a mental block of this sort, however childish and unrealistic it may be.

The best means of accomplishing this is a simple discussion of the problem, carried out in a casual, matter-of-fact attitude unencumbered by any element of self-consciousness. Obviously the two people best qualified to conduct such a conversation are the two people most involved, the husband and his wife, but in the great majority of cases a third person is needed. Since there is no one else to turn to, the person who is the next court of appeal is the gynecologist.

How Does the Physician Cope with the Problem?

Since the patient rarely offers information spontaneously, the physician (*a*) stumbles on her problem in the course of his attempts to discover the cause of her gynecologic complaints, (*b*) has a high index of suspicion that the gynecologic complaints are not the real cause for her visit, or (*c*) brings out the information as a result of gentle, sympathetic questioning.

To evaluate the situation properly it is important to obtain a complete history. To do this the physician must be prepared to devote a considerable amount of time and thought to his questioning. If he suspects the nature of the patient's difficulty, he will be wise if he schedules the patient for a visit at the end of his list of office appointments, so that he can devote all the time necessary.

When the gynecologist has the full confidence of the patient, he will have a more comprehensive insight into the cause of her marital unhappiness. Information must be gathered on many intimate details, touching on both her premarital and present experiences. For example, it is well known that from the time of puberty the actual center for sex sensation is localized in the area of the clitoris until she has had her first sexual experience involving penetration into the vagina. In the normal course of events the center for pleasurable impulses passes from the clitoris to the vagina. In many instances the transference of sensation from the clitoris to the vagina is completed only in part and frequently not at all. It is perhaps the main reason why some women obtain more satisfaction from preliminary love play than from the actual act of intercourse. This is the reason why the gynecologist should try to elicit information about such things as sex play in childhood, masturbation or petting experiences of varying degrees of intensity. If there has been much manual stimulation of the clitoris, it may be reluctant to abandon control, or the vagina may be unwilling to accept the combined role of arbiter of sensation and vehicle for reproduction. With this information at his disposal the gynecologist can then advise the husband to concentrate his preliminary caresses on this erogenous zone.

The gynecologist should also seek out all possible material on premarital sex experience, which may or may not have been happy and may even have been traumatic. These events may provide the background for her present attitude toward sex, particularly if she has come to have guilt feelings or has gained the impression that all sex life is simply an outrageous indignity. The gynecologist, through intelligent listening and simple advice, should be able to reassure the patient that her past experience is far less abnormal or degrading than she has come to believe. It is the physician's job to correct the patient's attitude toward sex, particularly when he sees that it has taken an unhealthy turn.

The information bearing on the marital experience should concentrate on such personal matters as her feeling toward her husband, her evaluation of him as a lover, his coital technique, the possibility of a love interest outside the family, her own attitude toward sex and its relation to her early upbringing, the attitude of her family toward sex matters, her relation to her mother and her father, and her present home environment and economic status.

It is in the field of reassurance and education that the physician can do the most good. By a sympathetic explanation it is frequently possible to re-educate the wife and bring about a more open and intelligent outlook toward her sex life. The mere reassurance that her desires have been normal for countless women through the ages and are not products of her own disordered emotions may accomplish a great deal. Both the patient and the gynecologist should have in mind that there is no quick cure to her problem, but with time and conversation the patient will gradually recognize that perhaps she bears some portion of blame for the disordered state of her marriage, and that it is not all her husband's fault, as she would like to have the physician believe. The chances of success are greater if the wife can be made to see that she is a main source of the difficulty.

As far as possible the interview should be carried on with the wife alone. If, however, the husband appears to be ignorant or inadequate in his love making, much can be accomplished by consultation with the husband alone. He may not be aware that his wife cares more for the preliminaries leading up to intercourse than she does for the act itself. It may be wise to suggest as part of the love play that gentle stimulation of the clitoris is important in preparing his wife for intercourse, particularly if such a suggestion has appeared in the gynecologist's interview with the wife. His resentment at his wife's lack of response may be resolved if his own inadequacies are made known to him. If the questioning suggests that he is impotent or the wife so dominant that overtones of homosexuality appear, psychiatric help is needed.

WHAT ABOUT THE USE OF DRUGS? From time immemorial various drugs have been used to stimulate erotic excitement in women. *Cannabis indica* (Spanish fly) is one undesirable example. Either ingested or applied to the clitoris, it sets up an intense local irritation which supposedly increases the woman's desire for relief through sexual intercourse. Alcohol has been used to relax women's inhibitions for centuries.

In more recent years the male sex hormone has been used because of the stimulating effect it seems to have upon the clitoris. Some women are more affected than others, but in all the effect is only temporary. In general it may be said that there is little excuse for the common practice of giving hormones for relief in the problem of frigidity. It is far better in the long run to reorient and re-educate the patient than to resort to any form of drug therapy, whether it be alcohol or testosterone.

DYSPAREUNIA

When sexual intercourse becomes painful or difficult to accomplish, the patient has dyspareunia. Primarily she is concerned with the pain, but in many instances the problem becomes complicated by other elements such as total lack of desire or failure to achieve any satisfaction from the act.

In What Forms Does Dyspareunia Manifest Itself?

Dyspareunia appears in various forms. It makes some difference when in the woman's marital life the symptoms first appear. Without previous experience dyspareunia in the early stages of marriage is usually due to some mechanical obstruction, which makes insertion of the penis difficult. The patient desires intercourse and wants intensely to consummate the marriage, but the acute pain denies intromission. With persistent efforts to carry out the act the problems are compounded by protective spasms which appear as a defense mechanism. Pain in the presence of a real obstruction from an imperforate or abnormally fibrous and resistant hymen or atresia of the lower portion of the vagina is so acute that coitus is often impossible. Rarely is the difficulty due to disproportion in the size of the organs. Not infrequently both partners by mutual consent or discouragement abandon all attempts to have normal intercourse and resort to coitus without vaginal penetration. Most patients consult the physician early in their marital careers, but in some instances this situation continues for years. We are aware of one patient who finally became pregnant seventeen years after a marriage that had not previously been consummated. In discussions of sterility problems it is not uncommon to find that the act of intercourse has never been carried out successfully.

VAGINISMUS EARLY IN MARRIAGE. In more complex situations no mechanical obstruction can be detected. Neurotic women, poorly adjusted to the process of normal living, are often emotionally unprepared for the act of coitus. The problem is more complicated when normal desire is present, but anxiety and fear of genital injury deny penetration. This fear may spring from earlier experiences in childhood or from an overemotional response to the advice of parents or friends who talk of the painful rupture of the hymen and the bleeding that follows. To the highly neurotic woman this may be enough to associate the sex act with a profound fear and dread.

The response to this marital complex is a spasm of the sphincter vaginae and superficial perineal muscles. This is called *vaginismus*. The mental element is evident before any contact is made. The physician is aware of this when he attempts to examine such a patient. The legs are separated with great difficulty and much persuasion. Digital contact with the external genitalia is followed by an immediate protective response on the part of the patient. The back arches, the buttocks rise from the examining table, and the patient pulls back as the thighs clamp together. To examine such a patient adequately an anesthetic will be necessary. Some form of authoritative reassurance, hypnotic suggestion or psychiatric help may be necessary before the marital act can be accomplished.

VAGINISMUS LATER IN MARRIAGE.   The patient who suffers dyspareunia years after successful marital relations presents a different problem. The same difficulty in penile insertion may be noted, but no medical reason can be found to explain it Again the sphincteric muscles of the vagina go into spasm and deny admission of the male organ. The phenomenon may be sporadic and probably reflects the emotional response of the woman at the time. This is particularly true in high-strung, neurotic women who are maladjusted to the process of living. It may also appear in women who for one reason or another have "tired" of their husbands.

Bizarre forms of vaginismus have been recorded in the literature. In well documented cases such severe spasm of the vaginal muscles has set in during the act of intercourse that the penis cannot be withdrawn. Anesthesia may be required to free the male organ.

PAIN ON DEEP PENETRATION.   Dyspareunia is not restricted to penetration of the vaginal outlet. In most instances a dull aching pain occurs high up in the vagina during the act and persists for hours after intercourse has been completed. Frequently examination will reveal an adequate cause. The patient may have an old episiotomy scar, the uterus may be in retroversion, the uterosacral ligaments are often tense and tender, evidence of pelvic infection—either acute or chronic—may be present, or an ovary can sometimes be felt prolapsed into the vaginal vault.

How Do You Treat Dyspareunia?

The patient who presents visible and palpable evidence of organic cause for the painful intercourse can usually be treated with every prospect of permanent relief. When there is no obvious reason, or the patient will not permit examination, the problem is more complex.

A tender episiotomy scar, fissure or urethral caruncle can and should be excised. Chronic urethritis or chronic inflammation in Skene's glands should be treated by dilation of the urethra or local destruction of the glands by cautery.

The rigid hymen can either be excised or gradually dilated. The latter method is preferred. It is our practice to teach the patient to use the rectal dilators herself. The abdominal muscles normally are opposed to the action of the sphincter muscles of the vagina. The patient is instructed to strain down with the abdominal muscles as she gently inserts one of the dilators, which are graduated in size, into the vaginal outlet. Straining of the abdominal muscles allows the vaginal muscles to relax.

This procedure has many advantages over excision. The patient realizes that it is possible to insert the dilator by pressing down on the posterior vaginal vault without producing any great pain. It convinces her that there is no anatomic obstruction or reason why intercourse cannot be accomplished. She also now has proof that there is no disproportion in size between the two sexual organs. Finally it shows the patient the direction of the vaginal canal so that she can assist her untrained husband in properly placing the penis.

Any obvious intravaginal or intra-abdominal cause may be treated according to the degree of disease or the severity of dyspareunia. In some instances it may be necessary to resort to surgical exploration and excision or suspension of an offending organ. If the uterus can be replaced in normal position, it may be held there between times by a pessary inserted in the vagina. In rare instances a surgical incision may be indicated that will divide the sphincter muscles of the vagina on one or both sides. The dilation thus obtained is maintained by the use of vaginal dilators for several weeks after the operation.

Much can often be accomplished by joint conversation with husband and wife about the technique of intercourse and the preliminary acts leading up to the actual act. Reassurance is frequently all that is needed for success. When the problem is more deep-seated, it may be necessary to seek intensive psychiatric therapy.

REFERENCES

Response of Female Partner

Ford, C. S., and Beach, F. A.: *Patterns of Sexual Behavior*. New York, Paul B. Hoeber, Inc., 1951.
Keiser, S.: Psychopathology of Orgasm. *Psychoanalyt. Quart.*, 16: 378, 1947.
Masters, W. H.: The Sexual Response Cycle of the Human Female. Vaginal Lubrication. *Ann. New York Acad. Sc.*, 83: 301, 1959.
Idem: The Sexual Response Cycle of the Human Female. I. Gross Anatomic Considerations. *West. J. Surg., Obst. & Gynec.*, 68: 57, 1960.
Masters, W. H., and Johnson, V. E.: The Human Female: Anatomy of Sexual Response. *Minnesota Med.*, 43: 31, 1960.

Marital Counseling

Abramson, M., and Martin, R. R.: Education for Marriage and Parenthood. *Obst. & Gynec.*, 9: 243, 1957.
Brill, N. Q.: Emotional Problems of Marriage. *Postgrad. Med.*, 28: 573, 1960.
Deutsch, H.: Psychiatric Component in Gynecology; in J. V. Meigs and S. H. Sturgis, eds.: *Progress in Gynecology*. New York, Grune & Stratton, Inc., 1946, Vol. 1, p. 152.
Griffith, E. F.,: Medical Aspects of Marriage Guidance. *Lancet*, 1: 165, 1947.
Johnson, C. A.: The Pre-marital Lecture. *South Dakota J. Med. & Pharm.*, 12: 91, 1959.
McCormick, C. O.: A Young Woman Seeks Premarriage Counsel. *Obst. & Gynec.*, 4: 355, 1954.
McCready, R. B.: Premarital Counseling: A Multidimensional Approach. *Obst. & Gynec.*, 13: 420, 1959.

Sexual Adjustment

Silverman, A. J.: Psychiatric Aspects of Sexual Disturbances. *Am. J.M. Sc.*, 224: 103, 1952.
Sinclair, D. A.: Marriage and Its Sexual Problems. *Urol. & Cutan. Rev.*, 42: 378, 1938.
Wortis, S. B.: Unsuccessful Sex Adjustment in Marriage. *Am. J. Psychiat.*, 96: 1413, 1940.

Frigidity

Burdine, W. E., Shipley, T. E., and Papas, A. T.: Delatestryl, a Long Acting Androgenic Hormone; Its Use as an Adjunct in the Treatment of Women with Sexual Frigidity. *Fertil. & Steril.*, 8: 255, 1957.
Heiman, M.: Reproduction: Emotions and the Hypothalamic-Pituitary Function. *Fertil. & S.eril.*, 10: 162, 1959.
Hitschmann, E., and Bergler, E.: *Frigidity in Women: Its Characteristics and Treatment*. Washington, D. C., Nervous and Mental Disease Publishing Company, 1936.
Kroger, W. S., and Freed, S. C.: Psychosomatic Aspects of Frigidity. *J.A.M.A.*, 143: 526, 1950.
Rutherford, R. N., Banks, A. L., Davidson, S. H., Coburn, W. A., and Williams, J.: Frigidity in Women, with Special Reference to Postpartum Frigidity; Some Clinical Observations and Study Programs. *Postgrad. Med.*, 26: 76, 1959.

Dyspareunia

Agnew, A. M.: Surgery in the Alleviation of Dyspareunia. *Brit. M.J.*, 1: 1510, 1959.

Bourne, A.: Discussion on Psychosomatic Gynaecology. *J. Obst. & Gynaec. Brit. Emp.*, 66: 769, 1959.

Dannreuther, W. T.: Vaginal Dyspareunia. *Am. J. Obst. & Gynec.*, 74: 747, 1957.

Frank, R. T.: Dyspareunia: A Problem for the General Practitioner. *J.A.M.A.*, 136: 361, 1948.

Novak, J.: Nature and Treatment of Vaginismus. *Urol. & Cutan. Rev.*, 52: 128, 1948.

Chapter 39

Premenstrual Tension

and Secondary Dysmenorrhea

A WIDE spectrum of symptoms of a general nature regularly manifest themselves to many women in the period immediately preceding the menstrual period. It is not easy to define the syndrome of premenstrual tension, nor to assess accurately its frequency, for the symptoms are many and varied, and women respond differently to the same stimuli. The problems involved in a discussion of the vague syndrome of premenstrual tension are closely allied to those observed in essential dysmenorrhea including the psychogenic component. It is this merging of symptoms that makes the treatment of dysmenorrhea so difficult.

One might expect women to feel better at this time, for all metabolic processes have been stimulated rhythmically in anticipation of pregnancy. Whether or not the symptoms appear because pregnancy does not take place is highly conjectural, but the fact of the matter is that many women complain during the ten-day span preceding menstruation of emotional instability, irritability, lack of concentration, insomnia, headache, painful breasts, abdominal distention, bearing-down pelvic discomfort, nausea, anorexia, constipation, urinary frequency and general weakness. Many have an acquired or secondary dysmenorrhea. In some patients these symptoms are present without palpable pelvic abnormalities, while others do have fibroids, endometriosis, pelvic relaxation or ovarian cysts, but are untroubled except during the ten days before the menstrual period.

PREMENSTRUAL TENSION

How Common Is Premenstrual Tension?

The response of the individual woman to these rhythmic changes varies widely and is in part dependent on her emotional adjustments. In some patients the symptoms are mild, while in others they are severe enough to produce serious problems both in the home and at work. The housewife is disturbed by little events in her home life that are not present only during this time, but now result in emotional outbursts without cause, constant nagging of the husband or screaming at the children. She is unable to explain to herself why she does it, but she cannot seem to stop it. She wonders whether mental illness is developing. This adds to her depression and general sense of malbeing. The office worker becomes inefficient, irritable and hard to get along with Extreme instances of emotional instability are evident from crime statistics. These indicate that 80 per cent of major crimes committed by women occur in the premenstrual phase of the cycle.

In all probability all women experience discomfort to a greater or lesser degree during this period, but in only about 60 per cent does it become evident to themselves or others. Women in general seem to expect to feel poorly and are far less ready to make an issue of symptoms that would send a man running to a physician.

In What Stage of a Woman's Life Do the Symptoms Appear, and How Long Do They Persist?

Although it is theoretically possible for premenstrual tension to appear any time after the first menstrual period, more women become noticeably plagued by the syndrome in the twenty- to thirty-year age group. It seems to have little relation to fertility and childbirth. Though there is some accentuation in the girl who is frustrated by her inability to marry or to conceive, tension is also noted in the patient who has had several children and fears further additions to the family.

No one knows exactly how long the symptoms persist. A recent study carried out in patients with symptoms severe enough to require treatment suggests that the span may be prolonged. Over 40 per cent had had symptoms of premenstrual tension from 1 to 5 years, while over 10 per cent had been severely troubled for 15 to 20 years.

What Are the Symptoms of Premenstrual Tension?

The symptoms of the oncoming period, called molimina, are usually a sense of fatigue, headache, irritability, inability to concentrate, and bearing-down discomfort in the pelvic area. Varying degrees of one or several combinations of these symptoms are common occurrences in the lives of many women.

Exaggeration in severity is often associated with an element of mental tension that begins about ten days before the period and gradually increases as the period approaches, reaching a climax with the onset of menses and gradually disappearing. In severe cases the woman literally becomes a witch against her will (Fig. 39–1). She actually undergoes a personality change far removed from her normal behavior pattern. Petty annoyances bring forth emotional outbursts out of proportion to the magnitude of the irritation. The husband and the children are amazed at the violence of the response, which is usually followed by seemingly uncontrolled weeping spells. These may occur without any cause at all. The patient is apprehensive and frightened by the possibility that she is headed for a nervous breakdown.

Headache, which frequently mimics migraine, is probably the most frequent complaint. Unlike true migraine, there is no constancy in the location pattern. It may appear as a unilateral headache, but frequently occurs on both sides and may be temporal or occipital. Commonly nausea and often vomiting accompany the headache, which begins several days before the period and reaches a climax with the onset of menstrual flow. During this time the headaches may be constant or come and go, seemingly without cause. It is possible that the patient may be allergic to her own hormones and that the headaches are actually a "menstrual migraine," or that it represents intermittent intracranial edema.

The most dramatic manifestation of the mounting premenstrual tension is the *emotional instability* of the patient during this phase of the cycle. Two extremes are present. In some, crying spells and violent bursts of temper make up the pattern, while others are lethargic, listless and depressed and show little desire to do anything. The profound personality change in the woman who has severe premenstrual tension suggests a possible psychogenic cause. Certainly there is a psychogenic component in the syndrome, just as there is in dysmenorrhea, but again it is difficult to tell which is the cart and which the horse. Thorough psychiatric study of this syndrome ascribes a primary psychogenic background to less than 10 per cent. Emotional unrest is present in a sufficient number of cases and in sufficient degree to raise a question in court trials for criminal acts committed during this time as to the mental competence.

Generalized *edema* is noted in a number of different regions, especially the breasts and the abdomen. The breasts are often full and very tender along the lateral borders, as are the nipples. Abdominal distention or "bloating" is common. The patient is aware of it, for her clothes become too tight during this period. Along with the abdominal distention come nausea, vomiting, and disturbances in bowel habit. Occasionally there are abdominal cramps. During the earlier phases constipation is the rule, but this changes to frequent watery movements as the process starts to clear up

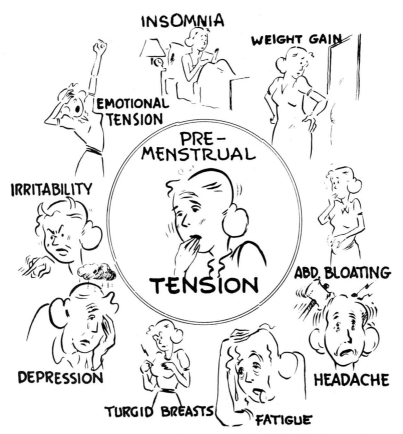

Fig. 39-1.   The aspects of premenstrual tension also include difficulties in mental concentration and pelvic discomfort. (Courtesy of Erle Henriksen.)

and body fluid is lost. For the same reason urinary frequency is noted toward the end of the ten premenstrual days. Storage of fluid within the tissues is noted in other areas. It can be seen in puffiness of the eyes and pitting edema of the hands and feet, and is the probable cause of the pelvic discomfort and bearing-down backache. Newspictures of some popular cinema actresses show the variable facial edema. Both generalized and pulmonary edema has been reported. Pulmonary edema can become a problem in a patient with congestive heart failure.

This tendency to store fluid is evident in the charting of the patient's weight during the premenstrual phase. Normally the patient gains from 2 to 3 pounds just before the period, only to lose it with the onset of menstruation. Patients with severe premenstrual tension may gain as much as 10 or 12 pounds. There appears to be a definite relation between the amount of weight gained and the severity of the symptoms. Little disturbance occurs in menstrual regularity. The majority of patients menstruate normally; approximately 20 per cent have foreshortened intervals consistent with anovulatory cycles and progestational deficiency.

Several interesting factors are noted in association with some but not all patients who have severe premenstrual tension. Excessive nasal discharge (rhinorrhea) is a source of annoyance in some instances during the premenstrual phase. On occasion the patient with premenstrual tension has troublesome areas of ulceration in the buccal mucosa and floor of the mouth (ulcerative stomatitis) which defy treatment. The occasional abnormal craving for sweets, and increased thirst and appetite are perhaps traceable to the hypoglycemia that some patients have at this time.

The symptoms outlined are not necessarily present in every patient who suffers from premenstrual tension, even in extremely severe cases, but varying combinations with different degrees of severity are usually found.

Why Do Patients Have Premenstrual Tension?

The actual cause of premenstrual tension has not been established. Some part of the explanation rests with the well documented observation that during the premenstrual phase of the cycle sodium, chloride and water are retained, to be excreted with the onset of menstruation. Whether storage and release of fluid are brought about by hormonal activity on the part of the adrenal gland and ovary or the altered production of antidiuretic hormone by the posterior pituitary is debatable. The theories as to cause are many.

EXCESSIVE ESTRIN SECRETION.   It has been suggested that these patients have a high estrin level in the blood, because of an inexplicably elevated renal threshold for estrin. Most investigators will subscribe to the relation of increased amounts of estrin as one factor in intercellular fluid storage, but not all will agree that the increase is due to a kidney threshold. Some authorities point out that the excess of estrin may be due to its faulty metabolism and utilization, which may be traced to deficient corpus luteal function. Endometrial biopsy studies in patients with severe premenstrual tension show a notable lack of progestin activity. Others have attributed the lack of estrin utilization and resultant high blood levels to a faulty metabolism of estrin in the liver, as a result of vitamin B deficiency. The vitamin B deficiency may be due to its inefficient absorption from the intestinal tract.

RETENTION OF SODIUM.   In all probability the retention of salt and water in the tissues is caused by estrin rather than progestin. The fluid is stored in the extracellular spaces and may be minimal or appear in large quantity. The neurologic symptoms, such as emotional instability, irritability and headache, are due to fluid retention within the brain. Fluid stored within the tissues of the intestinal tract explains the abdominal cramps, nausea and distention. Whether the edema is evident or not will depend on its magnitude.

OVERACTIVITY OF POSTERIOR PITUITARY.   Headache, edema and hypertension are often noted in toxemia of pregnancy. It is interesting that a high percentage of patients with toxemia have an antecedent history of premenstrual tension. This combination of symptoms has often been attributed to an overactive posterior pituitary lobe, producing an excess of antidiuretic hormone. This theory has not received general acceptance, for it is not clear whether the primary disturbance is in the kidney or liver, or whether the increased amount of antidiuretic hormone in the blood is due to increased production by the posterior pituitary or simply to a diminished rate of its destruction.

ALLERGY.   There is some suggestion that certain patients may be sensitive to their own hormones, particularly progestin. We know that many patients who have premenstrual tension also have various forms of dermatitis, asthma and hay fever. It is possible, then, that some such allergic phenomenon may operate with regard to progestin. An intradermal sensitivity test has been devised to detect such cases.

PSYCHOGENIC FACTORS.   As noted in dysmenorrhea, there is a large psychogenic component, but rarely is it possible to point to psychiatric cause as the sole trigger mechanism. It is true that highly emotional, tense women are more prone to store fluid and chloride and to suffer premenstrual tension.

Treatment of Premenstrual Tension

Based on the theory that storage of excessive sodium, chloride and water in the extracellular spaces of the body is the main basis of the symptoms, regardless of the activating cause, the accepted therapy calls for (*a*) the restriction of all factors known to produce water retention, and (*b*) the use of drugs to promote fluid elimination.

DEHYDRATION.   Beginning at the midinterval of a 28-day cycle, or 14 days before the expected period, a regimen is instituted that will (*a*) limit the fluid intake to 1000 cc. daily; (*b*) restrict salt intake to the amount used in cooking and eliminate table salt; (*c*) promote fluid elimination by diuretic drugs. Ammonium chloride, 0.5 gm. orally 4 to 6 times daily, has been used with success. Potassium chloride can be used on the same dosage schedule as ammonium chloride. Acetazolamide (Diamox), 250 mg. daily, has recently become popular. Neohydrin, one to four tablets daily, may give fewer distressing side effects.

PSYCHIATRIC TREATMENT.   Much can be accomplished by reassurance. The patient is prone to think that her abnormal behavior is a too obvious indication that she is losing her mind. It is a source of enormous relief to the patient to be told that there is nothing serious or unusual in her condition and that a cure can be expected from the simplest forms of therapy. It is the rare case that will need more intensive help from a psychiatrist.

TRANQUILIZING DRUGS.   The psychogenic element is present in the premenstrual syndrome despite the fact that there is a reasonable physiologic explanation. The mounting tensions seem to increase with each succeeding period as some patients become more and more concerned with their mental health. As a supplement to the restriction of fluid and salt intake, in combination with diuretic drugs, it is then rational therapy to give one of the tranquilizing drugs. A number have been tried, and successes in a high percentage of instances have been reported. Rauwolfia serpentina (Serpasil), used in a dosage schedule of 0.25 gm. once daily for 10 days before the period, has been a useful adjunct. Meprobamate (Miltown) has been used recently, and enthusiastic reports appear in the literature. Eighty per cent of patients obtained relief by taking one 400-mg. tablet of meprobamate at the first sign of tension and following each meal thereafter until the symptoms subsided with the next menstrual period. This drug is said to have minimal side effects and does not establish a habit or induce withdrawal symptoms.

DIETARY AND VITAMIN SUPPORTS.   Vitamins and food supplements to the normal diet are rational factors in successful therapy. Previously we noted that a deficiency in vitamin B interfered with the metabolism of estrin by the liver. Daily doses of vitamin B will improve the utilization of estrin. The addition of milk and cheese to the diet, between meals and at bedtime, will help the hypoglycemia noted in the menstrual period.

INTERMENSTRUAL TENSION

Some women apparently note an increase in tension both at ovulation and in the premenstrual period. The mechanisms are apparently similar. The original investigations linking sodium, chloride and water retention with the appearance of symptoms of mounting tension showed an increased body weight in the midcycle, corresponding to a high level of sodium and potassium. Electrolyte changes were actually more pronounced at the time of ovulation than in the premenstrual phase.

Despite these observations the majority of women show an increased sense of awareness and freedom from nervous tension rather than depression at the time of ovulation. This may simply reflect a normal anticipation of the possibility of pregnancy. A great many women are acutely aware of the ovulatory period, termed *Mittelschmerz* when associated with unilateral abdominal pain after the follicle has ruptured.

The treatment of the woman who has headache, obvious fluid accumulation and mental aberrations at the time of ovulation will logically be identical with that given in the premenstrual phase of the cycle, since the mechanisms are considered essentially the same.

MENSTRUAL BACKACHE

Many women complain more vociferously about the bearing-down pain and backache that accompany the menstrual period than they do about abdominal cramps. When one considers the frequency with which women have backache, it is obvious that the sole cause cannot be found in the pelvis. This is particularly true when no pelvic disease can be detected. Women are particularly prone to attribute such pains to pelvic disease or malfunction of pelvic organs, but better than 50 per cent of the time the true explanation may be an orthopedic or urologic condition. Whatever the true source, the discomfort is apt to be accentuated at the time of the period.

What Part Do Orthopedic Conditions Play in Backache?

Among the orthopedic situations that contribute to pelvic backache are poor posture, spinal disease or inflammatory processes that irritate the nerves in the region of and adjacent to the spine. Many such conditions cause referred pain in the lower portion of the abdomen as well as the back. Since the symptoms invariably become worse at the time of the menstrual period, the patient is convinced that her acquired dysmenorrhea is due to pelvic disease. The gynecologist should examine her back before attributing the source of the backache to pelvic abnormalities, especially when the findings are not very striking on vaginal and rectal examination. When adequate cause for the pain can be found both in the back and in the pelvis, either the orthopedic surgeon or the gynecologist should assume the primary responsibility for treatment. For example, a patient with a ruptured intervertebral disk may also have a uterine fibroid tumor impacted in the pelvis. Both may produce a pelvic backache which is more severe at the time of the period. Which operation is to be done first? In most instances the orthopedic surgeon will prefer to have the pelvic abnormality corrected before performing any operation on the back.

How Does Urologic Disease Contribute to Backache?

Other sources for chronic pelvic backache made worse by the onset of the menstrual flow can be found in lesions of the urinary tract. Ureteral strictures commonly produce such symptoms. Urethral disease and obstruction of the neck of the bladder are prone to produce pain localized in the perineum and back. Trigonitis and a stone in the lower ureter will do the same thing. These symptoms are made worse by the menstrual period and become part of the symptom complex of acquired dysmenorrhea. Before placing the blame on disease within the pelvic organs the bladder should be thoroughly investigated by cystoscopy and the ureters by pyelography.

What Role Does Relaxin Play in Menstrual Backache?

Many women in the course of pregnancy complain bitterly of pelvic backache. There are many possible explanations of the cause of this sort of discomfort. The same sort of pain is often present in the premenstrual and early menstrual phases. X-ray evidence tends to show that a temporary relaxation of the joints in the pelvis occurs at this time. This can be demonstrated both in the symphysis and in the sacroiliac region. There is experimental evidence to suggest that this relaxation is due to the action of the hormone "relaxin" produced by the corpus luteum. In guinea pigs the symphysis undergoes wide separation after injection of relaxin.

Support of the pelvis by a pelvic girdle or adhesive strapping often provides relief from a menstrual backache caused by separation of the symphysis.

SECONDARY DYSMENORRHEA

A high percentage of patients who complain of premenstrual tension experience severe lower abdominal pain before and during the period. At times the pain simulates the cramplike contraction noted in primary (essential) dysmenorrhea, but more often the patient describes a dull, nagging, bearing-down pain that spreads to the back and upper thighs. Through the rest of the month the patient may be relatively comfortable, but about the time the symptoms of premenstrual tension appear she begins to experience dull dragging pain. This has been called a "pelvic toothache." The symptoms increase in severity and persist to and through the menstrual period.

Why Does the Patient Have Pain?

The mechanism of pain production is not the same as in primary dysmenorrhea, for secondary or acquired dysmenorrhea is invariably associated with organic pelvic disease. In all probability a large part of the pain is produced by pelvic vascular congestion, secondary to the pelvic lesion. To this the generalized tissue edema common in the premenstrual phase may contribute. The combination of acquired dysmenorrhea and symptoms of premenstrual tension has often been called the "chronic pelvic congestion syndrome."

What Are the Pathologic Conditions Commonly Present in a Patient with Secondary Dysmenorrhea?

PELVIC INFLAMMATION.   One of the most common abnormalities that contribute to secondary dysmenorrhea is pelvic inflammatory disease, either tuberculous, gonorrheal or nonspecific. The pain may be due to adhesions or to chronic lymphangitis in the parametrial tissues. Since pelvic infections are prone to occur during the age periods of greatest sexual activity, it is not surprising that secondary dysmenorrhea is most common in women of the twenty- to thirty-year age group.

When pelvic inflammatory disease involves both the tube and the ovary, abnormal menstrual bleeding problems and sterility are often present. The pain may be low-grade through the rest of the month, but invariably becomes more severe as the period approaches, reaching its climax with the menstrual onset. The diagnosis is usually obvious on physical examination. The history may prove helpful in determining the kind of infection present. The cause can be traced to gonorrheal, streptococcal or tuberculous infection. The reader is referred to the later discussion of individual infections (Chaps. 43–45).

STRICTURES OF THE CERVIX.   Anything that will interfere with the easy passage of menstrual debris will produce both bearing-down pain and painful uterine contractions. Obstructions to the cervical canal frequently result from previous infection or surgical trauma. These may be suspected if the menstrual discharge is dark brown or black or if the patient complains of profuse leukorrhea.

ABNORMAL POSITION OF THE UTERUS.   Not infrequently pelvic examination of the patient with secondary dysmenorrhea will demonstrate a uterus in the retroverted position. Of itself this means little, and except in rare instances it can hardly be considered the explanation of the pelvic pain. If, however, the uterus cannot be displaced to a normal anterior position without considerable pain, or it seems to be fixed in retroversion, then it may well be the cause of pain. The important fact to remember is that pelvic disease is the reason why the uterus is fixed. It is the disease, not the position of the uterus, that accounts for the pain. Pelvic inflammation and external endometriosis are the most common entities that produce a fixed uterus.

ENDOMETRIOSIS.   The form of endometriosis which produces widespread dissemination of ectopic implants over the pelvic floor, cul-de-sac and ovaries is most common in the thirty- to forty-year age group. It may, however, begin in the teen-age patient and become well established in the twenties. A full description of this pathologic entity will appear in Chapter 47. The dense fibrotic adhesions that bind down the uterus and the swelling that occurs within the individual endometrial implants serve to explain the dysmenorrhea. The symptoms are present in greater or less degree during the other phases of the cycle, but become acute at the time of the onset of the menstrual flow. Severe dysmenorrhea, increasing with each succeeding period, is a diagnostic sign of external endometriosis. Adenomyosis (internal endometriosis) is so rare in this particular age group that it will be left for discussion in Chapter 49.

UTERINE AND OVARIAN TUMORS.   The patient in this age group may have either uterine or ovarian tumors. Because of their position, size, or accidents that may occur within them, they may contribute to pain at this time of the menstrual cycle. Pelvic pain is due in most instances to (1) distention within a hollow viscus and stretching of the capsule; (2) hemorrhage within the tumor or cyst wall due to alterations in its blood supply; (3) irritation of the surface peritoneal covering from infection within the tumor; (4) impingement upon nerves by fibrosis or inflammation. The increased vascularity of the pelvis may exaggerate any one of these factors. It is amazing how large a tumor may be present in the uterus or adnexa without producing any symptoms and what a tremendous amount of discomfort small tumors can sometimes produce.

OVARIAN DYSMENORRHEA.   A good example of the intense discomfort that can be produced by a small tumor is the "pelvic ache" that occurs with the polycystic ovary. The pain is referred to the suprapubic region and lower portion of the abdomen. This pain is exaggerated at the time of the menstrual period. Such ovaries have a heavy fibrous capsule which prevents the normal expansion of the developing follicles, thereby producing pain through stretching of the covering. This entity is commonly associated with chronic vascular congestion in the pelvis. The ovarian source of the pain can be identified sometimes by passing a probe into the uterus. Such a maneuver is painless when the ovary is the cause.

EXTRAGENITAL SOURCES.   A wide variety of extrapelvic disease processes seem to contribute to secondary dysmenorrhea. Chief among these are low-grade infections within a low-lying *appendix* that prolapses into the pelvis. Ordinarily such a recurrent appendicitis produces little in the way of symptoms, but pain appears during the period of premenstrual congestion.

The same factors are operative in diseases of the *lower urinary tract*. Bladder ulcerations, urethral strictures, infections in and around the lower ureter all tend to increase the severity of the dysmenorrhea by adding their own obstructive symptoms to those produced by pelvic vascular congestion. Dilatation of a urethral stricture has cured secondary dysmenorrhea in a number of instances.

Any disease process, whether local or general, will contribute to the degree of pelvic congestion. Inanition or any chronic debilitating disease such as cirrhosis of the liver, pulmonary tuberculosis or diabetes mellitus may increase the severity of the acquired type of dysmenorrhea. The effect is in part due to the congestive aspect, but perhaps more can be attributed to the action of a chronic disease in lowering the threshold for pain.

Allergies to certain foods or to the patient's own hormones have been suggested as causes of many of the associated symptoms of acquired dysmenorrhea and perhaps pain as well. The uterine muscle is said to be sensitive to many of the allergic properties in such foods as wheat, milk, eggs, fish, nuts, chocolate and a number of roughage vegetables. Elimination of foods proved to be a cause of the allergy has resulted in freedom from menstrual pain. Apparently a certain number of patients are sensitive to histamine and obtain relief from their dysmenorrhea by taking antihistaminic drugs. Such factors should be considered when secondary dysmenorrhea appears in a patient who has no demonstrable pelvic disease.

How Do You Treat Secondary Dysmenorrhea?

The treatment will naturally depend upon the cause. If there is no pelvic disease, a search should be made for possible allergy to foods or to histamine by proper sensitivity tests, eosinophil counts or therapeutic trials. The great majority will have ample cause in demonstrable pelvic lesions. Some may be candidates for psychiatric help if conservative supportive measures fail. Certainly in this age group one would prefer to be conservative. It is a simple matter to determine whether stenosis of the cervical canal is present and to dilate the canal if need be. One may try to replace a retroverted uterus in normal position and hold it there with a pessary. Dietary and vitamin supplements, combined with attempts to regulate living habits, may improve the general condition enough so that the patient can tolerate the periodic monthly pelvic discomfort. Antibiotic therapy combined with hot douches may help to relieve dysmenorrhea that is on an inflammatory basis.

Whether surgery is indicated will be influenced by the progression of the symptoms, the severity of the pain, the persistency, the extent of the disease, the age of the patient and the desire to have children. Operation should not be performed for the relief of pain alone if pelvic abnormalities cannot be demonstrated. Surgery should be conservative whenever possible. The symptoms on occasion may become so progressively disabling and the disease state so extreme that hysterectomy is indicated, even in the younger age group. Not infrequently the underlying disease process then is so extensive that the chances of pregnancy are practically nonexistent.

REFERENCES

Premenstrual Tension

Billig, H. E., Jr., and Spaulding, C. A., Jr.: Hyperinsulinism of Menses. *Indust. Med.*, 16: 336, 1947.

Cooke, W. R.: The Differential Psychology of the American Woman. *Am. J. Obst. & Gynec.*, 49: 457, 1945.

Döring, G. K., and Feustel, E.: Ueber Veränderungen des Differentialblutbildes im Cyclus. *Arch. f. Gynäk.*, 184: 522, 1954.

Eichner, E., and Waltner, C.: Premenstrual Tension. *Med. Times*, 83: 771, 1955.

Frank, R. T.: The Hormonal Causes of Premenstrual Tension. *Arch. Neurol. & Psychiat.*, 26: 1053, 1931.

Idem: Interrelations of Estrogen and the Nervous System. *J. Mt. Sinai Hosp.*, 9: 419, 1942.

Freed, S. C., and Kroger, W. S.: Psychologic Manifestations of the Menstrual Cycle. *Psychosom. Med.*, 12: 229, 1950.

Gillman, J.: The Nature of the Subjective Reactions Evoked in Women by Progesterone, with Special Reference to the Problem of Premenstrual Tension. *J. Clin. Endocrinol.*, 2: 157, 1942.

Greene, R., and Dalton, K.: The Premenstrual Syndrome. *Brit. M.J.*, 1: 1007, 1953.

Israel, S. L.: *Mazer's Diagnosis and Treatment of Menstrual Disorders and Sterility.* 4th Ed. New York, Paul B. Hoeber, Inc., 1959.

Kalz, F., and Scott, A.: Cutaneous Changes during the Menstrual Cycle. A Clinical and Experimental Study under Physiological Conditions after Therapy. A.M.A. *Arch. Dermat.*, 74: 493, 1956.

Macht, D. I.: Concerning the Chemical Nature of Menstrual Toxin. *Am. J. Obst. & Gynec.*, 57: 251, 1949·

MacKinnon, P. C. B., and MacKinnon, I. L.: Hazards of the Menstrual Cycle. *Brit. M.J.*, 1: 555, 1956.

Morton, J. H.: Premenstrual Tension. *Am. J. Obst. & Gynec.*, 60: 343, 1950.

Morton, J. H., and others: A Clinical Study of Premenstrual Tension. *Am. J. Obst. & Gynec.*, 65: 1182, 1953.

Rees, L.: Psychosomatic Aspects of Premenstrual Tension Syndrome. *J. Ment. Sc.*, 99: 62, 1953.

Robinson, F. H., Jr., and Farr, L. E.: The Relation between Clinical Edema and the Excretion of an Antidiuretic Substance in the Urine. *Ann. Int. Med.*, 14: 42, 1940.

Thorn, G. W., Nelson, K. R., and Thorn, D. W.: A Study of the Mechanism of Edema Associated with Menstruation. *Endocrinology*, 22: 155, 1938.

Zondek, B., and Bromberg, Y. M.: Endocrine Allergy. I. Allergic Sensitivity to Endogenous Hormones. *J. Allergy*, 16: 1, 1945.

Secondary Dysmenorrhea

DeVere, R. D.: The Problem of Dysmenorrhoea. *Practitioner*, 185: 308, 1960.

Kroger, W. S., and Freed, S. C.: The Psychosomatic Treatment of Functional Dysmenorrhea by Hypnosis. A Preliminary Report. *Am. J. Obst. & Gynec.*, 46: 817, 1943.

Pickles, V. R., and Clitheroe, H. J.: Further Studies of the Menstrual Stimulant. *Lancet*, 2: 959, 1960.

Snaith, L., and Ridley, B.: Gynaecological Psychiatry. A Preliminary Report on an Experimental Clinic. *Brit. M.J.*, 2: 418, 1948.

Theobald, G. W.: Discussion on Dysmenorrhoea and Unexplained Pelvic Pain. *Proc. Roy. Soc. Med.* 50: 246, 1957.

Wengraf, F.: Psychodynamic and Therapeutic Aspects of Functional Dysmenorrhea. *Am. J. Obst. & Gynec.*, 48: 475, 1944.

Chapter 40

Vaginal Infections and Leukorrhea

INFECTION in the genital tract, despite the new antibiotic and chemotherapeutic drugs, still occupies a frontline position among the gynecologic conditions that plague women in the twenty- to thirty-year age group. Some of these infections produce troublesome symptoms, but bear no serious consequences, while others affect the patient's reproductive capacity and may seriously impair her health. The more serious forms of pelvic inflammation often start as local vaginal infections, only to spread to the uterus and adnexa either directly, as in gonorrhea, or by the lymphatics, as in streptococcal infections. A few forms of vaginal infection, such as by *Trichomonas vaginalis*, produce symptoms that are distressing to the patient, but have greater significance in that they may closely simulate the picture of local gonorrheal infection.

The chief symptom produced by the local vaginal infection is a leukorrhea. Normally one expects to find some vaginal secretion, but in the presence of even minimal pathologic changes within the vaginal canal the secretion often becomes excessive and a considerable nuisance to the patient. More women complain of leukorrhea than of any other gynecologic symptom.

It is important from the viewpoint of determining the cause of leukorrhea to obtain from the history (*a*) how long the patient has had the discharge; (*b*) whether this is a new or recurring complaint; (*c*) how much it bothers the patient and why; (*d*) what are its characteristics, such as amount, color, odor and consistency. The physical characteristics should be checked by inspection and sampling before the discharge becomes contaminated by the lubricating jelly used in the vaginal examination. Many women prepare themselves for gynecologic examination by taking a douche before they arrive. Naturally this maneuver will destroy all evidence of the infection. To get the maximum of information the patient should not have taken a douche for several days.

What Does the Normal Vaginal Secretion Look Like?

The normal vaginal secretion is odorless, acid, nonbloody and colorless in its appearance. On examination it is found to contain little mucus and rare bacteria. Characteristically, one finds a distinctive, long thick bacillus which is nonmotile. When stained, the bacterium is gram-positive. It grows anaerobically and is close kin to the lactic acid bacillus and hay bacillus, *B. subtilis*. This is the *Döderlein bacillus* (Fig. 40–1, *A*).

This normal inhabitant of the vagina apparently has a protective function, for

518

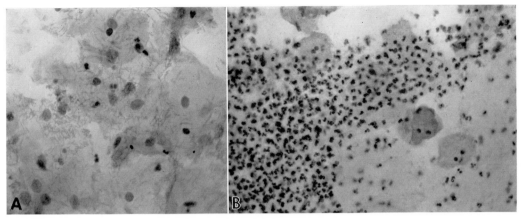

Fig. 40-1.   *A*, The large rod bacilli in the vaginal smear are Döderlein bacilli, usually an indication of normal vaginal acidity. *B*, Neutrophilic leukocytes in purulent exudate are an indication of inflammation, most commonly cervicitis, when found in the vaginal smear.

it tends to destroy the more pathogenic organisms such as the staphylococcus, probably because of its capacity to produce lactic acid. It does this by acting on the glycogen contained in the desquamating epithelial cells of the vagina. As long as the Döderlein bacillus is present, the vaginal secretion will remain acid. With the appearance of a normal pregnancy or introduction of an element of infection the acid concentration diminishes, and the vaginal reaction becomes alkaline.

What Is the Appearance of an Abnormal Vaginal Secretion?

As the vaginal pH approaches the alkaline side, the secretions change in their appearance, depending on the degree of infection. In the presence of an uninfected erosion of the cervix, for example, the discharge may be "mucoepithelial." It is then creamy white. No bacteria are found, but there is now a mixture of desquamating epithelial cells and mucus.

When there is a pathologic inflammatory basis for the discharge, the color changes to yellowish or greenish and may contain gas bubbles. Discharges of this sort are called "mucopurulent" or purulent, depending on the relative amounts of mucus and leukocytes, which in turn reflect the degree of infection (Fig. 40–1, *B*).

The Döderlein bacillus is no longer present, but in its place one finds all varieties and abundant quantities of organisms, from yeasts and trichomonads to staphylococci and streptococci. In most instances these organisms are not pathogenic, but the streptococcus is always potentially dangerous. If the local resistance of the vaginal tissue is lowered by any factor such as trauma, serious consequences can follow. This is particularly true when pregnancy is present. The vaginal pH tends to be alkaline during pregnancy, and streptococci are present in the vagina in approximately half of the patients. Streptococci are rare in the normal nonpregnant woman, but are found in nearly 30 per cent of those who have a frankly purulent discharge.

The *odor* varies considerably from scarcely noticeable to extremely foul. It does not necessarily reflect the seriousness of the vaginal infection. For example, the characteristic discharge of trichomoniasis may produce as distressing an odor as the watery discharge that follows the breakdown of a malignant neoplasm of the cervix.

The actual *amount of vaginal secretion* is dependent on the phase of the menstrual cycle as well as upon the individual patient. It was noted earlier that cyclic changes take place in the vaginal and cervical epithelia under the influence of estrin. One may then expect an increasing amount of discharge up to the time of ovulation and a decline thereafter until the menstrual period occurs. Regardless of the general state of health or local condition within the vaginal canal, individual variations occur in the amount of secretion produced. All are aware of the increased amount of secretion that follows sexual excitement and emotional disturbances. These are physiologic changes and may be regarded as normal.

What Are the Common Causes of Leukorrhea?

In the age group with which we are now concerned, twenty to thirty years, the most likely causes of leukorrhea stem from (1) Trichomonas vaginalis, (2) monilial infection (*Candida albicans*), (3) general constitutional disease, (4) foreign bodies, (5) bartholinitis, urethritis, cervicitis and endometritis secondary to infection produced by either gonococcus, streptococcus or staphylococcus.

TRICHOMONAS VAGINALIS INFECTION

This protozoan infection of the female genital tract is perhaps the most common of all vaginal infections. The actual incidence cannot readily be determined, for not all who have the infection have symptoms, but estimates of the frequency among American women run from 15 to over 50 per cent. It is more of a nuisance than a serious disease, but it has been implicated in sterility problems, largely because of the alterations it produces in the vaginal environment and the change in vaginal acidity. Because of the irritating symptoms it produces, chiefly burning and itching, it causes more disability through its effects on the patient's peace of mind than through any debilitating effect on her general health. Since the inflammation in the vaginal epithelium is often violent and the discharge profuse, the differential diagnosis between it and gonorrhea must be established.

Where Do These Trichomonads Come from, and How Do They Spread?

Despite the fact that the *Trichomonas vaginalis* was identified over 100 years ago, we still have only limited knowledge of how it gets into the vagina and why it seems to produce symptoms for a while, clear up and return again. We do know that it is transmitted by sexual intercourse, for this flagellate has been recovered from the male partner of a woman with the infection. It is equally obvious that this is not the only method of contamination. Women who have been isolated from sexual exposure in mental institutions have Trichomonas vaginitis fairly frequently (20 per cent). One can postulate that the Trichomonas has been present from birth, for it is known to be transmitted to the infant by passage through the vaginal canal at the time of delivery. It is possible, then, that it may remain latent. This brings out another observation that we recognize, namely, that the patient may carry the infection without having symptoms from it. Statistical observations on the number of asymptomatic carriers are inconclusive, but indicate that the organism is recovered in 20 to 60 per cent of cases. This could be the source of contamination, through sexual intercourse with noninfected persons.

As yet it has been impossible to prove that the patient becomes infected by using towels, toilet seats or bed linen. At times there appears to be circumstantial evidence that the infection can be acquired in this manner, but despite the fact that the organisms can be recovered from these sources, it is still an unsolved problem as to how they get into the vagina.

Other sources for the infection have been suggested, but there is little proof that transmission occurs from them. Origin from the rectum is unlikely, though closely related types of Trichomonas, such as *Trichomonas hominis* or *T. intestinalis*, are normal inhabitants of the intestinal tract. These organisms fail to survive when inoculated into the vagina. It is possible, however, that *Trichomonas vaginalis* may take up residence in either the bladder or rectum and serve as the locus of reinfection.

The Trichomonas has a predilection for the vestibular and urethral glands. Both Skene's and Bartholin's glands have served as a focal point for reinfection of the vaginal canal. In searching for the source of reinfection or explanation of failure of therapy, one must be convinced that the infection does not stem from these glands.

Therapeutically, we would like to know why some cases are difficult to cure and others tend to recur after an initial success. We are still uncertain whether the failures are due to a relapse or reinfection.

Why Do Some Patients Have Symptoms and Others Not?

It is surprising that the organisms can be recovered with such frequency in patients who have no symptoms, while others are made miserable by the irritating discharge. There is incomplete evidence that other organisms such as the streptococcus must be present with the Trichomonas to produce a real vaginitis. There is also the possibility that emotional stress and strain may be responsible factors in producing a persistence or a recurrence of the symptoms. The patients who complain of Trichomonas infection tend to be nervous and highly emotional. Whether any actual change occurs in the vaginal epithelium, such as vasodilation or hypersecretion secondary to emotional strain, is highly debatable. It is true that uncertainty as to the cause of the infection arouses a definite fear that the underlying explanation may be venereal disease or even cancer. Some observers contend that the symptoms of Trichomonas vaginalis infection rarely appear without accompanying psychosomatic symptoms as well.

What Are the Symptoms of Trichomonas Vaginalis Infection?

The infection is confined to the vaginal canal and practically never involves the uterine cavity or extends above the level of the cervix, either directly or by the lymphatics.

The chief symptom is a bubbly green-yellow or yellowish-white vaginal discharge which is very irritating and makes the patient unhappy, because of the local tenderness and intense itching that is usually localized to the vaginal canal, but often spreads to the external vulva. Because of the vaginal soreness intercourse is extremely painful (dyspareunia) or even impossible. The discharge has usually an unpleasant odor and is often so profuse that the patient must wear a protective pad. The symptoms are worse just before and just after the menstrual period when the vaginal pH is more alkaline.

On physical examination in the acute phase the introitus is bathed in a thin, frothy, bubbly discharge, and the surrounding vulva is much inflamed. The urethra

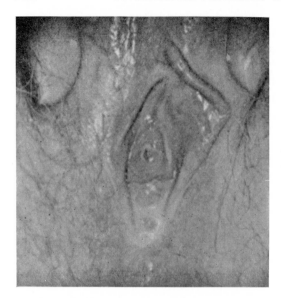

Fig. 40-2.   The vaginal discharge of trichomoniasis is thin and green, yellow or whitish. The reddening and granular appearance of the inflamed mucous membrane are evident.

looks reddened, but actually is so by contamination, rather than through its participation in the infectious process (Fig. 40–2).

On direct inspection of the vagina, using a speculum, a pool of discharge is found in the vaginal fornix that exhibits the same characteristic appearance. When this has been sampled for microscopic examination, the vagina is wiped out with a cotton applicator. It is then that the intensely inflamed vaginal epithelium is seen. The inflammatory process extends to the cervix, and many typical focal red granular areas are seen on both the upper fornix and the cervix. These have a characteristic "strawberry-like appearance" and may be regarded as pathognomonic, for they are never seen in any other kind of vaginal infection.

In the chronic or asymptomatic phase the same sort of discharge may be present without the accompanying inflammatory response.

How Do We Confirm the Diagnosis of Trichomonas Vaginitis?

In many instances it is possible to make an accurate diagnosis on the basis of the clinical impression. This can be confirmed by a simple laboratory test. To avoid contamination by lubricating jelly, a dry speculum is gently inserted into the vagina and a drop of the pus is taken from the vaginal pool or blade of the speculum and then placed on a microscope slide. To this is added a single drop of warm tap water or saline, and the wet preparation is covered with a coverslip to permit immediate low-power microscopic examination. There should be no delay in the examination, for the motile organisms become inactive when chilled or if the material is allowed to dry.

A definite diagnosis can be made when rounded or pear-shaped organisms are seen. These are somewhat larger than a pus cell, but less in diameter than an epithelial cell. On close examination they are found to have definite flagellae that whip about when examined under higher magnification. The whipping motion is accompanied by an undulating ameba-like motion of the cell membrane and jerky movements or whirling of the entire trichomonad. The organism must be motile to establish a diagnosis. The detection of active motion of the flagellae is important, for the

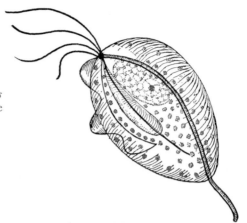

Fig. 40-3. Schematic drawing of *Trichomonas vaginalis*. The flagellae and undulating membrane are shown.

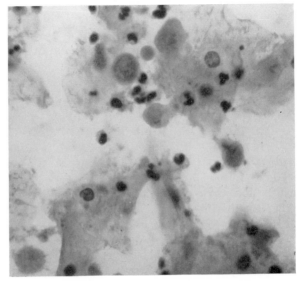

Fig. 40-4. The 5 ovoid, opaque blobs with faint internal details are dead trichomonads, mixed with cornified cells and exudate, from a vaginal smear. Usually they stain green with the Papanicolaou method.

Trichomonas is the only flagellate that one finds in the female genital tract. Experienced cytologists may be able to identify the dead trichomonads on Papanicolaou smears (Figs. 40–3, 40–4).

If the test gives negative results in the face of obvious infection, another specimen should be taken from the urethral pus and re-examined. If all results are negative, the patient should be questioned about the use of medications or the time of the last douche. The recent use of either may defeat the value of the wet-specimen test. When the clinical impression persists despite a negative examination, one may choose to take cultures. For routine use the culture technique is cumbersome and impractical. It is important, however, if one wishes to make a scientific study of the disease.

Treatment

The primary aim in therapy is to create a vaginal acidity unfavorable to the continued existence of the Trichomonas and to attack the Trichomonas directly by using some agent to act as a protozoacide. Multiple medications and techniques of therapy have been devised for the treatment of Trichomonas vaginalis infection. All have had a modicum of success, but none are 100 per cent efficacious. In all probability any one would be effective if we could be sure that all potential reinfective sources were reached and the Trichomonas completely destroyed. Unfortunately, relapses or recurrences of the infection are frequent.

The simplest form of therapy, which the patient may carry out at home, is the use of 5 tablespoonfuls of ordinary vinegar to 2 quarts of water as a douche. The douche should be taken lying down in the bathtub with the hips elevated on a folded towel. Before douching, the external vulva should be cleansed with water and the douche tip boiled. The labia of the vagina should be closed and released alternately as the water flows into the vagina and then is shut off. This allows the rugae of the vagina to become distended. The rationale of the use of vinegar (a poor man's lactic acid) is to create a vaginal acidity in the pH range of 4.5 to 5.0, at which the Trichomonas will not survive.

If treatment in the home does not suffice, office therapy is indicated. Perhaps the most effective part of the office treatment is the thorough mechanical cleansing with soap and water or the new detergent, pHisoHex, commonly used in preoperative cleansing of the hands. Several forms of powder are available to insufflate the vaginal canal and distend the vaginal folds, behind which the Trichomonas may lurk. Good results have been reported from the use of such preparations as Floraquin, Milbis powder and Powdex. Floraquin is a combination of lactose and dextrose with a protozoacide, Diodoquin. Milbis and Powdex are arsenical preparations that have a specific effect on the Trichomonas.

When any carbarsone or acetarsone preparation (arsenical preparations) is used, one should be on the alert for possible toxic reactions. These usually appear after prolonged and repeated treatment in the form of a local vulvitis, showing an urticarial, erythematoid or hemorrhagic eruption. Systemic reactions are not common, but any insufflation carries with it the danger of embolism. It is desirable to distend the vaginal folds, but the preparation should be blown in through a speculum or some outlet to air should be provided so that too much pressure does not develop within the vagina.

The initial office insufflation is followed by a vinegar douche thirty-six hours later. This regimen is repeated 4 times at 48-hour intervals in intractable cases. When the infection is less resistant to therapy, the initial insufflation is supplemented by an arsenical preparation in the form of suppositories inserted in the vagina. After the vinegar douche, each night one or two suppositories are placed as far back in the vaginal canal as possible, for at least one week. The following week the suppositories are used every other night.

Whether vinegar douches are used alone or in combination with Floraquin, Devegan or other arsenical suppositories, it is important that the regimen continue through the menstrual period. Sexual intercourse is contraindicated during the period of treatment in the severe cases or until improvement is noted in the less troublesome ones, and then only with a condom. One must persist in the treatment if the primary desire is to eradicate the Trichomonas. A permanent cure of the initial infection can be expected if the treatment is carried out for three months. In most cases the patient tires of the therapeutic routine and quits it once the distressing symptoms disappear.

When the symptoms persist or recur after a course of therapy, the cause can usually be traced to one or two sources: (a) the patient is being reinfected by her consort. Approximately 50 per cent of the male partners of patients who have a trichomoniasis that resists treatment carry Trichomonas in their prostatic fluid. Less than 20 per cent of these men have overt symptoms to indicate it. (b) The Trichomonads are probably resident in regions remote from attack by local vaginal therapy. To date no general systemic medication has been produced which will successfully reach these areas, in either the male or the female, without undesirable side effects. A new drug, Metronidazole, holds promise of being the most effective therapy yet available and is now being given an extensive clinical trial. It is effective when given orally but is even more useful when intravaginal inserts are used and oral medication is given to the man as well.

How Effective Are Antibiotics?   Since we are dealing with a protozoan rather than a bacterial infection, it is not surprising that chemotherapeutic drugs have not been particularly successful. Aureomycin, Terramycin and Triple Sulphacream have been tried, and successful reports have been recorded. With increasing knowledge of the sequelae that follow the systemic use of the antibiotics we become increasingly aware of the fact that they may actually destroy the normally protective Döderlein bacillus and increase rather than diminish the likelihood of vaginal protozoan infections.

What about the Treatment of Trichomonas Vaginalis Infection during Pregnancy?   With the advent of pregnancy the Döderlein bacilli tend to disappear and the vaginal pH approaches the alkaline side. Trichomonas, then, is a common finding in normally pregnant women. The presence of the infection makes many of these women miserable, because the intense itching keeps them awake at night. The treatment during pregnancy does not change materially from that carried out in the nonpregnant woman, and infection is frequently easier to cure, since the periods are absent. In some instances it may be necessary to continue the treatment until delivery is imminent, but for the most part it is wise to avoid treatment in the last month of gestation.

MONILIAL VAGINAL INFECTIONS CAUSED BY CANDIDA ALBICANS

The burning, itching type of leukorrhea is commonly attributed to *Trichomonas vaginalis*, but the same symptoms apply equally well to infections with Monilia, produced for the most part by the yeastlike organism, *Candida albicans*. Anything that will alter the normal vaginal flora will provide a suitable environment for Monilia to flourish in. Thus we commonly find monilial infections in diabetes mellitus, during pregnancy, in poor nutritional states and after prolonged use of antibiotics given systemically.

What Are the Symptoms and Physical Findings, and How Do They Differ from Those of Trichomonas Vaginalis Infection?

As in Trichomonas vaginalis infection, the patient may tolerate the fungus within the vagina without having any symptoms other than a thick, whitish, curdlike discharge. If the patient becomes pregnant, however, the vaginal epithelium under the stimulus of estrin stores increased quantities of glycogen. In this medium the fungi grow profusely. The same rich carbohydrate environment is also present when the patient has diabetes mellitus.

The chief difference between Trichomonas vaginalis infection and the mycotic infection produced by *Candida albicans* lies in the *amount and nature of the discharge*. The primary symptoms of burning, itching, localized soreness and pain, bladder frequency, dyspareunia and vaginismus are common to both, but in monilial infection there may be *far less vaginal discharge*. The nature of the discharge and the effect produced on the vaginal epithelium are fairly characteristic. Inspection of the external vulva gives no diagnostic clue, but when the speculum is introduced into the vaginal canal, the epithelium is found to be intensely inflamed and irritated. On this hyperemic background will be found varying quantities of white, cottage-cheese or curdlike discharge, which sometimes adheres tenaciously to the epithelium and can only be dislodged with difficulty and frequently with bleeding. The free flecks appear desiccated and have no moist or mucoid element.

There is another point of difference that may aid in distinguishing between the two entities. *Trichomonas vaginalis* tends to remain localized and can be recovered only from the genital tract, bladder and rectum. *Candida albicans*, on the other hand, has a more widespread distribution and can often be recovered from the mouth, skin and stool, as well as the genital tract. These areas may serve as a focus for subsequent vaginal infection.

How Is the Diagnosis Confirmed?

A fairly accurate diagnosis can be made on direct inspection of the vagina, but further confirmation may be had by smear or culture of the discharge or scrapings of the surrounding vulvar skin. Microscopic examination of the discharge, smeared on a glass slide and stained either with Gram stain, methylene blue or gentian violet, will demonstrate the fungus in the form of long, thin, bamboo-like threads (mycelia) with occasional minute budding cells coming off in branches. Also the yeast forms are found in Papanicolaou smears (Fig. 40–5). It is possible to identify these structures by simply examining under high power a bit of the discharge, to which a few drops of water have been added. If one chooses to culture the discharge for conclusive diagnosis, Nickerson's and Sabouraud's media have been used. Dark brown or black colonies appear after four or five days. The culture technique does help to distinguish *Candida albicans* from other pathogenic forms of Candida, but practically speaking, one may rely on the clinical impression and interpretation of the smear for an accurate diagnosis.

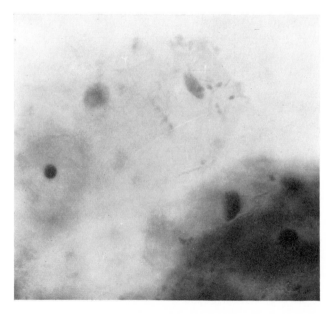

Fig. 40-5. Yeast forms of *Candida albicans* are seen to the right of the nucleus of the largest cornified vaginal epithelial cell.

Treatment

The primary aim in treatment is to eradicate the fungus. Fortunately the monilial infection produced by *Candida albicans* is far more suceptible to treatment than Trichomonas vaginalis infection. The history will prove more helpful in therapy, for from it one gets a lead as to whether the patient is pregnant, has diabetes or is under a therapeutic regimen of systemic antibiotics. Some of these agents, namely, Aureomycin and Terramycin, seem to be more likely to promote monilial infections than others. Elimination of the primary causative factors must go hand in hand with specific therapy for the Monilia.

The best treatment still seems to be the local application of 2 per cent gentian violet. Under direct vision the entire vagina with its many rugae and folds, as well as the clitoris and external vulva, are thoroughly covered with the dye. The heat from an ordinary examining light will expedite thorough drying. To prevent soiling the clothes, bed linen and everything else in sight, it is necessary to wear a protective pad. This treatment should be repeated every three days for three treatments. If it is inconvenient for the patient to return for office treatments, she can follow up the initial application by vaginal suppositories of gentian violet (Gentersal or Gentia-Jel). These should be inserted one each night after a cleansing douche. The regimen continues for two weeks.

Some patients are sensitive to gentian violet, and care must be taken that the patient is not overtreated. When confronted with this problem, one may prefer to use one of the therapeutic jellies, such as Gentia-Jel, Gentersal or PropionGel. Recently Mycostatin has proved effective when given in 100,000 unit doses as a vaginal suppository.

What Do You Do for the Persistent Case?   Usually the infection disappears after one or two weeks of treatment. Occasionally, and particularly during pregnancy, the Monilia may be more resistant. In this case one may wish to try oral Mycostatin tablets, 500,000 units, when local gentian violet treatments have not eliminated the infection. The dosage recommended is one tablet three times daily for a week or ten days, or as long as seems necessary. With pregnancy it is perhaps unwise to use douches, and Mycostatin vaginal tablets had better be given as a supplement.

Whenever a resistant infection is found or a recurrence is noted, the husband should be checked, for he may be the source of the reinfection. During therapy for the acute phase sexual intercourse is contraindicated.

From the point of view of prophylaxis one should stress cleanliness and proper vaginal toilet. The infection may be spread by intercourse, masturbation, towels, unclean toilets or bathtubs, douche tips and other instruments. The patient should be instructed not to touch the genital tract without previously washing her hands.

MIXED INFECTIONS

Another likely cause of refractory or recurrent vaginal infection is a combined infestation of both *Trichomonas vaginalis* and *Candida albicans*. It is a curious paradox that the two should exist together, for *Trichomonas vaginalis* grows best in alkaline media, while *Candida albicans* prefers an acid environment. A combined treatment using gentian violet with one of the arsenical powders will be more effective than either one alone. Douches will probably defeat the purpose and should be used sparingly, if at all.

SO-CALLED NONSPECIFIC INFECTIONS

For many years any vaginal infection that could not be specifically labeled with a causative agent such as Trichomonas, Monilia, streptococcus, staphylococcus or diphtheroid was said to be nonspecific. There is some recent evidence to suggest that such infections are actually due to *Hemophilus vaginalis*. The organism has been recovered by culture technique from both the male prostate and the female cervix.

The symptoms do not differ materially from those produced by *Trichomonas vaginalis* or *Candida albicans*, except that the burning and itching are less violent. There is some slight difference in the discharge, which takes on a grayish hue rather than the yellowish-white appearance characteristic of Trichomonas vaginalis infection. The vaginal epithelium is often red and edematous and has a smooth granular sensation to touch. Over these areas the epithelium may be absent. The diagnosis is usually confirmed by smears, which may be examined either as wet preparations or after staining with Gram's solution. The so-called clue cell is a common finding and reasonably pathognomonic of infection caused by the Hemophilus organism. These cells have an irregular outline and a coarsely granular cytoplasm. The organisms are minute (Fig. 40–6).

Treatment

This type of infection seems to respond well to local antibiotic therapy in the form of Triple Sulphacream. The patient can usually carry on this treatment at home, after the initial diagnosis has been made, by inserting a vaginal applicator well back in the vaginal canal and injecting the jelly nightly for about two weeks. Since the male may also harbor the infection in the prostate, he too should be treated to avoid reinfection. This can best be done by giving one of the broad-spectrum antibiotics such as tetracycline, in 250-mg. doses every 6 hours for several days.

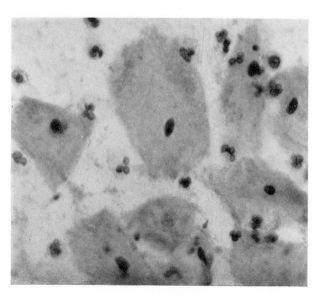

Fig. 40-6. The minute granules seen between and on vaginal cells are *Hemophilus vaginalis*. The granular appearance of these cornified cells on wet smear is termed the "clue cell."

FOREIGN BODIES

It is amazing how many different kinds of foreign bodies can be placed in the vaginal canal and forgotten. Sooner or later such objects produce a leukorrhea which is persistent, irritating and almost always malodorous. The most common cause is a neglected vaginal tampon inserted as protection at the time of the menstrual period. Similarly, the patient may forget to remove a contraceptive diaphragm. In the past, cervical pessaries constructed of gold or some other metal were inserted and left in the cervical canal to act as preventives to conception. Over a period of time these frequently set up a chronic cervicitis and produced a vaginal discharge. Occasionally one encounters such a pessary today.

The adolescent girl is not the only woman who inserts foreign objects in the vagina for purposes of sexual stimulation. A variety of such objects lost in the vagina has been recorded. In the presence of a persistent vaginal discharge one must consider the possibility of the presence of a foreign body before blindly advising douches for cure.

LOCAL PATHOLOGIC CONDITIONS IN AND AROUND THE VULVA

A variety of pathologic entities involving anatomic structures around the external genitalia can be responsible for or accompanied by a vaginal discharge.

What Are the Common Inflammatory Conditions Seen around the Vulva?

Most local infections near the vulva appear in the older age group and will be discussed later (Chap. 70). Even in the younger age group, however, it is possible for patients to have an acute vulvitis based on chemical irritation, such as from protective napkins used to control the menstrual flow, allergic response to nylon or rayon underclothing, or just plain neglect of ordinary hygienic principles.

An inflammation in and around the vulva that spreads to the skin of the adjacent thighs is particularly prone to appear in fat girls during the warm summer months. It may or may not be complicated by fungus infection. The prominence of the fat pads on the medial surfaces of the upper thighs in the act of walking results in chafing as the two skin surfaces are apposed (intertrigo). The intense itching often leads to scratching as the patient seeks relief. Excoriations and minor abrasions of the skin are produced, and secondary infection results. The source of the vulvar discharge may then be due to leukorrhea from a vaginal source, or it may be a purely local phenomenon.

Secondary infection often involves the hair follicles around the mons and vulva, leading to the formation of a widely disseminated papular and pustular eruption. This is the so-called *follicular vulvitis.*

Perhaps the most common type of vulvar irritation in this age group is that produced by diabetes mellitus. The picture presented is characteristic. The entire external vulva and mons look as though they had been beaten by a wire brush. A diffuse, dull red, raw, swollen skin covers the entire vulvar area. The patient complains of intense itching in this area, which is further aggravated by the secondary infection introduced by scratching. This is usually due to the monilial infection that frequently accompanies diabetes.

How Do We Treat Acute Vulvitis?

Whatever the type of vulvitis, the basic treatment consists in (1) eliminating the cause, (2) applying the simplest forms of local treatment. If vulvitis is caused by a vaginal infection, the treatment applied to the vaginal canal should also extend to the surrounding vulva. It will do little lasting good to treat diabetic vulvitis locally without first regulating the basic cause, diabetes, as well as the associated monilial infection.

Attention may then be directed toward local therapy for the inflamed vulva. In most instances these inflammations have already been overtreated with all manner of chemicals and ointments. The great majority will respond to a regimen of cleanliness, hot boric acid compresses and avoidance of further trauma. Every effort should be made to keep the area dry. After hot sitz baths or the application of boric compresses, the patient should gently dry the parts with linen or cotton. Coarse bath towels should be avoided. She should then lie down with her legs spread apart to permit thorough drying to occur. Only then should drying powders be applied. To use powder before the parts are dry is to encourage caking and more itching. Lotions are preferred to ointments. Simple calamine lotions are effective for minor degrees of pruritus, while 1 per cent cortisone lotion will relieve more intractable symptoms. It is amazing how the most acute inflammations of the vulva will respond to this sort of simple therapy within a matter of a few days.

INFECTIONS IN BARTHOLIN'S GLANDS

Perhaps the commonest site for infection to occur around the vulva is Bartholin's glands. These two glandular structures are situated within the vulvar tissue on either side of the fourchette and express their contents into the vaginal canal through ducts located laterally and posteriorly just above the midline. They are obvious only when infection occurs within the duct or gland itself. These glands through their secretion provide lubrication to the vaginal canal during sexual intercourse.

In the past, infection in Bartholin's glands was regarded as sound circumstantial evidence of the presence of gonorrhea. We now know that *Escherichia coli*, *Trichomonas vaginalis* and other pathogenic organisms, including both staphylococcus and streptococcus, can produce such infections, although gonorrhea is still the most probable cause.

How Does the Infection Enter the Bartholin Gland, and What Happens to It?

Infections enter the duct from a focus within the vagina. When the infecting agent is the gonococcus, the opening of the duct is readily recognized because of the intense erythema around it. The gland itself is palpable as a tender nodule, but it is not greatly distended, since the duct is patent. Usually pus can be expressed by pressure over it. On the other hand, a different train of events ensues when the duct becomes involved in infection caused by the *E. coli* or streptococcus. Since the duct is primarily involved, it responds by becoming swollen and edematous, and the gland can no longer extrude its contents because of the obstruction. The backed-up secretion rapidly becomes infected, and an acute Bartholin's abscess develops. Clinically, one recognizes it as a hot, tense, swollen, exquisitely tender mass. There is no place for the infection within the gland to go, for the exit is blocked. As the inflammatory process becomes more acute, both the overlying skin and the tissue deep to the abscess become involved, and the entire labium becomes diffusely swollen. It may still be possible to see pus at the duct opening or to express pus from it through pressure on the mass, but this exudate comes from infection within the plugged duct. The infection within the gland is trapped. Rarely does it subside without drainage. The patient is usually so intensely miserable, both sitting and walking, that surgical excision or drainage is performed for relief. If the patient has applied heat in an attempt to localize the infection, or if the process progresses rapidly, spontaneous evacuation of the abscess may occur.

The symptoms in this acute phase are more local than general. The temperature and leukocyte counts are only moderately elevated. After evacuation of the pus the acute symptoms promptly subside.

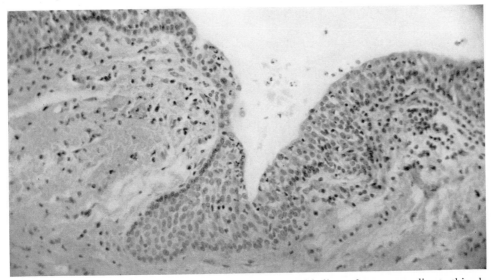

Fig. 40-7. The duct lining of a Bartholin cyst is intact epithelium of a type peculiar to this gland. Note the underlying fibrosis and leukocytic infiltrate, which lead to duct stenosis and obstruction.

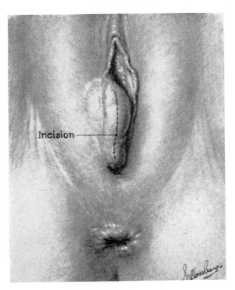

Fig. 40-8. Removal of infected Bartholin's gland. First, an incision is made over the most prominent part of the enlarged gland, usually in the mucous membrane. (Wharton: *Gynecology, Including Female Urology.*)

Incision

The process now enters the chronic phase. The gland epithelium is not usually altered to any great extent, or it undergoes rapid regeneration after the infection has subsided. The permanent inflammatory changes are localized to the duct, which becomes scarred and fibrosed (Fig. 40–7). The secretions produced by the undamaged epithelium of the gland proper now have no place to go, and a Bartholin's cyst develops. Such cysts vary widely in size up to that of a hen's egg (Fig. 40–8). At this stage the patient may be completely unaware of the presence of the cyst, or it may interfere with intercourse and become a nuisance.

Obviously, the extent of change to the duct is not constant. Some drainage may still be possible, and the chronic phase is manifested simply by a firm, nontender nodule noted by the examiner in the lateral vulvar tissues. Frequently the patient has not noticed it and may not even remember any previous acute episodes.

What Is the Best Treatment for the Acute Bartholin's Abscess?

There appears to be little reason to apply topical heat in the hope that the abscess will eventually subside or drain spontaneously. Such a course simply prolongs the patient's discomfort and provides inadequate drainage when spontaneous perforation does occur. It is far better to provide complete evacuation through early surgical drainage under the protection of antibiotic therapy.

If the process is seen early enough in its course, before widespread cellulitis has taken place in the supporting vulvar tissue, it may be good surgical judgment to excise the abscess in toto. The reason for this is that otherwise the residual gland and duct are prone to develop recurrent inflammatory states, and if possible it is thus better to excise the entire inflammatory focus. In most instances total excision is impossible, and drainage alone can be safely performed. To minimize the risk of recurrence the cyst wall should be marsupialized by suturing it to the edges of the skin incision.

What Is the Accepted Treatment of Chronic Bartholinitis?

Whether the chronic infection in Bartholin's gland manifests itself by a Bartholin's cyst or by simple nodular enlargement, the gland should be completely excised. The history of untreated cysts or chronic bartholinitis is one of repeated infection and recurrent abscess formation.

URETHRITIS AND INFECTIONS OF SKENE'S GLANDS FROM CAUSES OTHER THAN GONORRHEA

It is customary to regard infection of the female urethra and the adjacent Skene's glands as *prima facie* evidence of gonorrhea. The openings to Skene's glands are found in the urethral mucosa in close proximity to the meatus. Infection in the urethra will usually extend to these paraurethral glands. When infected, the urethral mucosa pouts outward, and pus can be seen oozing from the ducts when pressure is applied to the under surface of the urethra. Undoubtedly most urethritis and skenitis are caused by the gonococcus, but other infections, both specific and nonspecific, are implicated. Any infection within the vaginal canal can extend to the urethra. We have noted, for example, how *Trichomonas vaginalis* hides in the urethral mucosa out of the reach of local vaginal therapy. Because of its exposed position the urethra is also easily traumatized and readily infected. Many infections are probably brought to the female urethra from a male focus within the prostate, seminal vesicle or urethra through sexual intercourse. Not all of these infections are gonorrheal, but simply secondary infections which crept in after the gonococcus had disappeared. The discharge from nonspecific inflammation of the urethra, when cultured, usually shows nonhemolytic streptococcus, staphylococcus and the colon bacillus.

In the acute phase there is little to distinguish a urethritis caused by the gonococcus from that produced by nonspecific organisms. In both instances the urethral mucosa tends to evert and becomes red and swollen. The amount and nature of the discharge give no clue to the etiology, and the final diagnosis must depend on smear and culture. The chief symptoms in both, in addition to the discharge, are urinary frequency, and burning and pain on voiding. It is of the utmost importance that the identity of the infectious organism be established and not be falsely labeled as gonorrhea. In the past many patients were thought to have gonorrhea when the true cause was actually *Trichomonas vaginalis*. This was particularly true of the group in whom equivocal smears were not confirmed by culture.

In the chronic phase the diagnosis is even more difficult. In many of these patients the urethral discharge is minimal or absent and the pathogenic organisms cannot be identified, but the patient is extremely uncomfortable. Chronic nonspecific urethritis is the most common of all urologic complaints in women. The appearance of the urethra is fairly characteristic. Since infection may linger for long periods, the urethral mucosa and muscular walls respond to the chronic irritation by thickening of the mucosa and fibrosis of the wall. Within the urethral canal polypoid and papillary masses appear and tend to block it. The stenosis is aggravated by the increasing fibrosis in the wall. This thickening of the wall can readily be palpated in the lower portion of the vagina.

The symptoms produced are out of proportion to the physical findings and the seriousness of the infection. They are chiefly urinary frequency and painful micturition, which is both severe and persistent. Rarely, the patient notes the passage of blood toward the end of urination.

The diagnosis is usually suspected when the patient's local symptoms are severe, yet little or no pus or blood can be found on examination of the voided urine specimen. When attempts are made to obtain a catheter specimen, the patient complains bitterly of pain. A panendoscope readily demonstrates narrowing of the urethral canal and the presence of an irritated, red, granular mucosa along the floor. Occasionally papillary excrescences are present.

Since chronic urethritis may be produced by a variety of organisms, both specific and nonspecific, cultures should be taken from any discharge that may be expressed. When the organism can be identified, it is helpful in directing therapy, but in many instances no bacteriologic confirmation is possible.

Treatment of Chronic Urethritis

The treatment will depend in part on what causes the urethritis. The antibiotic drug specific for the organism should be given. Symptomatic relief can be obtained by urethral dilatation, massage of the urethra with the dilator in place and irrigation of the bladder with a mild solution such as 1:5000 silver nitrate.

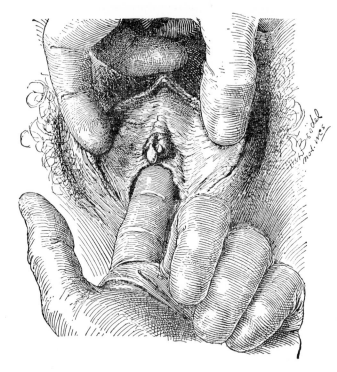

Fig. 40-9.   The urethra is compressed to express pus from Skene's ducts. Also one palpates the entire urethra and the region around it to detect any infiltration or evidence of infected posterior urethral glands. (Kelly and Burnam: *Diseases of the Kidneys, Ureters and Bladder*. New York, A. Appleton-Century Co.)

Treatment of Chronic Infection of Skene's Glands

Infection of the urethra spreads to the immediately adjacent paraurethral and Skene's glands and produces similar changes. It is harder to eradicate here because of the stenosis produced in the narrow ducts, which tend to form crypts. Sometimes pressure over the ducts will express a drop of pus that can be cultured. If this is possible, antibiotic therapy may be helpful, but by and large the only way to get rid of the infection is to destroy the glands by cautery. This maneuver can be expedited by introducing a blunt curved needle into the duct. Traction on the needle brings the duct into a position where it can be more thoroughly destroyed by the cautery (Fig. 40–9).

CERVICITIS AND ENDOCERVICITIS

Inflammation of the external cervix (cervicitis) and the cervical canal (endocervicitis) is one of the most common causes of leukorrhea. It exists in both an acute and a chronic state. The frequency of occurrence is not surprising when we consider that the cervix normally provides an effective barrier against the extension of any infection to the uterus and tubes. As such, it is bound to receive the full brunt of any infection that chooses to enter the vaginal canal. The various kinds of organism cultured from an infected cervix reflect this. Gonorrhea is still the most common bacterial invader, but the streptococcus activated by cervical trauma as the result of attempts at criminal abortion or injudicious instrumentation accounts for nearly as many acute and chronic cervical infections.

What Does the Acutely Inflamed Cervix Look Like, and Does the Appearance Vary with the Type of Infection?

In the acute phase the cervix, along with the rest of the vaginal canal, is red, swollen and edematous, and pus can be seen pouring from the cervical canal. The surface epithelium has been denuded for a variable distance around the external cervical os. There is usually a sharp line of demarcation between the raw granular area and the normal epithelium (See Frontispiece). This picture is common to all acute infections and is not pathognomonic of gonorrhea. The distinction between gonorrhea and other causative agents can be made only by wet or stained smears and by cultures when the smear examinations are equivocal.

The appearance of the cervix in the acute phase is not always constant. In most instances the patient with acute exocervicitis will also have infection in the cervical canal. Occasionally, however, one finds little derangement of the external surface epithelium, but mainly an acute inflammatory process in the cervical canal. The extent of endocervical involvement does have some relation to the infecting agent. Gonococcal infections are largely confined to the epithelial lining and the ducts of the racemose endocervical glands located deep in the cervical stroma. Streptococcal and staphylococcal organisms, on the other hand, tend to penetrate deeper into the cervical wall and involve the gland acini themselves. In this manner streptococcal infections reach the lymphatic channels and produce pelvic cellulitis. In contrast, gonorrhea usually spreads along contiguous mucous membrane surfaces as a superficial catarrhal infection.

There is nothing particularly unusual about the pathologic picture in the acute phase. There is an obvious loss of surface epithelium and an infiltration of leukocytes, particularly neutrophils, into the subepithelial tissue. There may be some low cuboidal epithelium replacing the high columnar type usually covering the endocervix (Fig. 40–10).

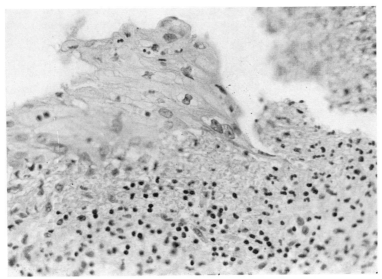

Fig. 40-10.   To the right is an eroded area infiltrated by neutrophils, as an indication of acute cervicitis. The exocervical cornified epithelium nearby is partially degenerated.

What Symptoms Appear in the Acute Phase?

The primary symptom is leukorrhea. It is usually purulent and profuse, particularly if the cause is gonorrhea. With less acute specific infections it can be mucopurulent, thick and tenacious. When gonorrhea is the causative agent, the rest of the vaginal canal is usually involved, and the patient frequently complains of urinary frequency, urgency and dysuria. At times the patient is troubled by external burning and itching of the vulva. This is more apt to come from the cervical infections caused by *Trichomonas vaginalis*, Monilia and gonorrhea rather than streptococcal cervicitis. With low-grade streptococcal cervical lesions the amount of discharge is apt to be less and the irritation factor minimal. There is little in the way of systemic reaction. There may be a slight elevation of body temperature, but most of the symptoms are concentrated in the genitalia. In many instances the only symptom is the purulent discharge.

What Treatment Do We Advise for Acute Cervicitis?

Since the cause may be ascribed to a variety of organisms, the treatment of acute cervicitis and endocervicitis will depend on isolation of the responsible agent. In any case and whatever the cause, there is no longer any place for local treatment of the disease. Overenthusiastic attempts to treat the local cervicitis by cauterizing agents in the acute phase present a real danger of dissemination of the infection to the pelvic lymphatics, which in turn leads to salpingitis and peritonitis.

The most likely cause is still the gonococcus, and its presence should either be established or ruled out by both smear and culture. When gonococci are present, penicillin in dosage of 600,000 units should be given daily for one week. A resistant gonococcal strain may be present, and recurrences are occasionally noted. Repeated smears and cultures should be done at regular intervals. If the problem is one of antibiotic resistance, it is common practice to give one of the broad-spectrum antibiotics, such as Chloromycetin or one of the sulfa drugs. In the acute phase when the discharge is profuse, the patient should be cautioned about personal hygiene, lest the infection spread to other areas of the body, particularly the eyes. Gonorrheal ophthalmitis is not confined to infancy and actually has no respect for the age of the patient.

The same antibiotic regimen will be helpful in acute cervicitis due to causes other than gonorrhea. In addition, bed rest, urinary antiseptics, forced fluids and adequate bowel elimination will serve to limit the spread of the infection, while making the patient more comfortable.

Cervicitis and Endocervicitis in the Chronic Phase

We have elected to discuss chronic cervicitis and endocervicitis in the twenty-to thirty-year age group, for this is the greatest period of sexual activity and reproductivity. Chronic cervical inflammation is not only a common sequel to normal delivery, but conversely it is one of the main causes of infertility, as noted previously. Also it may be precancerous. In the past the gonococcus was the principal factor in the etiology of chronic cervicitis, but present-day therapy with antibiotics and sulfa drugs is so effective in the initial phases of gonorrhea that the balance is now heavily weighted on the side of pregnancy and its complications as prime causes of cervicitis.

Thus in a normal delivery a certain amount of tearing is to be expected as the cervix dilates. Vessels as well as muscle fibers are stretched and ruptured, thereby giving rise to vascular thrombosis, which can be the focus for a low-grade inflammatory reaction. Cervical infection is also prone to occur in a pregnancy that terminates in abortion, particularly when there has been instrumentation in some form. Chemical agents such as potassium permanganate which are used by some women in the hope that abortion may follow more often result in cervical infection than in evacuation of the uterus.

These are not the only source of infection, for the past history of many patients who have chronic cervicitis fails to bring out any previous suggestion of infection, instrumentation or pregnancy. Congenital underdevelopment, constitutional disease, hormonal imbalance and malnutrition may contribute to the establishment of cervical infections by altering the normal environment of the upper portion of the vagina and destroying the protective Döderlein bacillus. Cervical infection is occasionally found in infancy, adolescence and virginal adult states.

What Does Chronic Cervicitis Look Like Grossly?

The cervix that harbors chronic infection does not offer any constant picture which may be regarded as characteristic. There is a variety of clinical manifestations. The most common is the so-called cervical erosion. Here the superficial epithelium has been lost from the area surrounding the external os. The line of demarcation between the central erosion and the surrounding normal squamous exocervical epithelium is well delineated, the infected, eroded area showing up as a red granular zone that tends to bleed easily on the slightest trauma. At times the reddish granulations are raised above the surrounding surface and give the impression of being papillary (See Frontispiece). Some pathologists call this a papillary erosion.

In the process of repair by upward growth of the squamous epithelium some of the ducts of the endocervical glands are pinched off, thereby producing a retention of mucus within the otherwise undamaged glands, which continue to function. These form readily visible translucent cysts that project above the surface and present mute evidence of a previous erosive cervical infection. They are called nabothian cysts. They

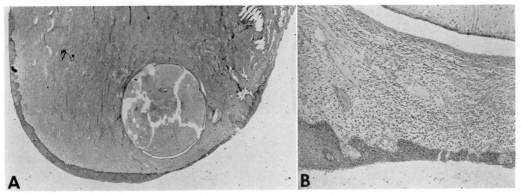

Fig. 40-11. *A*, The cervix contains a mucus-filled nabothian cyst, and the overlying epithelium is thin where it has grown along the surface as an erosion healed. *B*, At higher magnification the epithelium that has epidermized the cervical canal is shown on the surface. Beneath is the typical leukocytic infiltrate of chronic cervicitis. The mucus-producing epithelial lining of the cystic gland is artefactually detached from the stroma.

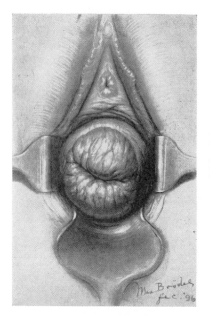

Fig. 40-12.   An ectropion or cervical eversion is covered by red mucous membrane of endocervical type. The covering epithelium is intact, and the vascular stroma shows through it. This may be examined by biopsy under the erroneous impression that it is a cervical erosion. (From a drawing by Max Brödel in T. S. Cullen: *Cancer of the Uterus*. New York, Appleton & Co., 1900.)

may be single or multiple and vary in size. Many are no bigger than the head of a match, while others are grape-size or larger (Fig. 40–11). When the cysts are opened, one usually finds clear mucus, but if there is much infection in the obstructed glands, the fluid may be pure pus or mucopurulent.

As a result of forceful or precipitous childbirth the cervical os may become severely lacerated. The streptococcus, which is present in limited numbers in the nonpregnant vagina, seems to proliferate in the vaginal secretion as the hormones of pregnancy alter the pH toward the alkaline side. The element of trauma during delivery plus the increased growth of streptococci adds up to produce cervical infection. As a result of the infection the mucous membrane lining the cervical canal becomes swollen and edematous and tends to pout out through the hypertrophied lips of the lacerated cervix. This is the so-called cervical eversion or ectropion. It differs from true erosion in that (a) the cervical lips are lacerated and hypertrophied; (b) the red, granular, vascular epithelium is thicker and spreads over a wider area than one normally finds with an erosion (Fig. 40–12). It differs from a "congenital erosion" in that (a) it occurs after childbirth; (b) it is associated with obvious inflammation, not merely a prolapse of the endocervical mucous membrane. The extent of the eversion becomes more apparent as the lacerated lips of the cervix are separated by the blades of the examining speculum. At times the thick, red granular eversion is so extreme that it is mistaken for carcinoma of the cervix. The impression is further strengthened by the fact that it bleeds readily after minimal trauma.

As we noted in the description of acute cervicitis, the external exocervical surface epithelium may be intact, but the cervix itself is hypertrophied and becomes barrel-shaped because of the inflammatory process going on deep in the cervical glands. The cervical canal itself is frequently obstructed by a thick, tenacious mucopurulent plug. When this is removed, the raw granulating endocervical epithelium can be seen bulging out into the canal. Usually the canal is patent, but if the process goes on long enough or inadequate attempts are made to destroy the endocervical infection by chemical or electric cautery, the end-result is apt to be a stenosis.

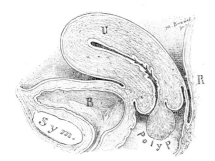

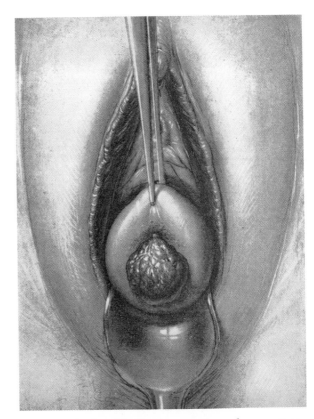

Fig. 40-13. Typical cervical or so-called endocervical polyps arise in the canal and may protrude through the external os. Smaller polyps or those attached higher up in the cervical canal do not present on examination of the external cervix. (From T. S. Cullen: *Cancer of the Uterus.* New York, Appleton & Co., 1900.)

The overgrowth of the inflamed endocervical epithelium sometimes becomes so pronounced in localized areas within the canal that it forms large polypoid accumulations which we know as a polyp. The polyp acts as a foreign body, and the uterus by muscular action tries to extrude it. As a result the polyp becomes dislodged from its primary location, and a pedicle is formed with the club-shaped polyp on the end (Fig. 40–13). A cervical polyp itself is enough to account for a vaginal discharge, but some part of the leukorrhea is due to the underlying infection that produced the polyp.

What Does Chronic Cervicitis Look Like Microscopically?

Leukocytes are collected in the stroma beneath the epithelium of the exocervix and endocervix. Lymphocytes, macrophages and plasma cells predominate. Sometimes lymph follicles with germinal centers occur, and this condition may be called *chronic follicular cervicitis.* The inflammation, whether slight or severe, usually involves both the exocervix and the endocervical canal, including the glands of the endocervix (Fig. 40–14, *A*).

The stratified squamous epithelium of the exocervix may appear microscopically normal or show slight thickening and hyperplasia. If an erosion is present, the surface consists of raw granulation tissue, composed of proliferating capillaries and young fibroblasts mingled with leukocytes. Healing of an erosion is indicated by a thin sheet of squamous epithelium partly covering the granulation tissue (Fig. 40–14, *B*). Overgrowth of this squamous epithelium up into the endocervix is recognized when some

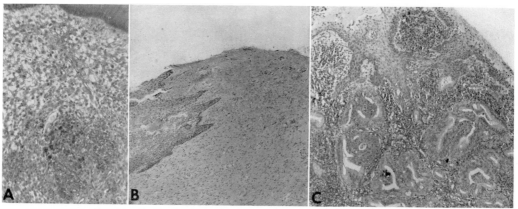

Fig. 40-14.　　*A,* The cervical stromal infiltrate of chronic cervicitis includes many lymphocytes and plasma cells. The lymph follicle present permits a diagnosis of chronic follicular cervicitis. *B.* Part of the cervical surface is eroded, and a finger of epithelium is growing along the surface from the left, as an attempt to heal the erosion. *C,* Epidermidization of cervical glands is proceeding by a downgrowth into the glands of surface epithelium. Also, independent foci of squamous metaplasia appear to be present in epithelium deeper in the glands. The stroma is inflamed.

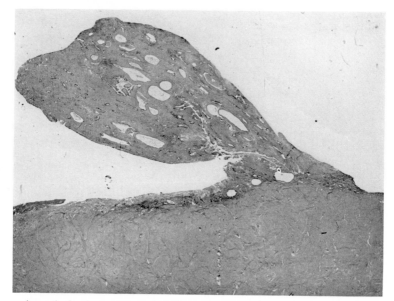

Fig. 40-15.　　A cervical polyp, composed of fibrous stroma and cystic endocervical glands. The surface epithelium has become partially eroded by friction in the canal.

of the endocervical gland mouths become covered by stratified squamous epithelial cells. This is called epidermidization, and as already mentioned, it causes mechanical obstruction of glands and leads to the formation of nabothian cysts.

Inflammation may produce a degeneration of the endocervical and glandular mucus-secreting epithelium. Regenerated foci of the endocervical mucosa microscopically are seen to have squamous cell characteristics in some cases. This aspect of chronic cervical inflammation is called squamous metaplasia of the endocervix. Epidermidization and squamous metaplasia often occur together (Fig. 40–14, *C*). Neither is considered to be a precancerous lesion.

Cervical polyps, which appear to arise from enlarged papillary erosions, are largely composed of granulation tissue, dilated blood vessels, nabothian cysts and leukocytes. Their surface is frequently eroded or shows localized epidermidization or squamous metaplasia (Fig. 40–15). This is attributed to damage and repair from frictional trauma in the cervical canal. The vast majority of cervical polyps are neither neoplastic nor show any indications of a precancerous process.

Specific infections of the cervix by tuberculosis or syphilis are considered elsewhere (Chap. 45). Nothing diagnostic of gonorrhea, trichomoniasis or moniliasis can usually be found on routine microscopic examination of a cervical biopsy.

Of What Does the Patient with Chronic Cervicitis Complain?

Chronic cervicitis is the most common cause of leukorrhea. The discharge is invariably thick, gelatinous and mucoid. If there is much infection, the mucoid content will be mixed with pus. Often a tenacious mucoid plug fills the cervical os and defies extraction.

Because the endocervical epithelium is swollen, edematous and exposed, it is readily traumatized, with the result that the patient frequently has slight, irregular intermenstrual bleeding. This is most noticeable when the process has progressed to polyp formation.

Backache is a common complaint in the patient who has chronic cervicitis. This is understandable when one considers that the lymphatic drainage from the cervix extends back along the uterosacral ligaments, which are often firm and tense. Men complain of the same sort of backache when they have chronic prostatitis. This is also the probable explanation of the "heaviness" in the pelvis that bothers many patients. It is in part the cause of dyspareunia. Contact of the penis with a tense, rigid cervix is enough to produce pain.

Many patients with chronic cervicitis complain bitterly of urgency and frequency of urination. The immediate cause is an infection of the trigone of the bladder. The primary source of the trigonitis is in the immediately adjacent cervix. The infection spreads along the lymphatic pathways to the floor of the bladder. This is also the probable explanation of the so-called honeymoon bladder, in which excessive stimulation and trauma have stirred up a low-grade inflammatory process. Any attempt to treat the trigonitis without first clearing up the infection in the cervix will be fruitless.

Though the infection spreads to nearby areas such as the bladder and parametrium, there is little evidence that it serves as a focus of infection for such entities as iritis, arthritis or neuritis. In earlier discussions we pointed out the importance of a normal cervix in solving the problems of sterility or relative infertility. Sterility indeed may be the patient's chief complaint.

On What Do We Base the Diagnosis of Chronic Cervicitis?

The diagnosis is made chiefly on the appearance of the cervix in a woman who may have a history of having borne a child or suffered an abortion, or who has given a story of some form of intracervical instrumentation. In most instances these factors operate to cause chronic cervicitis. Despite the efficiency of antibiotic drugs it is still possible that such a cervix may harbor the gonococcus. Smears and cultures should be taken before embarking on definitive therapy. Rarely are vigorous attempts made to eradicate chronic cervicitis without antibiotic drugs.

It is of the utmost importance that cancer of the cervix be ruled out before one undertakes any therapy that will result in tissue destruction. Many cervices that appear to represent benign cervicitis actually have either premalignant changes or frankly invasive cancer. The more one sees of cancer of the cervix, the more one biopsies any cervical lesion that shows any apparent departure from the normal variations. Clinically, it is often impossible to make an accurate differential diagnosis. The final measure must be expert microscopic examination of tissue removed not from one but several places in the area under suspicion. Then and only after the pathologic study should the cervicitis be cauterized or excised. This will be discussed in greater detail in the consideration of cancer of the cervix (Chap. 61).

What Forms of Treatment Are Commonly Used for Chronic Cervicitis?

When the suspicion of cancer of the cervix or gonorrhea has been satisfactorily eliminated, one may proceed with the therapy of choice. Because chronic cervical irritation is closely linked to the cause of cancer of the cervix, it is important from the viewpoint of prophylaxis to eradicate chronic cervicitis. In most instances this is done by some form of heat application, either electrocauterization or electric conization. In the older age group surgical repair is used. There is little excuse in this present day for topical application of chemical cauterizing agents such as silver nitrate, largely because they are ineffective and can be dangerous if improperly used.

Some form of electrocauterization is the treatment of choice. This should be done approximately one week after the completion of the menstrual flow. It requires no anesthesia and may be successfully carried out as an office procedure. The occasional patient may ask for a topical application of some anesthetic such as Pontocaine. If necessary, the cervix can be infiltrated with Novocain. In the vast majority one need only explain to the patient that the procedure is not painful and that at most she may have a local sensation of heat. This simple expedient will allay any fear she may have, and it minimizes the chance of inadvertently burning the vaginal wall because the patient makes a sudden move.

What Is the Technique for Cervical Cauterization? With the speculum in place and a good light available, the mucus plug is removed from the cervix. If this does not come away easily, one may apply Caroid powder or hydrogen peroxide on the tip of a cotton applicator. These agents dissolve the protein in the mucus, and after a few minutes the plug is easily dislodged.

Before applying a nasal-tip type of cautery, it is advisable to explore the cervical canal with a uterine probe to be sure that the canal is patent before you cauterize. There are a number of ways other than a preliminary explanation to protect the patient against a burn of the vaginal wall. Some gynecologists cover the blades of the speculum with a cylinder of rubber taken from the finger of a rubber glove. This prevents the redundant lateral vaginal folds from encroaching on the lumen. Others insert the cold cautery tip into the vagina after testing it for the proper amount of current.

Regulation of the amount of heat to be used is extremely important, for upon it depends the extent of tissue destruction. If the cauterization is too deep or too heavy, the patient may have a severe hemorrhage later as the slough separates. The description generally accepted as indicating a proper degree of heat is a cautery tip that is cherry-red.

The nature of the presenting lesion will determine how the cauterization is to be applied. If one is dealing with an erosion and the external cervical os is not patulous, the cauterization should be restricted to the external portion of the cervix. One may then proceed in one of two ways. Most gynecologists prefer shallow radial cauterizations running out from the os toward the periphery at spaced intervals. Others cauterize superficially all obviously diseased areas, including the nabothian cysts, leaving the entire external cervix covered with a yellowish-gray coat of coagulated tissue. However it is done, the cauterization need not extend deeply into the tissue, for the erosion itself is not very deep-seated.

The cervical canal should also be cauterized (*a*) when the primary disease lies within the canal, and the external portions are normal; (*b*) when an ectropion is combined with a deep endocervical infection in a lacerated cervix. When the involvement is extensive, one may prefer to do this under anesthesia or in a hospital operating room.

In either case the tip of the cautery, heated to the proper temperature, is inserted in the canal for about 1½ inches, to the level of the internal cervical os. One holds the cautery tip firmly against the anterior endocervical wall at about the 12 o'clock position and makes a linear incision out to the external os. This maneuver is repeated in rotation through 6 positions around the clock, 12–2–4–6–8–10. If there is an ectropion as well as endocervicitis, the excisions are extended onto the portio. After this the nabothian cysts are destroyed, and the entire external cervix is cauterized lightly with the flat blade of the cautery.

WHAT INSTRUCTIONS DO YOU GIVE THE PATIENT, AND HOW ESSENTIAL IS A FOLLOW-UP PROGRAM?   The patient should be told that there may be an appreciable increase in the amount of discharge for the next two or three weeks, until the slough finally separates. Frequently the discharge is foul, and it may become bloody. If the patient knows what to expect, she will be less disturbed by these unpleasant sequelae. For her comfort the patient may take hot sitz baths, but she should not resort to douches until three or four days after cauterization. If douching is done too early, distressing vaginal bleeding may follow. For the same reason intercourse is forbidden for two or three weeks, or until after the slough has separated. Even then there may be some bleeding, for a raw granulating area is left after the slough has come away. Complete epithelialization does not take place until two or three months have passed.

If the cervical cauterization is properly done, the end-result is often so perfect that the previously hypertrophied infected cervix cannot be told from normal. If the result is less than perfect, one may cauterize the external surface repeatedly without danger, but when endocervical disease is present, a repeated cauterization should not be done until after four months, and probably should not be repeated thereafter because of the danger of inducing a permanent stenosis of the canal. The most important feature of the follow-up program is concerned with preventing stenosis of the cervical canal as healing takes place. In the process of repair, adhesions form within the canal, and they should be broken up by gentle dilatation with a Hegar dilator at weekly visits for the next six weeks.

WHAT ABOUT HYAMS'S CONIZATION?   Electrocauterization may be carried out with a special cautery tip devised by Hyams. It consists of a metal rod with a fine tungsten wire at the tip shaped so that it comes to a point at the tip, but slopes off to the base to form a triangle. The tip is passed into the cervix up to the level of the internal os. As the instrument is slowly rotated the electric current resects a cone of tissue from the endocervical canal that resembles an apple core when a corer is used.

This is an excellent procedure when used properly, but it does have disadvantages. Some carry on the procedure in the office, but those of us who are less well tutored in its use prefer to do it with an anesthetic in a hospital operating room. There are two main disadvantages: (1) postoperative hemorrhage, (2) stenosis of the canal. To avoid hemorrhage the operator should take care that (a) the current in the wire is not too hot, and (b) that the cone is removed slowly and deliberately. He may choose to place a figure-of-eight stitch deep into the cervical musculature at the level of the internal os in order to constrict bilaterally the cervical branches of the uterine artery. To prevent cervical stricture one must be careful not to go up too far into the canal or to remove too much tissue. Repeated dilatations are necessary in the follow-up period to prevent stricture in the reparative stage.

ENDOMETRITIS

Though the cervix protects the other functioning parts of the genital tract against most infections that would invade from the vagina, occasionally the protection breaks down and an inflammatory process is set up within the endometrial cavity. This may then be the source of a vaginal discharge.

In the acute phase endometritis is usually caused by the gonococcus, which, as was previously noted, tends to spread superficially along contiguous mucous membrane surfaces. In this case the discharge is apt to be yellow and purulent. Another possible source of contamination is instrumentation. In this manner streptococcal and colon bacillus infections are introduced into the endometrial cavity. The response of the endometrium is in direct relation to the virulence of the infection. If an abortion has been attempted by instruments or chemical agents, the entire endometrium is transformed by streptococci into a greenish-gray slough. This is called a *diphtheritic* or *membranous endometritis*. Minor injuries produced through the introduction of instruments during a gynecologic procedure, on the other hand, cause only local reactions and a catarrhal form of endometritis, without much in the way of tissue destruction. Sometimes in the course of acute systemic infections the endometrium is involved by the hematogenous route and becomes so irritated that the discharge is bloody. This is the so-called *hemorrhagic* type of *endometritis*.

What Are the Symptoms of Acute Endometritis?

The reaction of the patient to the infection within the endometrial cavity bears a definite relation to the severity of the infection and the nature of the infecting organism. When the gonococcus is the culprit, there is little local or systemic reaction and frequently only a low-grade fever. The uterine cavity, however, does not tolerate infections caused by either the colon bacillus or streptococcus, particularly the latter. The intensity of the response is shown by a spiking temperature rise characteristic of severe infections. Locally the uterus is engorged, tense and extremely tender on motion of the cervix. Pressure usually produces a flow of foul discharge, which consists partly of blood, but is mostly pus. Since severe infections of the endometrial cavity usually spread to the fallopian tubes, the remaining symptoms are the same as those present with salpingitis and pelvic peritonitis. These entities will be discussed separately in all aspects, including treatment (Chap. 42).

Does Acute Endometritis Ever Become Chronic?

In the past many abnormal menstrual patterns were attributed to chronic endometritis. With our present knowledge of endocrinology we now recognize that most menstrual irregularities were and are due not to infection, but to hormonal imbalance. This is logical, for the endometrium is shed practically in its entirety with each menstrual period. There is little chance, then, so long as the endometrium is receiving an adequate hormonal stimulation, for most infections to progress to the chronic stage. This is less true as endocrine influences decline around the time of the menopause. Also, certain originally acute pathologic processes such as tuberculosis and septic abortions characteristically do set up a chronic endometritis. These will be discussed individually (Chaps. 41, 45).

REFERENCES

Bauer, A. C., Epifanio, A., and Redner, W. J.: Cytology of Vaginal Smears with Trichomonas. *Obst. & Gynec.*, 14: 381, 1959.

Bedoya, J. M., Rios, G., and Rico, L. R.: Trichomonadenbefall der Genitalien: venerische Erkrankung. Ergebnisse von Untersuchungen an Trichomonasleiden. *Geburt. u. Frauenh.*, 18: 989, 1958; *Internat. Abst. Surg.*, 108: 481, 1959.

Burch, T. A., Rees, C. W., and Kayhoe, D. E.: Laboratory and Clinical Studies on Vaginal Trichomoniasis. *Am. J. Obst. & Gynec.*, 76: 658, 1958.

Carter, B., Jones, C. P., Creadick, R. N., Parker, R. T., and Turner, V.: The Vaginal Fungi. *Ann. New York Acad. Sc.*, 83: 265, 1959.

Falk, H. C.: Practical Clinical Gynecology. Endocervicitis, Trichomonas Vaginalis Vaginitis. *Am. J. Surg.*, 39: 186, 1938.

Heltai, A., and Taleghany, P.: Nonspecific Vaginal Infections. A Critical Evaluation of Hemophilus Vaginitis. *Am. J. Obst. & Gynec.*, 77: 144, 1959.

Hesseltine, H. C.: Factors Relating to Mycotic and Trichomonal Infections. *Ann. New York. Acad. Sc.*, 83: 245, 1959.

Huffman, J. W.: Disorders of the External Genitals and Vagina. *Pediat. Clin. N. Amer.*, 5: 35, 1958.

Hunter, C. A., Jr., and Nicholas, H. J.: A Study of Vaginal Acids. *Am. J. Obst. & Gynec.*, 78: 282, 1959.

Jillson, O. F., and Lyle, J. S.: Yeast Vulvovaginitis. Its Successful Treatment with Nystatin (Mycostatin). *A.M.A. Arch. Dermat.*, 74: 489, 1956.

Kleegman, S. J.: Office Treatment of the Pathologic Cervix. *Am. J. Surg.*, 48: 294, 1940.

Lang, W. R.: Benign Cervical Erosion in Nonpregnant Women of Childbearing Age. *Am. J. Obst. & Gynec.*, 74: 993, 1957.

Lang, W. R., Israel, S. L., and Fritz, M. A.: Staphylococcal Vulvovaginitis; A Report of Two Cases Following Antibiotic Therapy. *Obst. & Gynec.*, 11: 352, 1958.

McGoogan, L. S.: Vaginal Discharge. *J. Michigan M. Soc.*, 55: 682, 1956.

McGruder, C. J., Jr.: Surgical Management of Chronic Pelvic Inflammatory Disease: A Study of 138 Cases. *Obst. & Gynec.*, 13: 591, 1959.

Trussell, R. E.: *Trichomonas Vaginalis and Trichomoniasis.* Springfield, Ill., Charles C Thomas, 1947.

Chapter 41

Septic Abortion

THE MOST likely causes of infection within the endometrial cavity, aside from gonorrhea, can be traced to complications incident to abortion or septic delivery. In the past severe intrauterine infections spread rapidly to the adnexa, invaded the peritoneum and blood stream and accounted for the great bulk of deaths occurring in pregnancy or the puerperium (puerperal sepsis, childbed fever). With the advent and widespread use of antibiotics and related therapeutic drugs, as well as blood transfusions, the consequences of intrauterine infections are far less grim.

It is hard to know exactly how many gynecologic patients admitted to hospital wards have had some mechanical interference with pregnancy. Approximately 40 per cent will show some evidence of infection in the uterine cavity. Uterine infection, however, is not *prima facie* evidence that an instrument has been introduced into the cavity to interrupt a pregnancy, for infection may occur after a spontaneous abortion without instrumentation. It is also well to keep in mind that a foolproof diagnosis of septic abortion cannot be made when an apparently pregnant patient enters the hospital, simply because she is running an elevated temperature and is bleeding from the uterus. These symptoms may be due to general systemic diseases, pelvic inflammations or urinary tract infections.

In most instances, however, some foreign body or substance has been introduced into the uterus with the main object of interrupting the pregnancy. The social and emotional stresses are so great that the patient does not stop to consider the consequences of her act. All manner of foreign bodies have been used, even by patients who because of their training should know better.

Infected abortion is a common complication in the pregnant patient today, regardless of the widespread use of antibiotics. It is impossible to determine the exact incidence, for only those who get into trouble enter the hospital. Despite the potent protective power of antibiotics, approximately one fifth of all gynecologic admissions to the wards of a metropolitan hospital will bear the tag of infected abortion.

There appear to be two groups of women who make up most of the patients having criminal abortions. The majority are married women who have become exhausted physically, emotionally and financially by repeated pregnancies. The probability of another child compounds their problems and is enough to derange their thinking and send them to an abortionist. The other main group is composed of young women who have become separated or divorced. They are forced through economic necessity not only to earn their own livings, but often also to support a previous child of the broken marriage. The occurrence of another pregnancy is a disaster both socially and

546

economically. Such girls are apt to go to extremes to obtain interruption of the pregnancy. With greater sexual promiscuity in the postwar years more unmarried girls have become pregnant. Undoubtedly many of these girls undergo criminal abortions, but more often they either do not recognize that they are pregnant or will not admit it until it is too late for the abortionist to accept them as patients.

We have already discussed complete, missed and incomplete spontaneous abortions in the absence of infection. Our present concern is now with the group in whom infection is either confined to the uterus itself or in whom spread has taken place to the fallopian tubes, peritoneum or blood stream.

How Do We Make a Diagnosis of Septic Abortion?

It is of fundamental importance in febrile patients to obtain information as to whether any attempt has been made to interfere with a pregnancy. The great majority will deny any such attempt, regardless of the evidence to the contrary, but approximately one quarter will admit that they have (*a*) inserted either a catheter, slippery elm sticks or some other foreign body into the uterus, or (*b*) have used some irritating douche such as Lysol, potassium permanganate, pine soap, or finally (*c*) have ingested some abortifacient pills such as quinine. We are primarily concerned here with the introduction of foreign bodies into the uterus.

HISTORY.   Since only one quarter of the patients will admit interference, the physician's suspicions may or may not be confirmed by an incomplete or misleading history. We are interested in the date of the last menstrual period and the duration of the suspected pregnancy. Most induced abortions will occur within the first trimester, usually at eleven weeks. Some idea of the timing of the suspected interference will be obtained from the history of the nature and duration of the vaginal bleeding. To obtain some idea of the localization of infection the patient should be questioned as to the nature and site of any lower abdominal pain and as to whether the fever, which is usually around 102°, has been accompanied by chills that might suggest septicemia.

PHYSICAL EXAMINATION.   Since extrauterine sources are often the cause of temperature elevations in the pregnant patient who is threatening to abort, a general physical examination is in order. Particular attention should be paid to examination of the lungs and urinary tract as the most likely sites of infection. The vaginal bleeding also may occasionally be due to such general systemic diseases as thrombocytopenic purpura.

When extragenital causes of fever and vaginal bleeding are ruled out, we then concentrate on the local pelvic findings. They may be minimal or exaggerated, depending on the severity of the infection. We are primarily interested in the size, contour and consistency of the uterus, and whether the uterus and pelvic floor are tender. The uterus could be enlarged by fibroids, or perhaps because the conceptus is still contained within the uterus, with the undelivered abortion either threatened or incomplete. The source of the pelvic infection could be extrauterine and be primarily located in the adnexa. Masses there may or may not be present.

Some infections will be confined to the uterus, while others will have spread to the tubes and peritoneum. The degree of extension of inflammatory disease beyond the uterus is best determined by a rectal examination. If spread has occurred to the parametrium and tubes, the patient may have local tenderness in both lower abdominal quadrants and also the suprapubic area on abdominal examination. With more widespread disease a localized or generalized peritonitis may be accompanied by paralytic ileus. The abdomen will be distended and intestinal peristaltic sounds absent.

LABORATORY FINDINGS.   The elevation in leukocyte count parallels the severity of the infection and the extent of its spread. If there is much parametrial involvement or actual thrombosis of the pelvic veins, the white blood cell count may be high. When the infection is confined to the uterus, the cell count is rarely over 12,000 to 14,000 per cubic millimeter. Variations in hemoglobin depend on the degree of blood loss; rarely is it less than 10 gm. per 100 ml. The red blood cell determinations frequently demonstrate little in the way of anemia.

It is customary to take blood cultures, but unless the patient has recurring bouts of fever to high levels, above 102° F. and accompanied by chills, bacteria rarely grow out. When they do, they are usually anerobic streptococci. By and large, blood cultures are useful only in the very sick patient or in one who does not respond to treatment. The same may be said of cultures taken from the vagina or cervix. Most of these cultures will show a mixture of organisms in combination with the predominant strains of alpha and beta streptococci. It would be helpful if these cultures could pinpoint the primary offending bacterial species and antibiotic sensitivity studies could provide a guide for the use of the proper antibiotic agent, but they rarely do so.

Tests of the urine for pregnancy, such as the frog test, give about the same results as for incomplete abortion in the absence of sepsis. A little over 20 per cent will be positive.

General Considerations in the Management of Septic Abortions

The primary consideration in management is based on proper evaluation of the location of the infection, its virulence and its spread. For this reason we shall discuss diagnosis and treatment, depending on whether the abortion is complete or incomplete and on whether infection has advanced beyond the confines of the uterus.

WHAT IS THE PICTURE OF INFECTION CONFINED TO THE UTERUS WITH INCOMPLETE ABORTION?   In any large series of cases between 75 and 90 per cent will have an incomplete abortion with the infection confined to the uterus. The patients are not acutely ill, but do have temperatures varying from 100 to 103° F. with a corresponding elevation of the pulse rate. The patient's last menstrual period is usually three months in the past, but there is a recent history of vaginal bleeding and abdominal cramps. The bleeding is rarely excessive. The cramps suggest that not all the products of conception have been passed. This is further confirmed on inspection of the cervical os, which is usually dilated and frequently contains placental remnants. The vaginal discharge is bloody and may be copious. The size and consistency of the uterus will depend on the duration of the pregnancy and on how much evacuation of its contents has occurred.

On bimanual examination one can elicit abdominal wall tenderness if the infected uterus is pushed up against the sensitive parietal peritoneum, but on moving the uterus with the examining finger only uterine tenderness will be present. When the uterus is examined by rectum, there will be no thickening or tenderness to either side of the cervix in the bases of the broad ligaments.

HOW DO YOU MANAGE AN INFECTED UTERUS CONTAINING AN INCOMPLETE ABORTION?   There is general agreement based on pathologic evidence that the primary site of infection in the septic abortion rests in the fetal membranes and

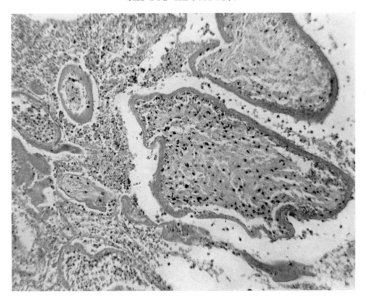

Fig. 41-1.   Chorionic villi from the placenta of a septic abortion are degenerated and infiltrated by neutrophilic leukocytes. Purulent exudate is mixed with the intervillous blood clot. Chorionamnionitis would also be present.

placenta (Fig. 41–1). Since the bacterial dissemination stems from this focus, the uterus should be evacuated as quickly as possible. Experience has shown that when there has been a delay in emptying the uterus, either because of a closed cervix or for whatever cause, infection has invariably spread beyond the uterus.

How rapidly operation is undertaken depends on the extent of the vaginal bleeding. In most cases the hemorrhage is not extreme, and one can afford to wait for twelve hours to obtain some protection from antibiotics. Penicillin and streptomycin are the chemotherapeutic agents most commonly used. Vaginal cultures take too long for completion and are of so little help that treatment should not be delayed to determine the predominant bacteria.

Penicillin, 600,000 units stat on admission followed by 300,000 units intramuscularly every 4 hours, combined with streptomycin, 0.5 gm. twice daily, will satisfactorily contain most septic abortions of this type. After twelve hours under the protection of these antibiotics the uterus is cleaned out, using either a sharp curet or placental forceps, depending on the size of the uterus. Rarely is it larger than a ten weeks' pregnancy. Some obstetricians give diluted Pitocin by intravenous drip to encourage the uterus to expel its contents. If the abortion is nearly complete, this treatment may suffice to evacuate the uterus thoroughly, but in the majority of instances it will be better to do this with a curet, particularly if the cervix is dilated.

When the uterus is larger, the vaginal bleeding is often profuse, and it may be necessary to pack the uterus to control the hemorrhage and to transfuse to replace the blood lost, before completing the evacuation by curettage.

After a complete cleanout of the endometrial cavity the patient's temperature usually returns to normal over the next 48-hour period, provided that antibiotic therapy is continued on the preoperative schedule. As a safeguard, the penicillin and streptomycin regimen is maintained either for a full five days or for forty-eight hours after the temperature has become normal.

INFECTION IN THE UTERUS WHEN THE ABORTION IS COMPLETE.   Since the primary source of infection—namely, the placenta and its membranes—is absent, the infection within the uterus is less severe, provided it has not already spread to the lymphatics in the parametrial regions or to the blood stream. The latter situation is far more common and far more dangerous than an infection confined to the uterus. The decisive factor in differential diagnosis is the degree of pelvic floor tenderness. Uterine infection alone also is accompanied by little fever and leukocytic reaction. Little vaginal bleeding is noted, and there is largely a vaginal discharge.

The treatment is tailored to the patient's less serious condition and physical findings. Supportive treatment and antibiotic therapy are usually sufficient.

PELVIC INFLAMMATION FOLLOWING INFECTION AFTER INCOMPLETE OR COMPLETE ABORTION.   The problem of spread of the infection beyond the confines of the uterus is much more serious than that of infection localized to the endometrial cavity. In the great majority the abortion is complete, but occasionally some placental fragments remain.

How Does the Spread of Infection Occur?   The primary site of infection will appear at the point of placental implantation or anywhere within the endometrial cavity if the integrity of the uterine wall has been impaired. This may be at the cervix or may occur within the uterine cavity as a result of the instrumentation. The wall may actually be perforated by the foreign body inserted in the uterus. Within the myometrium thrombosed veins and distended lymphatics are found, and they often contain pus. From these septic foci the streptococci spread by communicating veins and lymphatics to the main channels and tissue spaces in the broad ligaments. These are particularly prominent during pregnancy and aid in dissemination of the disease. As a result of this invasion several things may happen: (*a*) An extensive thrombophlebitis appears, as multiple septic thrombi fill the venous trunks. (*b*) The patient has a diffuse burning pelvic cellulitis. (*c*) The infection spreads along the veins and lymphatics to the fallopian tubes, setting up an extensive peritubal infection. (*d*) As a result of the tubal inflammation plus direct extension by way of the lymphatics the patient suffers an acute pelvic peritonitis.

What Are the Symptoms and Physical Findings?   The symptoms and physical findings are typical of acute pelvic inflammation from any cause. The preponderance of streptococci as the infecting organism explains the virulence of the infection. Since the pelvic peritoneum is affected, there is exquisite pelvic tenderness on rectal examination. Actually, there are varying degrees of pelvic peritonitis. This accounts for the lower abdominal tenderness, spasm and rebound tenderness noted on abdominal palpation and confirmed by bimanual examination. There is a considerable degree of systemic reaction. The temperature is consistently over 102° and often goes to 104° or 105°. The patient complains of abdominal pain, a direct result of the peritoneal irritation. This is the picture in most patients who have pelvic infection in association with an incomplete abortion.

Pelvic Inflammation after Complete Abortion.   The symptoms and physical findings in this instance are simply exaggerated manifestations of the picture outlined above and reflect the more overwhelming infection. The systemic reaction is more pronounced. The symptoms are actually identical with those of a generalized peritonitis. As one might suspect, the temperature falls below 103° with peaks to 105°. The pulse is rapid, may be thready and at times is out of proportion to the temperature elevation.

The abdominal findings are typical of severe peritoneal infection. The abdominal wall is tense and distended. Peristalsis is often absent, and no bowel sounds can be heard. The lower portion of the abdomen is extremely tender and rigid with protective spasm. On pelvic examination the exquisite pelvic tenderness is so extreme that it outweighs any other observation that may be made. Varying degrees of uterine fixation are noted, but the tenderness is such that it is often impossible to determine the size of the uterus or whether any pelvic masses are present.

How Does the Treatment of Pelvic Inflammation Differ from That of Infection within the Uterus Alone?   As long as the infection is confined to the uterus, it is both logical and effective therapy to empty the uterus at the earliest possible moment and to rely on antibiotics only as adjuvant therapy. In this manner serious complications and length of hospitalization are materially reduced.

When the infection has spread to the pelvis rather than resembling a localized abscess, the emphasis on therapy shifts from surgery to conservative management. The treatment is that given for generalized peritonitis. The antibiotic regimen of penicillin and streptomycin continues as long as the physical findings and condition of the patient require it. Transfusions are given to combat the toxic effects of sepsis, rather than to replace blood loss. In the acute phases of the infection, fluids are restricted by mouth, and electrolytes are replaced by intravenous therapy. Paralytic ileus is a common finding with generalized peritonitis and is combated by passing a Miller-Abbot tube into the small intestine for decompression. The head of the bed is elevated, and the patient rests in Fowler's position, which tends to localize the infection to the lower pelvis where the peritoneum has greater protective power. Sedatives and other supportive therapy are given as needed.

Several things may happen on this sort of regimen. In the majority of instances considerable improvement will be noted in the progress of the infection after the first week. In the course of the next two weeks the infection may entirely disappear. The pelvic tenderness, induration and uterine fixation subside, leaving a soft pelvic floor.

What Complications May Be Anticipated in the Course of Conservative Management? Not every case of pelvic peritonitis with an etiologic background of septic abortion clears up without any residual difficulty. Occasionally the patient has a later flareup of the infection, heralded by an elevation in temperature, a reappearance of an elevated white cell count and an increase in abdominal pain. One should be on the alert for any evidence of a broad ligament abscess. With the disappearance of the acute pelvic tenderness adnexal masses may become more obvious. Soft spots in these masses suggest fluctuating pus and provide an adequate indication for drainage. Pelvic examinations should be done every other day when this train of events exists.

What Are the Most Serious Complications of Septic Abortion?

There are two serious sequelae to pelvic infection caused by septic abortion, which have lethal implications. They are pelvic thrombophlebitis and septic shock.

PELVIC THROMBOPHLEBITIS.   The first line of defense against an overwhelming infection is the development of localized pelvic cellulitis. Occasionally, however, thromboses appear within the pelvic veins, starting in the uterine wall and gradually propagating to both uterine and ovarian veins. From there they may progressively involve the hypogastric and common iliac veins until the process finally reaches the inferior vena cava. As long as the clot is fixed to the vein wall there is no serious danger to the patient's life. Occasionally portions of the clot break off, enter the general circulation and produce death from pulmonary embolus.

The greatest challenge to the patient's life and good health appears when some of these clots become infected. Since the infection in abortion usually begins at the placental site, the veins in the uterine wall occasionally clot, but they also become infected. We are then faced with "suppurative pelvic thrombophlebitis." The same danger of fatal embolus to the lung exists, but there is the additional hazard that these infected emboli may enter the general circulation and produce a septicemia. Showers of these small infected clot fragments are set free and may lodge finally in the lung, brain, kidney or liver or even localize in the heart valves and skin. These septic foci, combined with the septicemia, contribute to the death of the patient.

How Do We Make a Differential Diagnosis between Pelvic Cellulitis and Pelvic Thrombophlebitis?   The striking and frightening fact about the diagnosis of thrombophlebitis is that there are no characteristic physical findings. The pelvic floor is usually too tender to determine much from palpation. The diagnosis of pelvic thrombophlebitis before death is made more by suspicion and conjecture than by any physical manifestation of its presence.

There are a few particular observations that arouse suspicion. Perhaps the most common symptom of thrombophlebitis is the appearance of shaking chills, which occur as showers of these small septic emboli are cast forth. These are usually accompanied by recurring bouts of a spiking kind of fever with peaks running to 105° or 106°. Blood cultures taken at this time will frequently show anerobic streptococci. There is a corresponding elevation of the pulse rate, which is sustained and does not drop with the fall in temperature. Pain is frequently absent, or at most the patient feels little discomfort.

These observations are somewhat in contrast to the findings in pelvic cellulitis, which is discussed more fully in Chapter 43. In the first place the pelvic floor is apt to be stony hard in pelvic cellulitis. The uterus and adnexa cannot be distinguished, for they are bound down in a fixed mass, but occasionally other masses can be felt. In pelvic thrombophlebitis tenderness alone is present. The fever in pelvic cellulitis is sustained and does not have the wide excursions common to thrombophlebitis. When the temperature does fall, it does so gradually, and the pulse rate follows it down. This is not true of thrombophlebitis. Chills are usually absent in pelvic cellulitis.

These differences apply only to the type of thrombophlebitis in which the thromboses are infected. Unfortunately, they give no clue to the uninfected thrombus that may become dislodged and kill the patient by pulmonary embolism. Here the swings in temperature, the chills, the elevated pulse rate are absent, and there is no clear-cut differentiation between thrombophlebitis and pelvic cellulitis.

What Is the Treatment for Pelvic Thrombophlebitis?   The majority of gynecologists prefer to step up the dosage of antibiotics, along with intensifying the rest of the supporting regimen in the patient who is suspected of harboring suppurative thrombophlebitis. Recognizing the potential danger, one should be careful not to order any anticoagulant therapy.

When the patient (*a*) fails to respond to antibiotic therapy after a week's trial or (*b*) suffers a pulmonary infarct while under antibiotic treatment, one should consider very carefully the advisability of ligating the inferior vena cava and ovarian veins to prevent a fatal outcome.

SEPTIC SHOCK.   This is the most serious and lethal complication encountered in septic abortions. In its presence immediate and drastic therapy is imperative. This calls for evacuation of the uterus under the protection of massive doses of antibiotics. Since the placenta is still in the uterus and the cervix is still closed, one may elect to do a hysterectomy rather than try to empty the uterus by curettage.

The clinical picture is fairly characteristic. The picture is that of typical shock in the absence of any external evidence of blood loss. The peripheral collapse is due to the toxic absorption from an overwhelming infection in the placenta and membranes retained within the uterus. All the elements of shock are present: (*a*) subnormal temperature, (*b*) fall in blood pressure, (*c*) rapid, thready pulse, (*d*) peripheral vascular collapse with cold, clammy, gray, pallid skin, and (*e*) apprehension.

It is not unusual to have the patient suddenly go into shock because of her critical condition while conservative therapy is being carried on in the ward. Occasionally she is brought to the hospital in shock. Transfusions are always given for the shock, since blood loss is suspected. Unfortunately blood replacement neither restores the blood pressure nor gets the patient out of her shocked state. Emergency measures must be instituted at once. After the blood pressure has been restored to normal and peripheral collapse has been overcome by intravenous fluids and Levophed (norepinephrine), the uterus should be emptied of its contents. Massive doses of antibiotics are given both before and after the operation.

Modern therapy calls for early evacuation of the uterus under the protection of antibiotics, rather than the more conservative management by antibiotics alone. Delay in emptying the uterus will almost invariably lead to spread of infection beyond the uterus. When the patient has been poorly treated or not treated at all to the point at which general peritonitis or thrombophlebitis has developed, the treatment of choice would be antibiotics combined with supportive therapy for the peritonitis. In the presence of septic shock the uterus should be emptied.

REFERENCES

Septic Abortion

Berry, L. J., Smythe, D. S., and Young, L. G.: Effects of Bacterial Endotoxin on Metabolism. *J. Exper. Med.*, 110: 389, 1959.

Bobrow, M. L., and Friedman, S.: Burns of the Vagina and Cervix Following the Use of Potassium Permanganate. *New York State J. Med.*, 58: 527, 1958.

Davis, A.: Two Thousand Six Hundred and Sixty-Five Cases of Abortion. A Clinical Survey. *Brit. M.J.*, 2: 123, 1950.

da Cunha, F. A. L., Lean, T. H., Blagg, C. R., and Parsons, F. M.: The Management of Renal Failure Following Septic Abortion. *J. Obst. & Gynaec. Brit. Emp.*, 67: 796, 1960.

Falk, H. C., and Blinick, G.: Management of Postabortal Peritonitis. *Am. J. Obst. & Gynec.*, 54: 314, 1947.

Knapp, R. C., Platt, M. A., and Douglas, R. G.: Septic Abortion; Five Year Analysis at the New York Hospital. *Obst. & Gynec.*, 15: 344, 1960.

Tenney, B., Jr., Little, B., and Wamsteker, E.: Septic Abortion. *New England J. Med.*, 257: 1022, 1957.

Turksoy, N.: The Management of Infected Abortion. *Obst. & Gynec.*, 13: 399, 1959.

Wall, L. A.: Abortions: Ten Years Experience at Kansas University Medical Center. *Am. J. Obst. & Gynec.*, 79: 510, 1960.

Complications of Septic Abortion

Adcock, L. L., and Hakanson, E. Y.: Vascular Collapse Complicating Septic Abortion. *Am. J. Obst. & Gynec.*, 79: 516, 1960.

Deane, R. M., and Russell, K. P.: Enterobacillary Septicemia and Bacterial Shock in Septic Abortion. *Am. J. Obst. & Gynec.*, 79: 528, 1960.

Dilworth, E. E., and Ward, J. V.: Bacteremic Shock in Pyelonephritis and Criminal Abortion. *Obst. & Gynec.*, 17: 160, 1961.

Fine, J.: Relation of Bacteria to the Failure of Blood-Volume Therapy in Traumatic Shock. *New England J. Med.*, 250: 889, 1954.

Melby, J. C., and Spink, W. W.: Comparative Studies on Adrenal Cortical Function and Cortisol Metabolism in Healthy Adults and in Patients with Shock Due to Infection. *J. Clin. Invest.*, 37: 1791, 1958.

Studdiford, W. E., and Douglas, G. W.: Placental Bacteremia: A Significant Finding in Septic Abortion Accompanied by Vascular Collapse. *Am. J. Obst. & Gynec.*, 71: 842, 1956.

Visscher, M. B.: Shock, with Particular Reference to Endotoxin Shock. *Postgrad. Med.*, 23: 545, 1958.

Chapter 42

Acute Pelvic Inflammation

from Causes Other than Pregnancy

It is obvious from a consideration of the spread of infection following septic abortion that several things may happen when the disease process extends beyond the confines of the uterus. There may develop a localized salpingitis, peritonitis either local or general, septicemia or an acute pelvic cellulitis. The final outcome will depend on the virulence of the infection and the resistance of the patient. The pattern of spread from whatever cause closely follows that commonly seen in postabortional or puerperal sepsis.

Among the many etiologic factors that produce nonvenereal streptococcal and staphylococcal infections other than those associated with pregnancy are (a) electrical and cold-knife cauterizations of the cervix, (b) hysterosalpingogram or endometrial biopsy, (c) high-pressure douches, (d) cervical stenosis, and (e) the use of metal or plastic stem pessaries.

How Do Cauterization and Dilation of the Cervix Produce Acute Pelvic Inflammation?

In earlier discussions we have pointed out that many patients carry potentially pathogenic bacteria within the cervical canal, particularly if the cervix happens to be lacerated and the endocervical epithelium is exposed externally or an erosion is present. Under normal conditions these bacteria are not pathogenic. When trauma is produced by instrumentation or cauterization and tissue is destroyed, the local environment is altered, resistance to infection is impaired, and spread takes place into the adjacent paracervical lymphatic channels. An ascending infection then follows with resultant pelvic cellulitis, salpingitis or peritonitis.

It is also possible that cauterization or cervical trauma incident to instrumentation may light up a pre-existing, asymptomatic, latent pelvic infection. Before advocating or utilizing cauterization or dilatation of the cervical canal, one should try to establish the presence of any evidence of pelvic inflammatory disease by both careful history and examination. An elevated sedimentation rate may provide a clue to a suspected but otherwise unidentifiable low-grade pelvic inflammation.

After conization, cauterization or too vigorous dilation of the cervix one may produce cervical stenosis. Because the drainage from the uterus is inadequate, the infection may be forced back into the lymphatic channels within the uterine wall and

555

spread from there to the collecting pathways in the pelvic connective tissue. To prevent this train of events the surgeon should dilate the cervical canal monthly for two or three months after surgical procedures of this sort.

Can Uterosalpingography or Insufflation or Endometrial Biopsy Produce Acute Pelvic Inflammation?

Uterosalpingography is used to test the patency and outline of the fallopian tubes in problems of sterility. Since many of the obstructive factors in the tubal lumen are traceable to infection, it is not surprising that occasionally an old infection may be reactivated and made acute by the introduction of iodized oil into the tubes. The same sequence of events has been known to follow simple gas insufflation in the presence of a pre-existing pelvic inflammation.

Though the risk is not great, endometrial biopsy will on occasion result in a sudden acute pelvic infection. This can be tragic, particularly if biopsy is being done as a part of a sterility investigation. The pelvic infection is probably secondary to the reactivation of a pre-existing process rather than a new one introduced by way of the endometrial cavity. Endometrial biopsy preferably should not be done in the three to five days preceding the menses.

What about Cervical Stenosis as a Cause of Acute Pelvic Inflammation?

We have previously mentioned that overenthusiastic surgical procedures may produce cervical stenosis, mild pyometra and acute pelvic inflammation. A mechanical stenosis can also be produced by pathologic lesions that arise within the endometrial cavity or endocervical canal, such as cervical polyps or fibroids. If they become wedged in the canal and lose some portion of their blood supply, they often become infected. From this septic focus an acute pelvic infection may develop, particularly if the uterus happens to be fixed in retroversion.

Are High-Pressure Vaginal Douches Dangerous?

It is possible to produce an ascending infection and acute pelvic inflammation by using a vaginal douche with too high a head of pressure, particularly if the cervical os is patulous and the uterus retroverted. It is possible to force pathogenic bacteria resident in the vagina or cervix into the endometrial cavity in this manner. In certain instances a pelvic cellulitis may be induced by dissemination of the infection into the broad ligament, veins and lymphatics from a septic focus within the uterus.

What Part Do Stem Pessaries Play in Acute Pelvic Inflammation?

In the old days stem pessaries made of a variety of forms of metal or rubber were inserted and maintained in position within the cervical canal for long periods of time as a means of contraception. Acting as a chronic irritant, they frequently produced a chronically infected cervix which on rare occasion served as the source for an acute pelvic cellulitis. One rarely sees a stem pessary used in modern gynecology, because of refinements in contraceptive technique that studiously avoid any trauma to the cervical canal.

What Kind of Disease Is Produced by Streptococcal and Staphylococcal Infection from These Sources?

The predominating organisms, such as the anerobic streptococci, hemolytic streptococci and the staphylococci, enter the extrauterine venous and lymphatic drainage system either by direct breaks in the normal tissue barrier of the cervix and vagina or from infection introduced into the endometrial cavity.

What Is the Picture within the Uterus?

This has been discussed previously under the heading of endometritis (Chap. 40). When examined under the microscope, the chronically inflamed endometrium shows a heavy infiltration of leukocytes, particularly lymphocytes and plasma cells. The degree of degeneration of the endometrial glands and stroma will depend on the severity of the infection and the response of the endometrium. If the infection is overwhelming, the necrosis may be extreme, while milder infections produce only local edema and infiltration without much loss of tissue substance. In the attempt to repair the damage when considerable tissue injury has occurred, many bizarre patterns of immature epithelial cells appear. To the unwary the picture may simulate malignant disease (Fig. 42–1).

If the infection is secondary to instrumentation of the endometrial cavity, local hyperplasia and edema appear and are confined to the endometrium, but when the septic process is severe enough to produce necrosis, the myometrial cells may likewise become swollen, edematous and infiltrated with leukocytes, including neutrophils.

When the pelvic infection stems from a primary source within the endocervix, the leukocytes such as lymphocytes and plasma cells are scattered through the

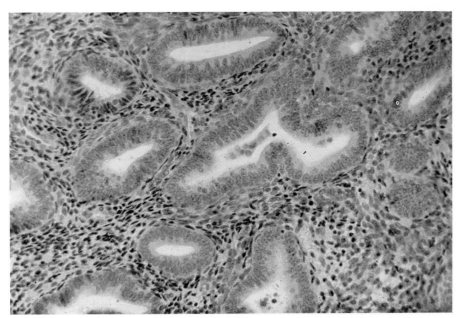

Fig. 42-1. Chronic endometritis is recognized by the identification of plasma cells in the stroma, as shown near the center of the illustration. In the presence of chronic inflammation the atypical epithelial changes that occur are generally discounted as of no precancerous significance.

edematous cervical stroma. Occasionally one finds nests of pus cells forming septic thrombi within the cervical tissue.

REFERENCES

Barrett, C. W., and Lash, A. F.: Pelvic Reactions to Infection. A Study of 493 Operative Cases. *Am. J. Surg.*, 64: 45, 1944.

Curtis, A. H.: The "Cellulitis Group" of Pelvic Infections; in *Textbook of Gynecology*. Philadelphia, W. B. Saunders Company, 1938, p. 163.

Fluhmann, C. F.: *The Cervix Uteri and Its Diseases*. Philadelphia, W. B. Saunders Company, 1961.

Gardner, G. H.: The More Common Pelvic Infections; Their Etiology, Pathology, Differential Diagnosis, Treatment and Prevention. *Northwest. Med.*, 34: 417, 1935.

Johnson, C. G., Collins, C. C., and Webster, H. B., Jr.: Pelvic Abscess. *South. M.J.*, 45: 926, 1952.

Penman, W. R., Kleppinger, R. K., Gaby, W. L., and Heller, E. M.; A Correlative Study of the Bacteriological and Clinical Results Observed in the Management of Common Pelvic Infections with a New Oral Penicillin-Sulphonamide Preparation. *Am. J. Obst. & Gynec.*, 65: 175, 1953.

Richardson, K. S.: The Diagnosis of Salpingitis. *M.J. Australia*, 12: 478, 1957.

Ringrose, C. A.: Clinical, Etiological, and Economic Aspects of Salpingitis. *Canad. M.A.J.*, 83: 53, 1960.

Walker, V. N., and Baker, A. S., Jr.: Surgical Management of Acute Pelvic Infection Refractory to Conservative Therapy. *Am. J. Obst. & Gynec.*, 82: 497, 1961.

Chapter 43

Pelvic Cellulitis

IN MOST instances after ascending infections caused by the bacteria already mentioned the patient will have pelvic cellulitis, since the spread is directly from the cervix or endometrium to the veins and lymphatics in the broad ligament (Fig. 43–1). Just as in postabortal or puerperal infections, one of several things may happen. Depending on the severity of the infection, there may be a diffuse inflammatory infiltration of all the pelvic tissues in and around the uterus, bladder or rectum, or only a minor degree of reaction in the pelvic tissues on one or both sides. In early stages the exudate is usually serous and the firm brawny hard pelvis has not yet developed. The vaginal vault or vaults feel hot and tender, and there is a sense of resistance at the base of the broad ligaments, but the unyielding rocklike masses found later are absent.

Pelvic cellulitis is apt to be more pronounced on the side the infection was introduced. There is a tendency then for it to be unilateral. The infection produces a brawny hard mass around the cervix and extending into the broad ligament on the affected side, but unless the infection is severe, the opposite side may be involved only to a minor degree.

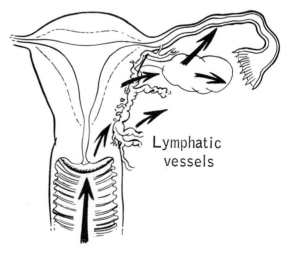

Fig. 43-1. The lymphatic and venous spread of streptococci and some other bacteria accounts for their tendency to produce a pelvic cellulitis.

Lymphatic vessels

Streptococcus

As the infection increases in severity the broad ligament becomes more involved. The cellulitis may extend (*a*) out toward Poupart's ligament, (*b*) upward above the symphysis to the level of the umbilicus, (*c*) into the iliac fossa and become palpable at the level of the anterior superior iliac spine, or (*d*) remain localized around the cervix, base of the bladder and rectum, in which case the cul-de-sac is free unless there is also a pelvic peritonitis.

Some element of thrombophlebitis is usually present. Its extent is often masked when there is heavy infiltration of the base of the broad ligament. The infected thrombus is more evident and is prone to shed septic emboli into the general circulation. A silent pelvic thrombus gives little indication of its presence and may be unsuspected until a fatal embolus lodges in the pulmonary circulation.

The cellulitis may respond rapidly to appropriate therapy or go on to the chronic phase with or without abscess formation.

Why Do Streptococci and Staphylococci Produce a Perisalpingitis?

When a pre-existing infection flares up or an ascending infection involves the fallopian tube, an acute perisalpingitis results. The infection is primarily in the lymphatic and venous channels around the tube and within its walls rather than in the tubal epithelium itself. This is in contrast to gonococcal infections, in which the organism ascends from the endometrium to produce an endosalpingitis as the tubal epithelium becomes involved. In most instances, then, in ascending infections other than gonorrhea the tubal mucosa is undamaged. If a streptococcal infection within the uterus is severe enough, it may spread to the tube, but usually so much edema is produced that the uterine isthmic opening to the tube is sealed early in the course of infection. Usually the fimbriated end of the tube remains open, but if the surrounding pelvic peritoneum is sufficiently involved, the abdominal tubal ostia are often closed by adhesions due to the inflammatory process. A hydrosalpinx results, though neither the mucosa nor fimbria is badly damaged.

The characteristic gross picture of the tube during the acute phase is one of

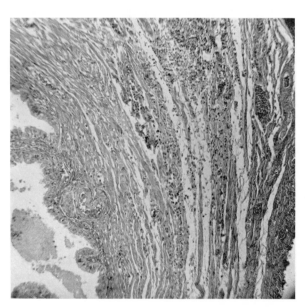

Fig. 43-2. Edema and leukocytes within the tubal subserosal and muscular layers indicate a bacterial perisalpingitis.

intense thickening of the mesosalpinx, together with a heavy infiltration of the tubal musculature while the mucosa remains relatively undamaged. The tubes are surrounded by a serous and fibrinous exudate, because one rarely finds any degree of tubal infection without an accompanying local pelvic peritonitis. It is almost an invariable sequel. It is these thin, filmy fibrinous bands that later become adhesions and account for the kinking and tortuosity of the tube so characteristic of perisalpingitis in the chronic stage. Infection is apt to linger in these adhesions without producing any suggestive symptoms. This probably explains unexpected flareups following instrumentation.

The microscopic picture shows infiltration of the tubal muscular wall with edema and leukocytes, and relatively minor edema in the tubal mucosa. The serosal surface of the tube and the adjacent pelvic peritoneum take part in the inflammatory response (Fig. 43–2).

To What Extent Does the Peritoneum Take Part in the Acute Infection?

One rarely sees an acute salpingitis from streptococcal infections without some reaction on the part of the pelvic peritoneum. Furthermore it usually becomes involved when there is any great degree of pelvic cellulitis or thrombophlebitis, as a result of lymphatic permeation. If the infection is at all severe, the peritonitis is usually widespread throughout the lower pelvis and extends, for example, to the appendiceal serosa. In the early phases the peritoneum is covered by a shaggy exudate that later organizes to form adhesions and binds all the pelvic structures into one solid irregular mass, often without recognizable anatomic landmarks. Within this mass lie the uterus, tubes, ovaries and not infrequently pelvic abscesses. Usually these abscesses lie between, rather than within, the major structures. Thus we have tubo-ovarian abscesses that surround both, but do not spread into the interior of either.

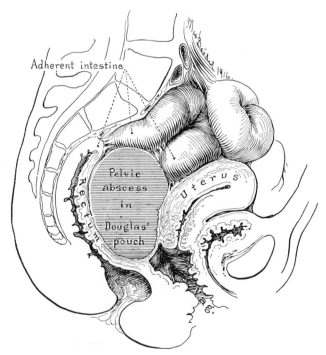

Fig. 43-3. Pelvic peritonitis with the formation of adhesions and a retrouterine abscess in the pouch of Douglas may complicate a severe salpingitis. (Cullen: *Surg., Gynec. & Obst.*, Vol. 25.)

Since the exudate binds the posterior peritoneum and back of the broad ligament to the tubal wall and mesosalpinx, the tube is drawn backward into the cul-de-sac, and the abscesses tend to localize there (Fig. 43–3). The omentum and intestine play their usual roles in the natural defense process, and fairly rapidly after the infection gets started they become intimately adherent to the pelvic mass. A certain amount of ascitic fluid is always present as the peritoneum reacts to the infection.

Does the Ovary Become Involved in Acute Pelvic Inflammation?

The ovary is exposed both by contiguity and lymphatic drainage to the same influences that produce infection in and around the fallopian tube, but it is implicated far less often. Because of its anatomic location it does frequently become surrounded by an infectious process, but actual penetration of the infection into the ovarian substance is relatively rare. Ovarian abscesses can occur in acute pelvic inflammation, but in the majority of instances the infection is a "peri-oophoritis" and the abscess is tubo-ovarian.

In response to the infection around it (peri-oophoritis) the ovary itself becomes edematous, swollen and covered with flakes of fibrin. In the early phases the ovary can readily be separated from the tube. Later the fibrin organizes and adhesions develop, while the cortex of the ovary may become thickened by fibrosis which prevents extension of inflammation into the interior. Because of these adhesions the ovary becomes fixed to the tube and often to surrounding structures. Adhesions tend to trap exudate produced in response to the peritoneal insult, and inflammatory peritoneal inclusion cysts may form that surround both the tube and ovary (Fig. 43–4).

It is possible for the patient to have an "interstitial oophoritis" in the course of an acute streptococcal infection. Blood stream invasion can cause this if the patient has a septicemia, but more often the invasion is direct. The infection gains access to the interior of the ovary by breaks in the continuity of its surface after rupture of either a follicle or a corpus luteum. The process tends to be confined to the developing corpus luteum, without involving the ovarian stroma. It does cause hyperemia, and not infrequently a hematoma develops that constitutes a fine culture medium for the infecting organisms. This is a true corpus luteum abscess, as shown by the fact that

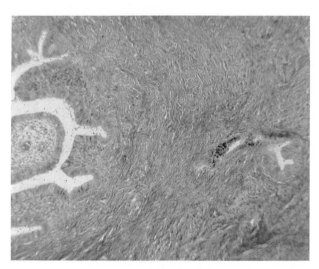

Fig. 43-4. The fibrous scar tissue in the center of the illustration is part of a tubo-ovarian adhesion with trapped foci of germinal epithelium within it.

lutein cells line the abscess cavity when it is excised early in the course of the infection. Follicular abscesses occur through direct spread into a recently ruptured follicle at the time of ovulation, although a primary septicemic cause is possible.

Multiple abscesses sometimes develop in the stroma of the ovary as a result of scattered septic emboli from the blood stream in the course of a general septicemia, but they do not occur from direct invasion of the ovary.

Once an ovarian infection becomes established, it is far harder to eliminate than from other pelvic structures such as the tube, for it responds indifferently to therapy that works effectively elsewhere.

What Symptoms Are Produced by Acute Pelvic Inflammation of Streptococcal Origin in the Absence of Pregnancy?

ENDOMETRITIS.   When the infection is confined to the uterus, the symptoms are not dramatic and are directly proportional to the virulence of the organism and the extent of necrosis produced. If there is a great deal of endometrial degeneration and inflammatory infiltration of the uterine wall, the patient will run a spiking temperature with an accompanying elevation of the leukocyte count. There is some increase in the amount of leukorrhea with a tendency of the discharge to become foul. A moderate amount of vaginal bleeding may be expected. On physical examination the foul discharge can be seen oozing from the cervical canal, and the uterus is often somewhat enlarged and is always tender when the cervix is moved.

In most cases the symptoms are both minimal and transient. The response to treatment is rapid, provided extension of infection has not already taken place to the tubes or pelvic connective tissue.

SALPINGITIS AND OOPHORITIS.   The symptoms of acute inflammation of the tube and ovary are not readily dissociated from those produced by the accompanying pelvic peritonitis. Later, in the chronic phase, when localizing signs appear such as definite masses or palpable tubes, the differentiation is easier. Symptoms depend in large part upon how virulent the infection is and how rapidly it spreads upward from its source to involve the tube. About all that can be told in the acute fulminating spread is that one is dealing with an "acute abdomen" without localizing signs. One must then exclude acute appendicitis, pyelitis, torsion of an ovarian pedicle and diverticulitis, among other entities that may produce evidence of a pelvic infection.

In the overwhelming acute phases the patient is acutely but not dangerously ill. The temperature usually spikes to 103° and 104° with an accompanying elevation of both pulse and leukocyte count. The lower quadrants of the abdomen are distended and acutely tender to palpation. The patient complains of pain through the lower portion of the abdomen, which is often made worse by voiding or defecation. All these factors point to pelvic peritonitis secondary to a variety of causes, but are not pathognomonic of acute infection of the fallopian tube. There is one important symptom lacking that is of material help in differentiating acute salpingitis from peritonitis due to other cause such as appendicitis. Vomiting is rare in acute salpingitis, but common in patients with appendicitis.

In most instances the onset is less dramatic, but pain and fever appear a few days after the instrumentation or other factor that precipitated the infection. The disease may progress to produce the symptoms described above, or it may subside rapidly, depending on the virulence of the affecting organism and the ability of the peritoneum to wall off and localize the infection. In some instances under proper therapy the fever and pain may subside rapidly, leaving no residue after a few days. In others the irregularly elevated temperature persists and not infrequently flares up as the infection breaks through the protective barrier and involves previously uncontaminated areas of the peritoneum.

Abscess formation may occur early in the course of the acute infection with or without any change in the symptoms. Repeated estimations of the total and differential white blood cell counts are important, particularly when increased band forms or young neutrophils appear. One should be suspicious that suppuration is developing when comparison of the leukocyte counts shows the total number of white cells to increase from 10,000 or 15,000 per cubic millimeter to 20,000 or more, particularly when the differential count shows an increasing proportion of polymorphonuclear leukocytes, 80 per cent or higher. This usually means that pus has collected or is being produced. The erythrocyte sedimentation rate is also helpful. In acute infection the rate may be four times the normal value or more. The increase of sedimentation is proportional to and reflects the severity of the infection. Used in combination with the white cell count and differential, it gives a fair idea of the progress of infection in the lower pelvis.

What Symptoms Do We Associate with Pelvic Peritonitis?

A more generalized pelvic peritonitis occurs with streptococcal infection than one customarily finds with gonococcal infection, in which peritoneal contamination is apt to be less widespread. It is usually ushered in by a sharp rise in temperature associated with acute pain over the lower portion of the abdomen, rapid pulse and vomiting if the infection is sufficiently widespread. The abdomen is distended at first in the lower portions, but distention becomes more generalized as the infection spreads. The abdomen is tender to touch, particularly over the pubic symphysis and in both lower quadrants, with spasm present throughout the same area. As in salpingitis, the symptoms are exaggerated by voiding and defecation.

In the acute phases there is usually so much induration secondary to pelvic cellulitis that it is impossible to distinguish the thickened tubes as a separate entity. Abscesses often form early in the course of the infection and sometimes can be felt as a tender mass behind the cervix in the cul-de-sac, bulging into the vagina and pushing the uterus forward.

What Are the Signs and Symptoms of Pelvic Cellulitis in the Acute Phases of Non-puerperal Streptococcal Infections?

In most instances pelvic cellulitis follows an infection that arises in lacerations of the cervix, vagina or lower uterine segments, from instrumentation or surgical procedures applied to these areas. It may of course be part of a pelvic peritonitis or salpingo-oophoritis. Since cellulitis is far more dangerous, it fortunately is rare, as compared with pelvic peritonitis. In evaluating the symptoms arising from pelvic cellulitis per se, we must be aware that it is often accompanied by varying degrees of thrombophlebitis.

Symptoms usually appear a few days after instrumentation or manipulation of the cervical canal. The first noticeable sign is a feeling of general malaise accompanied by a high sustained fever that shows little tendency to drop. The pulse rate in patients with pelvic cellulitis parallels the course of the temperature. As the fever declines, so does the pulse rate. This is a significant observation in distinguishing pelvic cellulitis from suppurative pelvic thrombophlebitis. In the latter the fever runs a spiking course with daily peaks rising to 105° or higher. The pulse rate, however, is sustained and does not follow the temperature downward.

Pain is a great variable in the acute phases. If the infection is extensive, the patient usually complains of pelvic pain, but if not, the pain may be minimal or absent. If the pain is extreme, it usually means that there is an accompanying pelvic peritonitis. Pain is an infrequent part of the picture of thrombophlebitis, but the presence of chills is most common. The chills occur periodically as septic emboli shower forth into the general circulation from the infected venous thromboses in the pelvic connective tissue. As one might suspect, the leukocyte count is elevated and the sedimentation rate increased. In estimating the persistence of the infection the sedimentation rate is a better guide, particularly in thrombophlebitis, since it will still show an abnormally increased value even though the white cell count has returned to normal levels.

On physical examination during the early phases of acute pelvic cellulitis, before the exudate organizes, the only physical findings may be a sense of resistance and exquisite tenderness in the vaginal fornices. Within a matter of days the exudate organizes on one or both sides, and rocklike masses can be felt around the cervix, extending out laterally or posteriorly in the direction of the rectum. The uterus becomes fixed, and the mass bulges into the vagina, thereby obliterating the usual fornix. The more pronounced findings are noted on the side that provided entry to the invading organisms, with relatively little induration on the opposite side.

The typical findings of pelvic cellulitis, then, are the tenderness at the base of both broad ligaments, together with uterine fixation and the presence of rocklike masses on one or both sides. Rarely one finds tenderness and palpably engorged veins on the pelvic floor, in the absence of the hard masses or fixation. Such patients usually have a predominant element of thrombophlebitis. This, however, is in sharp contrast to the usual findings, for cellulitis alone is much more common.

Differentiation between Pelvic Cellulitis and Pelvic Peritonitis

In the more complete discussion of streptococcal infections as they applied to septic abortions (Chap. 41) we attempted to point out the basic points of difference between pelvic cellulitis and thrombophlebitis. It is also important to distinguish pelvic peritonitis as far as possible from pelvic cellulitis. Recounting of the differences will serve as a summary:

(1) Although pelvic peritonitis is relatively common, pelvic cellulitis is relatively rare. (2) When it does appear, pelvic cellulitis usually follows some form of trauma to the endocervix, lower uterine segment or vagina. Pelvic peritonitis, on the other hand, usually has salpingitis as a precursor. (3) In the early phases of pelvic peritonitis there may be a considerable amount of lower abdominal pain. Pain is often lacking in pelvic cellulitis. (4) On vaginal or rectal examination one usually feels a fixed cervix surrounded by a band of indurated tissue that often extends out on one side and frequently posteriorly compressing the rectum when the infection has produced pelvic cellulitis. It is primarily a unilateral lesion. In pelvic peritonitis the cervix is not fixed, though it is painful on motion. The irregular masses are always felt bilaterally behind the cervix, and there is no tendency to encroach on the rectum.

Initially, pelvic cellulitis is more dangerous to the patient's life than localized pelvic peritonitis. As the infection responds to treatment, pelvic cellulitis leaves far less residual damage and has a much better prognosis for complete recovery than pelvic peritonitis. Although pelvic cellulitis usually disappears entirely, pelvic peritonitis often persists. The adhesions formed by pelvic peritonitis immobilize the uterus and interfere with the motility of the fallopian tube. Such patients are often made permanently sterile and may become chronic invalids because of persistent pelvic pain. The residual infection not infrequently flares up into acute activity with minimal trauma years after the initial infection.

Treatment of the Acute Phase of Streptococcal Infection of Nonpuerperal Origin

In the acute phases of streptococcal infection due to a cause other than septic abortion or puerperal infection, the treatment is largely a supportive regimen amply supplemented by antibiotic therapy. At the onset of the infection the patient should be put to bed and maintained in Fowler's position, which is designed to keep the infection localized to the lower pelvis. The peritoneum of the lower pelvis is far better equipped to deal with infection than is that of the upper part of the abdomen. The semisitting position with the legs bent also takes strain off the abdominal muscles and the inflamed parietal peritoneum. The patient is therefore more comfortable. The pain may be severe enough to require opiates for relief. Though the pain may be mild, discomfort and apprehension are sufficient to keep the patient awake and make her restless, unless sedatives in the form of barbiturates are given.

The most important direct attack upon the infection is the immediate use of antibiotics in large quantity. Before starting the therapy it is advisable to try to obtain a culture of any discharge. In most instances it will show some form of anerobic or hemolytic streptococcus and occasionally a staphylococcus. The rarer infections will arise from invasion by *E. coli*, *Cl. welchii*, pneumococci and occasionally gonococci. There is no occasion, however, to hold off the antibiotic therapy until the culture reports are received, for this may take twenty-four to forty-eight hours. It is customary to use penicillin and streptomycin. Penicillin, 600,000 units, is given on admission to the hospital, followed by 300,000 units intramuscularly every 4 hours. This is combined with streptomycin, 0.5 gm. twice daily. If one chooses, sulfadiazine in full doses may be given instead of the streptomycin. Occasionally the cultures indicate a mixed infection, which may call for the use of one of the broad-spectrum antibiotics. Sensitivity studies on cultures should be done to select the proper drug.

In the early phases the temperature is frequently elevated to 104° or 105°, and at times there may be nausea and vomiting. Dehydration should be combated and the electrolyte balance restored by intravenous administration of saline, glucose and the replacement of any electrolytes that may be deficient. Blood transfusions are given according to need. As soon as possible the patient should be encouraged to take fluids by mouth.

In the presence of abdominal distention secondary to pelvic peritonitis there may be a large element of paralytic ileus. The bowel should be decompressed by passing a Miller-Abbot tube into the small intestine. When there is no longer need to decompress the small bowel, the tube is withdrawn. A soft diet can be given as soon as it can be tolerated. It is also important to promote free bowel elimination and to prevent constipation. This had best be done by enema rather than cathartic. Warm enemas of saline, soap suds or oil are usually effective. With favorable progress of the dsiease, the patient later may be given mild laxatives.

The pelvic infection itself is best dealt with locally by the frequent use of large quantities of warm tap water or saline applied in the vaginal canal as a douche. Heat is more important than any ingredient placed in the douche water. It is customary to order a 6-quart douche. Whenever possible, it should be taken with the patient lying on her back with her buttocks slightly elevated. The douche should have a low pressure, easily regulated by the height of the douche bag above the patient.

Under this regimen the infection should respond, as judged by a fall in the temperature and pulse rate, improvement in the patient's general condition and a decline in the white cell count, with return to normal of the differential count and sedimentation rate. If the favorable progress is steady, it is best not to examine the patient vaginally or rectally during the acute phases of the infection.

Pelvic abscesses may point toward the rectum if there is much associated pelvic peritonitis or toward the groin if the process is primarily a pelvic cellulitis. If the patient does not respond satisfactorily, one should examine her to search for soft spots within the firm or hard areas of induration suggesting pus present that should be drained.

What Is the End-Result of Acute Pelvic Cellulitis?

With the advent of chemotherapy and antibiotics the natural course of pelvic cellulitis has changed appreciably. Suppuration is now relatively rare. In most instances the exudation subsides without leaving any residual that will interfere with normal function. The convalescent period, however, is apt to be prolonged, for the pelvic exudate absorbs slowly. The acute symptoms may subside, but the patient frequently runs a low-grade fever and complains of varying degrees of pelvic pain as well as local tenderness. The convalescence is often punctuated by bouts of flaring temperature rise accompanied by exacerbations of pain, which last about two or three weeks and recur at monthly intervals during the next twelve or eighteen months.

Treatment

Because of these recurring episodes of infection one is tempted to use some surgical procedure. If possible, it is better not to try to interfere too soon, because of the danger of stirring up a more severe infection. The longer one postpones operation in the absence of any indication of encapsulated pus, the more satisfactory will be the result. One may be forced to operate if (*a*) the attacks recur too frequently; (*b*) the pain is persistent and incapacitating; (*c*) the recurring episodes are accompanied by signs of peritonitis; or (*d*) signs of intestinal obstruction appear. One may then operate under the protection of heavy doses of antibiotics and chemotherapeutic agents, given both before and after operation.

Though suppuration is rare today, it does present a real problem in management when it does occur. Fortunately the pus usually seeks an external exit on the abdominal wall, and rarely perforates into the bladder, rectum or vagina. The majority of pus pockets will come to a point on the lower abdominal wall to either side of the pubic symphysis close to the inner end of the attachment of the inguinal (Poupart's) ligament. Less often the abscess will localize laterally on the outer portions of Poupart's ligament, around the kidney or in the gluteal region. Since the process of resolution is a slow one, the evidence of suppuration may not appear for two or three months. It is suspected by the presence of pitting edema or soft spots within the area of induration.

When the pus is evacuated and drained adequately, the patient usually recovers promptly.

REFERENCES

Curtis, A. H., and Huffman, J. W.: Chronic Pelvic Cellulitis; in *Textbook of Gynecology*. Philadelphia, W. B. Saunders Company, 1950.

Freed, C. R., and Chatfield, R. C.: Surgical Treatment of Pelvic Inflammatory Disease. *Rocky Mountain M.J.*, 54: 907, 1957.

Haddad, G. H., and Decker, W. H.: Superior Mesenteric Syndrome Following Pelvic Inflammatory Disease. *Am. J. Obst. & Gynec.*, 78: 1301, 1959.

Peel, J. H.: The Role of Major Surgery in Infertility; Pelvic Inflammatory Disease. *Am. J. Obst. & Gynec.*, 71: 712, 1956.

Robinson, S. C.: Pelvic Abscess. *Am. J. Obst. & Gynec.*, 81: 250, 1961.

Solomons, B.: The Conservative Treatment of Pathological Conditions of the Fallopian Tubes. *J. Obst. & Gynaec. Brit. Emp.*, 43: 619, 1936.

Vermeeren, J., and TeLinde, R. W.: Intra-abdominal Rupture of Pelvic Abscesses. *Am. J. Obst. & Gynec.*, 68: 402, 1954.

Wills, S. H., Jacobs, W. M., Lauden, A. E., and Fromhagen, C.: Cortisone and Tetracycline in Resistant Pelvic Inflammatory Disease; Further Observations. *Obst. & Gynec.*, 11: 112, 1958.

Chapter 44

Gonorrhea

IN THE not too distant past when an explanation was sought for the presence of any pelvic infection, gonorrhea and tuberculosis dominated medical thinking. Though both entities are still present in the community and continue to produce many tragedies, particularly in the field of infertility, they have declined steadily in incidence. Both have succumbed to a better understanding of public health problems in relation to the known life history of the diseases. By education of the public the contagiousness and serious consequences of these disease entities have become common knowledge. Most are now aware that the infection may be spread by carriers, who either do not know that they have the disease or believe themselves to be cured. There has been far greater emphasis on the need for segregating infected from uninfected persons. Antibiotic agents and chemotherapeutic drugs have materially increased the number of cures and arrested cases, thereby reducing the number of unsuspected carriers of both gonorrhea and tuberculosis.

Gonorrhea and tuberculosis in the genital tract both act upon the mucosal lining of the uterus and tube to produce lesions that are not clinically too dissimilar. In this they differ materially from streptococcal infections, which produce perisalpingitis rather than endosalpingitis. Although both gonorrhea and genital tuberculosis spread along mucous membrane surfaces rather than lymphatic pathways, they do differ in the direction of the spread. Gonorrhea is primarily an ascending infection, while tuberculosis usually infects the endometrial cavity only after a primary attack on the tubal mucosa.

As a form of venereal disease gonorrhea was known to the ancients of all countries, and there are reported references to it in biblical history. As early as the fourteenth century the disease was linked to the act of coitus, and its contagiousness suspected. For approximately two centuries considerable confusion existed as to whether syphilis and gonorrhea were one and the same disease with different manifestations. In the nineteenth century the true nature of gonorrhea was finally recognized. Gradually the present concept of its natural history developed. Originally gonorrhea in the female was thought to be a simple vaginitis. Later Noeggerath (1872) championed the observation that the disease existed in both acute and latent forms and was actually an ascending infection that affected the uterus, tubes, ovaries and pelvic peritoneum. Finally the causative organism was isolated by Neisser, grown on artificial culture media by Bumm and differentially stained by Roux.

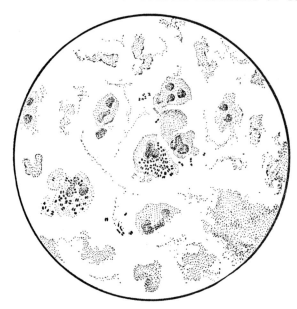

Fig. 44-1.   Drawing of smear of the cervical discharge in acute gonorrhea. The gram-negative intracellular diplococci (often reported as GNID) in neutrophils are typical of *Neisseria gonorrhoeae*.

How Does One Recognize the Gonococcus?

The gonococcus has readily recognizable characteristics on both smear and culture. Since special culture media are necessary to grow the gonococcus, initial efforts to identify the organisms are made by smear. The discharge to be smeared is obtained from the external urethra, Skene's glands or the uterine cervix. Customarily one tries to obtain the pus discharge by stripping the urethra from the neck of the bladder to the external meatus by pressure of the index finger. Pus, which is characteristically thick and light yellow, may be collected from the cervical canal after gentle cleansing of the external cervix with cotton. The previous use of a douche or any cleansing agent may interfere with the collection of a suitable sample of pus. When obtained, a drop of the discharge should be placed on a glass slide and stained by the Gram technique.

The gonococci tend to appear in pairs, though they may be found in groups of four or eight. They are recognized as large, rounded, biscuit-shaped diplococci. These are gram-negative organisms. One of the chief factors in differentiating the gonococcus from other organisms is the characteristic arrangement of the diplococci within the cytoplasm of the leukocytes. The intracellular position of the organism is important. G.N.I.D., the abbreviation for gram-negative intracellular diplococci, is used to report smears of bacteria that appear morphologically to represent gonococci (Fig. 44–1).

In some instances the disease is suspected, but smears of the discharge show only a few biscuit-shaped diplococci, which tend to be extracellular rather than intracellular. It is extremely important that such a patient not be labeled with a false diagnosis of gonorrhea. Many chronic cases of gonorrhea fail to show the gonococci on smear, yet demonstrate the organisms on culture of the discharge.

When there is any doubt about the diagnosis on smear examination, a drop of the discharge should be inoculated on chocolate (blood) agar or agar combined with ascitic or hydrocele fluid. The gonococcus does not grow readily on ordinary culture media. Even on chocolate agar the organisms die readily, particularly when exposed to heat or drying. Diagnosis by culture is far more accurate than by smear. It is unwise, however, to accept a single negative report as proof if there is clinical suspicion of the disease. Repeated cultures at spaced intervals are essential, particularly when they are being used as the final evidence to determine whether the patient has been cured of her disease.

How Does the Patient Acquire the Disease or Become Infected?

In most instances the patient becomes infected through direct sexual contact in the act of coitus. Since the organism has been found to be highly contagious in the human being, it is also possible for the disease to spread by indirect methods. Patients frequently give a history of acquiring the disease after using an infected toilet seat, but in all probability infection from this source is relatively rare, though it is still possible. It could be spread by instruments used in the physician's office. Since both heat and drying tend to kill the gonococcus very easily, one would have to presuppose that a fresh drop of pus was present in either instance.

It is true that the disease can be disseminated to other people and other mucous membrane surfaces in the same person by unclean hands. Children, for example, should be kept from contact with a known infected adult, for the disease may be spread by actual handling of the child or contamination of towels or bed linen. There is no better example of the contagious potential of gonorrheal infection than the bonfire-like spread of the disease through a children's hospital ward. Since this possibility is well recognized, such episodes are largely a thing of the past if adequate security measures are taken.

How Does the Disease Spread and Manifest Itself?

The destructive effects produced by the gonococcus are for the most part due to an endotoxin that sets up a severe inflammatory response in the mucosal-lined structures that it invades. The catarrhal exudate produced is largely made up of serum and pus cells with little or no fibrin. Frequently the infection spreads upward along the epithelial surfaces without producing any notable necrosis in the epithelium itself. Occasionally, because of the virulence of the infection or lowered local tissue resistance, destruction of the epithelium occurs and abscesses develop locally; or in extreme cases blood vessel invasion takes place with resultant gonorrheal septicemia. With the organisms in the blood stream one can expect widespread dissemination to joints, tendons, meninges and endocardium.

The incubation period usually ranges from three to eleven days in most instances. Gonorrhea remains in the acute phase for several weeks, but gradually passes into the chronic state. This is the stage when it is most commonly found. During the acute phase the disease is usually confined to the genital tract below the level of the cervix. Thus the urethra, Skene's glands, the cervix and Bartholin's glands are the areas primarily attacked in a fresh infection. There the infection tends to remain until the next menstrual period, when it ascends into the endometrial cavity and spreads to the tube and peritoneum. It is highly desirable that the disease be recognized when it is sharply localized to the lower genital tract, for at this point the areas are accessible and the organisms highly vulnerable to chemotherapeutic agents. Unfortunately the symptoms are often so minimal that the patient is hardly aware of any infection. If we are to prevent the ascending infection and subsequent tubal involvement, which is far more difficult to cure and frequently results in sterility, we must recognize and treat gonorrhea while it is still a local disease confined to the region below the cervix.

How Do We Recognize Gonorrhea in the Early Stages?

The chief symptoms, which may be only slight burning on micturition, urinary frequency and an increase in the amount of vaginal discharge, usually appear three or four days after a known exposure by sexual intercourse. The *urethra* is the most vulnerable area because of its exposed position. In response to the toxin produced by the gonococcus the mucosal lining rapidly becomes swollen, edematous and bathed in a greenish-yellow pus. It appears red and inflamed and frequently pouts outward. In many instances the infection passes upward along the entire urethral canal to the neck of the bladder. On direct inspection the red, swollen urethral mucosa can be seen covered with pus through its entire extent. With this degree of involvement there is a considerable degree of urinary frequency, accompanied by a dull cramplike pain as the patient tries to pass urine over the inflamed surfaces. Some women have a minimal degree of dysuria and hardly any increase in the amount of leukorrhea, but the great majority are sorely tried by the distressing pain on micturition.

Minor abrasions are frequent in and around the urethra because of its exposed position. If breaks are present in the epithelial lining, the gonococcus penetrates into the underlying connective tissue. The environment is favorable for its survival and proliferation, and a suppurative process is set up. Paraurethral abscesses and suppuration in Skene's glands are common findings in the acute phase of the disease. When gonorrheal penetration has occurred, the disease is much harder to cure, and latent infections persist for months after the gonococcal infection has passed into the chronic phase.

THE VULVA.   Since the urethra is commonly involved and is a major source of the acute exudative response to the gonorrheal infection, it is not surprising that the vulva becomes actively involved, since it is constantly bathed in pus. The situation is made worse if the infection sets up a suppurative process in the paraurethral (Skene's) or Bartholin's glands. The discharge is often abundant and intensely irritating. As a result the labia become edematous, red and swollen and frequently seem to be bound together. Excoriation may be present, and voiding is exquisitely painful. Occasionally the discharge is so irritating that the vulva responds by forming condylomata, which may be venereal warts (condylomata acuminata) due to a symbiotic virus. These occur anywhere on the perineum around the vulva, on the medial surfaces of the thighs, or extending up the entire length of the vaginal canal. They vary widely in appearance. Frequently they are pedunculated and have a fine stalk. They have a tendency to fuse. Thus there are all gradations from warty growths with a fine individual stalk to solid masses of tissue that cover the whole vulvar area (Fig. 44–2). As the acute infection subsides they usually disappear, but they may persist into the chronic phase if the disease is neglected or inadequately treated. Vulvovaginitis of gonorrheal origin is most severe in children.

VAGINAL INFECTION.   The principal method used by the gonococcus in its upward spread is to progress along mucous membrane surfaces. One would expect, then, that the vagina would be a common place for the gonococcus to proliferate in. Actually, except in children, pregnant women and the aged, vaginal infections are rare. The normal adult stratified vaginal epithelium, which is lacking in children, seems to provide protection against the penetrating power of the gonococcus. If the vaginal canal does appear to be red, swollen and edematous, it is probably because the cervix is infected and the vaginal epithelium secondarily irritated. (Fig. 44-3).

Gonorrheal infection in children has been discussed previously (p. 132). In the young pregnant patient, when hormonal stimulation has altered the vaginal epithelium from its normal keratinized state, gonorrheal vaginitis may occur. Similarly the parchment-like vaginal epithelium of older women may crack sufficiently to permit the gonococcus to gain a foothold in the subepithelial tissue.

When gonorrheal vaginitis does occur, it is exquisitely painful, owing to the extensive inflammatory reaction in the vaginal epithelium, which is red, swollen and edematous. Pus covers every crevice within the vaginal epithelium throughout the canal and spills over onto the vulva, which becomes intensely irritated and swollen. The labial folds are often obliterated and so eroded by the necrotizing action of the infection that they actually adhere. Voiding is extremely painful, and walking becomes a torture. The patient complains bitterly of pain and burning within the vaginal canal. This acute phase persists for two or three weeks, only to disappear thereafter, leaving little evidence except in the cervix that the vagina has ever been involved.

BARTHOLINITIS.   Although the vagina is implicated relatively infrequently, infection in Bartholin's glands is common. Since there are two such glands, situated one on each side of the vulva, bilateral involvement is to be expected. The first evidence

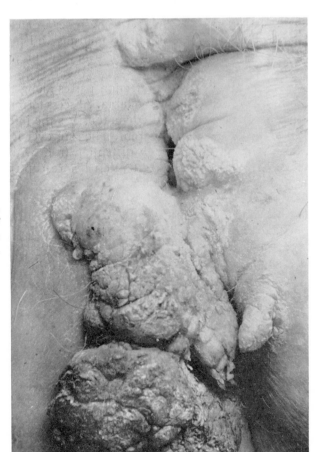

Fig. 44-2. Unusually large masses of condylomata acuminata of the vulva. These had no known relation to gonorrhea. (Courtesy of Dr. F. Ronchese, Providence, R.I.)

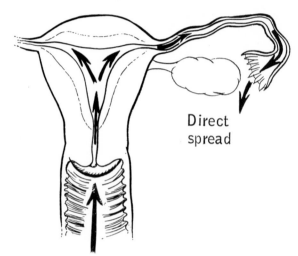

Direct spread

Staphylococcus and Gonococcus

Fig. 44-3. The surface spread of infection is characteristic of gonorrheal and staphylococcal pelvic inflammatory disease.

of Bartholin gland infection is noted at the opening of its duct into the vagina just above the fourchette on either side. The meatus is red and swollen and pouts out into the vaginal canal. Formerly this was regarded as pathognomonic of gonorrheal infection, but other nonspecific organisms will produce the same appearance. The diagnosis can be made only by smear and culture, using a drop of pus expressed from the duct.

In most instances the infection passes along the duct epithelium to involve the gland proper, deep within the labia. Abscess formation is common. The surrounding tissues become swollen and edematous. As the infected gland expands, the localized swelling becomes more apparent. The skin over it is placed on tension and becomes reddish-purple. After enough distention from within, the abscess will rupture spontaneously. While it is under tension before rupture, the patient complains of local soreness, pain on micturition and difficulty in walking or sitting. Occasionally these abscesses regress without drainage, either spontaneous or surgical, but the majority have to be evacuated surgically to relieve symptoms. Again, one should be careful about making a diagnosis of gonorrhea simply because the patient has a Bartholin's abscess. In the past such presumptive diagnoses were made, but we now know that other organisms can produce a similar picture.

THE CERVIX.   This is a common place for the gonococcus to lodge in during the acute phase of infection. With the predilection of gonorrhea for mucous membrane surfaces, the organisms attack the epithelium of the endocervix. The immediate reaction is edema and softening of the entire cervix, as well as swelling of the mucous membrane. The external os is bathed in pus and consequently loses its surface epithelium because of the necrotizing effect of the gonococcal toxin. An angry-looking erosion results, but unfortunately there is nothing about the appearance of the cervix that is pathognomonic of gonorrhea. Any severe infection will produce similar pathologic findings.

With more severe infections or in neglected cases the gonococcus follows the small ducts down into the deep racemose endocervical glands in the cervical musculature. Small abscesses may form in nabothian cysts. When the infection extends so deeply into the cervix, it is difficult to eradicate either by local or systemic treatment. The infected cervix, once the acute phase has passed, becomes the chief source of latent gonococcal infection. Approximately 95 per cent of the unsuspected carriers of gonococcus harbor the organisms in the cervix. The patient complains of little but a profuse, irritating discharge.

How Is the Diagnosis of Acute Gonorrhea Made in Areas below the Level of the Cervix?

It is apparent from the foregoing discussion that the gonococcus will set up an acute inflammatory reaction in all the areas described, but it is equally obvious that other severe infections will do the same thing. The disease is suspected when the patient has a vaginal discharge and complains of burning and frequency of urination three or four days after sexual intercourse. The diagnosis in the final analysis, however, rests upon evidence provided by smear and culture. The disease in this acute state can be arrested and eradicated, provided treatment is begun early enough and is adequate.

Unfortunately the symptoms are often so minimal that the patient either fails to consult her physician early enough or does not come at all. The organisms tend to disappear rapidly, often within a few days. Smears and cultures of the purulent discharge must be taken the first time the patient is seen. When the patient is late in visiting her doctor, neisserian colonies may be absent or few and far between. Frequently the cultures will be positive, though the smears are negative. If the clinical impression is a suspicion of gonorrhea, it is the part of wisdom to begin intensive chemotherapy without waiting for confirmation by either smear or culture.

How Do We Treat Acute Gonorrhea with Local Manifestations?

The time to treat gonorrhea is early, before it has had a chance to spread to the uterus and tubes, or to become chronic below the level of the cervix. The neglected or inadequately treated case will certainly progress by one of these paths. Early recognition and prompt treatment are the main factors in successful therapy.

In the past great reliance was placed on cleansing douches and hot baths. These probably did more harm than good, despite the fact that the patient's chief complaint was often simply an irritating discharge. Today all baths, douches and instrumentations are contraindicated. The chief reliance in modern therapy is placed upon the use of the sulfonamides, penicillin and streptomycin. Local therapy is restricted to the use of protective ointments for an excoriated vulva. The improvement in the results of therapy from the use of the antibiotics and chemotherapeutic agents has been dramatic.

With the first appearance of the sulfonamide drugs enthusiasm ran high for sulfonamide therapy. Now their use is largely restricted to the cases proved by repeated smears and cultures to be resistant to penicillin. Curiously enough, the initial interest in sulfonamide therapy waned because of the high incidence of women who became sensitized and refractory to the drugs. Modern therapy calls for the prompt intramuscular injection of large doses of penicillin. Though small doses may be adequate for some infections, there seems to be little contraindication other than expense for not giving massive doses. The usual plan of treatment calls for 300,000 units of procaine penicillin G daily for one week. Some clinics give one million units daily during this period of time. The response to therapy is usually prompt, and frequently the smears and cultures will be negative after two or three days.

Attempts have been made to carry out the penicillin regimen by oral medication. It is now possible to establish a high titer of penicillin in the blood promptly by utilizing dosage schedules three or four times larger than those commonly used for intramuscular injection, but the reports of cures fall short of the goals obtained by the injection method.

Supportive therapy still plays an important part in treatment. The patient should be put to bed, particularly if the menstrual period is imminent. Alcohol and sexual intercourse are forbidden, and the patient is advised to eat a light, bland, unspiced diet.

WHAT ABOUT THE PATIENT WHO CANNOT TOLERATE OR BECOMES RESISTANT TO PENICILLIN?   Just as some patients proved resistant to the sulfonamides, so others have failed to respond to intensive treatment by penicillin. These cases are fewer, however. It is also well known that certain persons are allergic to penicillin. Urticarial skin reactions and anaphylaxis occasionally appear in these women.

Two possible courses of action are available in the gonorrheal patient who is either sensitive or unresponsive to penicillin therapy: (1) Sulfadiazine has enjoyed some success when given orally in doses of 15 grains (1 gm.) 4 times daily for 5 days. The dose is reduced to 3 gm. a day over the next 4 days and finally to 2 gm. for the last 2 days of the prescribed course. The therapy can be better tolerated if fluids are forced and sodium bicarbonate is used as a buffer. (2) In recent years streptomycin and dihydrostreptomycin have been injected intramuscularly in 1-gm. doses, dissolved in distilled water. Successes in the neighborhood of 90 per cent have been reported. This has the advantage of convenience, for only one dose is given. For those resistant or intolerant to both sulfonamide and penicillin therapy this had been the last recourse until newer antibiotics were introduced.

How Do You DETERMINE WHETHER THE PATIENT HAS BEEN CURED?   In most instances the response to antibiotic or chemotherapeutic drugs is dramatic, and the majority, over 90 per cent, are cured in a matter of 3 or 4 days. It is difficult to get a positive smear or culture after a patient has been on intensive penicillin therapy for more than two days. Unfortunately one cannot rely on a single negative smear or culture, and clinical evidence is totally unreliable. The patient may carry the gonococcus in the absence of any discharge or may show a persistent discharge that contains no gonococci, but simply secondary invaders which have persisted after the gonococcus was destroyed. It is unwise to assume that any patient has been cured until repeatedly negative cultures and smears have been obtained over a period of at least three months. Cultures provide a far more accurate evaluation of the true status than do smears. The greatest accuracy is achieved when the cultures are taken either just before or after the menstrual period. If the cultures continue to be positive, or if there is any question of the completeness of the cure, the penicillin regimen necessarily must be repeated.

A word of caution should be introduced at this point. It is possible that the patient may have acquired syphilis as well as gonorrhea at the same time. The clinical evidence of syphilis may be masked or delayed by the use of penicillin early in the course of the gonorrheal infection. If there is any reason to suspect a combined infection, syphilis should be ruled out by proper serologic tests.

Is THERE ANY PLACE FOR SURGERY IN THE ACUTE STAGES OF GONORRHEA WITHIN THE VAGINAL TRACT?   The only place that surgery occupies in the treatment of acute gonorrhea is in the incision and drainage of abscesses, in either Skene's or Bartholin's glands, that may fail to respond to penicillin or sulfonamide therapy. Usually infection in these regions will be successfully treated by local applications of heat in the form of hot compresses, supplemented by mild sedatives, such as codeine and aspirin, for the relief of pain. Occasionally abscesses become so painful and persistent that incision is indicated. This is not the time for local excision of a Bartholin's abscess.

In the past it was customary to treat the cervix or urethra by dilation, application of silver nitrate or cauterization. Today all such therapy is contraindicated unless one chooses to use silver nitrate to irritate the urethral mucous membrane, in order to bring any deep-seated infection to the surface so that the persistence or absence of gonorrhea can be determined.

Does Acute Gonorrhea Ever Become Chronic Locally if It Fails to Respond to Treatment?   If local tissue resistance is powerful enough, the infection that is not cured may progress to the chronic stage either in the cervix or in Skene's or Bartholin's glands, rather than spreading above the level of the cervix. As a result of the chronic gonorrheal infection we may find urethral and cervical strictures, chronic cervicitis, abscesses or cysts in Skene's or Bartholin's glands, and vulvar condylomata.

CHRONIC BARTHOLINITIS

Infection in Bartholin's glands may last for months and produce recurring episodes of painful swelling and abscess formation. The symptoms and physical findings will depend upon the degree of obstruction to the duct that leads to the vaginal canal. If it is only partially obstructed, the gland may swell temporarily, but empties as the discharge escapes into the vagina. If the obstruction to the ducts is complete and the glands, which are lined by mucin-producing epithelium, continue to secrete, bilateral cysts are formed. In most instances the Bartholin's cysts produce little in the way of symptoms. Usually they are small, nontender and fluctuant. Occasionally they become so large that they interfere with intercourse or cause discomfort on sitting or walking. Not infrequently abscesses develop which do produce extreme discomfort and pain. If the ducts are partially open, they may discharge pus into the vagina only to flare up at the next attempt at coitus, or they may spread into the labia and become so enlarged that they bulge into the vaginal canal or distend the skin over the labia.

What Is the Treatment of Bartholin's Cyst or Abscess in the Chronic Stage?

When Bartholin's cysts are large enough to produce symptoms, they should be excised during the period when any acute inflammation they may have harbored is in abeyance. Some gynecologists prefer to marsupialize the cyst by suturing the lining of the cavity to the margins of the skin incision. Others incise, drain and cauterize the epithelial lining with either caustic solutions such as silver nitrate or the actual electric cautery. There are advocates of aspiration of the contents of the cyst by syringe and needle and replacement with penicillin solution. By and large it is better to excise the cysts surgically.

If the chronic gonorrheal infection has created large or recurring abscesses in Bartholin's glands, they should be treated by any of the methods mentioned above.

In some instances it may be wise simply to drain the gland during the acute phase of abscess formation and to delay total excision until later. Rarely will a complete cure follow either spontaneous or surgical evacuation alone. Almost invariably abscesses reappear at varying intervals. Extirpation of the glands is indicated. Surgical excision is the surest way of accomplishing this.

CHRONIC INFECTION IN SKENE'S GLANDS

Residual infection in Skene's or the paraurethral glands is common. When gonococci persist in the deep tissues, reinfection of the male partner is possible, though all clinical and bacteriologic evidence may suggest a cure. The gonococcus has now burrowed beneath the duct and gland epithelium, and it subsists in the sub-epithelial tissue. Sometimes minute nodular thickenings can be felt on either side of the urethral meatus. If one presses on the floor of the urethra, the pinpoint openings of the ducts are obvious, and when the urethra is milked, either pus or a gray gelatinous material oozes from the duct orifices. In most instances the gonococcus has been killed, and the chronic infection is due to secondary invaders. At times the ducts become completely obstructed, and miliary abscesses form.

Whether treatment is performed depends upon (1) the possibility that gonococci persist in these glands, and (2) the kind of symptom produced. If miliary abscesses are present, there will be enough dysuria to warrant destruction of the glands. Usually the symptoms are minimal, but occasionally the patient with chronic Skenitis complains of urinary frequency and urgency. The bladder irritability is due to infection ascending along the lymphatic pathways to the bladder neck from a primary source in these paraurethral glands.

How Do You Treat Chronic Skenitis?

There are a number of methods devised to bring about destruction of Skene's glands and their ducts. The area around the urethral meatus is anesthetized by a topical application of 10 per cent cocaine, followed by the injection of 1 per cent procaine or Novocain. If the operator will apply a little upward pressure on the floor of the urethra, the duct orifices can be seen. Each can then be entered by inserting a curved needle held under tension while an electrocautery is applied to the mucous membrane overlying it. This will destroy the duct and the epithelial lining of the gland. After this the urethral meatus is cauterized with radial striations. Micturition in the postoperative period is a problem best answered by having the patient void while taking a hot sitz bath. To avoid stenosis of the urethra weekly office visits are required to permit urethral dilatation.

CHRONIC CERVICITIS

Most patients who continue to harbor gonococci despite several courses of adequate penicillin therapy have chronic gonorrheal cervicitis. Usually there is some evidence of erosion or endocervicitis, but not infrequently the cervix appears entirely innocuous. There is, moreover, nothing diagnostic about the external appearance of a cervix infected with gonorrhea in the chronic state. The infection is resistant to treatment, for again the gonococci have taken up residence in the subepithelial tissue and the racemose glands deep in the musculature of the cervix. In this protected position they serve as the source of repeated infection of the partner in the act of coitus.

The symptoms again are minimal. A disturbingly profuse mucopurulent discharge may be present. Occasionally the patient complains of dyspareunia and low sacral backache, due to the spread of the secondary infection into the lymphatic network. If the cervix has become stenosed because of a severe endocervicitis, there may be enough obstruction to the menstrual flow to produce bearing-down discomfort and mild cramps.

What Treatment Is Offered for Chronic Cervicitis?

Because of the danger of lighting up a hidden infection and causing it to spread to structures above the level of the cervix, cauterization of the cervix is postponed for at least six months. Further delay may be in order if the cultures and smears for Neisseria remain positive. If an accompanying stenosis of the cervical canal is noted at the time of electrocauterization, Hegar dilators are inserted to overcome it. The dilatations should be repeated as an office procedure in the intermenstrual period for several months thereafter.

CHRONIC INFECTION IN THE URETHRA

Like the cervix, the urethra itself is a common place in which to find gonorrhea in the chronic state. When the infection has penetrated the protective epithelial cover and lodged in the tissue beneath it, the urethra often becomes thickened and is likened to a pipe stem. The urethral meatus also tends to narrow as the result of a fibrotic response to the deep infection. Stenosis of the urethra through its entire course is common after gonorrheal infection.

As one might expect, the symptoms of chronic urethritis are chiefly urinary. Delay in the passage of the urine stream, urgency, frequency and burning are common complaints.

The Treatment of Chronic Urethritis

If inspection of the urethral canal by endoscopy shows a red granular epithelial base, one may elect to attempt topical application of Argyrol or silver nitrate, 2 or 3 per cent. When the canal is strictured, it should be dilated with dilators or bougies of increasing diameter, after first applying some topical anesthetic such as Zylocaine or 0.5 per cent cocaine. The dilations must be repeated at weekly intervals for several months.

GONORRHEAL INFECTION ABOVE THE LEVEL OF THE CERVIX

The efficacy of the newer antibiotic and chemotherapeutic drugs and the greater emphasis on early diagnosis and treatment of gonorrhea have now reduced the number of cases we see in which the infection has spread beyond the level of the cervix to involve the endometrial cavity, tube or peritoneum. For the same reason there are far fewer women who are chronic carriers of gonorrhea. Nevertheless the different strains of gonococcus vary widely in their virulence. Some are known to be resistant to present-day therapy. These cases, together with those neglected or inadequately treated, provide the nucleus for a number of instances of acute and chronic pelvic inflammation that now present themselves for treatment.

How Does the Infection Spread to the Endometrial Cavity and Tube?

If the gonococcus is responsive to adequate modern drug therapy, it should disappear from its local habitus in three days to one week. There should be little reason in the majority of cases for it to spread beyond the cervix, provided (a) the patient has avoided intercourse during the course of therapy, (b) douches have not been taken, (c) there has been no ill-advised cauterization or instrumentation of the cervix during the acute phase, (d) menstruation has not taken place before completion of the treatment.

Normally the gonococcus prefers to pass along mucous membrane surfaces, but local trauma of any of the kinds mentioned will encourage the organisms to take up residence in the subepithelial tissue. The infection does not spread to the endometrial cavity at any other time than menstruation, for the endocervical canal is usually protected by mucus. With the onset of the menstrual flow, however, the cervix softens and dilates and the mucus plug disintegrates. There is always enough necrotic tissue and serum present to provide an ideal culture medium for propagation of the gonococcus. The organisms then present in the endocervix, either because the exposure took place just before the menstrual period or near enough to it so that therapy has not had a chance to eradicate them, have an easy time in transit to the endometrial cavity.

What Is the Course of the Disease Once the Cervical Barrier Has Been Broken?

Though the infection passes readily into the endometrial cavity at this time, it does not remain there long, nor does it leave much in the way of a residual. This is probably because the endometrium is constantly being shed and undergoing regeneration. One can usually find some evidence of endometritis in patients who have salpingitis, but gonococci are rarely recovered. The pathologic evidence of chronic endometritis is no different from that produced by any other invading organism. The duration of stay of bacteria is so short and the tubes become involved so rapidly that there are no symptoms associated with the intrauterine infection (Fig. 44–4). When infection is present, it is impossible to dissociate the symptoms from those produced by early salpingitis. There may be some increase in vaginal discharge or more profuse menstrual bleeding than usual, but these observations have little diagnostic significance. The patient usually runs a moderate fever, and if one chances to examine her during this early acute phase, a circumstance which is highly unlikely, the uterus will be extremely tender when one attempts to move it. This tenderness and the cramplike bearing-down pain that the patient usually has in the very early stages disappear rapidly.

Just as there is a natural barrier at the internal os of the cervix, so there is obstruction to the inner opening of the fallopian tube within the endometrial cavity, except at the time of menstruation. The gonococci have no propulsive power and can migrate

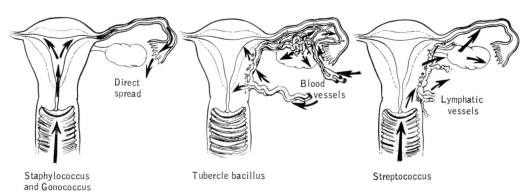

Direct
spread

Blood
vessels

Lymphatic
vessels

Staphylococcus
and Gonococcus

Tubercle bacillus

Streptococcus

Fig. 44-4. Comparison of the modes of invasion of 4 important bacterial infections of the female genitalia. The gonorrheal and staphylococcal infections spread upward along surfaces to reach the peritoneal cavity. Tuberculosis is blood-borne. Streptococci penetrate via lymphatics and veins to reach the parametrium.

only by growing and extending along the endometrial lining to enter the tube. This tendency to spread along mucous membrane surfaces is in sharp contradistinction to streptococcal infections, which disseminate widely through the lymphatics.

Infection of the mucosal lining of the tube usually shows up shortly after the period is over. If the exposure has taken place just before the period, there may be only a week's delay between the signs of acute gonorrhea and the appearance of tubal infection. The onset then may be relatively acute, but for the most part there is a delay of two or three weeks before the evidence of acute salpingitis appears.

What Are the Gross and Microscopic Pictures of Acute Gonorrheal Salpingitis?

Since gonorrhea tends to spread along mucous membrane surfaces, the first manifestation of infection will appear within the mucosa of the tube. It becomes hyperemic, congested and thickened. The tubal lumen fills with shaggy fibrinous exudate, and pus can either be expressed from or be seen dripping from the fimbriated ends of the tubes, which are usually open in this phase of the inflammatory process. As the infection progresses the lymphatics within the wall pick up the exudate and carry it to the serosal surface. This then becomes red, granular and covered with fibrin and pus, but with few filmy adhesions.

The infection is almost invariably bilateral, and both tubes become thickened, stiff and moderately distended. In the acute stage the tubes enlarge to perhaps twice their normal size, but rarely exceed that, unless the fimbriated ends seal off or become adherent to the adjacent ovaries or parietal peritoneum. Because of the weight of the exudate within the lumens, the tubes themselves tend to fall backward into the cul-de-sac and lie on the posterior leaves of the broad ligament. The adjacent peritoneum is contaminated both by direct contact and by the discharge of pus from the open ends of the tubes. If the tubal infection is sufficiently extensive, one of two things may happen in the acute phase; either the fimbriated end becomes involved, closed and adherent to the ovary or peritoneum, forming a pus sac or pyosalpinx within the tube, or the peritoneum lining the cul-de-sac becomes so contaminated that an acute pelvic peritonitis is created, which may become generalized or localize to form a pelvic abscess.

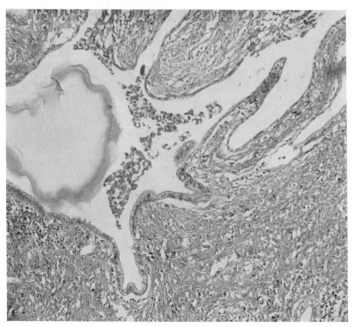

Fig. 44-5. In acute salpingitis there is purulent exudate and protein-rich fluid in the tubal lumen. As the inflammation becomes chronic, increased numbers of lymphocytes and plasma cells are found in the stroma.

In many instances the entire inflammatory process resolves within a ten-day period, leaving no residual. This is particularly true when adequate antibiotic therapy is provided early in the course of the disease. Many women have become pregnant after recovery from a mild or successfully treated gonorrheal salpingitis. Unfortunately not all are so lucky, for the disease tends to subside into the subacute or chronic state with a tendency toward re-exacerbation. Many recurrences can be traced to re-infection, either from an infected partner or from failure to eradicate completely foci of infection lying dormant within the cervix or lower vaginal canal.

Microscopically, the presenting picture is that of an acute response on the part of the tubal epithelium to the inflammatory insult. The blood vessels are engorged, and the tubal plicae are swollen and infiltrated with neutrophilic leukocytes. The extent of actual destruction of the tubal epithelium varies with the virulence of the infection. If it is mild, there may be only hyperemia, leukocytic infiltration and patchy loss of epithelium. With more serious infections when there is more pus and exudate, extensive destruction of the mucosa may take place. The infection, however, is not limited to the tubal mucosa, for the muscle wall becomes infiltrated with leukocytes as the infection spreads to the serosal surface of the tube. As the infection progresses to the chronic stage the neutrophilic leukocytes give way to lymphocytes and plasma cells (Fig. 44-5).

Whether the tube loses its functional capacity depends on the virulence of the infection and the degree of local tissue resistance supplemented by antibiotic therapy. It may recover completely if the tubal epithelium is not destroyed excessively, or it may be damaged beyond repair if there is widespread destruction of the mucosa or if the tubal ostia become closed.

What Are the Symptoms and Physical Findings in Acute Gonorrheal Infection above the Level of the Cervix?

The severity of the symptoms produced by gonorrheal infection above the level of the cervix depends upon the degree of contamination of the peritoneal cavity. The same symptoms can be produced by any other infectious process that involves the peritoneal cavity. If the organism can be recovered from the lower genital tract by smear or culture, there will be no question. If there is a history of sexual contact with a partner known to be infected, the diagnosis may be assumed to be gonorrheal in origin. In many instances one becomes suspicious when symptoms appear in a patient who gives no history of other causes, such as childbirth, abortion, endometrial biopsy or other operations involving the cervix or endometrial cavity. This is particularly true if the symptoms appear coincident with or directly after the menstrual period.

Since the onset of the spread of gonorrhea appears to be linked to the menstrual period, it is not surprising that the menses may be prolonged. This is rarely excessive. The uterus is simply trying to rid itself of a bacterial invader.

The most common symptom is pain. It is often unilateral during the early stages, but it subsequently centers over the pubic symphysis and invades both lower abdominal quadrants. If the infection is confined to the tube, the pain is caused simply by tubal distention by exudate. The pain then is mild to moderate and tends to be cramplike. As pus drips from the tube onto the peritoneum, or the tube becomes adherent to it, the pain becomes more severe and constant and is felt throughout the lower portion of the abdomen. As a result of the peritoneal insult the abdomen becomes distended, and muscular rigidity appears. The patient then has a pelvic peritonitis. The small intestine in contact with the inflamed pelvic peritoneum likewise becomes irritated, and nausea and vomiting make their appearance. Fever, which was low-grade as long as the infection remained within the tube, rises sharply to 102° or more, depending on the extent of the peritoneal inflammation.

As the infection spreads, the leukocyte count rises, the pulse rate becomes more rapid, and the patient is acutely prostrated. This is due to contamination of the upper abdominal cavity. If the infection spreads to the general peritoneal cavity, all the symptoms become more pronounced, and there is a true generalized peritonitis. Not infrequently the pain extends to the right upper quadrant. One later finds evidence of such spread in the form of adhesions between the superior surface of the liver and the diaphragm. They are separate and stringlike and sometimes have been called "violin-string" adhesions.

During this acute phase of disease, usually lasting from ten days to three weeks, the uterus is tender on motion of the cervix, and tenderness can be brought out on light palpation of the lower portion of the abdomen, particularly in the midline above the pubic symphysis. Some part of this is due to peritoneal contamination, which always produces tender parietes. Sometimes it is important to distinguish a lower abdominal tenderness and muscular rigidity due to uterine or adnexal disease from other inciting causes that will irritate the peritoneum. If one finds lower abdominal tenderness, the exact site of disease is not clear. On bimanual examination, if a normal uterus is pressed against a tender anterior abdominal wall, peritoneal pain may be produced. One may get the impression that the uterus is tender. If, however, pressure of the abdominal hand is released and the cervix gently elevated, the elicitation of pain suggests that the abnormality is truly centered in the uterus or adnexa. Rarely

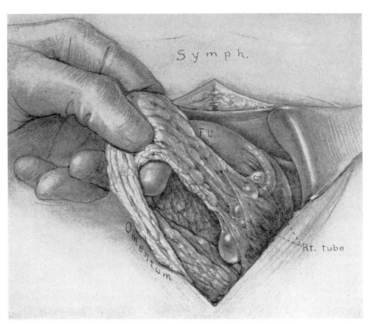

Fig. 44-6.   At laparotomy in pelvic inflammatory disease, adhesions may be found between the omentum and the fimbriated ends of the fallopian tubes. Adhesions due to pelvic peritonitis at deeper levels may be associated with a pelvic abscess. (Courtesy of Dr. T. S. Cullen.)

is it possible to palpate the swollen fallopian tubes as a distinct entity during the acute phase of the infection.

In the usual course of events one may expect the infection to subside in the next one or two weeks. Under appropriate therapy all evidence of the infection should disappear in about three weeks. If the symptoms become progressively more severe during this time, the patient has either a pyosalpinx or a tubo-ovarian or pelvic abscess. The severe pain throughout the lower portion of the abdomen is due to a combination of factors, including distention within a closed space and irritation of the pelvic peritoneum. The temperature spikes to peaks of 103° to 104° with a rise in the pulse rate and leukocyte count. The patient is acutely ill and prostrated. Though the infection is localized, there is enough reflex irritation of the intestine and abdominal peritoneum to cause increasing distention, nausea and vomiting.

At this phase one can usually palpate a bulging mass in the cul-de-sac on either vaginal or rectal examination (Fig. 44–6). Such abscesses are dangerous, for rupture into the general peritoneal cavity occurs not infrequently. The mortality rate in such instances approaches 25 per cent because of the general peritonitis and the sequelae such as septicemia or subhepatic and subdiaphragmatic abscesses.

What Is the Treatment of Acute Gonorrheal Salpingitis or Pelvic Peritonitis of Gono-coccal Origin?

Except for the finding of a pelvic abscess the treatment of acute gonorrheal salpingitis and peritonitis is strictly supportive. Many cases will subside on the simple regimen of bed rest with the head of the bed elevated (Fowler's position), light diet, proper bowel elimination and barbiturates for sleep. Demerol or codeine combined with aspirin is usually sufficient to relieve pain. In the more extreme cases of generalized peritonitis one may prefer to restrict fluids by mouth, supply fluid requirements by intravenous saline and glucose, and give morphine in some form on a four-hourly sedation (Ochsner) regimen.

Though review of the charts of patients treated with chemotherapy and antibiotics shows no great clinical improvement over those treated in the manner outlined above, modern therapy calls for antibiotic supplement. Early in the course of the infection 600,000 to 1,200,000 units of penicillin procaine G given daily will materially improve the chances of a prompt recovery and minimize the extent of tubal damage. After the first forty-eight hours little can be accomplished in the way of preventing destruction of the tubal mucosa, and when the abscess stage appears, the antibiotics will have little effect on the course of the disease. To be effective they must be given at the earliest indication that the infection has spread above the level of the cervix. As long as there is no suggestion that the pelvic infection is spreading, and the pain does not increase in severity, there is no rush about utilizing vaginal drainage. If an abscess becomes fixed to the vagina or the rectum and develops soft spots that can be felt, suggesting that the abscess has pointed, they may be incised and drained through either the vagina or rectum, depending on the presenting point.

What Other Pathologic Entities May Be Confused with Acute Gonorrheal Salpingitis?

Although the spread of infection is definitely different, the primary site of infection and the final target are similar in acute pelvic inflammation, both of gonorrheal and streptococcal origins. The past history of disturbed menstrual cycles, abortion, operative treatment of a nonpregnant cervix, or endometrial probing in the pregnant or nonpregnant, all would influence a decision in favor of pelvic inflammation caused by lymphatic dissemination of the streptococcus. The relation of infection to a recent menstrual period, known gonococcal disease in the past, recent sexual exposure with a recognized carrier, or the appearance of acute suppurative discharge after intercourse with an unsuspected partner would suggest gonorrhea as the cause.

APPENDICITIS.   Though the treatment of acute gonorrheal infection is primarily nonsurgical, there are several pathologic processes that must be ruled out, for their treatment calls for immediate surgery. The confusion with *acute appendicitis* usually appears with the onset of the spread of infection above the level of the cervix. Not infrequently the pain of acute salpingitis is unilateral or more pronounced on one side than on the other. If this happens to be on the right side, the differential diagnosis between salpingitis and appendicitis may be difficult. It is particularly difficult when pelvic peritonitis follows salpingitis or when appendiceal rupture occurs.

In differentiating acute appendicitis from early salpingitis or contamination of the pelvic peritoneum the most conclusive factors are the leukocyte count and the degree of pelvic tenderness on motion of the cervix. In most instances in the patient who has acute appendicitis the white blood cell count will be relatively much higher compared to the patient's temperature elevation, while there is absent to minimal tenderness on motion of the cervix. If the uninvolved appendix happens to be located deep in the pelvis, the degree of tenderness may be so definite that abdominal exploration should not be delayed. At operation one should not be tempted to interfere with the inflamed tubes, if an incorrect preoperative diagnosis has been made. Any associated disease should be corrected, and the appendix removed, but the infected tubes should be left alone.

When the appendix has ruptured, and pelvic or generalized peritonitis follows,

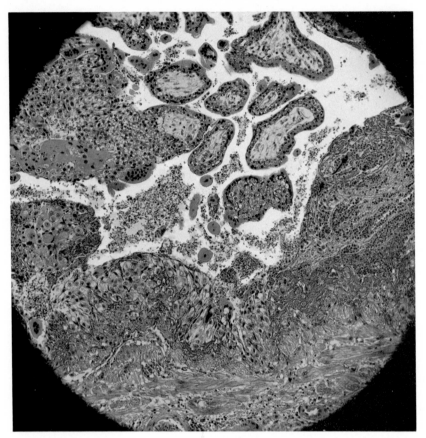

Fig. 44-7.   A tubal ectopic pregnancy may be associated with hemorrhage into the wall and tubal lumen that distends the fallopian tube and clinically simulates an acute salpingitis.

there are few clear facts that help in the differentiation. One is forced to go back to the history of the nature of onset of the infection. The flaring up of the process during or immediately after menstruation would favor salpingitis, while the onset of peri-umbilical pain with subsequent right lower quadrant localization, coupled with a history of previous attacks, would shade the diagnosis in the direction of ruptured appendicitis.

ECTOPIC PREGNANCY.   Since the appearance of gonorrheal pelvic infection coincides with the menstrual period and is ushered in by prolonged vaginal bleeding or spotting, it is not surprising that an occasion may arise when acute salpingitis simulates the picture of an *unruptured ectopic pregnancy*. Both will have pain, (a) from tubal distention and (b) from tubal leakage onto the pelvic floor. The main point of differentiation may prove to be the history of a slightly deranged menstrual pattern and the finding of unilateral pelvic tenderness or perhaps a palpable enlargement of one of the adnexa in the patient who has an unruptured ectopic pregnancy. The presence of fever would be supporting evidence for the diagnosis of salpingitis. The same observation may be made for an ovarian hematoma that follows sudden hemor-rhage into a graafian follicle or corpus luteum. Since the surgeon's hand is not forced, time will usually resolve the disturbing similarity of symptoms. (Fig. 44–7).

PELVIC CYST.   Ovarian cysts are usually unilateral and develop a pedicle which contains the blood supply. Torsion of this pedicle will produce lower abdominal pain, and a sudden distention by blood released within the cyst cavity causes further pain not unlike that of pelvic peritonitis. The weight of the hemorrhagic cyst will force it into the cul-de-sac, where it can be felt as a tender mass. Because of the altered blood supply, infection may become established in the twisted and infarcted ovarian cyst, but this happens infrequently.

ACUTE PYELITIS. Though the localization of pain is primarily high in the abdomen with acute tenderness localized in one or both costovertebral angles, generalized abdominal pain and tenderness may occur with acute pyelitis. The points of similarity with acute pelvic inflammation are the high fever, pain, abdominal distention and tenderness, nausea, vomiting and an elevated white blood cell count. Though the pulse rate may be rapid with acute pyelitis, it is less increased in proportion to the temperature rise than occurs in acute pelvic inflammation. Chills are present in both, but the history of onset is different.

With acute pelvic inflammation chills are an indication of the later spread of disease, while they frequently usher in an attack of pyelitis and actually precede the appearance of pain. The reverse is true in pelvic inflammation. Perhaps the most disturbing element in making the differential diagnosis is the frequently negative report of microscopic examination of the urinary sediment. This sometimes occurs when an acute pyelitis is due to inadequate urinary drainage secondary to ureteral block. In most instances, however, the patient will void frequently with pain and spasm. Tenderness will be present in the region of the kidneys, and pain radiates from there to the groin. The urinary sediment will then be full of pus, usually including leukocyte clumps and pus casts.

What Happens When Acute Salpingitis Does Not Heal Completely?

As we have noted, acute gonorrheal infection above the level of the cervix may subside, leaving a functional tube and little residue of the infection. In the past the majority of cases passed into the chronic stage, either in the form of minimal damage as seen in chronic interstitial salpingitis, a moderate chronic follicular salpingitis, or the more extreme pyosalpinx, hydrosalpinx or chronic inflammation of all the pelvic structures (the so-called P.I.D. or pelvic inflammatory disease). With a medically more alert population and superior methods of therapy fewer cases now reach the chronic stage.

It is obvious, however, that many patients will always pass into the chronic stages of the disease because (*a*) the initial infection may be overwhelming, (*b*) the infection above and below the level of the cervix proves resistant to the best of modern therapy, (*c*) the treatment is inadequate, or (*d*) the plan of therapy is well conceived, but the patient refuses to complete the course outlined for her. Such patients become carriers.

RECURRENT SALPINGITIS. Before discussing the various manifestations of chronic pelvic inflammatory disease, a word should be said about *recurring attacks* of acute salpingitis. Unless the acute gonorrheal infection subsides completely, the patient usually gives a history of repeated attacks and flareups of pelvic infection, similar to the initial event. These recurring infections usually take the form of "acute pus tubes," i.e. bilateral pyosalpinx mixed with varying degrees of inflammation of the pelvic peritoneum. Pyosalpinx is rarely seen in association with an initial infection unless it is overpowering, but it is a common finding with recurring bouts of infection.

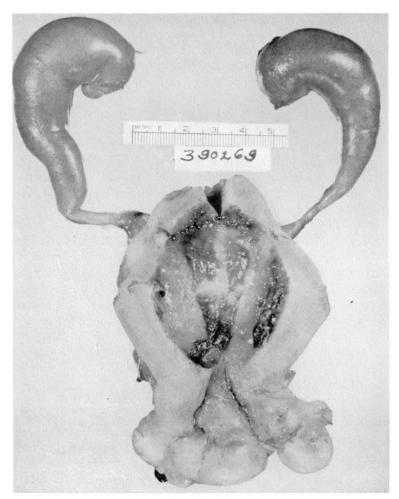

Fig. 44-8.   Typical advanced bilateral salpingitis with pyosalpinges, or retort-shaped tubes. The uterine cavity also contained pus, a pyometra secondary to cervical stenosis.

How May Recurring Attacks Be Prevented?   We have noted the reasons why many primary cases do not experience a complete and permanent cure. The devastating effects of repeated infections are well recognized. This is why so much emphasis is placed upon measures to prevent reinfection. Any suggestion of persistence of infection in Skene's or Bartholin's glands, the urethra or the cervix calls for definitive therapy and vigorous attempts at eradication. Intensive antibiotic therapy may be required, and at times surgical or electrocautery resection of the affected areas is indicated. Since the disease can be reactivated through sexual intercourse, coitus is forbidden for at least six weeks after all evidence of the original infection has completely disappeared.

WHAT IS THE MECHANISM OF THE DEVELOPMENT OF A PYOSALPINX?   The end-result of repeated infections is not only local loss of the epithelial lining of the tubes and interadherence of the plicae within, but also hyperemia, congestion, inflammation and fibrosis that tend to seal off both the uterine and fimbriated ends of the fallopian tube. At times occlusion of the lumen may take place anywhere along the course of the tube. Less often the inflamed fimbriae so irritate the adjacent peritoneum that the outer end of the tube becomes adherent to the ovary, and a *tubo-ovarian abscess* develops. The ovary itself is very resistant to gonorrheal infection, but a severe peri-oophoritis is common.

When the tube is sealed at both ends, the intense suppurative process is confined within a closed space. In response to the inflammatory reaction within the tube and the increasing amounts of exudate and pus, the tube becomes distended. It may exceed 10 cm. in greatest diameter. The greatest distention occurs at the fimbriated end, gradually diminishing as it approaches the uterus. In appearance it then closely resembles the glass retort once commonly used by chemists. The term "retort tube" is often applied to a pyosalpinx (Fig. 44–8).

What Organisms Are Cultured from a Pyosalpinx? Unless the pyosalpinx occurs as the result of the original attack, it is unlikely that the gonococcus will be recovered on culture of pus from within. This observation is well substantiated by several bacteriologic investigations. In the great majority of cases secondary invaders, *E. coli* and streptococcus, are found. Both are prone to produce pelvic peritonitis.

What Symptoms Appear in Recurring Salpingitis and Pyosalpinx?

It is the secondarily invading organisms that account for the severity of symptoms. When the "pus tube" is the result of an overwhelming gonorrheal infection, there is a constant, severe pain that spreads over the entire lower portion of the abdomen. This pain is due to distention of the tube with pus as well as to irritation of the adjacent peritoneum. The pulse rate is elevated, and the temperature spikes to 103° or 104°. Abdominal distention, nausea and vomiting may be expected, for the parietal peritoneum takes part in the infection, which is generalized throughout the lower portion of the abdomen. Some improvement in the symptoms follows the use of intensive chemotherapy in the acute phase of the disease.

In recurring infections, however, the inflammatory process does not respond to antibiotic therapy in the same manner as the original infection. The patient is usually much sicker, because there is more extensive peritoneal involvement. Abdominal distention due to paralytic ileus, nausea and vomiting are more pronounced. Despite massive doses of antibiotics the lower abdominal pain and fever persist. The white blood cell count is in the range of 20,000 per cubic millimeter, and the sedimentation rate is increased. Not infrequently the patient has abnormal uterine bleeding, particularly when there is infection around the periphery of the ovary.

What Is Found on Pelvic Examination?

The secondary invaders such as *E. coli* and streptococcus also influence the degree of pelvic abnormality. When a pyosalpinx develops as part of an initial gonorrheal infection, we may suspect it because the symptoms persist longer than the usual ten days to three weeks usually required to produce a cure. Gradually on vaginal and rectal examinations the tubes can be felt to become enlarged, lateral to and behind the cervix. They are palpable as tender, cystic, irregularly shaped masses, characteristic of distended fallopian tubes. Some improvement may be expected by increasing the dose of antibiotics or by combining penicillin and streptomycin.

The pelvic findings in the patient who has recurring attacks of gonorrheal infection are much more pronounced, largely because of the ravages of the streptococcus and *E. coli* organisms. The tube has already been severely damaged by the gonococcus, but more extensive invasion and destruction take place with the appearance of the secondary invaders. Because of the tendency of these organisms to produce peritoneal inflammation, the tube and ovary become adherent to the bladder and rectum, as well as the small intestine. The uterus is bound down in the pelvis by extensive adhesions, and pelvic abscesses are common.

In contrast to the pyosalpinx that results from the primary gonococcal infection, neither sulfonamide drugs, combinations of penicillin and streptomycin, nor any of the broad-spectrum antibiotics appreciably influence the resolution of these pelvic masses once they have developed as a result of repeated infections. The explanation is found in the presence of coliform bacteria and the streptococcus. Tubo-ovarian abscesses give the most trouble and are slowest to respond to any kind of treatment. It is true that subjectively the patients feel better after intensive chemotherapy. Whatever success chemotherapy has had may be traced to the eradication of foci of infection within the lower genital tract. It has little or no effect on resolving the large pyosalpinges or tubo-ovarian abscesses.

What Treatment Is Required for Pyosalpinx and Tubo-ovarian Abscess?

Experience has shown that surgical treatment should be avoided in the acute stages of gonorrheal salpingitis and pelvic peritonitis. When the symptoms increase in severity, and there is evidence of a spreading pelvic infection, the tubo-ovarian abscess may have to be drained through the vagina or rectum. The drainage site will depend on the localization of the fixed mass and the obvious point of fluctuation. Abdominal surgery should be avoided during the acute phase. In rare instances abdominal exploration may be required, particularly when in differential diagnosis there is a question of some pathologic entity whose treatment demands surgery. In such a case the surgeon may be tempted to take out one tube, particularly in a young woman whose other tube appears to be grossly normal. Since the disease is invariably bilateral, this so-called conservative surgery proves to be anything but that, for the tube left untouched will flare up and develop a pyosalpinx. Either both tubes and the uterus should be removed, sparing the ovaries whenever possible, or the operation should be concluded without doing any more than evaluating the situation. Later, under combined intensive medical management and chemotherapy with the natural processes of repair, the infection will either resolve or localize to an area that may be safely excised should the patient's symptoms require it.

By and large it is better to postpone operation and rely on conservative methods of treatment when the symptoms do not tax the patient unduly. Many such women have moderately severe dysmenorrhea, bearing-down pain and increased menstrual flow, but are not greatly incapacitated.

When Should Operation Be Performed?   When the process passes into the subacute or chronic phase, marked by recurring attacks of fever and pain at increasingly frequent intervals, together with palpable evidence of tubal or tubo-ovarian disease, surgery may be required to prevent the recurrent episodes or to relieve disabling symptoms.

Operation should not be done during the acute inflammatory phase, whether it be primary or recurrent disease. Unless symptoms indicate impending rupture of a pyosalpinx or tubo-ovarian abscess that might produce a generalized peritonitis, the surgeon can afford to select the proper time for operation. Results will be better and the morbidity less if conservative measures, including antibiotics, are used until the temperature has remained normal for at least two weeks. Then, if there is no tendency for the temperature to flare up after a pelvic examination and the white blood cell count and sedimentation rate are not elevated, operation may be done with minimal risk.

WHAT OPERATIVE MEASURES SHOULD BE CONSIDERED? No generalizations can be made as to the proper operation for pyosalpinx or any of the residual manifestations of gonococcal infection in the pelvis. The sort of operation must be tailored to the individual needs of the patient. Since the patient is nearly always young, her potential infertility problem is of primary concern. Both tubes are implicated to a greater or lesser degree. Though some may have minimal damage, the great majority have serious damage. The likelihood of restoring these tubes to adequate functional activity by any of the plastic operations now in vogue has no better than a 5 per cent chance of success. Similarly, one tube may appear to be hopelessly involved on gross inspection, while the other seems less severely damaged. One may choose to leave the latter, recognizing that it can and will get into trouble later. This fact should be explained to the patient, as well as the chances of success of any of the plastic procedures. She may elect to assume the risks because of her profound desire to become pregnant.

WHAT OPERATIONS ARE POSSIBLE WHEN THE PATIENT DESIRES FUTURE PREGNANCY? *Plastic Procedures.* The kind of plastic operation performed will depend upon the nature and location of the obstruction. If there is reason to suspect that damage to the epithelium and tubal wall is minimal, the surgeon may elect to free up adhesions around the tube with the main object of improving tubal motility. The patency of such a tube would likely have been determined previously by gas insufflation or hysterosalpingography, using an aqueous medium. When these examinations have pinpointed the site of obstruction within the tube, the surgeon must choose the operation that will best deal effectively with an obstruction in that area.

The obstruction may occur at the cornual, or uterine, end of the tube, as evidenced by the fact that no gas or radiopaque substance enters the tube. The tube may be blocked at its midportion or anywhere else along its course, depending on the site of maximum destruction of the tubal epithelium. In most instances the fimbriated end of the tube is completely closed. In addition to the information acquired in the preoperative investigation through tubal insufflation, much knowledge can be obtained by planning the operation so that the tube may be artificially distended while the abdomen is opened and the tube is in direct view. This is done by fixing an insufflation apparatus in the cervix in such a manner that the uterine cavity and tube can be injected with saline or carbon dioxide at will by the surgeon.

Block at the Uterine End. When the block occurs at the uterine end, and the fimbriated end is open and apparently normal, the median portion of the tube is excised. The lateral portion of the incised tubal lumen is then split longitudinally, and the end "fish-mouthed." The freshly incised tube is then sutured within the uterine cavity by mattress sutures placed in each of the split ends of the tube. To ensure patency of the canal during the healing process a polyethylene catheter is placed in its lumen, fixed to the serosa after passing it through the fimbriated end and then led through the uterine cavity and into the vagina. It is further immobilized by suturing it to the cervix. Six weeks later the catheter is removed from below as an office procedure.

The results are less favorable when the obstruction is localized to the cornual end, as compared to fimbrial occlusions. If success is measured by patency of the tube, approximately two thirds will achieve it. When judged by subsequent pregnancy, this figure will be roughly 10 per cent.

Obstruction at the Midportion of the Tube.   It is an unusual finding to have only the middle portion of the fallopian tube involved. In most instances the fimbriated end will also be damaged. When it does occur as a solitary area of occlusion, this portion of the tube can be excised and continuity re-established, again using a polyethylene catheter as a splint to maintain patency while the reparative process is taking place.

The Fimbriated End.   If the remaining portion of the tube is undamaged, it should be possible to perform a successful plastic operation on the fimbriated end of the tube, provided the surgeon uses delicate instruments and fine suture material and is careful in his dissection and handling of tissue. Unfortunately in the past the most delicate operations that embodied these cardinal principles were fraught with failure. Newer methods have been devised, utilizing the principle of the polyethylene catheter splint, but also adding another factor of protection during the repair process to prevent tubal occlusions by adhesions. A square sheet of polyethylene film is used to fashion a hood that will fit over the newly formed fimbrial ostia. The protective hood is tailored to the size of the tube and tubo-ovarian ligament before fixing it to the serosa. At a second abdominal operation six weeks later the protective cover is removed.

Preliminary figures from this experimental approach to the problem of tuboplasty have been most encouraging. Approximately 75 per cent of tubes remain patent, while one third of the patients have become pregnant. In evaluating the effectiveness of plastic operations it is only fair to point out that the results quoted are not limited to damage produced by the gonococcus alone. Since the primary point of attack in gonorrheal infection is upon the tubal epithelium, the over-all results will be far less favorable.

Salpingostomy.   Though the chances of subsequent pregnancy are not great, the surgeon may choose to form a window in the tubal wall if the fimbriated end is hopelessly fixed. In this manner an artificial opening is made, which could conceivably permit the entrance of an ovum.

WHAT OPERATIVE PROCEDURES SHOULD BE DONE IF THERE IS NO STERILITY PROBLEM?   *Total Hysterectomy and Salpingectomy.*   The primary lesion lies in the tubal epithelium. When the damage is extensive and there is either no chance or no desire for further pregnancies, the most acceptable procedure is a total removal of the uterus and tubes, rather than salpingectomy alone. Since the disease involves the entire genital tract, including the cervix as well as the tubes, the entire uterus should be removed whenever possible. Except when technical difficulties are encountered, there is little excuse for performing a supracervical hysterectomy, for the remaining cervix may continue to harbor disease.

Should the Ovaries Be Preserved?   The ovaries should be left in whole or preserved in part, unless they are seriously implicated in the infectious process, regardless of whether or how the uterus is removed. Involvement by infection of the interior functioning portion of the ovary is rare, while peri-oophoritis is common. Unless the blood supply to the ovary is hopelessly compromised, as much of the ovary as possible should be left behind.

The Falk Procedure.   Since many of the patients are young, preservation of menstrual function may be desirable. The primary aim of total hysterectomy is to remove all uterine sources of infection and to prevent distressing symptoms, chiefly pain and abnormal uterine bleeding. If reinfection of the tubes could be prevented, the patient might prefer to put up with symptoms as the price she might have to pay for retaining the menstrual cycles. This objective can be achieved with reasonable success by the Falk procedure, which simply is to resect the tube at the point of its insertion into the uterus. The pathway of infection through the uterus to the tube along membrane surfaces is permanently interrupted, but the blood supply to the ovary is not disturbed. In the absence of recurring episodes of infection the tube will eventually sterilize itself, even though a pyosalpinx will be present. Should the ovary itself be part of the abscess, cornual resection of the tube alone would be advisable.

CHRONIC GONORRHEAL SALPINGITIS (CHRONIC PELVIC INFECTION)

From the foregoing discussion it would seem that the gonococcus is responsible for the initial infection of the tube, but the ravages of repeated infections are more often due to the streptococcus or colon bacillus. Chronic salpingitis is the end-result of a mixed infection within the tube. The degree of chronic pelvic inflammation depends upon the extent of involvement of the pelvic peritoneum.

Several things may happen to the tube infected with gonorrhea: (*a*) If the attack has been mild, the entire episode may pass without doing any permanent damage to the tube. (*b*) If it is more severe, or recurring infections appear, the tubal epithelium

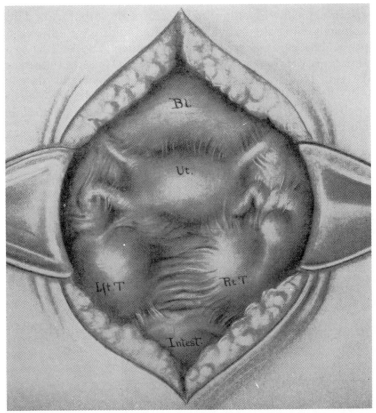

Fig. 44-9. A plastic type of peritonitis in which fibrinous and fibrous adhesions bind all the pelvic organs more or less firmly together characterizes chronic pelvic inflammatory disease. (From Graves: *Gynecology.*)

may be damaged in patchy areas, while the fimbriated end remains open. (*c*) With more virulent forms of infection the muscle wall becomes thickened by fibrosis, with lymphocytes and plasma cells. It loses some of its motility. This is called *chronic interstitial salpingitis*. (*d*) With overwhelming infection or repeated incidents of re-infection, a pyosalpinx develops when the fimbriated end closes. (*e*) The pus within the closed sac (pyosalpinx) may gradually disintegrate through the processes of proteolytic digestion, leaving a tube distended by clear serous fluid. This is called a *hydrosalpinx*. (*f*) When the infection has been severe in its initial stages or there have been repeated incidents of recurring infection caused by the streptococcus and coli-form bacilli, extensive pelvic peritonitis results. The tube, ovary, rectum, bladder, small intestine and omentum then adhere to a greater or lesser extent, depending on the magnitude of the insult to the peritoneum (Fig. 44–9). This is chronic pelvic inflammatory disease (P.I.D.).

Chronic Interstitial Salpingitis

A moderate initial infection by the gonococcus will destroy varying amounts of the tubal epithelium. The fimbriated ends may be either partially closed or untouched by the infection. As the acute process subsides, the polymorphonuclear infiltration of the connective tissue and muscle gives way to lymphocytes and plasma cells. They can be seen microscopically invading the depths of the tubal wall. The loss of tubal epithelium is obvious, since the individual plicated folds have adhered and produced localized blind pouches and pockets within the lumen (Fig. 44–10). As a result of the infection and repair within the tubal musculature the wall becomes thickened, tortuous and rigid. Though the tubal lumen may be partially patent throughout, there is little likelihood that pregnancy will occur, for the motility of the tube is definitely impaired. In the end-stages there are usually no symptoms. The chief problem is infertility.

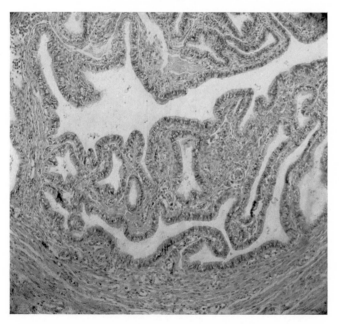

Fig. 44-10. In chronic salpingitis the inflamed mucosal folds, or plicae, become adherent. This process forms follicles and pouches with blind ends in the tubal lumen, which is called follicular salpingitis.

Hydrosalpinx

This is the end-stage of a pyosalpinx. Unable to escape from the enclosed cavity, the pus absorbs and is replaced by clear, serous fluid totally free of bacteria. It is truly a "burned out" salpingitis. The degree of tubal distention varies. The tube may become so large as to be confused with an ovarian cyst, with a diameter in excess of 15 cm. The greatest portion of the distention is at the fimbriated end, gradually tapering down as it approaches the uterus. The wall thins out in proportion to the degree of distention. It is often so thin that the tube is actually translucent (Fig. 44–11). Frequently the tapered, sausage-shaped masses lie free in the lower pelvic

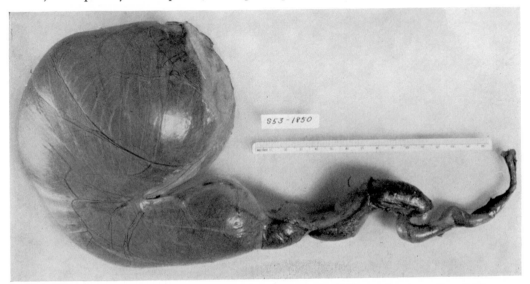

Fig. 44-11.   Massive distention of the fallopian tube with clear fluid stretches the wall until it becomes translucent, producing a typical hydrosalpinx. The average case is only about half this size.

Fig. 44-12.   A portion of the wall of a hydrosalpinx shows the stretched epithelial lining and an occasional focus of healed follicular salpingitis. The tubal muscle is replaced by fibrous tissue.

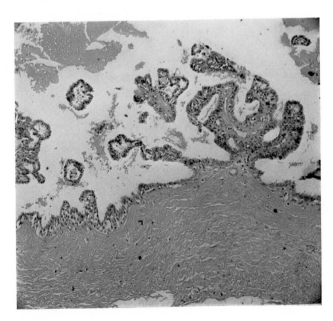

cavity bilaterally, but equally often there are adhesions to the ovary and pelvic peritoneum.

Microscopically, two types of hydrosalpinx can be recognized. The larger tubes with their thin walls distended by the accumulation of fluid within have a single cavity. The plicae are few and widely separated. Both single and braided plicae have a thick fibrous tissue core that makes them appear stunted or stubby. Though the tubal epithelium is intact, the folds have disappeared, and the epithelium appears to be flattened out. No evidence of inflammatory change can be seen in either the epithelium or the thinned-out wall. This is the so-called *hydrosalpinx simplex*.

The *hydrosalpinx follicularis* has no central cystic cavity. The tubal lumen is broken up into compartments, as the result of fusion of the tubal plicae. The wall is less thin, for there is not the same degree of distention. Again the tubal epithelium is intact, and evidence of any previous infection has completely disappeared (Fig. 44–12).

CHRONIC PELVIC INFLAMMATION

After a severe initial infection by the gonococcus or recurring infections produced by the streptococcus, staphylococcus or *E. coli*, the entire pelvic peritoneum is intensely irritated. The outpouring of protective serous fluid is followed by the formation of fibrous adhesions. The more virulent the infection, the more cellular the exudate and the less likely is it that adhesions will form. As the infection spreads away from its site of origin, the virulence of the infection diminishes, fibrin is deposited, and adhesions are produced to wall off the septic process. It is a well known fact that the gonococcus is mildly irritating to the peritoneum. As a result, large quantities of fibrin are produced, which do not absorb, but do bind the tubes, uterus and ovaries as well as the bladder, rectum and small intestine, into one indistinguishable mass. The uterus is firmly fixed in retroversion, but the tubes and ovaries cannot be identified. Repeated secondary infections serve to produce more peritoneal irritation and accentuate the pelvic inflammatory response.

What May Be Found in the Chronic Inflammatory Pelvic Mass?

The tube and ovary lie somewhere in the mass. It is a well known clinical observation that the adhesions which follow gonorrheal infection are far less tenacious than those that arise secondary to tuberculous infection, endometriosis or those produced by secondary bacterial invaders. It will depend upon how virulent the invasion by the secondary organisms has been, but in most instances a plane of cleavage can easily be developed in the seemingly inextricable mass that follows a widespread pelvic peritonitis of gonorrheal origin (Fig. 44–13).

After the omentum and small intestine have been dissected free and a line of cleavage has been developed between rectum, bladder and uterus, several pathologic entities may be uncovered.

INFLAMMATORY PERITONEAL CYSTS.   It is not uncommon to find inflammatory cysts filled with clear serous fluid. The cysts represent encapsulation of the original serous exudate thrown out in response to the peritoneal insult, or resorption of pus and its replacement by fluid, as seen in hydrosalpinx. The inflammatory cyst may completely envelop the tube and ovary and extend down into the cul-de-sac.

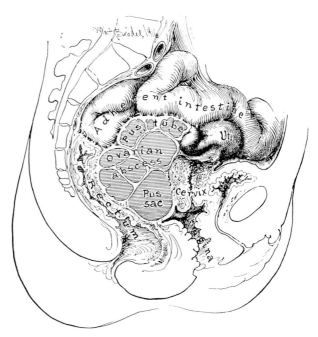

Fig. 44-13. In severe pelvic inflammatory disease the adhesions may enclose a pyosalpinx, a tubo-ovarian abscess and an abscess of the pouch of Douglas. These may or may not intercommunicate. (From Cullen: *Surg., Gynec. & Obst.,* Vol. 25.)

CHRONIC PERI-OOPHORITIS. If the original or recurring infections have been mild, the ovary can usually be separated from the tube. The interior portions of the ovary are not involved, but usually the external capsule thickens as a sort of protective response. The ovary is apt to have increased in size because of the presence of multiple follicle cysts that develop within its substance. The heavy, protective outer cover prevents normal development of the follicles, producing changes much like those in the polycystic ovary syndrome. It is interesting in this respect that the abnormal menstrual cycles which frequently accompany chronic pelvic inflammation are associated with a proliferative endometrium.

TUBO-OVARIAN ABSCESSES. When some or all of the interstitial portion of the ovary is in communication with the inflamed tube, a true tubo-ovarian abscess develops. The surface of the ovary normally prevents the spread of infection to its interior, but bacteria can and occasionally do gain entrance. The spread is direct and not via the blood stream. Grossly, the interior of such tubo-ovarian abscesses may have a yellowish appearance, and sometimes luteinized cells can be detected microscopically among the granulation tissue lining the cavity. In contrast to the pyosalpinx, these abscesses are not sterile, even though they may have been present and under treatment by antibiotics for a long time. Because of this, the rupture of a tubo-ovarian abscess is always dangerous, owing to the possibility of generalized peritonitis.

What Symptoms Result from Chronic Pelvic Inflammation?

In the absence of any evidence of active infection the patient may have an astonishing amount of disease in the pelvis with a minimum amount of discomfort. This is true even in the presence of tubo-ovarian masses and extensive pelvic adhesions. There is little relation between the size of the mass palpable in the pelvis and the severity of symptoms. Conversely, many patients with chronic pelvic inflammation are made miserable by constant burning, bearing-down pain, dysmenorrhea, disturbances in bowel function, partial intestinal obstruction, dysuria, urinary frequency and abnormal uterine bleeding. The most serious consequence of the residue of gonorrheal infection in this younger age group is sterility. Although the majority of these complaints are distressing, the patient may be willing to put up with a life of semi-invalidism rather than come early for treatment.

PAIN.   The constancy and severity of the pain vary and seem to be independent of the amount of inflammation or the size of the masses. The pain is described as burning and bearing down, localized in both lower quadrants and extending down the legs. It is often worse just before the menstrual period. Women who have jobs that require long hours on their feet complain particularly of the bearing-down sensation. These women are also particularly prone to have backache.

DYSMENORRHEA AND ABNORMAL BLEEDING.   These are common. The dysmenorrhea is apt to be the more troublesome, with pain that is boring rather than the cramplike pain experienced in essential dysmenorrhea. It does not disappear a few hours after onset of the menses, but continues through the first few days of the period and is often severe enough to keep the patient away from work and frequently forces her to bed.

The periods are inclined to come at more frequent intervals, and the amount of blood loss is increased, because of excessive bleeding and prolongation of the flow. The explanation lies in the peri-oophoritis that prevents normal maturation of the graafian follicles. Menstruation is therefore anovulatory, and bleeding occurs from a proliferative endometrium.

DYSPAREUNIA AND RECTAL DISCOMFORT.   These are occasional complaints. In most instances they are due to uterine fixation and pressure on the rectal wall. Some of the rectal discomfort may come from *erosions* in the *anal canal* secondary to chronic gonorrheal infection. Occasionally they lead to stricture, perirectal abscesses and on rare occasions fistulas. Gonorrheal proctitis, though rare, may occur.

PARTIAL INTESTINAL OBSTRUCTION.   In massive pelvic inflammation the small intestine is frequently a part of the pelvic mass. Disturbances in intestinal motility are not infrequent, and if there is enough angulation of the loops, the patient may have bouts of partial obstruction manifested by cramps, abdominal distention and occasional vomiting.

DYSURIA AND FREQUENCY.   These are the chief urinary symptoms. Usually they are due to the presence of the pelvic mass and irritation of the bladder wall. Some portion, however, may be traced to residual infection in the paraurethral glands at the neck of the bladder.

STERILITY.   Inability to conceive may be the only symptom that disturbs the patient to any great degree. Except in the stage of interstitial salpingitis, there is little hope that pregnancy will ever be possible.

ASSOCIATED SYMPTOMS.   Anything that produces congestion and fibrosis of the pelvic connective tissue is inclined to bring out a characteristic train of symptoms. Premenstrual tension, irritability, mental depression, sleeplessness, distaste for food and weight loss are secondary to the persistent pelvic discomfort sometimes called a "pelvic toothache." It must be clearly pointed out that women who have seemingly equal amounts of disease do not respond with the same symptoms. Some are annoyed rather than distressed, and others eke out a weary existence and are virtually semi-invalids.

Gonorrheal Septicemia

Gonorrheal infection can have serious sequelae. Invasion of the blood stream occurs on occasion, the bacteremia leading to gonococcal tenosynovitis, arthritis, meningitis and endocarditis. Septicemia from the gonococcus alone is rare. In most instances it is a mixed infection, combining the gonococcus with staphylococcus, streptococcus and *E. coli*. The association of streptococcus with gonorrheal organisms produces the most serious complications. The mixed infection is interesting, for the attacks are prone to appear when the disease has disappeared from the lower genital tract and become chronic in the tubes and pelvic peritoneum.

Gonorrheal organisms in the general circulation are prone to affect serous, endothelial and synovial surfaces. The commonest manifestation of gonorrhea in regions remote from the genital tract is a predilection for joint surfaces. Usually the infection is monoarticular, but it may be widespread, affecting a number of joints. It has an affinity for the knee, though the wrist is particularly susceptible in women. Joint effusions are common when the gonococcus alone affects the synovial surface. If the infection is mixed, the effusion becomes purulent, and the chance of permanent ankylosis is increased. Since attacks are apt to recur, there is excellent reason for removing the primary focus in both upper and lower genital tracts.

What Are the Pelvic Findings?

In the previous discussion it was noted that the symptoms have little relation to the extent of palpable abnormality. The pelvic findings are equally variable. In most instances the uterus is fixed in retroversion, and motion of the cervix produces pain. The uterosacral ligaments are stiff and extremely tender to palpation. Lateral to the uterus, in the base of the broad ligament, one may feel enlarged masses adherent in the cul-de-sac, which are unmistakably tubo-ovarian abscesses. If they are soft and compressible, the abscess is attempting to point in the direction of the vagina or rectum, or the softer consistency is due to an inflammatory cyst. The degree of lateral induration varies widely. It may be stony hard and extend out to the lateral walls of the pelvis; on the other hand, there may be no palpable enlargement of the adnexa and only minimal thickening of the bases of the broad ligaments on one side or the other.

The evaluation of the extent of disease is in part determined by the patient's physique and emotional response. If she is obese, the delineation of the masses and the extent of induration may be difficult to assess. The patient may be in such a highly nervous condition that it is impossible to gain a true estimate of the amount of disease or the degree of tenderness.

Finally, the residue of the infection presents a picture that is not pathognomonic for gonorrhea alone.

What Pathologic Entities Simulate Chronic Pelvic Inflammation of Gonorrheal Origin?

PUERPERAL SEPSIS.   Because of the role played by the secondary invading organisms, the end-result of the pelvic infection does not differ materially from that following puerperal sepsis. To establish the differential diagnosis it will be wise to reconstruct the history of the onset of the infection.

ECTOPIC PREGNANCY.   When the pelvic findings are localized to one side, the differential diagnosis between a localized pyosalpinx with or without tubo-ovarian abscess and ectopic pregnancy may be difficult. In the chronic state the inflammatory elements have disappeared. The points of similarity are (*a*) the disturbed menstrual cycles, (*b*) tenderness on motion of the cervix, and (*c*) the presence of a unilateral mass.

The two entities differ in (*a*) the pain, which is usually unilateral and cramplike in ectopic pregnancy, while it is bilateral, constant and boring in pelvic inflammation; (*b*) the history of onset of the symptoms differs materially; (*c*) the opposite broad ligament is apt to be nodular and tender in pelvic inflammation; (*d*) the Friedman or other pregnancy test may be positive in ectopic pregnancy.

ACCIDENT IN AN OVARIAN CYST.   Pelvic infection may follow loss of the ovarian blood supply of a cyst through torsion of its pedicle. Hemorrhage frequently occurs within the cyst cavity after the acute episode. This provides an excellent culture medium for infection. A dermoid cyst (benign cystic teratoma) may rupture and spill its contents on the pelvic floor. This is highly irritating chemically to the peritoneum. The defense response is similar to that produced by the gonococcus and mixed organisms. These cysts become adherent in the cul-de-sac and walled off from the general peritoneal cavity by adhesions, omentum and small intestine. By and large these adherent cysts are more mobile than the tubo-ovarian masses of gonorrheal infection, and not infrequently they have a contour that aids in distinguishing between the two.

ENDOMETRIOSIS.   Pelvic thickening, tender nodular uterosacral ligaments, adherent broad ligament cysts, and fixation of the uterus appear both in endometriosis and pelvic inflammation. The past history is helpful. If no germane history can be obtained, it may not be possible to differentiate the two conditions. From a practical point of view nothing is lost, for the therapeutic indications and the kind of treatment of one are equally good for the other.

MALIGNANT DISEASE.   Firm or hard nodular masses with minimal symptoms are also found with ovarian cancer, in the absence of any other physical finding. If there is any question about the diagnosis, abdominal exploration is imperative.

What Is the Treatment of Chronic Pelvic Inflammation?

Before embarking on a surgical approach to the problem of pelvic inflammatory disease, every effort should be made to try relieving the symptoms by the intensive use of heat, in the form of 8-quart douches twice daily, using warm water and vinegar, in the proportion of 5 tablespoonfuls of vinegar to a quart, or the use of diathermy. By improving the circulation through the use of heat, the chronic inflammatory process may subside to a certain extent, with corresponding relief of symptoms.

Any regimen of heat therapy should be amply supplemented by intensive antibiotic therapy. Penicillin in daily dosage ranging from 300,000 to 1,200,000 units continued for one week may be given at intervals. Mixed infections call for combination therapy with streptomycin, 1.0 to 2.0 gm. per day, along with penicillin or heavy doses of the broad-spectrum antibiotics. A general supportive medical regimen is also indicated. Anemia should be corrected by blood replacement and iron therapy. A diet high in vitamin and protein content is advisable to combat the depletion incident to any long-standing infection.

Recently cortisone therapy, in 75-mg. doses daily to a total of 3 gm., has been given to patients who have stony hard pelvic masses that show no indication of resolution under a regimen of heat and antibiotics. Some resorption of the pelvic induration has been reported under cortisone therapy. This has also been used as a preliminary step preceding radical pelvic surgery, with the idea of reducing the technical difficulties of surgical extirpation of the pelvic organs.

WHAT ARE THE ADVANTAGES OF SURGICAL TREATMENT? The symptoms of chronic infection in the pelvis vary widely. One is justified in trying medical management for a reasonable time, but the process is chronic, and if no improvement is noted after repeated courses of adequate therapy, this approach should be abandoned and a surgical attack instituted.

When the patient is incapacitated or rendered semi-invalid by pelvic inflammation in its chronic phase, a total hysterectomy with removal of both tubes is indicated, regardless of her age. Ovarian conservation is important in the younger age group, for physiologic as well as psychologic reasons. The problem has been discussed under the heading of treatment for recurring salpingitis above. A small residual portion of normal ovarian function is far better than large doses of a synthetic estrin supplement.

REFERENCES

Curtis, A. H.: Adhesions of the Anterior Surface of the Liver. *J.A.M.A.*, 99: 2010, 1932.

Davidson, N. R.: One Hundred and Fourteen Cases of Cornual Resection in Chronic Gonorrheal Salpingitis. *West. J. Surg.*, 59: 319, 1951.

Editorial: Gonorrhea in Women. *Clin. Med.*, 53: 262, 1946.

Falk, H. C.: Interpretation of the Pathogenesis of Pelvic Infection as Determined by Cornual Resection. *Am. J. Obst. & Gynec.*, 52: 66, 1946.

Goodman, H.: Public Health Aspects of Social Hygiene in New York City; Treatment of Gonorrhea Past and Present. *New York State J. Med.*, 57: 3695, 1957.

Keefer, C. S.: Gonococcic Infections; in *Oxford Medicine*. New York, Oxford University Press, 1949, Vol. V, p. 39.

King, A. G.: An Evaluation of the Criteria of Diagnosis and Cure of Gonorrhea in the Female. *Am. J. Obst. & Gynec.*, 53: 829, 1947.

Noeggerath, E.: Latent Gonorrhea, Especially with Regard to Its Influence on Fertility in Women. *Am. J. Obst. & Gynec.*, 62: 726, 1951.

Peters, H.: Gonorrhea in Gynecology. *Am. J. Obst. & Gynec.*, 54: 517, 1947.

Chapter 45

Other Specific Infections That
May Produce Pelvic Inflammation

TUBERCULOSIS

GENITAL tract tuberculosis in women is not a common form of gynecologic disease in the United States, yet it has tremendous significance for the person who happens to have it, especially in the childbearing age. Tuberculosis of the tube and endometrium is intimately bound to the problem of sterility. Tuberculous infection in the reproductive organs seems to occur chiefly when the uterus and ovaries are in a state of activity. Rare examples are found before puberty, and an occasional patient may have tuberculosis in the menopause, but over 80 per cent of cases appear between the ages of 20 and 40 years.

Genital tuberculosis derives its significance as a clinical entity because of this tendency to focus on the reproductive age group. It poses a clinical problem, for unless it is detected and treated adequately in its earliest phases, tuberculosis will render a large percentage of these women incapable of conception or of achieving a successful pregnancy.

Unfortunately tuberculosis of the genital tract gives rise to few symptoms in its mild or moderate phase. Discovery is usually made unexpectedly, most often by endometrial biopsy in the course of investigative studies to explain infertility.

How Common Is Genital Tuberculosis?

The actual incidence is not easy to determine. From a review of the world literature it is apparent that tuberculosis of the reproductive tract is much more common in India, the Middle East and the British Isles than in Australia and the United States. The figure commonly quoted is 5 per cent of all types of salpingitis examined pathologically. When this criterion is used, the total incidence in the world literature shows little variation. It is only when the incidence is computed on the basis of proved diagnoses in relation to the number of gynecologic admissions that discrepancies are noted. Frequently the pathologically distinctive tubercles are not apparent grossly. Unless careful studies are done both on the endometrium and fallopian tubes at the proper time in the menstrual cycle, a certain number of cases will be missed.

602

Two developments have led to an increased interest in the problem of the frequency of genital tuberculosis. The first of these is the growing number of cases of unsuspected tuberculous endometritis uncovered in the last ten years, paralleling the more widespread use of curettage and endometrial biopsy in sterility studies. Between 2 and 5 per cent of such patients show evidence of previously unsuspected tuberculosis. Since the disease is usually primary in the tube and only 50 per cent of the cases involve the endometrium, the number of cases of tubal tuberculosis is thus appreciable. With clinical tuberculosis in other areas such as lung, kidney or peritoneum, the incidence of genital involvement rises to 8 to 13 per cent. It is evident that tuberculosis is a real factor in the sterility problem. The second reason for the heightened interest is the fact that the new antituberculous drugs such as streptomycin, para-aminosalicylic acid (PAS) and isonicotinic acid hydrazide (isoniazid) have provided possible improvements in therapy for a process that was formerly fairly hopeless.

What Organism Causes Genital Tuberculosis, Why Does It Appear in the Genital Tract, and How Does It Spread?

Tuberculosis of the genital tract is a chronic infection produced in most instances by the human type of tubercle bacillus. A few cases can be traced to the bovine strain. Pasteurization of milk has done much to eliminate the bovine type as a factor in genital tuberculosis.

There are three recognized methods of spread: (*a*) hematogenous dissemination of the tubercle bacillus from a focus elsewhere in the body; (*b*) a direct spread of the bacilli and caseous material from primary disease in the intestinal tract that has produced tuberculous ulcers or mesenteric nodes. A breakdown of these sources would set up tuberculous peritonitis and secondary involvement of the tubes. (*c*) A few primary genital cases have been recorded in which the infection seemingly came from inoculation through sexual contact with a husband known to have active tuberculous lesions in some part of his genitourinary system. In one reported series only one case of proved transfer to the wife was found among 500 married men with tuberculosis in the genitourinary tract. It is surprising that there are not more cases of this sort, since tubercle bacilli are not infrequent findings in the male urine, semen and epididymis.

In most cases tuberculosis in the genital tract is secondary to disease elsewhere in the body and is but one manifestation of a generalized systemic infection. The most likely source is the lung, from which bacilli disseminate by the hematogenous route to involve the pelvic organs. Approximately two thirds of the cases can be traced to pulmonary involvement. How rapidly the disease spreads through the blood stream is not known. There is some suspicion that the genital tract becomes infected shortly after the primary infection in the lung. The symptoms suggesting genital involvement are often delayed for a year or more, or may never be apparent unless infertility requires investigation. It is also possible that the tube and endometrium may escape the initial onset, but fall before a fresh blood-stream infection secondary to a breakdown in a previous lesion in lung or lymph node.

A less common source is via lymphatic spread from generalized tuberculosis of the peritoneum implicating the tubes. When the fallopian tubes are primarily infected, there is usually some degree of local extension to the immediately adjacent peritoneum. Many observers feel that peritoneal tuberculosis stems from primary disease in the tubes. Miliary tubercles on the peritoneum appear and persist as long

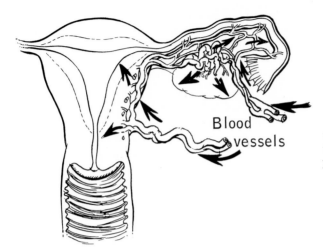

Blood
vessels

Fig. 45-1. Tuberculosis reaches the genital tract via blood stream infection and localizes primarily in the fallopian tube.

Tubercle bacillus

as the tubes are open. Nevertheless it is reasonable to expect that the tubes also might become infected by lymphatic spread after the breakdown of a caseating mesenteric node, though the occasions may be rare.

In genital tuberculosis the fallopian tubes are invariably involved. The endometrium is probably infected more often than statistical study would lead us to believe. Much of the evidence is based on endometrial sampling, which provides the pathologist with little material for accurate evaluation. The reported incidence of 50 to 75 per cent is undoubtedly too low, for the reason stated.

The primary source of the infection within the genital tract lies in the fallopian tubes. Since the spread of infection is downward rather than upward, one can be sure if the endometrium is affected that the patient also has tuberculosis in both tubes as well. Unilateral tubal involvement is rarely encountered. It is surprising, in view of the downward spread of the disease and the presence of tuberculosis in the genital tract of the male consort that more cases of tuberculosis of the cervix, vagina and vulva are not found. The reported incidence is in the range of 2 to 3 per cent of all tuberculous infections.

In the past tuberculous oophoritis secondary to tuberculous salpingitis was thought to be uncommon. Most recent careful histologic studies have indicated that some degree of tuberculous ovarian involvement is present in 25 to 40 per cent of the cases. When it does occur, it is often bilateral and usually appears as granulomas on the surface of the ovary (tuberculous peri-oophoritis). With more extensive disease caseation may take place within the ovarian substance. The spread to the interior of the ovary possibly occurs by way of ruptured follicles.

SUMMARY OF THE NATURE OF SPREAD OF TUBERCULOSIS IN THE GENITAL TRACT. Tuberculosis of the female genital tract is classically secondary to a primary focus situated elsewhere. The reproductive organs become implicated when the primary infection takes place near the menarche or in early childbearing years when these organs are undergoing their greatest period of functional activity. Minute foci of infection are set up as the result of hematogenous spread from the primary site, usually the lung. Both the primary site and the remote infectious metastases may heal or remain dormant for several years, only to flare up later.

The initial point of attack in genital tuberculosis is in the tube. After or during more extensive involvement of the tubes the infection spreads downward into the endometrial cavity and occasionally through the cervix to infect the lower genital tract. Contiguous spread occurs to the pelvic peritoneum and ovary (Fig. 45–1). Dense adhesions are formed in response to the localized peritonitis. As a result, in some cases there may be hydrosalpinx, tubo-ovarian abscesses, collections of pus in the cul-de-sac, and rarely fistulas form to the bladder, small intestine and rectum. Ascites is often present.

What Are the Gross Characteristics of Tuberculosis of the Tubes?

The gross appearance of tuberculosis of the fallopian tubes at operation varies widely. The only departure from normal may be a seeding of grayish-white miliary tubercles over the surfaces of the tubes and uterus, roughly following the superficial lymphatic channels in these organs. These findings are not to be confused with the small follicular-like plaques often seen with chronic salpingitis. Frequently the rest of the pelvis is normal, and the tubes themselves may be only slightly thickened, with perhaps a few adhesions to the adjacent uterus, ovary or bowel. Straw-colored ascitic fluid may be present.

As the disease becomes more extensive two types of tubal alteration are apparent: the adhesive type and the exudative type.

ADHESIVE TYPE.   Because of the localized peritoneal involvement the tubes are often buried in extremely dense adhesions, making exposure difficult. The initial appearance of the pelvic mass may not be much different from that encountered in chronic pelvic inflammatory disease. There are four observations that are helpful in differentiating the two entities: (*a*) The adhesions encountered in tuberculous infections are much tougher, and a plane of cleavage is not readily established, as it is in pelvic inflammation of gonorrheal origin. (*b*) When the tubes are finally uncovered, they are usually thickened either segmentally or diffusely. This may be true in gonorrheal salpingitis, but in tuberculosis the pathologic process in most instances does not involve the interstitial or isthmic portions of the tube. (*c*) In chronic gonorrheal salpingitis the fimbriated ends of the tube are almost invariably closed, the ostia wide open and the fimbria everted in nearly half of the cases with tuberculous infection. This kind of tuberculous salpingitis has been compared in shape to an old-fashioned tobacco pouch with a drawstring. (*d*) The tuberculous lesions can often be distinguished from gonorrheal salpingitis by pallor of the tissues, which is characteristic of tuberculosis.

Except for these differential points, on inspection there is little to distinguish tuberculosis from chronic salpingitis due to gonorrhea, unless gross tubercles are seen or caseation is evident.

The infection is primarily within the tubal lining, as it is in gonorrhea. Both produce interstitial damage within the tube. On cross section of the tuberculous tube minute yellow or gray tubercles are frequently seen within the mucosa, and occasionally extension occurs into the muscle wall of the tubes. At other times only the use of a microscope can establish the diagnosis. Irregular attempts at regeneration of the epithelium explain the segmental thickenings found in the tuberculous tubes.

EXUDATIVE TYPE.   When the ostia are closed, the tuberculous tubes grossly resemble the typical pyosalpinx seen in gonorrheal infections. Such tubes may be large and fill the pelvis. In this form dense adhesions are rarely seen, and the tubes

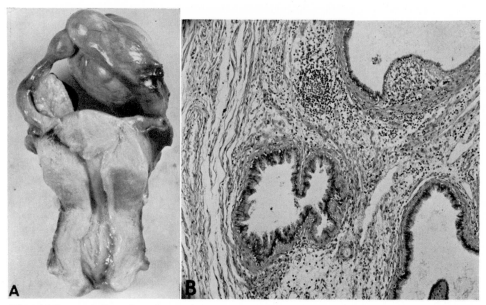

Fig. 45-2.   *A,* In tuberculous salpingitis the tubes may be bound together and irregularly, moderately or greatly swollen. As usual, the uterus shows no gross evidence of tuberculosis. *B,* Epithelial hyperplasia in the tube affected by tuberculosis is common. Much of the inflammation often appears nonspecific, with only occasional tubercles, as seen at the upper right.

are readily mobilized. The serosal surfaces are usually smooth. The true nature of the disease is noted only on sections of the tubes. They are filled with yellow caseous material of putty-like consistency (Fig. 45–2, *A*). When this material has become contaminated by a mixed infection, the contents become more fluid, but there is rarely a true hydrosalpinx. Frequently no gross tubercles are seen, and reliance must be placed on microscopic examination of the tubal epithelium and muscle wall.

How Do We Recognize Tuberculosis within the Uterine Cavity?

Though shallow ulcerations may be seen in the cornual portions of the endometrial cavity immediately adjacent to the entrance of the tubes, one is unlikely to make an accurate diagnosis of tuberculosis on the basis of gross inspection of the endometrium. Occasionally there may be a yellowish or green cast of endometrium, but in most instances the diagnosis is based on microscopic interpretation of the curettings.

It makes a great deal of difference when such curettings are obtained in the menstrual cycle. With each menstruation the uterus largely sheds its endometrium. With it may go the evidence of tuberculous involvement. With each cycle the endometrium becomes reinfected. This will be most evident in a fully developed endometrium. The reinfection usually comes from the tubes, but it is also possible that foci of tuberculous infection may remain in the persisting basal endometrial layer. Evidence of this is found in the cyclic reappearance of tubercles within the endometrium of a patient who has had both tubes removed.

By and large in the uterus the endometrium alone is concerned in the tuberculous process. The myometrium confines the infection, but is rarely invaded.

What Is the Microscopic Picture in Tubes and Endometrium?

The microscopic picture in tubes and endometrium is not usually so obvious as in other tissues, such as lung and lymph nodes. A chronic inflammatory exudate with abundant plasma cells and lymphocytes is present, but the characteristic tubercles are found only after some searching. Frequently there is no caseation, but only focal accumulations of epithelioid cells packed into tubercles. Occasional giant cells are present, either with their nuclei in horseshoe arrangement (Langhans giant cells) or with the nuclei scattered throughout the cell. Both in the uterus and tube special acid-fast stains as a rule will demonstrate recognizable tubercle bacilli.

In the tube a striking epithelial hyperplasia commonly accompanies tuberculous salpingitis (Fig. 45–2, *B*). This may even arouse a suspicion of tubal cancer, although there is no real precancerous tendency present. Any tube that shows an unexplained epithelial hyperplasia with intraluminal adhesions of the plicae should be studied by further sectioning in the expectation of finding active or healed tuberculosis.

Endometrial glands are not altered in appearance and may show proliferative or secretory activity. Increased numbers of leukocytes are present in the endometrial stroma, including nests of lymphocytes and plasma cells. Tubercles as a rule are few, small and widely separated (Fig. 45–3, *A*). Often no caseation is present, but tubercle bacilli usually can be demonstrated with acid-fast stains (Fig. 45–3, *B*).

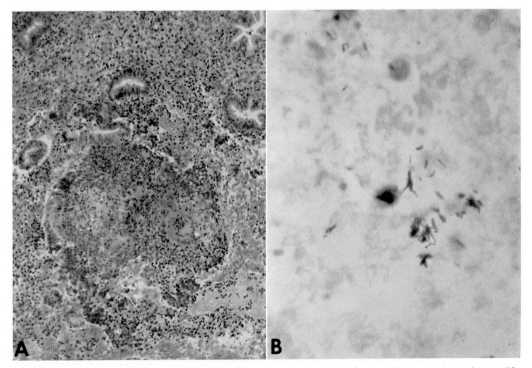

Fig. 45-3.   *A,* This focus of tuberculous granulomatous inflammation was the only specific pathologic finding in an otherwise ordinary case of chronic endometritis investigated by curettage. It is frequently necessary to search through the tissue in chronic endometritis in order to find the scattered, small, noncaseous tubercles. *B,* Acid-fast staining usually demonstrates some bacilli in tuberculous endometritis.

What Conditions May Imitate Tuberculosis?

Uncommonly, granulomas may be inflammatory reactions to infestations caused by pinworms or the ova of Schistosoma. Such foci may imitate tuberculosis both grossly and microscopically, but the responsible parasites or their ova are usually recognizable. Lipoid granulomas that develop after oil hysterosalpingography may be confusing grossly, but small round droplets of lipid are evident microscopically. Sarcoidosis does not seem to involve the female genital tract.

Other Genital Sites

Tuberculous infections of the cervix, vagina and vulva are rare. When seen on the cervix, a shallow tuberculous ulcer with indurated, punched-out borders may closely resemble early cervical carcinoma. The lesions in the vagina or vulva have similar characteristics of ulceration and induration. The diagnosis is made by biopsy and bacteriologic study.

What Are the Symptoms of Tuberculosis of the Genital Tract?

The disease varies in severity and extent. In many instances, as in some patients with generalized pulmonary tuberculosis, the patient may appear perfectly well with a minimal amount of genital disease present. It is unwise, however, to regard a mild case as of no particular consequence. Sudden exacerbation may disseminate the tuberculosis widely, causing disintegration of the patient's health in a relatively short time.

The onset of the disease is apt to be insidious. Genital tuberculosis may develop within a year after the initial manifestations of pulmonary tuberculosis, or be delayed several years. Not infrequently a history of previous infection cannot be obtained. The disease has usually been present for long periods of time without giving rise to symptoms.

STERILITY.   Patients with genital tuberculosis are rarely fertile. The diagnosis of tuberculosis is frequently made by endometrial biopsy on a patient apparently well and complaining only that she has been unable to conceive. Full-term pregnancies are rare when tubercle bacilli have been isolated. Ectopic pregnancies have been reported in the world literature, though in no great number.

PAIN.   Lower abdominal pain is a common symptom. The pain is not necessarily severe, and there is little to distinguish it from the pain of other chronic pelvic inflammations. The dense adhesions are the likely source of pain, which is constant, dull and like a toothache. Some part of the pain may be attributed to distention of the tube due to the caseating process within its lumen. When pelvic masses are palpable, the patient commonly has pain.

A greater degree of suspicion should be aroused when lower abdominal pain of long duration is noted by a woman in the childbearing age who has either never been able to become pregnant or who seeks a second child. This is particularly true if she also has lower abdominal tenderness or complains of unusual fatigue, weight loss, night sweats, chills or fever, cough or menstrual irregularity. The associated symptoms usually point to a more advanced stage of tuberculosis. A prolonged fever of over 100° is usually a poor prognostic sign.

DYSMENORRHEA.   The patient with tuberculous salpingitis or endometritis is no more likely to have dysmenorrhea than a patient with any other disease. Frequently she does have an exacerbation of pain at the time of her period. When this is accompanied by an elevation of body temperature, tuberculosis should be considered, for other tubal infections do not produce this picture. The explanation is not clear, but may have something to do with regurgitation of tubal contents through the open ends of the tube onto the pelvic peritoneum.

ALTERATIONS IN THE MENSTRUAL PATTERN.   Approximately half of women with genital tuberculosis have no change in the menstrual pattern. Whether menstrual disorders occur depends upon how much local disease is present. The form the disorder takes will parallel the extent of local disease, but it is influenced profoundly by the degree of general systemic infection.

Excessive menstrual bleeding is far more common than amenorrhea, when associated with local disease in the genital tract. Amenorrhea is more likely to be a manifestation of active pulmonary tuberculous infection, as indicated also by fatigue, lassitude and loss of both weight and appetite. One would then expect a low-grade fever that is not associated with any rise in the leukocyte count or progression of an anemia.

How Is the Diagnosis of Tuberculosis in the Genital Tract Made?

There is little in the physical examination to distinguish tuberculous infection from any other kind of pelvic inflammation. Depending on the extent of disease, the pelvic findings may be completely negative, or one may palpate bilateral inflammatory masses, firm hard tubes and a fixed uterus. In the absence of masses the uterosacral ligaments may seem to be foreshortened on one side or the other, and the uterus is drawn to that side. None of these observations are pathognomonic of tuberculosis. The abdomen is often tender and resistant to palpation, or it gives a "doughy" feeling when examined. These factors are present with other forms of intra-abdominal disease besides tuberculosis. The finding of ascites is of some significance and may accompany tuberculous peritonitis. The actual physical signs are difficult to interpret even with the abdominal contents exposed. To make the diagnosis accurately on physical examination before surgical intervention is an accomplishment.

How Can Tuberculous Salpingitis Be Distinguished from Chronic Gonorrheal Pelvic Inflammation?

The most likely explanation of failure to diagnose tuberculous pelvic infection correctly is the difficulty in distinguishing it from the various forms of chronic pelvic inflammation. There are several helpful bits of information that may be obtained from the history, as well as observations of the course of the disease.

1. The family history may prove illuminating. Approximately 20 per cent of patients with genital tuberculosis have a family history of tuberculosis. In many instances there will be a suggestion that the patient as an infant or child had been exposed to an infected adult. Approximately half will have had pleurisy, pulmonary lesions, or renal or osseous tuberculosis.

2. The physician should be strongly suspicious of tuberculosis when symptoms of chronic pelvic inflammation appear in a virgin or infertile woman who has no past history of postabortional or venereal infection.

3. Similarly, one may suspect tuberculosis if the pelvic inflammatory process

does not respond to antibiotic therapy as one would expect if the principal abnormality were due to the gonococcus or streptococcus.

4. Although an elevated sedimentation rate and increased leukocyte count may be expected in gonorrheal salpingitis, results are frequently within the normal range in tuberculosis. There is some elevation of the white cell count in approximately one third of the patients who have tuberculous pelvic peritonitis.

How Helpful Is X-ray in the Differential Diagnosis?

Suggestive evidence of tuberculosis is sometimes brought forth on routine examination or in the interpretation of hysterosalpingograms performed in the course of sterility studies. Observations that may lead to a possible diagnosis of tuberculosis are (1) a smooth, rigid "lead pipe" kind of tube with straight contours and dilated regions distal to the isthmus and a tubal lining that is irregular and shaggy; (2) a normal isthmus, but closed ostium from which no dye escapes. Small saccular dilations or fistulous tracts extend out from the ampulla like a "bunch of currants." (3) Filling defects in the tubal shadows, or fistulous tracts in the region of uterus or tube; (4) the presence of calcification in the position of either the tube or ovary; (5) a small uterine cavity and elongated cervix. The outline of the cavity is shaggy and irregular and gives a sawtooth appearance.

The information obtained is useful but not conclusive evidence and alone could hardly provide a basis for definitive therapy. Usually salpingography is used as a diagnostic tool when there has been no suspicion of tuberculosis. This is not without its dangers, for it is possible that unrecognized tuberculous disease might be disseminated by its use.

What Other Tests Are Available as a Diagnostic Tool?

The tuberculin or Mantoux test may be useful in ruling out tuberculosis in the presence of a pelvic mass of unexplained etiology. A negative test is presumptive but not absolute evidence that the patient is free of tuberculosis.

The Mantoux test consists in the intradermal injection of graded amounts of tuberculin to see whether a local skin reaction results. If active tuberculosis is present, a positive skin test will be evident from as little as 0.001 mg. of tuberculin. More concentrated doses are used if no reaction is observed from the smaller amounts. If the patient does not register a response to 0.01 mg. of tuberculin, she probably does not have tuberculosis. Reactions to either old or purified types of tuberculin do not localize the infection. They simply mean that the patient has had tuberculosis and that the infection is producing active hypersensitivity. The focus may be in lung, bone, kidney or lymph node. Lymph nodes affected may be cervical, bronchial or mesenteric.

A careful review of the surgical specimen is in order if there is any clinical suspicion of tuberculosis. Sometimes the diagnosis of tuberculosis is missed in cursory examination if there has been no prior suspicion of tuberculosis. Incomplete removal of tuberculous intestinal or pelvic tissue can result in the appearance of spontaneous fistulas into bladder, rectum or to the abdominal wall, particularly if the operative wound has been drained. When this happens, one should re-evaluate the initial pathologic interpretation and suspect tuberculosis.

Upon What Does the Final Diagnosis Depend?

Since suspicion of genital tuberculosis before operation is aroused by the history, yet cannot be confirmed by physical examination or x-ray study, the final diagnosis must depend on pathologic and bacteriologic study of tissues or secretions.

There are three methods available: (1) histologic study of endometrium removed by biopsy curet or total curettage; (2) culture of tissue or menstrual discharge; (3) guinea pig inoculation of endometrial samples. A combination of these means of study is desirable to provide the most reliable information, for no single method is over 50 per cent accurate, according to recent reports.

HISTOLOGIC STUDY. Certain histologic changes in the endometrium are suspicious of tuberculosis. The finding of tubercles or giant cells in the endometrial stroma surrounded by lymphocytes and plasma cells adjacent to the endometrial glands is presumptive evidence of tuberculosis. The tubercles are usually identifiable, provided the endometrial sample is taken in the week preceding the menstrual period. They will then be present in the superficial layers, although the pathologist may have to hunt for them. If the endometrium has recently been shed, they may still be found in the basal layers, but discovery is more difficult. One should beware of making a diagnosis of tuberculosis on the basis of such observations without positive acid-fast stains, particularly if the patient has had a recent injection of iodized oil in the course of sterility studies (Fig. 45–3, *B*).

There has been some reluctance to perform a curettage for fear of disseminating the tuberculous disease widely. Certainly the pathologist is in a better position to render an accurate diagnosis when presented with adequate material for study. He may or may not obtain this from an endometrial sample. The disadvantages of curettage are more theoretical than real. In most instances a discovery of endometrial tuberculosis is made by accident. If there is real suspicion, the patient can be protected against possible spread by prophylactic injections of streptomycin.

BACTERIOLOGIC STUDY. Two methods are available: (1) culture on special egg media and (2) guinea pig inoculation. Of the two, guinea pig inoculation is the more conclusive. The chief disadvantage is the time required, for it takes six weeks from the time of inoculation before the animal can be sacrificed. Smears are then taken from the regional and lumbar nodes and spleen. These are stained for the tubercle bacillus. The strain may also be typed to determine whether it is human or bovine. Sensitivity determinations complete the study. It is possible to make the inoculation from secretions of menstrual discharge, but endometrial specimens provide the best material for accurate study.

Treatment

Tuberculosis of the uterus and adnexa varies widely in severity and in extent of pathologic change. The treatment, then, must depend on the age of the patient, coupled with the extent of the disease.

Since genital tuberculosis is but a localized manifestation of a general systemic disease, an integral part of any therapeutic regimen must incorporate a program to improve general health. Adequate rest, both physical and mental, must be combined with a properly balanced diet. This is true whether an active extragenital source of infection is demonstrable or not. Since tuberculosis of the endometrium and tube is rarely primary, the basic foci, such as lung and mediastinal lymph nodes, should either be pinpointed or ruled out as far as possible by x-ray study. It is of utmost importance that minimal evidence of the disease should not be regarded lightly and the symptomless patient be left untreated.

In the past there were three methods of therapy available: (*a*) sanatorium care, (*b*) radiation in the form of x-ray or radium, (*c*) surgery, either conservative or radical.

How Effective Were the Older Methods of Therapy? *Sanatorium Care.* Though sanatorium care per se proved very helpful in arresting tuberculosis in lung, bone and kidney, it did little in the long run for genital tuberculosis. The disease progressed slowly and steadily under this passive form of treatment until the patient finally came to operation.

Radium and X-ray. The use of irradiation, whether by x-ray or radium, has been largely abandoned, not only because the newer methods of therapy are more effective, but also because of complications that often followed its use. In many instances radiation seemed to break down the process of repair, permitting further dissemination of the disease, as well as encouraging fistula formation and intestinal obstruction. Because of the deleterious effect of radiation upon the ovary and endometrium, this form of therapy destroyed rather than aided the chances for future pregnancy.

Surgery. Before the advent of the newer drugs, surgery for genital tuberculosis carried a mortality rate of 3.7 per cent, regardless of whether supportive medical care preceded it or not. It was also unfortunate that the highest mortality rate seemed to occur in the younger age group, in whom conservative measures were used. Complications of surgery were also frequent. Chief among these was fistula formation, which ran as high as 14 per cent.

What Does Present-Day Therapy Have to Offer? Today we have the newer drugs, isonicotinic acid hydrazide (isoniazid), para-aminosalicylic acid (PAS) and streptomycin. When these are used alone or in various combinations, the chances of cure are improved dramatically. Enthusiastic reports in the literature suggest that 70 to 80 per cent of patients receiving some combination of these drugs will be cured, and a minimum number will recur.

What Are the Criteria of Cure? The results of therapy from the newer drugs are encouraging, but should be scrutinized closely. To obtain a clearer idea of what it is hoped to accomplish in therapy we should decide what we mean by cure. There are two fundamental aims: (1) eradication of the disease, and (2) the achievement of pregnancy in the nonfertile patient. At present we are able to judge the effectiveness of therapy for the cure or control of the disease by (*a*) the disappearance of symptoms, (*b*) a decrease in the size of the pelvic masses, and (*c*) a failure to grow organisms from material obtained from menstrual discharge, biopsy specimens and endometrial scrapings after curettage.

It is obvious that these criteria are at best an estimate. A patient may have active genital tuberculosis and be asymptomatic, for example. Moreover, the failure to discover tuberculosis on pathologic examination or to grow bacteria from the endometrium does evaluate the effect of drug therapy upon the uterus, but gives no indication of the condition of the fallopian tube. If the tubes are not healed, there is a continuing danger of recurrence.

Achievement of pregnancy is the best proof of the value of the newer drugs in the problem of infertility. A small but increasing number of cases of successful pregnancy following the use of the antibiotic drugs is beginning to appear in the literature.

To apply the drugs effectively on an individual basis and to acquire a true estimate of their value, it is essential that we know how extensive the genital tuberculosis was before treatment. There are reports in the literature suggesting that medical treatment will cure 70 to 80 per cent of endometrial lesions, but only 5 or 10 per cent of tubal tuberculosis.

WHAT IS THE OPTIMUM TREATMENT FOR PATIENTS WITH A MINIMAL AMOUNT OF GENITAL TUBERCULOSIS? For the young patient with minimal disease discovered by endometrial biopsy or curettage, optimum therapy calls for the use of (*a*) isonicotinic acid hydrazide (INH), (b) para-aminosalicylic acid (PAS), and (c) streptomycin. There is encouraging evidence from controlled studies that any combination of these three chemotherapeutic agents may hold the disease in abeyance, or even eradicate it. These results are based on endometrial biopsy studies made at three-month intervals. Ninety per cent of patients showed no reappearance of tubercles within the endometrium after one to three years. A few recurrences have been noted after twelve to eighteen months.

Drug therapy seems to be more effective when only two of the three drugs are combined. The third component is held in reserve for use if the chosen combination fails to control the disease. For example, isonicotinic acid hydrazide is effective in the management of many cases of tuberculosis. Other cases develop a bacterial resistance to it after a time. Para-aminosalicylic acid (PAS) reduces the tendency for the tubercle bacilli to become resistant. This is reduced further when streptomycin is added.

Experience with the use of these drugs has suggested that the therapy should be continued longer than was formerly believed necessary. Excellent results were reported to follow the combined use of either streptomycin and INH, or INH and PAS, given over a three-month period. In every series, however, there were always a few cases that reactivated after one to three years. For this reason therapy has now been prolonged to cover a two- or three-year period.

The dosage schedule varies widely. The following schedule has been recommended by the Committee on Therapy of the American Trudeau Society for the treatment of genital tract tuberculosis:

1. Streptomycin and PAS: (*a*) 1 gm. of streptomycin given intramuscularly 2 or 3 times a week. (*b*) 12 gm. of PAS taken daily by mouth, in 3 or 4 divided doses.

2. Isoniazid alone: 5 mg. or more per kilogram of body weight per day, in 2 or 3 divided doses.

3. Isoniazid plus streptomycin given daily: (*a*) 5 mg. of INH or more per kilogram of body weight. (*b*) 1 gm. of streptomycin daily.

4. Isoniazid daily plus streptomycin twice weekly: Same doses as in *3*.

5. Isoniazid and PAS daily: (*a*) 5 mg. or more of INH per kilogram of body weight. (*b*) 12 gm. of PAS in 3 or 4 divided doses.

6. Isoniazid–PAS–streptomycin: (*a*) 5 mg. or more of INH per kilogram of body weight. (*b*) 12 gm. of PAS in 3 or 4 divided doses. (*c*) 1 gm. of streptomycin given once or twice daily.

The last regimen is very effective, as shown by the fact that renal tuberculosis has practically disappeared after using it. Although some gynecologists prefer to use all three drugs at the same time, most physicians would prefer to withhold streptomycin to cover the patient during surgical therapy, should reactivation appear.

The measure of success of chemotherapy has been based on studies of the endometrium. The effect on the tubes is not known. Enough information is available to state that radical surgery is no longer indicated on every patient with genital tuberculosis. The surgeon can afford to try an intensive regimen of chemotherapy before advocating surgery in the young patient who desires a family. A few successful pregnancies have now been reported following chemotherapy.

SURGERY.   Operation still has a prominent place in modern therapy partly (1) because the diagnosis is frequently not made preoperatively, and (2) because the symptoms from anything more extensive than the earliest phases of the disease stem from the presence of dense adhesions that can hardly be resolved by medical forms of therapy. Surgery is reserved for (a) the patient with pelvic masses that either do not decrease in size or perhaps increase under a regimen of chemotherapy; (b) the girl whose disease is reactivated after years of successful chemotherapy; (c) women in whom the diagnosis has been made at or after the menopause; (d) severe menstrual bleeding that is undermining the patient's general resistance; (e) fistulous tracts that do not heal.

Under the protection of chemotherapy it is now possible to operate on the tuberculous patient without fear of setting up a generalized systemic infection that might lead to death or a serious complication. Operations may help the patient, over and above the actual removal of diseased organs, for it has been a clinical observation for years that many complete cures from peritoneal tuberculosis have followed abdominal exploration alone, without the removal of anything.

With chemotherapy as a protection, one may now safely remove the fallopian tubes, which represent the main genital focus of tuberculous infection, and spare the uterus and ovaries in a young girl who continues to have symptoms of enlarging adnexa. If the disease is too extensive for conservative surgery of this sort, it will still be acceptable therapy to remove the uterus and tubes and leave the ovaries, unless there is actual caseation in their substance. In the woman over forty whose symptoms warrant surgery, it is wise to remove the entire uterus, tubes and ovaries.

Although it is too early to evaluate conclusively the newer therapeutic agents, there is ample reason to predict a more conservative approach to surgery in the near future, provided the disease has not passed into the phase of caseation. The effect of chemotherapy upon the problems of fertility will be determined by the accumulated experience of the future.

SYPHILIS

Syphilis is an infectious venereal disease caused by *Treponema pallidum*. It is a serious disease that develops insidiously and may cause irreparable derangement in function in a variety of organs throughout the body if its true nature is unrecognized. This point is stressed, for the advent of penicillin has naturally reduced the number of cases of syphilis seen in either private practice or hospital outpatient clinics. Through unfamiliarity with its varied manifestations, the physician may well overlook the diagnosis and fail to obtain specimens of blood or spinal fluid for serologic examinations.

Women are usually infected in one of these ways: (1) sexual or osculatory contact with a person who is actively carrying the disease. The contact is customarily either genital or oral. (2) Transmission of the disease through impregnation by a male partner who is in the tertiary stage of the disease. The infectious agent ostensibly passes from the sperm to the fertilized ovum and thence to the maternal blood.

(3) Accidental infection through contaminated blood transfusion. This is a rare occurrence, due to the routine serologic tests of blood donors.

Transmission of the disease to the mother by impregnation of the ovum requires a brief explanation. In the male partner with tertiary syphilis there are no open lesions harboring active *Treponema pallidum*. In order that the female partner be infected, the sperm containing Treponema must actually impregnate the ovum. The spirochete cannot otherwise survive, for it cannot invade normal epithelium as the gonococcus does. Once the ovum is impregnated, the blood of the mother becomes contaminated. The manifestations of the disease are allegedly so mild that she is frequently unaware of it and may even nurse the syphilitic child she has borne without exhibiting any signs of the disease in herself. This was formerly regarded as evidence of the apparent immunity of a mother with a syphilitic child. This was called "Colles's Law of Immunity." In all probability such immunity does not exist. The woman, because of the pregnancy, has mild syphilis. It is said to be impossible to confirm its existence by serologic study of the blood until years later when the late manifestations of maternal syphilis appear.

Course of the Disease

The primary lesion most often appears on the labia majora, but may arise anywhere on the external genitalia. The cervix, formerly disregarded as a primary site, may be directly infected, but this is unrecognized more often than it should be. The vaginal epithelium is rarely affected.

External Genital Manifestations of the Disease

THE PRIMARY LESION.   The primary lesion usually develops on the vulva three or four weeks after exposure. Despite the fact that the disease is transmitted by sexual contact, primary lesions in women in the earliest phases are not commonly encountered. This would seem to indicate that the primary lesion, usually a small papule, superficial crack or minute abrasion, passes unnoticed. Any abraded surface on the external genitalia should be regarded with suspicion. Later on the painless, oval, indurated ulcer with a gray, sluggishly oozing base and a cartilaginoid border becomes unmistakable (Fig. 45–4, *A*). This is a *chancre*. The *swelling* is due to the induration of the surrounding area, and the *discharge* to the weeping from the open ulcer. Unless secondary infection enters the picture, the chancre is painless.

It is obvious that every open sore on the vulva should be investigated, regardless of whether it seems to be healing rapidly and may or may not have the typical appearance of lues. This is best done by wiping the surface of the ulcer with a cotton pledget, followed by gentle squeezing of the lesion to get clear serum, which is placed on a slide. This should be promptly examined by an expert under a darkfield microscope, and a search made for active spirochetes.

When the characteristic chancre develops on the labia, evidence of infection frequently appears in a number of different areas. Glands develop in the groins. Though these glands enlarge, they are rarely tender and never break down into abscesses. The surrounding tissues are not affected. The inflammatory process is confined to the lymph node. The rate of spread to the regional node from the primary site is rapid and occurs before other lesions become evident.

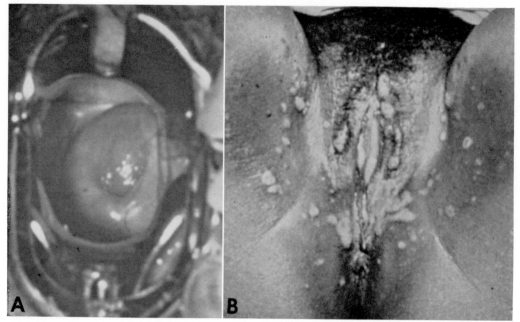

Fig. 45-4.   *A*, A chancre of the cervix has an indurated quality approaching the consistency of cartilage. It is usually eroded or ulcerated and painless. To make a gross diagnosis of chancre here is more difficult than on the lip, penis, or nipple. *B*, Secondary syphilis with condylomata lata and mucous patches on the perineum and thighs. (*B*, Courtesy of U.S. Public Health Service Museum.)

Mixed infections of gonorrhea and syphilis are not uncommon. Since the symptoms of gonorrhea appear earlier and the initial lesion of syphilis is often innocuous, the diagnosis of syphilis may be missed. In any patient with recently acquired gonorrhea, syphilis must be ruled out.

THE SECONDARY STAGE.   As the result of the continually irritating discharge passing over the vulva, syphilitic condylomata (condyloma latum) or mucous patches may develop. The individual warty-like growths tend to run together to form masses scattered over the entire vulva, perineum, arms and the inner surfaces of the thighs (Fig. 45–4, *B*). These broad-based excrescences have moist surfaces and tend to be ulcerated, producing a particularly foul discharge. Spirochetes are frequently present in the discharge. By darkfield examinations and biopsy the syphilitic condylomata are distinguished from condylomata acuminata, which resemble them fairly closely, but are not luetic in origin.

Concomitant with the development of the mucous patches in vulva and mouth, the patient may have a generalized reaction. A maculopapular rash appears on the trunk, and the patient complains of sore throat, headache, fever and malaise. The initial lesion on the vulva has disappeared, but the regional lymph nodes continue to be enlarged. This sequence of events typically follows the initial exposure by seven to ten weeks.

To establish the diagnosis the physician may smear the serous discharge on a slide for darkfield examination or excise the base of a condyloma for pathologic examination (Fig. 45–5). The blood serologic tests, Wassermann, Kahn, Kline, Hinton or VDRL, usually become positive at five weeks and are always strongly positive at this stage.

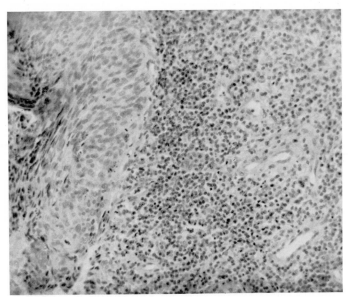

Fig. 45-5.   A syphilitic condyloma, like the other lesions of syphilis, is characterized by vascular endothelial proliferation and an abundant perivascular leukocytic exudate rich in plasma cells. Hyperplastic epithelium covers the surface of the condyloma.

Syphilis of the Cervix

The cervix may be the primary inoculation site, but the initial phases frequently pass unrecognized, for there are no pathognomonic symptoms. The preliminary papillary or superficial ulceration rapidly gives way to a red granular area practically undistinguishable from a simple erosion. There is no obvious induration at this time. Later the cervix frequently exhibits a painless ulcer with overhanging cartilaginoid edges. Induration of the tissue around the ulcer base occurs. The ulceration may appear in more than one area, with seemingly normal cervical epithelium noted between the margins of ulcers. When the superficial discharge is removed from the ulcer crater, the base has a characteristic yellow color that is said to be pathognomonic

The differential diagnosis from cancer of the cervix may necessitate biopsy in the early phases, when it resembles a cervical erosion, and again in the presence of an ulcerating chancre. The two entities are known to coexist. Leukoplakia is thought to arise sometimes on a syphilitic background and later be a precursor of cancer of the cervix.

Treatment

With the advent of penicillin and its proved efficacy in the treatment of syphilis, a tremendous advance was made in the management of a serious disease. Because of the reported results, which are encouraging, the treatment of syphilis has passed from the hospital to the individual physician's office. With it has come a tendency to belittle the potential dangers, which are still present. The syphilitic patient is known to be unreliable. For the treatment to be entirely successful the initial course of therapy must be adequate, and the patient must be followed up for at least one year after the first negative serologic test.

Penicillin in the form of procaine penicillin is the treatment of choice. Many clinicians continue to supplement the penicillin regimen with bismuth and arsenic in an uncomplicated early case of syphilis. To forestall the patient who may fail to appear for the complete course of therapy, a regimen has been devised whereby she receives 1,200,000 units of penicillin G procaine in 4 injections at different sites. If the patient does report for further injections, 600,000 units are given daily for 10 consecutive days.

Syphilis in Pregnancy

Excellent results in infant and mother have been obtained by institution of penicillin therapy as soon as the diagnosis has been made. In all probability a repeat course of treatment should be given with each pregnancy, though one may debate the necessity when a satisfactory response was obtained from an adequate initial course. In a case first diagnosed when the patient is approaching term, 1,200,000 units of penicillin are advised, followed by 600,000 units daily for 10 days. In the earlier trimesters the initial booster dose can be avoided and 600,000 units given daily for 10 days.

Some patients are sensitive to penicillin. The antihistaminic drugs in doses of 75 to 100 mg. daily should then be given as a supplement. If the patient acquires an exfoliative dermatitis or demonstrates uncontrollable intolerance to penicillin, it should be discontinued. Reliance must then be placed on Mapharsen and bismuth subsalicylate.

It would be well to keep in mind that many patients may have been inadequately treated or have not been properly followed up. The late manifestations of syphilis may appear in them years after treatment.

CHANCROID, OR SOFT CHANCRE

Chancroid is primarily a venereal infection, but may be acquired accidentally, particularly by physicians, nurses or orderlies in contact with a patient. It will not penetrate a healthy epithelial cover and infects through a previously existent abscess or skin crack. The causative agent is the Ducrey bacillus. The incubation period is short. Usually chancroid appears in three to five days, but if an open abrasion is present, it may appear in twenty-four hours.

Course of the Disease

The initial lesion is usually a vesicopustule that breaks down rapidly to form a circumscribed saucer-shaped ulceration with a surrounding zone of inflammation and edema. The uneven base of the ulcer is covered with a grayish slough. It is usually painful and very tender to touch. From the ulceration comes a profuse, foul, purulent discharge, which is highly infectious. Infection, however, is characteristically caused by sexual intercourse rather than contamination by contacted articles. Multiple ulcerations are common, tend to become larger and may recur over the years.

The ulcer edge lacks the firm cartilaginous quality of the syphilitic primary chancre. For this reason it is called a "soft chancre." Because of the frequency of the two in combination, it is important to rule out syphilis by darkfield examination.

Approximately half of the cases will develop enlarged inguinal lymph nodes, anywhere from a few days to two weeks later. These are usually unilateral. A characteristic bubo develops as the nodes fuse and become matted together. The mass frequently breaks down into an abscess and may drain spontaneously through the overlying skin. About half, however, will subside.

Diagnosis

Recovery of the Ducrey bacillus may be achieved by smears or culture of material taken from the open lesion. The best method of establishing a diagnosis is by aspirating the pus and culturing on rabbit-blood-agar plates. An intradermal skin test with bacillary vaccine is effective. Although it is said that the typical extensive superficial necrosis of exuberant granulation tissue may permit a correct biopsy diagnosis of chancroid to be made, this is not a generally useful method of diagnosis.

Syphilis, granuloma inguinale and lymphopathia venereum are to be ruled out by darkfield examination, biopsy for Donovan bodies and the Frei test, respectively.

Treatment

The sulfonamide drugs seem to be specific, with a complete cure expected in approximately two weeks. Streptomycin has been used in recent years with considerable success. Hot sitz baths and applications of heat relieve the local discomfort, in anticipation of final cure. If breakdown of the inguinal glands is imminent, it is better to aspirate the nodes rather than incise them.

LYMPHOPATHIA VENEREUM

Lymphopathia or lymphogranuloma venereum differs from granuloma inguinale and other common venereal diseases in that it is caused by a filtrable virus, related to that of psittacosis. The disease is acquired through intercourse with an infected partner. It is a disease of lymph channels and lymph nodes. Lymphatic spread carries the virus to the regional nodes, where a chronic inflammatory process is set up, not only in the glands themselves, but in the adjacent connective tissue as well.

In contrast to granuloma inguinale, it appears not infrequently in the white population. In fact, it may occur in any race at any age, but is seen most commonly in tropical and subtropical countries.

Course of the Disease

The initial lesion, usually a small blister, appears on the genitalia after an incubation period of seven to twelve days. It is often so small and disappears so rapidly that the primary site may be unrecognized. A low-grade inflammatory process develops in the groin within ten to thirty days after exposure. The process usually develops on the same side as the primary lesion. Bilateral groin involvement is uncommon. In the earliest stages a discrete, tender, movable gland can be felt. As the process progresses, all the lymph nodes become involved, as well as the surrounding connective tissue. This results in a firm, tender, bulging mass commonly called the *inguinal bubo.*

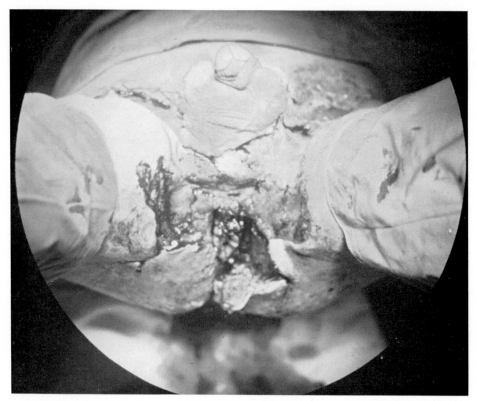

Fig. 45-6.   An advanced case of esthiomène in a male. The extremely destructive nature of the process in the perineal region is evident.

Because of the connective tissue extension, the skin becomes adherent and typically undergoes a color change to purplish-blue. Soft spots develop within the indurated areas, which often drain spontaneously, forming multiple fistulas. In women, actual abscess formation is rare.

Depending on the site of the primary lesion in women, it is common to have direct lymphatic spread to the deep lymph nodes in the pelvis around the rectum. This form of extension follows the appearance of a primary infection in the region of the fourchette; more anterior lesions tend to extend to the inguinal regions.

Perianal and rectal involvement is common. Lymphatic spread extends up along the rectum as far as the sigmoid. Lymphatics in the broad ligaments are implicated, and a "frozen pelvis" may result. The uterus and tubes show some evidence of inflammation, but this is more probably due to an associated gonococcal infection than to the virus of lymphopathia venereum. The urethra is rarely destroyed, or strictures appear. The entire length of the rectum is involved by a deeply penetrating rubbery induration. The rectal mucosa becomes edematous, fibrotic and ulcerated. The end-result is a stiffened tubular rectal structure that tends to stenose later and produce rectal strictures. Formerly these were believed to be secondary to gonorrhea or syphilis.

Because the spread is by lymphatic channels, vulvar elephantiasis is a natural sequel to the perianal and rectal ulcerations. These manifestations are grossly identical with esthiomène or anorectal syphiloma. The late appearance of cancer in these ulcerations occurs more often than can be attributed to chance. (Fig. 45–6).

Symptoms

The clinical course varies. It may be minimal with spontaneous regression. More often the chronic perineal ulceration progresses over a period of years, leaving the patient utterly miserable. The pronounced ulceration and subsequent vulvar elephantiasis make ordinary walking or sitting down a problem. Because of rectal involvement, defecation is accompanied by pain and bloody discharge. As the disease progresses, and in its advanced stages, constitutional symptoms such as fever, headache, chills and abdominal and joint pains are not uncommon. The fever is never high, and leukocytosis is not commonly present. Because it is a virus disease, other systemic manifestations may appear, such as meningitis, arthritis, pleurisy or peritonitis. Occasionally skin rashes are noted.

How to Make a Diagnosis

The most important routine procedure is the Frei test. It usually has become positive when the test is made from twelve to forty days after the appearance of the primary lesion. It is felt to be specific. Once it becomes positive the Frei test remains so for the life of the patient. The test depends on the sensitivity of an infected patient to an antigen prepared by growing the filtrable virus in the yolk sac of embryonated chicken eggs. An intradermal wheal of injected Frei antigen is made on the flexor surface of the forearm. The reaction is read after forty-eight hours. The appearance of a nodule and surrounding erythema, with or without vesicle formation or necrosis of its central portion, is regarded as positive.

Because the test cannot rule out chancroid or granuloma inguinale, and does not

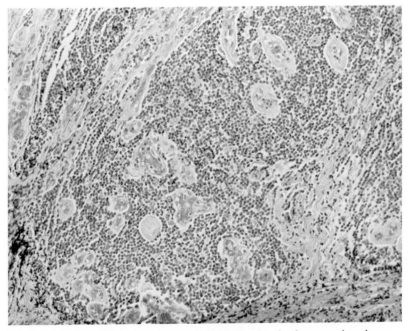

Fig. 45-7. In chronic lymphopathia venereum the involved connective tissues may become infiltrated by sheets of plasma cells. Occasional tuberculoid granulomas may occur, and the combination of these findings around the rectum or in pelvic tissues suggests the correct diagnosis.

give a true index of the activity of the disease process, other tests are sought. The complement-fixation test gives promise of far greater accuracy. Investigators have also noted a reversal in the serum albumin-globulin ratio.

Biopsy characteristically shows a granulomatous process somewhat resembling tuberculosis. The tubercles present have central fibrinoid or nonspecific necrosis rather than caseation, and polymorphonuclear leukocytes collect in their necrotic centers. Between these tuberculoid granulomas there are dense masses of plasma cells (Fig. 45–7). The same microscopic picture characterizes the genital, rectal and lymph node lesions.

The differential diagnosis commonly lies between granuloma inguinale and lymphopathia venereum. Syphilis and chancroid can be eliminated by darkfield examination or cultures for chancroid bacilli, respectively. It is helpful to remember that lymphopathia venereum spreads by lymphatic channels to invade lymph nodes, but granuloma inguinale spreads through the skin itself. When deep sinuses are present, lymphopathia venereum should be suspected. When an open lesion exists, a biopsy may be taken to look for the Donovan bodies of granuloma inguinale or the giant cells of tuberculosis. When there is no open lesion, it is unwise to incise and drain the inguinal bubo. The process may spread to the entire abdominal wall. The bubo should be aspirated, not incised. Proctoscopy and biopsy of rectal lesions should be undertaken to rule out cancer or schistosomiasis.

Treatment

Unlike in other virus infections, sulfonamide therapy seems to be useful, particularly for the inguinal nodes. Aureomycin and particularly Chloromycetin give increasing promise of effective control of the early cases, as well as palliation for the more advanced ones. When the rectum is involved, less satisfactory results are obtained. A colostomy may eventually be necessary because of rectal stricture. In the quiescent stages of vulvar elephantiasis a complete vulvectomy may be indicated.

GRANULOMA INGUINALE

This is a chronic granulomatous ulcerative process that commonly involves the external genitalia and particularly the inguinal region. It is probably venereal in origin, with an associated element of uncleanliness. The etiologic agent is a Klebsiella bacterium, visible as the Donovan bodies, which are encapsulated inclusion bodies in large mononuclear cells. The disease is common in Negroes, but is rare in the white population. The racial incidences are about 10 to 1. It may occur at any age, but is common between twenty and forty years. The incubation period varies from eight days to twelve weeks.

Course of the Disease

The primary lesion is commonly found on the external genitalia. It may occur on the cervix. Rarely cases involving the uterus and ovary have been reported, perhaps acquired through blood stream dissemination. Areas remote from the customary extragenital sources have been noted. A few cases of osteomyelitis have occurred.

The initial lesion rapidly ulcerates. The ulcerations are usually raised above the surface and are nontender. Frequently there is an exuberant growth of soft granulating tissue, which becomes necrotic and bleeds easily. When the lesion is ulcerated, the discharge is profuse and malodorous, partly because of contamination by fusiform bacilli and spirochetes. If secondary infection does not enter the picture, one finds an ulcerating lesion with sharply defined borders and a soft granulating base.

The local sites of infection show little tendency to heal. Extension is usually slow. Daughter lesions develop, and coalescence takes place, forming an extensive chronic ulceration. The advancing border has a characteristic rolled edge. There may be scar tissue at one margin and chronic advancing disease at the other. Spread occurs by way of the superficial layers of the skin and not by lymphatic extension. In rare instances Donovan bodies have been aspirated from lymph nodes, but the customary extension occurs within the skin itself. In this manner the inguinal region becomes involved, but it is not a true gland involvement. Inguinal swellings are common, and abscesses are present. A biopsy of the mass will show involvement of all layers of the skin and the subcutaneous tissue, but classically not of the lymph nodes themselves. This type of swelling carries the name "pseudobubo."

Diagnosis

The diagnosis is confirmed by the finding of Donovan bodies in smears made directly from the surface of the ulcerating lesion. Occasionally the characteristic large phagocytic mononuclear cells with their encapsulated inclusion bodies containing the gram-negative bipolar Donovan bodies are located too deeply within the lesion to appear on the smears. Biopsy of the lesion should be done if smears are negative. Tissue is removed from the central portion of the ulceration, and part may be rubbed between two glass slides. It is then stained with ordinary Wright's or hematoxylin and eosin stain, and the Donovan bodies are identified.

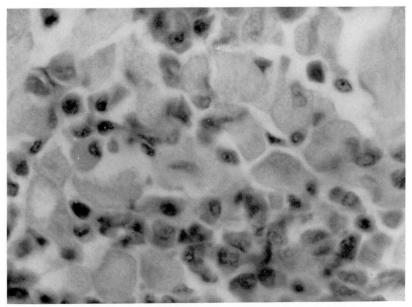

Fig. 45-8.   Large macrophages containing encapsulated inclusions, or Donovan bodies, are the characteristic pathologic finding in granuloma inguinale.

Histologically, granuloma inguinale is recognized by sheetlike proliferations of swollen pale macrophages or Mikulicz cells. Careful scrutiny shows rod-shaped cytoplasmic inclusions with clear capsules. They are gram-negative and resemble minute bacilli (Fig. 45–8). These Donovan bodies are generally considered to represent phagocytosed bacteria related to Friedländer's bacilli, and called *Klebsiella donovani*. Some believe that there is a symbiotic virus infection.

Symptoms

The extensive, chronic spreading ulceration with its concomitant element of secondary infection gives rise to a painful tender mass that exudes a foul discharge. Since the ulceration encroaches on both the urethra and the anus, acts of elimination are most uncomfortable. Contraction of the vagina and the tenderness of the ulceration make intercourse impossible. Sitting or walking may become an ordeal.

Treatment

Streptomycin, 4 gm. daily for 2 to 4 weeks, has proved effective. This has supplanted the time-honored treatment using tartar emetic or antimony salts, which worked well for the early lesions, but did not prevent relapses. Sulfonamides and penicillin preparations have been useless. Failures after streptomycin therapy have been satisfactorily handled by electrosurgical excision, removing wide margins around the lesion.

REFERENCES

Pelvic Tuberculosis

Auerbach, O.: Pulmonary Tuberculosis after Prolonged Use of Chemotherapy. *Am. Rev. Tuberc.*, 71: 165, 1955.

Bloch, R. G., Buchberg, A. S., Permutt, S., and Neumann, G.: The Bacteriology of Tuberculous Lesions Resected after Chemotherapy. *Am. Rev. Tuberc.*, 77: 245, 1958.

Bobrow, M. L., Posner, A. C., and Friedman, S.: A Successful Pregnancy after Endometrial Tuberculosis. *Am. J. Obst. & Gynec.*, 74: 1136, 1957.

Bromberg, Y. M., and Rozin, S.: Pregnancies in a Case of Endometrial Tuberculosis Treated by Streptomycin. *J. Obst. & Gynaec. Brit. Emp.*, 61: 121, 1954.

Burns, W. T., and Burns, F. D.: Extrauterine Pregnancy Complicating Tuberculous Salpingitis. *Am. J. Obst. & Gynec.*, 66: 429, 1953.

Coletta, S.: A Case of Primary Tuberculosis of the Uterine Cervix. *Arch. Ostet. e Ginec.*, 63: 83, 1958.

Halbrecht, I.: Tuberculosis of the Female Genitalia and Pregnancy. *Obst. & Gynec.*, 6: 174, 1955.

Idem: Tubal Missed Abortion in Active and Healed Genital Tuberculosis. *Obst. & Gynec.*, 14: 127, 1959.

Henderson, D. N., Harkins, J. L., and Stitt, J. F.: Pelvic Tuberculosis. *Am. J. Obst. & Gynec.*, 80: 21, 1960.

Kistner, R. W., Hertig, A. T., and Rock, J.: Tubal Pregnancy Complicating Tubercular Salpingitis. *Am. J. Obst. & Gynec.*, 62: 1157, 1951.

Krohn, L., Priver, M. S., and Gotlib, M. H.: New Etiological Factor in Ectopic Pregnancy. *J.A.M.A.*, 150: 1291, 1952.

Lattimer, J. K., and others: Transmission of Genital Tuberculosis from Husband to Wife via the Semen. *Am. Rev. Tuberc.*, 69: 618, 1954.

Magnusson, W.: Further Experience in Roentgen Diagnosis of Tuberculous Salpingitis. *Acta Radiol.*, 28: 824, 1947.

Malkani, P. K., and Rajani, C. K.: Pelvic Tuberculosis. *Obst. & Gynec.*, 14: 600, 1959.

Nogales, F., and Vilar, E.: Clinical and Therapeutic Study of Tuberculosis of the Uterine Cervix; Report Based on Study of 102 Cases. *Rev. Fr. Gyn. Obst.*, 52: 275, 1957.

Rozin, S.: The X-ray Diagnosis of Genital Tuberculosis. *J. Obst. & Gynaec. Brit. Emp.*, 59: 59, 1952.

Ryden, A.: The Treatment of Tuberculous Salpingitis. *Acta Obst. & Gynec. Scand.*, 37: 114, 1958.

Schaefer, G.: Antimicrobial Treatment of Tuberculous Salpingitis. *Am. J. Obst. & Gynec.*, 77: 996, 1959.

Sharman, A.: Genital Tuberculosis; in J. V. Meigs and S. H. Sturgis: *Progress in Gynecology*. New York, Grune & Stratton, Inc., 1957, Vol. III, p. 397.

Studdiford, W. E.: Pregnancy and Pelvic Tuberculosis. *Am. J. Obst. & Gynec.*, 69: 379, 1955.

Sutherland, A. M.: Tuberculosis of the Endometrium. A Report on 250 Cases with the Results of Drug Treatment. *Obst. & Gynec.*, 11: 527, 1958.

Idem: Genital Tuberculosis in Women. *Am. J. Obst. & Gynec.*, 79: 486, 1960.

Syphilis and Chancroid

Binkley, G. W., and Levin, E. A.: The Yearly Admissions of Four Genitoinfectious Diseases at Cleveland City Hospital, with Special Reference to Syphilis. *Am. J. Syph.*, 22: 588, 1938.

Brown, W. J., Sellers, T. F., and Thomas, E. W.: Challenge to the Private Physician in the Epidemiology of Syphilis. *J.A.M.A.*, 171: 389, 1959.

Fiumara, N. J., Appel, B., Hill, W., and Mescon, H.: Venereal Diseases Today. *New England J. Med.*, 260: 863, 1959.

Morgan, H. J.: Factors Influencing the Course of Syphilis. *Am. J. Syph.*, 25: 233, 1941.

Neilson, A. W.: Today's Physician and Venereal Disease. *Missouri Med.*, 57: 591, 1960.

Weiss, R. S., and Joseph, H. L.: *Syphilis*. New York, T. Nelson & Sons, 1951.

Lymphopathia Venereum

Barber, W. H., and Murphy, W. B.: Lymphogranuloma Venereum. *Ann. Surg.*, 113: 30, 1941.

Greenblatt, R. B.: Management of Chancroid, Granuloma Inguinale, and Lymphogranuloma Venereum in General Practice. U.S. Public Health Service Publ. No. 255, 2nd Ed., 1953.

Koteen, H.: Lymphogranuloma Venereum. *Medicine*, 24: 1, 1945.

Mathewson, C., Jr.: Inflammatory Strictures of Rectum Associated with Venereal Lymphogranuloma. *J.A.M.A.*, 110: 709, 1938.

Weinstock, H. L., and Keesal, S.: Lymphogranuloma Venereum. Report of a Case in a Child. *Urol. & Cutan. Rev.*, 50: 520, 1946.

Granuloma Inguinale

D'Aunoy, R., and von Haam, E.: The Pathology of Granuloma Venereum. *Am. J. Path.*, 14: 39, 1938.

Greenblatt, R. B., and Barfield, W. E.: Newer Methods in the Diagnosis and Treatment of Granuloma Inguinale. *Brit. J. Ven. Dis.*, 28: 123, 1952.

Hare, P. J.: Granuloma Inguinale. *Proc. Roy. Soc. Med.*, 53: 564, 1960.

Hester, L. L., Jr.: Granuloma Venereum of the Cervix and Vulva. *Am. J. Obst. & Gynec.*, 62: 312. 1951.

Pariser, H., and Beerman, H.: Granuloma Inguinale. *Am. J.M. Sc.*, 208: 547, 1944.

PART IV

Special Problems in the Later Reproductive Period (Age 30 to 40 Years)

Chapter 46

Abnormal Uterine Bleeding

THE PROBLEMS of diagnosis and management of the patient who gives a history of abnormal menstrual bleeding can be most difficult, particularly in the age group between thirty and forty years. Whereas the predominant cause of abnormal uterine bleeding in the twenty- to thirty-year age span rested with some abnormality of pregnancy, either inside or outside the uterus, abnormal menstrual patterns in the thirties may appear because of (1) derangements of endocrine balance, (2) blood dyscrasias or (3) organic disease within the uterus.

The problems are by no means made less onerous by the fact that there is incomplete agreement as to the basis of normal menstruation. We are, therefore, less well equipped to interpret and direct therapy for the abnormal. We know that much of the bleeding is functional and that the gonadotropic hormones are involved, but there is increasing evidence to indicate that local conditions within the uterus and other bodily systems, as well as the emotional state of the patient, are also implicated.

The history as given by many patients follows no standard pattern and must be evaluated on an individual basis, for it will be modified by each woman's temperament, reaction to life's problems and the circumstances of her surroundings. This is particularly true when one tries to estimate the severity of the vaginal bleeding and the amount of blood loss. The amount of blood actually lost varies from an inconsiderable amount involving daily staining over a prolonged period to excessive amounts noted at regular intervals. The estimate of blood loss is based on the patient's history of the number of pads required daily and the degree of their saturation. Although it is possible for a woman to bleed excessively without the loss being reflected in her blood picture, many women give such a frightening account of excessive bleeding that the hemorrhages hardly seem possible, particularly when no organic disease can be detected. It is always interesting to try to figure out just what any individual patient's periods are like. Some patients record complete data, others have no idea when their period occurred, much less what went on, and still others seem to rely on their husbands to supply the essential details. Furthermore, it is difficult for the gynecologist to decide just when a menstrual period can be considered abnormal. What may be normal for one patient may be totally abnormal for another. As long as the patient's health continues to be unimpaired, there is little reason to regard the bleeding phase as pathologic. Moreover, any attempts to change it are apt to be unsuccessful.

Before any true clinical evaluation can be made of the abnormal bleeding pattern, the history obtained from the patient must be checked against the physical and laboratory findings, as well as consideration given to the patient's temperamental and emotional status. The most important factors in the history are the amount and duration of the flow.

What Types of Abnormal Bleeding Are Noted in This Age Group?

The types of menstrual flow have limitless variations as concern the frequency, duration of the period and the amount of actual blood loss. Among the common patterns of menstrual flow noted in this age group are (1) irregular or continuous bleeding, (2) frequent and often profuse periods occurring at regular intervals, (3) profuse regular periods that appear at normal intervals, (4) periods that come infrequently, but are profuse when they do.

Many terms are used to describe the menstrual flow. Patients with *menorrhagia* make up the largest group with abnormal vaginal bleeding patterns. The flow occurs regularly, but is profuse and may be prolonged. The cycle may be either ovulatory or anovulatory. *Metrorrhagia* is the term used when bleeding occurs at other times than the normally expected date. Various types of vaginal bleeding are encountered: (1) The bleeding may be prolonged for several weeks after a normal period. (2) The flow may occur at any time without regard to the normal cycle. (3) Intermenstrual spotting may appear at irregular intervals or be continuous throughout the cycle. It is apt to occur just before the period.

What Are the Possible Causes of Abnormal Uterine Bleeding in This Age Group?

The principal causes of bleeding in the thirty- to forty-year age group are functional ones. They may or may not be associated with palpable organic abnormalities. When vaginal bleeding is associated with palpable gross lesions, the bleeding is far more likely due to endocrine imbalance than to either tumor or an aftermath of infection, statistically speaking.

Cancer is not unknown in this age group, but it is not a prime consideration as a cause of uterine bleeding. Papillary cystadenocarcinoma of the ovary can occur in any age group. Carcinoma of the cervix occurs occasionally, and cancer of the endometrium rarely. Though malignant tumors appear infrequently, they occur often enough for one to keep the possibility constantly in mind before accepting a diagnosis of benign disease.

Though we have discussed abnormal bleeding in the twenties and suggested that pregnancy and its complications provide the most logical explanation, the problem is by no means restricted to that age group. There are simply fewer functional explanations of vaginal bleeding at that time. As long as a woman remains reproductive, there is always the chance that the bleeding may be secondary to retained products of gestation, miscarriage, ectopic pregnancy or abortion, whether threatened or real.

Tumors or infection within the endometrial cavity may be the explanation of abnormal uterine bleeding. Chronic endometritis often follows an abortion or miscarriage. Submucous fibroids, intramural fibroids that encroach on the endometrial cavity, or polyps are frequent causes of excessive vaginal bleeding in this age group.

Profuse and prolonged uterine bleeding can be due to clotting disturbances or other alterations in blood or blood cells, as well as to tumors or endocrine imbalances. Blood dyscrasias such as leukemia and aplastic anemia have always to be considered possible indirect explanations of the cause of menorrhagia. Usually, however, the main cause of vaginal bleeding from these entities is either some associated uterine disease or a functional one. In *thrombocytopenic purpura* the cause is more direct, for the defect can be traced to the reduction in the number of platelets. Iron deficiency anemia is another example of a hematologic cause of menorrhagia. A vicious circle seems to develop, for the excessive blood loss at the time of the period causes a chronic iron deficiency, which in turn produces further and more intensive bleeding. Less common hematologic causes of menorrhagia are vascular purpura and a recently discovered type of *pseudohemophilia* peculiar to women.

Systemic diseases occasionally may account for persistent bleeding. Perhaps the most likely constitutional causes for excessive bleeding are hypertension and cardiovascular disease, particularly when they manifest themselves by cardiac decompensation and chronic passive venous congestion. Cirrhosis of the liver is another relatively rare cause of persistent and excessive uterine blood loss. The most common metabolic disturbance that produces a pronounced increase in menstrual flow is *hypothyroidism*.

The evaluation of the patient's psyche and emotional state in relation to the vaginal bleeding problem is receiving increasing support to explain some of its bizarre manifestations.

Although disturbances in hormonal balance explain most abnormal uterine bleeding patterns in this age group, the spectrum of causes is so broad that therapy often seems empirical and carries with it little physiologic background. Before instituting treatment it is of the utmost importance that differentiation be made between functional and organic causes for the bleeding picture.

WHAT ROLE DOES INFECTION PLAY IN THE ETIOLOGY OF ABNORMAL UTERINE BLEEDING IN THIS AGE GROUP? It is well known that many women date the onset of their irregular menstrual pattern from the time of a previous miscarriage. The explanation may lie in the retention of placental fragments, placental polyps or subinvolution of the uterus, but it is far more likely that inflammatory changes have occurred in the epithelial lining and possibly the muscle around the endometrial cavity. When the infection has involved the basal layer of the endometrium, it will show, on histologic examination, focal or diffuse infiltration with plasma cells and lymphocytes, sometimes with polymorphonuclear leukocytes as well. Normal cyclic development of the inflamed uterine mucosa may take place, but the sloughing of this endometrium is often accompanied by profuse and prolonged menstrual bleeding. Intrauterine infections that appear post delivery or secondary to abortions are apt to interfere with the normal regenerative processes in the superficial or functional layers of the endometrium, with the result that the subsequent periods are both excessive and prolonged.

The diagnosis of chronic endometritis based upon examination of endometrial scrapings has recently been revived and is now being reported increasingly frequently. The histologic diagnosis depends on the presence of lymphocytes, plasma cells and other leukocytes in adequate quantity to substantiate the diagnosis of inflammatory change. Typically the maturation and secretory functional changes of the inflamed endometrium are so altered that no dating of such specimens is possible (Fig. 46–1). Though the majority of patients who show chronic endometritis on endometrial biopsy sampling will give an antecedent history of pregnancy or its complications, there are many recorded instances in which the diagnosis is made in the absence of any history suggesting previous pregnancy. To date bacteriologic studies, both in aerobic and anaerobic media, have not progressed to the point at which it can be stated with any certainty whether the isolated areas of endometritis are due to bacterial infection or to other causes, such as viruses, hypersensitivity or autosensitization.

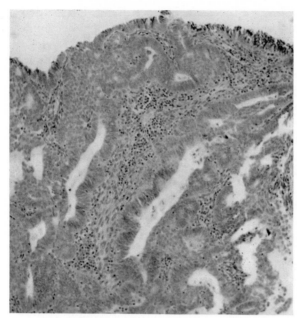

Fig. 46-1. Chronic endometritis is recognized by the presence of plasma cells, as well as lymphocytes and macrophages, in the endometrial stroma. The glandular changes are not classifiable as either normal proliferative or secretory phase endometrium.

In addition to actual infection within the endometrial cavity, it is also evident that extrauterine infections may be responsible for the changes noted in the endometrium. This would be particularly true of postabortal infections and tuberculosis. Miliary tubercles are sometimes found when the curettage or endometrial biopsy has been carried out in the latter half of the menstrual cycle. They are almost invariably secondary to primary disease in the fallopian tube. Such lesions may be silent, however, and the first manifestation of tuberculosis in the genital tract may be abnormal vaginal bleeding that calls for endometrial sampling or curettage. Postabortal infections, on the other hand, are ascending in nature with the endometrium primarily involved and the tubal infection a secondary manifestation. Periodic sloughing of the endometrial lining takes place, however, leaving the residuum of infection in the tube and ovary. Such patients may have both a profuse and irregular vaginal bleeding that is atypical in timing.

WHAT INTRAUTERINE ORGANIC LESIONS PRODUCE EXCESSIVE UTERINE BLEEDING IN THE THIRTY- TO FORTY-YEAR AGE GROUP? The two most common pathologic entities within the uterus which account for excess bleeding at regular intervals are (a) endometrial polyps and (b) submucous fibroids. Neither one can be felt on physical examination.

Endometrial Polyps. Localized hyperplastic overgrowths of endometrium are called polyps. They vary in size from 0.5 to 3 cm. in diameter and may be either single or multiple. In most instances they are small, flat, smooth sessile growths that have little clinical significance. Some are located in the uterine cornua, where they are rarely detached by curettment (Fig. 46–2). Occasionally they produce an unbelievable amount of bleeding. The actual mechanism is not clear, but it is a clinical fact that many patients are cured of menorrhagia when small polyps have been removed. Pedunculated polyps are larger. Microscopically, they closely resemble the pattern of the surrounding hyperplastic mucosa. The stroma is edematous or fibrous, and the histologic picture typically is that of cystic hyperplasia.

Sometimes adenomatous hyperplasia, carcinoma in situ or invasive carcinoma is found in endometrial polyps. True polyps are generally regarded as neoplastic, whether benign or malignant. Because the larger polyps are pedunculated, they often prolapse through the external os (Fig. 46–3, *A*). The distal end may become ulcerated either because of the exposed position or because it has outgrown the blood supply. Profuse bleeding may occur from the necrotic tip. Generally speaking, endometrial polyps are considered to be precancerous lesions, but only a few ever develop into cancer.

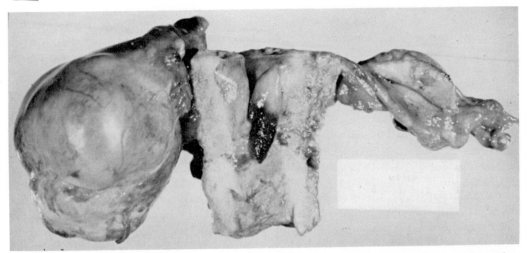

Fig. 46-2.   A cornual endometrial polyp with a hemorrhagic distal portion is shown, so located as to be difficult to remove by curettage. The large ovarian mass proved to be a fibroma.

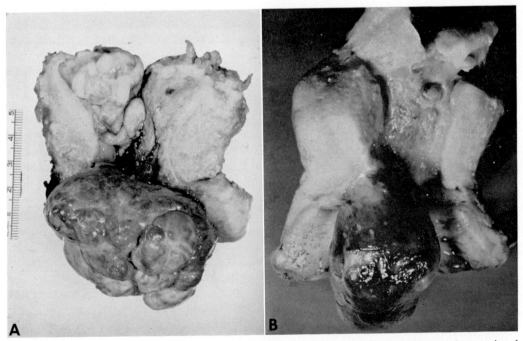

Fig. 46-3.   *A*, Prolapse of a massive endometrial polyp through the cervical os may be associated with considerable vaginal bleeding. *B*, A submucous fibroid tumor of the myometrium may protrude through the cervix into the vagina. Whether prolapsed or not, submucous uterine fibroids often bleed excessively from their peripheral blood vessels, which are seen beneath the surface of this specimen.

Submucous Fibroids (Leiomyomas). Excessive hemorrhage, occurring at the regular time of the menstrual period, particularly when the patient speaks of "flooding" or "gushing," is in all probability due to the presence of a submucous fibroid (leiomyoma), or an intramural fibroid tumor that encroaches on the uterine cavity (Fig. 46–3, *B*). The patient bleeds so profusely that additional sanitary pads are necessary during the day and protective covering of the bed linen at night. Many women never leave their home during the period because of fear of embarrassing incidents when sudden flooding occurs. Large clots are common, and the patient has a "washed-out feeling" after the completion of the menstrual flow, which normally is not prolonged. If successive menstrual periods of hemorrhagic proportions occur, the hemoglobin frequently falls to the range of 6 or 8 gm. per 100 ml. Whenever this sort of history is encountered, one thinks immediately of either a submucous fibroid tumor or hypothyroidism.

The majority of fibroid tumors, other than the submucous fibroid, bleed because of estrin stimulation unbalanced by progestin. The vaginal bleeding is anovulatory. The patient with a submucous leiomyoma usually has ovulatory cycles. She does not bleed from endometrial hyperplasia, but rather from thinning out of the endometrium overlying the fibroid tumor. The normal rhythmic contractions of the uterine musculature are impeded by the presence of the tumor, the exposed, coiled arterioles cannot contract, and they continue to bleed excessively. The mechanism is not unlike the bleeding one notes in the postmenopausal age group, when hemorrhage may occur from an atrophic, nonfunctioning endometrium.

WHY DO PATIENTS WITH CHRONIC IRON DEFICIENCY ANEMIA BLEED EXCESSIVELY? The mechanism of bleeding in patients with iron deficiency anemia is similar to that of the submucous fibroid, namely, atrophy of the endometrium. The mucous membranes throughout the body are thought to become thinned out and unusually friable, particularly at all mucocutaneous junctions, of which perhaps the endometrium may be regarded as one.

It is important to distinguish between a normochromic anemia, which results simply from chronic blood loss, and a hypochromic anemia due to iron deficiency. The treatment is obviously to administer iron if a deficiency exists, while one must find the principal source if anemia is simply due to blood loss.

The cause of an iron deficiency anemia in women may be (*a*) a diet inadequate in iron, (*b*) gastric achlorhydria, which prevents the proper digestion of iron-containing foods, (*c*) poor intestinal absorption, and (*d*) menorrhagia. Menorrhagia is rarely the only factor, but when it is combined with achlorhydria and an inadequate diet, an iron deficiency hypochromic anemia may be expected.

Clinically, one may suspect iron deficiency anemia in a woman who demonstrates pallor, particularly of mucous membranes and nail beds, lassitude and indifferent appetite, and who gives a history of frequent or excessive menstrual periods, or both.

WHAT ROLE DOES PSYCHIATRY PLAY IN THE ABNORMAL BLEEDING PATTERN? There can be little doubt that emotional unrest can disturb the menstrual pattern. Usually this is in the direction of amenorrhea, but excessive bleeding episodes are not uncommon. The actual mechanism of uterine bleeding is not known, but the action may be mediated through either the release or blockage of the pituitary gonadotropins by the hypothalamus, or perhaps via direct action on the uterine vascular system through the sympathetic nerves. Fear manifesting itself in many guises seems to figure prominently in the history of patients who have psychogenic menorrhagia. Emotional stress, nervous and personality disorders, psychoses and sexual perversions have all been listed as possible causes.

In most instances the bleeding is excessive and prolonged, though the interval is not disturbed. The cycle would appear to be associated with ovulation in most instances. This is not always true, however, for at times the endometrium appears to be hyperplastic. Furthermore, it has been noted that emotional stress may inhibit ovulation and the uterine bleeding be painless, though excessive, in contrast to the pattern preceding the psychiatric episode, when dysmenorrhea was to be expected.

Occasionally the vaginal bleeding occurs at times other than the time of the expected period (metrorrhagia). The same initiating causes are present, namely, emotional shock, stress or fright. There is much we do not understand of the mechanisms involved, for it is a well known observation that many kinds of therapy, including curettage, have proved ineffective. Final cure has come about only when the psychiatric cause has been removed.

WHAT ENDOCRINE FACTORS ARE CONCERNED IN THE MECHANISM OF ABNORMAL UTERINE BLEEDING BETWEEN THIRTY AND FORTY YEARS? *Hypothyroid State.* One important example of endocrine imbalance that produces an excessive degree of uterine bleeding is hypothyroidism. The same gushing, flooding sort of flow is noted in patients who have a submucous fibroid tumor. The true myxedematous patient does not bleed at all, but the less extreme thyroid malfunction does produce an excessive menstrual flow. These patients frequently do not perspire in the summer heat and are apt to complain of cold hands and feet. Constant and pronounced fatigue is usually noted, together with a tendency to gain weight. In most instances the hypothyroid patient will also have anovulatory bleeding. Relatively few will show secretory changes in the endometrium.

Endometrial Hyperplasia. Although true functional bleeding and anovulatory cycles from endometrial hyperplasia are most common at puberty and just preceding the menopause, it is still a common explanation of abnormal bleeding problems between these ages. The difference between anovulatory bleeding and hyperplasia is simply one of duration and degree of estrin stimulation and the intensity of the endometrial response in the thirty- to forty-year age group. Microscopically, excessive cystic or adenomatous overgrowths of the endometrial glands, in the proliferative phase, are noted (Fig. 46–4). This histologic picture of endometrial cystic or adenomatous hyperplasia is sometimes referred to clinically as *metropathia*. Inspection of the ovaries may reveal polycystic changes. Many follicles are as yet unruptured with no evidence of corpus luteum development, either recent or old. The abnormalities present were discussed previously with the Stein-Leventhal syndrome (Chap. 35). The proximate endocrine defect lies in the ovary, which produces excessive amounts of estrogen unbalanced by progestin. It is possible that some of the fault lies in the pituitary, which fails to produce the normal rhythmic output of the FSH and LH gonadotropins. FSH may be secreted exclusively.

Functional bleeding of this sort is common also to such conditions as intramural and subserous fibroid tumors, endometriosis, adenomyomas and pelvic inflammation. There is a common misconception that the patient with a fibroid tumor bleeds because of the tumor. This is true only of the submucous fibroid, which cannot be felt. A patient may have many fibroids in the uterus or a large fibroid rising to the umbilicus and have normal, uncomplicated menstrual periods. When the patient with a fibroid tumor bleeds, she commonly does so because of the ovarian dysfunction associated with the tumor. The same mechanism explains the excessive bleeding that sometimes appears in patients with pelvic inflammation or endometriosis.

The actual mechanism is not known. It is probable, however, that (a) the con-

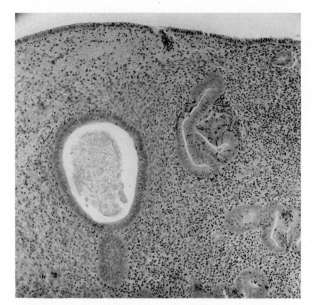

Fig. 46-4. Endometrial hyperplasia, here partially cystic and partially adenomatous, may arise from continuous estrogenic stimulation and lead to functional bleeding, as shown in the superficial layers.

tinuous stimulation by estrin eventually causes the endometrium to outgrow the blood supply locally, become necrotic and break down in patchy areas. This is called "breakthrough" bleeding. (*b*) At higher levels of estrogen found with endometrial hyperplasia, smaller changes in estrogen concentration than would be effective with a normal endometrium may lead to necrosis. This is called "teetering of the titer" of estrogen. (*c*) The estrin stimulation from the ovary falters and finally ceases, producing a withdrawal type of bleeding.

Irregular Endometrial Maturation in Ovulatory Cycles. A far less common type of functional vaginal bleeding occurs from an endometrium that contains both proliferative and secretory elements (Fig. 46–5). The cycles themselves are of normal duration, and obviously ovulation has taken place, for some of the endometrium is secretory. In contrast to the true functional uterine bleeder, in whom no ovulation occurs, irregular maturation of the endometrium is most common in the thirty- to forty-year age group and is rarely encountered at puberty or immediately before the menopause.

Clinically, the entity may be suspected when the patient gives a history of constantly recurring periods that are normal in interval, but both excessive and prolonged. The period, instead of stopping within four or five days, continues on for ten or twelve.

The basis of irregularity of the endometrial development is believed to be irregular ripening or maturation of the secretory endometrium. In normal women curetted as part of a sterility investigation or for other reasons, it is not uncommon to find a small quantity of proliferative endometrium mixed with a large amount of normal secretory-phase curettings. Usually it is thought that a small part of the uterine lining for unknown reasons had not responded to the normal hormonal stimulation. Also in secretory endometrial specimens it is often observed that different portions show changes characteristic of a spread of three or four different days of the cycle, such as a mixture of 18-day, 21- and 22-day secretory endometrium. This is believed to be within normal limits, and the date assigned for diagnostic purposes is the furthest advanced day that is recognized. The reason is that this is found to give the best clinical correlation with the menstrual history and basal body temperature data.

Irregular maturation and shedding of the endometrium is an exaggerated variation similar to what has just been described. Perhaps half of the endometrium is found in proliferative phase, however, and the other half in secretory phase. Or portions of secretory endometrium are found that vary in maturation by 7 days or more, such as foci of 17-day and 24- or 25-day endometrium side by side. If a double or bicornuate uterus, or confusion with lower uterine segment endometrium can be excluded, such a wide variation in endometrial maturation is recognized as abnormal, and bleeding from it is ascribed to irregular maturation.

Ostensibly, failure of the endometrium to react correctly to normal hormonal stimulation is to be blamed. If abnormal hormonal factors are involved, there is no evidence to prove this. The condition of genuine abnormal irregular maturation and shedding of endometrium is so rare that it should be diagnosed only after elimination of several more likely possibilities discussed in this section.

Irregular Endometrial Shedding. The histologic picture in a patient who sheds her endometrium irregularly, so that secretory changes are noted at a time when reparative proliferation is to be expected, is similar to the typical pattern observed during the desquamation that accompanies normal menstruation and the resulting attempts at regenerative repair. It is simply the timing that is wrong. This process is normally usually completed by about the third day of menstruation. With the entity of irregular shedding the same observations are made beyond the fifth menstrual day. If we are to attribute abnormal bleeding to irregular shedding, the endometrial sample, preferably a curettage specimen, must be taken on or after the fifth day of bleeding.

There is complete lack of any surface covering epithelium and a great variation in the thickness of the mucosa. The endometrial glands are for the most part collapsed, though they continue to show evidence of secretion. The reason for the collapse probably can be attributed to the stroma, which has become condensed through fluid loss. The dense stroma is seen compressed between the secretory glands. Leukocytes infiltrate into the stroma, and the coiled arteries have not involuted, though they have

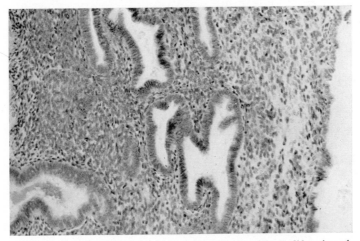

Fig. 46-5. Irregular endometrial maturation is evident, with proliferative phase glands in the center, and a gland with secretory vacuoles at the lower left. This uncommon condition may be associated with menorrhagia.

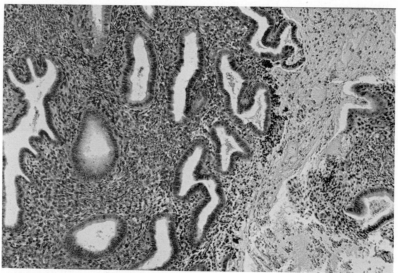

Fig. 46-6.   The coexistence of fragments of proliferative, secretory and menstrual endometrium in the same curettage specimen constitutes evidence of chronic menstruation.

begun to contract and lose their elastic fibers. Along with the exhausted secretory glands one finds some short straight tubules indicating early regenerative proliferation. Thus we have evidence of secretory glands, menstrual desquamation and early repair going on at the same time. These changes are not uniform throughout the endometrium, but tend to occur in isolated areas.

In essence, then, irregular shedding of endometrium involves a prolonged menstrual phase, with histologic evidence of late secretory endometrium, exhausted secretory endometrium, menstrual fragmentation and early regeneration.

CHRONIC MENSTRUATION.   This term, or chronic menstrual endometrial bleeding, is applied particularly when a period of uterine bleeding continues for more than ten or twelve days, and lasts up to forty days. The flow may be slight, moderate or severe enough to require transfusions. Most of these women are otherwise healthy and fertile.

Curettage provides endometrium portions of which are typical of the mid or late proliferative, the secretory and the menstrual phases of the normal cycle. This mixture is paradoxical, and the problem is resolved by the diagnosis of chronic menstrual endometrium (Fig. 46–6).

The actual cause of vaginal bleeding in the patient who matures and sheds her endometrium in this irregular and delayed fashion is not completely understood. There appears to be some defect in corpus luteum function. Normally one would expect the corpus luteum to regress promptly at the end of a cycle when pregnancy is not forthcoming. In these cases there appears to be a persistence of luteal secretion, so that one finds an active secretory endometrium in some areas while menstrual changes occur elsewhere, and the regeneration of the proliferative phase is noted in still others. This may be due to faulty secretion of gonadotropins on the part of the anterior pituitary. Evidently there is enough residual corpus luteal activity to maintain some secretory endometrium intact so that we can recognize it microscopically, but progesterone is not present in sufficient quantity to keep the entire endometrium from menstrual bleeding followed by local regeneration. Whatever the cause, curettage alone usually cures chronic menstruation, and nothing need be done to the ovary. This suggests some functional interdependence between endometrium and ovary beyond the usual target-organ status of the uterus.

What Are the Histologic Characteristics of the Different Types of Endometrium Found in This Age Group?

A wide variety of patterns of menstrual flow has been recognized in the thirty- to forty-year age group. Unfortunately there appears to be no constant relation between the histologic pattern in the endometrium and the type of vaginal bleeding. This is particularly true of this age group.

Endometrial Hyperplasia

All grades of endometrial proliferation are noted, depending on the degree of hormonal stimulation and the duration of its activity. There appears to be little relation between the thickness of the hyperplastic endometrium and the extent of the vaginal bleeding. In most instances curettage produces a copious amount of thick endometrium which has a moist, velvety texture for the most part, but can be granular. The color varies from gray to yellow. The more yellow and mucoid, the more likely the diagnosis of hyperplasia (Fig. 46–7).

The final analysis depends on the histologic examination. The microscopic picture varies, depending on whether or not the patient is bleeding at the time curettage is performed. Among the many histologic patterns encountered two principal types are commonly seen: (1) cystic hyperplasia and (2) adenomatous hyperplasia.

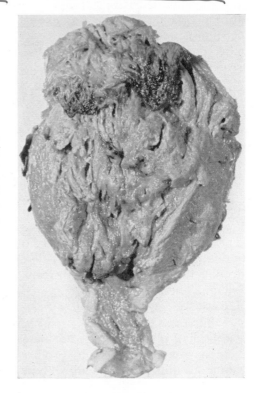

Fig. 46-7. Hysterectomy specimen of extreme endometrial hyperplasia, removed because of prolonged, severe vaginal bleeding. The shaggy overgrowth of the uterine lining and the darker hemorrhagic areas are evident. This diabetic patient had received depot estrogen injections to assist in maintaining pregnancy. (Courtesy of Dr. A. T. Hertig, from the Warren Museum.)

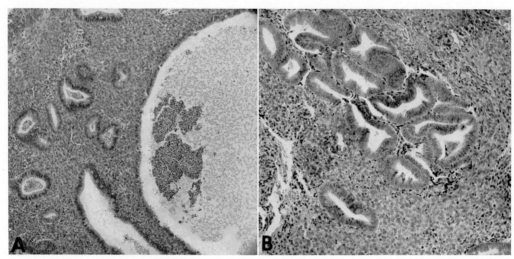

Fig. 46-8. *A,* The endometrial glands are slightly or greatly spherically dilated and lined by crowded columnar cells. It is an equal proliferative growth of the epithelium all along the glands that results in cystic hyperplasia. The largest gland contains pus, indicating pyometra, which commonly complicates endometrial hyperplasia. *B,* Irregular epithelial proliferation results in the crowded, distorted glandular pattern of adenomatous endometrial hyperplasia. The stromal pattern is not of diagnostic value.

CYSTIC HYPERPLASIA IN THE NONBLEEDING PHASE.   Histologic evidence is sought in both the glands and the stroma.

The Glandular Pattern.   On microscopic section cystic dilatation of the glands is the most characteristic finding. Evidence of such change is apparent on examination of the prepared slide with the unaided eye. This is what one means when the endometrium is said to resemble "swiss cheese." Only a few of all the glands may have undergone cystic dilatation, but the remainder appear crowded and present in increased numbers. The epithelial cells lining the glands are compressed together, are tall and columnar and follow a well oriented pattern. There is no evidence of normal secretory changes within the cells (Fig. 46–8, *A*). This picture is a pathologic exaggeration of that observed normally during the stage of proliferation, and it follows perhaps after four to six months of continuous uninterrupted endometrial proliferative growth. True secretion is usually absent, beyond that small amount of seromucoid produced by all glands and ducts that are not completely inactive.

When the cystic glands become stabilized and their active growth phase ends, the epithelial lining changes to the cuboidal type and achieves the characteristic appearance of a fully developed "swiss cheese" endometrium. Since glands of this type are apt to appear in the inactive or senile endometrium, a diagnosis of cystic hyperplasia cannot be entertained simply on the finding of cystic glands. In obsolete cystic hyperplasia the epithelial cells are locally flattened and stretched, and in cystic atrophy the endometrial epithelium is so flattened as to resemble vascular endothelium. The finding of secretory activity will in most instances rule out true hyperplasia.

Appearance of the Stroma.   When one looks at the stroma, particularly in the nonbleeding phase, there is an increase in both its density and cellularity. In fact there may sometimes be more proliferation of the stroma than the glandular element. Numerous mitotic figures are seen in the proliferating spindle-shaped cells. Another important observation is the presence of numbers of large sinusoidal vessels which, instead of being confined to the basal layers, as they are in a normally developing endometrium, extend throughout the full thickness and can be identified in the superficial layers. This phenomenon occurs in response to estrin stimulation, in all probability.

Lymph follicles composed of lymphocytes with or without germinal centers are found in all proliferative endometria, and may be prominent in hyperplastic endometrium. The old diagnostic term "hyperplastic endometritis" did not refer to inflammation, but to the triad of cystic glandular hyperplasia, dilated vascular sinusoids, sometimes with thrombi, and the presence of lymphocytic follicles.

CYSTIC HYPERPLASIA IN THE BLEEDING PHASE. There are two added elements that appear in patients with cystic hyperplasia who are bleeding at the time curettage is performed: (a) The presence of patchy areas of necrosis can be identified, within which there is thrombosis of sinusoidal blood vessels. (b) Leukocytic infiltration of the tissues is more extensive.

With or without vaginal bleeding, cystic endometrial hyperplasia has some precancerous significance. Most women with this type of hyperplasia never have endometrial cancer, so that the change to cancer is anything but inevitable. In a few cases, however, perhaps 5 or 10 per cent of the entire group, endometrial cystic hyperplasia does eventually progress to carcinoma. Investigation of previous curetted specimens in women with proved endometrial carcinomas has showed that it is most often about eight to twelve years between the stage of endometrial cystic hyperplasia and the later diagnosis of carcinoma. Some of the cystic hyperplastic changes are found in endometrial polyps.

ADENOMATOUS HYPERPLASIA. Endometrial proliferation depends on the amount and degree of unbalanced estrin stimulation. It is therefore not surprising to find more atypical growth patterns, in addition to excessive cellular proliferative activity. There is some evidence that adenomatous hyperplasia may be a more immediate forerunner of endometrial carcinoma than cystic hyperplasia. The true explanation for the presence of the overactive endometrium may well be due to the unremitting effects of unopposed estrin, but there is a recent suggestion that the pituitary may also be implicated, as the ovaries receive an abnormal stimulation from the pituitary gonadotropins. On gross examination adenomatous hyperplasia presents much the same appearance that was noted with cystic hyperplasia, except that there is a greater tendency for it to be irregular and granular, as well as finely nodular. Some evidence of true or pseudopolyp formation may be present.

The microscopic picture is a distinct contrast to that seen in cystic hyperplasia. The stroma is similar, but there is a notable overgrowth of the glandular elements, which have a multiplicity of growth patterns. Changes may occur diffusely throughout the endometrial lining or appear in patchy areas. In many places the glands are so closely packed together that they appear almost back to back with little intervening stroma. Papillary projections are frequently seen, some of them extending into the gland lumens, while others appear to project outward into the surrounding stroma. The glands are no longer cylindrical, but are irregularly formed, with shapes like clover-leaves or the fingers of a glove (Fig. 46–8, B). This is what is meant by adenomatous. At all points, however, the basement membrane is intact.

The epithelial cells themselves vary in size and shape and may contain mitoses. In most instances the cells are properly oriented to each other, but in the areas where they seem to pile up and project into the stroma the arrangement is not always so clear. There is a tendency for nuclei of the cuboidal or columnar cells lining the glands to be hyperchromatic. It is evident that there are often some of the histologic characteristics of anaplasia present in adenomatous hyperplasia. Invasion is absent, but in the most atypical instances the histologic pattern approaches that of intraepithelial cancer (carcinoma in situ). Anaplasia and carcinoma in situ will be discussed later in relation to endometrial carcinoma (Chaps. 58, 68).

As with cystic endometrial hyperplasia, adenomatous hyperplasia is to some extent a precancerous condition, but the fact is that in most women adenomatous hyperplasia never develops into carcinoma. In many one curettage is curative, and in others repeated curettements will control the condition until the menopause, when atrophy ensues. Probably at the most 10 per cent of women with adenomatous hyperplasia may later have endometrial carcinoma. Thus the condition usually is not irreversible and can be managed successfully with conservative therapy.

In women who have been proved to have endometrial carcinoma, re-examination of previously curetted material has shown adenomatous hyperplasia to be most common about three to eight years before carcinoma was recognized.

What Is Meant by an Underdeveloped Secretory Endometrium?

Much interest has recently been aroused in the so-called underdeveloped secretory endometrium. This could be an important factor in infertility. Unfortunately it is not easy to confirm the histologic evidence of progesterone deficiency by clinical methods. We know that the progestational response in the gland epithelium and stroma is linked to glycogen and the activity of the enzyme, alkaline phosphatase. Phosphatase apparently increases sharply in the proliferative and early secretory phases of the cycle, but drops rapidly after the eighth postovulatory day. Unfortunately, varying quantities of the enzyme are recovered from different endometria, and we are sure of the ovulatory date only if the basal body temperature is a true indication of this event. The vacuoles containing glycogen can be seen in the basal levels of the glandular epithelium after ovulation and can be traced into the lumen of the gland and surface thereafter, but unfortunately variations in the quantity of glycogen cannot be determined by the histochemical methods so far used. The evidence for the underdeveloped secretory endometrium thus is based on histologic interpretation (Fig. 46–9).

This appears to be a real entity, for it has been said that 20 per cent of the endometria will appear to be retarded in their development if biopsies are taken late in the cycle, after the basal body temperatures have suggested that ovulation has occurred. It is important that the histologic evidence be sought in the most highly developed areas of the endometrium and that no conclusions be made on material obtained from the lower uterine segment. It is uncertain whether the underdeveloped secretory endometrium appears because of corpus luteum failure or whether the endometrium is simply sluggish in its own response.

Some deficiency of glycogen is evidently important in both sterility and habitual abortion. It would be useful to correct the progestational deficiency by substituting the proper hormone in effective doses. We know that sufficient estrin will prevent the progestational phase from developing and that chorionic gonadotropin will augment it, but unfortunately even large doses of progesterone, either alone or in combination with estrin, do not seem to alter the endometrial pattern when given in the latter half of the cycle. There is some evidence that the newer progestational drugs may be more effective in improving the development of the secretory endometrium.

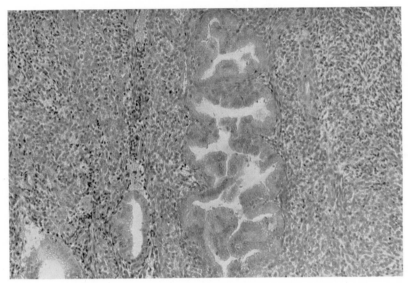

Fig. 46-9.   Example of a secretory endometrium with glandular secretory exhaustion and leuko-cytic infiltration of the stroma. No predecidual reaction is present, such as would be expected in an endometrium approximately 3 days before menstruation. This is evidence of progestational hypoplasia in a secretory endometrium.

How Do We Go About Making a Diagnosis?

The primary step in the investigation of the cause of abnormal uterine bleeding in this age group is the recording of the clinical history. In so doing, some information is acquired about the amount of blood lost, the duration of the periods, the timing of the bleeding within the cycle, the nature of the bleeding, the number of pads used and the manner in which the abnormal period differed from the preceding normal periods. The most important of all these factors is the duration of vaginal flow. Any extension of the bleeding beyond a week should be regarded as pathologic. This information must then be evaluated after making due allowance for the patient's temperament and the likelihood of exaggeration in the recounting of the experience. An effort should be made to unearth any suggestion of emotional stress that might adversely affect normal endocrine function.

The physical examination will provide useful information. This should be a complete general examination and not simply a pelvic and rectal examination. Evidence of blood dyscrasia, anemia, systemic disease and metabolic disturbances may appear and serve as possible causes. The local pelvic and rectal examinations will disclose or rule out local pelvic disease. It is extremely important to differentiate between functional and organic causes before instituting therapy. It is not enough to base treatment on the simple fact that the patient is having abnormal vaginal bleeding.

Laboratory aids in diagnosis are not as helpful as they might be. A complete study of the blood is useful in establishing the degree of anemia and confirming the patient's estimate of blood loss. It is helpful in ruling out blood dyscrasia. The serum cholesterol and the protein-bound iodine or basal metabolic rate must be measured to determine the level of thyroid function. Tests are available to help evaluate the levels of the circulating female hormones. Unfortunately they are not sensitive enough to reflect small variations in quantity of either estrin or progestin. They are, therefore, impractical and far too time consuming and expensive.

The endometrial biopsy and vaginal smear can be used to measure the effect of hormone activity on the target organs present in the endometrium and vagina. Unfortunately the vaginal smear gives no clear indication of the amount of hormone being secreted. The endometrial biopsy is helpful in estimating whether ovulation has occurred, but in an obscure case of bleeding it provides only a sample of the total endometrial lining. Frequently the response of the endometrium is not uniform throughout. Isolated samples obtained by biopsy will hardly give full data upon which therapy can be based.

The final diagnosis depends for the most part on a curettage under anesthesia. In this manner the presence of gross pathologic lesions in the uterus is confirmed or refuted, and the pathologist obtains all the endometrium for histologic review. The curettage should be performed in the latter half of the cycle, unless one has reason to believe from the history that the patient is shedding her endometrium irregularly. In this case the curettage should be performed at some point after the fifth day of the onset of menstruation.

Treatment

As we have tried to point out, the treatment of abnormal bleeding depends on the underlying cause.

If the symptoms and laboratory findings suggest hypothyroidism, thyroid extract supplements in dosage according to need will often produce a dramatic improvement. Since many patients with low thyroid secretion bleed in frightening quantity, with hemoglobin levels that fall to the range of 6 to 8 gm. per 100 ml., blood transfusions are often necessary.

When anemia is present, it is necessary to determine whether this is due to blood lost at the time of the menstrual period, blood loss from elsewhere as from the urinary and gastrointestinal tracts, or whether blood dyscrasia is in the background. With thrombocytopenia, for example, the treatment may involve splenectomy, not hormone therapy or hysterectomy. Iron deficiency anemia may be the result of blood loss or it may contribute to repeated menorrhagia. Since some of the defect may be in the diet or the manner in which iron is either absorbed or metabolized, the patient should be given iron compounds, either orally or intramuscularly. Improvement may be expected after 2 weeks to a month when 1 to 1.5 gm. of iron is given daily. A diet high in protein and low in fat can often be used, together with vitamins. Liver extract and vitamin B_{12} could be given when liver disease is suspected or a secondary anemia is present, but this is not good practice in cases that might actually have pernicious anemia. Cobalt is also not recommended in the therapy of anemia with menorrhagia.

The patient who gives a history of abnormal vaginal bleeding associated with a strong suspicion of psychic unrest as a possible cause usually does poorly when attempts are made to regulate the bleeding with either hormones or curettage. The abnormal blood loss will continue until the underlying psychiatric defect is eliminated.

Hormone therapy for abnormal uterine bleeding should be ideal for this age group, since it is desirable to avoid drastic therapy. Unfortunately, hormones often prove disappointing, for it is in this age span that one encounters the more bizarre forms of abnormal endometrium. They are still a satisfactory form of treatment when there is evidence of anovulatory bleeding and progestin lack. The substitution of progestin by intramuscular injection, or by mouth if the newer progestational drugs are used, will frequently stop the bleeding and return the menstrual cycle to normal.

Hormone therapy based on less well defined histologic evidence is unpredictable. Gynecologists have become increasingly aware of the fact that abnormal uterine bleeding may take place from a variety of types of endometrium, independent of the phase of the cycle. Much of the hormone therapy today is given empirically. A number of different hormones, alone or in combination, are frequently given at varying periods of time during the cycle.

It is small wonder that the results are not rewarding. It must be constantly kept in mind that all hormone therapy is simply a substitution. If a deficiency does exist and proper supplements are provided, the patient will receive relief from a temporary upset. The final cure may occur spontaneously or follow the elimination of the fundamental cause.

How Should the Steroid Hormones Be Used? All three types of steroid hormones, estrin, progestin and androgen, will influence the bleeding abnormality, particularly if there is a progestin deficiency or if endometrial hyperplasia is present.

Estrin. The primary place for the estrogens is in the immediate control of uterine bleeding of hemorrhagic proportions. In the last ten years there have been a number of enthusiastic reports in the literature suggesting that the intravenous use of estrogenic substances will prove to be a satisfactory method of controlling uterine hemorrhage. The actual mechanism through which an estrogen exerts its effect is little understood.

The chief explanation has to do with raising the blood level of estrin, which was believed to have fallen below that critical point beyond which bleeding occurs, just as is supposed to happen at the onset of menstruation. The only trouble with this explanation is that investigators have not been able to demonstrate any sudden fluctuation in the level of urinary estrogens. Estrin given intravenously will raise the blood levels, but this is rarely maintained for longer than two hours and is usually recorded at minimum levels after four hours. What happens to the estrin after the intravenous injection is incompletely understood. After four hours only 10 per cent can be recovered in the urine. It seems likely that the estrin is deactivated and rendered inert so far as the target organs are concerned by its passage through the liver. Investigators have been unable to observe any cornification of the vaginal epithelium or change in the urinary electrolytes when estrogen is given by vein to castrate female subjects.

The other theories advanced to explain the action of estrogen in the control of hemorrhage also lack laboratory and experimental support. Evidently it does not work by altering the blood coagulation mechanism, nor by affecting either the blood vessels in the endometrium or the contractility of the uterus.

One cannot deny that there are reports of the successful use of estrogen in the control of uterine hemorrhage. Kelly points out that in these clinical trials the successes reported have followed the use of a preparation obtained from the urine of pregnant mares (Premarin). This is not a pure estrogen, but a complex containing as many as six estrogenic components. There may well be some factor, then, other than estrin that explains the clinical results obtained.

The dose recommended is Premarin, 5 cc., containing 20 mg. of conjugated estrin, intravenously every 4 hours as required.

Progestin. The primary aim in the use of progesterone is so to influence the endometrium that it will shed completely rather than in patchy areas after discontinuation of the hormone. This produces a so-called medical curettage. It is particularly useful in patients with anovulatory bleeding and endometrial hyperplasia, for in this instance there is a true hormonal deficiency that the progestin replaces.

The recommended dosage schedule follows: (1) progesterone, 25 mg., intramuscularly daily for 5 days; (2) Colprosterone, 50 mg., vaginally for 5 days. Withdrawal bleeding may be expected three or four days after discontinuation of the hormone, and the patient should be so informed. It is customary to repeat the series at monthly intervals for three or four months, starting each series approximately eighteen days after the onset of the last menstruation.

New Progestational Agents. Despite the availability of the new synthetic progestins, progesterone continues to be the best of the endometrial hemostatic hormonal preparations. The action of progesterone is twofold: (a) Changes are brought about in the endometrium. Enlargement and differentiation of the stromal cells with decidual cell formation take place, together with glycogen storage and increased alkaline phosphatase activity in the cells of the endometrial glands (b) A direct action on the myometrium makes the muscle less sensitive to the stimulating effect of the oxytocin elaborated by the posterior pituitary.

The reason the synthetic relatives of hydroxyprogesterone, such as Delalutin and Provera, are less effective in controlling bleeding of hemorrhagic proportions is in all probability the need for estrogen priming, despite the fact that action is noted just as promptly and progestational effect is anywhere from two to four times as powerful as with pure progesterone. To get the desired effect estrogen must either be available naturally or be given with the intramuscular injection of either Delalutin or Provera.

Norethynodrel (17 alpha-ethinyl-17-hydroxy-5 (10) estren-3-one), which has been given the name Enovid, is more effective, for it contains an estrogen in its complex. When given orally for 10 days in 10-mg. doses in the latter half of the cycle to women who have proved anovulatory cycles, it will produce a secretory endometrium. It should not be given early in the cycle, for it can inhibit ovulation and compound the problem when given over a prolonged period. Enovid has the disadvantage of creating nausea that will disappear if the hormone is given for long enough, but it also tends to increase fluid storage, as shown by the tendency of some women to gain weight at an alarming rate.

Another useful progestational agent much like ethisterone (Pranone) has recently become available for clinical use and bears the name Norlutin. It is a powerful progestin when given orally, and because of its powerful antiestrogenic effect it acts much like the androgens.

The chief value of the newer progestational agents rests in their ability to bring about changes in the endometrium and a more physiologic balance in hormonal activity after the excessive vaginal bleeding has been controlled. Artificial cycles with proper estrin priming can be created and maintained then by:

(a) Progesterone—50 mg. intramuscularly on day 24, or 20 mg. daily beginning on day 18. Withdrawal bleeding occurs two to six days later.

(b) Delalutin—250 mg. intramuscularly on day 14. Withdrawal bleeding can be expected in eight to ten days.

(c) Norlutin
    Provera } — 10 mg. daily as oral medication given from day 5 through 25.
    Enovid

Androgen. The effect of testosterone on the management of abnormal uterine bleeding is unpredictable and frankly disappointing. It may be used in the form of methyltestosterone linguets, 10 mg. daily, for 14 days. Unless the patient is unusually sensitive to androgen, she is unlikely to have any of the undesirable side effects such as facial hirsutism, clitoral enlargement or enlargement of the larynx. These are apt to appear if the dose exceeds 300 mg. per month. If hormones are to be used, the gynecologist will be well advised to rely on the progestins rather than testosterone, whether given orally or parenterally.

WHAT IS THE BEST METHOD OF MANAGING THE UTERINE BLEEDING PROBLEM? Curettage is by far the most logical and practical answer to the abnormal bleeding *Note* problem in this age group. As we have previously stated, bleeding can take place from almost any type of endometrium. Hormone therapy can therefore not be based on anything other than a hit-or-miss philosophy. Curettage is not only the best method of controlling hemorrhage, but also it is curative as well as diagnostic for the group in which vaginal bleeding is excessive and prolonged without being alarming. When intrauterine pathologic entities, such as endometritis, polyps, or retained products of conception, are present, curettage will remove the cause. It is amazing how much bleeding can be caused by a small endometrial polyp. The curet is also useful in detecting the presence of a submucous fibroid tumor, which often produces bleeding of hemorrhagic proportions. Such fibroids cannot be felt on pelvic examination and can only be suspected from the history. Curettage is curative as well as diagnostic in the large group of functional bleeders with a persistent proliferative endometrium or hyperplasia. Diagnosis is improved by providing a complete specimen of the endometrial lining for histologic review.

It is a little difficult to understand why this is curative, for the curet simply removes the endometrium then present in the uterus. It does nothing to prevent or influence the regeneration of that endometrium. Why the endometrium is not again replaced by the same kind of endometrium that previously produced the abnormal bleeding is not clear. It could be entirely a psychologic cure, but in all probability the removal of all the endometrium leads to a hormonal readjustment and permits the ovarian hormones to act on a clean base. Whatever the cause, curettage is far more effective than hormone therapy for both hyperplasia of the endometrium and irregular shedding. The only disadvantage is economic. The cost of hospital admission, anesthesia, and operating room is often formidable and would hardly be justified if other methods were effective. In this age group, in whom there is only a small chance of cancer, it is possible to bring the patient to the hospital on a six-hour admission program. A complete curettage can be done under light anesthesia with a minimum of preoperative preparation. The patient is discharged home on her recovery from anesthesia. This reduces the cost to a certain extent. The patient is far more likely to achieve permanent relief and a return to normal existence much sooner if curettage is performed, rather than resorting to the use of hormones, which are not inexpensive.

IS THERE ANY PLACE FOR HYSTERECTOMY? Curettage is better therapy than the administration of hormones, but it is not 100 per cent curative. Even when the surgeon has explored the endometrial cavity with common duct forceps after curettage, it is possible to miss a polyp. The patient can have a submucous fibroid tumor that cannot be detected with the curet. Moreover, not all cases of functional bleeding respond equally well to curettage. Many patients repeat the abnormal bleeding pattern after a short period of remission following a careful curettage.

When the patient has been subjected to two or three curettages without permanent success, the gynecologist will be well advised to remove the uterus, sparing the ovaries. When functional bleeding is associated with pelvic diseases such as leiomyomas, endometriosis, pelvic inflammation or fixed uterine retroversion, the gynecologist may well elect to perform a hysterectomy. In this decision, however, bleeding is only one factor. The nature of the disease, its extent and the likelihood of further progression are equally important elements in the choice of hysterectomy as a form of treatment. Hysterectomy is far better than intrauterine radium or external x-ray therapy, for radiation would accomplish its purpose more directly by its action on the ovary, not the endometrium. Irradiation of the endometrium for benign conditions has a bad reputation, because of various complications within the uterus and sometimes in adjacent organs. More uterine cancers develop after irradiation therapy for uterine bleeding than can be accounted for by chance. After ovarian irradiation the bleeding is controlled and cure established at the price of radiation castration, which is altogether too much to pay, particularly when the target organ can be removed and ovarian function preserved.

REFERENCES

Aaro, L. A.: Endocrine Therapy in Obstetrics and Gynecology. *Proc. Staff Meet., Mayo Clin.*, 35: 555, 1960.

Abel, S.: Causes of Abnormal Uterine Bleeding. *Clin. Obst. & Gynec.*, 1: 741, 1958.

Allen, W. M.: Functional Uterine Bleeding. *Clin. Obst. & Gynec.*, 1: 825, 1958.

Baldwin, R. M., Whalley, P. J., and Pritchard, J. A.: Measurement of Menstrual Blood Loss. *Am. J. Obst. & Gynec.*, 81: 739, 1961.

Barnes, A. C.: The Relationship between the Hemorrhagic Blood Dyscrasias and Hypermenorrhea. *Am. J. Obst. & Gynec.*, 58: 570, 1949.

Barr, R. W., and Sommers, S. C.: Endocrine Abnormalities Accompanying Hepatic Cirrhosis and Hepatoma. *J. Clin. Endocrinol.*, 17: 1017, 1957.

Bayly, M. A., and Greene, R. R.: Ovarian Tumors and Abnormal Uterine Bleeding. *Am. J. Obst. & Gynec.*, 72: 143, 1956.

Birnberg, C. H., Livingston, S., and Davis, J. G.: Large-Dose Oral Progesterone Therapy in Menstrual Disorders. *Obst. & Gynec.*, 11: 115, 1958.

Biskind, L. H., and Biskind, J. I.: Functional Uterine Bleeding, a Modern Approach to Therapy. *Missouri Med.*, 53: 843, 1956.

Blaikley, J. B.: Psychogenic Menorrhagia. *J. Obst. & Gynaec. Brit. Emp.*, 66: 786, 1959.

Cohen, M. R., and Hankin, H.: The Inadequate Luteal Phase. *Internat. J. Fertil.*, 4: 58, 1959.

Copeland, W. E., Nelson, P. K., and Payne, F. L.: Intrauterine Radium for Dysfunctional Bleeding. A Long-Term Follow-up Study. *Am. J. Obst. & Gynec.*, 73: 615, 1957.

Dalton, K.: Menstruation and Accidents. *Brit. M.J.*, 2: 1425, 1960.

Davis, M. E., and Fugo, N. W.: The Diagnosis and Treatment of Menstrual Disorders. *M. Clin. North Amer.*, 45: 3, 1961.

DeWatteville, P. H.: Androgen Therapy in Gynecology. *Clin. Obst. & Gynec.*, 3: 1032, 1960.

Faulkner, R. L.: Endometrial Diagnosis. *Am. J. Obst. & Gynec.*, 62: 321, 1951.

Fluhmann, C. F.: *The Management of Menstrual Disorders.* Philadelphia, W. B. Saunders Company, 1956, Chap. 21.

Greenblatt, R. B.: Hormonal Control of Functional Uterine Bleeding. *Clin. Obst. & Gynec.*, 2: 232, 1959.

Greenblatt, R. B., Clark, S. L., and Lord, J. A.: The Thyroid in Obstetrics and Gynecologic Disorders. *Clin. Obst. & Gynec.*, 3: 1006, 1960.

Haden, R. L., and Singleton, J. M.: Disturbances of Menstruation Due to Simple Achlorhydric Anemia. *Am. J. Obst. & Gynec.*, 26: 330, 1933.

Hamblen, E. C.: The Use of Estrogens in Obstetrics and Gynecology. *Clin. Obst. & Gynec.*, 3: 1021, 1960.

Harris, C.: The Vicious Circle of Anemia and Menorrhagia. *Canad. M.A.J.*, 77: 98, 1957.

Haskins, A. L.: Adjunctive Estrogen Therapy. *Obst. & Gynec.*, 11: 49, 1960.

Heiman, M.: The Role of Stress Situations and Psychological Factors in Functional Uterine Bleeding. *J. Mt. Sinai Hosp.*, 23: 775, 1956.

Henriksen, E.: Disorders of the Ovulatory Phase. *Clin. Obst. & Gynec.*, 2: 180, 1959.

Holmstrom, E. G.: Dysfunctional Uterine Bleeding. *Clin. Obst. & Gynec.*, 1: 187, 1958.

Idem: The Newer Progestational Compounds. *Clin. Obst. & Gynec.*, 2: 247, 1959.

Holmstrom, E. G., and McLennan, C. E.: Menorrhagia Associated with Irregular Shedding of the Endometrium. A Clinical and Experimental Study. *Am. J. Obst. & Gynec.*, 53: 727, 1947.

Hughes, E. C.: Irregularities of the Corpus Luteal Phase of the Menstrual Cycle. *Clin. Obst. & Gynec.*, 2: 190, 1959.

Israel, S. L., and Weber, L. L.: Methods Used in Diagnosis of Abnormal Uterine Bleeding. *Clin. Obst. & Gynec.*, 1: 774, 1958.

Jacobson, B. M.: Menometrorrhagia Due to Generalized Hemorrhagic Disorders; in J. V. Meigs and S. H. Sturgis, eds.: *Progress in Gynecology*. New York, Grune & Stratton, Inc., 1957, Vol. III, p. 50.

Kellar, R., Matthew, G. D., MacKay, R., Brown, J. B., and Roy, E. J.: Some Clinical Applications of Oestrogen Assay. *J. Obst. & Gynaec. Brit. Emp.*, 66: 804, 1959.

Kelly, J. V.: Intravenous Estrogen Therapy, an Assessment. *Obst. & Gynec.*, 17: 149, 1961.

Kistner, R. W.: The Use of Progestational Agents in Obstetrics and Gynecology. *Clin. Obst. & Gynec.*, 3: 1047, 1960.

Leventhal, J. M., Ronan, F. F., and Wotiz, H. H.: Pregnanediol. Its Determination and Occurrence in the Proliferative Phase of the Normal Menstrual Cycle. *Boston Univ. M. Quart.*, 11: 46, 1960.

Lock, F. R.: Psychosomatic Aspects of Uterine Bleeding. *Clin. Obst. & Gynec.*, 1: 819, 1958.

McKay, D. G., Hertig, A. T., Bardawil, W., and Velardo, J. T.: Histochemical Observations on the Endometrium—Abnormal Endometrium. *Obst. & Gynec.*, 8: 140, 1956.

McKelvey, J. L., and Samuels, L. T.: Irregular Shedding of the Endometrium. *Am. J. Obst. & Gynec.*, 53: 627, 1947.

McLennan, C. E.: Current Concepts of Prolonged or Irregular Endometrial Shedding. *Am. J. Obst. & Gynec.*, 64: 988, 1952.

Idem: The Major Types of Dysfunctional Uterine Bleeding. *Clin. Obst. & Gynec.*, 2: 218, 1959.

Menzer-Benaron, D., and Sturgis, S. H.: Relationship between Emotional and Somatic Factors in Gynecologic Disease; in J. V. Meigs and S. H. Sturgis, eds.: *Progress in Gynecology*. New York, Grune & Stratton, Inc., 1957, Vol. III, p. 235.

Moore, C. V., and Dubach, R.: Metabolism and Requirements of Iron in the Human. *J.A.M.A.*, 162: 197, 1956.

Munnell, E. W., and Flick, F. H.: The Surgical Diagnosis and Management of Dysfunctional Uterine Bleeding. *Surg., Gynec. & Obst.*, 106: 321, 1958.

Noyes, R. W.: Underdeveloped Secretory Endometrium. *Am. J. Obst. & Gynec.*, 77: 929, 1959.

Parsons, L.: The Causes and Management of Uterine Hemorrhage. *M. Clin. North Amer.*, 37: 1497, 1953.

Parsons, L., and Tenney, B., Jr.: Endocrine Therapy in Menstrual Disorders. *M. Clin. North Amer.*, 34: 1537, 1950.

Pritchard, J. A.: Management of the Gynecologic Patient with Anemia Due to Chronic Blood Loss. *Texas J. Med.*, 56: 112, 1960.

Radman, H. M.: Blood Dyscrasia as a Causative Factor in Abnormal Uterine Bleeding. *Am. J. Obst. & Gynec.*, 79: 1, 1960.

Rock, J., Garcia, C. R., and Pincus, G.: Use of Some Progestational 19 Nor-steroids in Gynecology. *Am. J. Obst. & Gynec.*, 79: 758, 1960.

Rothchild, I.: Amenorrhea. *Clin. Obst. & Gynec.*, 1: 173, 1958.

Salvatore, C. A.: Arterioles of the Endometrium in the Etiopathogenesis of Dysfunctional Hemorrhage. *J. Internat. Coll. Surg.*, 29: 599, 1958.

Seaman, A. J., and Benson, R. C.: Coagulation Studies of Patients with Abnormal Uterine Bleeding. *Am. J. Obst. & Gynec.*, 79: 5, 1960.

Smith, O. W., Smith, G. V., and Gavian, N. G.: Urinary Estrogens in Women. *Am. J. Obst. & Gynec.*, 78: 1028, 1959.

Southam, A. C.: A Comparative Study of the Effect of the Progestational Agents in Human Menstrual Abnormalities. *Ann. New York Acad. Sc.*, 71: 666, 1958.

Stander, R. W.: Irradiation Castration, a Follow-up Study of Results in Benign Pelvic Disease. *Obst. & Gynec.*, 10: 223, 1957.

Sutherland, A. M.: Functional Uterine Bleeding; in J. V. Meigs and S. H. Sturgis, eds.: *Progress in Gynecology*. New York, Grune & Stratton, Inc., 1957, Vol. III, p. 167.

Taymor, M. L.: Laboratory and Clinical Effects of Nortestosterone—The Endometrial Response. *Am. J. Obst. & Gynec.*, 81: 95, 1961.

Taymor, M. L., and Sturgis, S. H.: Synthetic Progestins in the Management of Anovulatory Dysfunctional Uterine Bleeding. *Obst. & Gynec.*, 17: 751, 1961.

Taymor, M. L., Sturgis, S. H., Goodale, W. T., and Ashbaugh, D.: Menorrhagia Due to Chronic Iron Deficiency. *Obst. & Gynec.*, 16: 571, 1960.

Word, B.: Current Concepts of Uterine Curettage. *Postgrad. Med.*, 28: 450, 1960.

Chapter 47

Endometriosis

ENDOMETRIOSIS is one of the most mysterious and fascinating disease entities in the entire field of gynecology. By definition, the presence of ectopic implants of tissue composed of endometrial elements, endometrial stroma and endometrial glands in regions remote from the endometrial cavity is called endometriosis. These implants respond to cyclic hormone stimulation in much the same manner as the normal endometrium. It is therefore a pathologic process that is most commonly encountered during the years of menstrual activity. The growth pattern of the endometrial implants is unique in that it is the only known instance other than pregnancy in the pathology of human beings of a benign proliferative process having the propensity to invade the normal surrounding tissue.

It has been the custom to distinguish two clinical types of endometriosis. The term *internal endometriosis* (adenomyosis) refers to endometrial ingrowths formed within the uterine myometrial wall. The patient has true or *external endometriosis* when the lesions are found on the serosal surface of the uterus, as well as in more remote areas, such as the pelvic peritoneum, ovary, appendix and sigmoid. Though the two have many properties in common and may have a similar etiology, the age groups in which they appear, their pathogenesis and the problems presented in therapy are entirely different. Internal endometriosis is an undesirable term that should be replaced by the designation of *adenomyosis*, leaving genuine endometriosis to refer to the process now being discussed. In the thirty- to forty-year age group we are primarily interested in the external type, in which widespread dissemination of ectopic endometrium occurs.

Why Is There Such Widespread Medical Interest in Endometriosis?

External endometriosis is becoming a more common rather than a rarer disease, particularly among the more fortunate economic groups. As such, it falls into the province of the general practitioner as well as the general surgeon and pathologist, and it is no longer the private problem of the gynecologist alone.

The pathologist is fascinated by the many theories advanced to explain how the implants manage to arise in such a wide variety of locations, as well as the stimuli that must serve to activate and maintain the growth of the implant and the self-limited nature of the process. In addition, he is intrigued by the growth pattern and its invasive propensity, as well as the evidence for cyclic activity within the components of the implant and its complications.

Surgeons and gynecologists are presented with many perplexing problems in therapy. There is a high index of infertility in patients who have external endometriosis. Therapy must then be tailored to the patient's age and parity and be balanced with the extent of disease as well as the severity of the symptoms. Since it is well known that the growth elements in the implant depend on ovarian function, fine judgment is required to make the decision for or against castration.

The general practitioner is concerned, because he is aware that he is seeing more patients who have sterility problems and present symptoms that are progressively more severe and incapacitating.

The increasing awareness of the disease as a pathologic entity is praiseworthy, but with it have come some disadvantages. Since there are many questions as yet unanswered, concerned not only with the etiology, but also with the life history of endometriosis, every surgeon, gynecologist and practitioner forms his own clinical impressions, which are often more fanciful than factual.

Is There a True Increase in Incidence, and Does It Operate in Particular Economic Groups?

There can be little doubt that the medical profession has become more aware of external endometriosis as a disease entity with protean manifestations. Before Sampson's classic paper in 1921 there were fewer than 20 studies of endometriosis in the world literature. Though the first report of involvement of the small intestine was presented by Meyer in 1908, no note of bladder involvement appeared until 1925, when Keene noted such an extension. In the era immediately following the appearance of Sampson's article a voluminous literature piled up, concerned chiefly with the etiology of the disease. In recent years, as the profession has become more conscious of its presence and has learned more of its behavior, an equally substantial number of reports has appeared, dealing chiefly with the different types of therapy as they apply in the different age groups. The treatment of the disease in the last thirty years has run the gamut from extremely radical surgery to the present trend toward ovarian conservation.

The present-day surgeon unquestionably takes greater pains to inspect the lower pelvis, cul-de-sac and uterosacral ligaments and is better able to recognize endometrial implants when he sees them. Clinical recognition, however, is not always accompanied by a pathologic confirmation. The true incidence of the frequency of endometriosis is therefore hard to determine. It will definitely be increased if the surgeon will take the trouble to mark the area he suspects in a resected specimen with a safety pin or a black silk suture. This maneuver calls the pathologist's attention to the suspicious area. If this is not done, the clinical impression will not be confirmed histologically, simply because these areas do not stand out with equal clarity in the excised specimen when it is examined in the laboratory. Nevertheless the increase in the number of patients with external endometriosis seems to be a true one and cannot be attributed simply to a greater sense of awareness on the part of the physician. The explanation for the greater number of cases now seen and recognized is not entirely clear. Meigs first noted discrepancy between the number of cases encountered in private practice as compared with the incidence in the hospital ward population. This was particularly true when the ward patients included members of the colored race. These observations have been confirmed by many observers. In most of the reported series external endometriosis is found in

Note approximately 25 per cent of all private gynecologic operations, as opposed to 5 per cent in ward patients. The disproportion may be due to the fact that pelvic inflammatory disease, which closes the fimbriated end of the fallopian tubes, is found with greater frequency in the ward population and particularly the colored race. The tubes are almost invariably open in patients with external endometriosis, which may or may not be a coincidence.

Many physicians interested in the reason for the apparent increase in the incidence of endometriosis have suggested that early and repeated pregnancies are important in preventing its development, particularly in the patient who manifests some of the stigmata of underdevelopment, such as an infantile uterus with congenital erosion. Early pregnancy has been more common among the less fortunate economic groups, and this may account for the discrepancy in incidence between the ward and private patients. Evidently this is not the complete explanation, for in recent years the trend has been reversed with more early marriages and pregnancies. During the depression years of the 1930's the professional and college graduate groups were reproducing themselves at a rate 9 per cent less than the number needed for replacement. At present the birth rate is 27 per cent above the required number. Despite this, the incidence of external endometriosis continues to rise. TeLinde notes a threefold increase in incidence in the last fifteen years. Though the true explanation for the increase is not yet evident, one may postulate that the pressures and stresses of modern living adversely affect the hormonal balance.

In What Age Group Is Endometriosis Usually Found?

External endometriosis is a disease of the reproductive years. One may also find it in the adolescent age group and again after the menopause. The symptoms begin to appear in the early twenties and disappear after the cessation of menstrual activity. The great preponderance in numbers among the patients who come with complaints *Note* due to external endometriosis is in the age group between thirty and forty years.

We are not accustomed to looking for the early phases of endometriosis in the adolescent girl, but unquestionably the process begins shortly after the onset of menstruation. The literature records an incidence in teen-age girls in the neighborhood of 5 per cent of all cases. Clinical symptoms for the most part are lacking in the early phases of the disease. Many cases of dysmenorrhea, however, which we believed were primary because no palpable lesions could be found, are actually secondary and due to small endometrial implants on the pelvic floor or uterosacral ligaments.

Note 2 Endometriosis, previously unrecognized, was present in 15 per cent of patients with essential dysmenorrhea who were subjected to exploration with the primary purpose of performing a presacral neurectomy for the relief of pain. Since endometriosis is intimately linked to infertility, it is important to recognize the early manifestations and deal with the disease at a time when its correction can be accomplished with minimal trauma. The possibility of endometriosis as a cause of symptoms should be considered in planning the operative approach in many young girls. For example, a midline incision might better be made so that one can get a better view of the pelvis, provided localizing signs do not demand a right pararectus or McBurney incision.

The disease is progressive, subject to individual variations, so that the symptoms become more severe and the physical findings increasingly evident as the patient passes into the forties. Beyond the menopause, however, the reported incidence drops sharply, and the identification of endometriosis and evidence of functional activity in the implants recognized as being endometriosis is minimal. It is rather surprising that there are not more reported instances of endometriosis in this postmenopausal age group. If endometriosis is as frequent as it appears to be during the reproductive years, there should later be more evidence of its presence in some form. We do see white striate scars, dense adhesions, kinking and knuckling of the colon, but one rarely sees or hears about old chocolate cysts of the ovary. It may be that such cysts become simple serous cysts as the degenerated epithelial debris and blood are absorbed. Such cysts may collapse, leaving little that can be interpreted as obsolete endometriosis. Occasionally one does find nodular thickenings within the wall of the sigmoid or rectovaginal septum that point to pre-existent endometriosis. Rarely do such implants exhibit any evidence of activity.

Where Are the Ectopic Implants Found?

The ectopic growth of endometrial-like tissue, including epithelium, glands and stroma, is found widely dispersed throughout the lower pelvis. The *ovaries, serosal surface* of the uterus and the *posterior cul-de-sac* are the regions most often involved. Far less frequently one encounters the implants on the round ligaments, tubes, rectosigmoid, sigmoid, terminal ileum, appendix, cecum, anterior cul-de-sac, bladder and retroperitoneal lymph nodes. The ectopic endometrium is found but rarely above the umbilicus, and almost never in the anterior abdominal wall, unless after a previous abdominal operation. After operations it has been found in the umbilicus, tubal amputation stumps, abdominal incisions and scars in the vulva and perineal area. By direct extension, or subsequent to operative trauma, it is occasionally found in the cervix and vagina, particularly the posterior fornix. These are the most common areas and are recorded in their relative order of frequency of occurrence (Fig. 47–1).

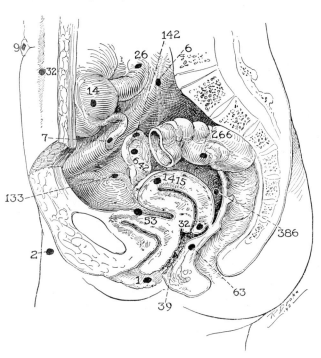

Fig. 47-1. Sites of endometriosis, with the number of cases observed. The 5 most common sites in order are uterus, ovary, pouch of Douglas, rectosigmoid colon and fallopian tube. (From Masson and Cariker.)

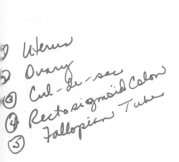

The most fascinating remote sites where endometriosis has been detected are in the pleura, lung, extensor carpi radialis, thigh and posteriorly in the buttock. Reams of literature and much research have accumulated in attempts to explain how these endometrial implants happen to be found in such distant areas, far removed from their proper site in the genital tract.

How Do You Recognize These Implants Grossly?

Ovary.   Approximately 60 per cent of the patients with external endometriosis have ovarian involvement in some form. The great majority are found on the lateral and under surfaces of the ovary. The lesions vary in size from small pinhead-sized implants to large cysts measuring 20 or more cm. in diameter. Rarely, however, are they larger than an orange.

The small lesions usually are either bluish, dusky red or brownish black, depending on how long they have been present and how much fresh or old blood they contain. They resemble small blood blisters. Some puckering of the surrounding tissue is noted, but they do not appear to have any great power of invasion and tend to remain superficial throughout their existence (Fig. 47–2). Rarely do they serve as the point of development of the larger hemorrhagic cysts. Such implants appear to be part of the general picture of pelvic endometriosis, although they may occur without evidence of involvement elsewhere. The small lesions do not contribute to the symptoms, but are recognized when pelvic laparotomy is done for other causes.

The typical gross picture of ovarian endometriosis is that of bilateral ovarian cysts of varying size that are filled with a characteristic tarry, thick, chocolate-colored fluid (Fig. 47–3). This gives them the name of "chocolate cysts." There is nothing pathognomonic about the nature of the contents, however, for the same kind of thick fluid may be found in the so-called tarry lutein or old hemorrhagic corpus luteum cysts. The diagnosis of endometriosis should therefore not be made on the clinical impression gathered from the appearance of the cystic contents without other confirmatory evidence.

There is one characteristic of such cysts of the ovary that is peculiar to endometriosis. Usually one notes a depressed, scarred, puckered, blue-black area on the surface of an ovary which contains a larger cyst directly below it. As this cyst enlarges periodically under the cyclic influence of the hormones the surrounding capsule is placed under tension. Not infrequently and usually immediately before or just after the menstrual period the cyst ruptures at some point, spilling its highly irritating contents onto the sensitive pelvic peritoneum. The distention and subsequent spillage explain much of the pain associated with endometriosis. The irritative discharge sets up a local chemical peritonitis. This is followed by an immediate protective fibroblastic tissue response that typically seals the defect and plasters the ovary against the posterior wall of the broad ligament. It is a well known clinical observation that the true chocolate cyst associated with endometriosis cannot be mobilized from its fixed position on the back of the broad ligament without rupturing it and spilling its contents. This observation is extremely helpful in differentiating the chocolate cyst of endometriosis from the other cysts that contain old blood.

The presence of dense adhesions, which are much finer than those encountered in pelvic inflammation, radiation reaction or even tuberculosis, is characteristic of the more extensive lesions of external endometriosis. Adhesions are in all probability the cumulative response to repeated peritoneal insults produced by the periodic escape of the irritating contents of the cyst.

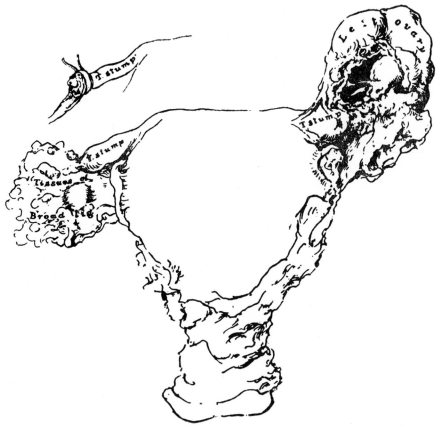

Fig. 47-2.   Original unpublished drawing by Sampson of puckered and scarred ovaries involved by endometriosis, following a previous attempt at operative removal of the implants.

WHAT DOES ENDOMETRIOSIS LOOK LIKE IN OTHER AREAS?   The large endometrial cysts that we associate with endometriosis are characteristic of its growth within the ovary. On the posterior surface of the uterus, uterosacral ligaments and pelvic peritoneum, particularly the posterior cul-de-sac, the appearance is different.

The characteristic appearance of ectopic implants in these areas is that of varying numbers of blueberry-like spots, surrounded by a puckering scar that seems to be intent on drawing other tissue into it. When excised and examined histologically, the obvious endometrial lesion is small in proportion to the amount of surrounding fibrous tissue, which may be several centimeters in over-all diameter. Sometimes the isolated bluish spots coalesce to form solid nodules that become one of the most readily recognizable stigmata of the disease.

The epithelial lining of the implants attempts to mimic the regular menstrual cycle under the influence of the estrogenic hormones. In a sense the ectopic endometrium menstruates into its own cavity, but only so long as the surrounding fibrous tissue will permit it. For that reason many of those puckered clawlike areas are in their end-stage and no longer active. The damage, however, may be considerable, as the scarring draws more tissue and adjacent organs inward before the end-stage is reached (Fig. 47-4). The implant continues to swell with each menstrual cycle, though menstruation no longer occurs within it. Because of the unyielding nature of the surrounding fibrous tissue the swelling within the implants is accompanied by pain.

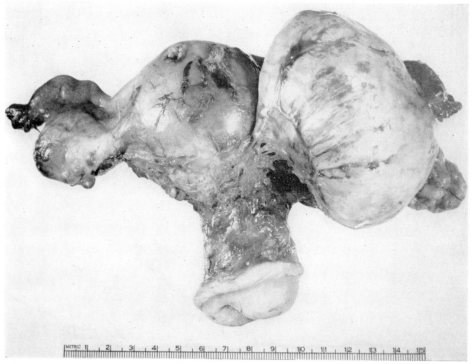

Fig. 47-3.   Large endometriotic ovarian cyst filled with chocolate-colored thick material due to menstrual hemorrhage. The adhesions between tube, ovary and uterus also commonly accompany ovarian endometriosis.

The posterior cul-de-sac is a common place in which to find endometrial implants. The nodular thickening noted on palpation of the posterior cul-de-sac and uterosacral ligaments is one of the outstanding findings on vaginal and rectal examinations.

Widespread isolated implants are frequently observed throughout the lower peritoneal cavity. They are found in hernial sacs, on the vesical or uterine peritoneum, the round ligaments and in the serosa of sigmoid, ileum and appendix (Fig. 47–5). They are never seen on the previously untraumatized anterior peritoneum and are unknown above the level of the umbilicus. In many instances endometriotic implants are present without any suggestion of ovarian involvement and only exhibit evidence of minimal local invasion.

WHAT ABOUT FOCI OF ENDOMETRIOSIS THAT DEMONSTRATE INVASIVE PROPERTIES? Lesions found in the pelvic cavity that do show evidence of the power to invade are almost invariably associated with ovarian involvement. Endometriosis in the cul-de-sac may exist without disease in the ovary, but when the rectovaginal septum is invaded and the growth process continues in such a way as to (*a*) penetrate the vaginal fornix, where it can be seen on direct inspection of the vaginal vault; or (*b*) invade the serosal surface of the anterior rectal wall and produce a firm dense mass in which the cervix and rectal wall are implicated, then the ovaries as a rule are also a part of the more generalized dissemination of endometriosis.

Because of the inflammatory peritoneal reaction set up by recurrent spillage from the ruptured endometrial cysts both in the peritoneum and ovary, the lower pelvis is full of dense fibrotic adhesions that cannot be readily separated. There are no cleavage planes resembling those found in pelvic inflammation. Great care must be exercised in separating the normal tissue of the functioning organs from that of the invasive endometriosis, for the adhesions are far more resistant than normal tissue, and tearing of the normal tissues may result.

The structures most frequently involved, in addition to the rectovaginal septum and posterior fornix of the vagina, are the rectum, sigmoid, urinary bladder and small intestine.

WHAT ARE THE CHARACTERISTIC FEATURES OF ENDOMETRIOSIS IN THE INTESTINE? *Large Intestine.* By far the commonest sites of endometrial implants in the bowel are the sigmoid and rectosigmoid. The gross lesions, when viewed at abdominal exploration, can hardly be distinguished from carcinoma in the same areas. The bowel wall is invaded in endometriosis, but unlike in carcinoma, the invasion begins from the serosal surface and gradually invades deeper into the muscular and submucosal layers. The implants tend to burrow into the muscular layers and tunnel up and down in the long axis of the large intestine to a far greater extent than is apparent on gross palpation. Unlike endometriosis in the terminal ileum and cecum, the endometrial glands and stroma are found deep in the muscular layers of the lower large bowel.

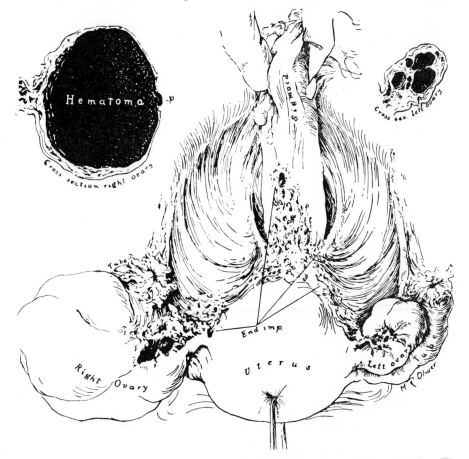

Fig. 47-4. Demonstrating the appearance of retrouterine endometriosis at operation. The pouch of Douglas, the parametrial regions and ovaries, as well as the sigmoid colon, show multiple, superficial endometriotic implants (*End imp.*). Cross sections of the ovaries in the inserts reveal the chocolate-type endometriotic cysts.

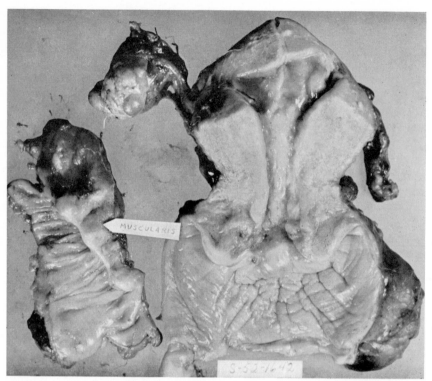

Fig. 47-5.   Implants of endometriosis are visible in the thickened colonic muscularis, the ovary, parametrium and posterior vaginal fornix. They present as either scars or small bluish cysts. There is a coexisting cancer of the cervix.

Though the lesions in the muscular and submucosal layers may be enough to present a tumor that occludes the lumen of the large intestine and produces either acute or chronic intestinal obstruction, the mucosa is rarely invaded either grossly or microscopically (Fig. 47–6). The "endometrioma" may be adherent and cause puckering of the colonic mucosa, but the mucous membrane is not ulcerated.

There is a widespread impression that endometriosis is a common cause of rectal bleeding. This is an error. Recognizable bleeding from the large bowel must be attributed to ulcers, polyps or cancer and not to endometriosis, for the simple reason that the lesions of endometriosis do not produce mucosal ulcerations. In rare instances the patient with endometriosis in the sigmoid or rectum may note some bleeding at the time of the period, probably due to excessive congestion of the mucosa. The bleeding, if any, appears only at this time. Cancer of the large intestine is far more likely to be the true explanation.

The symptoms produced by endometriosis in the lower large bowel are those of increasing constipation, aggravated at the time of the menstrual period and frequently accompanied by tenesmus, but only rarely by the passage of blood. With further progress in the growth of the lesions the patient's colon may become acutely obstructed.

Small Intestine.   The behavior of endometrial implants in the terminal ileum and cecum is somewhat different from that of endometrial growth in lesions of the sigmoid and rectum. As in the large intestine, the serosal surface is primarily invaded, but the extent of muscle penetration is much less. The mucosa is rarely if ever involved. Intestinal obstruction, either partial or complete, is produced by the kinking and angulation of several loops of terminal ileum, rather than by tumor narrowing the bowel lumen. The scarring and puckering of the serosa are readily noted. Unlike endometriosis of the sigmoid, the ileum may become involved without a widespread dissemination of pelvic endometriosis or chocolate cysts in the ovary. Endometriosis of the ileum tends to appear in younger people, who have far less associated disease to confuse the symptomatology.

The symptoms of intermittent small bowel obstruction with lower abdominal pain, distention and vomiting have usually been present for a year or two and are less often aggravated by the menstrual cycle. The differential diagnosis usually rests between endometriosis, carcinoma, carcinoid tumor, acute appendicitis, Meckel's diverticulum, ileus and pelvic inflammatory disease caused by adhesions.

WHAT DOES ENDOMETRIOSIS LOOK LIKE IN THE BLADDER, AND HOW DOES IT BEHAVE? Endometriosis in the urinary tract is uncommon. In 90 per cent of such cases, ectopic implants appear in the bladder while the remaining patients have involvement of the ureter. Ureteral lesions undoubtedly result from lateral extension of the fibrosis secondary to lesions arising in the cul-de-sac and pelvic peritoneum.

Endometriosis of the bladder manifests itself by (a) implants on the serosal surface that produce little in the way of symptoms, and (b) a coalescence of implants in the musculature of the bladder wall to form a recognizable mass that is tender when palpated. The mass bulges into the bladder interior, but is almost invariably covered by normal bladder epithelium. The symptoms will depend on the extent of the invasion and the site of the implants. When they are located near the trigone, the patient may have dysuria and frequency as well as occasional bleeding on or about the time of menstruation. The bleeding is due to congestion of the overlying mucosa rather than to ulceration.

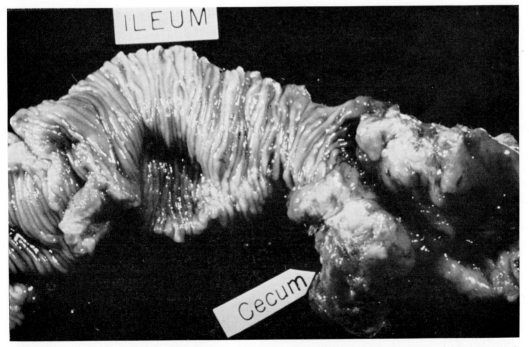

Fig. 47-6. Thickening by endometriosis of the wall of the cecum produces dense scarring, but as is characteristic in this condition, the mucosa is intact.

Endometriosis involving the ureter probably occurs more often than the paucity of reports in the literature would indicate. Obstruction to the ureter usually appears only on one side and always in the lower third. It may come about in one of two ways: (1) Endometriosis within the bladder wall encroaches upon the intravesical portion of the ureter, thus producing a block at the outlet. (2) Invasion of the ureteral wall with projection into the lumen of the ureter may occur from an endometrial implant on the lower pelvic peritoneum. More often the obstruction is due to compression of the ureter from an external implant that is part of widespread endometriosis. We have seen this happen from a solitary nodule or group of implants that coalesced in a local area.

Rarely is the diagnosis made before operation. In most instances some other pathologic entity is suspected, such as inflammatory stricture or nonopaque calculus.

The symptoms are chronic and not very specific. Hematuria does not appear unless the lumen is involved or multiple bladder implants exist. Pain in the flank radiating to the groin that becomes more pronounced before and during the menstrual period should arouse suspicion.

WHAT ARE THE GROSS CHARACTERISTICS OF THE VISIBLE REMOTE LESIONS, AND HOW DO THEY BEHAVE?   "Endometriomas" (solitary non-neoplastic nodules containing endometrial tissue) that respond cyclically to the stimulus of the ovarian hormones are often found in abdominal and perineal scars after operations. These lesions have evidently or obviously been transplanted through trauma incidental to either operation or delivery. The interval between the trauma and the subsequent appearance of the implant varies considerably. They have been reported as early as four weeks and as late as sixteen years postoperatively. The great majority appear in less than two years.

In the region of the umbilicus similar nodules are found, but frequently there is no antecedent operative trauma. A few isolated cases of endometriosis have appeared on the pleura, in the lungs, thigh, gluteal and axillary folds and the muscles of the forearm. The etiologic explanation as to why the lesions occur in these remote areas is complicated and speculative, but they do respond with menstruation and to hormonal stimulation in the same manner as the endometrial implants in abdominal incisions and perineal scars.

Wherever these lesions appear, they present similar patterns of growth. A firm or hard, fibrotic mass is usually fixed to the underlying tissue. Such masses vary considerably in size and are usually tender to touch at any time, but particularly when they enlarge in the few days preceding the menstrual period. Pain is present most of the time, but it becomes appreciably worse as the period approaches. The lesions that appear in the region of the umbilicus or the vulva often show a discoloration indicating that blood has accumulated. Occasionally if the overlying tissue is thin and in an area easily traumatized, bleeding may occur at the time of greatest activity within the implant, namely, at the time of the period. This is one form of vicarious menstruation. The more remote endometriotic implants and those in the scars of abdominal incisions rarely show any color change.

What Is the Microscopic Picture of These Ectopic Endometrial Implants?

The microscopic picture varies widely, depending on (a) the location of the implant, (b) the extent of the fibrotic response in the normal tissue surrounding the implant, and (c) the duration of the disease.

Since endometrial implants contain the same type of epithelium, glands and stroma as the uterine endometrium and respond in the same way to hormonal stimulation, one might reasonably expect the epithelium within the cyst to duplicate the phases of the normal endometrium within the uterus. Occasionally in a relatively young implant this is true, and one may find secretory endometrium, as well as decidual reaction within stromal cells in the cyst wall. One is far more likely to find a proliferative epithelium when a progestational response is normally due. For the most part, the epithelial cells appear cuboidal rather than cylindrical, and it is often practically impossible to correlate the activity of the normal endometrium with that of the endometriotic cyst. The fact that the correlation is not easy is probably due to the presence of an expanding cyst working against the constricting fibrosis that surrounds the implant. This is less true of endometrial cysts within the ovary, for there is less connective tissue present to stifle their expansion. Occasionally, cyclic changes are found in patchy areas of the lining of endometrial cysts in the ovary after considerable expenditure of effort in sampling and histologic examination. More often the expansion of the cyst and degeneration in response to the presence of the retained

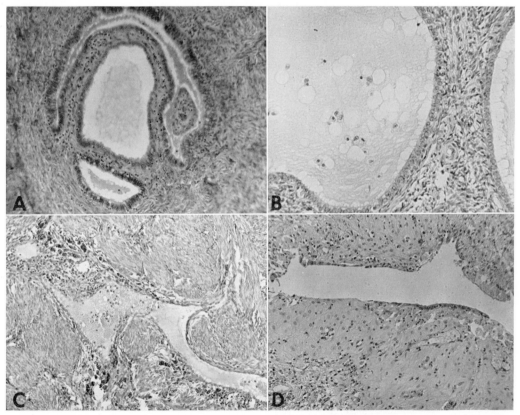

Fig. 47-7.   *A*, Endometriosis in ovarian tissue shown mostly in the proliferative phase. *B*, Ovarian endometriosis with a cystic glandular hyperplasia, secretory activity and edema of the endometrial stroma. *C*, Sometimes, as in this sigmoid focus, hemorrhage into endometriosis results in destruction of the glands, so that only the endometrial stroma and pigmented macrophages filled with hemosiderin remain. *D*, Decidual reaction of the stroma of endometriosis may be striking, as in this ovarian implant. Decidua may be present with or without pregnancy, and in the ovary it may occur in the absence of other criteria for the diagnosis of endometriosis.

blood are enough to destroy almost the entire endometrial lining (Fig. 47–7, *A, B*).

For diagnosis histopathologically, three features are sought: *(a)* endometrial glands, *(b)* endometrial stroma, *(c)* hemorrhage, either fresh or remote. Old hemorrhage is evident partly as foci of macrophages containing hemosiderin pigment absorbed from degenerated red cell hemoglobin (Fig. 47–7, *C*). Since endometriosis is a self-destructive process, a diagnosis is permissible in the presence of any two of the three characteristic findings. If only one is present, such as the endometrial glands, a diagnosis of epithelial inclusion cyst or peritoneal mesothelial inclusion cyst might be made. If only decidual reaction of the endometrial stroma is found, as occurs in the appendiceal subserosa or ovarian cortex during pregnancy or in the ovaries of older nonpregnant women, the diagnosis is simply decidual reaction, and full-fledged endometriosis is not regarded as having been established (Fig. 47–7, *D*).

How Does One Make the Clinical Diagnosis of Endometriosis?

It has been demonstrated that endometriosis is a disease of the active reproductive years and will be found most frequently in the age group between twenty-five and forty years. A few cases will appear in the late adolescent period, but they are usually discovered incidentally in the course of a laparotomy for another cause. There is such a variety of pathologic changes associated with endometriosis from the age of forty years on through the time of the menopause that endometriosis again is apt to be found mainly incidentally. The symptoms that commonly appear in these older patients with endometriosis can hardly be considered pathognomonic of the disease.

We are primarily concerned, then, with making a clinical diagnosis of endometriosis in the reproductive age group, when treatment will be more productive than destructive.

The diagnosis of endometriosis per se will be made by a careful evaluation of the symptoms and pelvic findings with occasional help from x-rays. If the patient has extrapelvic lesions, such as endometriomata in the umbilicus or vulva, one can observe directly the changes that occur in relation to menstruation, but when the lesions are entirely intraperitoneal, the diagnosis must be made on the basis of the history and physical findings.

There appear to be two groups of patients who are likely candidates for the development of endometriosis: *(1)* the patient who has the stigmata of underdevelopment, such as the so-called infantile uterus with congenital erosion of the cervix. When these patients have increasing dysmenorrhea, pelvic pain that becomes progressively worse as the menstrual period approaches, dyspareunia or a complaint of sterility, endometriosis should be suspected. *(2)* Patients who have been able to have one or two children, but have been unsuccessful in their efforts to have more, may have their difficulties traced to endometriosis, particularly if they have the train of symptoms mentioned above. Secondary infertility has endometriosis as one major cause.

What Is the Most Common Symptom of Endometriosis?

Pelvic pain that bears a direct relation to the menstrual period is the most common symptom associated with endometriosis. In general there are two types: *(1)* Lower abdominal pain which comes on just before the onset of the period. Its severity varies between a vague, heavy bearing-down pain and a sudden severe pain that may precipitate an emergency surgical exploration. *(2)* Acquired dysmenorrhea, which becomes progressively more incapacitating. The important fact is not that the patient has a pain which she had not had before, but that the pain, once acquired, increases in severity with each subsequent menstrual period.

The nature and severity of both types of pain vary, depending on the location of the implant and the amount of disease present. In certain locations there may be no pain at all. Approximately 25 per cent of patients in whom the diagnosis is finally made have no pain, regardless of the stage of the disease. Certainly in the early stages patients have little pain, but the process is progressive, and the vague pains associated with menstruation in adolescence or the early twenties may later become recognizable as evidence of endometriosis.

Peritoneal implants, even when the lesions are small, usually produce more pain than the larger cysts found in the ovary. It is possible, for example, to have extensive disease within the ovary with little discomfort, until rupture disseminates the contents of a chocolate cyst throughout the lower pelvis.

What Is the Mechanism of Pain Associated with the Lesions of Endometriosis?

The explanation as to why the small lesions produce so much pain, while a minimal amount of pain may be present with extensive lesions, is not entirely clear, but it is probably related to the extent of fibrosis that surrounds the implants and the degree to which the peritoneum is subjected to repeated insults through the escape of the cyst contents.

THE SMALL PERITONEAL LESION.   The peritoneal lesion may manifest itself as either an indefinite or severe pain in the right or left lower abdominal quadrant, as a bearing-down pain, or as pain in the back or rectum on defecation. In the early phases of the disease the endometrial implant menstruates into its own cavity, and the physiologic activity simulates that of the uterus itself. Either as the result of minute ruptures and spillage of the contents onto the sensitive peritoneum immediately adjacent or because of a natural attempt on the part of the peritoneum to resist invasion of any tissue foreign to it, a protective fibrous tissue response develops around the implant. As this process progresses, the implants have an increasingly difficult time in the monthly expansion stimulated by the ovarian hormones. Distention of a cyst that has nowhere to go because of peripheral constriction fibrosis invariably produces pain that becomes more severe with each menstrual cycle.

This is the principal reason for the pain, but there is an additional factor. Patients with small peritoneal implants usually have ovulatory cycles. It is well known that the cerebral cortex at the time of the menstrual period becomes more sensitive to stimuli that would produce little response at any other time of the month. This is apparently due to the action of progesterone, which produces cerebral ischemia and edema. As the endometriosis progresses, the cerebral pain pattern becomes more firmly established with each passing month. Not only is there aggravation from the progression of disease, but also there appears to be a gradual decrease in the pain threshold. The site of the implant accounts for the location of the pain. Thus involvement of the uterosacral ligaments produces backache.

The same mechanism is operative when lesions are present in small intestine, rectosigmoid, sigmoid colon, bladder or the remote sites of endometriosis.

THE LARGER OVARIAN LESIONS.   Growth within the ovary, on the other hand, is much slower, and the constricting fibrosis is absent. The patient then has pain only as the cyst distends. The progression is so gradual that the visceral nerve endings are able to adjust to the painful stimuli produced by distention of the peritoneal surface cover. It is also true that the patient with the large ovarian lesion tends to have anovulatory cycles, as evidenced by the amount of menstrual irregularity noted in such patients with endometriosis. Without the progestin element the threshold for pain in the cerebral cortex is perhaps much higher.

Acute excruciating pain may appear suddenly when the endometrial cyst ruptures and spills its contents onto the sensitive pelvic peritoneum. The nature of this pain is similar to that observed in a ruptured ectopic pregnancy. This train of events occurs not infrequently. Fifteen per cent of patients who have a final diagnosis of endometriosis enter the hospital with a diagnosis of an acute abdominal emergency.

PAIN ASSOCIATED WITH PELVIC ADHESIONS.   With continued spillage of the contents of endometrial cysts, both small and large, extensive adhesions develop in the lower peritoneal cavity. The natural course of the disease and the progressive formation of adhesions tend to bind the adjacent organs, such as the bladder, small intestine and rectum, to the uterus. As a result the patient has a fixed pelvis which is unyielding to any sort of pressure. The pain is similar to that found in pelvic inflammation, whatever the cause.

What Characteristic Forms of Pain are Noted?

ACQUIRED DYSMENORRHEA.   The most common symptom of endometriosis is an increasingly severe dysmenorrhea of the acquired type. Pain begins before the onset of the period and builds up constantly in severity as the menstrual flow begins, but stops shortly thereafter. It may continue throughout menstruation if the disease process is extensive. This is in contrast to the symptoms of pelvic inflammation, which tend to improve during menstruation. The pain is steady, dull and boring rather than cramplike. This fact should be kept in mind in operating for what is believed to be essential dysmenorrhea because no abnormality can be felt. Fifteen per cent of these patients have peritoneal endometriotic implants. Since the parietal peritoneum is not innervated by the presacral nerves, little help can be expected from excision of these nerves.

In general one may say that any patient who begins to have dysmenorrhea for the first time between the ages of twenty-five and thirty-five years should be considered a likely candidate to have endometriosis. It would be unwise, however, to diagnose endometriosis on the basis of dysmenorrhea alone, for approximately one quarter of the patients have no pain at all.

DYSPAREUNIA AND BACKACHE.   Nodular thickening of the uterosacral ligaments and widespread dissemination of endometrial implants through the posterior cul-de-sac tend to fix the uterus in the pelvis. This frequently results in severe backache Motion of the cervix produces pain, which explains the dyspareunia that many patients note. It may be so severe that intercourse becomes infrequent. Dyspareunia could be the explanation of some of the lowered fertility so common in endometriosis.

RECTAL LESIONS AND DYSURIA.   When the rectal wall is involved, defecation may be accompanied by pain, particularly at the time of the menstrual period. This is particularly true when the rectovaginal septum is involved. If the lesion in the sigmoid or rectum is large enough to bulge into the lumen, or is annular, the patient may have severe intestinal cramps and intermittent intestinal obstruction.

Lesions of the bladder wall, particularly in the region of the trigone, often produce dysuria because of the swelling within the implant and the edema of the surrounding bladder mucosa that occurs at the time of the menstrual period.

Is There a True Infertility Problem with Endometriosis?

The true incidence of sterility in patients with endometriosis cannot be accurately determined, for we can never know how many may have an endometriosis that produces little in the way of symptoms, nor do we have accurate information on the fertility index of the husbands of the patients with symptoms. There appears to be, however, an associated sterility problem in patients who have proved endometriosis. The figure quoted in the literature is in the neighborhood of 40 per cent. This is chiefly concerned with the ability to achieve pregnancy. Once the patient becomes pregnant, she has as good a chance as her sisters to go through to the delivery of a normal infant. There are many instances in the literature, and more that are unreported, of the coexistence of normal pregnancy with extensive endometriosis in both ovary and pelvic peritoneum, particularly the ovary. Patients who have extensive endometriotic disease of the rectovaginal septum have been known to deliver normal babies without any particular complications.

It is strange that the patient with endometriosis has such a hard time becoming pregnant. Unlike in other forms of pelvic disease, the fallopian tubes are almost always open, and though a few cases have endometriosis present in the muscle walls of the tubes, which might alter their mobility, the majority appear fairly normal. When the tubes have become involved in extensive adhesions, the chances of pregnancy are materially reduced, despite the fact that the fimbriated ends may still be patent. It is stranger yet that many of the patients have one or two children, but are unable to produce more, however hard they try.

The fact that about 40 per cent of patients with endometriosis are sterile and that the remainder have an average family of two suggests that endometriosis is associated with a relative infertility factor, at least. It is by no means clear that endometriosis per se actually causes this, but we have noted that patients who have endometriosis tend to have rather underdeveloped uteri with congenital erosions, particularly in the group who have never been pregnant. This suggests that the anatomic substrate is unsound.

Meigs has suggested that the reason lies in the restriction of the family size and the late marriages that take place for economic reasons. A large number of women who prove to have endometriosis have married after the age of twenty-five years and had their first child shortly thereafter. If a girl is actually normal in the development of her genital organs, late marriage and pregnancy probably may have little part in the etiology of endometriosis, but for the patient with any of the stigmata of underdevelopment, postponement of marriage may play a decisive role. Such patients likely should marry early and have at least one child every five years. It is a rather striking clinical observation that many patients who have endometriosis have spaced their pregnancies at wider intervals. Nearly three quarters of the patients will have such a history.

Dyspareunia may be an important factor in the fertility problem. No one quite understands why patients who have nodular uterosacral ligaments or cul-de-sac implants have so much pain on sexual contact. This is also a notable observation on vaginal examination. It seems to be far more pronounced in endometriosis than in other forms of pelvic disease that cause fixation of the pelvic floor. It may be enough to discourage intercourse.

Another factor that may have a bearing on sterility is the high percentage of patients who have anovulatory cycles, particularly when the ovaries are involved.

Is Abnormal Menstrual Bleeding Due to Endometriosis?

Patients who have endometriosis frequently have an abnormal menstrual bleeding pattern. The association is reported in the literature, varying in frequency from one half to two thirds of all the patients with endometriosis. Nevertheless it is an erroneous clinical impression that the patient bleeds because of the endometriosis. Certainly one's accuracy in clinical diagnosis will not be improved if one depends on variations in time and the amount of menstrual flow. The patient bleeds because of ovarian dysfunction, in all probability. We have noted the occurrence of anovulatory cycles. In addition there is the factor of other lesions associated with endometriosis. If one excludes uterine polyps and fibroids, which usually cause dysfunctional bleeding, somewhat less than 20 per cent of patients with endometriosis will have abnormal vaginal bleeding. The younger patient, who is far less likely to have other pelvic disease, does not list abnormal menstrual bleeding as one of the complaints when questioned.

What Are the Prominent Findings on Physical Examination?

The gross and microscopic findings of endometrial implants as found on abdominal exploration and in the regions of the body remote from the genital tract have been described. When suspicion of the presence of endometriosis has been aroused by the history of an acquired dysmenorrhea of increasing severity, or dyspareunia and relative infertility, what physical findings lend support?

The most constant factor on bimanual examination, which tends to distinguish endometriosis from other lesions such as pelvic inflammation and tuberculosis that give the same symptoms and exhibit similar pelvic fixation, is the presence of shotty noduar thickenings of the uterosacral ligaments. These are best felt by rectum. Tenderness on palpation of these areas is exquisite and out of proportion to the extent of the abnormality present. Palpation of the pelvic floor usually demonstrates similar areas of induration, which are likewise very tender to touch. When these findings are associated with a fixed retroverted uterus that cannot be dislodged and with bilateral

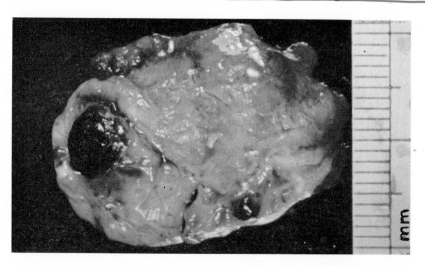

Fig. 47-8.   Endometriosis in the broad ligament has resulted in the formation of these blue cysts filled with altered blood, a relatively unusual form of this disease.

masses in the adnexal regions, the diagnosis of endometriosis can usually be made with fair certainty.

When the isolated, indurated, nodular areas coalesce in this region, one or two types of lesions tend to develop. (1) By far the most common finding is the presence of a nodular mass that results from the fixation of the anterior wall of the sigmoid to the posterior wall of the uterus in the area between the two uterosacral ligaments. This is called endometriosis of the rectovaginal septum. When felt by rectum, it is firm, nodular, hard and fibrotic. Cancer could arise in this region, but the fact that the mucosa is intact over the lesion in endometriosis helps to establish the correct diagnosis. If there is any doubt, the patient should have a proctoscopy, and the suspicious area should be biopsied. (2) Occasionally, but far less often, the accumulation of implants produces one large or several small blue-domed cysts that invade the posterior vaginal fornix and can actually be seen behind the cervix (Fig. 47–8).

One of the most difficult problems in the physical diagnosis of endometriosis is the well documented fact that it is frequently associated with other forms of pelvic disease. Pelvic inflammation, for example, may fix the uterus in retroversion and produce bilateral adnexal enlargements. Approximately 20 per cent of patients with endometriosis also have pelvic inflammation. Nearly three times that number have fibroids.

Because of the associated disease the diagnosis of endometriosis cannot be made solely on the basis of palpation of fixed adnexal masses. They may well be due to endometriosis, particularly when isolated tender nodules are also felt on the pelvic floor and uterosacral ligaments, but in many instances it is difficult to distinguish between endometriosis and pelvic inflammation. The percentage of diagnostic accuracy increases when the physical findings are considered with the history and symptoms.

Are Any Laboratory Aids Helpful in Making the Diagnosis?

Little help can be obtained from the laboratory or x-ray department to establish the diagnosis. The most helpful and definitive are (a) biopsy with microscopic interpretation of the tissue removed; (b) x-ray studies of the lower colon and terminal ileum; (c) cystoscopy and retrograde or intravenous pyelography.

BIOPSY. By definition, endometriosis is an ectopic implant of endometrial tissue in regions remote from the uterine cavity. Since it contains stroma and glands that respond in the same way as normal endometrium to the ovarian hormones, microscopic examination of the tissue is essential to a final diagnosis of endometriosis, whether it is found at abdominal operation or in regions of the body where it can be seen either directly or by such visual aids as the cystoscope or proctoscope.

X-RAY. Endometriosis of the sigmoid colon or rectosigmoid—where most of the bowel lesions occur—occasionally encroaches on and narrows the lumen of the large intestine either by the tumor bulging into the bowel or by annular constriction of it.

Since the gross picture in the areas on the surface and within the muscular walls of the intestine that can be seen and felt, as well as the symptoms, is not very different from that produced by carcinoma of the colon, some help in differentiation is necessary. Little help can be obtained from proctoscopy and biopsy, for the mucosa is rarely ulcerated. Biopsy reports of the constricted area usually indicate only chronic inflammation, which simply adds to the confusion. The barium enema may provide the information needed to establish a diagnosis, since cancer grows from within outward and characteristically disturbs the mucosal pattern of the bowel, while endometriosis does not.

What Is the Characteristic Picture Seen on Barium Enema That Suggests Endometriosis? When the intestine is completely obstructed, the barium enema simply localizes the lesion within the bowel. No further differentiation can be made. The block could be due to carcinoma, diverticulitis or endometriosis.

The outline of the mucosal pattern, however, is significant when the colonic obstruction is incomplete. The principal points are as follows: *(a)* The bowel is fixed and is tender at the point of fixation; *(b)* the mucosa is intact; *(c)* a long, inconstant filling defect with sharp irregular borders seems to be the prevailing pattern.

The x-ray evidence for endometriosis of the terminal ileum, after a small-bowel study, is far less definite than the information derived from barium examination of the lower colon. Fixation, kinking and an intact mucosa tend to rule out carcinoma on the one hand, and a postoperative obstruction due to adhesions on the other, but these signs do not help in differentiating endometriosis from pelvic inflammation. In the acute phases, when the symptoms simulate acute appendicitis, a barium study of the small intestine would be contraindicated.

WHAT IS THE TYPICAL CYSTOSCOPIC PICTURE OF ENDOMETRIOSIS? The cystoscopic picture varies, depending on the phase of the menstrual cycle during which the investigation is carried out. Earlier in the discussion it was noted that the bladder mucosa is intact, even when a tender mass can be felt at the bladder neck.

The typical picture of endometriosis within the bladder will appear with the greatest clarity when a cystoscopy is performed when the menstrual period occurs. At that time a definite elevation of the intact mucosa can be seen, pushed upward from beneath into the bladder lumen. The bladder mucosa around the tumor is edematous and appears in folds. In the region of the main tumor mass there are small transparent cysts, together with other cysts that appear blue or black, depending on the amount of blood contained within them. All these factors are exaggerated if the cystoscopy is performed during menstruation. After the period the congestion of the bladder mucosa is less, fewer blue-domed cysts are found, and the numerous transparent cysts are not as evident. The tumor beneath the mucosa remains unchanged in size, regardless of the time of the month the cystoscopy is done.

The Treatment of Endometriosis

From the foregoing discussion of the life history, resultant symptoms, and physical findings of patients who have endometriosis, obvious factors appear that have a direct bearing on therapy.

In brief, we recognize the following facts:

1. Endometriosis is a disease process common to the reproductive age group, with its maximum incidence in the early thirties.

2. Its life history is intimately related to ovarian function and the action of its hormones. Rarely is endometriosis encountered in adolescence, and it becomes largely inactive after the menopause. Its growth activity is therefore limited to the years of ovarian function.

3. Endometriosis is a benign disease, though it has a propensity to invade the peritoneum and adjacent organs. Such growth is said to be progressive.

4. The symptoms commonly associated with endometriosis are varied. Many

symptoms that are attributed to endometriosis are due to the associated pathologic changes and cannot be considered pathognomonic of endometriosis alone. Furthermore, the patient may have endometriosis without symptoms.

5. There appears to be an infertility factor in patients with endometriosis that seems to be independent of the extent of the disease.

WHAT FACTORS INFLUENCE TREATMENT? *General Observations.* The observations listed above are all true, but their significance and interpretation have been badly distorted and have led to considerable confusion as to the proper therapy for the individual case.

The terms *invasion* and *progression* have been intimately linked with endometriosis and have been the greatest offenders in obscuring clear thinking. As soon as the words "invasion" or "progression" are used, the surgeon automatically begins to think in terms of malignant neoplastic disease, not in the sense that endometriosis is a neoplastic process or becomes malignant, but simply that it acts like malignant disease. This tends to influence the rationale of treatment toward the side of radical extirpation, which the life history of endometriosis does not warrant.

Realizing that the endometriosis, in its growth pattern, is under the influence of the ovarian hormones and accepting the word "invasion" on the same terms that apply to cancer, surgeons formerly practiced radical removal of all ovarian tissue, regardless of the age of the patient or extent of the disease. We now recognize that this approach was in error, and conservative management is the therapy of today. Nevertheless endometriosis continues to have a malignant connotation that influences therapy.

The suggestion that the disease is always progressive should come under close scrutiny. Much endometriosis, particularly that found in the peritoneum and cul-de-sac, has run its full course and is no longer active. It may still be felt as a nodule in the uterosacral ligaments and on the pelvic floor, but in many instances it is found in the absence of any symptoms. The same may be said of foci on the serosa of the bowel or minimal invasion of the muscle wall. At times progression of the disease does appear to be rapid, but this usually occurs when the ovaries are involved with endometrial chocolate cysts. Sudden rupture of such cysts may disseminate endometrial fragments and produce new implants on the pelvic peritoneum. But when cul-de-sac or rectovaginal septal endometriotic lesions are present without ovarian involvement, the progression is limited to coalescence of the adjacent nodules.

There is one similarity in the growth pattern of endometriosis which imitates that of malignant tumors. Endometriosis may rarely spread along lymphatic channels. Dissemination to distant areas, such as lung and extremity, occurs so rarely that such instances are medical curiosities.

How Often Are Ovarian Cancer and Endometriosis Associated? The proved cases are rare. This may occur in one of two ways: (*a*) Malignant changes may arise in the mixed type of epithelium present in the nonendometrial portions of ovarian cysts. Thus serous cystadenocarcinoma may arise close to an area of endometriosis within an ovary. (*b*) Malignant transformation of the endometriotic epithelium of the chocolate cyst. The endometrial cyst of the ovary is less likely to be associated with carcinoma than the more common serous and mucinous types of ovarian cyst. Criteria of the diagnosis of ovarian adenocarcinoma arising in endometriosis are discussed later. The danger lies not in the fact that the endometriotic cyst has become malignant, but that any ovarian enlargement that is felt may be due to carcinoma.

This is the limit of the extent that endometriosis parallels the life history of malignant disease. The discussion has been prolonged in an attempt to dispel the lingering misconception that endometriosis, though benign, behaves like malignant cancerous disease. Unless this is established, the case for conservative management is less strong.

WHAT ARE THE INDICATIONS FOR TREATMENT IN THE YOUNGER WOMAN? The primary objective in the treatment of the woman in the early reproductive years is to (a) relieve pain, (b) correct menstrual irregularities, (c) improve fertility, and (d) prevent further destruction of tissue when the ovaries are involved. Whether or not treatment is undertaken, and the nature of the therapy that is given will depend on the severity of the symptoms and the extent and location of the endometriosis. Treatment will be modified by the age of the patient and the size of her family, as well as her desire to maintain menstrual function. It will be further altered by the amount of coexisting tissue abnormality and the symptoms associated with it.

The treatment of endometriosis in the young patient may be (1) observation, (2) medical, or (3) surgical, with the emphasis on the side of conservatism.

WHEN SHOULD THE PATIENT BE LEFT UNTREATED AND OBSERVED? Since pelvic endometriosis in the absence of ovarian involvement progresses slowly, if at all, there would seem to be no danger in postponing surgical intervention. The patient with mild pain and minimal physical findings to go with her infertility should be left alone or be treated medically.

There are two main reasons for operating on patients who have minimal amounts of endometriosis: (1) relief of pain, and (2) the possibility that the infertility problem may be improved.

Acquired dysmenorrhea, increasing in severity, is one of the chief symptoms suggestive of endometriosis, when it is accompanied by the palpation of tender nodules on the pelvic floor. We know that we can relieve the pain produced by extensive endometriosis by taking out the uterus and removing ovarian tissue. This approach is manifestly impractical for the young patient who has minimal disease and has an infertility factor in addition to her pain. This patient may prefer to put up with her discomfort rather than subject herself to surgery. Before advising operation the surgeon would do well to consider what he hopes to accomplish by operating on the patient. Unfortunately the conservative operations with excision of peritoneal implants do not always relieve pain, whether or not a presacral neurectomy is done in combination with the local excision. Pain-relieving drugs might well be given before resorting to operation.

The indications for operation are far greater when ovarian masses are felt than when nodules are palpated on the pelvic floor or uterosacral ligaments for the following reasons: (1) The adnexal masses may not be endometriosis; (2) the process is more likely to be progressive in the face of ovarian involvement, because of the chance of secondary dissemination as the cysts rupture; and (3) the gradual expansion of the chocolate cyst within the ovary is bound to result in the replacement of increasing amounts of normal ovarian tissue.

Besides pain relief, the second reason for advising operation is the possibility of improving the relative infertility factor present in endometriosis. The patient who has been unable to become pregnant and has endometriosis limited to the pelvic floor in all probability has little to gain from an abdominal exploration. The sole exception to this observation rests with the patient who has such severe dyspareunia, because of tender pelvic nodules, that she tends to avoid intercourse. The surgeon should be cautious of operating on any patient with the idea of improving her fertility if she has symptoms suggestive of endometriosis, but no palpable evidence of it.

The chances of a subsequent pregnancy are higher and the indications for surgical intervention are greater if the patient has had one or two children, but has been unable to have more.

IS HORMONAL TREATMENT INDICATED IN THE PATIENT WITH MINIMAL ENDOMETRIOSIS? It is well known that the growth factor in endometriotic foci, as well as the symptoms, is held in abeyance when the periods become anovulatory for any reason, or if pregnancy is established. One may, therefore, elect to use hormonal therapy for the suppression of ovarian activity in general and ovulation in particular.

The hormones usually given are estrogens, the newer progestational drugs, and androgens.

Estrogens. The rationale for the use of the estrogens is based on the regression of activity in endometriosis noted during pregnancy, when high concentrations of estrin as well as progesterone are noted in urinary assays. In all probability the improvement noted from the use of the estrogens in endometriosis is due to the suppression of ovulation. The primary aim is to produce amenorrhea for an interval of three to six months. Since endometrial hyperplasia tends to develop under continuous estrogen therapy, this treatment should be interrupted after at most six months. Also, the dosage of estrogen must be increased at regular intervals to prevent breakthrough or withdrawal bleeding.

The following dosage schedule has been suggested. One may substitute any one of the forms of estrin in common use, provided the dosage levels are comparable.

One milligram of diethylstilbestrol is given on the first day of the period. This is increased by 1 mg. every 3 days to a total of 5 mg. daily. Thereafter the dosage is increased by 5 mg. each 3 days until 100 mg. becomes the daily dose. This dosage level is maintained for 3 months. After this period the dosage is reduced by 5 mg. daily until the patient is off the drug.

The results are good but somewhat unpredictable, probably because the pathologic elements that go to make up the endometriosis are not constant. The response in the epithelial lining does not always follow that of the uterine endometrium. The lesions are said to become smaller and atrophic and the pelvic floor softer and more pliable. Although this is frequently true during the period of medication, recurrences are often noted when the hormone is discontinued.

The Newer Progestational Drugs. The theory behind the use of the new progestin-like drugs is that they produce not only amenorrhea and inhibit ovulation, but also a decidual response in the endometriosis, thereby effecting a state of pseudopregnancy (Fig. 47–7, *D*). We have noted that normal pregnancy improves the symptoms and retards the evidence of growth in the lesions. The drug most commonly used at present is norethynodrel, available commercially as Enovid. The dosage schedule recommended is 10 mg. daily, taken with a glass of milk on retiring, for 2 weeks beginning on the fourth day of the menstrual period. The daily dosage is increased by 10 mg. every 2 weeks until the daily dosage is 40 mg.

Because of the estrin contained in the preparation, the patient rarely has breakthrough bleeding, but nausea, weight gain and breast soreness appear and are often troublesome. The improvement during medication is obvious clinically, and evidence of its suppressive activity is apparent in the endometriosis when it is seen in patients who for one reason or another have had abdominal exploration while undergoing this treatment. The drug has not been in use long enough to permit any deductions on the chances of reactivation of the endometriotic foci.

Androgens. Sublingual linguets of small doses of methyltestosterone have been used with varying degrees of success. The larger doses inhibit ovulation through their action on the pituitary, but have the definite disadvantage that they, too, often produce hirsutism, acne and deepening of the voice. Unfortunately these undesirable side effects may not disappear when the drug is discontinued. Smaller doses may produce the same changes in sensitive women. The effect of the smaller 5- or 10-mg. daily doses would appear to be by direct action on the endometriosis itself, rather than acting through the pituitary to suppress ovulation. The basis for this statement rests on the number of reported instances of pregnancy that have occurred under this treatment.

The dosage of methyltestosterone (Metandren; Oreton-linguets) usually is 5 mg. daily for 100 days. Occasionally a dose of 10 mg. daily has been used. If the results have been satisfactory and the side effects insignificant, the course may be repeated after a two-month period.

WHEN IS SURGERY INDICATED?   As we have tried to indicate, the diagnosis of endometriosis does not automatically call for abdominal exploration. The primary indication for surgical intervention will depend in the final analysis on the location and extent of the endometriosis in relation to the severity of the symptoms it produces. This is true regardless of age, for the young patient may have extensive disease with severe symptoms, while her older sister may have minimal disease. We speak of conservatism in the treatment of endometriosis because of our desire to maintain menstrual and childbearing functions. This term applies to what is done at operation, not to whether the patient should or should not be operated on. It could hardly be called conservative to postpone operation in a young girl who has severe symptoms and fixed adnexal lesions. By denying the patient surgical assistance because of her youth you may force her into a position in which only radical extirpation of the uterus and all the ovarian tissue is possible.

Operation is indicated when (1) the patient's symptoms and palpable lesions become increasingly noteworthy while under observation or medical therapy; (2) there is extensive fixation of the uterus and pelvic floor, and nodular masses are palpable in the uterosacral ligaments or rectovaginal septum; (3) fixed ovarian cysts are palpable on one or both sides; (4) the symptoms of rectal tenesmus or hematuria appear cyclically in a patient who has a tender mass palpable either in the rectovaginal septum or at the base of the bladder; (5) the patient has an infertility problem in the presence of pelvic disease that gives the clinical impression of endometriosis; (6) the dysmenorrhea and low abdominal pain, associated with palpable abnormalities, become increasingly severe with each ensuing menstrual period; (7) blue-domed cysts are encountered in the vaginal vault, vulva, perineum, round ligament or umbilicus; or (8) acute abdominal pain appears suddenly in a patient who has fixed adnexal lesions.

HOW MUCH SURGERY IS REQUIRED?   The treatment of endometriosis must be highly individualized to comply with the many and varied problems that these patients present. We know that endometriosis depends on ovarian function and that ovarian ablation by either radiation or surgery will induce regression within the implants. In the past many combined hysterectomies and oophorectomies were done for minimal amounts of endometriosis. This can hardly be any answer for the patient who wants to preserve either childbearing or menstrual function.

The primary aim of modern surgery for endometriosis is conservative preservation of ovarian and reproductive functions in the young patient or ovarian tissue alone in the older patient who has passed the time when pregnancy can reasonably be expected. To what extent one practices conservative surgery depends more upon the extent of the disease than any other factor, such as age, that may modify the planned surgical attack. Thus a patient with extensive endometriosis at the age of thirty years may have to be treated more radically than her sister with less disease at the age of forty. One would like to save the uterus and as much ovarian tissue as possible in such a patient; good surgical judgment must be exercised and the likelihood of a subsequent pregnancy seriously considered.

The problem of whether or not all ovarian tissue should be sacrificed also depends on the extent of disease and the surgical judgment of the operator. Unless we are dealing with widespread endometriosis of such degree that local excisions of the endometriomata are impossible without incurring a risk of morbidity or malfunction in the organs from which they are excised, there is no good reason for removal of the ovaries.

WHAT DO WE MEAN BY CONSERVATIVE SURGERY? One generally means here the excision of all gross endometriosis whenever possible, with preservation of the uterus and as much ovarian tissue as possible. One may elect to cauterize the localized areas on the peritoneum rather than to excise them. This is true whether the endometriomas are seen on the serosal surface of the bowel or on the uterosacral ligaments. These involved areas are often confined to the parietal peritoneum and frequently show no tendency to invade the adjacent tissue. Bowel should be separated from the uterus and the adhesions excised in order to restore motility to the tubes and ovaries. If the raw areas are extensive, they may be covered with patches of excised omentum. Though it is generally believed that endometriosis is accompanied by invasion, endometrial cysts can be shelled out of the ovary, leaving some portion of normal ovary. Even a nubbin of ovarian tissue is better than none at all, and it is notably superior in its endocrine effects to synthetic estrin given by tablet or injection. It is amazing at times how fertile such patients can be.

Presacral neurectomy, together with suspension of the retroverted uterus, has been performed frequently in association with the excision or destruction by cautery of the peritoneal implants. The main object of the resection of the presacral nerves has been to minimize the dysmenorrhea and to eliminate the pain problem, should endometriosis recur after conservative surgery has been performed. Although suspension of the uterus continues to be regarded as a reasonable procedure in conjunction with the excision of peritoneal foci of endometriosis, presacral neurectomy is performed far less often. Neurectomy may provide a better blood supply to the ovary and uterus and thus increase fertility, but there is less evidence that it improves the pain problem. Many patients will have no pain anyhow, and the percentage of recurrences after conservative surgery is low. As far as fertility is concerned, the extent of the endometriotic disease bears only a slight relation to the fertility index. Furthermore, the presacral nerve has little to do with the innervation of the pelvic peritoneum.

Rather than perform presacral neurectomy, we have preferred to excise Frankenhauser's plexus, including the endometriotic implants on the posterior wall of the uterus, rectovaginal septum and uterosacral ligaments and to follow by doing a uterine suspension. If the disease is more extensive and the patient either has completed her family or is too old to expect to have children, hysterectomy should be done with salvage of as much ovarian tissue as possible, even though obvious disease is left behind in such areas as the rectal wall.

HOW WELL DO WE DO WITH CONSERVATIVE SURGERY? The test of how successful conservative surgery may be rests with (1) the number of patients who require further operation and (2) the degree of influence such surgery has on subsequent fertility.

In general the number of secondary operations following conservative surgery for endometriosis is low, certainly no greater than 10 to 15 per cent. The removal of the uterus does away with much of the train of symptoms associated with endometriosis, such as pain and abnormal bleeding. Many of the implants in the bowel wall or pelvic peritoneum are no longer active, so that conservative surgery without removal of the uterus is frequently successful in eliminating the pain factor. The excision of ovarian endometriosis minimizes the danger of further spread of the endometriotic lesions. When one leaves ovarian tissue in the face of known endometriosis, there is a calculated risk that no further progression will follow, but the history of the disease amply justifies the assumption of this risk. This is far superior to carrying out castration in any age group.

How Well Do We Do with the Infertility Problem after Conservative Surgery?   There are two schools of thought as to how much fertility is influenced by conservative surgery: (1) Some gynecologists believe that fertility is not increased by conservative surgery and that one had best tide the patient over her most fertile period without resorting to surgery, unless the symptoms become too severe. This may be done by analgesics, sedatives, hormones or small doses of codeine. Surgery is postponed until the time when the likelihood of childbearing is minimal and the definitive excision can be more radical.

2. Others are of the opinion that fertility is improved and that one may expect up to 40 per cent of pregnancies and approximately one third to have living children after conservative procedures. There does appear to be a relative infertility factor in endometriosis. Some patients are destined never to have children regardless of the extent of the disease. Others have one or two children, but no more, regardless of their tenacity and their desire. It would seem logical that the patient who has palpable evidence of disease, adnexal involvement, symptoms and the desire to have more children should be given whatever chance conservative surgery has to offer.

What Should Be Done if Symptoms Recur or the Process Advances after Conservative Surgery?   There are three possible avenues of therapy that may be taken if the process does not regress or remains stationary after conservative surgery. The patient may be subjected to (1) further surgery, (2) hormonal therapy or (3) x-ray treatment.

If further surgery is indicated, all ovarian tissue should be removed with the uterus. Since endometriosis is frequently accompanied by the formation of dense adhesions and the agglutination of intestine, either small or large, to the uterus, there is better rationale for re-exploration than x-ray treatment. Damage to adherent normal structures may be the price one has to pay for castration by x-ray.

In the poor-risk patient who may have a history of several abdominal interventions it may be wise to ablate all ovarian activity by x-ray treatment. The risks of damage to normal tissues must be considered and compared with those that might result from further surgery.

Hormone therapy, designed (a) to suppress ovarian activity and (b) to inhibit ovulation, may be given cyclically and at repeated intervals. As long as the patient can be made amenorrheic and anovulatory there can be no progression of disease. When this is established, symptoms are relieved. As with all forms of hormone therapy designed to suppress ovulation, the ovary becomes increasingly refractory to the effect of externally administered hormones to the point at which it becomes harder and harder to prevent ovulation. There is little doubt that pain can be relieved by suppressing ovarian activity with hormones, but there is some question as to whether the endometriosis actually diminishes in size and remains so after the discontinuation of treatment. In the experience of many the palpable masses reappear along with the symptoms when hormonal therapy is given up.

By and large the patient whose endometriosis does not regress or reappears after conservative surgery should be re-explored rather than be treated by hormone therapy or x-ray castration.

Huffman has provided a working outline that relates the amount of surgery required to the stage of the disease. The extent of the operation must be modified by the age of the patient and the desire to maintain reproductive, ovarian or menstrual function.

Stage I: Simple excision of the areas of endometriosis.
    a. Limited to the uterosacral ligaments.
    b. In one ovary.
    c. Superficial on peritoneum.

These may exist alone or in combination.

Stage II: Simple excision of the implant with or without dissection of the chocolate cyst from the ovary.
    a. Extensive involvement of one ovary with less in the other.
    b. Superficial on the pelvic peritoneum.
    c. On the serosal surface of the bowel.
    d. Infiltration of the uterus or uterosacral ligaments.

Whether the uterus is removed will depend on the degree of its involvement by endometriosis or other diseases and on the amount of pain or abnormal bleeding the patient experiences. The decision for or against hysterectomy must also consider the age of the patient, the size of her family and the psychologic importance of preserving the menstrual flow.

Stage III: Excision of the local endometriosis and dissection of the cysts from the ovaries, leaving as much ovary as possible. Hysterectomy should be done in most instances.
    a. Extensive endometriosis in both ovaries.
    b. Bilateral large cysts.
    c. Deep invasion of the rectovaginal septum.
    d. Infiltrations that do not obstruct the intestinal lumen.

Since endometriosis, for practical purposes, never invades the intestinal mucosa, solitary endometriosis may be excised from the bowel wall. If the surgeon is reluctant to take the risk, he may safely leave the implant in the bowel, even though he leaves ovarian tissue.

If the uterus is not removed because the patient is young and wants to have a family, the surgeon must balance carefully her chances of achieving pregnancy against the possibility of disabling discomfort in the future.

Stage IV: The uterus and tubes and ovaries should be removed, leaving the offending endometriosis untouched.
    a. Obstruction of the large or small intestine.
    b. Large endometriomata at the bladder neck.
    c. Ureteral involvement.

In the young patient who has not had her family the bowel, large or small, should be resected and end-to-end suture be performed, provided the uterus and ovarian tissue are not hopelessly compromised. Likewise, segmental resections of the bladder and dissection of the ureters from the bed of endometriosis surrounding them should be considered.

Etiology of Endometriosis

IMPLANTATION THEORY.   In the United States endometriosis was popularized by the pioneer work of Sampson, who held that the cause of the condition was a reflux of menstrual endometrium upward through the fallopian tubes and the subsequent implantation and growth of fragments of endometrium on the pelvic peritoneum and nearby structures. Examination of the copious illustrations that accompanied Sampson's articles reveals many pictures purporting to show stages of endometrial implantation that would today be regarded as technical artefacts. So-called wipe-on artefacts are produced when bits of tissue present on the instruments or cutting board used in the laboratory become adherent to the blocks cut for histologic study.

Markee implanted endometrial fragments in the anterior chamber of monkeys' eyes and studied the changes during more than 1000 menstrual cycles. In regard to endometriosis, these studies showed that human and monkey endometrium was transplantable, but when menstrual necrosis developed and the fragments of endometrium fell down into the lower levels of the anterior eye chamber, no regrowth ever occurred. This indicated the small chance of menstrual endometrium becoming reimplanted and growing thereafter.

Rarely, human cases are reported with an imperforate hymen or cervical atresia and whose menstrual flow for months or years has escaped upward into the peritoneal cavity. These women whose retrograde menstruation has been habitual and voluminous have pelvic endometriosis that may be derived from endometrial implants. TeLinde and others have imitated this situation experimentally by turning the monkey's uterus upside down surgically, so that menstrual flow characteristically is directed upward into the peritoneal cavity. By this technique peritoneal endometriosis has been achieved in monkeys, apparently owing to a retrograde menstruation and endometrial implantation.

METASTASIS THEORY.   Since the distribution of endometriosis in the pelvic peritoneum, adnexa of the uterus, and retroperitoneal lymph nodes in general is along lymphatic or vascular lines of drainage, it has been proposed that endometrial fragments reach these sites by embolization from their origin in the menstrual endometrium. Cancer cells spread in a similar way from the uterus to the various sites where endometriosis occurs. During pregnancy trophoblastic cells embolize and spread even farther, reaching the pulmonary capillaries. These trophoblastic cells degenerate and disappear after delivery, but rarely they are thought to proliferate and produce a primary lung choriocarcinoma.

This theory depends upon a similarity of the distribution of endometriosis and analogy with embolism of other living cells. It suffers from the lack of any direct supporting evidence. Endometrial emboli are so far unknown in nonpregnant human beings, and the endometriotic foci in lymph nodes morphologically appear more likely to have developed primarily there, rather than to have embolized from the uterus (Fig. 47–9, *A*).

METAPLASTIC THEORY.   According to Schiller and other workers, endometriosis arises chiefly by metaplastic changes of nests or infoldings of the peritoneal mesothelium and from other tissue cells or embryonic rests that are responsive to hormonal stimuli. All of the peritoneum and immediately underlying connective tissue below the level of the umbilicus was at one time during embryonic life closely related to the retroperitoneal mesenchyma from which the müllerian ducts arose. It is thought that some potentiality of reactivity resembling müllerian tissue is retained by the lower abdominal mesothelium and the adjacent connective tissue stroma.

In the ovary small infoldings frequently produce cysts formed from the germinal epithelium that normally covers the surface. Many germinal inclusion cysts degenerate and leave minute, laminated calcified bodies to mark the spot. Other such cysts enlarge, and these may undergo various types of metaplasia. Serous or ciliated cells, mucous or goblet cells, and metaplastic cells with secretory activities like endometrial epithelium are all observed. Sometimes a metaplastic epithelial change of one of these types affects only part of the lining of a cyst that elsewhere is seen to be composed of germinal epithelium. At other times closely adjacent cysts show different types of metaplasia. Some of them are endometrial cysts, others serous or mucinous, and still others retain the germinal epithelial lining; all may occur together in the same ovary. These observations favor a metaplastic origin of ovarian endometriosis.

Occasionally hundreds of small mesothelial inclusion cysts filled with clear fluid develop in the pelvic peritoneum. Some of these cysts degenerate and leave calcified laminated bodies behind, identical with those found when ovarian germinal inclusion cysts break down. In some of these mesothelial inclusions a metaplastic change of the lining simulates the endometrial epithelium; in others which are lined by flattened mesothelium the surrounding stroma resembles that of the endometrium. By the ususal criteria of pathologic diagnosis they do not meet the minimum requirements for designating such cysts as endometriosis. It is notable, however, how closely many such mesothelial inclusions resemble endometriosis (Fig. 47–9, *B*). In the presence of more active hormonal stimulation during pregnancy, such epithelial implants, or their stroma, may show sufficient changes, such as a decidual reaction, to permit the pathologist to diagnose endometriosis.

Experimental production of uterine subserosal endometriosis has been possible in rabbits injected with estrogen in a form that produces a long-continued hormonal stimulation.

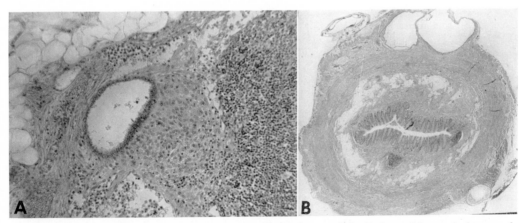

Fig. 47-9. *A*, Endometriosis in a lymph node is characteristically located beneath the capsule in the region of the sinusoids. To this extent it behaves like an embolic metastasis. But the relation of the endometrial focus to adjacent tissues suggests its primary origin here. *B*, Several subserosal mesothelial cysts are shown in the appendix. Some meet the diagnostic requirements for endometriosis, but others are merely cystic inclusions.

In the human cervix and vagina metaplastic alterations of some endocervical or vaginal glands may be responsible for the development of endometriosis. At present it would appear fair to state that the metaplastic theory of endometriosis is in greatest favor with pathologists to explain the majority of lesions. A minority of the cases of endometriosis may arise by mechanisms of implantation or metastasis.

REFERENCES

Cullen, J. S.: Adenomyoma of the Broad Ligament. *Bull. Johns Hopkins Hosp.*, 7: 112, 1896.

DeStefano, N. M., and Clough, D. M.: The Enigma of Endometriosis. *Am. J. Surg.*, 100: 122, 1960.

Fallon, J., Brosnan, J. T., and Moran, W. G.: Endometriosis; Two Hundred Cases Considered from the Viewpoint of the Practitioner. *New England J. Med.*, 235: 669, 1946.

Henriksen, E.: Endometriosis. *Am. J. Surg.*, 90: 331, 1955.

Huffman, J. W.: External Endometriosis. *Am. J. Obst. & Gynec.*, 62: 1243, 1951.

McCall, M. L., and Dolan, W. G.: Experiences with Pelvic Endometriosis. Review of Private Cases and Patients at the Charity Hospital of Louisiana at New Orleans. *J. Louisiana M. Soc.*, 108-43, 1956.

Meigs, J. V.: Endometriosis; The Occurrence of Endometriomata in the Abdominal Wall. Four Cases Following Operations in the Female Pelvis. *New England J. Med.*, 200: 1020, 1929.

Idem: An Interest in Endometriosis and Its Consequences. *Am. J. Obst. & Gynec.*, 79: 625, 1960.

Melody, G. F.: Endometriosis: Half-Century of Progress. *Stanford M. Bull.*, 13: 125, 1955.

Scott, R. B., and TeLinde, R. W.: External Endometriosis— The Scourge of the Private Patient. *Ann. Surg.*, 131: 697, 1950.

TeLinde, R. W.: Endometriosis. *Clin. Obst. & Gynec.*, 4: 788, 1961.

Ulfelder, H.: Pelvic Endometriosis. *New England J. Med.*, 254: 12, 1956.

Endometriosis of Colon

Cattell, R. B.: Endometriosis of the Colon and Rectum with Intestinal Obstruction. *New England J. Med.*, 217: 9, 1937.

Colcock, B. P., and Lamphier, T. A.: Endometriosis of the Large and Small Intestine. *Surgery*, 28: 997, 1950.

Hauck, A. E.: Endometriosis of the Colon. *Ann. Surg.*, 151: 896, 1960.

Kratzer, G. L., Salvati, E. P., and Hamandi, W. J.: The Problem of Endometriosis of the Colon. *Am. J. Surg.*, 100: 381, 1960.

Lane, R. E.: Endometriosis of the Vermiform Appendix. *Am. J. Obst. & Gynec.*, 79: 372, 1960.

MacCafee, C. H. G., and Greer, H. L.: Intestinal Endometriosis. A Report of 29 Cases and a Review of the Literature. *J. Obst. & Gynaec. Brit. Emp.*, 67: 539, 1960.

Rogers, H. L., Jr.; The Management of Endometriosis of the Colon. *Am. Surg.*, 25: 654, 1959.

Sampson, J. A.: Intestinal Adenomas of Endometrial Type. Their Importance and Their Relation to Ovarian Hematomas of Endometrial Type (Perforating Hemorrhagic Cysts of the Ovary). *Arch. Surg.*, 5: 217, 1922.

Spjut, H. J., and Perkins, D. E.: Endometriosis of the Sigmoid Colon and Rectum. A Roentgenologic and Pathologic Study. *Am. J. Roentgenol.*, 82: 1070, 1959.

Wolfe, S. A.: Endometriosis of the Vagina. Discussion and Report of a Polypoidal Form Associated with Rectovaginal Endometriosis. *Obst. & Gynec.*, 15: 612, 1960.

Endometriosis of Urinary Tract

Abeshouse, B. S., and Abeshouse, G.: Endometriosis of the Urinary Tract. Review of the Literature and Report of Four Cases of Vesical Endometriosis. *J. Internat. Coll. Surg.*, 34: 43, 1960

Beacham, C. T., and McCrea, L. E.: Endometriosis of Urinary Tract. *Urol. Survey*, 7: 2, 1957.

Beahrs, O. H., Hunter, J. S., Jr., and Sloss, P. T.: Intramural, Obstructing Endometriosis of the Ureter. *Proc. Staff Meet., Mayo Clin.*, 32: 73, 1957.

Chinn, J., Horton, R. K., and Rusche, C.: Unilateral Ureteral Obstruction as Sole Manifestation of Endometriosis. *J. Urol.*, 77: 144, 1957.

Fitzgerald, W. L., and Kuhn, M. A. R.: Endometriosis of the Bladder. *J. Urol.*, 62: 467, 1949.

Grayburn, R. W.: Ureteric Obstruction Due to Endometriosis. *J. Obst. & Gynaec. Brit. Emp.*, 67: 74, 1960.

Lichtenheld, E. R., McCauley, R. T., and Staples, P. P.: Endometriosis Involving the Urinary Tract. *Obst. & Gynec.*, 17: 762, 1961.

Ratliff, R. K., and Crenshaw, W. B.: Ureteral Obstruction from Endometriosis. *Surg., Gynec., & Obst.*, 100: 414, 1955.

Endometriosis of Other Areas

Asherman, J. G.: The Myth of Tubal and Endometrial Transplantation. *J. Obst. & Gynaec. Brit. Emp.*, 67: 228, 1960.

Barnes, J.: Endometriosis of the Pleura and Ovaries. *J. Obst. & Gynaec. Brit. Emp.*, 60: 823, 1949.

Dormandy, T. L.: Inguinal Endometriosis. *Lancet*, 1: 832, 1956.

Javert, C. T.: The spread of Benign and Malignant Endometrium in the Lymphatic System, with a Note on Coexisting Vascular Involvement. *Am. J. Obst. & Gynec.*, 64: 780, 1952.

Jimenez, M., and Miles, R. M.: Inguinal Endometriosis. *Ann. Surg.*, 151: 903, 1960.

Kirk, E. W.: Endometriosis in Posterior Half of the Labium Major. *J. Obst. & Gynaec. Brit. Emp.*. 57: 237, 1950.

Lane, R. E.: Endometriosis of the Vermiform Appendix. *Am. J. Obst. & Gynec.*, 79: 372, 1960.

Meyer, R.: Adenomatous Proliferation of the Serosa in an Abdominal Scar. *Ztschr. f. Gebursh. u. Gynäk.*, 49: 32, 1903.

Novak, E. R., and Hoge, A. F.: Endometriosis of the Lower Genital Tract. *Obst. & Gynec.*, 12: 687, 1958.

Nunn, L. L.: Endometrioma of the Thigh. *Northwest. Med.*, 48: 474, 1949.

Overton, D. H. J., Wilson, R. B., and Dockerty, M. B.: Primary Endometriosis of the Cervix. *Am. J. Obst. & Gynec.*, 79: 768, 1960.

Williams, G. A.: Endometriosis of the Cervix Uteri—A Common Disease. *Am. J. Obst. & Gynec.*, 80: 734, 1960.

Wolfe, S. A., Mackles, A., and Greene, H. J.: Endometriosis of the Cervix. Classification and Analysis of 17 Cases. *Am. J. Obst. & Gynec.*, 81: 111, 1961.

Symptoms

Bayly, M. A., and Gossack, L. L.: External Endometriosis and Abnormal Uterine Bleeding. *Am. J. Obst. & Gynec.*, 72: 147, 1956.

Dailey, H. R., and Tafel, R. E.: Superior Hypogastric Sympathectomy for the Relief of Pain Associated with Endometriosis. *Am. J. Obst. & Gynec.*, 64: 650, 1952.

Fleishman, S. J., and Davidson, J. F.: Vicarious Menstruation. A Likely Case of Pulmonary Endometriosis. *Lancet*, 2: 88, 1959.

Forman, I.: Fever in Endometriosis. *Am. J. Obst. & Gynec.*, 63: 634, 1952.

Green, T. H., Jr., and Meigs, J. V.: Pseudo-menstruation from Post-hysterectomy Vaginal Vault Endometriosis. *Obst. & Gynec.*, 4: 622, 1954.

Kempers, R. D., Dockerty, M. B., Hunt, A. B., and Symmonds, R. E.: Significant Postmenopausal Endometriosis. *Surg., Gynec. & Obst.*, 111: 348, 1960.

Norwood, G. E.: Sterility and Fertility in Women with Pelvic Endometriosis. *Clin. Obst. & Gynec.*, 3: 456, 1960.

Pappas, H. J.: Endometrial Adhesions and Endometriosis. Report of a Case. *Obst. & Gynec.*, 13: 714, 1959.

Roddick, J. W., Jr., Conkey, G., and Jacobs, E. J.: The Hormonal Response of Endometrium in Endometriotic Implants and Its Relationship to Symptomatology. *Am. J. Obst. & Gynec.*, 79: 1173, 1960.

Scott, R. B.: Pelvic Pain in Association with External Endometriosis—Mechanism of Reproduction and Relief and Treatment by Conservative Surgery. *Clin. Obst. & Gynec.*, 2: 1107, 1959.

Stevenson, C. S., and Campbell, C. G.: The Symptoms, Physical Findings and Clinical Diagnosis of Pelvic Endometriosis. *Clin. Obst. & Gynec.*, 3: 441, 1960.

Sturgis, S. H., and Call, B. J.: Endometriosis Peritonei—Relationship of Pain to Functional Activity. *Am. J. Obst. & Gynec.*, 68: 1421, 1954.

Treatment in General

Beacham, C. T.: Changing Concepts in the Treatment of Endometriosis. *J. Michigan M. Soc.*, 59: 164, 1960.

Brewer, J. I., and Mahar, F. M.: Conservatism in Endometriosis. *Am. J. Obst. & Gynec.*, 68: 549, 1954.

Bruser, M.: The Common Occurrence of Endometriosis in Young Women. *Canad. M.A.J.*, 72: 190, 1955.

Greenblatt, R. B., and Suran, R. R.: The Conservative Management of Endometriosis. *S. Clin. North Amer.*, 29: 583, 1949.

Malone, C. M.: Treatment of External Endometriosis. *West. J. Obst. & Gynec.*, 64: 243, 1956.

Meigs, J. V.: Endometriosis: Age of Occurrence, Ovarian Conservation, Atrophy and Growth in the Operative Scar. *New England J. Med.*, 202: 672, 1930.

Randall, C. L.: Management of Complications of Endometriosis. *J.A.M.A.*, 139: 972, 1949.

Medical Treatment

Andrews, M. C.: Medical Treatment of Endometriosis. *Clin. Obst. & Gynec.*, 3: 492, 1960.

Andrews, M. C., Andrews, W. C., and Strauss, A. F.: Effects of Progestin-Induced Pseudopregnancy on Endometriosis: Clinical and Microscopic Studies. *Am. J. Obst. & Gynec.*, 78: 776, 1959.

Dito, W. R., and Batsakis, J. G.: Norethynodrel-Treated Endometriosis—A Morphologic and Histochemical Study. *Obst. & Gynec.*, 18: 1, 1961.

Douglass, C. F., and Weed, J. C.: Endometriosis Treated with Prolonged Administration of Diethylstilbestrol. Report of a Case. *Obst. & Gynec.*, 13: 744, 1959.

Kistner, R. W.: Conservative Treatment of Endometriosis. *Postgrad. Med.*, 24: 505, 1958.

Idem: The Treatment of Endometriosis by Inducing Pseudopregnancy with Ovarian Hormones. A Report of Fifty-Eight Cases. *Fertil. & Steril.*, 10: 539, 1959.

Meigs, J. V.: The Medical Treatment of Endometriosis and the Significance of Endometriosis. *Surg., Gynec. & Obst.*, 89: 317, 1949.

Ober, W. B., Grady, H. G., and Schoenbucher, A. K.: Ectopic Ovarian Decidua without Pregnancy. *Am. J. Path.*, 33: 199, 1957.

Roddick, J. W., Jr., Conkey, G., and Jacobs, E. J.: The Hormonal Response of Endometrium in Endometriotic Implants and Its Relationship to Symptomatology. *Am. J. Obst. & Gynec.*, 79: 1173, 1960.

Scott, R. B., and Wharton, L. R., Jr.: The Effect of Testosterone on Experimental Endometriosis in Rhesus Monkeys. *Am. J. Obst. & Gynec.*, 78: 1020, 1959.

Swyer, G. I.: Effects of Norsteroid Progesterone on the Endometrium. *Proc. Roy. Soc. Med.*, 52: 515, 1959.

Thomas, H. H.: Conservative Treatment of Endometriosis—Use of Long Acting Ovarian Steroid Hormones. *Obst. & Gynec.*, 15: 498, 1960.

Surgical Treatment

Gray, L. A.: Surgical Treatment of Endometriosis. *Clin. Obst. & Gynec.*, 3: 472, 1960.

MacLeod, D.: Endometriosis. A Surgical Problem. *Brit. J. Surg.*, 34: 109, 1946.

Whitehouse, D. B., and Bates, A.: Endometriosis—Results of Conservative Surgery. *J. Obst. & Gynaec. Brit. Emp.*, 62: 378, 1955.

Etiology

Allen, E., Peterson, L. F., and Campbell, Z. B.: Clinical and Experimental Endometriosis. *Am. J. Obst. & Gynec.*, 68: 356, 1954.

Fallas, R. E.: Endometriosis. Demonstration for the Sampson Theory by a Human Anomaly. *Am. J. Obst. & Gynec.*, 72: 557, 1956.

Gardner, G. H., Greene, R. R., and Ranney, B.: The Histogenesis of Endometriosis. *Am. J. Obst. & Gynec.*, 78: 445, 1959.

Markee, J. E.: Menstruation in Experimental Endometrial Implants. *Carnegie Contrib. Embryology*, 28: 223, 1940.

Meigs, J. V.: Endometriosis: Etiologic Role of Marriage, Age and Parity—Conservative Treatment. *Obst. & Gynec.*, 2: 46, 1953.

Mey, R.: Experimental Investigations in Animals on the Pathogenesis of External Endometriosis. *Obst. & Gynec. Surv.*, 15: 120, 1960.

Ridley, J. H., and Edwards, I. K.: Experimental Endometriosis in the Human. *Am. J. Obst. & Gynec.*, 76: 783, 1958.

Sampson, J. A.: Perforating Hemorrhagic (Chocolate) Cysts of the Ovary. Their Importance and Especially Their Relation to Pelvic Adenomas of Endometrial Type (Adenomyoma of the Uterus, Rectovaginal Setpum, Sigmoid, etc.). *Arch. Surg.*, 3: 245, 1921.

Idem: Ovarian Hematomas of Endometrial Type (Perforating Hemorrhagic Cysts of the Ovary) and Implantation Adenomas of Endometrial Type. *Boston M. & S.J.*, 186: 445, 1922.

Schiller, W.: Embryology of the Female Genital Tract; in J. V. Meigs and S. H. Sturgis, eds.: *Progress in G necology.* New York, Grune & Stratton, Inc., 1950.

Scott, ʋR. B.: External Endometriosis; Mechanics of Origin, Theoretical and Experimental. *Clin. Obst. & Gynec.*, 3: 429, 1960.

Scott, R. B., and TeLinde, R. W.: Clinical External Endometriosis; Probable Viability of Menstrually Shed Fragments of Endometrium. *Obst. & Gynec.*, 4: 502, 1954.

TeLinde, R. W., and Scott, R. B.: Experimental Endometriosis. *Am. J. Obst. & Gynec.*, 60: 1147, 1950.

Chapter 48

Carcinoma in Situ of the Cervix

CLINICAL cancer of the cervix most often occurs in women in their forties, but the noninvasive form of cervical carcinoma is most common between thirty and forty years of age.

Carcinoma in situ is the earliest form of cancer arising in the uterine cervix. It is a pathologic entity proved only by microscopic examination of material obtained from (1) biopsy, (2) diagnostic curettage, (3) surgical specimens removed for other causes, or (4) colpomicroscopy. There is nothing characteristic about its appearance on gross examination, and it gives rise to no pathognomonic symptoms. Its presence may be suspected when vaginal smears are studied or special stains are applied by the clinical examiner to the cervical and vaginal epithelium, but the final confirmation awaits histologic examination.

What Do We Mean by Carcinoma in Situ?

To the clinician and the pathologist carcinoma in situ anywhere in the body means that morphologic changes which meet all the criteria of malignancy except the element of invasion are found in the epithelium usually covering a surface. In the cervix carcinoma in situ arises most commonly at the squamocolumnar junction between the stratified exocervical epithelium and the glandular epithelium that lines the endocervical canal and its crypts or ducts. Carcinoma in situ also may arise purely in the squamous epithelium of the exposed exocervix or within the endocervical canal. Involvement, first, of the surface epithelium and, second, of the epithelium lining the glands represents the earliest two stages of developing carcinoma in situ. The first sign of progression of the morphologic epithelial changes toward true clinical carcinoma appears when the stroma is invaded.

It is the local quality of the process that led to a variety of synonyms used interchangeably with carcinoma in situ. The most common are intraepithelial carcinoma, preinvasive cancer, precancerous anaplasia, noninvasive carcinoma, and Bowen's disease of the cervix. Though carcinoma in situ receives the most attention, a few pathologists feel that precancerous anaplasia provides a more accurate biological and morphologic description, since the epithelium is undifferentiated, but will ultimately invade. This is a point of philosophy, since to some a neoplasm is not a cancer unless it invades and kills.

682

Is the Recognition of Carcinoma in Situ a Relatively New Observation?

Though the interest in carcinoma in situ has become intense in recent years, the true significance of the pathologic changes in the cervical epithelium in relation to the subsequent development of cervical cancer has been suspected for many years. In the monograph of Friedell, Hertig and Younge interesting historical data are given. Waldeyer, for example, as early as 1872 recognized that carcinoma of the cervix was epithelial in nature and that different types of carcinoma did arise from many anatomic areas within the cervix. Sir John Williams made intraepithelial cancer the subject of his Harveian Lecture in 1886. It is worth while to record that he noted the following characteristics which we now associate with carcinoma in situ: (1) The process may arise at one or several points within the cervix. (2) It is a superficial growth and may remain so for long periods of time. (3) The spread often occurs to the vaults of the vagina. (4) Its appearance is often innocuous and smooth to palpation. (5) All his patients were married and had had children. (6) There were no symptoms that could be considered pathognomonic.

The foregoing observations are basic and as true today as they were then. No further important contributions were made until 1912, when Schottlaender and Kermauner made the additional discovery that the surface epithelium immediately adjacent to a frankly invasive cervical cancer demonstrated the same cellular changes that were noted in the true carcinoma, with the sole exception that the basement membrane was intact. Controversy today still rages around the question of whether the intraepithelial changes seen around the periphery of an ordinary cervical cancer simply represent spread from the primary tumor, or are actually remains of the initial stages in the development of the advanced cancer.

In recent years, particularly since 1946, when emphasis in the treatment of malignant disease has focused on the detection of cancer in its earliest stages, the role of carcinoma in situ and its relation to the later appearance of cancer within the cervix have come in for much intensive study and discussion.

What Is the Significance of Carcinoma in Situ, and Why Is It Discussed among the Problems Bearing on the Thirty- to Forty-Year Age Group?

We have elected to discuss carcinoma in situ in this age group, for this is the period when the true significance of the epithelial changes becomes of prime importance in relation to therapy. If the pathologic material is thoroughly studied and the findings are those of a true epithelial cancer without invasion, repeated biopsies at spaced intervals may be used as a check on the status of the cervix in younger women who desire children. A number of women may have some deliveries without harm, provided they are carefully studied clinically and systematically re-examined, including the use of repeated vaginal smears and biopsies. A total hysterectomy is indicated and will provide adequate treatment for the woman who has completed her family or is in the forties, when no further children may be either wanted or reasonably expected.

There appears to be a time element in the progression of carcinoma in situ both during the intraepithelial phase and from that to stromal invasion. We recognize either surface epithelial proliferation or surface plus glandular epithelial involvement as comprising the earliest stages of carcinoma in situ. In a recent intensive study of 235 cases of cervical carcinoma in situ from the pathology laboratory of the Free

Hospital for Women the average age for this early stage was thirty-eight years, whereas glandular and early stromal invasion appeared later, at the average age of forty-three years. Other investigators have noted this same time lag.

The latent phase would seem to indicate that the growth pattern of cervical cancer may be relatively slow in its incipient stage. This must be taken into consideration in therapy. Whereas hysterectomy is a satisfactory solution for the woman who has completed her family, it is not a happy one and perhaps may not be a necessity for the patient who wants to have more children or who is married and nulliparous. It is interesting to note that the average age of the married but childless women who had cervical carcinoma in situ was thirty-two years as against a general average age of thirty-eight years.

Since there does appear to be a slow progression to definitive invasive cancer, one may logically consider the possibility of repeated biopsies or local excision of the carcinoma in situ rather than hysterectomy in the thirty-year-old woman who wants to have a child or more children.

The true significance of carcinoma in situ lies in its relation to invasive cancer. When encountered early in its development, carcinoma in situ may be destroyed or eliminated by far less drastic measures than will be necessary for a cure when invasion has taken place. The extent of the prophylactic treatment will depend on the histologic findings in relation to age, parity and the desire of the woman to have children.

What Signs and Symptoms Are Commonly Believed to be Associated with the Finding of Carcinoma in Situ?

SYMPTOMS.   It is customary to consider intermenstrual and postcoital bleeding as suspicious signs of possible cervical cancer. This continues to be true, despite the fact that at most only 33 per cent of women who are found to have carcinoma in situ ever had any abnormal vaginal bleeding or postcoital spotting. In the age group in which cervical carcinoma in situ is most common, namely the thirties, only 25 per cent noted intermenstrual bleeding or spotting as a symptom.

The same may be said of other pelvic complaints in women who also show intraepithelial changes consistent with the diagnosis of carcinoma in situ. The symptoms vary widely in nature and severity. In many instances carcinoma in situ is found incidentally after a hysterectomy for other cause, in some hospitals in about 2 or 3 per cent of such cases. It may be found in biopsy specimens of the cervix taken when the primary complaint is infertility or perhaps a uterine prolapse or a skin rash unrelated to any gynecologic problem. It may be truly stated that there are no pathognomonic symptoms of carcinoma in situ, but one would be remiss if the cause of any intermenstrual or postcoital vaginal spotting were not thoroughly investigated.

SIGNS.   Unfortunately, there is nothing on gross inspection or palpation of the cervix that can truly arouse a definite suspicion of the possible presence of this earliest of malignant changes. We have noted that most of the women have married and had one or more children. Some degree of abnormality in the appearance of the parous cervix may then be expected. Most of the patients with carcinoma in situ (85 per cent) will have some abnormality, either a laceration, eversion of the cervix or cervical erosion. (See Frontispiece.) These are common findings, however, in patients who show, when biopsied, only chronic cervicitis, with a variety of manifestations to indicate nature's attempts to repair the damage.

Approximately 15 per cent of patients with carcinoma in situ will have cervices that appear grossly normal, showing no disturbance of the squamous epithelial covering and feeling smooth to the examining finger. A few will give a history of intermenstrual or postmenstrual vaginal spotting, and the cervix may bleed easily when lightly traumatized, but the majority do not do so. One should be suspicious of the patient who does bleed during the cycle, and attention should focus on the endocervix, which can be neither seen nor palpated. Such a patient should have several biopsies from different areas within the endocervical canal. About 15 per cent of carcinomas in situ arise wholly within the endocervical canal. The vaginal smear will provide the most useful information in the patient who has a normal cervix and no symptoms.

How Is the Diagnosis of Carcinoma in Situ Made?

In the preclinical phase of cancer of the cervix there are no pathognomonic symptoms. The symptomatology attributed to cancer of the cervix applies to the disease in well established, even advanced stages. The diagnosis of carcinoma in situ is made when the index of suspicion is high. Not only are there no specific symptoms, but also there is little in the gross appearance or palpation of the cervix that characterizes the earliest form of cancer. With suspicion aroused, however, there are diagnostic tests which are of the utmost help in establishing a diagnosis. The most important tool is the biopsy, for the final diagnosis must depend on the microscopic picture. There are other tests which are used in conjunction with the biopsy. They will be described in the order in which they should be taken when the possibility of cancer of the cervix comes to mind.

How Valuable Is the Vaginal Smear?   Papanicolaou and Traut have given the medical profession a most useful implement for the early detection of cervical carcinoma. The vaginal smear is by all odds the most effective method of screening for cells that may exfoliate from an area not obvious to inspection and unlikely to be biopsied. Approximately 1 per cent of normal women will have a positive smear, while less than 0.5 per cent will give positive findings on repeated examinations of smears.

The chief value of the vaginal smear is to alert the physician to the possible presence of malignancy. The vaginal smear is but one of a series of tests that must be taken before the diagnosis of cancer can be established. It is axiomatic that a positive smear must be confirmed by histologic review of material obtained by biopsy before definitive therapy is initiated. If the smear continues to be positive in the face of negative pathologic findings from the initial biopsy, the investigation should continue. There is no great need for haste, for cancer at this phase has a leisurely pace, but clinical persistence should take the place of speed of action. It does place the problem squarely in the hands of the examiner, who must make every effort to assure himself that the patient does not have cancer. If there is to be the proper degree of correlation between the findings of the vaginal smear and the cervical biopsy, the physician must provide the pathologist with adequate tissue upon which to base a diagnosis.

The vaginal smear is a basic part of the vaginal examination for the woman of today. There is mounting evidence that the incidence of cervical cancer will be materially reduced by a routine yearly checkup consisting of a vaginal examination and smear in the complete absence of symptoms.

How Do You Take a Vaginal Smear?   The vaginal smear is so widely known through the medium of press and radio that nearly every woman now expects

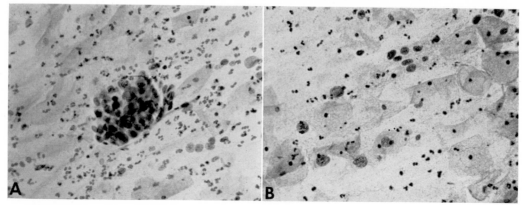

Fig. 48-1. *A*, Malignant tumor cells in a vaginal smear (so-called Class V Papanicolaou smear). *B*, Atypical cells, consistent with tumor cells of carcinoma in situ (Class V or Class IV, depending upon the opinion of the cytologist).

to have a Papanicolaou smear before she considers that an adequate examination has been performed. This test involves a cytologic diagnosis based on the known fact that cancer cells are constantly being shed into the vaginal secretion. The smear may be made in a number of ways.

The simplest and quickest method of collection is to aspirate the secretion pooled in the vaginal fornix with a suction pipet. It has the added advantage that the material in the vaginal pool is an accumulation of exfoliated cells. More painstaking techniques involve scraping the entire circumference of the cervix in the area of the junction of the cervical epithelium and endocervical canal. This is done with the sharp edge of a wooden spatula or tongue depressor.

The smear is useful only to the extent that care has been taken (1) to aspirate sufficient cells for adequate evaluation, (2) to smear them over the slide surface so that the smear is not an opaque mass of piled-up cells, (3) to fix the smear promptly in the proper fluid, since otherwise the cells become so distorted as to be unidentifiable, and (4) to label the specimen correctly before sending it to the laboratory.

Technique of Aspiration from the Vaginal Pool. This is described because of its simplicity and universal applicability. It is the first step to be taken in the vaginal examination of the patient. Lubricant should not be used in the vagina, for it interferes with the proper reading of the smear. The steps are as follows:

1. Using *no* lubricant, the examiner depresses the posterior vaginal wall, separates the labia, and inserts a blunt-end bent glass drinking tube with an Asepto rubber bulb attached to the outer end.
2. The glass tube is introduced upward into the proximal vagina by exerting light pressure on the posterior vaginal wall. The secretions from the vaginal pool are aspirated, and the tube is removed.
3. Squeezing of the bulb deposits the secretions evenly on a frosted-end glass slide marked with a pencil for identification.
4. The slide is immediately immersed in a bottle containing equal parts of 95 per cent ethyl alcohol and ether.
5. The slide is then sent to the laboratory. If it is necessary to send the slide through the mail to a distant laboratory, this may be done by air drying and then adding glycerin lubricant to the slide after it has been fixed and applying another slide over it for protection.

Evaluation of vaginal smears involves special training and knowledge. In some places technicians evaluate or "screen" all smears and mark the unusual or suspicious cells for later scrutiny by the chief cytologist or a pathologist. Elsewhere pathologists may review all the material. Reports may include mention of the presence of estrogen effect, bacteria or fungi, parasites or blood, sperm and leukocytes. Tumor cells may be reported as present or absent, or "suspicious cells" noted, usually with a request for another smear.

Papanicolaou has classed smears as class I, benign; class II, benign with some atypical cells; class III, benign but atypical; class IV, some atypical cells, but not conclusive for cancer; class V, malignant neoplastic cells present (Fig. 48–1, *A*).

The skilled cytologist examining a vaginal smear may find tumor cells in cases of carcinoma in situ that are indistinguishable from the cells of invasive cancer. Nevertheless it is often possible to suspect cervical carcinoma in situ on the basis of finding neoplastic cells with large, rather pale folded or notched nuclei that are not seen in invasive carcinoma (Fig. 48–1, *B*). Thus sometimes it is possible to recognize not only the presence of cancer cells, but also their preinvasive status. In about 70 per cent of carcinoma in situ of the cervix the first vaginal smear is positive for tumor cells.

THE VALUE OF THE SCHILLER TEST. This test with a solution of iodine and potassium iodide that is painted on the cervix is a most useful diagnostic tool, for it aids the gynecologist in his decision as to where to take a cervical biopsy. The test depends upon the amount of glycogen present in the superficial layers of the squamous epithelium that normally covers the external portion of the cervix and the vagina. When glycogen is present, the normal epithelium is stained a deep mahogany color by the iodine, with gradations from brown to light yellow, depending on the amount present. The columnar epithelium of the endocervix will not take the stain. One may of course observe a carcinoma in situ within the canal of a cervix whose external cervical epithelium stains normally. Only a few patients will actually prove to have carcinoma in situ when cervical biopsies are taken from the "Schiller-positive" areas that do not take the stain, but the important fact remains that all areas of carcinoma in situ which involve the external cervix and vagina do fail to take the stain (see Frontispiece).

TECHNIQUE OF APPLYING SCHILLER'S SOLUTION. The cervix and vaginal fornices should be cleared of all mucus and detritus by gentle cleansing of the area with cotton moistened with a mild alkaline solution such as Alkalol. The entire area should then be carefully inspected. This is most important, for the proper interpretation of the test is based on the contrast between the way the epithelium looked before the Schiller's solution was applied and its appearance afterward. It does not depend solely on how the epithelium looks immediately after staining. The Schiller's solution, made up of one part of iodine, 2 parts of potassium iodide and 300 parts of water, is then gently painted over the surface of the cervix and upper part of the vagina with a cotton pledget liberally saturated with the solution.

INTERPRETATION OF THE SCHILLER TEST. The suspicious areas that should be biopsied are those that fail to take the stain. They remain the same color as they were before the stain was applied. Grossly abnormal areas obviously will not take the stain, for the superficial overlying epithelium is either immature, metaplastic, hyperkeratotic, or it has been destroyed. It is well known that ulcerated areas remain red and they will not change when the solution has been applied. Any area immediately adjacent to an ulcer or erosion that appears otherwise normal, but does not stain, is suspected.

It must be kept in mind that a positive Schiller test means only that the area that fails to take the stain is abnormally deficient in the amount of glycogen it contains.

Other pathologic changes than neoplasia may produce the same appearance. The test is good only for those areas of the cervix that can be seen. Consequently a negative test does not rule out cancer, for the true focal area of carcinoma in situ may rest entirely in the endocervix. A positive vaginal smear would mean that the patient had a cervical cancer, in all probability. This is not true of a positive Schiller's test. On the other hand, the smear gives no indication of the location of the carcinoma in situ, while the Schiller test is useful in delineating the area that should be biopsied. When the Schiller test is used in conjunction with the smear, the accuracy runs as high as 80 per cent. Though a few well differentiated invasive carcinomas or cases of carcinoma in situ contain some glycogen, as shown by the periodic-acid-Schiff stains, most patients with carcinoma in situ have Schiller-positive areas on the cervix.

3. How Valuable Is the Biopsy?　A positive vaginal smear and suggestive Schiller test are invaluable diagnostic aids, but they are not positive proof that carcinoma is present in the cervix. Before any definitive therapy is instituted the suspicion of malignancy must be confirmed by tissue biopsy. Only after the pathologist has had an opportunity to review the histologic appearance of the tissue in question can the true diagnosis be established. Biopsy is reliable, provided the examiner takes an adequate amount of tissue from the proper place and keeps in mind the all-important fact that a negative biopsy means only that no cancer was found in the specimen submitted. This points up the necessity of taking more than one biopsy, for a single biopsy is often not enough. It is possible, for example, to have carcinoma in situ in one specimen and invasive cancer in an area immediately adjacent.

How and Where to Take the Cervical Biopsy?　Any suspicious area should be biopsied regardless of its appearance before or after the application of Schiller's solution. Carcinoma in situ is particularly prone to appear in areas where cervical erosions are present. All such eroded areas should be biopsied, for it is impossible to tell from the gross appearance whether carcinoma in situ is present. If the smear is reported as suspicious, yet the cervical epithelium outwardly appears entirely normal, the biopsies should be taken from (a) the border where the normal pink squamous epithelium covering the portio joins the deep red columnar epithelium of the endocervix; (b) the endocervical canal. These are the places where carcinoma is most frequently found. If Schiller's solution has been used, the biopsy should be taken at the junction of normal and abnormal tissue, taking tissue in continuity so that the pathologist can compare the two.

The examiner does not have to be surgically trained to take a biopsy. The procedure is painless and is rarely followed by any troublesome bleeding that cannot be controlled by pressure or the application of a pledget of cellucotton.

There are no contraindications to and no dangers in taking a biopsy. The known fact of pregnancy need not deter one, for nothing untoward will happen. A suspicious lesion in a pregnant cervix is added reason for doing a biopsy, since the epithelium of the cervix in pregnancy is prone to exhibit changes that closely resemble cancer. The interpretation of such biopsies, however, must be evaluated with extreme care, because there are many borderline changes in this type of epithelium. There should be no reluctance in repeating the biopsy if the initial findings are suspicious or inconclusive.

The biopsy may be done in one of two ways: (1) punch biopsy from four quadrants and the endocervical canal; or (2) surgical conization.

Punch Biopsy.　Any suspicious area evident to the naked eye or demarcated by Schiller's solution should be selected as the site. A punch biopsy forceps grasps the area to be excised with a twisting motion. Some experts prefer a square-jawed biopsy punch, since the pieces are easier to orient for microscopic examination. If the cervix is high in the vagina, it may be necessary to grasp it with a tenaculum and steady it as the specimen is taken. Several bites should be taken from four quadrants on the external portion of the cervix and again from the endocervical canal. One may elect to scrape the canal with a curet rather than biopsy it blindly. If the procedure is carried out in this manner, there is little chance that occult cancer will be missed, regardless of whether there are any suspicious areas or not. When clinical leukoplakia is noted close to an area of erosion or near the external os, it is just as important to biopsy the areas adjacent to it as it is to biopsy the leukoplakia itself. The punch biopsy is an office procedure.

Surgical Conization.   When the Papanicolaou smear is positive or repeatedly suspicious, or if the punch biopsy does not clearly indicate whether the patient has a true carcinoma in situ and not an invasive cancer, she should be hospitalized and have a cone of cervical tissue removed under anesthesia. The specimen should include the outer border of any erosion and the full extent of the endocervical canal, not only upward to the internal os, but also laterally into any sulci that may have been caused by lacerations of childbirth. This will provide the pathologist with adequate tissue from all the areas potentially implicated. The cone should not consist of multiple whittled-out tissue fragments that may be impossible to orient properly.

This relatively simple operative procedure oddly enough is a most difficult one to do properly. It should be performed by the more experienced gynecologist and not be delegated to a less well trained subordinate.

Carcinoma in situ grows both laterally and longitudinally, progressively involving the surface epithelium of the external cervix and mucosa of the endocervical canal. It has been known to grow over the epithelium lining the entire endometrial cavity. The upper portion of the vagina may also become involved. From its superficial position within the endocervical canal it may follow down into the crypts and crevices to grow and line the glandlike spaces. Single biopsies often do not give the pathologist a true picture. Multiple biopsies improve the diagnostic accuracy, but material from a well taken surgical cone is most likely to be truly representative.

The tissue should be removed surgically with a knife and not an electric current. There is a great temptation to use diathermy, for the surgical procedure is frequently accompanied by troublesome bleeding. Stitch ligatures placed in the cervical musculature on either side at the level of the internal os will secure the cervical branches of the uterine artery and minimize any blood loss. This is far better than electric conization, since otherwise the coagulated tissue specimen obtained makes it difficult, if not impossible, for the pathologist to interpret the histologic picture.

The biopsy is the all-important factor in making the diagnosis of cancer of the cervix. It is most valuable in the early, unsuspected case. The clinician does not need it in fully developed lesions except to confirm the diagnosis.

4. COLPOMICROSCOPY.   In Vienna for some years observations of the surface of the cervix have been possible with a special microscope, as part of a vaginal examination. The epithelial covering is examined both unstained and stained, at magnifications comparable to those used in interpreting vaginal smears. Ulcers, areas of epithelial hyperplasia and carcinoma in situ are recognizable.

The most experienced European operators carry out therapy without prior biopsy confirmation when the colpomicroscopic findings are characteristic. At present in the United States the instrument has been used mainly as an experimental accessory to diagnosing cervical diseases.

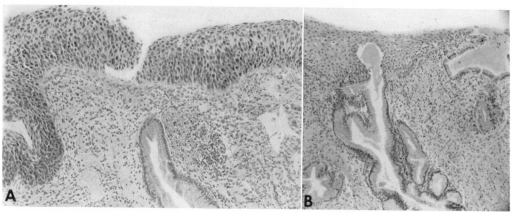

Fig. 48-2.   *A*, Carcinoma in situ of the cervix has full-thickness dedifferentiation of the surface epithelium, with anaplasia and relative increase in nuclear size and chromatin content. *B*, Epidermization overgrows part of the endocervical surface. The surface epithelium is well differentiated, however, and orderly, and the cells are of uniform sizes and staining qualities in each stratum.

WHAT IS THE MICROSCOPIC PICTURE OF CARCINOMA IN SITU?   With some dissenting voices, there is a fairly complete agreement on the histologic criteria for the diagnosis of carcinoma in situ. To be called carcinoma in situ the microscopic picture usually must fill two requirements: (1) It must involve the entire thickness of the squamous epithelium; (2) it must have all the criteria of malignancy, minus evidence of invasion beneath the basement membrane.

WHAT IS THE NORMAL PICTURE OF CERVICAL EPITHELIUM?   The normal cervical epithelium encountered at the squamocolumnar junction on microscopic examination shows a transition of cell types from the base to the surface area. The basal cell layer is usually one cell thick, progressing through parabasal and pre-cornified stages of maturation in the middle zone, where three to ten layers of cells are normally found. The outer zone is made of clear cornified cells rich in glycogen and with pyknotic nuclei. Normally there is no superficial keratinization, though a parakeratotic type of cell that retains its pyknotic nucleus may be found at the surface.

Within each of these zones (*a*) the cells and their nuclei are all similar in size and shape; (*b*) they are all well oriented toward the basement membrane and to each other; (*c*) the mitoses seen are usually found in the basal cell layers, with occasional mitotic figures in the lower precornified cell layer.

WHAT ALTERATIONS IN THE MICROSCOPIC PICTURE ARE SEEN IN CARCINOMA IN SITU?   The histologic pattern is that of carcinoma, with the same cellular changes as are noted in an invasive carcinoma and with the sole difference that extension does not occur into the underlying stroma. The most pronounced and readily recognized difference is the disappearance of the normal stratification pattern. No longer is there an orderly transition or maturation of the cells from base to superficial layer. This is called dedifferentiation and is associated with a loss of individual cellular polarity. The cells one normally expects to find have been replaced by atypical immature cells that vary widely in size and shape. Both the cells and their nuclei are likely to be hyperchromatic, for they absorb more of the hematoxylin stain than normal cells. In general the nuclei are abnormally large in relation to the amount of cytoplasm. Increased numbers of normal or abnormal mitotic figures are seen at all levels in the epithelium. Not infrequently abnormally large and bizarre nuclei are seen (Fig. 48-2, *A*).

The transition between normal and neoplastic epithelium in most instances is abrupt and striking. Once the dividing line was thought to be oblique ("Schiller's oblique line"), but there is now general agreement that the line of demarcation between the two types of epithelium may be either oblique or vertical. Less often there appears to be a gradual transition between an overactive but benign hyperplastic epithelium and its malignant counterpart. This occurs often enough to suggest that the transition zone may be important, since malignant changes appear to arise in these marginal areas of atypical epithelium.

The histology of carcinoma in situ varies widely, and the epithelium may be well or poorly differentiated. Attempts are made to grade carcinoma in situ, but there appears to be little correlated difference in the prognosis, provided the lesion is adequately treated. All variations in growth pattern may appear in the same specimen. The grading may change, depending on where the specimen is taken from. If the biopsy comes from the external cervix at the squamocolumnar junction, more differentiation is often noted than is seen when the specimen is removed from a point higher in the endocervical canal. Since it is not known whether the less differentiated carcinoma in situ has any more rapid rate of growth than the more highly differentiated carcinomatous epithelium, the gradations are at present of more interest to the pathologist than to the clinician.

What Pathologic Conditions Resemble Carcinoma in Situ?

There are certain benign pathologic changes that appear in the cervical epithelium which must be differentiated from true carcinoma in situ to ensure an accurate diagnosis and before proper therapy can be instituted.

EPIDERMIDIZATION.   One of the most common types of epithelial change which on cursory examination might present some of the histologic attributes of carcinoma in situ is *epidermidization.* Here the squamous epithelium grows upward in the healing of a cervical erosion and with more or less success attempts to cover the exposed areas of the endocervix. The exocervical cells as they cover the endocervical surface and the mouths of the glands, however, are mature, retain their polarity and have no tendency to vary in size and shape (Fig. 48–2, *B*).

SQUAMOUS METAPLASIA.   The clinician frequently receives a report of squamous metaplasia after biopsy of the suspicious cervix. In this instance a local proliferation of squamous epithelial cells can be seen either replacing or lying beneath the columnar epithelium of the endocervix or its glands. This gives rise to a characteristic scalloped appearance histologically. In some areas the columnar epithelium is present, but in others, particularly in the later stages, it has completely disappeared. At times the squamous epithelium may appear relatively undifferentiated, and when it involves the glands the distinction between squamous metaplasia and carcinoma in situ, or even invasive carcinoma, sometimes may be difficult (Fig. 48–3, *A*). In most instances the differentiation between squamous metaplasia and carcinoma is easily made, since anaplasia and invasion are lacking. Squamous metaplasia is distinguished from epidermidization because it arises locally, not as part of a sheet of epithelium that grows upward over the endocervical surface.

Neither of these benign conditions appears to have any clear relation to the development of carcinoma. Squamous metaplasia is common in cervical polyps and in pregnancy. In pregnancy it is more often anaplastic and makes for a difficult

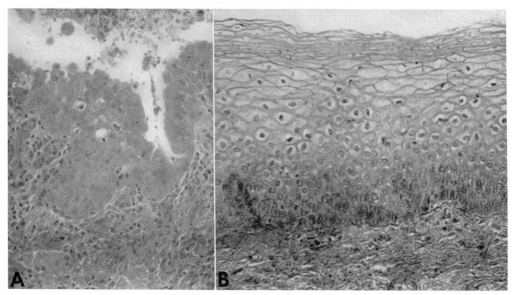

Fig. 48-3.   *A*, Squamous metaplasia is a focal epidermoid alteration of glandular endocervical epithelium, of no known neoplastic significance. *B*, Leukoparakeratosis of the cervix presents as an opaque white and Schiller-positive area because of the superficial, adherent parakeratotic scale.

differential diagnosis. Some pathologists in this situation, when no obvious carcinoma is found, prefer to wait until after delivery, and then ask for another biopsy.

3.   LEUKOPARAKERATOSIS.   These lesions present as whitish plaques on the squamous epithelium covering the external cervix and do not take the Schiller stain, for the cells of the surface layer contain no glycogen. Characteristically, one finds a sharp line of demarcation between the normal epithelium and the stratified layers containing superficially close-packed layers of parakeratotic cells without glycogen. Leukoparakeratosis is an innocent change that helps to explain some Schiller-positive areas (Fig. 48–3, *B*).

4.   LEUKOPLAKIA.   This entity will be discussed in more detail in relation to invasive carcinoma of the cervix (Chap. 61). Histologically and clinically, it somewhat resembles leukoparakeratosis, except that layers of excessive keratinization are superimposed on layers of glycogen-deficient cells like those present in leukoparakeratosis. Sluggish and irregular epithelial maturation is also present. It is possible that the conditions are related and that leukoplakia is a late and more serious stage in the development of dyskeratosis.

5.   BASAL CELL HYPERPLASIA.   It is sometimes difficult to differentiate between basal cell hyperplasia and carcinoma in situ of the cervix. Many instances of intraepithelial cervical cancer appear to represent extreme variations in the degree of hyperplastic activity of the basal or precornified cell layers. It is probably the partly mature cells rather than the basal cells that proliferate, so that this intermediate zone becomes many layers thick and contains a varying number of mitotic figures. The surface stratification remains unchanged, and the fact that some cell maturation does occur superficially is a strong point against the diagnosis of carcinoma.

The degree of proliferation of the partially matured cells has a definite bearing on the percentage chance of the epithelial changes progressing after some time to true carcinoma in situ. A relatively few cases that show precornified cell hyperactivity will regress completely, but in approximately 17 per cent of such cases a carcinoma

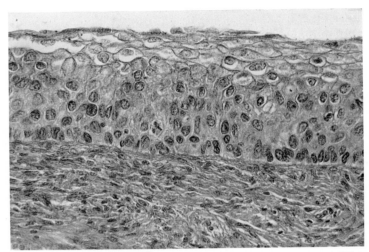

Fig. 48-4. Cervical dyskeratosis with basal cell hyperplasia has some degree of atypicality, nuclear hyperchromatism and enlargement. Cellular maturation, however, occurs in the surface layers, which is not found with carcinoma in situ.

in situ will eventually develop. When the extent of epithelial hyperplasia is excessive, 65 per cent later become carcinoma in situ.

Since there are many histologic patterns of intraepithelial growth that simulate carcinoma in situ to some extent, it is of vital importance that the true diagnosis of carcinoma in situ be established before outlining a plan of therapy. In most instances close scrutiny of the lesions that superficially resemble carcinoma in situ will reveal stratification and cellular maturation to some degree, and here the cells show only minor departures from the normal pattern (Fig. 48–4).

Studies, both published and unpublished, by pathologists and epidemiologists throughout the United States strongly suggest that there has been some tendency to overdiagnose squamous metaplasia and atypical hyperplasia as carcinoma in situ of the cervix, and thereafter to treat these benign conditions as if they were cancer. Such an undesirable practice is best prevented by resorting to consultation with other pathologists known for their interest in this field.

By this means the pathologist who sees perhaps six carcinomas in situ annually profits from the experience of someone who may have seen hundreds of such cases. This is in the interests of improving the care and conservative management of the patient.

Does Carcinoma in Situ Invariably Progress to Invasive Cancer?

Just as there is doubt about the transition from basal cell or precornified cell hyperplasia in the cervical epithelium to the stage of carcinoma in situ, so the direct link between intraepithelial cancer and a finally invasive carcinoma has not yet been established with absolute certainty. On the one hand there is evidence that carcinoma in situ may regress to the normal state spontaneously, particularly in pregnancy. As yet we are unable to determine which cases may revert to normal. In contrast, increasing numbers of recorded instances appear in which proved cases of carcinoma in situ have become invasive cancers. No mass statistics are available to support the contention that untreated carcinoma in situ will inevitably lead to invasive carcinoma

Though the rate of progression from carcinoma in situ to invasive carcinoma apparently is rather slow, it takes courage to allow a carcinoma in situ to go untreated. When this has been done by plan, 4 per cent became invasive carcinoma in one year, 9 per cent in 5 years and 22 per cent in 9 years.

Much of the information available is based on a second retrospective look at the cervical biopsies taken some years before a final diagnosis of invasive cancer was made. A high percentage of these cases reveal previously unrecognized carcinoma in situ in the original specimens. This is suggestive evidence, but one cannot overlook the possibility that the biopsy may have been taken from an area remote from the spot where the final invasive carcinoma appeared, or even that a focus of invasive cancer may have been present at the time the biopsy was taken.

A drawback has been that one cannot both remove a biopsy for diagnosis and leave the epithelium to grow undisturbed. Small carcinomas in situ have apparently occasionally been completely removed and cured by a biopsy, or by cauterization without biopsy confirmation. Now by colpomicroscopy it is said to be possible to recognize carcinoma in situ and other epithelial abnormalities and to follow their growth without the necessity of repeated biopsies. This promises to provide an important new tool for research and the management of cervical lesions.

Since definite proof is lacking that all carcinomas in situ eventually become invasive cancer, and the life history suggests a slow rate of progression that takes approximately ten years when it does occur, there is no overpowering need to initiate immediate therapy. There is ample evidence to support the contention that carcinoma in situ is clinically precancerous, but less that it is a true irreversible cancer from the beginning. When there is doubt about the diagnosis of carcinoma in situ, or if it is diagnosed before invasion has taken place, the gynecologist has ample time to carry out a thorough clinical and pathologic appraisal. We must, as already discussed, first establish that the histologic picture is truly that of carcinoma in situ.

Has Invasion Taken Place?

With the diagnosis firmly established as carcinoma in situ, the next important question is whether it is actually in situ or whether perhaps extension has occurred beyond the basement membrane at any point. The two crucial areas to examine are the surface epithelium and the cervical glands. The question of invasion is vital, for the therapy is entirely different when invasion is present.

With enough material and sufficient study the pathologist can be reasonably certain as to whether stromal invasion has taken place when the superficial epithelium of the external cervix is the only portion involved. The problem becomes more complicated when carcinoma in situ arises within or extends to the endocervix, as it may do with or without implicating the squamous epithelium of the external cervix. Carcinoma in situ may start in or adjacent to either the covering epithelium of the endocervix or the lining of its glands, crypts or ducts. Since the epithelial lining of the ducts is continuous with the surface epithelium, the glands may become involved by direct extension from the surface, and this is a natural route of spread of carcinoma in situ. The ducts of these glands or crypts, as they are now believed to be, have their external openings close together on the surface of the endocervix. In this manner the carcinoma in situ may easily spread to several glands (Fig. 48–5, A).

When extensive glandular involvement has taken place, the columnar epithelium may be destroyed by the carcinoma in situ as it fills the glands. If only single biopsy sections are available for study, it is hard to tell whether the basement membranes around these glands that are partly or completely filled with carcinoma in situ have been disrupted and stromal invasion has taken place. The presence of other glands is often essential for comparison, and multiple biopsies are necessary. For this reason electrocoagulation should be avoided, since it destroys the glands.

There are three fundamental patterns of growth of carcinoma in situ that involves the endocervix: (1) The anaplastic cells tend to proliferate in the zone between the basement membrane and the columnar epithelium. The columnar epithelium is elevated, split off, and one obtains the impression that the malignant cells are growing down into a gland in a sheet. (2) Instead of undermining the columnar epithelium, the malignant epithelium seems to destroy the normal cells as it spreads. (3) If the tumor cells in the superficial epithelium are growing rapidly, they may extend as finger-like processes into the gland lumen rather than down along the gland wall.

The distinction between carcinoma in situ with gland involvement and invasive carcinoma is relatively easy if the carcinoma is minimal or the invasive carcinoma is widely disseminated. It is more difficult when glandular involvement is extensive, and there are no other less affected glands present for comparison. Further complications arise when the pathologic sections are cut tangentially. One then has difficulty in deciding whether the nests of cells seen in stroma are there because it has been invaded, or whether they represent the advancing end of a prong of tumor cells surrounded by an intact basement membrane that appears pushed out into the stroma because of the plane of section.

When there is doubt about the invasion, the pathologist may decide to diagnose "carcinoma in situ with gland involvement and questionable early stromal invasion." The accuracy of diagnosis will depend on the number of sections available for study and the diligence of the pathologist's search. Approximately one third of the specimens believed to have questionable stromal invasion will actually have this proved when multiple serial sections are reviewed.

What Does Early Stromal Invasion Look Like Microscopically?

Evidence of invasion is sought by scrutinizing both the basement membranes and stroma. The most common type of early stromal invasion is from the bottoms of endocervical glands filled with carcinoma in situ, and presents as downgrowths of buds of rather well differentiated malignant squamous epithelium that may retain their intercellular bridges. The next most common type is characterized by prongs of poorly differentiated cells that seem to infiltrate the stroma and have no basement membrane over the advancing tips. The carcinoma cells at this point are poorly defined with indistinct borders, the nuclei are pleomorphic, and the cytoplasm of the cells is scanty as well as amphophilic (Fig. 48–5, B). This is still regarded clinically and prognostically as a League of Nations stage 0 carcinoma.

There are several factors to look for in the stroma. Directly beneath the point where the basement membrane is lost and invasion takes place there is likely a heavy infiltration of lymphocytes and plasma cells in the stroma. This phenomenon is more rarely seen beneath nonmalignant squamous epithelium, but it is commonly present at the site of invasion when cancer arises on a background of atypical epithelial hyperplasia. In addition to the infiltration of plasma cells and lymphocytes, a heavy concentration of neutrophils is sometimes also noted in the stroma. They are present

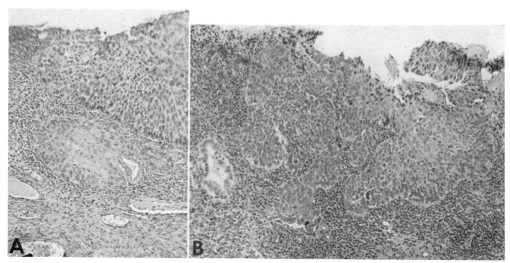

Fig. 48-5.   *A,* Carcinoma in situ involving the surface epithelium and almost all of an underlying endocervical gland. No stromal invasion is evident. *B,* Early stromal invasion involves breaking out into the connective tissue of single or multiple prongs of malignant epithelium. A heavy local leukocytic infiltrate is commonly present.

because of the tumor, not sepsis, in an invaded area. Apparently the presence of neutrophils does not reflect the ability of the stroma to resist invasion.

It is interesting to note that the histologic picture at the point of invasion does not necessarily resemble the pattern of growth observed in the main field of carcinoma in situ.

Treatment of Carcinoma in Situ

It is evident from the preceding discussion that carcinoma in situ may not inevitably progress to invasive cancer. Yet there is too much evidence that it frequently does so to consider the lesion clinically not truly precancerous. If the lesion is not a surgical cancer in this stage, but only precancerous, one might ideally elect to follow up patients with carcinoma in situ and postpone therapy until the lesion gives evidence of invasive malignant change. This presupposes close and continual supervision over many years. Practically we are often forced to make a diagnosis and then to treat the patient. It seems doubtful whether more than a few cases will revert to normality even in pregnancy. The majority will become ordinary cancers of the cervix. It becomes a question of how extensively the lesion should be treated, not whether it should be treated. When a definite diagnosis of carcinoma in situ has been made, it is unwise to postpone all treatment simply because we know that it may take years before the intraepithelial cancer becomes invasive, for we actually do not know how long the lesion has been present in the individual case.

In outlining therapy, two important questions must be answered. We have discussed the more important question of whether invasion has taken place. The next vital question is whether the specimen presented for study is truly representative of the pathologic condition in the cervix. Treatment cannot be outlined on the basis of a single biopsy specimen unless frank invasion is found in it. Evidence of carcinomatous invasion calls for intensive therapy, but carcinoma in situ per se can be adequately treated by far less drastic measures. When doubt exists, multiple biopsies or cold-knife conizations are necessary in order to provide the pathologist with enough material to establish the presence or absence of invasion.

Two pitfalls remain that must be recognized and satisfactory answers obtained before treatment can be instituted: One must be assured (1) that the section under microscopic study has not been taken from the advancing border of an ordinary invasive carcinomatous lesion; (2) that there are no other areas of microscopic invasion anywhere else in the cervix. Carcinoma in situ is frequently present at the periphery of an advanced cancerous lesion of the cervix. The biopsy specimen may show only noninvasive cancer in this section, while invasive carcinoma remains unbiopsied adjacent to it. There is ample evidence to support the contention that carcinoma in situ has multicentric points of origin (Fig. 48–6). The pathologic picture may vary in the different foci.

If the foregoing criteria are satisfied, a workable plan of therapy may be presented:

1. In the young woman who desires to have a family or augment the one she has, if the lesion is truly in situ, the cervix should be treated by surgical conization, removing all the endocervical lining as high up in the cervical canal as the internal os. Great care must be taken to include all the tissue lining the lateral crypts within the canal that may have been formed at the time of a previous delivery. Some recent studies of hysterectomies performed after conization have shown persistent carcinoma in situ in these areas.

This is not an operation to delegate to the less experienced members of the gynecologic staff. In many instances a junior surgeon will do a better hysterectomy than a conization. Cauterization and electrical conization should be avoided when the diagnosis of carcinoma in situ has been established. The heavily coagulated tissue cannot be adequately evaluated by the pathologist. These patients should be followed up at regular intervals for many years to anticipate any further change in the cervical

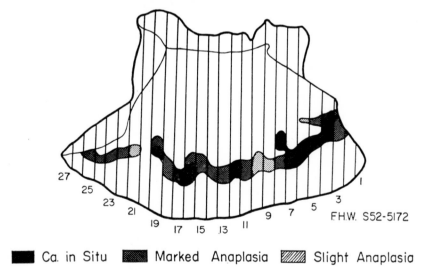

Fig. 48-6. When the entire cervix is blocked and a slide is made at least from each block, areas of carcinoma in situ with varying degrees of extension or invasion may be found, as well as peripheral benign abnormalities. (From Friedell, Hertig and Younge: *Carcinoma in Situ of the Uterine Cervix*, Chas. C Thomas, 1960. Springfield, Illinois.)

epithelium. If close supervision is impossible for any reason, the gynecologist had best recommend hysterectomy, regardless of the status of the family.

2. When the patient has completed her family, has passed beyond the child-bearing age, or has no desire to have children, a total hysterectomy should be done. Since carcinoma in situ may extend from the cervix to involve the vaginal fornix, it is important to remove a sufficiently wide cuff of vaginal epithelium to minimize the risk of recurrence. The ovaries should be left undisturbed, for there is no valid evidence that cervical carcinomas are hormone-dependent. The hysterectomy specimen should be surveyed by enough step sections or serial sections to be sure that no unsuspected area of invasion has been overlooked. Such information is of value only in alerting the surgeon in the follow-up period, for little can or should be done about it unless the carcinoma in situ or invasive cancer encroaches on the line of surgical excision. Watchful expectancy is better than immediate postoperative irradiation.

3. If the patient is pregnant and the lesion is not invasive, she may be allowed to continue with the pregnancy. This is a calculated risk, based on the known fact that many bizarre forms of epithelial response are seen during pregnancy and that some changes regarded as carcinoma in situ seem to revert to normal in the post-partum period. Repeat smears and biopsies should be taken at intervals to anticipate any further change. The obstetrician need have no fear that the course of the pregnancy will be disturbed by the trauma incident to biopsy. The advantages of waiting far outweigh any theoretical disadvantage. The cervix should be re-evaluated in the postpartum period to determine whether the epithelium has reverted to normal or whether intraepithelial cancer remains. If a truly invasive carcinoma is present, treatment adequate for the disease and appropriate for the trimester of pregnancy must be carried out.

REFERENCES

Antoine, T.: Early Diagnosis of Cancer of the Cervix. *Am. J. Obst. & Gynec.*, 68: 466, 1954.

Cullen, T. S.: *Cancer of the Uterus.* New York, D. Appleton & Co., 1900.

Decker, D. G.: Invasive Carcinoma of the Uterine Cervix—General Considerations. *Proc. Staff Meet., Mayo Clin.*, 35: 505, 1960.

Fanger, H., and Murphy, T. H.: Carcinoma in Situ of the Uterine Cervix. *Surg., Gynec. & Obst.*, 111: 177, 1960.

Friedell, G. H., Hertig, A. T., and Younge, P. A.: *Carcinoma in Situ of the Uterine Cervix.* Springfield, Ill., Charles C Thomas, 1960.

Gusberg, S. B.: The Relative Efficiency of Diagnostic Techniques in the Detection of Early Cervical Cancer. A Comparative Study with Survey of 1000 Normal Women. *Am. J. Obst. & Gynec.*, 65: 1073, 1953.

Hamperl, H.: Definition and Classification of the So-Called Carcinoma in Situ; in G. E. W. Wolstenholme and M. O'Connor, eds.: *Cancer of the Cervix.* Ciba Foundation Study Group No. 3. Boston, Little, Brown & Co., 1959, p. 2.

Kaufmann, C., and Ober, K. G.: The Morphological Changes of the Cervix Uteri with Age and Their Significance in the Early Diagnosis of Carcinoma; in G. E. W. Wolstenholme and M. O'Connor, eds.: *Cancer of the Cervix.* Ciba Foundation Study Group No. 3. Boston, Little, Brown & Co., 1959 p. 61.

Kottmeier, H. L., and others: Histopathological Problems Concerning the Early Diagnosis of Carcinoma of the Cervix; in G. E. W. Wolstenholme and M. O'Connor, eds.: *Cancer of the Cervix.* Ciba Foundation Study Group No. 3. Boston, Little, Brown & Co., 1959, p. 20.

Krieger, J. S., and McCormack, L. J.: The Individualization of Therapy for Cervical Carcinoma in Situ. *Surg., Gynec. & Obst.*, 109: 328, 1959.

Morton, D. G.: Carcinoma in Situ of the Uterine Cervix. *Clin. Obst. & Gynec.*, 1: 1003, 1958.

Younge, P. A.: Cancer of the Uterine Cervix. A Preventable Disease. *Obst. & Gynec.*, 10: 469, 1957.

Idem: Problems Concerning the Diagnosis and Treatment of Carcinoma in Situ of the Uterine Cervix. *Am. J. Roentgenol.*, 79: 479, 1958.

Cytologic Diagnosis

Bauer, A. C., Epifanio, A., and Redner, W. J.: Cytology of Vaginal Smears with Trichomonas. *Obst. & Gynec.*, 14: 381, 1959.

Bechtold, E., and Reicher, N. B.: The Relationship of Trichomonas Infestations to False Diagnoses of Squamous Carcinoma of Cervix. *Cancer*, 5: 442, 1952.

Elevitch, F. R., and Brunson, J. G.: Rapid Identification of Malignant Cells in Vaginal Smears by Cytoplasmic Fluorescence. *Surg., Gynec. & Obst.*, 112:3, 1961.

Fennell, R. H., Jr., and Graham, R. M.: Serial Section Study of Cervix in Cases with Positive Vaginal Smears and Negative Biopsies. Report of 10 Cases. *Cancer*, 8: 310, 1955.

Ferguson, J. H., and Lozman, H.: Fate of Women with Positive Cervical Cytology. *South. M. J.*, 51: 296, 1958.

Ferguson, J. H., and Offen, J. A.: Management of Women with Positive Vaginal Cytological Findings. *J.A.M.A.*, 170: 1892, 1959.

Fremont-Smith, M., and Graham, R. M.: Early Diagnosis of Uterine Cancer by Vaginal Smear. *S. Clin. North Amer.*, 27: 1215, 1947.

Fremont-Smith, M., Graham, R. M., and Meigs, J. V.: Vaginal Smears as an Aid in Diagnosis of Early Carcinoma of the Cervix. *New England J. Med.*, 237: 302, 1947.

Graham, R. M.: The Prognosis of Cancer of the Cervix by Vaginal Smear. Correlation with Five Year Results. *Surg., Gynec. & Obst.*, 93: 767, 1951.

Koss, L. G., and Durfee, G. R.: Cytological Changes Preceding Appearance of in Situ Carcinoma of the Uterine Cervix. *Cancer*, 8: 295, 1955.

Liu, W.: Basal Cells in Vaginal Smears of Patients with Carcinoma of the Cervix. *Cancer*, 10: 522, 1957.

MacFarlane, C., Sturgis, M. C., and Fetterman, F. S.: Results of an Experiment in the Control of Cancer of the Female Pelvic Organs and Report of a 15-Year Research. *Am. J. Obst. & Gynec.*, 69: 294, 1955.

MacKenzie, L. L.: The Cytology of Early Squamous-Cell Carcinoma of the Cervix. *Am. J. Obst. & Gynec.*, 69: 629, 1955.

Martin, P. L., Higgins, L. W., Slate, T. A., and DeSanto, D.: Five Year Community Study of Papanicolaou Screening for Cervical Cancer. *West. J. Surg.*, 63: 223, 1955.

Papanicolaou, G. N.: *Atlas of Exfoliative Cytology*. Cambridge, Harvard University Press, 1954.

Papanicolaou, G. N., and Traut, H. F.: The Diagnostic Value of Vaginal Smears in Carcinoma of the Uterus. *Am. J. Obst. & Gynec.*, 42: 193, 1941.

Soule, E. H., and Dahlin, D. C.: Cytodetection of Preclinical Carcinoma of the Cervix. Twelve Years Experience with Initial Screening and Repeat Cervical Smears. *Proc. Staff Meet., Mayo Clin.*, 35: 508, 1960.

Swinton, N. W., and Lehman, G.: The Management of Patients with a Postive Papanicolaou Smear. *S. Clin. North Amer.*, 39: 825, 1959.

Vincent Memorial Laboratory Staff: *The Cytologic Diagnosis of Cancer*. Philadelphia, W. B. Saunders Company, 1950.

Histologic Diagnosis

Ashworth, C. T., Luibel, F. J., and Sanders, E.: Epithelium of Normal Cervix Uteri Studied with Electron Microscopy and Histochemistry. *Am. J. Obst. & Gynec.*, 79: 1149, 1960.

Beacham, C. T.: Quadrant Cervical Biopsy. *S. Clin. North Amer.*, 34: 1653, 1954.

Broders, A. C.: Carcinoma in Situ Contrasted with Benign Penetrating Epithelium. *J.A.M.A.*, 99: 1670, 1932.

Carson, R. P., and Gall, E. A.: Preinvasive Carcinoma and Precancerous Metaplasia of the Cervix. *Am. J. Path.*, 30: 15, 1954.

Carter, B., and others: Clinical Problems in Stage 0 (Intraepithelial) Cancer of the Cervix. *Am. J. Obst. & Gynec.*, 71: 634, 1956.

Christopherson, W. M., and Parker, J. E.: A Critical Study of Cervical Biopsies Including Serial Sectioning. *Cancer*, 14: 213, 1961.

Coppleson, M.: The Value of Colposcopy in the Detection of Preclinical Carcinoma of the Cervix. *J. Obst. & Gynaec. Brit. Emp.*, 67: 11, 1960.

Crossen, R. J.: Wide Conization of Cervix. Follow-up of 1000 Cases, 600 from Two to Fourteen Years. *Am. J. Obst. & Gynec.*, 57: 187, 1949.

De Alvarez, R. R., Figge, D. C., and Brown, D. V.: Long-Range Studies of the Biologic Behavior of the Human Uterine Cervix. II. Histology. Cytology and Clinical Course of Cervical Disease. *Am. J. Obst. & Gynec.*, 74: 769, 1957.

Decker, W. H.: Minimal Invasive Carcinoma of the Cervix with Lymph Node Metastasis. Report of a Case. *Am. J. Obst. & Gynec.*, 72: 1116, 1956.

Fennell, R. H., Jr.: Carcinoma in Situ of the Uterine Cervix. A Report of 118 Cases. *Cancer*, 9: 374, 1956.

Fluhmann, C. F.: Epidermidization of the Cervix Uteri and Its Relation to Malignancy. *Am. J. Obst. & Gynec.*, 15: 1, 1928.

Idem: Carcinoma in Situ and the Transitional Zone of the Cervix Uteri. *Obst. & Gynec.*, 16: 424, 1960.

Foote, F. W., Jr., and Stewart, F. W.: The Anatomical Distribution of Intraepithelial Epidermoid Carcinomas of the Cervix. *Cancer*, 1: 431, 1948.

Foraker, A. G., and Reagan, J. W.: Nuclear Mass and Allied Phenomena in Normal Exocervical Mucosa, Squamous Metaplasia, Atypical Hyperplasia, Intraepithelial Carcinoma and Invasive Squamous Cell Carcinoma of the Uterine Cervix. *Cancer*, 12: 894, 1959.

Friedell, G. H., Hertig, A. T., and Younge, P. A.: The Problem of Early Stromal Invasion in Carcinoma in Situ of the Uterine Cervix. *A.M.A. Arch. Path.*, 66: 494, 1958.

Galvin, G. A., Jones, H. W., and TeLinde, R. W.: The Significance of Basal-Cell Hyperactivity in Cervical Biopsies. *Am. J. Obst. & Gynec.*, 70: 808, 1955.

Gray, L. A., Barnes, M. L., and Lee, J. J.: Carcinoma in Situ and Dysplasia of the Cervix. *Ann. Surg.*, 151: 951, 1960.

Greene, R. R., and others: Preinvasive Carcinoma of the Cervix during Pregnancy. *Surg., Gynec. & Obst.*, 96: 71, 1953.

Gross, S. J., and Danziger, S.: Histochemical Techniques Applied to the Study of Benign and Malignant Squamous Epithelium of the Cervix Uteri. *Am. J. Obst. & Gynec.*, 73: 94, 1957.

Gross, S. J., and Kinzie, G.: Cytochemistry of Benign and Malignant Squamous Epithelium of the Cervix Uteri. *Obst. & Gynec.*, 15: 261, 1960.

Gusberg, S. G., and Moore, D. B.: The Clinical Pattern of Intraepithelial Cancer of the Cervix and Its Pathologic Background. *Obst. & Gynec.*, 2: 1, 1953.

Hahn, G. A.: Carcinoma in Situ. Errors in Interpretation. *S. Clin. North Amer.*, 34: 1657, 1954.

Hopman, B. C.: Histochemical Methods Applied to Benign and Malignant Squamous Epithelium of the Cervix Uteri. *Am. J. Obst. & Gynec.*, 79: 346, 1960.

Howard, L., Jr., Erickson, C. C., and Stoddard, L. D.: A Study of the Incidence and Histogenesis of Endocervical Metaplasia and Intraepithelial Carcinoma. *Cancer*, 4: 1210, 1951.

Huey, T. W., Jr., Large, H. L., Jr., and Kimmelstiel, P.: Preinvasive Carcinoma of the Cervix: Correlation of Findings in Biopsy and Hysterectomy Specimens. *Am. J. Obst. & Gynec.*, 68: 761, 1954.

Jones, H. W., Jr., Calvin, G. A., and TeLinde, R. W.: Re-examination of Biopsies Taken Prior to the Development of Invasive Carcinoma of the Cervix; in *Proceedings of Third National Cancer Conference.* Philadelphia, J. B. Lippincott Company, 1957, pp. 678-81.

Kaufman, W., Adham, M., and Tardif, L.: An Evaluation of Colpomicroscopy in the Diagnosis of Carcinoma in Situ of the Cervix. *Surg., Gynec. & Obst.*, 114: 261, 1962.

Koss, L. G., and Wolinska, W. H.: Trichomonas Vaginalis Cervicitis and Its Relationship to Cervical Cancer. A Histocytological Study. *Cancer*, 12: 1171, 1959.

Kottmeier, H. L.: *Carcinoma of the Female Genitalia.* Baltimore, Williams & Wilkins Company, 1953.

Lamb, E. J., Fucilla, I., and Greene, R. R.: Basement Membranes in the Female Genital Tract. *Am. J. Obst. & Gynec.*, 79: 79, 1960.

Lombard, H. L., and Potter, E. A.: Epidemiological Aspects of Cancer of the Cervix; Hereditary and Environmental Factors. *Cancer*, 3: 960, 1950.

McKay, D. G., Terjanian, B., Poschyachinda, D., Younge, P. A., and Hertig, A. T.: Clinical and Pathologic Significance of Anaplasia (Atypical Hyperplasia) of the Cervix Uteri. *Obst. & Gynec.*, 13: 2, 1959.

Martzloff, K. H.: Carcinoma of the Cervix Uteri. A Very Early Case. *Bull. Johns Hopkins Hosp.*, 33: 221, 1922.

Meyer, R.: The Basis of the Histological Diagnosis of Carcinoma, with Special Reference to Carcinoma of the Cervix and Similar Lesions. *Surg., Gynec. & Obst.*, 73: 14, 1941.

Idem: The Histological Diagnosis of Early Cervical Carcinoma. *Surg., Gynec. & Obst.*, 73: 129, 1941.

Nolan, J. F.: Response of Carcinoma in Situ of the Cervix to Radiation Therapy. *Am. J. Obst. & Gynec.*, 79: 914, 1960.

Novak, E.: Pseudomalignant and Precancerous Lesions of the Cervix. *J.A.M.A.*, 108, 1145, 1937.

Peightal, T. C., Brandes, W. W., Crawford, D. B., Jr., and Dakin, E. S.: Conservative Treatment of Carcinoma in Situ of Cervix. A Clinical Cytopathological Study. *Am. J. Obst. & Gynec.*, 69: 547, 1955.

Pemberton, F. A., and Smith, G. V.: The Early Diagnosis and Prevention of Carcinoma of the Cervix. A Clinical Pathological Study of Borderline Cases and Treatment at the Free Hospital for Women. *Am. J. Obst. & Gynec.*, 17: 165, 1929.

Petersen, O.: Precancerous Changes of the Cervical Epithelium in Relation to Manifest Cervical Carcinoma. *Acta radiol.* (supp. 127), 1, 1955.

Idem: Spontaneous Course of Cervical Precancerous Conditions. *Am. J. Obst. & Gynec.*, 72: 1063, 1956.

Reagan, J. W., and Hamonic, M. J.: The Cellular Pathology in Carcinoma in Situ. A Cytohistopathological Correlation. *Cancer*, 9: 385, 1956.

Riva, H. L., Hefner, J. D., and Kawasaki, D. M.: Carcinoma in Situ of the Cervix: A Review of 156 Cases. *Obst. & Gynec.*, 17: 525, 1961.

Schiller, W.: Early Diagnosis of Carcinoma of the Cervix. *Surg., Gynec. & Obst.*, 56: 210, 1933.

Schiller, W., Daro, A. F., Gollin, H. A., and Primiano, N. P.: Small Preulcerative Invasive Carcinoma of the Cervix: The Spray Carcinoma. *Am. J. Obst. & Gynec.*, 65: 1088, 1953.

Schottlaender, J., and Kermauner, F.: *Zur Kenntnis des Uteruskarzinoms*. Berlin, Verlag von S. Karger, 1912.

Stoddard, L. D.: The Problem of Carcinoma in Situ with Reference to the Human Cervix Uteri; in J. F. A. McManus, ed.: *Progress in Fundamental Medicine*. Philadelphia, Lea & Febiger, 1952.

Studdiford, W. E., and Decker, W. H.: The Role of Cervical Biopsy in the Detection and Evaluation of Early Carcinoma of the Cervix. *Am. J. Surg.*, 87: 268, 1954.

Takeuchi, A., and McKay, D. G.: The Area of the Cervix Involved by Carcinoma in Situ and Anaplasia (Atypical Hyperplasia). *Obst. & Gynec.*, 15: 134, 1960.

TeLinde, R. W., Galvin, G. A., and Jones, H. W., Jr.: Therapy of Carcinoma in Situ. *Am. J. Obst. & Gynec.*, 74: 792, 1957.

Wheeler, J. D., and Hertig, A. T.: The Pathologic Anatomy of Carcinoma of the Uterus. I. Squamous Carcinoma of the Cervix. *Am. J. Clin. Path.*, 25: 345, 1955.

Younge, P. A., Hertig, A. T., and Armstrong, D.: A Study of 135 Cases of Carcinoma in Situ of the Cervix at the Free Hospital for Women. *Am. J. Obst. & Gynec.*, 58: 867, 1949.

Chapter 49

Fibromyomata of the Uterus
(Uterine Fibroids—
Leiomyomata Uteri)

THESE benign tumors represent the most common form of uterine growths that appear in women. They vary widely in size, shape and point of origin within the uterus. Their actual incidence is difficult to establish, for many tumors are either too small or inaccessibly placed to be palpated. It has been said that one out of five women over the age of thirty years will have fibroids.

There appears to be a definite age incidence, for leiomyomata are not found before the onset of puberty and rarely exhibit growth activity after the menopause. The fibroid thus makes its appearance within the reproductive age of the woman. For this reason the etiology of leiomyomatous fibroid tumors has been linked to estrin stimulation, though the exact cause is unknown. The highest incidence is noted in the middle and in the latter half of the menstrual life. In the Negress, who seems to be peculiarly susceptible to fibroid tumors, the peak incidence occurs earlier.

Where Do the Tumors Arise?

The fibroid is a solid encapsulated tumor growing in the muscular walls of the uterus, usually in the fundal portion and rarely in the cervix. The presence of a capsule sharply demarcates the growth from the surrounding myometrial musculature. The primary point of origin is within the muscle wall itself, where a small interstitial smooth muscle growth appears. The tumors may be single or multiple. As long as they are confined to the wall they are called *intramural* fibroids. The great majority of fibroid tumors are of this type.

From this site the leiomyomatous tumors may expand, pushing muscle aside in the direction either of the peritoneal covering of the uterus, where they become *subserous* or *subperitoneal* fibroids, or they may encroach on the endometrial cavity, growing beneath the epithelium as *submucous* fibroids. These last are much less common than the others (Fig. 49–1, *A*).

1) Intramural
2) Subserous
3) Submucous

702

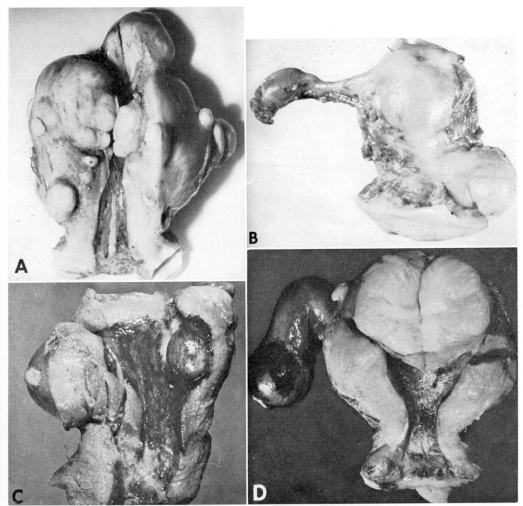

Fig. 49-1. *A*, Multiple uterine leiomyomata of various sizes protrude from the cut surfaces of the myometrium. In this uterus some of the fibroids are subserous, others intramural or submucous. *B*, Cervical fibroid tumor, already illustrated as a cause of difficult delivery. *C*, To the right is a subserous leiomyoma bulging into and distending the endometrial cavity. *D*, A fibroid tumor of the uterine fundus is protruding from the cut surface in the characteristic way. It also has the typical white, whorled appearance of leiomyomata. A pyosalpinx is present.

How Do They Continue to Grow?

INTRAMURAL FIBROIDS. Multiple small smooth-muscle tumors are usually found scattered throughout the walls of the uterine fundus. The uterus is usually symmetrically enlarged, sometimes more through hypertrophy of the surrounding musculature than the presence of tumors. If the tumors within the uterus grow to any size, there may be disturbances in the general contour, and the endometrial cavity becomes deep and sometimes distorted. Not infrequently there is a large solitary fibroid that completely occupies the anterior or posterior wall. The intramural fibroid, because of its location within the muscular wall, keeps its capsule intact. Since the blood supply lies within the capsule, nourishment is usually adequate, and the tumors rarely become cystic or calcify. Red degeneration, however, does occur in intramural fibroids, frequently during pregnancy, and at other times as well.

If the tumor grows in the direction of the peritoneal surface, the restricting myometrial cover thins out. Continued growth causes the fibroid to project beyond the normal contour of the uterus into the peritoneal cavity. It may progress to considerable size. Frequently multiple protruding tumors are present in varying stages of development. Because of their tendency to expand beyond the muscle wall, the actual size of the main body of the uterus is not disturbed. The subserous fibroids appear to grow as excrescences upon it. The tumor is covered with peritoneum, but as growth continues, the only connection with the uterus may be a peritoneum-covered pedicle or stalk within which lies the only blood supply to the tumor. This is the so-called *pedunculated* fibroid.

Because of the mobility provided by the pedicle the tumor may rise into the abdominal cavity or fall down behind the uterus into the cul-de-sac. The pedicle may be broadened, and the blood supply to the fibroid remains adequate for continued growth. The stalk, on the other hand, may become thin and attenuated. The weight of the tumor supported by a thin base makes such a fibroid easily subject to torsion or twist. Inadequate blood supply produces necrosis within the tumor. Usually the subserous tumors are free of any peritoneal attachments. With the inflammatory change that follows necrosis the omentum may attempt to wall off the tumor. In rare instances the blood supply from the uterine side is lost, and the tumor is forced to subsist on whatever nourishment it can pick up from the omentum. Such leiomyomata are called *parasitic* fibroids.

Depending upon the location of the primary site within the uterus, its continued growth may force the tumor out into the space between the leaves of the broad ligament. Such fibroids are called "*interligamentary* or *broad ligament*" tumors. In this instance there is no potential covering of its own. Uncontrolled lateral expansion causes the leaves of the broad ligament to distend so that the tumor dissects upward beneath the peritoneal surface as a "*retroperitoneal fibroid*." The cecum or sigmoid, depending upon the side from which the tumor arose, may be found stretched across the top of the fibroid together with the tube and ovary. If the fibroid has its primary origin in the lower uterine segment, lateral expansion may produce compression of one or both ureters or displace the bladder upward. Disturbances in urinary function may follow pressure on either the urethra in the midline or the ureter laterally. This is one pattern of growth that one finds from a "*cervical fibroid*."

In addition to the lateral extension of the cervical fibroid, tumors of this site of origin sometimes remain confined to the cervical musculature as small intramural growths. The musculature becomes stretched out over the tumor, which pushes up into the uterine cavity, thereby elongating the cervix and distorting the canal. Rarely the tumor becomes pedunculated and extends into the vagina on a thin stalk. Unlike the fibroid tumors of fundal origin, the cervical fibroid is both a solitary tumor and a relatively rare one (Fig. 49–1, *B*).

From its interstitial origin the fibroid exerts its growth potential less frequently in the direction of the endometrial cavity. The submucous fibroid then develops. Usually these are single smooth-muscle tumors that occupy the entire uterine cavity, which becomes increasingly distended as growth progresses (Fig. 49–1, *C*). The uterus enlarges symmetrically, however, and the tumors cannot be palpated. Less commonly there may be smaller pedunculated tumors that take the form of fibroid polyps.

Unlike with the intramural or subserous fibroids, the uterus does not tolerate the submucous fibroid well. These tumors seem to act like foreign bodies which the uterus tries to expel with each menstrual period. Severe dysmenorrhea continuing through the entire bleeding period is common to the patient with a submucous fibroid.

As a result of the growth pattern and the continued uterine contractions these tumors tend to become globular and pedunculated. They often take the shape of a bell clapper, fill the uterus, dilate the cervix and present in the vagina. Ordinarily they have a broad fibromuscular base, actually the former capsule of the tumor. The blood supply to these tumors comes from both the stalk and the endometrium spread over the surface. Since the endometrium becomes flattened out over the tumor or is absent in some areas as the growth progresses, the blood supply from this source often fails adequately to supplant that from the pedicle, which is poor at best. The distal portion of the submucous fibroid tends to become necrotic, particularly when it presents through the cervix and is subjected to frictional trauma.

In addition to the element of hemorrhage from necrosis, submucous fibroids tend to produce excessive menstrual flow of the gushing type, probably because of the distortion of the endometrial mucosal pattern and the inability of the uterus to contract because of the tumor. The fibroid polyp has similar characteristics and is subject to the same influences as the submucous fibroid. The stalk is longer and contains less blood supply. Not infrequently it prolapses through the cervix and presents at the introitus. Because of its exposed position and scanty blood supply, the fibroid polyp readily bleeds and becomes infected after trauma. Since the cervix has become dilated by the descent of the polyp, it is often possible to secure and clamp its base. Because the blood supply is limited, the polyp can be removed without danger of hemorrhage.

What Does a Fibroid Feel and Look Like?

Normally the fibroid tumor is made up of a mass of interlacing smooth-muscle fibers within a connective tissue framework. It is primarily a myoma and not a fibroma. The more fibrous connective tissue that is present, the firmer and harder the tumor becomes. It makes some difference where the tumor arises. The submucous and intramural fibroids contain more muscle than fibrous tissue, while the subserous tumors show the reverse picture.

The uncomplicated uterine fibroid varies widely in its consistency. Usually it is solid and unyielding. Some tumors are stony hard. When fully developed, they are surrounded by a well formed capsule, which is highly vascular and carries the blood supply of the fibroid. There is a sharp line of demarcation between the tumor and the surrounding myometrium. This fact distinguishes the fibroid from adenomyosis, which also arises within the uterine muscle wall, but tends to involve it diffusely. The presence of the capsule allows the tumor to be shelled out of its encapsulating muscle bed.

Once the leiomyomatous tumor is removed, transection of the fibroid presents a characteristic picture. One is immediately impressed with the manner in which the tumor pops out as the edges of the severed capsule retract. The cross section shows a shiny, glistening white surface, with the tissue arranged in whorls resembling a sample of watered silk. The color varies, depending on the blood supply and the amount of fibrous tissue it contains. The more fat content, the more yellow the surface of the tumor. The contrast with the reddish myometrial fibers of the uterus is striking (Fig. 49–1, *D*).

The microscopic picture adds little, for the same interlacing smooth-muscle bundles mixed with connective tissue strands are evident. The smaller tumors have less connective tissue and are relatively pure leiomyomata. These are more cellular, and the smallest are called "seed leiomyomata." For the most part this tumor has few blood vessels. The softer the tumor and the greater the muscle cell component, the more vascular it becomes. The capsule shows the same interwoven arrangement of muscle and fibrous tissue, both adjacent to the tumor and on the periphery. Between the two layers lie the vessels that make up the blood and lymph supply of the tumor.

NOTE The fact that the blood supply to the tumor is peripherally placed is of great importance. As the tumor enlarges or becomes more pedunculated, the central portion receives less and less nourishment. It is not surprising that degenerative changes take place. This is why there is no characteristic feel to all fibroids. Many will be stony hard, but others will develop soft spots and feel spongy and cystic. It is difficult to find a fibroid that does not show some element of degeneration. This varies from spotty hyalinized areas within the tumor to a complete cystic change. Clinically, one may have difficulty in distinguishing a soft fibroid made up of myomatous elements from a fibroid that has undergone complete disintegration.

NOTE SECONDARY CHANGES IN THE FIBROID.   Elements of degeneration are so common in all but the smallest leiomyoma that such findings may be regarded as the rule, not the exception. They may be secondary to circulatory change, infection or regression. The fibrosis that develops in all the larger tumors, with fibroblastic overgrowth of the smooth-muscle cells, may indeed also be regarded as a degenerative alteration.

(1) HYALINE DEGENERATION.   This is the most common change found in a fibroid of any size. The degree of hyaline degeneration has a direct relation to the decreased amount of blood supply within the tumor. It is greatest in pedunculated tumors, when the growth pattern has restricted the amount of blood reaching the tumor.

The process usually begins in a small area among the collagen fibrils of the connective tissue surrounding the muscle bundles. The connective tissue is replaced by a mass of acellular hyaline material that presses on the muscle cells and gradually destroys them. Grossly, the hyalinized areas have a dull "boiled" appearance that corresponds to the acidophilic acellular glassy foci seen microscopically. Here the muscle cells and fibrous tissue have lost their fibrillar nature, probably owing to hydrolytic changes (Fig. 49–2).

(2) CYSTIC DEGENERATION.   The result of extensive hyaline degeneration is more or less massive liquefaction. This may occur uniformly throughout the tumor or as multiple small cystic regions separated from one another by connective tissue trabeculae. The color of the fluid content varies with the constituents that go to make it up. Because of the impaired blood supply, elements may be present that change the straw-colored fluid commonly found to dark brown. No mucin is present, and these cysts are not true cysts, but the end-result of liquefaction necrosis following the hyaline change.

(3) RED DEGENERATION.   This may occur in any type of fibroid, but it is chiefly encountered in the larger, single intramural tumors. It seems to be related to acute alterations in the blood supply and is common in pregnancy, though it may occur in its absence and has even been reported in nulliparous patients.

The clinical onset is ushered in by sudden pain and tenderness in the region of the tumor, accompanied by a temperature elevation. The fibroid is soft. The degeneration is a rapidly developing form of necrosis. On cut section the tumor may be malodorous and give the impression of raw beefsteak. The fishy odor is due to decomposition products. Dilated and thrombosed veins appear in the capsule and within the tumor. The red color is of no prognostic significance and probably reflects hemolysis. This is thought to be due to the reaction of blood leakage to lipoid substances that are always present (Fig. 49–3, *A*).

This red degeneration is called a *necrobiosis*, for the destruction of tissue may be partial, and occasionally a fibroid so affected may retrieve its vitality.

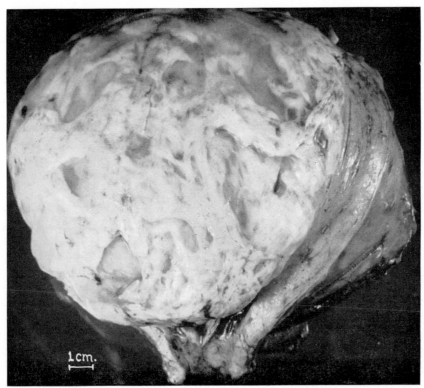

Fig. 49-2.   Hyaline and cystic degeneration of a large fibroid is characterized by a dull shiny appearance of the cut tumor. Multiple foci of liquefactive degeneration account for the cystic change.

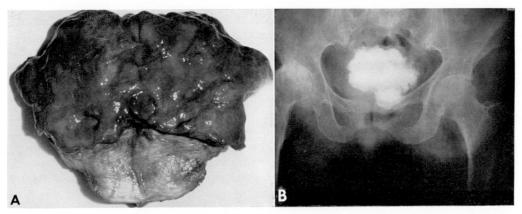

Fig. 49-3.   *A,* Red degeneration with liquefactive alterations may involve infarctive necrotizing degeneration of a fibroid tumor, illustrated here in a severe form. *B,* A calcified pelvic mass shown by x-ray study proved to be a large, completely calcified uterine fibroid.

(4) NECROSIS.   Elements of total tissue destruction within a tumor may follow interference with its blood supply. This may appear in the central portion of a large tumor. It is common in pedunculated tumors arising in subserous locations or within the uterine cavity. Torsion of the tumor pedicle and infection play definite roles. The necrotic portions of the tumor usually appear as dark hemorrhagic areas, often sharply demarcated from the surrounding viable tissue. At times, depending on the degree of vascular impairment, the regions may blend into one another.

(5) FATTY DEGENERATION.   This is a true degenerative process. It usually appears about the time of the menopause. The cut surface shows a homogenous surface without the characteristic whorl-like arrangement of the muscle fibers. The muscle fibers are replaced by small fat droplets. This gives the surface a pale yellow color. Its chief point of importance is that it invariably presages both necrosis and calcification.

(6) DEGENERATION WITH CALCIFICATION.   After fatty degeneration or necrosis, lime salts are deposited in the fibroid tumors of some elderly patients. The fat breaks down into glycerin and fatty acids, which in turn unite with the calcium in the blood to form insoluble calcium soaps. These are further transformed into calcium carbonates and phosphates. The process may take place around the periphery of the tumor, in which case an outer shell of calcium is noted on x-ray, or the entire tumor may become calcified (Fig. 49–3, *B*).

(7) CHANGES DUE TO INFECTION.   The fibroid tumor may be involved by way of the endometrium, by infectious processes adjacent to the tumor, or via the blood stream. Rarely does suppuration occur within a large fibroid tumor, but it may become involved when implicated in a generalized pelvic infection, such as a pelvic inflammation secondary to gonorrhea or septic abortion. In this case the infection probably spreads by lymphatic channels from both the endometrial cavity and the tube. When infection does attack the tumor, the resultant swelling further impairs its blood supply, thereby aggravating the degree of necrosis.

Sloughing of a pedunculated submucous fibroid is a fairly common finding. If the protective capsule has been penetrated, infection enters the degenerating tumor with further loss of its blood supply. The entire tumor may become detached and disappear. This process is often accompanied by a temperature elevation and frequently by a profuse bleeding episode approaching vaginal hemorrhage. Occasionally the pedunculated subserous fibroid may slough, separate and become parasitic as the omentum seeks to protect it.

(8) FIBROIDS WITH ADHESIONS.   Unless the fibroid tumor becomes involved in other extragenital pathologic processes, adhesions are not often found with intraperitoneal fibroid tumors. Pelvic inflammation, postpuerperal infection or endometriosis may produce adhesions in a patient who also has fibroids, but rarely is the fibroid alone responsible.

Symptoms Associated with Uterine Fibroids

There are no pathognomonic symptoms of leiomyomata of the uterus. A patient may have a uterus with a single small or multiple fibroid tumors without symptoms of any sort. She may also have a fairly large tumor without being aware of it. Many such fibroids are discovered only when routine vaginal examination is performed as part of a general checkup. Eventually the average fibroid gives rise to symptoms of some sort, though it may previously have been dormant for a number of years.

The symptoms commonly associated with fibroids within the uterus are (1)

NOTE

vaginal bleeding, (2) discharge, (3) localized abdominal pain, (4) pressure symptoms, and (5) the presence of a palpable abdominal mass or abdominal enlargement. The symptoms, either singly or in combination, will depend on the life history of that particular tumor, with additional complaints based on the associated pathologic state.

For example, consider what may happen to the two types of fibroid that may become pedunculated (the location of the tumor may be more important than the size): (a) The *submucous fibroid* may outrun its blood supply, become necrotic and produce either a foul bloody vaginal discharge or active gushing hemorrhage. Nature's attempt to extrude the foreign body produces a cramplike uterine pain as the cervical os tries to dilate. (b) The *subserous fibroid*, on the other hand, may twist on its pedicle, thereby shutting off its blood supply and producing necrosis. The pain is colicky, typical of torsion of any intra-abdominal viscus or tumor. Bleeding and vaginal discharge are not part of the symptoms, as they were in the submucous variety.

In addition, fibroids may be associated with cancer of the cervix, endometrium or ovary, pregnancy either in or outside the uterus, pelvic inflammation, endometriosis or benign adnexal abnormalities such as an ovarian cyst. The protean nature of the symptom complex associated with the fibroid uterus becomes evident.

VAGINAL BLEEDING. This is the most common symptom attributed to the *NOTE* fibroid uterus. The menstrual cycle is rarely disturbed, though the duration of the period may be prolonged and the interval shortened. Intermenstrual bleeding is rare and cannot be attributed to the presence of the leiomyomatous tumor. The nature and amount of the bleeding depend more on the location of the fibroid than its size. A small submucous fibroid may bleed excessively, while an intramural fibroid of greater size may produce no disturbance in the menstrual pattern.

Why Does the Fibroid Uterus Bleed? The submucous fibroid, or fibroid polyp, bleeds because of the presence and anatomic location of the tumor. The remainder of fibroids do not. This is an important observation, for many of the pitfalls of therapy for uterine bleeding stem from the misconception that the presence of a palpable fibroid is an adequate explanation of an abnormal vaginal bleeding pattern.

Mechanism of Vaginal Bleeding in the Common Types of Uterine Fibroid. The intramural, subserous, interligamentary, cervical or retroperitoneal leiomyomata may not be associated with vaginal bleeding at all. When patients with them do bleed, which usually happens, they bleed because of ovarian dysfunction. The ovaries in such patients may contain follicular cysts, but no active corpora lutea. The continued estrin stimulation, unopposed by progestin, produces a proliferative or later a hyperplastic endometrium. The bleeding is therefore anovulatory. This explains the shortened interval between periods, the rare instances of intermenstrual bleeding and the prolonged flow commonly seen.

The finding of a uterine fibroid on physical examination is an associated ob- *NOTE* servation, not an explanation of the vaginal bleeding. In all probability the cause of the bleeding is functional, but an organic cause such as cancer or pregnancy must first be ruled out.

Mechanism of Vaginal Bleeding in the Submucous Fibroid. When the tumor arises close to the endometrial cavity primarily or encroaches on it through growth from the initial point of origin within the uterine musculature, excessive bleeding may occur. Because of the tumor's location, the endometrium becomes thinned out over its surface. In addition, the tumor interferes with normal contraction of the uterine muscle, which ordinarily aids in the arrest of blood loss at the time of menstruation. Thus one may have an abnormal amount of bleeding from a small submucous fibroid or fibroid polyp. Since such fibroids are prone to become necrotic, additional causes for hemorrhagic incidents are present.

How Does the Type of Fibroid Influence the Bleeding?   The amount of blood lost at the menstrual period will depend on the location of the fibroid. If it is submucosal in location or becomes submucosal through growth, the amount of blood loss likely is excessive. The "flooding" episodes which often occur with embarrassing and unheralded suddenness can usually be attributed to submucosal fibroids. The flow tends to come in gushes, and the patient frequently prefers not to leave the house because of the possibility of hemorrhagic accidents. The hemoglobin may drop to 5 or 6 gm. per 100 ml. This type of vaginal bleeding is also common to the patient who has symptoms of hypothyroidism. Since the submucous fibroid usually cannot be felt, thyroid dysfunction must first be ruled out. Fatal hemorrhage is almost unknown, but the patient may be severely depleted.

Bleeding from functional cause in a patient with a fibroid uterus rarely approaches the magnitude of the loss commonly encountered in the submucous fibroid. It is a progressive depletion of moderate severity operating over a succession of menstrual cycles. Chronic secondary anemia is a common sequel. The patient feels dragged out and listless after the menstrual period and barely recovers before the onset of the next period. Increasing nervousness and faulty digestion and elimination are parts of the train of symptoms that appear secondary to regularly recurring episodes of moderate blood loss.

VAGINAL DISCHARGE.   There are many explanations for the presence of vaginal discharge. Though patients with leiomyomata often complain of leukorrhea, the symptom is in no sense pathognomonic. Pelvic congestion and proliferation of the endometrial lining are the basic causes. Usually the discharge is mucoid. With degeneration of a submucous fibroid the discharge becomes mucopurulent and frequently blood-tinged. Necrosis and infection in a sloughing submucous or intramural fibroid change the nature of the vaginal discharge to the thin, watery, brownish, malodorous variety.

PAIN.   The uncomplicated fibroid does not produce pain. When the patient with a leiomyoma complains of pelvic pain, one of three factors is usually present: (1) Primarily one suspects that something has happened to the tumor itself. This is particularly true when tenderness is present together with pain. Normally a fibroid is nontender. Necrosis of the tumor due to a faulty blood supply must be considered. The nature and location of the pain will depend on the location of the fibroid. (a) If the tumor is intramural, red degeneration or infection may explain the accident. When infection is present in a degenerating fibroid, the patient usually has an elevated temperature. The pain may come on suddenly over a localized area in the lower abdomen. Pain is usually severe, gradually subsiding into a constant, dull pelvic "toothache." (b) A pedunculated subserous fibroid may undergo torsion which first produces an obstruction to the venous return, leading later to necrosis and hemorrhage within the interior of the fibroid and an inflammatory reaction on its surface. The pain is sudden, severe, colicky, prostrating and typical of the kind of pain produced by infarction in any solid viscus. (c) Cramplike uterine pain that approaches the magnitude of labor pains suggests that the uterus is trying to expel a necrotic submucous fibroid or fibroid polyp through the cervical canal. This is most pronounced at the time of the period. (d) Rarely, after abdominal injury, rupture of the surface veins of the fibroid may produce an intraperitoneal hemorrhage and a severe lower abdominal pain.

(2) As a secondary factor, necrosis and inflammation in a twisted subserous fibroid can produce a severe peritoneal reaction, with the formation of adhesions that fix the uterus in the pelvis or to adjacent structures. The normal tube and ovary become implicated in the inflammatory process. Pre-existing abnormalities such as pelvic inflammation, endometriosis or ovarian cysts may contribute to and increase the pelvic and lower abdominal pain produced by the impacted fibroid. The lower abdominal or back pain is usually constant. Mildly acute to severe exacerbations are frequently noted just before and with the onset of menstruation.

(3) The fibroid may produce discomfort through pressure, owing to its position or size. Through size alone the fibroid can produce pressure on the stomach and diaphragm, resulting in disturbances in gastric function and at times in respiration. Similarly, pressure of the fibroid on the venous channels in the pelvis may cause obstruction to the return flow with resultant varicosities (varicose veins) of one or both lower extremities, as well as hemorrhoids.

PRESSURE DUE TO LOCATION AND SIZE. Owing to both location and size either the bladder or ureter is compressed. (*a*) If the fibroid occupies a lateral position within the broad ligament or grows retroperitoneally, the ureter may be either completely or partially obstructed, thereby producing hydronephrosis. The patient likely has pain in both flank and kidney area on the obstructed side. (*b*) On occasion the pressure of the fibroid may interfere with evacuation of feces from the rectum. Constipation is a common symptom, though actual intestinal obstruction is rare. (*c*) When the fibroid becomes impacted in the pelvis or arises in the cervical region beneath the bladder floor, the patient often suffers from urinary retention. The obstruction to bladder outflow can be chronic and partial, or it may suddenly become complete and require catheterization for relief. The latter is said to occur most often at the time of the menstrual period when pelvic congestion produces an increase in the tumor size. Overdistention of long standing often leads to incontinence, as the bladder spills over. An overdistended bladder with residual urine is a common source of infection. Painful micturition may then be due to cystitis.

The location and radiation of pain caused by the pressure of the fibroid will depend on the nature and direction of the growth in the tumor itself, as well as the complications it produces. Usually the pain is located in the back, lower portion of the abdomen or thighs. Prolonged standing, particularly at the time of the period, exaggerates the discomfort.

How Is the Diagnosis of a Fibroid Made?

The diagnosis of the intramural, subserous, interligamentary, cervical and retroperitoneal leiomyoma is made by physical examination of the patient. The presence of a submucous fibroid cannot be determined by palpation. The mere enlargement of the uterus or its endometrial cavity is not sufficient evidence for the diagnosis of a submucosal fibroid. The nature of the symptoms often arouses suspicion. The actual diagnosis can be made only by curettage, endometrial biopsy or roentgenologic interpretation of the appearance of the endometrial cavity after injection of an opaque dye such as Lipiodol.

The majority of fibroids are discovered by palpation.

ABDOMINAL EXAMINATION. Many women first complain of abdominal enlargement or the presence of a mass, in the absence of other symptoms. When the abdomen is palpated, a firm, smooth, centrally placed tumor can often be felt rising out of the pelvis. When the consistency is in doubt, the tumor may actually prove to be a distended bladder or an ovarian cyst which, through partial torsion of its pedicle, has come to occupy a midline position. If the contour is irregular and nodular, the chances are highly in favor of the diagnosis of fibroid. There is still a possibility that the nodularity may be due to solid portions within the wall of a large ovarian cyst. It is unwise to proceed with therapy on the basis of symptoms and abdominal examination alone.

BIMANUAL PELVIC EXAMINATION.   Bimanual examination by both vagina and rectum should be done to check the abdominal findings. Many large leiomyomata are so placed in the pelvis that they are not evident on abdominal examination. By bimanual palpation the examiner has the best chance of determining the size, contour, location, consistency, degree of fixation and areas of tenderness. In this manner he also has the best opportunity of evaluating the extent of associated disease, such as pelvic inflammation or endometriosis. It is often difficult to differentiate between pregnancy or adenomyosis and a uterus symmetrically and diffusely enlarged by the presence of a solitary intramural fibroid. One cannot tell with certainty whether a laterally placed tumor is a pedunculated or broad-ligament fibroid, or perhaps a solid or cystic ovarian tumor. If the differential diagnosis is made, it will be largely determined by palpation.

SIZE OF THE PELVIC MASS.   The size of the pelvic mass varies widely. The tumor may be small, and the size of the uterus not appreciably altered. The tumor may fill the entire pelvis or rise well out of it to distend the upper portion of the abdomen. It is important to note the size of the uterus as evidence of the growth rate of the tumor. An increase in size is often the determining factor in initiating therapy.

CONTOUR OF THE UTERUS AND LOCATION OF THE FIBROID.   A large fibroid may symmetrically enlarge the entire uterus. If the tumors arise within the walls, the enlarged uterus often feels smooth and rounded. Subserous fibroids usually are felt as smooth, rounded nodular projections upon the surface of the uterus, which may or may not be enlarged. Laterally placed fibroids may extend into the broad ligament from a broad base or assume a variety of positions when pedunculated. Usually they are felt posterior to the uterine fundus, but at times they assume a position anterior to the bladder. Occasionally the cervical os may be dilated, and the advancing edge of a prolapsing submucous fibroid can be felt.

CONSISTENCY AND AREAS OF TENDERNESS.   Normally the irregular tumors are firm, hard and nontender. If the pelvic mass feels soft, either the diagnosis is in error or something has happened to the tumor. One should become suspicious that one is dealing with either a pregnant uterus or an ovarian cyst. If there are tender soft spots within the substance of a firm tumor mass, degeneration of some of the fibroids has probably taken place. One should not overlook the possibility of an ectopic pregnancy that may occur with a fibroid uterus. A generalized softness of the tumor and the presence of edema may suggest sarcomatous change in the fibroid, if pregnancy is excluded.

DEGREE OF FIXATION.   Normally the fibroid uterus is movable. If the tumor mass cannot be dislodged from its position, one of the following conditions is usually present: (1) The uterus is fixed by such associated conditions as endometriosis or pelvic inflammation. Palpation by rectum of tender shotty nodules on the pelvic floor or uterosacral ligaments will help to establish the diagnosis of endometriosis. A generalized parametrial thickening suggests pelvic inflammatory disease. (2) Repeated accidents to the superficially placed or pedunculated fibroid may have set up a pelvic inflammatory process with resultant adhesive fixation. ③ The tumor by its size often molds itself to the contour of the true pelvis and becomes firmly lodged there. ④ The cervical or broad-ligament fibroid may be fixed by the anatomic limitation of the pelvic floor or bladder.

Differential Diagnosis

Most of the disturbing factors that cloud the diagnosis of leiomyomata uteri have been mentioned in the foregoing discussion. The most important are ① pregnancy, either in the uterus or in the tube; ② change in the consistency of the tumor, which may be due to pregnancy, sarcoma or disintegrative changes; ③ differentiation of a pedunculated subserous fibroid from a solid or a semisolid and semicystic ovarian tumor. Such ovarian tumors carry a high potential of malignant change. ④ Proper evaluation of bloody vaginal discharge, which may due to degeneration within a submucous fibroid or carcinoma of the endometrium; ⑤ infectious diseases, such as pelvic inflammation and tuberculosis, as well as other pathologic conditions that manifest themselves by either the presence of a mass or fixation of the pelvis, namely, endometriosis and ovarian tumors.

ADENOMYOMA OR ADENOMYOSIS. Benign permeation of the muscular walls of the uterus by islands of endometrial glands together with their stroma produces a uniform solid enlargement of the uterus which on palpation is indistinguishable from a solitary intramural fibroid of symmetrical proportions. The difference can be detected only when the extirpated uterus is sectioned. Grossly, the adenomyotic process blends into the surrounding musculature and lacks the distinguishable appearance of a capsule that serves to demarcate the leiomyoma from the adjacent myometrial tissue. Tiny blue or brown dots may mark the blood content of the buried glands. Microscopically, islands of endometrial glands and the characteristic associated

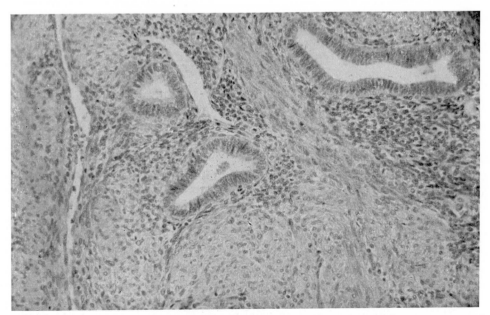

Fig. 49-4. In adenomyosis the basal endometrial glands as well as endometrial stroma penetrate into the myometrium to varying depths. No tumor is formed, but rather a diffuse myometrial thickening.

stroma are found abnormally deep in the muscle walls of the uterus (Fig. 49–4). On physical examination there are no distinguishing features. The diagnosis may be suspected when there is a history of continuous boring uterine pain that begins with the onset of menstruation and persists through its full extent.

NOTE   True adenomyoma represents the infiltration of endometrial glands and stroma into a leiomyoma. The tumor grossly may be marked by brown or blue cystic spaces and flecks like those of adenomyosis. Since the growth pattern and physical characteristics of adenomyosis and the adenomyoma closely parallel those of the uterine fibroid, expediency links them inseparably in management.

Treatment

There are three main forms of treatment for the patient with a uterine fibroid: (1) She is kept under observation, and nothing is done to the uterus and its tumor. (2) The patient is operated on, and either a myomectomy is performed or the uterus is removed. (3) She receives either radium or x-ray treatment.

The decision for or against therapy for the tumor depends upon whether (a) the patient's symptoms are severe enough to require treatment; (b) the growth pattern and location of the tumor are such that they present a threat to future health and happiness; (c) the associated disease is of sufficient importance to warrant operative intervention, independent of the presence of the fibroid. This in turn will be modified by the age of the patient, her general health and her desire to have children.

How Does One Treat a Fibroid in Women of the Childbearing Age? The patient in the childbearing age, forty years old or younger, who has a fibroid uncomplicated by the presence of other associated abnormalities is treated conservatively whenever possible. The discovery of a small asymptomatic fibroid in the fundal portion of the uterus of a woman in this age group requires no immediate treatment. The patient should be told that she has a fibroid and that periodic checkup examinations are both desirable and important.

Should the tumor arise in or near the cervix, this is an indication for its operative removal. Such tumors frequently produce urinary retention and occasionally cystitis. Dysmenorrhea is common. They also become a menace to the management of labor and may interfere with conception.

The location and growth pattern of the tumor play important roles in the decision for or against operative intervention. Large tumors may distort the uterine cavity and are prone to undergo degeneration. Pedunculated tumors frequently undergo torsion and become necrotic. They complicate the course of pregnancy. The fact that they are often indistinguishable from solid adnexal tumors that have a high malignant potential is an important consideration. The submucous fibroid can interfere with conception or pregnancy and often degenerates. In any one of these situations one may justifiably offer surgery in the absence of symptoms.

The severity of the symptoms is an important factor. Any change in the nature of growth in the tumor should be regarded with grave suspicion. A rapid increase in size or the sudden appearance of pain or local tenderness suggests that a sarcomatous change or some form of degeneration has taken place. Unless vaginal blood loss is excessive and prolonged, the physician may prefer to control the bleeding by giving progesterone therapy and to correct the anemia with oral administration of iron tablets. The excessively copious menstrual period of normal duration can produce a chronic anemia when this pattern persists. The shortened interval suggests an anovulatory type of bleeding, which frequently reverts to a normal menstrual bleeding pattern and requires no treatment. Should it persist, it will respond better to hormone therapy in the form of progesterone than it will to surgery.

Bleeding of hemorrhagic proportions that persists longer than ten days or appears in gushes demands investigation and appropriate therapy. The medical explanation is frequently hypothyroidism, in which case bleeding will be controlled by thyroid medication. Organic cause usually points to the submucous fibroid, fibroid polyp or intramural tumor encroaching on the endometrial cavity. After blood replacement by transfusion these tumors should be removed surgically.

WHAT TYPE OF SURGERY IS INDICATED IN THE CHILDBEARING AGE?   Whether she is married or not conservative surgery should be the procedure of choice in a woman under the age of thirty-five years, when there are no contraindications and the location of the tumor permits. In the nulliparous woman the age limit may be extended to forty years, to give her every chance to have a child. The majority of women like to feel that they can conceive, whether they actually want to or not.

Myomectomy is the procedure of choice.   Multiple myomectomies are compatible with conception and the successful maintenance of subsequent pregnancies. This is true despite the fact that the endometrial cavity is often entered in surgical removal of the fibroid. The mortality rate of myomectomy (1.3 per cent) is slightly higher than for hysterectomy. Recurrence of fibroid tumors after myomectomy is infrequent. Myomectomy may be carried out through either the vagina or abdomen, depending on the location of the tumor. Since other pelvic disease is often present, the abdominal approach is preferred.

Myomectomy is a particularly useful procedure in the woman under thirty-five years old who wants to have children, but has (1) a pedunculated fibroid, (2) a cervical fibroid or (3) a submucous fibroid. It should not be attempted in the presence of a rapidly growing tumor. Red degeneration, however, is no contraindication to myomectomy. There is little danger that a sarcoma will be removed in error. Myomectomy should never be done unless the remainder of the uterus and the adnexa are in a healthy state. It may be gainfully done when associated lesions such as endometriosis require surgical intervention. Since the full extent of the pathologic process cannot be adequately appraised preoperatively, the patient should be warned that hysterectomy may be required.

PREGNANCY AND THE FIBROID UTERUS.   The fibroid uterus may affect a young woman's ability to have children in one of two ways: (a) she may have difficulty in conceiving; (b) complications, both early and late, may arise in the pregnant fibroid uterus.

Infertility.   There appears to be a definite relation between the presence of fibroids within the uterus and sterility. The fibroid alone, however, is not solely to blame. The chief source of trouble is often pelvic inflammatory disease with severe tubal damage. Both endometriosis and salpingitis are frequently present in association with uterine fibroids. There can be little doubt that an ovum implanted on endometrium thinned out over a submucous tumor will have difficulty in surviving, owing to a faulty blood supply. If it does implant, there is a tendency for abortion to occur.

Only those fibroids located primarily within the uterine cavity or secondarily implicating it should be considered a cause of sterility. There is no indication for the removal of a fibroid situated elsewhere in the uterus, when conception is the main consideration.

Early and Late Complications of Pregnancy in the Fibroid Uterus.   The great majority of pregnancies occurring in a fibroid uterus will proceed normally without any serious complications, even when multiple large tumors are present. Fibroids rarely cause obstruction to normal vaginal delivery of a full-term child unless they occupy a position in the cervix, the lower uterine segment or in the posterior cul-de-sac. After noting the position of such tumors and in anticipation of difficulties that may possibly be encountered should pregnancy occur, one may elect to perform prophylactic myomectomy in the woman who is having trouble in establishing a family.

Once the pregnancy is established, several things can happen to the fibroid that may alter the normal course. Abortion may occur in the patient who has a retroversion, adenomyosis or a submucous fibroid in a uterus in normal position. In rare instances the submucous leiomyoma may be extruded during the course of the pregnancy. Abortion usually occurs early, probably because of irregular contractions induced by irritation from the fibroid and the inadequate blood supply to the implantation site of the ovum. The retrodisplacement of the uterus and its tumor predisposes to repeated abortions, largely through interference with the normal mobility of the uterus. The fibroid can become incarcerated in the cul-de-sac. Myomectomy is indicated in the young primipara if a pessary fails to improve the position of the uterus.

Red degeneration, occasionally seen in the nonpregnant fibroid uterus, occurs more frequently when the patient is gravid. Conservative treatment should be carried out unless the symptoms become progressively more severe. If the tumor is laterally placed, the indications for operative intervention are more urgent, for the tender mass may represent torsion in either a pedunculated fibroid or an ovarian cyst. If possible, the myomectomy should be delayed until the fourth or fifth month, when the fetus is both obviously viable and less likely to be dislodged. The incidence of abortion following myomectomy is lowest at this time.

The change in size of a leiomyoma during pregnancy cannot be evaluated. The apparent increase in size of some tumors seems to be less concerned with their more rapid growth rate than with the appearance of extensive degenerative changes and the accompanying edema within the fibroid. When there are no symptoms, any enlargement is more apparent than real. Some observers feel that they become smaller and even disappear. That fibroids can no longer be felt in a normally enlarging uterus is at best incomplete evidence of their disappearance.

The complications of pregnancy in the fibroid uterus that are related to problems of delivery at term fall in the province of obstetrics and will not be discussed here.

How Does One Treat a Fibroid in the Premenopausal Age Group?   After the age of forty there is no longer the problem of balancing the need for therapy against the desire to preserve childbearing function. The decision for or against treatment and the choice of the method are now based on the severity of symptoms plus the importance of associated disease, as modified by the patient's general condition.

A Critical Review of the Symptomatology.   A closer scrutiny of the symptomatology is essential, for many of the symptoms attributed to the presence of the uterine fibroid in the younger patient can now be due to malignant neoplastic disease. This is particularly true of the various types of vaginal bleeding that one encounters with the fibroid uterus. Bloody vaginal discharge and intermenstrual spotting in the woman under thirty-five years old could be attributed with reasonable accuracy to a fibroid polyp or submucous fibroid. After the age of forty years it is imperative that carcinomas of the external cervix or the endocervical canal be ruled out before instituting therapy for the fibroid.

Probably the greatest source of clinical error in this age group is the misconception that fibroids are the principal cause of abnormal uterine bleeding. As noted previously, the fibroid uterus bleeds not because of the presence of the fibroid, but from effects of ovarian dysfunction. The sole exception is the submucous fibroid, which gives a characteristic train of symptoms and cannot be palpated. Functional uterine bleeding is common in the age group from forty years to the menopause, but an abnormal bleeding pattern at this time also is associated with the presence of cancer in both the cervix and the fundus. The nearer to the menopause, the greater the chance of cancer. It is therefore imperative that the cause of the bleeding be clearly established before proceeding with therapy. Every pelvic laparotomy should be preceded by a diagnostic curettage and either a frozen section diagnosis or gross inspection of the curetted material.

With the cause of bleeding thoroughly established, one may elect to treat the functional causes with hormone therapy in the form of progesterone or testosterone. Excessive and prolonged periods have a more serious connotation in this age group. Failure to respond to the hormone therapy or recurrent similar episodes upon its discontinuance are adequate reasons for resorting to surgery in the patient with either a palpable tumor or a history that suggests that the fibroid may be submucous.

In this age group there is also less reason to delay abdominal surgery in the patient who has a lateral wall fibroid. Too frequently tumors in this location are indistinguishable from solid ovarian tumors. The onset of ovarian cancer is insidious, and the prognosis is poor largely because of delay in diagnosis. Benign fibroma of the ovary is the most common solid ovarian tumor, but the remainder are likely to be highly malignant. If there is any doubt about the diagnosis, surgical intervention is indicated.

The symptoms of abdominal enlargement, lower abdominal pressure and interference with the function of adjacent organs, such as bladder, rectum or ureter, must be judged on their severity and the inconvenience to the patient. The same factors apply to the tumors that produce venous obstruction, lower leg varicosities and hemorrhoids.

Many of the symptoms attributed to the fibroid are actually due to associated conditions such as endometriosis, pelvic inflammation, ovarian tumors and uterine cancers. Others are associated with a variety of manifestations of prolapse or with functional uterine bleeding. The indications for therapy are based less on the presence of the fibroid than the extent of discomfort and disability produced by the coexistent pathologic alteration or anatomic derangement.

Any indication of change in symptomatology or change in the size of a fibroid tumor that has been kept under observation should serve as an indication for therapy. In large fibroid tumors quiescent for years, degenerative processes may appear suddenly.

What Kind of Treatment Is Indicated in the Menopausal Age Group? Since there is no longer the need to preserve the childbearing function, myomectomy, which carries with it a somewhat higher risk in both morbidity and mortality, should give place to either total removal of the uterus or to irradiation.

Operative Treatment. When indications for therapy have appeared, total removal of the uterus is preferable to radiation. This may be done either abdominally or vaginally. When other factors are present that require surgery on the vaginal canal, the uterus may be removed by this route. In general the abdominal approach is preferred, for it gives far wider latitude to deal with associated adnexal disease that may be entirely unsuspected. In every instance the vaginal or total abdominal hysterectomy should be preceded by a curettage. Total removal of the uterus is a far better operation than simple subtotal removal of the fundal portion. Supravaginal hysterectomy should be done only when great technical difficulties are encountered. The disadvantages of total hysterectomy formerly advanced to support the advocates of supravaginal hysterectomy are not valid. These were increased morbidity and mortality, prolapse of the vaginal vault, foreshortening of the vagina and dyspareunia. Total hysterectomy removes the cervix, which frequently harbors infection and occasionally cancer. There is little excuse today for not removing the entire uterus when hysterectomy is indicated.

Hysterectomy is preferred to radiation for two reasons: (1) preservation of the ovary is possible with hysterectomy; (2) the entire uterus is removed.

Preservation of Ovary.   The effect of radiation, except for the local cauterizing effect upon the endometrium, is directly upon the ovary. Vaginal bleeding is controlled at the price of radiation castration. The effect on the tumor is entirely secondary, based on the theory that the fibroid will regress when estrin stimulation is withdrawn. Healthy ovaries may be left undisturbed at the time hysterectomy is performed, regardless of the age of the patient at the time.

If the surgeon follows prescribed techniques, there is little reason to fail to recognize a cystic change or cystadenoma. The possibility that cancer will develop later in the retained ovary is remote. So many ovarian tumors are developmental in origin that if they have not manifested evidence of tumor growth at the age when hysterectomy is performed, they are unlikely to do it later. If doubt exists, wedge-shaped sections should be removed from the ovaries for pathologic review.

Removal of the Entire Uterus.   The uterus that has grown leiomyomata may retain the potential to develop other tumors. Carcinosarcoma and endometrial carcinoma have been reported with increased frequency following irradiation for benign uterine bleeding associated with fibroids. Perhaps the carcinoma has developed on a background of previous radiation reaction, but in all probability the second tumor developed because the uterine substrate was inherently abnormal. Intrauterine irradiation has no direct effect upon later tumor development unless the tumor arises within the uterine cavity. The effect, as in the use of external x-ray therapy, is otherwise upon the ovary. Total hysterectomy eliminates all chance that cancer will develop later in the female pelvic organ that is most prone to produce it.

Irradiation.   This is reserved for the patient past the childbearing age who is too poor a risk to withstand the rigors of surgical intervention. Since the effect of radiation is partly on the ovary, directly or indirectly, there is no place for its use in the younger age group. Radiation is administered in the form of (a) implantation of radium (or radon needles) or (b) external irradiation (x-ray). The former has the definite advantage of ensuring that (1) the patient is examined under anesthesia and (2) that the endometrial cavity will be curetted to rule out cancer. Despite the fact that radiologists are more and more insistent that curettage should precede x-ray therapy, there are still too many instances when this is not routine procedure.

Radiation carries with it no immediate mortality and little morbidity. In the dose that is sufficient to produce ablation of ovarian activity, there is little danger of serious damage to small intestine or rectum.

There are, however, contraindications to the use of radiation. Intrauterine irradiation is definitely contraindicated in the presence of a submucous fibroid. A sloughing effect upon the fibroid follows direct contact with the radium applicator. Bleeding is increased, and infection further complicates the problem. It is unlikely that large fibroids will regress after ovarian function has ceased, and there is great danger that a further impairment of the leiomyoma's blood supply may increase the chances of degenerative change. The same factors apply to pedunculated fibroids. Localized pain, pelvic infection, ovarian tumors, rapid increase in the size of the tumor and the element of uncertainty concerning the seriousness of associated diseases may all be regarded as contraindications.

Since the effect of radiation is obtained only at the expense of castration, and there are so many contraindications to its use, it is far better to perform operation than to resort to radiation in the woman who is having an active menstrual life. *NOTE* Radiation should be reserved solely for the patient who for physical reasons cannot undergo surgery.

How Does One Treat a Patient with Fibroids at or after the Menopause? As the patient approaches the menopause, the chances of malignant neoplastic disease increase. Excessive and prolonged periods are frequent at this time. There is a common impression that the fibroids will regress after completion of the menopause. This encouraging misconception delays the investigation of symptoms that call for explanation. Again, one should keep in mind that the patient does not bleed because she has a fibroid. The cause may be functional, but at this age the most important source is cancer. It is not important whether the fibroid remains or disappears. A diagnostic curettage is indicated, followed by total hysterectomy. Since there is a definite possibility that the curettage may miss a carcinoma hidden behind polyps or in the cornual angles of the endometrial cavity, hysterectomy is preferred to irradiation.

The fibroid may undergo some regression in the postmenopausal state. Whether this is due to lack of estrin activity or simply to reduction in blood supply is debatable. It is unwise to be lulled into a sense of serenity that fibroids will inevitably regress at this time. There is increasing evidence that some estrin activity continues long after menstruation has ceased. As long as estrin is being produced, the fibroid will not only maintain its size, but also may grow. If the patient has no symptoms and continues to be observed, there is no need for surgery. Postmenopausal patients rarely require treatment of their fibroids. When symptoms do appear, the patient should be operated upon. This is particularly true of large fibroids, in which the reduction in blood supply can produce central degeneration of the tumor. The secondary changes that brought about the new train of symptoms in a tumor previously quiescent have increasingly severe implications. The operation should not be delayed in the hope that such a tumor will go away.

LEIOMYOSARCOMA

Sarcomatous changes may appear in a uterine leiomyoma. This is by far the most important alteration that may occur. Though such development is possible, the incidence is so low that the possibility of such change cannot be advanced as a valid reason for recommending that surgical removal of all fibroids be done routinely. The *NOTE* reports of its frequency vary from less than 1 per cent to 4 per cent of leiomyomata. This discrepancy is due to variation in the criteria used in histologic differentiation. If the diagnosis is based on individual cellular changes, the incidence will be higher, in contrast to requiring evidence of myometrial invasion. Rapidly growing benign cellular leiomyomata are common. Some of them may show an occasional mitotic figure among normally growing smooth-muscle cell groups. Others may show variation in the sizes and shapes of cells, with many mitoses.

The diagnosis of sarcoma has sometimes been made on the basis of certain numbers of mitoses noted per high-power field. This was more common when thicker histologic sections (25 or 30 microns) were made from blocks embedded in celloidin. Most patients with this kind of tumor (as high as 90 per cent) will continue to live for many years without ever having a recurrence. Others who reportedly showed more minimal changes have died promptly with widespread metastases. This emphasizes the difficulty of making an accurate diagnosis of sarcoma on the basis of the cellular changes alone. In the past pathologists were prone to call such fibroids "leiomyosarcoma, clinically benign," or "only histologically malignant."

Obviously this terminology should be abandoned. As in any cancer, the diagnosis of leiomyosarcoma should be based upon observing invasion or definite anaplasia, or both. When doubt exists as to sarcomatous changes in a cellular myoma, it should probably be termed an atypical leiomyoma. Time alone may establish the final diagnosis. When there is definite evidence of gross or microscopic myometrial invasion, the prognosis is uniformly bad, and the initial microscopic diagnosis of sarcoma is likely to be confirmed, most often by clinical indications of invasive spread or metastasis. Some leiomyosarcomata, either early tumors or those of low grade malignancy, are cured by simple hysterectomy.

Occasionally one finds an area of leiomyosarcoma in an otherwise necrotic or calcified fibroid. In all probability this represents invasion of the fibroid from a primary sarcoma arising in the adjacent myometrium. Sarcomatous alteration is usually a primary process and does not develop because of degeneration of a "dead" fibroid.

How Is Leiomyosarcoma Suspected Clinically and Grossly?

Unless the sarcoma arises in a submucous fibroid, when occasionally help may be had from the vaginal smear or curettage, there is little in the history, physical examination or resources of diagnostic aids that will distinguish leiomyosarcoma from a rapidly growing benign leiomyoma. Bleeding, fever, pain, local tenderness and increase in size of the uterus are too often simply the symptoms of ordinary degenerative changes in a benign fibroid.

At operation one should be suspicious of a soft fibroid that shows evidence of edema. The tumor should promptly be sectioned. Obviously, it will be impossible to detect early microscopic leiomyosarcomatous change without a frozen section, but a well established sarcoma has a characteristic gross appearance. The leiomyosarcoma will cut more readily than the benign leiomyoma and reveal a smooth, even, cream- or maple yellow-colored cut surface that is not whorled, does not grate against the knife and is far softer. It is sometimes said to look like raw pork (Fig. 49–5). The whorls of smooth muscle and fibrous tissue, characteristic of the benign fibroid, have disappeared. When further advanced, the leiomyosarcomatous mass may show ischemic degeneration and become cystic. This is particularly true of the central portions of a large sarcoma, where the blood supply is more limited. Bloodstained hemorrhagic streaks, which are simply collections of blood or bloodstained fluid, are one characteristic of leiomyosarcomatous change in a fibroid.

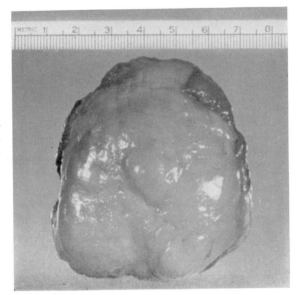

Fig. 49-5. A leiomyosarcoma typically has a smooth, slick, yellow or cream-colored cut surface, and it is poorly demarcated from the surrounding myometrium.

How Is Leiomyosarcoma Recognized Microscopically?

The benign leiomyoma, as mentioned, has a rather regular whorled or herringbone pattern formed from intertwined bundles of proliferating smooth muscle. Beyond a size of about 1 cm. in diameter, fibrous tissue rich in collagen tends to overgrow the more delicate smooth muscle, accounting for the clinical designation of the larger tumors as fibroids. Even during phases of rapid growth, such as in the pregnant uterus, the architecture and cytologic arrangement remain regular, although mitoses may be found in relative abundance (Fig. 49–6, *A*).

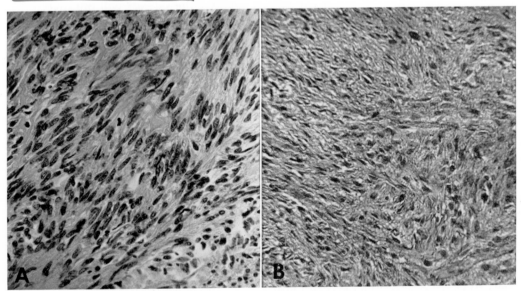

Fig. 49-6. *A*, The cellular benign leiomyoma has a regular structure of close-packed and locally palisaded smooth muscle cells. A mitosis is seen near the center. *B*, A leiomyosarcoma of medium-grade malignancy manifests an irregular pattern of growth and staining qualities, some abnormally hyperchromatic nuclei and occasional mitotic figures.

In leiomyosarcoma the structure of interwoven smooth muscle and fibrous stroma within the tumor is locally or generally replaced by irregular masses of poorly oriented, usually large, smooth-muscle cells. Often fingers of such cells invade the adjacent myometrium or blood vessels, or both.

NOTE Under higher magnification in these regions the cells, and particularly their nuclei, vary abnormally in size, and also in their interrelations, so that individual malignant cells grow at right angles to their neighbors. Giant hyperchromatic nuclei with abnormal lobulations may be identified. In such well marked instances of anaplasia, mitotic activity provides further evidence of leiomyosarcoma (Fig. 49–6, *B*).

Invasive growth and anaplasia are more important than simple cytologic and nuclear variations in size and staining. The latter may occur in locations that are ischemic and verge upon degeneration.

Leiomyosarcomata, as mentioned, may be either focal or diffuse, and of various degrees of malignancy. Some are so undifferentiated that it is difficult to be certain of their smooth-muscle origin unless special stains are used.

What Is the Best Treatment for Leiomyosarcoma of the Uterus?

The basic treatment, regardless of the pathologic diagnosis, is total removal of the uterus. Whether or not the ovaries are removed depends on the age of the patient, not upon the possible influence of hormonal stimulation of the tumor. If the fibroid *NOTE* is a cellular myoma or a leiomyosarcoma without invasion, approximately 80 per cent of the patients will be permanently cured. When myometrial invasion is present, few, if any, will survive, and no further salvage will appear if the ovaries are removed as well as the uterus.

In rare instances x-ray therapy, for patients who have myometrial invasion or local recurrences in the pelvic area, will prove helpful, but it should be offered simply in hope, rather than with any great expectancy that the salvage will improve.

NOTE There is no excuse for prophylactic hysterectomy based on the premise that because any fibroid can undergo sarcomatous change the uterus should be removed to prevent the possibility. The incidence is far too low to support such reasoning.

REFERENCES

Bigby, M. A. M.: Intraperitoneal Haemorrhage from a Vessel on the Surface of a Uterine Fibroid. *Brit. M.J.*, 2: 580, 1960.

Brown, A. B., Chamberlain, R., and TeLinde, R. W.: Myomectomy. *Am. J. Obst. & Gynec.*, 71: 759, 1956.

Copeland, W. E., Nelson, P. K., and Payne, F. L.: Intrauterine Radium for Dysfunctional Bleeding. *Am. J. Obst. & Gynec.*, 73: 615, 1957.

Corscaden, J. A.: Failures Following the Treatment by Irradiation of Cases of Benign Uterine Bleeding and Fibromyoma. *Am. J. Roentgenol.*, 45: 661, 1941.

Corscaden, J. A., Fertig, J. W., and Gusberg, S. B.: Carcinoma Subsequent to the Radiotherapeutic Menopause. *Am. J. Obst. & Gynec.*, 51: 1, 1946.

Everett, H. S.: Effects of Uterine Myomas on the Urinary Tract. *Clin. Obst. & Gynec.*, 1: 429, 1958.

Faulkner, R. L.: Blood Vessels of the Myomatous Uterus. *Am. J. Obst. & Gynec.*, 47: 185, 1944.

Idem: Red Degeneration of Uterine Myomas. *Am. J. Obst. & Gynec.*, 53: 474, 1947.

Finn, W. F., and Muller, P. F.: Abdominal Myomectomy: Special Reference to Subsequent Pregnancy and to the Reappearance of Fibromyomas of the Uterus. *Am. J. Obst. & Gynec.*, 60: 109, 1950.

Israel, S. L., and Mutch, J. C.: Myomectomy. *Clin. Obst. & Gynec.*, 1: 455, 1958.

Kurland, I. I., and Rosengart, M.: Problems Encountered in Bicornuate Uterus. *Fertil. & Steril.*, 11: 597, 1960.

Lardaro, H. H.: Extensive Myomectomy. Review of 157 Cases. *Am. J. Obst. & Gynec.*, 79: 43, 1960.

Macer, G.: Management of Uterine Fibromyomas. *Postgrad. Med.*, 28: 503, 1960.

Montgomery, J. B., Long, J. P., and Hoffman, J.: A Clinical Evaluation of the Use of Radium Therapy in the Control of Benign Uterine Bleeding. *Am. J. Obst. & Gynec.*, 64: 1011, 1952.

Idem: Radiation Therapy for Myoma Uteri. *Clin. Obst. & Gynec.*, 1: 445, 1958.

Morton, D. G.: Symptoms and Signs of Fibromyomas of the Uterus. *Clin. Obst. & Gynec.*, 1: 407, 1958.

Novak, E. R.: Benign and Malignant Changes in Uterine Myomas. *Clin. Obst. & Gynec.*, 1: 421, 1958.

Palmer, J. P., and Spratt, D. W.: Pelvic Carcinoma Following Irradiation for Benign Gynecologic Diseases. *Am. J. Obst. & Gynec.*, 72: 497, 1956.

Rubin, I. C.: Uterine Fibromyomas and Sterility. *Clin. Obst. & Gynec.*, 1: 501, 1958.

Sampson, J.: Blood Supply of Uterine Myomata. Based on the Study of 100 Injected Uteri Containing These Tumors. *Surg., Gynec., & Obst.*, 14: 215, 1912.

Sehgal, N., and Haskins, A. L.: The Mechanism of Uterine Bleeding in the Presence of Fibromyomas. *Am. Surgeon*, 26: 21, 1960.

Seidner, H. M., and Thompson, J. R.: Fibroma of the Fallopian Tube. *Am. J. Obst. & Gynec.*, 79: 32, 1960.

Stander, R. W.: Irradiation Castration. A Follow up Study of Results in Benign Pelvic Disease. *Obst. & Gynec.*, 10: 223, 1957.

Taylor, H. C.: Standard Practices at Sloane Hospital. The Management of Uterine Fibroids. *Bull. Sloane Hosp. for Women*, 2: 115, 1956.

Zeigerman, J. H., Valdes-Dapena, A. M., and Fettig, L.: Submucus Myoma in the Normal Sized Uterus. A Study of Endometrial Curettings for Its Detection. *Am. J. Obst. & Gynec.*, 73: 1286, 1957.

Leiomyosarcomas

Aaro, L. A., and Dockerty, M. B.: Leiomyosarcoma of the Uterus. *Am. J. Obst. & Gynec.*, 77: 1187, 1959.

Bell, H. G., and Edgehill, H.: Sarcomas Developing in Uterine Fibroids. Review of Literature and Presentation of Three Cases. *Am. J. Surg.*, 100: 416, 1960.

Crane, A. R., and Decker, J. P.: Sarcoma of the Uterus. A Study of 42 Cases. *Lab. Invest.*, 9: 28, 1960.

Davis, G. H., Howe, J. S., and French, W. G.: Leiomyosarcoma of the Uterus. A Report of 16 Cases, 1917 to 1948. *Am. J. Obst. & Gynec.*, 56: 1048, 1948.

Drake, E. T., and Dobben, G. D.: Leiomyosarcoma of the Uterus with Unusual Metastases. *J.A.M.A.*, 170: 1294, 1959.

Finn, W. F.: Sarcoma of the Uterus. A Review of Thirty-Three Cases. *Am. J. Obst. & Gynec.*, 60: 1254, 1950.

McEachern, C. G., Gitlin, M. M., and Sullivan, R. E.: Lobectomy for Metastatic Leiomyosarcoma of the Uterus. *J.A.M.A.*, 174: 1734, 1960.

Radman, H. M., and Korman, W.: Sarcoma of the Uterus. *Am. J. Obst. & Gynec.*, 78: 604, 1959.

Thornton, W. N., Jr., and Carter, J. P.: Sarcoma of the Uterus, a Clinical Study. *Am. J. Obst. & Gynec.*, 62: 294, 1957.

Wheelock, M. C., and Warren, S.: Leiomyosarcoma of the Uterus. *Ann. Surg.*, 116: 882, 1942.

Chapter 50

Physiologic Enlargements

of the Ovary

THE OVARY, by virtue of its anatomic structure and functional nature, is basically a cystic organ. As such it can be expected to vary in size as (*a*) the graafian follicles are stimulated to develop through the action of the gonadotropic hormones of the pituitary during the preovulatory phase, and (*b*) the corpus luteum comes into being upon maturation of the ova. Under normal conditions only one of the many follicles stimulated actually goes on to full maturation monthly, while many of the remaining follicles become atretic. If the follicle, for a variety of reasons that may be hormonal, circulatory or inflammatory, fails to rupture and give off the ovum or another follicle fails to regress to the atretic state, a follicle cyst of the ovary may develop. Similarly the corpus luteum under normal nonpregnant conditions should undergo regression after fourteen days, but if it fails to do so, a cyst may develop and persist.

Palpation of an adnexal enlargement, therefore, does not mean that the patient has an ovarian neoplasm. The distinction must be made, however, for if it is a neoplasm, immediate operative intervention is mandatory, but if simply a physiologic enlargement, it should be left alone and kept under observation, since in the majority of instances it will rupture spontaneously and disappear. In some instances a physiologic cyst, whether it takes origin from a follicle or arises in a corpus luteum, will produce alterations in the menstrual pattern. The majority, however, do not. When the menstrual period is changed, either the patient has foreshortened cycles with persistent bleeding, which may be heavy, or the period will be delayed. This is in contrast to the true ovarian neoplasm, which, except for functional tumors, has little influence on the menstrual flow or the rhythm of the cycle. Follicle cysts and corpus luteum cysts are by all odds the most common of all the ovarian tumors.

NOTE

FOLLICLE CYSTS

These cysts occurring in the ovarian cortex or immediately below the surface are so common that they can almost be regarded as normal. The size of the cyst or cysts, for there may be a number of them, varies widely. For the most part they rarely exceed 1.0 to 1.5 cm. in diameter, particularly if they are multiple. The larger retention cysts, which may acquire the dimensions of a 6- to 8-cm. lemon, are usually single.

724

If the cyst is large enough to undergo torsion of its pedicle and interruption of the blood supply, it may contain bloody fluid, but clear serous fluid is the normal finding.

If the cyst is of no great size and the intraluminal pressure is not too pronounced, the thin wall of the follicle cyst will show a lining of granulosa cells on histologic examination (Fig. 50–1, *A*). More often these have undergone pressure atrophy and are unrecognizable. In all probability it is the pressure within the cyst wall that prevents further production of fluid and greater enlargement.

How Should the Follicle Cyst Be Treated?

The natural life history of follicle cysts involves (*a*) gradual resorption of fluid or (*b*) spontaneous rupture. At any rate they tend to disappear spontaneously, while the ovary returns to its normal size. This happens so frequently that the surgeon who plans to operate upon a patient in whom he has palpated a tense, cystic adnexal structure will be well advised to check his office findings by a preoperative vaginal examination. All too frequently this is not done, the abdomen is explored with negative findings, and far too often an otherwise normal ovary is removed because it is said to contain cysts. In some ways the ovary is the most abused organ of the body, largely because it is bilateral and hidden within the abdominal cavity. The testicle enjoys a far happier and protected existence, despite or because of its exposed position.

The main problem is the decision as to whether the ovarian tumor is truly a physiologic enlargement and not a neoplasm. If the cyst is larger than 5 cm. in size, it had best be investigated, particularly if it is still present after one or 2 menstrual periods have gone by. It then becomes a space-occupying tumor that is replacing normal ovarian tissue, and there is always the chance that it may be a neoplasm and not a physiologic cyst. In either case it can usually be resected out of the ovary, leaving some normal tissue behind. If the cyst is small, there is no great need for haste, and the patient can be managed conservatively by repeated examinations in successive

NOTE

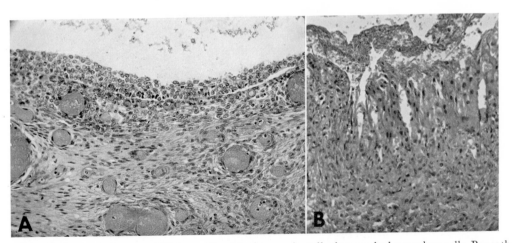

Fig. 50-1. *A*, Ovarian follicle cyst lined by layers of small, close-packed granulosa cells. Beneath is the theca interna, of about the same thickness, and beyond it is the theca externa. Dilated blood vessels are seen in the thecal zones in this case. *B*, The corpus luteum cyst is lined by a membrane composed of organizing blood clot, and its wall is made up of relatively large, acidophilic luteinized theca and granulosa cells lying in a vascular stroma.

menstrual cycles. In most instances it will disappear. Many women experience sudden sharp abdominal pain at periodic intervals much like the pain of *Mittelschmerz*. On examination little can be felt except slight tenderness in the vaults. Spontaneous rupture of physiologic follicle cysts or their absorption is a common occurrence.

CORPUS LUTEUM CYSTS

Under normal conditions the corpus luteum contains a moderate amount of fluid, but the persistence of a corpus luteum in the form of a cyst occurs less often than do follicle cysts. They do have a greater tendency to produce alterations in the menstrual cycle, and a delayed period is commonly observed. The corpus luteum cyst is apt to be larger than the follicle cyst. The size varies, depending on the amount of hemorrhage that takes place within its interior. Hemorrhage into a fresh corpus luteum is an entirely natural phenomenon, but on occasion it becomes excessive and assumes the proportions of a hematoma. If the corpus luteal hematoma is of long standing, some absorption of the blood element may take place, leaving the content of the cyst clearer and more fluid, but still bloodstained. Under normal conditions the fluid absorbs and the functional element declines as the interior of the cyst becomes fibrosed, stifling the luteal cells that line the cyst wall. They are still recognizable on gross inspection by the yellow-colored membrane (Fig. 50–1, *B*).

At times the corpus luteum persists and may produce a dull aching sensation or discomfort in one side of the pelvis. These symptoms are common to any cyst and give no indication of its nature. The persistence of corpora lutea, however, may be re-

NOTE

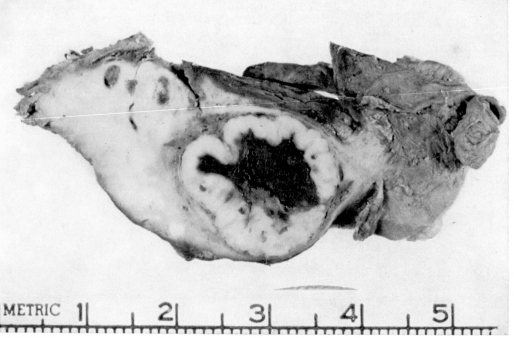

Fig. 50-2. A corpus luteum cyst with recent hemorrhage and rupture. This was a corpus luteum of pregnancy accompanying a tubal gestation, with peritoneal irritation by bleeding from both sites. The convoluted, yellow cyst wall is characteristic of a corpus luteum.

flected in the menstrual cycle producing (a) amenorrhea or (b) irregular persistent NOTE
bleeding of the types described as irregular ripening, shedding, or chronic menstruation.

Treatment

The corpus luteum cyst occasionally ruptures. The bloody contents of the cyst
prove irritating to the peritoneal cavity, and the patient has all the symptoms of
intraperitoneal hemorrhage. This often produces a difficult problem in the differential
diagnosis between a rupture of a corpus luteum cyst and an ectopic pregnancy. This
is a common problem, as attested by the reports in the literature. The two entities
have the following things in common: (a) amenorrhea, (b) slight bleeding, (c) a
palpable tender adnexal mass, (d) progestational changes in the endometrium, and
(e) the symptoms of intraperitoneal hemorrhage. Abdominal exploration may be
necessary to establish an accurate diagnosis. Even large corpora lutea may be excised
from the ovary if persistent bleeding warrants it. Otherwise they should be left alone.
There is absolutely no reason to take out the ovary as is all too frequently done 'Under
normal conditions the corpus luteum involutes and the ovary returns to its normal
size and shape (Fig. 50–2).

THECA LUTEIN CYSTS

An exaggerated form of persistently luteinized cysts often occurs in association
with a hydatidiform mole, chorioadenoma destruens or a chorionepithelioma, or
spontaneously in less dramatic form. The cysts are usually bilateral, and ovaries reach
sizable proportions—25 to 30 cm. Their appearance is due to the stimulating action
of the chorionic gonadotropin elaborated by the proliferating trophoblast upon the
theca lutein cells of the atretic follicles.

The clinical recognition and management have been discussed previously
in Chapter 33.

INFLAMMATORY CYSTS

At times after inflammatory episodes in the lower pelvis residual cysts may
develop that are clinically indistinguishable from benign neoplasms or physiologic
cysts of the ovary. They occasionally appear after local pelvic peritonitis secondary to
appendicitis, gonorrheal or streptococcal peritonitis, or any process occurring within
the abdomen that will permit an accumulation of material in the cul-de-sac.

ENDOMETRIAL OR CHOCOLATE CYSTS

Endometrial cysts are common in pelvic endometriosis and have been discussed
in detail in Chapter 47. It is frequently impossible to differentiate between a benign
cyst or physiologic tumor and a chocolate cyst of the ovary, particularly when the
endometriosis is confined to the ovary without dissemination to the adjacent peritoneum.

REFERENCES

Frank, I. L.: The Significance of Cystic Enlargement of the Ovary with Respect to Treatment. *M. Clin. North Amer.*, 32: 1611, 1948.

Garcia, C. R., and Rock, J.: Ovulation; in J. T. Velardo, ed.: *Essentials of Human Reproduction*. New York, Oxford University Press, 1958, p. 22.

Herbut, P. A.: *Gynecological and Obstetrical Pathology*. Philadelphia, Lea & Febiger, 1953.

Hertig, A. T., and Gore, H.: Non-Neoplastic Cysts of Graafian Follicle Origin; in *Tumors of the Female Sex Organs*. Washington, D. C., Armed Forces Institute of Pathology, 1961, Part 3, p. 11.

Hetlage, L. P., and Berry, P. T.: Giant Ovarian Cyst. *Missouri Med.*, 56: 158, 1959.

Kotz, H. L., and Herrmann, W.: A Review of the Endocrine Induction of Human Ovulation. *Fertil. & Steril.*, 12: 375, 1961.

Leatham, J. H.: Biochemistry of Cystic Ovaries; in G. E. W. Wolstenholme and M. O'Connor, eds.: *Hormone Production in Endocrine Tumours*. Ciba Foundation Colloquia on Endocrinology. Boston, Little, Brown & Co., 1958, p. 173.

Lynch, F. W., and Maxwell, A. F.: Mammoth Ovarian Tumors; in *Pelvic Neoplasms*. New York, Appleton & Co., 1922, p. 403.

Pearse, W. H.: Physiologic Ovarian Cysts. *Ohio State M.J.*, 55: 200, 1959.

Sharnoff, J. G., and Lisa, J. R.: Theca-Cell Cystoma of the Ovary. *Am. J. Obst. & Gynec.*, 51: 253, 1946.

Vara, P., and Niemineva, K.: Small-Cystic Degeneration of Ovaries as an Incidental Finding in Gynecological Laparotomies. *Acta Obst. & Gynec. Scand.*, 31: 94, 1951.

Velardo, J. T.: The Anatomy and Endocrine Physiology of the Female Reproductive System; in *The Endocrinology of Reproduction*. New York, Oxford University Press, 1958, p. 101.

Chapter 51

Clinical Behavior of

Neoplasms of the Ovary

THE TERM "neoplasm of the ovary" has been selected, rather than "tumor," for we now wish to discuss new growths within the ovary rather than physiologic enlargements. Physiologic cysts tend to vary in size periodically and frequently manifest themselves by recognizable symptoms, such as alterations in the menstrual pattern. Neoplasms produce few symptoms, none of which are distinctive, and tend to persist or increase in size rather than become smaller. Some are slow-growing, while others increase in size at an alarming rate.

Ovarian neoplasms may be either benign or malignant, and they are either cystic or solid, or a combination of both. The tumors may be large or small, but are usually mobile and displaceable from the positions in which they are found, unless accidents such as hemorrhage, necrosis or calcification have occurred within them or they are immovable because of their own weight. The pattern of growth in both benign and malignant neoplasms in the early stages of their development is similar. For the most part they are unilateral, but certain tumors such as the serous cystade-noma and dermoid (cystic teratoma) have a greater tendency to be bilateral. A few *NOTE* produce hormones and are considered to be functional, since they influence the regular cyclic menstrual flow in the direction of either excessive bleeding or amenorrhea, depending on whether and how much they produce of the male or female hormones.

What Is the Usual Age Incidence?

Certain ovarian tumors have a predilection for particular age groups. Granulosa cell tumors may appear in childhood and after the menopause. Sarcomas are seen most often in childhood and at the time of puberty. Dermoids (cystic teratomas) may *NOTE* be found in any age group, but are common in childhood, adolescence and in the twenties. Because of their apparent association with pseudohermaphroditism, dysgerminomas are commonly discovered in late adolescence or shortly thereafter. Benign tumors, either cystic or solid, have their greatest concentration in the years preceding the menopause. Cancers can develop at any time during the reproductive years, but the majority are diagnosed after the climacteric.

The problems of the clinical diagnosis and treatment of ovarian neoplasms in the forties or postmenopausal years are not very exacting. The question of whether the tumors found are malignant or even have a neoplastic potentiality is of no great moment, because the treatment of patients who have no desire for, or are no longer capable of, reproduction will usually involve total hysterectomy and bilateral salpingo-oophorectomy, whatever the diagnosis.

In the reproductive years, particularly in the thirties, the correct clinical diagnosis and treatment of ovarian tumors are both more complicated and more important, for it is at this time that the emphasis is on ovarian and uterine conservation in the interests not only of reproduction, but also of endocrine function. Such a policy is justified only if the possibility of malignant disease has been excluded. Proper management calls for mature clinical and surgical judgment. Because of their complicated nature we have elected to discuss the general problems of ovarian neoplasms here, in the thirty- to forty-year age group.

Classification of Ovarian Neoplasms

The study of the origin and behavior of ovarian neoplasms continues to fascinate the embryologist, the pathologist and the clinician. A number of classifications have been devised. To simplify further investigations it is customary to classify ovarian neoplasms according to (a) their histologic structure or (b) their clinical behavior. The embryologist and the pathologist are primarily interested in the origin, structure, function and relation of the ovarian neoplasm to other tumors. The clinician, on the other hand, is mostly concerned with the diagnosis, treatment and prognosis following therapy. The classifications in use reflect these diverging interests. Present knowledge of the embryologic origin of these tumors is too incomplete to work out a practical classification based on histogenesis alone. To have a complete understanding of the adult ovary one would have to be well versed in the intricacies of embryology as well as comparative anatomy. One outstanding gynecologic pathologist has stated that it is manifestly impossible to work out a completely successful practical classification of ovarian tumors. To attempt to list every ovarian tumor, as he suggests, is not very practical either.

Why Do Ovarian Neoplasms Have Such Varied Characteristics?

The mature adult ovary is a complex structure that has evolved through many embryologic stages. It is not surprising, then, to find vestigial remnants of various stages in its embryologic development which are useful no longer, but still persist. It is difficult to find a normal ovary that does not contain some fetal remnants or embryonic rests. Early in fetal life the ovary is indistinguishable from the testis. The ovary is simply like an overdeveloped testicle at this stage, and contains all its basic structure. When the final feminine differentiation is established, the testicular elements tend to disappear, for there is no longer any need for them, but the disappearance is not complete, and some embryologic remnants of the testis remain. It is not surprising, then, that arrhenoblastomas may develop in the ovary.

Early in its embryologic development the ovary rests in a mass of mesenchyma behind the peritoneum in close proximity to the primitive adrenal cortex and kidney. We may then expect to find on rare occasions ovarian neoplasms such as the adrenal rest tumor, renal cell carcinoma or mesonephroma. The ovum is a primordial cell that has an almost limitless potential for new growth. There is practically no limit to the variety of tissues that may appear from the ovum if some suitable stimulus is applied. Dysgerminomas, dermoid cysts, struma ovarii, teratomas and choriocarcinomas may develop when the ovum takes on an abnormal growth pattern. Finally, the ovary contains both connective tissue and reticuloendothelial cells capable of initiating solid new growths, as shown by the appearance of the fibroma, thecoma, granulosa cell tumor and various sarcomas.

A Workable Clinical and Pathologic Classification

It is apparent from the limited discussion above that the ovary has an enormous potentiality to develop cystic and solid growths of all kinds. For practical purposes it is possible to divide ovarian neoplasms arbitrarily into cystic and solid tumors. The epithelial tumors are primarily cystic, while the connective tissue tumors tend to be solid. It is obvious that many cystic tumors will have solid components, while many solid tumors undergo cystic degeneration. Certain rare types of tumor will defy such a classification. Despite these various objections this simple classification has a clinical value of practical nature. It is given in Table 7.

Table 7. A Simple Clinical and Pathologic Classification of Ovarian Neoplasms

BENIGN	MALIGNANT
Cystic:	
Germinal epithelial inclusion	Undifferentiated adenocarcinoma
Serous cystadenoma	Serous cystadenocarcinoma
Papillary serous cystadenoma	Papillary serous cystadenocarcinoma
Pseudomucinous cystadenoma	Pseudomucinous cystadenocarcinoma
Endometrioma (endometriosis)	Adenocarcinoma arising in endometriosis
Dermoid (cystic teratoma)	Malignant dermoid, most often epidermoid carcinoma; several other types
Solid:	
Fibroma	Fibrosarcoma
Thecoma-granulosa-cell tumor	Granulosa-cell-carcinoma with thecomatous foci
Luteoma	——
Brenner tumor	Malignant Brenner tumor
Hilar cell (Leydig cell) tumor	——
Solid teratoma	Teratocarcinoma
	Dysgerminoma
	Embryoma
	Chorionepithelioma
Arrhenoblastoma, Pick adenoma type	Arrhenoblastoma, intermediate and sarcomatous types
Gynandroblastoma	Malignant gynandroblastoma
Struma ovarii	Malignant struma ovarii
——	Mesonephroma
——	Grawitz carcinoma, of renal cell type
Adrenal rest tumor	Carcinoma of adrenal type
——	Metastatic carcinoma (Krukenberg tumor)
Leiomyoma, hemangioma, etc.	Leiomyosarcoma, angiosarcoma, etc.

Clinical Behavior of Neoplasms of the Ovary

Before beginning the detailed discussion of the various types of ovarian neoplasms, their clinical manifestations, diagnosis and treatment, it will be well to discuss the clinical behavior of neoplasms of the ovary in general. Both benign and malignant neoplasms have the same physical findings and growth patterns during the early phase of their development. It is the insidious nature of growth in ovarian neoplasms and the fact that it is almost impossible to distinguish a clinically benign tumor from one that is malignant that make these tumors so dangerous.

Cancer of the ovary appears to be on the increase. In 1930 the death rate from cancer of the ovary was about four in 100,000 women as opposed to 8 in 100,000 in 1955. These figures have been adjusted and corrected for the increase in the number of patients who reach the older age category. It is interesting that this increase was noted while the death rate from cancer of the uterus was falling. Cancer of the ovary was the fifth most common cause of death from cancer in women in 1956, and was only exceeded by malignant disease in the breast, uterus, intestine and stomach. The chances of cancer of the ovary developing today are about one in 100, and only 20 per cent of patients will be salvaged.

NOTE

Since the differentiation cannot be made on the history and physical findings, it is important to keep in mind that every ovarian neoplasm is potentially malignant.

Do Ovarian Neoplasms Produce Symptoms?

Except for the so-called functioning ovarian neoplasms such as the feminizing tumors of the granulosa cell, theca cell or its variant the luteoma, and the masculinizing tumors such as the arrhenoblastoma and adrenal-like neoplasms, ovarian growths, whether benign or malignant, rarely produce any symptoms that are pathognomonic of neoplastic disease. When they do, there is nothing about the symptoms that will permit differentiation between a benign and a malignant tumor, much less give any indication of the pathologic nature of the growth.

Symptoms of Cystic Ovarian Tumors

The type and severity of the symptoms depend largely on the size and position of the cyst and whether the tumor, by the manner of its growth, is prone to accidents that may occur within it. The symptoms are chiefly (*a*) enlargement of the abdomen, (*b*) a sense of fullness and bearing-down discomfort in the abdomen and pelvis, (*c*) pressure on adjacent organs, such as bladder and rectum, and (*d*) varicosities and edema of the lower extremities, secondary to obstruction of the venous or lymphatic return. Vaginal bleeding is rarely a symptom unless the tumor has a functional component. Painful symptoms appear only if the tumor becomes impacted in the pelvis or the blood supply of the cyst becomes compromised.

NOTE

In most instances the patient is unaware of the presence of an ovarian neoplasm until some complication arises within the tumor to direct attention to it. This holds true whether the tumor is large or small. It is amazing how large some of these tumors become without the patient's suspecting it. Often the first thing the woman notices is that she can no longer put on a new suit or dress because of her enlarging girth. This distresses her to such an extent that she seeks medical advice to find out the reason for her embarrassing predicament. If the neoplasm, because of its size, remains confined to the pelvis, the patient may have frequency of urination as the tumor presses on the bladder. Rarely is the bowel habit altered. When the tumor rises out of the pelvis, embarrassment of respiration and heart action may occur as the enlarging tumor presses on the diaphragm. A cyst often impacts in the lower pelvic cavity and blocks the venous return to such an extent that the patient has engorged veins on the abdominal wall, as well as hemorrhoids. The lymphatics may become obstructed in the same manner, producing edema of the lower extremities and of the vulva.

Pain is rarely a symptom of ovarian neoplasm as long as the regular pattern of growth is not altered and free expansion is possible. Normally, small ovarian cysts drop into the pelvis as their weight increases. As the tumor grows, it rises out of the pelvis when there is a sufficiently long pedicle, which is usually the case. Occasionally the tumor lacks a pedicle or adhesions are present as a result of a previous pelvic inflammation, and the tumor can no longer rise up into the abdominal cavity. The patient may then have pain, as well as the same pressure symptoms that one notes when large tumors are impacted in the pelvis. In most instances pain means that an accident has occurred in the tumor after constriction of its blood supply.

What Complications Arise in Cystic Ovarian Neoplasms That Will Produce Symptoms?

Both benign and malignant cystic neoplasms in the early stages of their existence not only develop along the same lines, but also actually look alike on gross external inspection. The neoplasms tend to be unilateral, lie relatively free in the abdominal cavity and derive their blood supply through a pedicle. These growth characteristics tend to make cystic tumors vulnerable to several complications that will produce symptoms severe enough to call attention to the presence of an abdominal or pelvic mass.

① TORSION OF THE PEDICLE.   Interference with the blood supply in the pedicle of either a benign or malignant cystic tumor will produce pathologic changes within the neoplasm and varying amounts of pain. The restriction of blood supply to the tumor can produce *(a)* hemorrhage and congestion within the cyst cavity, *(b)* necrosis, *(c)* infection, and finally *(d)* rupture, depending on the extent of torsion of the pedicle. **NOTE** Whenever the patient or physician suddenly becomes aware of the presence of an abdominal or pelvic mass, or a known tumor dramatically increases in size, one should suspect that torsion of the pedicle has occurred, particularly if the rapid enlargement is accompanied by acute abdominal pain. The moderate-sized tumors that rise out of the pelvis and have a relatively thin pedicle are more likely to get into trouble than the larger cysts that tend to drop into the pelvis and remain fixed because of their increased weight.

The severity of the symptoms produced depends not only on the extent of the torsion, but also on how rapidly it occurs. In the majority of instances little in the way of symptoms will be noted if only a partial twist occurs in the pedicle. A full turn of the pedicle is possible, if it does not occur too suddenly. The embarrassment to the circulation will cause a slow hemorrhage in the tumor and an increase in its size, but it will frequently produce only minor discomfort, though the tumor will be sensitive to palpation. Acute and severe pain appears with drastic suddenness when obstruction is complete and occurs rapidly. The patient will then have vomiting, along with the pain, abdominal distention, local tenderness, and fever. The acute symptoms usually develop more gradually and become more distressing over the next few days as the abdomen gets larger.

② HEMORRHAGE AND CONGESTION IN THE CYST.   When the twist in the pedicle of the neoplastic cyst is incomplete, only the venous return is affected, and arterial circulation is unimpaired. The veins in the pedicle and in the tumor itself become engorged, and hemorrhage occurs both in the cyst wall and within the cavity. This

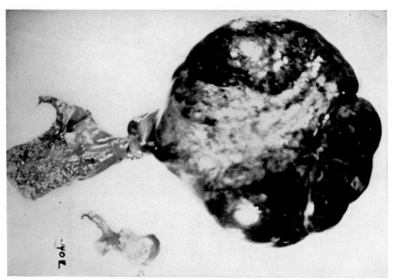

Fig. 51-1.   A twisted pedicle has resulted in hemorrhagic infarction of this ovarian cyst. Microscopically, it was too necrotic for accurate classification.

causes the cyst to enlarge, and the resulting pain is similar to that which follows the distention of any hollow viscus. If the hemorrhage is extensive and the cavity distends too rapidly, rupture of the cystic neoplasm may take place.

The gross appearance of the partially infarcted cyst, adjacent fallopian tube and broad ligament is both striking and characteristic. The cyst itself is dark purple, and the serosal surface is no longer shiny, but rather dull and inert (Fig. 51–1). The veins in the pedicle are distended and frequently thrombosed on both sides of the twist. The process is so extensive that the veins of the broad ligament and uterus are also distended. Edema is noted in the fallopian tube and the adjacent parametrium.

③ NECROSIS.   When the process progresses to the point at which the arterial blood supply also is compromised, necrotizing disintegration takes place within the cyst wall. The cyst and its contents then form an excellent culture medium and frequently become infected. If the arterial occlusion occurs gradually, the tumor may pick up a sufficient blood supply from the omentum to prevent infarctive necrosis of the cyst wall. Actually, it may become totally detached from the ovarian blood vessels and exist as an isolated tumor in the omentum, from which it acquires its blood supply. Sudden severe twists cause such rapid and profound disturbance in the main blood supply that necrosis takes place before the tumor has a chance to acquire any collateral circulation.

④ RUPTURE OF OVARIAN CYSTS.   On rare occasions the intracystic tension becomes so intense, because of hemorrhage or infection, that the weakened tumor capsule gives way, and the irritating contents either leak or are spilled in quantity into the abdominal cavity. Rupture of an ovarian cystic neoplasm can be a serious complication, particularly if one of the large distended veins is torn. Fatal intraabdominal hemorrhage can occur. The symptoms would be similar to those of any severe intraperitoneal hemorrhage. Immediate operative intervention is indicated.

Rupture of the cystic tumor may occur with a completely adequate blood supply. Cysts have been known to rupture in the course of an abdominal delivery, for example, as the fetus produces pressure on the wall. Also, ovarian cysts have been known to rupture after a fall or a direct blow on the abdominal wall. If the ovarian neoplastic cyst is malignant, the invasion by carcinoma of the restraining outer capsule of the ovarian cyst may weaken a vulnerable point through which spontaneous rupture may take place.

What Happens If a Cyst Ruptures? The patient's response to rupture of a cystic tumor depends primarily on the nature of the cyst contents and how much they irritate the peritoneum. One would expect little reaction from the thin serous fluid that escaped from a simple serous cyst or serous cystadenoma. On the other hand, the hair and fatty contents of a dermoid cyst or the gelatinous mucinous secretion of a pseudomucinous cyst may irritate the peritoneum so that a localized pelvic peritonitis usually results. As long as the cyst contents are not infected at the time of rupture, a general peritonitis should not be anticipated. The escaping material tends to accumulate in the cul-de-sac or gravitates along the lateral gutters to localize in the subphrenic regions above the kidneys. In both places the presence of such a foreign material creates a protective response, and the collection becomes walled off by adhesions. Organized collections of this sort are often tender to touch and give rise to such symptoms as pain upon exertion or intercourse. The symptoms will be those accompanying any pelvic abscess.

⑤ INFECTION IN THE CYST. When the blood supply of the pedicle of an ovarian cyst has been compromised, the viability of the cyst wall naturally is jeopardized. Coils of small intestine, omentum and adhesions attempt to wall off the damaged cyst. The cyst may then become infected, as bacterial contaminants pass through the bowel wall into the cyst contents, which provide a perfect culture medium. Small cysts are far more likely to become infected, particularly the dermoid (cystic teratomatous) variety. Sepsis is rarely overwhelming, but more often of a low-grade smouldering variety. Not infrequently the pus drained from such cysts is found to be sterile. It is an interesting observation that only a portion of the cyst cavity may be infected, particularly when the growth pattern of the tumor tends to set up loculated compart-

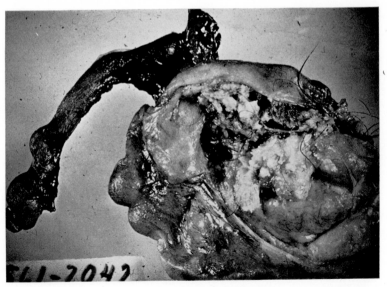

Fig. 51-2. Degeneration and rupture of an ovarian dermoid cyst release the sebaceous contents, which are extremely irritating to peritoneal surfaces. The abundant hair within the cystic teratoma is also evident.

ments within the cysts, such as one sees in the dermoid. The protective adhesions that develop in response to infection within the cyst may bind it to adjacent organs such as the bladder, rectum, small intestine or vagina. In this position the cyst may rupture through the wall of the attached viscus and discharge its contents into the lumen. Rarely do they rupture into the general peritoneal cavity. Dermoids may rupture into the rectum, but they seem to have a particular affinity for the bladder (Fig. 51–2).

If the neoplastic cyst does not rupture, but simply becomes incarcerated in the pelvis by the adhesions resulting from the pelvic peritonitis, the patient may have pelvic pain, dyspareunia, constipation or frequency of urination secondary to the pressure of the tumor mass. If the infectious process is acute, the patient may have an elevated temperature and be ill, but for the most part the symptoms are those of chronic pelvic inflammatory disease.

What Are the Physical Findings of Neoplastic Ovarian Cysts?

The physical findings in cystic ovarian neoplasms vary with the size of the actual tumor, its position and whether the cyst is bound down by adhesions.

SMALL CYSTS.   The smaller cysts are best felt by rectum. A tense elastic swelling is usually felt in the cul-de-sac posterior to the uterus, which moves independently

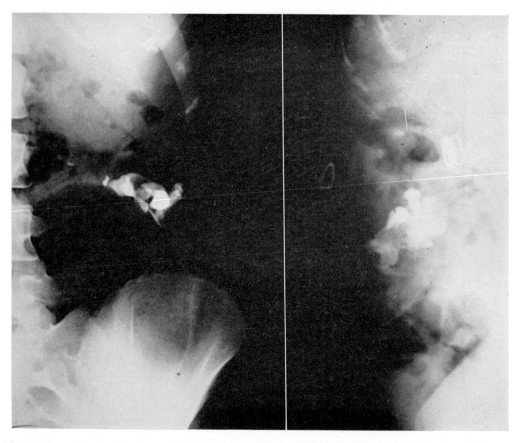

Fig. 51-3.   Anteroposterior and lateral x-ray films show the teeth and associated bone sometimes present in cystic ovarian teratomas (dermoid cysts).

of the cyst. Because these cysts are usually pedunculated, their point of origin often does not correspond to the position in which the cyst is palpated. A pedunculated left ovarian cyst, for example, may fall into the pouch of Douglas, partially rotate on its pedicle and lie in the right vault. Because they usually are free of adhesions, the tumors are movable without pain and are readily displaced from their pelvic position. If the cysts are trapped in the cul-de-sac by adhesions, palpation will produce tenderness, and the cyst cannot be moved. For the most part cysts are smooth walled, but solid knoblike prominences may be felt.

Any solid area within a cyst should be regarded with grave suspicion. The firm portion of the cyst may be simply a loculated area in a dermoid, but one cannot exclude the possibility of malignant disease. An x-ray film of the pelvis may be helpful in establishing the true nature of the tumor, particularly if it contains bone, teeth or cartilage (Fig. 51–3). The likelihood that the palpable tumor is a dermoid (cystic teratoma) will be heightened if it occupies a position anterior to the uterus overlying the bladder, for dermoids are prone to appear there.

NOTE

NOTE

MODERATE-SIZED CYSTS.   Larger cysts may be felt on abdominal as well as pelvic examination. Occasionally the upper border may be outlined lying in a midline position, but more often the cyst occupies one flank or the other. Sometimes it is possible to introduce the examining fingers between the symphysis and the lower border of the tumor, but the majority will descend into the pelvis, where the lower border of the tumor can be felt filling the cul-de-sac. Any irregularity or solid area within the tumor should raise the index of suspicion of the possibility of cancer, though the protuberance may simply be a sacculated area in either a benign serous or pseudomucinous cystadenoma.

How Does One Make a Diagnosis of Accompanying Ascites?

Many ovarian cysts are accompanied by the production of ascites. The association in gynecologic patients is more common with malignant ovarian neoplasms, but the presence of ascites cannot be considered pathognomonic, for it occurs with many benign solid and benign cystic tumors. It can be a difficult point in differential diagnosis to distinguish between a large ovarian cyst that occupies the patient's flank and a moderate-sized tumor with ascites.

Percussion of the flank usually gives a resonant sound when ovarian cysts are unaccompanied by ascites. Demonstration of a fluid wave may be so definite that there can be no question but that ascites is present; however, occasionally the disturbance of the fluid content within the cyst may produce a thrill that cannot be distinguished from free abdominal fluid.

The evaluation of minimal degrees of ascites is even more complicated and often unsatisfactory. Demonstration of the so-called puddle sign is said to be effective in detecting small amounts of intra-abdominal fluid.

TECHNIQUE OF ELICITING THE PUDDLE SIGN.   The patient is permitted to lie in a prone position for five minutes before being placed on all fours with the abdomen dependent. A stethoscope is then placed on the lowest position on the abdominal wall as the surgeon snaps the flank with thumb and forefinger. This method of percussion is continued as the stethoscope is gradually advanced toward the opposite flank. Fluid is believed to be present when the observer notes an increase in the intensity and nature of the percussion note as the stethoscope is moved toward the opposite flank. The patient is then placed in a sitting position, and the stethoscope is replaced in the original spot of greatest dependence. The percussion note should now be loud and clear. By this maneuver it is possible to differentiate between free intra-abdominal fluid and that trapped in an ovarian cyst.

Large Ovarian Cysts

In this present day one rarely sees the hugely distended abdomen due to excessively large ovarian cysts. Several hundred giant ovarian cysts weighing over 60 pounds are recorded in medical history. They can achieve their size only through the patient's neglect. The skin of the abdomen is tense, and the umbilicus is almost invariably everted. A dull percussion note is found over the entire area of the abdominal wall, except in the flanks and in the upper portion of the abdomen near the sternum, where the stomach becomes compressed. Dilated veins and lymphatics often course over the distended abdominal wall. The cul-de-sac is usually full and tense on vaginal and rectal examinations. With so much fluid in the cyst itself, it is difficult to decide whether the fluid wave is due to intrinsic or extrinsic accumulation.

Interligamentous Cysts

When the cyst has no pedicle, it may expand in its growth between the leaves of the broad ligament. If it is large enough, it may impinge on the iliac vessels and produce venous stasis in the veins of the lower extremity. As it grows in this confined space, the uterus is usually displaced to the opposite side. By its nature the neoplasm cannot ascend into the abdominal cavity, and the lower border of the cyst completely fills the pelvis and obliterates the cul-de-sac. Because of its position it cannot be displaced on vaginal or rectal examination.

Solid Neoplasms of the Ovary

The solid tumors—either benign or malignant—like the neoplastic cysts just considered, produce nothing in the way of symptoms that one may regard as pathognomonic. Though they also tend to be unilateral and to grow on a pedicle that contains their blood supply, they are far less likely to twist on the pedicle. Because of their solid nature the patient often becomes aware of their presence earlier than she might if the tumor were cystic; simply because they are so heavy the patient notices the discomfort sooner. They are far more dangerous than their cystic neoplastic counterparts, for all except the fibroma, thecoma and Brenner tumor have significant malignant potentialities. Clinically, the benign tumor cannot be distinguished from the malignant neoplasm. A few have distinctive features, but the majority do not. The fibroma of the ovary may be associated with ascites and right-sided hydrothorax (Meigs's syndrome); the dysgerminoma of the ovary may be associated with an enlarged clitoris and other suggestions of pseudohermaphroditism; but neither tumor has a distinctive train of symptoms. Other ovarian neoplasms produce ascites, and the enlargement of the clitoris could be due to a masculinizing neoplasm of the ovary, such as an arrhenoblastoma. Since the differentiation between the benign and malignant solid tumors is so difficult and the incidence of cancer is so high, practically speaking, we must assume that all solid ovarian neoplasms are malignant until proved benign by histologic review after excision.

The physical findings are not very helpful, except in distinguishing a solid from a cystic neoplastic tumor. In most instances the former have a firmer consistency that suggests their solid nature. For this reason the outline of the tumor is much more definite. Many of the solid neoplasms have cystic components in them, however, and it may be impossible to determine on examination which is the predominant element. They can only be classified grossly as being semisolid and semicystic.

In many instances it is impossible to decide whether the solid tumor felt on vaginal or rectal examination is a laterally placed pedunculated fibroid or a solid tumor of the ovary. If ascites can be demonstrated, the solid adnexal tumor is probably ovarian, not a fibroid, but the surgeon has so little else to go on that it should be an invariable rule that patients with solid, laterally placed tumors should have an abdominal exploration. Not only is the incidence of cancer high, but the salvage rate for solid tumors is appreciably lower than for cystic or semicystic ovarian neoplasms.

How Does the Gynecologist Make the Distinction between Benign and Malignant Ovarian Neoplasms?

It is evident from the previous discussion that there are no characteristic symptoms or clinical signs to aid in the separation of benign from malignant ovarian neoplastic growths. They have the same origin and are subject to the same complications. Moreover, they look absolutely alike when they are seen grossly at the time the abdomen is opened. Of course there is no particular problem in making the distinction at operation when papillary carcinomatous projections are seen on the external surface of the tumor or when carcinomatous seeding has occurred in the omentum and throughout the peritoneal cavity. We are primarily interested here in the early carcinoma that lies hidden within the interior of a cystic neoplasm or beneath the capsule of a solid one. The final diagnosis of both cystic and solid tumors awaits histologic scrutiny.

WHAT CAN WE LEARN FROM INSPECTION OF THE CYST WALL AND ITS CONTENTS? Since there is no other way of making a differential diagnosis between a benign and a malignant tumor, it is axiomatic that all tumors should be sectioned in the operating room after their removal. If the tumor is cystic, the contents may provide a lead and a strong index of suspicion that malignancy may be present. The two most common cystic tumors with malignant potential are the serous cystadenoma and the pseudomucinous cystadenoma. The former is said to have a malignant potential approximately seven times greater than that of the pseudomucinous cyst. Thus the index of suspicion is higher. Since the serous cystadenoma appears anywhere in the reproductive life of women, even in infancy, and occurs bilaterally in roughly 33 per cent, it is important to rule out cancer before leaving the uterus and the other ovary, which we would like to do in the young patient who never has had a chance to produce a family.

The distinction, based on the content of the cyst, is obvious. The serous cystadenoma will have clear serous fluid, in contrast to the thicker, sticky gelatinous secretion found in the pseudomucinous tumors. Fluid colored with blood is suggestive of cancer.

The internal surface of the walls of most ovarian cystic neoplasms is predominantly smooth, gray and glistening, whether the cyst is unilocular or multilocular. Places where sessile or pedunculated papillary granular white processes project internally are of the most interest. If the pedicles and bases of the adenomatous or papillary projections are resilient, rubbery or fibrous, this gross observation favors a

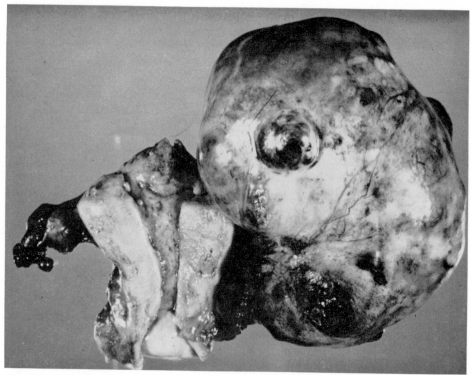

Fig. 51-4.   A large ovarian tumor, partly cystic and partly solid, of suspicious appearance. The granular and hemorrhagic areas in the tumor capsule, such as near the bottom, are suggestive of carcinoma that has penetrated from inside the mass.

benign neoplasm. If they are hard, gritty or fixed, carcinoma is likely. Papillary processes growing in continuity from within the cyst through its wall and projecting externally also almost inevitably represent carcinoma with invasion.

OF WHAT SIGNIFICANCE ARE THE SOLID COMPONENTS WITHIN A CYST AS THEY APPLY TO MALIGNANT DISEASE?   It is a general observation that the more solid the tumor, the greater the chance of malignancy and the worse the prognosis. If cancer is present, it will be found in the firm hard areas at the base of the papillary projections within the cyst cavity (Fig. 51–4). In the normal progress of development malignant disease in the ovary begins in these trabeculations, and goes on to spread along the inner surface before finally invading the capsule. Finally the papillary excrescences appear on the external surface and seed from there throughout the peritoneal cavity, including the omentum (Fig. 51–5). It must be kept in mind that the patient, however, may have a large cyst with only a small area of malignancy in its interior.

A biopsy should be taken from any hard area within a cyst cavity and the material subjected to frozen section examination. If the foci of malignant change are microscopic or cytologic, it may be too much to expect the pathologist to make the differentiation without permanent sections for review. Frozen section has its limitations, but it is far better than submitting the entire cyst unopened to the pathologist for routine reports after leaving the uterus and other ovary intact.

If cystic areas are seen within the substance of a solid tumor after it has been sectioned, it would be unwise to assume that such areas simply represent cystic

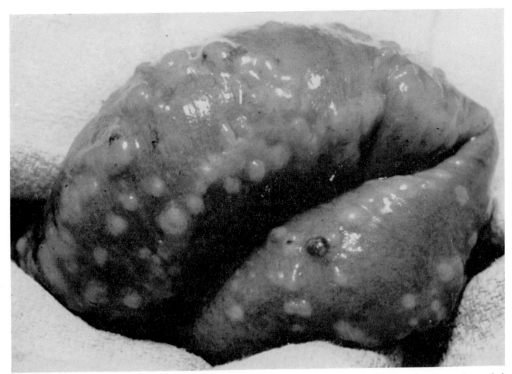

Fig. 51-5.   Widespread peritoneal metastases from ovarian carcinoma on the serosal surface of the small intestine.

degeneration in a benign tumor, for such findings are noted in both benign and malignant neoplasms. Many cystic ovarian neoplasms contain solid portions, while cysts are found within otherwise solid ovarian tumors. Whenever solid areas are found in an ovarian neoplasm, cancer must be ruled out. It is a sad commentary on modern gynecologic surgery that so many ovarian neoplasms are found to be malignant only when the operation has been completed and the pathologist has made his final report.

How Frequently Are Psammoma Bodies Found in Malignant Ovarian Tumors?   Another factor that may help at least in raising the index of suspicion of carcinoma is the presence of psammoma bodies or, more properly, calcospherites. These areas appear in the x-ray films of the pelvis as granular, flaky or fingernail-sized patches of calcium scattered throughout the tumor. These are usually found in actively proliferating growths and do not represent degeneration with calcification. Psammoma bodies are not pathognomonic of malignant disease, for they may appear in benign tumors such as ovarian cystadenofibromas and uterine fibroids, but when they are seen, one should become suspicious. Grossly, they may manifest themselves as local hard areas whose consistency varies in proportion to the amount of calcium they contain.

Microscopically, typical psammoma bodies appear as small, concentrically laminated, rounded objects with basophilic staining qualities due to their calcium content. They are approximately twice the size of a capillary in diameter, and lie individually scattered through the stroma of cystadenomas, cystadenocarcinomas and solid adenocarcinomas. They are also termed "calcospherites" to distinguish them from the true psammoma bodies originally described in the meninges (Fig. 51–6).

Calcospherites occur with germinal inclusion cysts, endometriosis and cyst-

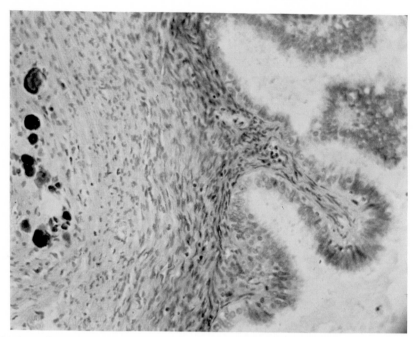

Fig. 51-6.   Laminated calcified bodies of psammoma type in the stroma of a papillary ovarian cystadenocarcinoma. The epithelium in this area is not definitely malignant, although the cells are piled up in a suspicious manner. Both psammoma bodies and epithelial palisading are indications that further search may demonstrate an invasive ovarian carcinoma.

adenofibromas, as well as with the benign and malignant ovarian tumors mentioned above. It is because they are generally more abundant in carcinomas that occasionally an x-ray study may be of assistance in diagnosis. Of course, not all ovarian tumors of any type mentioned necessarily contain psammoma bodies. Also, such objects are found in papillary tumors of other organs, such as the thyroid, lung and pancreas. The basis of their formation is unknown.

REFERENCES

Abel, S.: Ovarian Carcinoma; Diagnosis and Treatment. *Missouri Med.*, 54: 423, 1957.

Beck, R. P., and Latour, J. P. A.: A Review of 1019 Benign Ovarian Neoplasms. *Obst. & Gynec.*, 16: 479, 1960.

Corscaden, J. A.: *Gynecologic Cancer.* 2nd Ed. Baltimore, Williams & Wilkins Company, 1956, p. 472.

Davis, B. A., Latour, J. P. A., and Philpott, N. W.: Primary Carcinoma of the Ovary. *Surg., Gynec. & Obst.*, 102: 565, 1956.

Dockerty, M. B.: Ovarian Neoplasms. Collective Review of Recent Literature. *Internat. Abst. Surg.*, 81: 179, 1945.

Dougherty, C. M., Aucoin, R., and Cotten, N.: Diagnosis of Cystadenocarcinoma of the Ovary. *Obst. & Gynec.*, 18: 81, 1961.

Gardiner, G. A., and Slate, J.: Malignant Tumors of the Ovary. *Am. J. Obst. & Gynec.*, 70: 554, 1955.

Griswold, M. H., Wilder, C. S., Cutler, S. J., and Pollock, E. S.: Cancer in Connecticut 1935–1951. Hartford, Connecticut State Department of Health, 1955.

Hesseltine, H. C., and Smith, R. L.: Ovarian Malignancy. *Am. J. Obst. & Gynec.*, 72: 1326, 1956.

Javert, C. T., and Rascoe, R. R.: Serous Cystadenocarcinoma of the Ovary. A Review of 127 Cases. *S. Clin. North Amer.*, 33: 557, 1953.

Kent, S. W., and McKay, D. G.: Primary Cancer of the Ovary. An Analysis of 34 Cases. *Am. J. Obst. & Gynec.*, 80: 430, 1960.

Kerr, H. D., and Elkins, H. B.: Carcinoma of the Ovary. *Am. J. Roentgenol.*, 66: 184, 1951.

Kottmeier, H.L.: The Classification and Treatment of Ovarian Tumors. *Acta Obst. et Gynec. Scand.*, 31: 313, 1952.

Marks, J. H., and Wittenborg, M. H.: Results of Treatment of Carcinoma of the Ovary with Data on the Age Incidence of This Disease. *Surg., Gynec. & Obst.*, 87: 541, 1948.

Meigs, J. V.: Cancer of the Ovary. *Surg., Gynec. & Obst.*, 71: 44, 1940.

Idem: Medical Progress: Gynecology: Neoplasms of the Ovary. *New England J. Med.*, 228: 52, 1943.

Munnell, E. W., and Taylor, H. C., Jr.: Ovarian Carcinoma. A Review of 200 Primary and 51 Secondary Cases. *Am. J. Obst. & Gynec.*, 58: 943, 1949.

Pearse, W. H., and Behrman, S. J.: Carcinoma of the Ovary. *Obst. & Gynec.*, 3: 32, 1954.

Pemberton, F. A.: Carcinoma of the Ovary. *Am. J. Obst. & Gynec.*, 40: 751, 1940.

Taylor, H. C., Jr.: The Diagnosis and Treatment of Ovarian Carcinoma. *Clin. Obst. & Gynec.*, Dec., 1958, p. 1078.

Ullery, J. C., and Boutselis, J. G.: Gross Pathology, Diagnosis and Clinical Management of Ovarian Enlargements. *Obst. & Gynec. Surv.*, 14: 635, 1959.

Wharton, L. R.: Two Cases of Supernumerary Ovary and One of Accessory Ovary, with an Analysis of Previously Reported Cases. *Am. J. Obst. & Gynec.*, 78: 1101, 1959.

Wheelock, F. C., Fennell, R. H., Jr., and Meigs, J. V.: Carcinoma of the Ovary: Clinical and Pathological Evaluation. *New England J. Med.*, 245: 447, 1951.

Chapter 52

Cystic Tumors of the Ovary

SEROUS CYST OF OVARY

THE SIMPLE serous cystoma is the most common of all the benign cysts of the ovary, excluding the functional types such as follicular and corpus luteum cysts. Clinically, it is indistinguishable from any other ovarian cyst, either benign or malignant, for they all have the same gross external characteristics. Because it derives its blood supply from a pedicle, it tends to float around in the pelvis, occupying many positions. Normally one feels it behind the uterus in the cul-de-sac, but it is easily displaced from this position, for it lies free in the abdominal cavity with little to hold it. For this reason it may escape detection even when of fair size. Because the tumor is pedunculated, it is subject to torsion of the pedicle. Acute pain may arise suddenly as the blood supply to the cyst is cut off. The extent of the pain and its duration depend on how rapidly and completely spontaneous relaxation of the torsion occurs. These benign neoplasms are often large and tend to be bilateral.

Treatment

NOTE

When a cyst is discovered, immediate operation is advised for two reasons: ① The cyst may occupy only a portion of the ovary. If this is true, the cyst can be excised without removing the ovary completely. Eventually if no attempt is made to save it the entire ovary will be destroyed by the cyst. ② It is impossible to distinguish between a benign and a malignant cyst on the basis of history or palpation alone. This distinction also cannot be made at the time of abdominal exploration by holding the cyst in your hand. The surface cover of the large tense cyst is smooth and pearly white, with dilated veins running over it. The cyst may be thin-walled, but it is usually tough, and no firm portion, other than that representing the normal ovary, can be felt on it (Fig. 52–1).

On opening the cyst in the operating room after its removal clear watery, pale yellow serous fluid appears, and the typical unilocular cyst cavity has a smooth, shining internal surface epithelium. There are no papillary projections or solid areas in evidence to suggest malignant disease. On microscopic section the epithelium is low cuboidal in type and devoid of any sign of anaplasia.

Pathologically, serous cysts are recognized by epithelial linings composed of cells resembling fallopian tubal epithelium. Germinal inclusion cysts also contain serous fluid, but their cuboidal epithelium lacks tubal characteristics. Simple cysts may con-

744

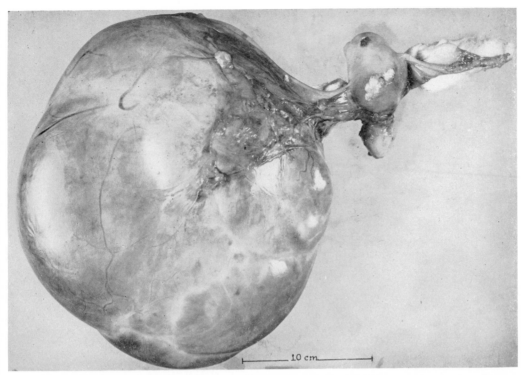

Fig. 52-1. A large serous cyst, or cystoma, of the ovary is typically spherical, smooth and translucent. Near its hilus, toward the top, is a nubbin of uninvolved ovary. The uterus and contralateral tube and ovary are of normal size, but appear small by comparison.

tain serous fluid, but their lining is so stretched or degenerated that the cell type cannot be identified. Hilar or rete ovarian cysts are lined by epithelium that resembles the male vas deferens.

There is nothing complicated about the treatment. If the cysts are bilateral and large and have destroyed all normal ovarian tissue, total hysterectomy and bilateral salpingo-oophorectomy should be done. If the serous cyst has replaced practically all ovarian tissue, the affected ovary should be removed entirely. The cyst should be excised from the rest of the ovary if there is sufficient uninvolved ovarian tissue.

NOTE

PARA-OVARIAN CYSTS

These tumors are relatively common among benign neoplasms in the 30- to 40-year age group, since they tend to occur at this time and do make up about 10 per cent of all adnexal growths. They rarely are subject to the complications noted in other ovarian cysts, simply because they expand into the leaves of the broad ligament and do not have a pedicle. Any symptoms produced are secondary to the displacement of the uterus caused by the expansive growth of the tumor, which pushes the uterus up and away from the cyst. There are no peculiar characteristics that permit a differentiation before operation between a primary ovarian neoplasm that has invaded the broad ligament and a true cyst of para-ovarian origin.

NOTE

The gross appearance of the tumor at operation is characteristic. The tumor elevates the uterus and forces it laterally away from the cyst. The tube is always

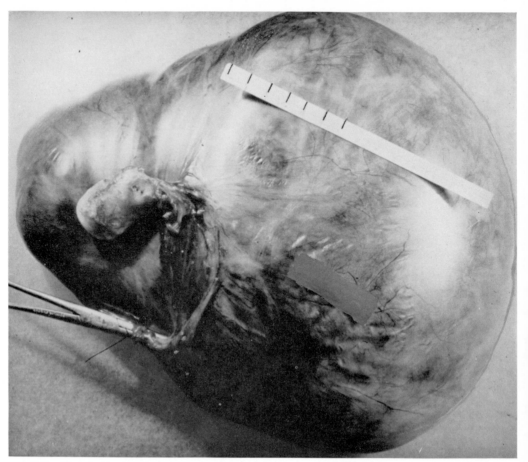

Fig. 52-2.   An unusually large para-ovarian cyst, oriented to demonstrate the fallopian tube stretched over its surface near the hemostat. The müllerian and wolffian subtypes appear grossly indistinguishable.

elongated and is always stretched out and movable over the surface of the tumor (Fig. 52–2). On opening the cyst the fluid content is exactly like that found in a serous ovarian cyst. The cavity contains no compartments or trabeculations, and the lining epithelium is smooth and glistening.

NOTE   Pathologically, the para-ovarian cyst may be lined either by müllerian epithelium that resembles fallopian tube or by wolffian epithelium that is less regular and less acidophilic and imitates renal tubules. Normally, from the lateral end of the tube there hangs a hydatid of Morgagni, in essence a pedunculated müllerian cyst. An enlarged variant of this, called a Kobelt cyst, is sometimes classed with the other para-ovarian cysts.

Treatment

Simple excision of the cyst is all that is required, but this may be technically more difficult than removal of a pedunculated serous ovarian cyst. These cysts are initially blended with the peritoneum overlying the broad ligament, particularly in the region of the uterus. The cyst almost invariably ruptures when attempts are made to remove it. The serous fluid content is nonirritating, and no sequelae follow inadvertent spillage. Para-ovarian cysts are not precancerous in their ordinary life history.

PSEUDOMUCINOUS CYSTADENOMA

The pseudomucinous ovarian cyst is found almost as often as the serous cystadenoma. In most series it represents approximately 25 per cent of ovarian tumors. For the most part there is nothing about its outer appearance, pattern of growth, physical findings or symptomatology to distinguish it from other common cystic tumors, such as the simple or serous cyst or a serous cystadenoma in the early stage of development. Mucinous cysts do tend to have a more nodular and lobulated appearance than the serous cystadenoma, largely because the majority are multilocular. This is due to the formation of daughter cysts within the cavity (Fig. 52–3, *A*).

NOTE

These tumors vary in size, but may expand to huge proportions. Since they are unilateral for the most part and receive their blood supply through a pedicle, they frequently undergo torsion and are prone to circulatory changes in parts of the cyst. Such accidents produce the adhesions that attach the omentum, small intestine and sigmoid to the tumor, particularly on its under side.

This tumor may be found in any age group, but it is rarely encountered before puberty. Approximately 40 per cent are found after the climacteric. The malignant potential is in the range of 5 per cent. Most of these occur in patients after the menopause. This fact, plus the observation that the pseudomucinous tumors are apt to be unilateral, makes the problem of surgical management in the patient who is still in the reproductive age group less complicated. Since the chance of malignancy is less, and the other ovary is unlikely to be the site of another tumor, one can afford to be more conservative and avoid removal of the uterus and other ovary.

NOTE

The contents of the pseudomucinous cyst are characteristic. The nature of the fluid content varies from a stringy, sticky mucoid secretion to that having the consistency of wet glue. The gelatinous material is tenacious and sticks to everything it touches. It is, however, water-soluble and can be washed from the surgeon's gloves. It is this adhesive property that creates the pseudomyxoma peritonaei described sometimes following rupture or spillage from the cyst. The color of the mucus ranges from yellow to brown, depending upon how much hemorrhage has occurred within the cyst cavity. It tends to be pale near the capsular lining where it is produced, but becomes darker as one approaches the center of the cyst.

NOTE

The interior of the cavity of the pseudomucinous cystadenoma is also different from that of the serous cystadenoma, in contrast to their similarity in appearance before the cyst is opened. The pseudomucinous cyst is frequently multilocular, with varying numbers of components containing isolated accumulations of gelatinous mucoid secretions. These are the daughter cysts. Though there is a wide variety of compartments, both large and small, usually one central cavity predominates. The formation of loculated cavities within a central cyst may be an indication of the proliferative capacity of the lining epithelium. Less often one finds a single large cavity. The inner surface of the cyst cavity is smooth, but covered by adherent gelatinous secretions. The cyst wall varies in thickness. In general it is fairly thick and fibrous, but in other areas it thins out appreciably, and bosses are seen on the external surfaces. It is not an uncommon finding to note firm or hard areas in the external capsule.

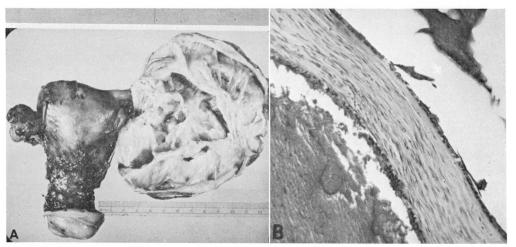

Fig. 52-3.   *A,* Multilocular mucinous or pseudomucinous cystadenoma of average size, after the extremely sticky cyst contents have been removed. The outer surface may be bosselated, but it has a smooth, shining appearance. *B,* The basophilic mucinous secretion is seen in the cyst spaces, which are lined by flattened epithelial cells that contain mucous droplets.

These areas are dangerous, for it is here that the pathologist is most likely to discover malignant changes. Unlike in the serous cystadenoma, papillary projections are relatively uncommon. Approximately 10 per cent of the pseudomucinous cystadenomas are papillary. Such cystadenomas are apt to represent a conglomeration of small cysts covered with papillary growths, together with the characteristic mucinous fluid contents. Rarely the pseudomucinous cyst appears in solid form.

The microscopic appearance is characteristic. The chief feature is a single layer of cylindrical cells with the nuclei at the bases. Often these cells assume a goblet shape, owing to distention of the cytoplasm by mucus (Fig. 52–3, *B*). An adenomatous pattern occurs when the cells are actively proliferating. To make room for more cells the lining tends to pile up and form ridges that invaginate into the wall of the original cyst, thus creating daughter cysts. These are the firm areas that arouse the clinical suspicion of malignant alteration.

The secreted material is true mucus. The old name "pseudomucinous" referred to chemical changes of the mucus now recognized as representing simply staleness. Nowadays many prefer to call these tumors "mucinous cystadenomas."

Malignant Change in a Pseudomucinous Cystadenoma

Carcinoma appears in an otherwise benign ovarian neoplasm as a result of local malignant alterations. The first sign of neoplastic growth most often appears in the form of papillary projections within one of the locules. The malignant potential of the pseudomucinous cystadenoma is therefore not great, for fundamentally it is not a papillary tumor. Approximately 90 per cent show no evidence of papillary growth. Carcinoma is said to occur in only 5 per cent of all pseudomucinous cystadenomas. This figure is appreciably less than for the other common cystic ovarian neoplasm, the serous cystadenoma, which is primarily a progressively proliferating tumor.

We have noted that a benign cyst cannot be distinguished externally from its malignant counterpart so long as cancer is confined to the interior. It is likewise impossible to differentiate a pseudomucinous cystadenoma from a serous cystadenoma on external gross appearance. The pseudomucinous cystadenoma and carcinoma tend to attain a larger size than any other cystic tumors of ovarian origin. The average size is greater than 15 cm., and occasionally they occupy most of the abdominal cavity. The more solid portions there are in a pseudomucinous cystadenoma, the greater the chance of carcinoma. The tumor is usually cystic, rarely solid, but it is common to find neoplasms that can only be classified as semicystic and semisolid. The pseudomucinous cystadenocarcinomas are bilateral far less often than the serous cystadenocarcinomas. The reported incidence of their bilateral occurrence is approximately 15 per cent of all pseudomucinous carcinomas.

15%
bilateral

On opening the cyst the same gelatinous secretions are noted in both the benign and the malignant mucinous cystadenomas. The multilocular nature of the cyst cavity is obvious at once, but malignant change manifests itself either by papillary projections rising from, or more commonly by hard solid regions within, the fibrous trabeculations. The malignant area may be confined to a single locule or it may spread throughout the cyst cavity.

The varying degrees of malignancy within these ovarian cysts are evident on microscopic study. Whatever the degree of anaplasia, mucinous epithelium tends to maintain a glandular pattern. Most often the epithelium of pseudomucinous cystadenocarcinoma forms invasive glands that vary in their histologic appearance. Some are lined by a single layer of cylindrical mucin-producing anaplastic cells, and others by many layers of irregularly shaped, undifferentiated carcinoma cells (Fig. 52–4). The average pseudomucinous cystadenocarcinoma has a histologic appearance not much different from that of an adenocarcinoma of the colon. The more malignant tumors are completely undifferentiated, and the normal cell pattern is lost in a diffuse growth of cells in sheets with occasional nests of mucinous tumor cells. Stains for mucus may show occasional droplets in isolated "signet ring" carcinoma cells.

NOTE

Whenever papillary projections appear on the external surface, the prognosis

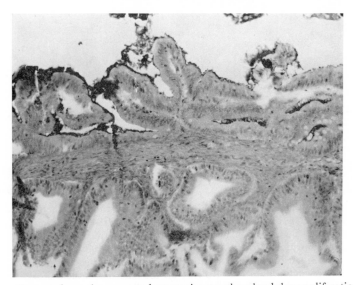

Fig. 52-4. In pseudomucinous cystadenocarcinoma the glandular proliferation is abnormally close-packed, with invasion and cytologic anaplasia. Darkly stained basophilic mucinous secretion is being produced by the carcinoma.

worsens. Since the pseudomucinous cystadenoma is infrequently papillary, the carcinomatous change is less likely to manifest itself in this fashion unless the carcinoma is versatile and rapidly growing.

SEROUS CYSTADENOMA

NOTE

This type of benign ovarian neoplasm occurs more frequently than the pseudomucinous variety. Because it is primarily a papillary growth, the tumor is far more dangerous, for its malignant potentiality is greater. It is this factor, plus the facts that these tumors are more heavily concentrated in the reproductive years and tend to occur bilaterally more often than the pseudomucinous cyst, that makes serous cystadenomas such a problem in therapy. If the uterus and ovary are to be left behind,

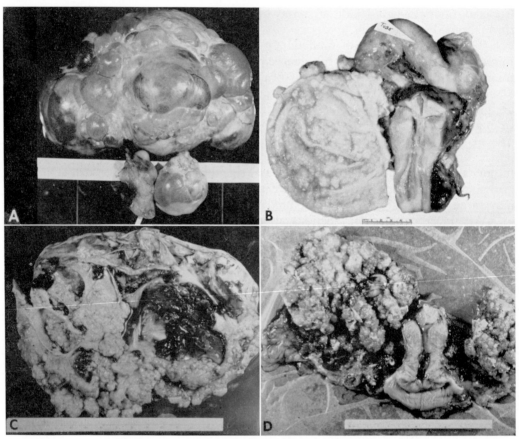

Fig. 52-5. *A*, Multilocular serous cystadenoma about 15 cm. in diameter of one ovary, together with the uterus and a smaller contralateral serous cystadenoma. The shining outer capsules and translucent walls of the locules favor benign neoplasms. *B*, When multiple granular papillomas cover the internal surface of a serous tumor, it is likely locally invasive and malignant. Microscopically, this was a papillary serous cystadenocarcinoma. If not ruptured, removal of such a carcinoma may be curative. *C*, Papillomatous masses both within and growing on the external surfaces of a serous ovarian tumor might be benign, but most of them, like this case, are papillary serous cystadenocarcinomas. *D*, Sometimes papillary adenocarcinoma is so extensive, and perhaps involves both ovaries as in this case, that its origin from papillary serous cystadenocarcinoma is obscured.

and only the cyst removed in the younger age patient who wants to have more children, it is of the utmost importance that the true nature of the tumor be known. Roughly one third of all ovarian serous cystadenomas will be found to be malignant. This makes their malignant potential approximately seven times greater than in pseudomucinous cystadenomas.   *NOTE*

The true nature of the tumor can be suspected only when the cyst is excised and opened, for the gross characteristics, growth pattern, history and physical findings are no different from those offered by the pseudomucinous cystadenoma. The difference in the fluid content is immediately apparent when the cyst is opened. The thin, clear, yellow serous fluid is completely different from the sticky gelatinous material found within the pseudomucinous cystadenoma. On inspection of the cyst cavity one may find either a single cystic space or many compartments. Arising from the epithelium lining the cyst, papillomatous outgrowths are commonly seen, either scattered throughout the cavity or concentrated in solitary areas with a localized overgrowth noted at this point (Fig. 52–5, *A*). The normal progression of growth in this neoplasm is to have papillary projections begin to develop on the internal surface and then enlarge and spread until they fill the cavity (Fig. 52–5, *B*). Either benign or malignant papillary projections may later appear also on the external surface as the capsule of the cyst becomes involved (Fig. 52–5, *C, D*).

For the most part, the serous cystadenomas are cystic tumors, but they may contain varying amounts of solid tissue. The primary cystic tumor that contains solid elements in it and may be classified as semicystic is far more dangerous than the *NOTE* so-called *serous cystadenofibroma* or the mixed Brenner tumor and pseudomucinous cyst. These are benign fibrous tumors with cystic elements in them that secrete either serous or mucinous fluid respectively.

The Microscopic Picture of the Serous Cystadenoma

There is no sharp line of demarcation between the histologic picture of the serous cystadenoma and the serous cystadenocarcinoma. The papillary appearance on gross examination immediately makes them cancer suspects. In the majority of instances the histologic evidence of anaplasia when present is obvious, but there are many borderline cases that make the differentiation difficult.

The typical benign serous cystadenoma contains two types of papillomata: ① The more benign type is simply a connective tissue core covered by a single layer of columnar cells resembling fallopian tubal epithelium. The small rounded masses of cauliflower-like papillomas jut into the cyst (Fig. 52–6, *A*). ② When proliferative activity of the cyst is more pronounced, the same central core is present, but more branching tends to occur, and the epithelial covering is often several layers thick and is composed of low columnar and occasionally large rounded vesicular cells, some desquamating. Intervening smoother areas are usually covered by epithelium one layer thick. These cells may be tall and ciliated with clear cytoplasm or nonciliated and secretory, and the latter are either low columnar or cuboidal. However profuse the papillary formation, the epithelial cellular pattern in benign tumors continues to be a regular one without palisading or piling up.

How Does Carcinoma Change the Histologic Picture?

Malignant changes appear when ⓐ the epithelial covering of the papillae piles *NOTE* up into several palisaded layers; ⓑ greater variation is noted in the size of the cells;

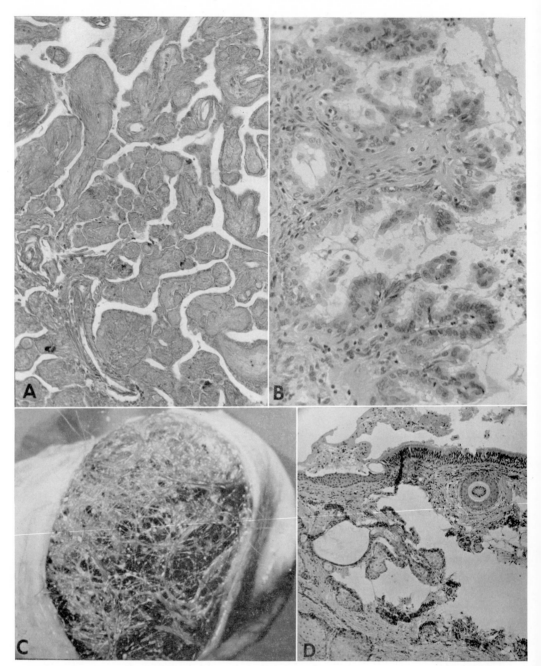

Fig. 52-6.   *A*, Benign papillary cystadenoma microscopically may appear largely as papillary overgrowths of connective tissue covered by a thin layer of epithelium that secretes a serous fluid. *B*, Conversely, in papillary serous cystadenocarcinomas there is greater epithelial overgrowth, with irregular layering of the cells covering the papillae, moderate or marked variation in cell sizes and staining, and invasion of the stroma. This example is not very anaplastic, but is invasive with a poor prognosis for surgical cure. *C*, The dermoid cyst is typically filled with coiled hair and rather rancid sebaceous material. *D*, Histologically, the most common features in the wall of the ovarian dermoid cyst are skin and skin adnexa, such as hair follicles and sebaceous glands, respiratory epithelium, and fat and fibrous tissue. Practically any tissue may be present.

(c) the growth pattern in the epithelial cells may have become totally irregular; (d) the cells are more hyperchromatic, and the nuclei reveal more mitoses; (e) the connective tissue cores and the cyst wall become invaded, and large, solid epithelial invasive masses are formed (Fig. 52–6, B). Within these solid cellular areas one can still see some papillary cystadenomatous growth and remnants of gland lumens. There is a change from the lighter lacy appearance of the benign serous cystadenoma to the heavy solid masses of cystadenocarcinoma cells.

When only the first two indications of likely malignant neoplastic change occur in the epithelial cells of papillary serous cystadenomas, namely, palisading and irregularity in cell size, definite evidence of invasive carcinoma is often absent. For this situation the pathologist may diagnose papillary serous cystadenoma, potentially malignant. This means that if the cyst was removed intact and unruptured, further trouble is unlikely. But if during its removal the cystadenoma was ruptured and its contents were spilled onto the peritoneum, the epithelial cells appear capable of progressive growth. Consequently there would be the likelihood of a later recurrence in the form of papillary cystadenocarcinomatous implants spread over the peritoneal surfaces.

If definite anaplasia and invasion are seen, the pathologic diagnosis of papillary serous cystadenocarcinoma can be made, and the outcome probably will depend on the depth of invasion and particularly whether carcinoma has grown through to the outside of the cyst. Some papillary processes on the outside of cystadenomas are benign, but the vast majority are papillary carcinomatous masses, representing invasive extensions of a cancer that started inside.

Within serous cystadenomas and cystadenocarcinomas tiny calcium deposits are found scattered throughout the stroma. These are called psammoma bodies or calcospherites. They are an integral part of the serous cystadenoma and are not evidence of unusual degeneration. Visible by x-ray, they suggest the papillomatous nature of the cyst and consequently raise the suspicion of malignancy, particularly since they accompany serous cystadenocarcinoma more commonly than benign serous cystadenoma.

NOTE

DERMOID CYST OF OVARY

The dermoid cyst, which is really a cystic teratoma, is one of the more common benign cystic tumors in the ovary. If one excludes the follicular and corpus luteum cysts, which are not neoplasms, the dermoid comprises about 20 per cent of all ovarian tumors. The incidence will be higher if one includes another 20 per cent of tumors that theoretically may be associated, such as the pseudomucinous cystadenoma. A dermoid cyst may appear anywhere in the reproductive age span and is actually the most common ovarian tumor of childhood.

NOTE

Despite the teratomatous nature of these tumors, which by definition include all three germ layers, the malignant potential is very low. Ninety-seven per cent are said to be benign. The growth process is a slow one, and the tumors rarely are larger than 6 inches (15 cm.) in diameter. They are pedunculated and tend to be unilateral, but appear often enough in the opposite ovary to present a real problem in conservative therapy in the early reproductive years. Not only do these tumors occur bilaterally in 25 per cent of cases, but also more than one dermoid cyst may be present in a single ovary. Occasionally they are so small as to go unrecognized until the ovary is actually bisected and the interior inspected.

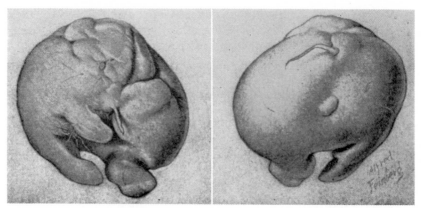

Fig. 52-7.   Two drawings of a homunculus found inside an ovarian dermoid cyst. Rudimentary limbs, hair and a tail are identifiable. (From A. Plaut: *J. Mt. Sinai Hosp.*, Vol. 12.)

What Do They Look Like Grossly?

The appearance of dermoids is fairly characteristic, though they cannot be distinguished from any other pedunculated tumor on pelvic examination. In the majority of instances the cyst lies free in the abdominal cavity except for the ovarian attachment and may be found in a number of positions as the tumor swings on its pedicle. The incidence of pedicle torsion in dermoid cysts is placed as high as 15 per cent. Occasionally the wall of the ovary is blended with the wall of the cyst, and less often encapsulated tumor masses may be found within the interior of an otherwise normal-appearing ovary.

The dermoid cyst usually has a spherical or elliptical contour with a smooth, grayish-white external covering. They rarely exceed moderate size. The wall of the cyst tends to be thick and fibrous, but when thin, there is a yellowish-white color that reflects the fatty content of the tumor.

The makeup of the cyst wall is variable, since all the germ layers—entoderm, mesoderm and ectoderm—are represented. The *ectodermal* elements appear in the form of skin, hair, sebaceous glands, teeth and fingernails. The *mesodermal* derivatives are bone, cartilage, fatty tissue, fibrous tissue and muscle. The *entodermal* components are less abundant, but are recognized as thyroid, intestinal mucosa and tissues derived from the bronchial tree. The relative frequency with which any particular one of this wide assortment of tissues is encountered is said to decrease as one proceeds from component tissues of the scalp to those of the pelvis. The bony elements and teeth are frequently detected on x-ray examination of the lower portion of the abdomen and pelvis (Fig. 51–3). The heavy concentration of sebaceous glands is responsible for the butter-like appearance and consistency of the rancid oily fluid in the fresh cyst, which solidifies as it cools. Hair, varying in length and color, may make up the bulk of the contents (Fig. 52–6, *C, D*). Teeth are present in nearly 50 per cent of dermoids and are frequently set in bone resembling a rudimentary jaw. Rudimentary portions of the eye, central nervous system, respiratory and intestinal tracts are less often seen. Sometimes parts of extremities such as fingers or caricatures of fetuses, called homunculi (little men) are formed (Fig. 52–7).

The cyst wall is partially lined with skin and often partially with granulation tissue, owing to the irritative and damaging quality of the contents. The cyst cavity is usually unilocular, but there may be several smaller loculated areas within the main cyst. Occasional warty protuberances are noted in an otherwise smooth interior, and usually one major ridge where the hair and any teeth are anchored. It is obvious that the dermoid is more of a retention cyst than a proliferating tumor. This accounts for its slow enlargement and relatively low malignant potentiality. They can be clinically dangerous, however, because of their propensity to undergo torsion and rupture. Occasionally the thin-walled dermoid ruptures and sets up a severe plastic pelvic peritonitis. Less often they discharge their contents by rupturing into the bladder and intestine.

When cancer develops in a dermoid cyst, it is most often a low-grade, locally invasive epidermoid carcinoma arising from the cyst lining. Various rarer malignant tumors have occurred, such as carcinoids and malignant melanomas.

What Is the Objective in Treatment of the Dermoid?

The underlying philosophy in the treatment of the dermoid cyst should be conservatism. These tumors have a low malignant potentiality and do have a tendency to be bilateral, but unless the patient is in her late forties there is no reason to perform a total hysterectomy and bilateral salpingo-oophorectomy. In the early forties, just as in the early reproductive years, every effort should be made to shell out the dermoid from the ovary. Normal ovarian tissue may make up part of the wall of the cyst, but it can usually be seen spread out over the surface and can easily be dissected free from the dermoid. Examination of some of the ovarian tissue that is to be preserved usually shows normal follicles and frequently corpora lutea. Plastic surgical reconstruction of the remains of the ovarian tissue can readily be accomplished, leaving a useful, normally functioning ovary.

The opposite ovary should always be inspected. The ovary must be split and the interior surveyed, because small and often multiple dermoids may be present without changing the outward appearance of the ovary.

NOTE

SOLID TERATOMA

This tumor is similar in origin to the cystic ovarian dermoid. There is usually a wide mixture of representative elements from all three germ layers. It is the benign solid teratoma that likely contains more of the recognizable organic structures such as thyroid, and bronchial and central nervous system tissue, while in the dermoid cyst ectodermal structures such as hair, teeth and skin predominate.

When seen grossly, they resemble the dermoid cyst to a certain extent, but are far more likely to be larger, bulky tumors, many of them enormous. When they are sectioned, the solid surface is interrupted by cystic regions where the tumor has differentiated or degenerated. The color and consistency vary, depending on the complexity of the structures that go to make up the tumor. It is often yellow and rubbery, but may be reddish-brown and firmer if much muscle or thyroid tissue is present. Teratomas also tend to be fixed to adjacent structures rather than lying free as the dermoid cysts do. This is due to the tendency of the solid teratoma to break through its restraining capsule.

On histologic review there is often a hodge-podge of recognizable adult structures mixed with some in embryonic stages of development (Fig. 52–8, *A*). These areas are widely dispersed throughout the loose connective tissue stroma. The organoid dif-

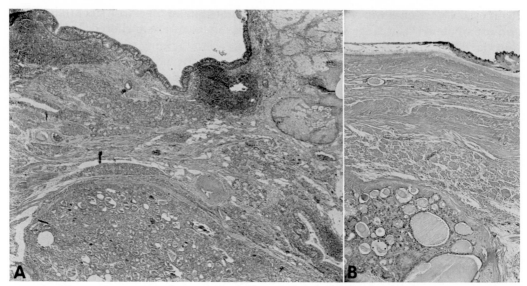

Fig. 52-8.   *A,* Part of a solid ovarian teratoma, showing the various tissue components, including respiratory epithelium, lymphatic tissue, sebaceous glands, colonic epithelium and thyroid. In this area all appear mature, but elsewhere undifferentiated or malignant growth patterns may be found. *B,* Struma ovarii, so sectioned as to illustrate its origin in the wall of a partly cystic teratoma. Many struma cases are not associated with any other recognizable teratomatous features.

ferentiation is rarely complete, though one may recognize teeth, bone and cartilage. Because the tumor often proliferates actively, the bulk of it may be composed of immature cells that tend to be sarcomatous rather than carcinomatous. Some teratomas are either wholly benign or only of low-grade malignancy.

Perhaps one third of patients treated only by surgical excision are well after five years. X-radiation is considered useless.

Struma Ovarii

This form of solid teratoma is for all practical purposes a benign lesion, though occasionally some portion of the tumor may prove to be malignant, when the tissues have undergone complete pathologic study. Five per cent of struma ovarii are said to be carcinomas. Thyroid tissue may be a single component of either the cystic or solid teratoma or may be found in a multilocular pseudomucinous cystadenoma, but the true struma ovarii is composed almost entirely of thyroid tissue.

These tumors appear in the early reproductive years, but have their greatest concentration in the late thirties and early forties. They occur not infrequently as bilateral tumors and vary greatly in size. The more poorly differentiated tumors usually tend to be larger than the average of 10 to 15 cm. The preoperative diagnosis is rarely made, although such tumors should concentrate radioactive iodine.

There is little in the gross appearance of these tumors to distinguish them from other solid teratomata, except that the capsule is not invaded. On section the soft or mushy interior is usually reddish brown, translucent and gelatinous when thyroid tissue predominates. The same cystic spaces that one sees in any solid teratoma are also present, owing to degeneration and necrosis.

The microscopic picture is that of a typical thyroid, predominantly made up of large follicles containing abundant colloid, but with occasional small fetal types of follicles present. Most often there are degenerative and regenerative changes, with nodularity, as in a nodular adenomatous goiter (Fig. 52–8, *B*). In the rare cases in which the thyroid tissue is hyperfunctional, there usually is evidence of unusual epithelial activity with tall columnar cells, vacuolated colloid and papillary projections into the follicular spaces. There may be areas of carcinoma in the tumor, but as often occurs in the thyroid, the rate of growth is usually relatively slow both in the primary adenocarcinoma and in any metastatic areas. The peritoneum is the most common site when metastases appear. Patients have been known to survive for long periods of time after metastatic disease to the peritoneum has been proved histologically.

The symptoms produced are not very different from those of any ovarian neoplasm. The thyroid tissue is usually not abnormally functional, but in rare instances, approximately 5 per cent of cases, the patient may present symptoms of thyrotoxicosis, secondary to overactivity of the functional thyroid tissue within the ovary, rather than the thyroid. Sometimes a thyroidectomy is performed without benefit before it is realized that a struma ovarii is responsible.

Treatment

In most instances simple excision of the solid tumor is adequate therapy, particularly when it is found in the reproductive years. The index of malignancy is low at best, and clinically significant carcinomatous changes are rare. One can afford to take a calculated risk, provided the capsule has not been invaded. In the older age group a total hysterectomy and bilateral salpingo-oophorectomy are indicated.

WHAT IS THE FUNDAMENTAL TREATMENT FOR AN OVARIAN NEOPLASM?

The treatment of ovarian neoplasm is mainly surgical. In the early phases of the growth period the benign ovarian tumors cannot be distinguished from those with a malignant component. They cannot be differentiated on the basis of the history or physical findings. The final diagnosis rests on the pathologist's interpretation of tissue presented to him. This often cannot be done accurately on small biopsy specimens unless the disease has already spread to accessible regional lymph nodes. The true nature of the neoplasm at times can be accurately diagnosed only when the entire tumor mass is available for review. Abdominal exploration is therefore essential if there is any doubt about the diagnosis. When there is powerful evidence of extensive carcinomatosis from an ovarian source, one may elect to give x-ray treatment in cancericidal dosage as a preliminary to the abdominal surgical intervention, but otherwise the earliest possible abdominal exploration is indicated.

It is unwise to tap a large ovarian cyst before subjecting the patient to operation, just as it is most important to avoid rupturing the cyst in the process of its removal. Dissemination of tumor cells from a ruptured cyst throughout the pelvic cavity may serve as a basis for metastatic growth. Ordinarily patients tolerate the removal of even large cysts with considerable equanimity. The operative removal of a malignant neoplasm of the ovary carries a mortality of 3 to 5 per cent. The only major danger is postoperative urinary suppression, brought about by change in intra-abdominal tension following the removal of a large cyst. If the patient has severe cardiac disease and suffers embarrassment in heart action because of the pressure of the large ovarian tumor against the diaphragm, one might consider tapping the cyst as a preliminary step, to achieve temporary relief, provided the cyst is to be removed surgically shortly thereafter.

NOTE

The principal treatment of cancer of the ovary is total hysterectomy with removal of both tubes and ovaries. There is no indication for extensive dissection of the regional nodes, for the simple reason that extension is far more likely to be directly to the retroperitoneal lymph node chain that lies along the aorta, renal veins and celiac axis. The uterus must be removed because of the extensive intercommunications of the lymphatic pathways between ovary, tube, uterine muscle and the opposite ovary. The other ovary should be removed because (1) many ovarian neoplasms arise primarily in both ovaries, (2) it may become involved by lymphatic spread from the involved ovary.

Is Simple Oophorectomy Ever Proper Therapy?

The primary problem when dealing with a unilateral encapsulated neoplasm of the ovary is to establish by pathologic study whether the tumor is or is not malignant. One becomes suspicious of cancer if the tumor is wholly solid or if solid portions are felt within a cystic tumor, but the clinical impression is not accurate enough to make a diagnosis. Moreover, the cyst that appears outwardly benign may harbor malignancy within its interior. Since the differentiation between benign and malignant cysts cannot be made on clinical grounds, the cyst must be removed and then opened in the operating room. If the pathologist cannot make the diagnosis with certainty after inspecting the interior of the cyst and doing frozen section examinations on any suspiciously firm areas within the cavity, one might elect to take a calculated risk that (*a*) there is no cancer present, or (*b*) that only microscopic foci of invasion exist, and leave the uterus and other ovary. This is adequate therapy if the patient is young, has no children or, having children, wants to have more. If there is gross evidence

NOTE

of cancer within the cyst cavity, the entire uterus and opposite ovary should be removed, regardless of age.

The nature of the tumor has some bearing on the advisability of leaving the uterus and other ovary. Some tumors are benign as well as unilateral. Others have a malignant potentiality of varying degrees and tend to be bilateral. A majority of solid tumors are malignant, but the single most common solid neoplasm, the fibroma, is benign and usually unilateral. One should not be confused by the presence of ascites with these fibromatous tumors, for there is no malignant connotation; simple excision is adequate therapy. The dermoid cyst (cystic teratoma), on the other hand, has a low malignant potential (3 per cent) and tends to be bilateral. If only one side is involved, the opposite ovary should be bisected and the interior of the ovary inspected for possible dermoid cysts. If none are found and there is no obvious malignancy on the involved side, a simple oophorectomy will suffice.

The granulosa cell tumor is another example. Late metastases do occur after simple excision of the solid tumor. This is far more likely to be the case when the tumor is discovered in the older patient who is well advanced in her reproductive life. If the tumor occurs in childhood, early adolescence or in the twenties, one may simply remove the tumor with comparative safety. In older patients the uterus and both ovaries should be removed.

Simple oophorectomy is indicated only when the neoplasm is known to be benign or has such a low malignant potentiality that the chances of cancer are minimal. If the index of suspicion of cancer is high, but the gross appearance and available pathologic confirmation are doubtful, the surgeon will be justified in doing a simple oophorectomy in the younger patient who wants children and then awaiting final pathologic interpretation.

What Is the Chance of Another Neoplasm Developing in the Ovary That Has Been Left Behind?

An important consideration in the discussion of whether or not to leave the uterus and the opposite ovary is the possibility that another tumor, either benign or malignant, may develop in it.

There is some tendency on the part of the gynecologist today to remove the ovaries when pelvic surgery is indicated for benign genital causes in a woman past the age of forty, on the theory that the risks of developing benign cysts or possibly carcinoma will be avoided. Certainly nothing will subsequently develop in the uterus or other ovary if it is not there, but if this type of thinking were carried into all areas of the body, the patient would be a hollow shell without breast, stomach or bowel.

NOTE

Many gynecologists believe that the ovary ceases to function within a few years after the uterus has been removed, even when the operation is done in the late thirties or forties. There is an increasing body of evidence to suggest that the ovaries do continue to function after operation and even after the menopause. There is some individual variation, but Randall finds that only one third of patients unoperated upon had estrogen deficiency five years after the menopause and that half still showed evidence of estrogen activity fifteen years thereafter.

The importance of preserving ovarian function is being increasingly expressed in recent reports. Not only are the atrophic changes that follow castration a source of discomfort and disability to the patient, but there is also evidence which suggests that there is a greater likelihood that the patient will have hypertension, myocardial disease or even a fatal coronary attack. One may argue that estrogen can be supplied to the patient or that extragenital sources will correct the deficiency. It is a well known fact, however, that many women will not take synthetic estrogens until after they have symptoms. Since no one yet knows which of the estrogen fractions is the most important biologically, and since the output of estrogen from extragenital sources is neither consistent nor predictable, the surgeon will be well advised to preserve ovarian function unless there is imperative need to ablate it.

When the patient is being operated on for removal of an ovarian cyst, there might appear to be good reason to sacrifice the uterus and other ovary. This is based on the possibility that a benign tumor or cancer may appear in subsequent years. No one will argue the fact that the uterus should be removed together with both ovaries if the diagnosis is malignant. To preserve the uterus and opposite ovary when the operation is being done for a benign neoplasm in a woman in the years immediately preceding the menopause is to run the risk of the development of cancer in the other ovary. It is important to have some idea of how great a risk is involved.

Randall, in reviewing the subsequent course of 310 women who had had a unilateral oophorectomy, found 21, or 7 per cent, who had to have the opposite ovary removed at a subsequent operation. Fourteen of these had benign tumors (4.5 per cent), while 7 were malignant (2.3 per cent). Approximately half had their tumor within five years, while the remainder appeared from five to twenty years later.

The surgeon, then, takes a calculated risk if he removes one ovarian tumor and leaves the opposite ovary. The decision revolves around the following conditions: (1) What is the nature of the tumor? (2) What is the likelihood that the patient will have another neoplasm, either benign or malignant? For example, there is little chance of malignancy when the primary tumor is a dermoid, benign teratoma, simple cystoma or pseudomucinous cystadenoma. The chances are far greater when the original diagnosis was a serous cystadenoma. (3) How much will the patient be disturbed if all ovarian tissue is removed?

Our personal feeling is to take a calculated risk for all tumors, other than serous cystadenoma, up to the time of the menopause, but to reduce that risk by bisecting and inspecting the interior of the ovary that it is planned to leave behind. Most ovarian carcinomas are developmental in origin, and if they have not manifested themselves by the time of the menopause, they are unlikely to do it later. The life history of cancer of the ovary and its male counterpart, the testicle, differs sharply from malignant disease in other areas. The incidences of carcinoma of the ovary and testicle reach a peak at the age of fifty-five and drop sharply thereafter, in contrast to many other forms of cancer, which increase steadily with advancing years. Serous cystadenomas are so variable and unpredictable that we would be willing to take the risk of leaving the opposite ovary only in the younger age group, in which they often occur; after the age of forty we would feel better if the uterus and other ovary were removed.

NOTE

To those who would sacrifice the uterus and other ovary, regardless of age or of the pathology in the involved ovary, Randall introduces the thought that although 7, or 2.3 per cent, had cancer in the remaining ovary and are dead, another 7 women in his series, during the same time, also had cancer of the breast, of whom 3 are dead.

HOW DOES EXTENSIVE CARCINOMA OF THE OVARY BEHAVE?

Most of the symptoms and physical findings commonly attributed to ovarian carcinoma are based on the spread of the tumor beyond the confines of the ovary. The manner of metastatic extension follows no set pattern, but may occur in a number of different ways: (1) In the normal progress of its growth carcinoma in an ovarian cyst begins somewhere in the trabeculated portions of the loculated cystadenoma cavity. Papillary tumor then fills the cavity, preceding invasion of the investing fibrous capsule. Finally, cauliflower-like excrescences appear on the external surface of the cyst, break off and seed throughout the pelvic cavity. (2) Less often the papillary growth develops on the inner or outer surface of the cyst wall, transforming a relatively small cystoma or cystadenoma into a large conglomerate mass made up of the original cyst and extensive overgrowths of papillary cystadenocarcinomatous tumor.

(3) Usually ascites appears along with the penetrating invasive growth of papillary tumor, but occasionally this is absent, and the peritoneum becomes diffusely infiltrated with adenocarcinoma by way of the lymphatics. In this situation the primary carcinoma in the ovary is usually very hard, solid and not large.

(4) The first indication of spread from the primary site may be the appearance of widely disseminated, minute globular swellings on the peritoneum or serosal surfaces of the small intestine, bowel mesentery and omentum, which look very much as

though they had been scattered over these areas with a salt shaker. They are grossly not unlike the miliary tubercles of peritoneal tuberculosis.

5. Metastases may occur by dissemination along lymphatic channels and by blood stream to appear in lymph nodal areas in the upper portion of the abdomen, mediastinum and supraclavicular regions, as well as in liver, lung and bone. Solid carcinomatous tumors are more prone to metastasize in this manner, for the local tumor usually remains encapsulated. Lymphatic spread also occurs in this manner from malignant ovarian cystomas and cystadenomas in the later stages of growth. It is also a common occurrence to have ovarian cancer spread to the fallopian tube and endometrium and thence by lymphatic channels within the uterus to the hilus of the opposite ovary. 6. Papillary spread of tumor usually appears as the result of natural growth process, but may occur from rupture of a malignant cyst.

WHAT UNIQUE CHARACTERISTICS ARE NOTED IN METASTASIS OF PAPILLARY OVARIAN CARCINOMAS?

The papillary type of metastatic spread is more often seen with serous cystadenocarcinoma than with pseudomucinous carcinoma. When metastatic papillary carcinoma is present, it is usually found on the pelvic peritoneum, particularly in the cul-de-sac of Douglas. It is not uncommon to find plaques over the peritoneum on both anterior and posterior walls, spreading along the lateral gutters as far as the superior surface of the liver and the under surface of the diaphragm. Implants frequently are found in the mesentery of the small intestine and in the omentum.

These secondary extensions appear to be true surface implants, for although they may grow into large blocks of tumor tissue, invasion of the subperitoneal layers is minimal. The omentum may be a solid cake of tumor, yet it is rare to have the muscle wall of the transverse colon invaded. This pattern of growth makes it possible in many instances to remove these metastatic deposits, which seem to have little blood supply of their own, without doing serious damage to the patient. It is this fact also that makes these secondary extensions so sensitive to intraperitoneal perfusion with such chemotherapeutic agents as radioactive gold, hemisulfur mustard or nitrogen mustard. *NOTE*

The superficial manner in which these metastases grow may explain in part the occasional documented observations that peritoneal metastases may completely disappear after (a) opening the abdomen, (b) repeatedly tapping large cysts, or (c) after removal of the primary cancer site. In the majority of instances such tumors are of low-grade malignancy. This is one of the human cancers most often spontaneously cured, but in any individual case the chance of this happening is very small.

WHAT IS THE PATTERN OF LYMPHATIC SPREAD FROM OVARIAN CANCER?

As previously noted, metastatic spread of ovarian carcinoma can occur by dissemination of tumor cells along lymphatic pathways, particularly when the primary tumor is solid or malignant. Papillary cystadenocarcinomatous tumors grow widely on the serosal or peritoneal surface. Once the peritoneum is involved, the spread of the malignant disease may be rapid.

The regional, obturator and inguinal lymph nodes are not involved as often as

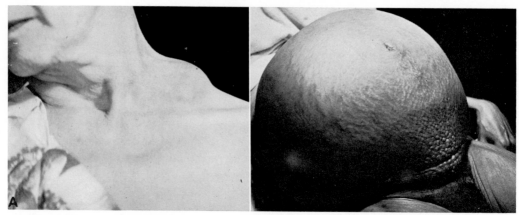

Fig. 52-9.   *A*, Supraclavicular lymph node metastasis from an ovarian adenocarcinoma. *B*, Extreme abdominal distention from fluid with metastatic ovarian carcinomatous spread onto the peritoneal surfaces.

NOTE the retroperitoneal nodes in the upper portion of the abdomen, particularly those located around the duodenum, kidney and celiac axis. This is due to the anatomic distribution of the ovarian veins, which empty into the inferior vena cava and left renal vein. The lymphatic channels from the ovary tend to follow this same pattern. From these lymph nodal areas further extension takes place to the mediastinal and supraclavicular regions. Enlargement of the lymph nodes in the left supraclavicular area occasionally provides the first indication of a small solid carcinoma primary in the ovary (Fig. 52–9, *A*). The secondary metastases may actually be larger than the original tumor and appear early, rather than late, in the disease. At times the spread may occur in retrograde fashion, and lymph node metastases are noted in the groin. We have previously noted that the peritoneum itself may be invaded directly via lymphatic channels, particularly when papillary carcinomatous foci are noted in the absence of ascites.

NOTE   Metastases to the liver are common in ovarian carcinoma. Also metastases may appear in lung or bone and are occasionally found in the brain.

WHAT PHYSICAL FINDINGS ARE NOTED IN ADVANCED CARCINOMA OF THE OVARY?

NOTE   The most common place for carcinoma of the ovary to deposit, once it has extended beyond the ovary itself, is in the pouch of Douglas. Irregular, firm, fixed masses can be felt in this area on both vaginal and rectal examinations. Frequently one can also delineate the primary tumor as well, but occasionally only the peritoneal metastases are palpable. The suspicion of malignant disease will be increased if the tumor is either solid or semicystic and semisolid.

In the absence of symptoms the pelvic nodularity may be indistinguishable from (1) pelvic inflammatory disease with an accompanying benign cyst, (2) a benign ovarian neoplasm that has undergone inflammatory change through interruption of its blood supply or infection within it, (3) diverticulitis with localized pelvic peritonitis, or (4) carcinoma of the sigmoid colon, which has penetrated the serosa and grown in its mesentery. This may occur without any bowel symptoms. A barium enema may be necessary to rule out colonic cancer.

Ascites is noted with about 50 per cent of malignant ovarian tumors, but its presence does not establish the diagnosis or rule cancer out if it is absent. Fluid does contribute to the abdominal enlargement. It is often difficult to differentiate between massive ascites and a large abdominal cyst. The ascites may mask the presence of intra-abdominal tumor masses other than the cyst itself (Fig. 52–9, *B*). The same may be said for the extensive involvement of the omentum, which frequently produces a thick solid plaque of metastatic disease. Both may be more easily palpated after paracentesis. If no tumor can be felt after the abdominal tap, examination of the removed fluid for tumor cells, either by the Papanicolaou technique, by histologic study of paraffin blocks made of the centrifugally spun sediment, or by the convenient Millipore filter method may differentiate between benign and malignant ovarian neoplasms, particularly if a papillary tumor is present, but inaccessible to palpation.

Since the liver is a common site for metastasis to appear, irregularity of the surface of an enlarged liver should be looked upon with grave suspicion. If there is much ascites present, it may be difficult to feel the liver edge until after the fluid has been withdrawn.

The presence of a pelvic mass with irregularities on the pelvic floor, ascites and palpable lymph nodes in the left supraclavicular area or groin should suggest advanced ovarian carcinoma. It is possible to have metastatic lymph nodal enlargement in these areas in the absence of any palpable abdominal tumor.

Finally, the patient may appear perfectly healthy and yet have widespread abdominal carcinomatosis from ovarian cancer.

WHAT SYMPTOMS MAY BE ATTRIBUTED TO ADVANCED OVARIAN CARCINOMA?

Even with extensive intra-abdominal spread of ovarian cancer the patient's only complaint may be abdominal enlargement or a sense of fullness low in the pelvic area. The symptoms are no different from those produced by benign tumors. Only 10 per cent of malignant ovarian tumors disturb the menstrual rhythm or alter the menstrual flow.

In the more advanced cases *pain* becomes the most important symptom. Malignant metastatic deposits tend to produce pain in one of two ways: (1) infiltration of nerve sheaths by tumor cells, or (2) the involvement of adjacent organs and peritoneal surfaces by adhesions. In most instances the pain is centered in the lower portion of the abdomen, but the most severe pains may be in the midback or epigastrium, owing to the rapid enlargement of the metastatic masses in lymph nodes. The metastatic deposits in the neck or groin may become very painful.

With the appearance of pain and a rapidly enlarging abdomen the patient begins to deteriorate rather suddenly. Anuria, cachexia and weight loss become appreciable as the patient's appetite drops off.

The most frightening thing about ovarian cancer is its insidious growth and lack of symptoms. The patient may be totally unaware that anything is wrong, only to be found completely inoperable when surgical exploration is performed two weeks after the rapid appearance of symptoms and physical signs.

WHAT IS THE BEST METHOD OF TREATING OVARIAN CARCINOMA THAT IS NO LONGER CONFINED TO THE OVARY?

The patient should be subjected to exploration even though one feels extensive induration and palpable tumor in the cul-de-sac or large masses within the abdominal cavity. The entire uterus, both ovaries, complete omentum and as much of the peritoneal extension as possible should be removed within the restrictions of common sense. Much of the papillary tumor grows on, rather than into and behind, the peritoneum. It frequently can be removed without danger to the patient or risk of jeopardy to the function of the abdominal viscera. Ovarian carcinoma has such variable characteristics, based on the multipotential growth possibilities inherent in the ovary, that one is justified in removing as much of the tumor as possible, provided the primary source is also excised, even though tumor is obviously left behind. Such a policy would be completely unjustified when operating for any other form of cancer anywhere else in the body. Patients have been known to live for years after incomplete removal of the tumor, if x-ray treatment is used in conjunction with the surgery. Kottmeier, with an extensive experience in the treatment of ovarian carcinoma, prefers to leave the uterus in position when he finds that it is impossible to remove all the tumor in the lower pelvis. The uterus then serves as a receptacle for radium, which is given as a supplement to external roentgen therapy. This procedure has not been used in this country to any extent.

Mature surgical judgment is needed to decide how much of the widely extensive tumor should be removed. Little will be gained by performing a bilateral pelvic lymphadenectomy, and it is an extremely rare case that will benefit from either partial or total exenteration of the pelvic organs. If tumor in the cul-de-sac completely surrounds the rectosigmoid and cannot be excised, the surgeon may justifiably perform a sigmoid colostomy to forestall almost certain intestinal obstruction. Tumor masses found in the small bowel mesentery should be left alone unless they are sharply localized and represent the only tumor deposits present in this area. It is rarely advisable to short circuit or to excise small intestine in anticipation of a possible obstruction.

What Is the Role of X-ray Therapy?

The majority of gynecologic surgeons give x-ray treatment as a standard adjunct to surgical therapy when the disease has spread beyond the confines of the ovary. There is little evidence that it improves the prognosis, if the tumor is entirely confined to the interior of the ovary. One cannot predict the response for obvious reasons: (1) There is a great variation in the postirradiation growth pattern in ovarian neoplasms. Some are apparently very sensitive like dysgerminoma, while others appear to be indifferent to radiation. (2) Not all tumors with the same pathologic diagnosis respond in the same way. Some patients go rapidly downhill after external radiation, while others seem to learn to coexist with their tumors and lead active lives for twenty or more years after the combination of surgery and x-ray therapy. (3) The extent of spread is often so great that it is practically impossible to subject the entire abdomen to a radiation dosage adequate to destroy the tumor deposits. The dosage levels customarily used are in the range of 7000 to 12,000 roentgens measured in air, given carefully through many portals (a) to reach the various areas where tumor is known to be located and (b) to avoid damage to vital structures such as the stomach and small intestine. The newer high-voltage x-ray therapy machines, cobalt units and cyclotrons are increasingly effective in delivering cancericidal radiation to tumor areas deep in the body without damaging the skin or jeopardizing the normal functions of important viscera. Treatment is usually begun two to four weeks after operation has been completed.

X-ray treatment used in conjunction with surgical excision will not cure all patients whose disease has spread beyond the ovary. Some will be made worse, but we have no yardstick to determine which individual patients will benefit, and enough are helped to justify its continued use. It has been said that approximately 20 per cent of patients who receive x-ray treatment for ovarian cancer that is left behind after operation will be alive at 5 years. If nothing further is done, all will be dead before that time.

X-RAY TREATMENT BEFORE OPERATION. The majority of gynecologists give radiation two to three weeks after completion of the operation. In advanced disease, when there is occasionally no question about the diagnosis of ovarian cancer, radiation has been used as a preliminary step preceding abdominal exploration. In some recorded instances the tumor has regressed in size, and in a few cases it has entirely disappeared. The reduction in the size of the tumor and the partial sterilization of the remaining cancer cells provide a greater opportunity to remove bulky tumors without disseminating them further in so doing. Surgery should follow the completion of the course of external radiation, for it is unwise to rely on x-ray treatment alone to cure the disease.

What Are the Other Types of Therapy That May Be Used for Advanced Cancer of the Ovary?

With recognition that much of the papillary growth beyond the confines of the ovary is a surface implantation phenomenon, various types of therapy have been developed in recent years in an attempt to destroy the carcinomatous implants wherever they occur.

RADIOACTIVE GOLD. Isotopic colloidal gold with radioactive properties, in salt solution, has been placed in the abdominal cavity after surgical extirpation of the primary carcinoma, uterus, omentum and as much of the involved peritoneum as possible. One must be assured that the solution will circulate freely in the abdomen as the patient is rotated, for otherwise local concentration of the radioactive material will seriously damage the intestine or anything else with which it is in constant contact. Its ability to destroy tumor, other than the most superficial implants, is doubtful, since it is capable of only a few millimeters of penetration. It does seem to be useful in reducing the collection of ascites and the frequency of the paracentesis required to remove the distressing fluid accumulations.

ADJUVANT CHEMOTHERAPY. Unfortunately, in far too many instances, the principal modes of therapy for ovarian carcinoma, i.e. surgery and radiation, do not produce the percentage of total salvage that we would like. All surgeons have had the discouraging experience of encountering persistent or recurrent disease after carrying out the best therapy. Secondary surgery or re-irradiation produces a limited increase in the number of patients who survive. Our surgical techniques improve and widen in scope, while more precise radiation is given from machines capable of producing higher tumor doses without damaging the skin or viscera. Despite this the anticipated improvement in therapeutic results has not been forthcoming. Chemotherapy offers some hope of increased benefit to the patient who has not responded to the principal forms of therapy. It is truly an adjuvant therapy, since it will be inadequate, except as palliation, if attempts are made to use it as the sole form of treatment.

Why Is Chemotherapy Effective?   The actual mechanism by which this new form of drug therapy obtains results is not clear. There seem to be two possible modes of action: (1) It may operate by altering the chemical processes within the tumor itself, thereby disrupting its metabolism so that it can no longer survive, or (2) the effect may be obtained by increasing the resistance of the host. There is little question that toxic agents, properly selected, can destroy cancer cells. The problem comes in the discovery of an agent that can achieve this in a manner that the patient can tolerate. The range of safety in these chemotherapeutic agents is not very great, and doses of too high concentration often lead to severe toxicity or even death, as the patient's normal cells are destroyed. The problem of finding ways and means of increasing host resistance is far more complex, and as yet is little understood.

The agents now used are classified as (*a*) alkylating agents, (*b*) antimetabolites, and (*c*) antibiotics. As yet no one understands just why the antibiotics obtain their effects. The alkylating agents, so-called because they bind a methyl or ethyl radical to a "susceptible receptor substance," apparently act by disorganizing the cellular metabolic processes. The intracellular enzymes or nucleic acids are examples of receptor substances.

The antimetabolites are frequently similar in chemical structure to the normally present purines, pyrimidines and vitamins. When added, they tend to compete with these substances in their normal metabolic functions. In addition to the toxic action of these chemotherapeutic drugs on the hematopoietic system, as manifested by leukopenia, thrombocytopenia and anemia, which arise because of bone marrow effects; there are other toxic manifestations stemming from the gastrointestinal and central nervous systems. As a result the patient may have nausea, vomiting, abdominal pain, diarrhea and frank gastrointestinal bleeding as the mucous membranes of the oral cavity and gastrointestinal tract ulcerate. These symptoms along with skin eruptions and vulvitis are particularly common when antimetabolites and antibiotics are given. One may note nausea and vomiting after administering the alkylating agents, probably because of central nervous system irritation, but the primary effect is bone marrow depression.

Not all patients respond in the same way, but in general it may be said that the more highly concentrated the dose, the greater the degree of toxicity. It may be possible to avoid toxic manifestations by giving smaller doses at spaced intervals or by using different routes of administration. When toxic symptoms appear, the drug should either be reduced in amount or be given up entirely. There are variations in individual response, and one may therefore elect to resume therapy after the toxic symptoms have subsided, utilizing a lower dose. It is unfortunate that toxicity and effective therapy seem to go hand in hand.

It would be ideal if there were a drug available that could be given either by mouth, intramuscularly or intravenously and which would have a selective action on the tumor wherever it was located. Since none is available, we are obliged to use chemotherapeutic agents by oral or parenteral routes or by instilling the drug in a body cavity or into an artery supplying the area.

Intracavitary Instillation.   The intracavitary method has experienced a mild degree of success. Pleural effusions as well as abdominal ascites have been shown to disappear entirely or to collect much more slowly after instillation of certain drugs into the pleural or abdominal cavity. The drugs most commonly used are alkylating agents such as nitrogen mustard or Thio-TEPA. The results are comparable to those obtained by giving radioactive gold or phosphorus (P^{32}).

Why it is effective continues to be a bit of a mystery. The drug may act directly on the tumor or perhaps be absorbed in part and exert its effect systemically. There is a suggestion that the latter may truly be the mode of action, since the same drug given systemically is equally effective in minimizing fluid collection.

Intra-arterial Perfusion. Recently there has been much enthusiasm for intra-arterial regional perfusion. Using the same technique for extracorporeal perfusion that is now commonly used for cardiac problems, attempts are made to shut off the general circulation by temporarily clamping the inferior vena cava and aorta while the drug is injected into the arterial circulation through catheters placed in the hypogastric or external iliac artery. Return flow takes place through a catheter in the external iliac vein. The motivating force is supplied by an extracorporeal pump. Theoretically, the drug fixes rapidly to the tissues supplied by the arterial circulation, and none escapes into the general circulation in quantity sufficient to produce systemic effect, such as depression of the bone marrow. This is not easily accomplished. To counteract the effect of the toxic agents other drugs are administered systemically to neutralize their action on the bone marrow and central nervous system. This new departure has been reasonably effective when such drugs as Methotrexate have been given for metastatic uterine choriocarcinoma, but so far the improvement in the technique of administering the drug has not produced any notable benefit in patients who have ovarian carcinoma.

Infusion. Despite the obvious limitations it is probably better to give the alkylating agents and antimetabolites either intravenously or intramuscularly when dealing with carcinoma of the ovary.

What Patients Are Suitable Candidates for Chemotherapy? These are powerful drugs, and not all patients who have persistent or recurrent carcinoma of the ovary after surgery or radiation are suitable candidates. To attempt to use chemotherapy is to run the risk of accentuating the downward course of the patient.

There are contraindications that have been established as the result of observation of definite deleterious effects of drugs. For example, patients who have bone marrow depression following x-ray therapy do badly when chemotherapy is added. It is likewise inadvisable to try to give any chemotherapeutic agent that is likely to induce leukopenia to a patient who has an active infection. On the other hand, one can give alkylating drugs to patients who have hepatic metastases or liver disease, provided vomiting is controlled. Since the antimetabolites do tend to produce gastrointestinal symptoms in any case, they should be used with caution in the presence of ureteral obstruction or liver disease.

Rather than treat recurrent disease, it would be of enormous benefit to give the chemotherapeutic drugs to prevent cancer development in the future when there is no clinical suggestion at the time of the initial operation that distant cancer spread has occurred. Unfortunately there is no evidence that the agents now available have this power, and the possibilities of disaster due to the toxic action of the drugs are serious enough to condemn the use of chemotherapeutic agents as a prophylactic measure, so far as carcinoma of the ovary is concerned.

What Drugs Are Commonly Given? **Nitrogen Mustard.** The first and still one of the most effective chemotherapeutic drugs to be used in the treatment of carcinoma of the ovary is nitrogen mustard. It has been injected or instilled in the abdominal and chest cavity as well as given intravenously. When it is instilled into cavities, the calculated dosage is about 0.4 mg. per kilogram of body weight. Hreshchyshyn cuts this dose in half (0.2 mg. per kilogram of body weight) when he gives the nitrogen mustard (Mechlorethamine, HN_2 or Mustargen) intravenously. Since the drug is irritating to tissue if it leaks out of the vein, the drug is injected into the tubing of an intravenous set which carries saline solution to prevent tissue necrosis. Two treatments on successive days are recommended, to be followed at weekly intervals by a maintenance dose of 0.1 mg. per kilogram of body weight.

TEM and Thio-TEPA. There are many reports on the effect of triethylene-melamine (TEM) in ovarian carcinoma. As an oral medication TEM proved too unpredictable because of the variation in its absorption from the gastrointestinal tract. Triethylene thiophosphoramide (Thio-TEPA), given intravenously in a dose of 0.4 mg. per kilogram of body weight on 2 successive days, has been much more satisfactory. Tissue necrosis does not appear at the site of injection, and there are far fewer side effects. A maintenance dose of 0.2 mg. should be given weekly, beginning 2 weeks after the initial dose.

Hemisulfur Mustard. There have been cautiously enthusiastic reports of the use of hemisulfur mustard, which has all the advantages and lacks the undesirable effects that follow the use of nitrogen mustard, such as the depressing effect on the bone marrow. When given intravenously through a catheter inserted in the inferior vena cava, it does produce some nausea, vomiting and general weakness, but more often neurologic manifestations such as temporary confusion, mild convulsive attacks and tremor. The dosage recommended by Green is 200 mg. repeated on 3 occasions at 48-hour intervals. The favorable effects, chiefly suppression of ascites and the improvement noted in comfort, sense of well-being and ability to eat and return to gainful occupation, are most noticeable when the drug is given by the intravenous route. There appears to be a limited effect on the size of the palpable tumor masses.

When it is given intraperitoneally, most of the systemic effects, including the neurotoxic symptoms, are minimized, probably because the action is local and the blood stream is not implicated; 300 mg. are injected through a trocar into the abdominal cavity. The patient is rotated through a series of positions to ensure widespread dissemination.

Chlorambucil and Cytoxan. Chlorambucil is one of the newer alkylating agents in the treatment of ovarian carcinoma. Its chief advantage lies in the fact that it can be given by mouth in daily doses of 0.2 mg. per kilogram of body weight. The usual course runs for about a month and may be repeated after a two-week respite.

The results in a limited group of patients, with such widespread dissemination of carcinoma that any other treatment was deemed inadvisable, have been encouraging. Two thirds of the patients demonstrated a favorable response to therapy, as shown by a diminution in the size of palpable tumor masses. Histologic review of the specimens taken from tumor plaques after chlorambucil therapy showed changes similar to those noted after radiation. It may therefore be unwise to use both radiation and chlorambucil at the same time. As yet an insufficient number of patients with less formidable disease have undergone chlorambucil therapy, but enough have been seen to encourage its use as adjuvant therapy. The best effects are noted with pleural effusion.

Cytoxan is the newest of the alkylating agents. If it is given by mouth, the dosage schedule is the same as that of chlorambucil. The intravenous dosage is 15 mg. per kilogram of body weight, given at weekly intervals. It has far fewer undesirable side effects than the other agents, but introduces a new one, *alopecia*, which may be partial or complete and appears in approximately one quarter of all patients exposed to the drug.

An antimetabolite, *5-Fluorouracil*, has been tried and has been of some benefit in patients who have lung metastases from a primary lesion in the colon, but is of little help in the treatment of ovarian malignancy. The toxic effects and the limited margin of safety are enough to discourage its use for cancer of the ovary.

Recently there has been a suggestion that the beneficial effects can be obtained while the toxicity is diminished by giving the same dose over a longer period of time by the intravenous route. A regimen of 15 mg. per kilogram of body weight on a schedule of 8 hours each day for 5 days seems to produce the best results.

Theoretically, the cells in any given tumor undergo cell division at different times. By giving the drug over a longer period it may be possible to obtain greater objective improvement, since more of the drug will reach cells in the phase of division when they are most ready to receive it. Concentrated doses given over a short period of time reach only a few cells in the favorable state of development. The respite lasts only a short time, and may have to be repeated in six weeks to two months.

There is also the interesting speculation that 5-Fluorouracil given in this manner may so sensitize the tumor that a more favorable response can be anticipated from irradiation therapy given subsequently.

What Effects Can Be Anticipated from Use of the Alkylating Agents? It is difficult to measure the palliative effects that follow the use of alkylating agents. Most of the metastases are remote or can only be seen by x-ray film. Rarely does one have the opportunity actually to measure the amount of regression in tumor size. At best, tumor regression can only be estimated. This is the ultimate objective goal, for most of the patients, in the absence of drug toxicity, experience subjective improvement such as an improved sense of well-being, increase in appetite, weight, activity, and decrease in fluid accumulation in the chest and abdominal cavity.

Approximately 25 per cent will also show appreciable reduction in the size of tumor masses that can be either felt or measured. This effect persists for as long as three months.

What about the Length of Survival after Chemotherapy? In general, patients who receive adjuvant therapy live longer than those with recurrent carcinoma of the ovary who do not. If the patient has a good subjective or objective response, she may be expected, on the average, to survive one year, as against four months if she does not.

In a limited group of patients Hreshchyshyn, at the Roswell Park Memorial Institute, finds that (*a*) patients with ovarian carcinoma who had no treatment of any sort failed to survive one year. (*b*) If the patient received radiation or chemotherapy, only approximately 10 per cent survived one year. (*c*) Finally, patients who received chemotherapy as additional treatment to the initial radiation can expect a 70 per cent chance of living one year. Rarely, however, does the patient survive longer.

Summary of Adjuvant Therapy. It is obvious that though patients under chemotherapy for recurrent carcinoma of the ovary feel better, exhibit some degree of tumor regression and live slightly longer, alkylating agents are not yet the answer to the problem of treating ovarian cancer. Further advances may be expected in the future when an agent is discovered that has a selective effect on tumor tissue alone and is not so highly toxic that the patient cannot tolerate it.

WHY IS THE GROWTH PATTERN OF OVARIAN NEOPLASMS SO UNPREDICTABLE?

A number of clinical manifestations exhibited by malignant ovarian neoplasms are little understood. One of the most bizarre is the documented observation that some histologically proved areas of metastatic carcinoma disappear after removal of the primary growth. Taylor has reported thirty-six such cases. The role of ascites in tumor spread is little understood. Some patients have ascites and no dissemination of their cancer, while in others the fluid seems to serve more as a culture medium than as a vehicle for the spread of detached cells. Despite the fact that the medium is poor in oxygen and contains little nutrient material, one can observe ascitic proliferation of cells containing many mitoses. We would also like to know why some patients suddenly take a turn for the worse and rapidly go downhill. In this instance does the tumor take on an increased rate of growth, or is it that metastatic cancer of the ovary behaves differently from localized tumor? In this regard it would be interesting to know whether all parts of the tumor have the same growth pattern and whether growth is constant throughout its life span. Taylor has good evidence that a tumor does have a consistent growth pattern for all its parts.

SPONTANEOUS REGRESSION OF TUMOR GROWTH

In reviewing the specimens known to have undergone spontaneous regression, Taylor finds that histologically they represented an intermediate stage between benign and malignant growth. They have the appearance of either a benign metastasizing adenoma or a regressing carcinoma. Such tumors can apparently grow rapidly, metastasize and proliferate in ascitic fluid, but they lack the power to invade or to maintain themselves after once initiating growth in a remote area. Apparently they need the primary tumor as a further impetus to progress, for they tend to disappear when it is removed. Taylor suggests that malignancy is not actually an entity, but a quality which varies with different tumors. The regressing tumor lacks the quality of persistent growth.

IS THERE ANY RELATION BETWEEN PATHOLOGIC GRADE AND THE ABILITY TO INVADE AND METASTASIZE?

A definite relation has been shown between the pathologic grade and the eventual prognosis in cancer of the ovary. Taylor finds that there is excellent correlation between the histologic appearance of the tumor and its eventual outcome. The patients with borderline ovarian malignancies almost invariably survived. Approximately 65 per cent of patients with low-grade carcinomas classified as grade I also survived, but three quarters of those with a histologic grade of II and III were dead within two years. It has been suggested by Taylor that cytologic characteristics vary with the degree of malignancy. If one counts the number of nuclei and measures their size, there appears to be excellent correlation with the degree of malignancy.

It has also been shown, by autoradiographic techniques after injection of radioactive phosphorus (P^{32}) into benign and malignant tissues, that the degree of incorporation into the RNA of the nucleolus closely parallels the nucleolar dimensions.

In all probability the nucleolar size and numbers are not only a measure of the RNA content of the cell, but also may reflect the grade of malignancy. Considering the number and size of the nucleoli, the malignant cell has far more RNA than the benign one. By quantitative cytology of this sort the quality of malignancy can perhaps eventually be prophesied.

REFERENCES

Clinico-pathologic Aspects

Benson, R. C., Sherman, R. S., Jr., and Lucia, E. L.: The Factors Influencing Prognosis in the Treatment of Papillary Cystadenocarcinoma of the Ovary. *West. J. Surg.*, 61: 387, 1953.

Broders, A. C.: The Grading of Carcinoma. *Minnesota Med.*, 8: 726, 1925.

Cariker, M., and Dockerty, M.: Mucinous Cystadenomas and Mucinous Cystadenocarcinomas of the Ovary: A Clinical and Pathological Study of 355 Cases. *Cancer*, 7: 302, 1954.

Corscaden, J. A.: *Gynecologic Cancer.* 2nd Ed. Baltimore, Williams & Wilkins Company, 1956.

Farrar, H. K., Jr., and Bryan, R.: Equilateral Distribution of Ovarian Tumors. *Am. J. Obst. & Gynec.*, 80: 1085, 1960.

Fisher, E. R.: "Pseudomucinous" Cystadenoma: A Misnomer? Histochemical Studies on Pseudomucinous Cystomas and Cystadenocarcinomas, with Special Reference to Their Apparent Mucopolysaccharide Secretions. *Obst. & Gynec.*, 4: 616, 1954.

Gaudrault, G. L.: Papillary Carcinoma of the Ovary. Report of a Case with Prolonged Dormancy and Spontaneous Regression of Metastases. *New England J. Med.*, 264: 398, 1961.

Giacobine, J. W., and Siler, V. E.: Evaluation of Diagnostic Abdominal Paracentesis with Experimental and Clinical Studies. *Surg., Gynec. & Obst.*, 110: 676, 1960.

Hertig, A. T., and Gore, H.: *Tumors of the Ovary and Fallopian Tube.* Washington, D. C., Armed Forces Institute of Pathology, 1961, p. 76.

Lawson, J. D., and Weissbein, A. S.: The Puddle Sign—An Aid to the Diagnosis of Minimal Ascites. *New England J. Med.*, 260: 652, 1959.

Lee, A. B. H., and Bowers, P.: Bilateral Primary Ovarian Carcinomas. A Case Report. *Am. J. & Gynec.*, 80: 1083, 1960.

Randall, C. L., and Gerhardt, P. R.: The Probability of the Occurrence of the More Common Types of Gynecologic Malignancy. *Am. J. Obst. & Gynec.*, 68: 1378, 1954.

Reagan, J. W.: Histopathology of Ovarian Pseudomucinous Cystadenoma. *Am. J. Path.*, 25: 689, 1949.

Sampson, J. A.: Implantation Peritoneal Carcinomatosis of Ovarian Origin. *Am. J. Path.*, 7: 423, 1931.

Schiller, W.: Concepts of a New Classification of Ovarian Tumors. *Surg., Gynec. & Obst.*, 70: 773, 1940.

Taylor, H. C., Jr.: Studies in the Clinical and Biological Evolution of Adenocarcinoma of the Ovary. *J. Obst. & Gynaec. Brit. Emp.*, 66: 827, 1959.

Turner, J. C., Jr., ReMine, W. H., and Dockerty, M. B.: A Clinicopathologic Study of 172 Patients with Primary Carcinoma of the Ovary. *Surg., Gynec. & Obst.*, 109: 198, 1959.

Whitelaw, R. G.: Pathology and the Conserved Ovary. *J. Obst. & Gynaec. Brit. Emp.*, 66: 413, 1959.

Woodruff, J. D., Bie, L. S., and Sherman, R. J.: Mucinous Tumors of the Ovary. *Obst. & Gynec.*, 16: 699, 1960.

General Treatment

Chu, F. C. H.: The Results of Treatment of Ovarian Cancer with One Million Volt X-ray. *Surg., Gynec. & Obst.*, 104: 45, 1957.

Ellis, F.: Malignant Disease of the Ovary and Radiotherapy. A Survey of 168 Cases with 10 Year Followup. *J. Fac. Radiologists*, 7: 1, 1955.

Henderson, D. N., and Bean, J. L.: Results of Treatment of Primary Ovarian Malignancy. *Am. J. Obst. & Gynec.*, 73: 657, 1957.

Kottmeier, H. L.: Radiotherapy in the Treatment of Ovarian Carcinoma. *Clin. Obst. & Gynec.*, 4: 865, 1961.

Krolin, L., Jaffee, H. L., and Izenstark, J. L.: Postoperative Radiation Therapy for Ovarian Carcinoma. Indications for Newer Types of Irradiation. *Obst. & Gynec.*, 9: 111, 1957.

Latour, J. P. A., and Davis, B. A.: A Critical Assessment of the Value of X-ray Therapy in Primary Ovarian Carcinoma. *Am. J. Obst. & Gynec.*, 74: 968, 1957.

Meigs, J. V.: The Surgical Treatment of Cancer of the Ovary. *Clin. Obst. & Gynec.*, 4: 846, 1961.

Munnell, E. W., Jacox, H. W., and Taylor, H. C., Jr.: Treatment and Prognosis in Cancer of the Ovary, with a Review of a New Series of 143 Cases Treated in the Years 1944-1951. *Am. J. Obst. & Gynec.*, 74: 1187, 1957.

Randall, J. H.: Treatment of Ovarian Carcinoma. Evaluation of Results at State University of Iowa Hospitals. *Obst. & Gynec.*, 5: 445, 1955.

Schanks, W.: Survey of Cases of Carcinoma of the Ovary Treated at the Radiotherapy Department, London Hospital 1943-1950. *J. Fac. Radiol.*, 7: 11, 1955.

Schmitz, H. E., and Majewski, J. T.: End Results in the Treatment of Ovarian Carcinoma with Surgery and Deep X-ray Irradiation. *Radiology*, 57: 820, 1951.

Taylor, H. C., Jr., and Greeley, A. V.: Factors Influencing the End-Results in Carcinoma of the Ovary. Report of a Series of 138 Patients Treated from 1910 to 1935. *Surg., Gynec. & Obst.*, 74: 928, 1942.

Tod, M. C.: Place of X-ray Therapy in Treatment of Malignant Ovarian Tumours. *J. Obst. & Gynaec. Brit. Emp.*, 58: 385, 1951.

Palliative and Adjuvant Therapy

Bateman, J. C.: Chemotherapeutic Management of Advanced Ovarian Carcinoma. *M. Ann. District of Columbia*, 28: 537, 1959.

Bateman, J. C., and Winship, T.: Palliation of Ovarian Carcinoma with Phosphoramide Drugs. *Surg., Gynec. & Obst.*, 102: 347, 1956.

Brunschwig, A.: Attempted Palliation by Radical Surgery in Pelvic and Abdominal Carcinomatosis Primary in the Ovaries. *Cancer*, 14: 384, 1961.

Clark, R. L., Jr., and Sutow, W. W.: Neoplastic Diseases (Tumor Chemotherapy). *Ann. Rev. Med.*, 10: 251, 1959.

Coonrad, E. V., and Rundles, R. W.: Mustard Chemotherapy in Ovarian Carcinoma. *Ann. Int. Med.*, 50: 1449, 1959.

Creech, O., Jr., Krementz, E. T., Ryan, R. F., Reemtsma, K., and Winblad, J. N.: Experiences with Isolation-Perfusion Technics in the Treatment of Cancer. *Ann. Surg.*, 149: 627, 1959.

Englander, O., and Sarangi, A.: Effect of Thio-TEPA on Advanced Malignant Ovarian Tumours. *Brit. J. Cancer*, 14: 28, 1960.

Green, T. H., Jr.: Hemisulphur Mustard in the Palliation of Patients with Metastatic Ovarian Carcinoma. *Obst. & Gynec.*, 13: 383, 1959.

Hatiboglu, J.: Prevention of Toxicity of Nitrogen Mustard (HN$_2$) by Sodium Thiosulfate (ST). *Proc. Am. A. Cancer Res.*, 3: 117, 1960.

Horwitz, H.: Intra-arterial Therapy. A Review of Its Clinical Applications in Malignant Disease. *Brit. J. Radiol.*, 33: 659, 1960.

Hreshchyshyn, M. M.: A Critical Review of Chemotherapy in the Treatment of Ovarian Carcinoma. *Clin. Obst. & Gynec.*, Sept., 4: 885, 1961.

Kligerman, M. M., and Habif, D. V.: The Use of Radioactive Gold in the Treatment of Effusion Due to Carcinomatosis of the Pleura and Peritoneum. *Am. J. Roentgenol.*, 74: 651, 1955.

Knock, F. E.: Perfusion of Chemically Modified Antibodies for the Therapy of Cancer. *Surg., Gynec. & Obst.*, 111: 322, 1960.

Masterson, J. G., Calame, R. J., and Nelson, J.: A Clinical Study on the Use of Chlorambucil in the Treatment of Cancer of the Ovary. *Am. J. Obst. & Gynec.*, 79: 1002, 1960.

Müller, J. H.: First 5 Year Results of Routine Intracavitary Administration of Colloidal Radioactive Gold (Au 198) for the Treatment of Ovarian Cancer. *Progr. Nuclear Energy* VII, 2: 265, 1959.

Rundles, R. W., and Barton, W. B.: Triethylene Melamine in the Treatment of Neoplastic Disease. *Blood*, 7: 483, 1952.

Shingleton, W. W., Reeves, J. W., Jr., Keppel, R. A., Mahaley, S., and Taylor, H. M.: Studies on Abdominal Organ Perfusion for Cancer Chemotherapy. *Ann. Surg.*, 151: 741, 1960.

Sholes, D. M., Jr.: Pelvic Perfusion with Nitrogen Mustard for Cancer: A Neurological Complication. *Am. J. Obst. & Gynec.*, 80: 481, 1960.

Stehlin, J. S., Jr., and others: Regional Chemotherapy for Cancer: Experiences with 116 Perfusions. *Ann. Surg.*, 151: 605, 1960.

Sullivan, R. D., Miller, E., and Sikes, M. P.: Antimetabolite-Metabolite Combination Cancer Chemotherapy. Effects of Intraarterial Methotrexate Intramuscular Citrovorum Factor Therapy in Human Cancer. *Cancer*, 12: 1248, 1959.

Teng, C. T., and Han, S. Y.: Intracavity Radiogold Therapy. A Critical Appraisal of Its Value. *Am. J. Roentgenol.*, 85: 62, 1961.

Ultmann, J. E., Hyman, G. A., Crandall, C., Naujoks, H., and Gellhorn, A.: Triethylenethiophosphoramide (Thio-TEPA) in the Treatment of Neoplastic Disease. *Cancer*, 10: 902, 1957.

Weisberger, A. S.: Direct Instillation of Nitrogen Mustard in the Management of Malignant Effusions *Ann. New York Acad. Sc.*, 68: 1091, 1958.

Chapter 53

Solid Benign Tumors of the Ovary

WHETHER a neoplasm grows as a cystic or solid tumor depends on its rate of growth and on its differentiation or lack of it. A cyst is normally slow and centrifugal in its growth process, which allows time for the lining cells to differentiate. Consequently they tend to become more like the parent cell, whose main function is secretory. The cystic neoplasms are therefore less likely as a group to be malignant or to undergo neoplastic change. The solid areas within the cyst will always be a potential source of danger, for it is in these areas that cancer first appears.

Unlike the cystic neoplasms that are only occasionally malignant, the basically epithelial solid ovarian tumors are almost invariably malignant. Only the fibroma, thecoma and Brenner tumor are benign.

OVARIAN FIBROMA

The fibroma is a relatively common form of solid ovarian neoplasm. Although nearly 20 per cent of all solid ovarian tumors are fibrous, they represent only 5 per cent of all tumors of the ovary. They are connective tissue tumors and arise in all probability from the ovarian cortical stroma. There seems to be some relation with the thecoma, and many pathologists believe that the fibroma is simply a burned-out thecoma that has no remaining hormonal function.

For the most part the fibroma is both unilateral and pedunculated. It is therefore subject to many of the same complications that appear in cystic tumors which derive their blood supply through a pedicle. Because of the pedicle the solid fibroma may occupy a number of different positions and is clinically and sometimes grossly indistinguishable from a subserous fibroid that has become pedunculated. Of far greater importance is the fact that fibromas have no special characteristics or physical findings and produce no symptoms that will permit clinical differentiation of a benign fibroma from a solid ovarian cancer.

The symptoms are those that go with any pelvic tumor. The patient may have pressure effects which disturb the function of bladder or bowel. She may have pain as torsion of the pedicle occurs and the tumor becomes distended by interstitial edema and hemorrhage. One characteristic physical finding sometimes noted with ovarian fibromas is the presence of ascites. For the most part the fibromas are unilateral tumors (90 per cent) and rather small, but they may appear bilaterally as diffuse fibromata and become fairly large. When this type of bilateral fibrous tumor growth

774

in the ovary occurs, the fibroma in one ovary may be appreciably larger than the other.

What Is Meigs's Syndrome?

The combination of a solid pelvic tumor, ascites and right hydrothorax has been ~Note~ called Meigs's syndrome (Fig. 53–1). The complete syndrome appears far less often than the combination of ovarian fibroma and ascites, without hydrothorax. Approximately 40 per cent of all ovarian fibromas over 6 cm. in size will be accompanied by excessive peritoneal fluid. The added element of fluid in the right pleural cavity appears with only 3 per cent of fibromas. On rare occasions fluid may appear in the left plural cavity.

There are two pertinent questions that to date have been inadequately answered. It is interesting to speculate on (1) why the fibroma secretes so much fluid and (2) how the fluid arrives in the pleural space.

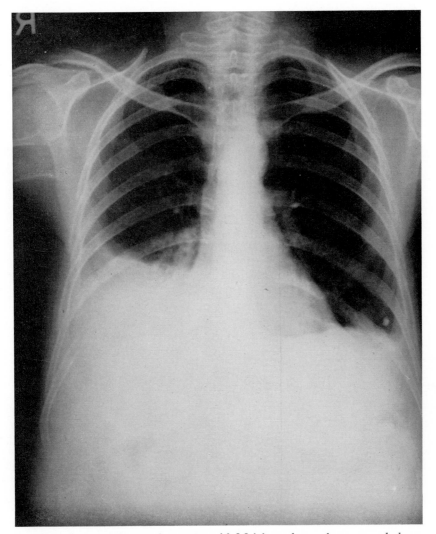

Fig. 53-1. X-ray film of abdomen of a woman with Meig's syndrome shows ground-glass appearance due to ascites. A right pleural effusion is also present.

It has been said that venous congestion within the fibroma brought on by repeated torsions of the vascular pedicle is the true explanation of the ascites. It has also been suggested that transudation takes place between the dilated lymphatics in the tumor and the free peritoneal cavity, owing to the pedicle twist.

The pleural fluid has the same characteristics as the abdominal ascites. Theoretically it arrives there by way of the transdiaphragmatic lymphatics. Meigs showed that India ink injected into the peritoneal fluid will accumulate in the thoracic cavity. The migration through the lymphatics of the diaphragm seems to be in one direction only, for ink injected in the pleural fluid does not appear in the abdominal cavity.

The fibroma is not the only ovarian tumor that is accompanied by ascites or even hydrothorax. Many other ovarian neoplasms, particularly those with a malignant component, also have the same association, though to a lesser degree. The important contribution made by Meigs was to show that the combination of pelvic mass, ascites and hydrothorax may be due to a benign cause that is curable, and hence these findings do not invariably add up to cancer with a poor prognosis because of metastases to peritoneum and pleura.

What Do Ovarian Fibromas Look Like When Transected?

Just as it is important to open ovarian cysts in the operating room before closing the abdomen, so the transection of solid ovarian tumors is indicated, and to an even greater extent, because so many solid tumors are malignant.

Fibromas are not only solid, but also hard, and many contain areas of calcifi-

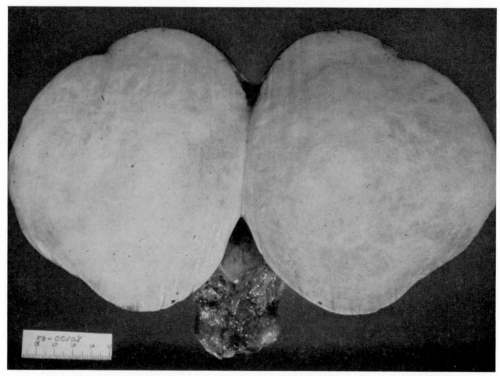

Fig. 53-2.   The dense white, whorled cut surface of a solid ovarian tumor is typical of benign fibroma. Only the more yellow thecoma and Brenner tumor have a similar gross appearance.

cation. These may be due to repeated episodes of vascular occlusion brought on by torsion of the pedicle.

The external surface of the fibroma is not distinctive. It is usually smooth and in general maintains the contour of the ovary as it enlarges. At times it is lobulated. The majority of fibromas are in the 5- to 10-cm. diameter range, though they may become larger. They are freely movable in the abdominal cavity because of the pedicle and are rarely bound down by adhesions, despite repeated degenerative episodes within the tumor secondary to incomplete vascular occlusion.

The cut surface resembles that of the uterine fibroid. It is customarily white and has the same whorled appearance (Fig. 53–2). Rarely there is a yellow tinge, which might be due to fatty degenerative products or perhaps suggests its thecomatous origin. Because of repeated accidents in the tumor, secondary to disturbance in the blood supply, the solid portions occasionally also contain cystic spaces with a liquefied hyaline content.

What Is the Microscopic Appearance?

The histologic picture of the ovarian fibroma varies and will depend greatly on its stage and rate of growth. For the most part the fibroblasts are mature and well differentiated with abundant intercellular collagen. Fat stains are negative (Fig. 53–3, A).

Occasionally one sees more cellular forms of fibroma with young spindle-shaped fibroblasts that closely resemble a fibrosarcoma. Approximately 2 per cent of fibromas will present this disturbing picture, and some actually are malignant tumors with a destructive life history. It is important, then, to distinguish between the fibrosarcoma, which is highly anaplastic and invasive, and the cellular fibroma, which is no more dangerous than a fibroma that is so well differentiated and inactive that calcification is seen in it. This is one reason why frozen section of all solid ovarian tumors is indicated.

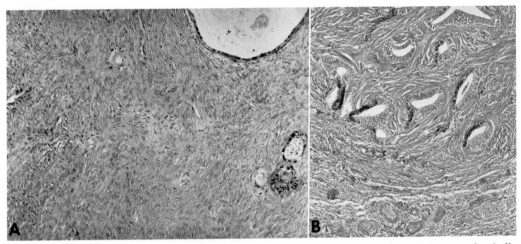

Fig. 53-3.   *A,* The cellular fibroma of the ovary is composed of compactly arranged spindle cells, and occasionally is associated with germinal inclusion cysts. *B,* An ovarian cystadenofibroma typically contains glandular nests of germinal epithelium in a dense fibromatous stroma. This is usually a functional neoplasm with estrogenic secretion.

What Is the Proper Treatment of the Ovarian Fibroma?

If the frozen section reveals no questionable elements within what is obviously a benign fibroma, the surgeon may safely excise the unilateral tumor from a patient in the reproductive or hormonally active age group. If the patient is postmenopausal, bilateral salpingo-oophorectomy and total hysterectomy are indicated.

It is interesting to watch the fluid in the pleural cavity and abdomen disappear after the removal of the primary tumor in the ovary.

OVARIAN CYSTADENOFIBROMA

Although many fibromas of the ovary may contain cystic spaces that result from hyaline degeneration, occasional tumors which resemble fibromas actually have glandlike cystic areas lined with cuboid or columnar epithelium (Fig. 53–3, *B*). They are usually small tumors and are customarily found within the substance of the ovary, but the cyst spaces may coalesce and form one large cyst. The tumor is usually of softer consistency than the true fibroma. These tumors are called "cystadenofibromas." Though these tumors have a large cystic component in an otherwise solid fibrous tumor and may be classified as semisolid and semicystic, they are benign neoplasms. The stroma often has some estrogenic functional activity like a thecoma.

BRENNER TUMOR

Like the thecoma, this is primarily a solid tumor of the ovary. A few present themselves grossly as cysts, but by and large these cysts simply represent degeneration

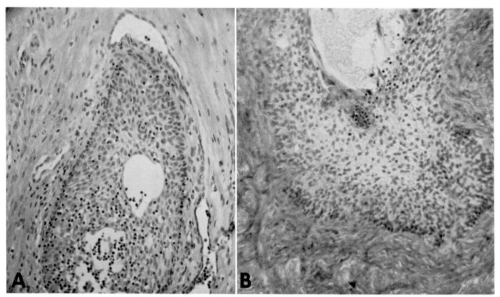

Fig. 53-4.   *A,* The Walthard rest is a minute focus of urinary-tract-type of wolffian epithelium commonly found in the paraovarian and paratubal stroma. Note the associated microscopic cysts. *B,* In the Brenner tumor analogous islands of the same type of epithelium are scattered through a fibromatous stroma. The same cystic alteration is seen occasionally as occurs in Walthard rests.

in the tumor, just as the thecoma or granulosa cell tumors may undergo cystic transformation. These tumors, again like the thecoma, tend to appear in the late reproductive period and are rarely encountered before the age of thirty years. The majority appear after the menopause, but enough are found in the thirty- to forty-year age group to discuss them here.

The tumors are usually small, though considerable variation in size has been reported. When they occur as individual entities, they are encapsulated and closely resemble fibromas. They are usually unilateral, solid fibrous tumors. Not infrequently they are found in the wall of a pseudomucinous cyst. This well documented observation raises some speculation as to their origin. Most pathologists believe that the tumors arise from Walthard rests, which are simply solid localized collections of wolffian urogenital epithelium commonly seen beneath the ovarian capsule at the hilus and in the subserosa of the fallopian tube (Fig. 53–4, *A*). Nevertheless it is also well known that Brenner tumors tend to undergo pseudomucinous transformation. Some authorities believe that large pseudomucinous cysts are actually the end-result of such changes occurring in a tumor that was originally basically a Brenner tumor. These tumors are usually benign, though the solid epithelial elements somewhat resembling squamous cells that are seen microscopically may arouse a transient suspicion of malignant disease.

What Do They Look Like on Histologic Examination?

Microscopically, the typical picture of a Brenner tumor is that of a primarily fibrous tumor with interspersed islands of squamous-like epithelial cells that stand out sharply in the fibrous tissue background. The cells are not keratinized, however, and have a distinctive nuclear peculiarity, in that the nuclear chromatin is arranged in

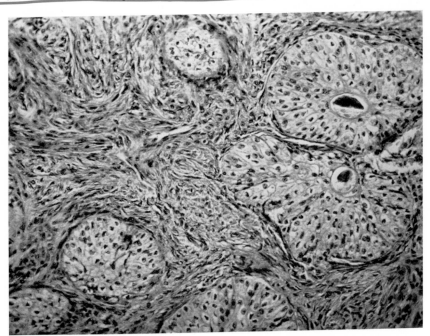

Fig. 53-5.   At lower magnification the nests of distinctive epithelium of the Brenner tumor are scattered through its dense fibromatous stroma.

a line down the long axis of each nucleus (Fig. 53–4, *B*). It is not an uncommon finding to note metaplasia within these cell nests that results in the formation of cystic spaces filled with mucus. There are typical goblet cells producing the mucous secretion. Around the cystic spaces the lining cells may become columnar such as those one sees in a pseudomucinous cystadenoma (Fig. 53–5).

The presence of squamous-like epithelial cells in the ovary may raise in passing the question of possible ovarian metastases from an epidermoid carcinoma of the cervix. Certainly this would be an unusual place for cervical cancer to metastasize anyway, and on closer inspection all mitoses are found to be lacking and the cells show no anaplastic change, aside from the cytologic distinctions mentioned above. The tumor grossly occasionally resembles a granulosa cell tumor. It has the same yellow tinge on cut section that one sees in both granulosa and theca cell tumors. It is also true that some theca cells may be found within a predominantly Brenner tumor pattern. The mucous and wolffian cells characteristic of Brenner tumors are not found in the granulosa cell tumor. Rarely, Brenner tumors are malignant.

It is of interest that Dr. Brenner wrote about his tumor in a thesis and when discovered recently practicing general medicine in South Africa was surprised that his work had attracted any attention.

What Symptoms Are Produced?

The only reason for bracketing the Brenner tumor with either the theca cell, granulosa cell tumor or luteoma among the causes of excessive menstrual flow is the fact that vaginal bleeding and Brenner tumors are sometimes associated. In all probability the explanation lies in the extent of the theca cell component in the tumor, for a pure Brenner tumor is nonfunctional.

There is nothing distinctive about the symptoms produced by a Brenner tumor. Except for the relatively few that may produce menorrhagia, the symptoms are similar to those associated with a fibroma or any other solid nonadherent ovarian tumor.

Is Any Special Treatment Indicated?

Since these tumors are essentially benign and well encapsulated, they need only be excised to produce a cure. The element of potential malignancy will simply be that of any pseudomucinous cyst that might also demonstrate neoplastic changes within its interior. When Brenner tumors are large, they are usually believed to be pseudomucinous cysts and are treated according to their size and the age group in which they are encountered. In the older age group total hysterectomy and bilateral salpingo-oophorectomy would be justified, and a simple ovarian excision would be adequate in the earlier reproductive years.

REFERENCES

Fibroma of the Ovary

Collingsworth, C. J.: Fibroma of Both Ovaries. *Tr. Obst. Soc. London*, 21: 276, 1879.
Dockerty, M. B., and Masson, J. C.: Ovarian Fibromas. A Clinical and Pathologic Study of 283 Cases. *Am. J. Obst. & Gynec.*, 47: 741, 1944.

Meigs, J. V.: Fibroma of the Ovary with Ascites and Hydrothorax. Meigs' Syndrome. *Am. J. Obst. & Gynec.*, 67: 962, 1954.

Idem: Pelvic Tumors Other than Fibromas of the Ovary with Ascites and Hydrothorax. *Obst. & Gynec.*, 3: 471, 1954.

Meigs, J. V., and Cass, J. W.: Fibroma of the Ovary with Ascites and Hydrothorax, with a Report of 7 Cases. *Am. J. Obst. & Gynec.*, 33: 249, 1937.

Meigs, J. V., Armstrong, S. H., and Hamilton, H. H.: A Further Contribution to the Syndrome of Fibroma of the Ovary with Fluid in the Abdomen and Chest, Meigs' Syndrome. *Am. J. Obst. & Gynec.*, 46: 19, 1943.

Mokrohisky, J. F.: So-called Meigs' Syndrome Associated with Benign and Malignant Ovarian Tumors. *Radiology*, 70: 578, 1958.

Owen, A. W.: Fibroma of the Ovary with an Account of a Case. *Lancet*, 1: 1211, 1923.

Rhoads, J. E., and Terrell, A. W.: Ovarian Fibroma with Ascites and Hydrothorax (Meigs' Syndrome); Report of a Case. *J.A.M.A.*, 109: 1684, 1937.

Ritvo, M.: Pleural Effusion and Ascites in Association with Fibroma of the Ovary (Meigs' Syndrome). *Am. J. Roentgenol.*, 48: 152, 1942.

Salmon, U. J.: Benign Pelvic Tumors Associated with Ascites and Pleural Effusion. *J. Mt. Sinai Hosp.*, 1: 169, 1934.

Schenck, S. B., and Eis, B. M.: Papillary Cystadenocarcinoma of Ovary with Hydrothorax. *Am. J. Obst. & Gynec.*, 38: 327, 1939.

Cystadenofibroma

McNulty, J. R.: The Ovarian Serous Cystadenofibroma. A Report of 25 Cases. *Am. J. Obst. & Gynec.*, 77: 1338, 1959.

Reddy, D. B.: Cystadenofibroma of the Ovary. *J. Indian M. A.*, 25: 319, 1955.

Scott, R. B.: Serous Adenofibromas and Cystadenofibromas of the Ovary. *Am. J. Obst. & Gynec.*, 43: 733, 1942.

Smith, E. B., Beamer, P. R., Vellios, F., and Schulz, D. M.: *Principles of Human Pathology*. New York, Oxford University Press, 1959, p. 937.

Brenner Tumors

Bland, P. B., and Goldstein, L.: Granulosa Cell and Brenner Tumors of the Ovary. Report of a Case with a Review of Those Cases Already Recorded. *Surg., Gynec. & Obst.*, 61: 250, 1935.

Farrar, H. K., Jr., and Greene, R. R.: Bilateral Brenner Tumors of the Ovary. *Am. J. Obst. & Gynec.*, 80: 1089, 1960.

Freda, V. J., and Montimurro, J. A.: Coexistence of Mucinous Cystadenoma and Brenner Tumor of the Ovary. Report of Two Cases. *Am. J. Obst. & Gynec.*, 77: 651, 1959.

Jondahl, W. H., Dockerty, M. B., and Randall, L. M.: Brenner Tumor of the Ovary: A Clinicopathologic Study of 31 Cases. *Am. J. Obst. & Gynec.*, 60: 160, 1950.

Kendall, B., and Bowers, P. A.: Bilateral Brenner Tumor of the Ovaries. Case Report and Review of the Literature. *Am. J. Obst. & Gynec.*, 80: 439, 1960.

Richardson, G. S., and Ulfelder, H.: Problems Presented by Benign Solid Ovarian Tumors. *Clin. Obst. & Gynec.*, 4: 834, 1961.

Chapter 54

Solid Malignant

Tumors of the Ovary

MOST solid ovarian neoplasms have a malignant potentiality of some degree. Since they can be differentiated from benign solid tumors only by histologic examination, the palpation of any adnexal mass that appears firm and solid should be a definite indication for the patient to be surgically explored. Only the fibroma, thecoma and Brenner tumor are practically exclusively benign.

NOTE

PRIMARY CARCINOMA (ADENOCARCINOMA)

This is an epithelial tumor that basically contains the same type of tissue encountered in the serous or pseudomucinous cystadenocarcinoma, yet on cut section the tumor is solid and contains no cystic spaces. It has been suggested that these tumors were originally cystadenocarcinomas in which the epithelial proliferation has become so great that the cystic or glandular spaces have been obliterated.

NOTE

These tumors are bilateral in approximately 50 per cent of cases. Grossly, they are usually of moderate size and tend to maintain the normal contours of the ovary. The capsule is usually well defined, though the smooth external surface is frequently nodular and the tumor lobulated. When the restraining capsule has been invaded, granular excrescences appear on the smooth outer surface. From this primary source on the surface the tumor then spreads widely by seeding throughout the peritoneal cavity.

On cut section the surface is composed of grayish friable tissue with areas of hemorrhage scattered throughout its substance. There are many foci that have undergone necrosis and cystic degeneration (Fig. 54–1).

On microscopic inspection the picture is far from a homogeneous one. This is due to the great variability in the proportion of the stroma to epithelial cells. When there is little stroma and a heavy proliferation of malignant epithelial cells, the tumor may be said to be of the *medullary* type. The tumor tends to grow in sheets and cords of relatively undifferentiated cells, without serous or mucinous secretion, cilia or much attempt to assume a papillary or glandular pattern. Such a tumor is said to be of the *plexiform* type. When the fibrous elements are in the ascendency, the cells can be seen

NOTE

in columns streaking through the surrounding fibrous tissue stroma. This is the *scirrhous* type. On occasion here one can still see papillary elements and ill-defined glandular spaces. This suggests a common origin with the serous cystadenocarcinomas that do not assume a papillary form (Fig. 54–2).

At present the descriptive terms "medullary" and "scirrhous" are no longer in common usage, and such tumors are called adenocarcinomas grade II to IV, or carcinoma simplex, after Ewing. Psammoma bodies, also called calcospherites, seen histologically may be the only clear indication of their ovarian origin.

These tumors are highly malignant and carry a poor prognosis. Fortunately they are less common than the cystadenocarcinomas whose growth pattern and meta- static potentialities they imitate. Solid adenocarcinomas make up about 10 per cent **NOTE** of all the malignant tumors of the ovary. Because they are usually bilateral and are highly malignant, the treatment must obviously include total hysterectomy and removal of both tubes and ovaries, regardless of the age group in which they are found. It matters little whether the adenocarcinoma arises primarily in one ovary and spreads to the other by lymphatic channels or whether the tumors appear simul- taneously in both ovaries. The solid adenocarcinoma is extremely lethal, however

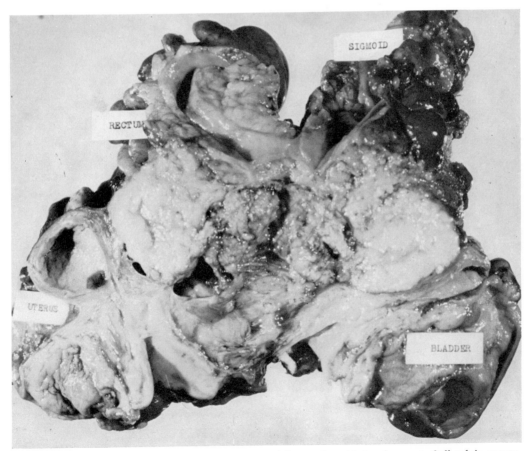

Fig. 54-1.   Advanced solid adenocarcinoma of the ovaries with involvement of all pelvic organs, removed by exenteration. Both grossly and microscopically, it had destroyed all remaining ovarian tissue.

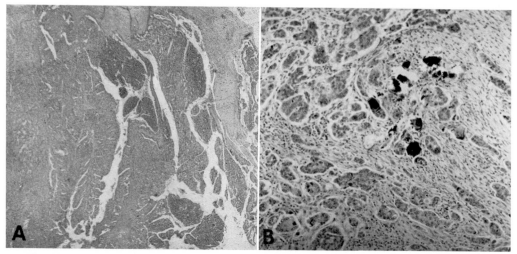

Fig. 54-2.   *A*, Solid ovarian adenocarcinoma may grow partly with a papillary pattern that suggests an origin from papillary cystadenocarcinoma. *B*, Psammomatous calcospherites are often found mixed with less well differentiated ovarian adenocarcinomas. In pelvic carcinomas of undetermined origin the psammoma bodies are thought to indicate the likelihood of a primary ovarian tumor.

widely it is excised. X-ray treatment after surgery may be useful if there is evidence of spread beyond the capsule of the tumor.

SOLID MALIGNANT TERATOMATOUS TUMORS

A number of different types of solid malignant tumors of the ovary apparently arise from the totipotential germ cells. They are not common and have varying degrees of poor prognosis. Many occur late in adolescence. Others occur in early middle age.

The pathologic terminology of malignant germ cell tumors of the gonad is rather confused. The fascicle of Hertig and Gore provides a useful, simple classification:

> Dysgerminoma
> Primary choriocarcinoma
> Malignant teratoma
> Teratocarcinoma

DYSGERMINOMA

This is an uncommon form of solid ovarian tumor, of which over 400 cases have been reported. It has its counterparts in the seminoma and embryonal carcinoma of the male testis. It appears most frequently before puberty and during adolescence, and is rarely encountered after the menopause. This is a functionally neutral tumor with no endocrine significance, despite the fact that one may occasionally in the seminoma of the testis obtain a positive pregnancy test. This simply means that active chorionic tissue is present somewhere in the tumor.

The fact that the dysgerminoma has no endocrine significance is important, for there is a definite association with sexual underdevelopment, and particularly with pseudohermaphroditism. One may find clitoral enlargement and evidence of gonadal deficiency. This is not due to any masculinizing influence on the part of the tumor, but rather to its association with pseudohermaphroditism. The diagnosis thus should be suspected when a solid pelvic tumor is found in a patient who also presents some evidence of sexual maldevelopment. *Note*

The underdevelopment is relative, however, for several cases have occurred during pregnancy, and a recent case of bilateral dysgerminoma with an enlarged clitoris first came to our attention after delivery of a normal infant. Also one should keep in mind that the "pseudohermaphrodite" may truly be a male with poorly differentiated secondary sex organs. A study of the nuclear sex pattern by skin biopsy or buccal smear should be done before assuming that the patient has a dysgerminoma.

When palpated within the abdomen at the time of exploration, these tumors are softer than fibromas, but they do have a rubber-like quality. The external surface is smooth. They have a tendency to be bilateral and usually lie freely movable in the abdominal cavity without adhesion to any other structure. The size of the tumors varies widely. Usually they are of moderate size, up to 12 cm. in diameter, but they may fill the entire pelvic cavity. On cut section the tumors are encapsulated, pulpy and solid with focal necrosis and degeneration. The color tends to be a grayish-pink with yellow patches scattered through the tumor. *Note*

The microscopic picture is as distinctive as the gross appearance is undistinguished. The over-all structure closely resembles the old-fashioned term, "large round cell carcinoma or sarcoma." The cytoplasm is abundant and watery; the nuclei are relatively large. The cuboidal clear cells are arranged in bundles with an alveolar pattern surrounded by thin connective tissue septa. Within these septa are scattered nests of lymphocytes, other leukocytes and giant cells, composing the so-called lymphoid stroma (Fig. 54–3). The histologic appearance of mixed teratomatous elements tends to darken the prognosis. One may find a cell pattern suggesting teratocarcinoma or choriocarcinoma in a predominantly dysgerminomatous tumor. Such neoplasms tend to behave like the most malignant component. All dysgerminomas are considered malignant neoplasms, of various grades of clinical behavior.

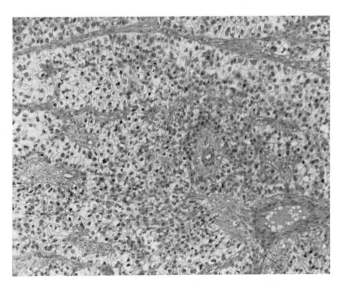

Fig. 54-3. Clear cells arranged in cords, with intermingled lymphocytes and other types of leukocytes, characterize the ovarian dysgerminoma microscopically.

Treatment

The age of the patient is important in outlining therapy. Approximately one third of dysgerminomas are highly malignant. This is more likely to be true of the tumors discovered in older women than in the prepuberal or adolescent age group. Proper treatment also depends on whether or not the capsule has ruptured. If the patient is under thirty years of age and a unilateral tumor has an unruptured capsule, simple excision of the ovary should suffice. If the tumor is bilateral or if the capsule has been penetrated, a total hysterectomy and bilateral salpingo-oophorectomy should be performed, regardless of age or parity. The bilateral tumor is usually malignant.

If the tumor is obviously malignant and has perforated its capsule, rapid dissemination throughout the peritoneal cavity occurs. The recurrence rate after removal of all clinically evident disease is about 75 per cent, and the over-all cure rate at 5 years is about 27 per cent. If the tumor is histologically malignant, but still encapsulated, the prognosis is good. These tumors are very sensitive to x-ray treatment, which should be given routinely when there is evidence of capsule rupture.

Chorionepithelioma of the Ovary

Most of these rare tumors appear as secondary metastases from chorionepithelioma within the uterus. Choriocarcinoma may arise primarily in the ovary, and this is simply another form of malignant teratoma. The origin is in doubt, but it probably arises from trophoblastic tissue developing within an ovarian teratoma, pointing up the heterogenous nature of these tumors. The gross and microscopic pathology and prognosis are like those of similar neoplasms that arise in the uterus.

Precocious puberty occurs in about one third of the children affected. No cure has been reported.

Malignant Teratoma

Only 1 per cent of ovarian teratomas are found to contain cancer, but if solid teratomas alone are considered, aside from the much more common dermoid cysts, nearly half may contain some malignant component. These are tumors of girls below twenty years of age, with rapid neoplastic growth.

Grossly, the malignant teratoma is not clearly distinguishable from the benign solid variety, except that an expert may detect foci of hard granular carcinoma or smooth, slick sarcoma.

Microscopically, sarcomatous elements usually predominate, particularly connective tissue overgrowths too immature to classify as fibrosarcoma or myosarcoma cell types. Occasionally mixed mesodermal sarcomas occur, not unlike those elsewhere in the female genital tract except for the presence of ectodermal and entodermal elements, either benign or malignant, indicating that a teratoma is present.

No five-year cure is known.

Teratocarcinoma

The term is more often applied to testicular than ovarian neoplasms. By it is meant a histologic structure resembling early embryonic growth. Differentiation occurs beyond the dysgerminomatous watery cells in cords, with the formation of

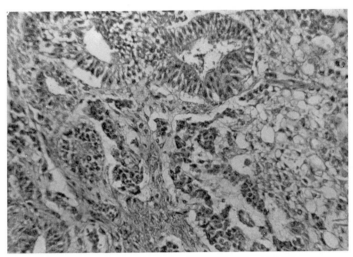

Fig. 54-4. In ovarian teratocarcinoma with so-called somatic differentiation primitive epithelial and connective tissues are formed that simulate early embryogenesis.

epithelial duct structures resembling the primitive neural canal, and the enteric, wolffian or müllerian ducts. Such differentiated foci lie in a mass of embryonal carcinoma. Sometimes cysts are formed that imitate the primitive chorion, amnion or yolk sac (Fig. 54–4).

Grossly, teratocarcinoma has the same appearance as a dysgerminoma. Actually, both grossly and microscopically there is an overlapping of these two tumors, as well as transitions to choriocarcinoma.

Treatment

These malignant teratomatous tumors have such a high lethal potential that there is no place for conservatism in therapy. Their recognition calls for a total removal of the uterus and both adnexa regardless of the age group in which they are found.

MESONEPHROMA OF OVARY

This uncommon malignant neoplasm is said to have teratomatous origin, though the histogenesis is in doubt. Most pathologists believe that it arises from the vestigial remnants of the mesonephric ducts or metanephric tubules. The tumors are only rarely found in adolescence and tend to appear when ovarian function has fully matured. Many of the patients have been unable to conceive, thereby suggesting that a basic maldevelopmental factor may be present.

Grossly, the smooth-surfaced tumors are unilateral and lie freely movable in the abdominal cavity. They are frequently large, and since they are pedunculated, they may twist and are subject to such complications as intracavitary hemorrhage, rupture and spillage. The symptoms then are no different from those produced by any ovarian neoplasm which has a pedicle. This semisolid, semicystic tumor is endocrinologically inert. Though the neoplasm itself tends to be unilateral, it is not unusual to find other related neoplasms like dysgerminoma in the same ovary, or unrelated tumors such as fibroma, Brenner tumor or papillary cystadenoma in the opposite ovary.

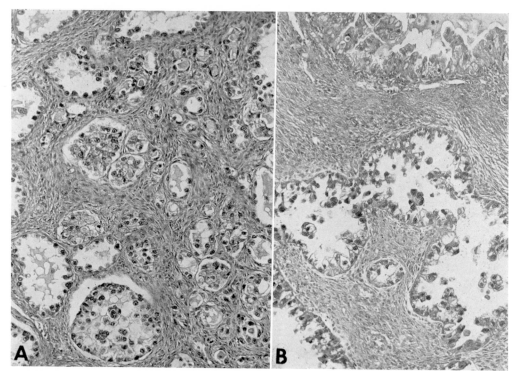

Fig. 54-5.   *A*, Malignant ovarian mesonephroma is characterized by tubules lined by a hydropic, irregularly hobnail type of mesonephric epithelium. In places, shown near the center of the illustration, there are growth patterns that resemble renal glomeruli. *B*, A more hypernephroid growth pattern occurs in other mesometanephric ovarian tumors, with closer simulation of renal tubules by the mesonephroma.

Histogenetic Considerations

The tumor, except for its lethal potential, has far more interest to the pathologist than to the clinician. Its origin is one chief point of discussion. There appear to be three varieties: (*a*) that described by Schiller, who believed that the tumor was mesonephric because of its local resemblances to the kidney glomerulus and tubule, (*b*) Teilum's mesoblastoma, or germ cell mesonephroma, and (*c*) the large clear cell tumors that look more like adrenal or lutein cell neoplasms.

The striking thing about the histologic picture of the Schiller type is the tubules, which may be small and closely packed and have an alveolar pattern or at times are dilated and cystic. The epithelium lining the tubules resembles that seen in the immature kidney (54–5, *A*). The low, irregularly cuboidal pale epithelium frequently piles up and sometimes forms buds that project into the tubal lumens to give the appearance of a renal glomerulus. When this type of proliferation is extensive, the pattern may approach that seen in a papillary cystadenoma. The large cuboidal cells are supposed to have a characteristic "hobnail" type of nucleus. The amount of supporting tissue varies. Usually it is scanty, but at times there may be such overgrowth on the part of the stroma that the tubular pattern is partly obscured.

The clear cell type, or metanephroma, has some of the tubular pattern, but it is less striking. The characteristic finding here is the presence of large, polyhedral, pale-staining cells with such abundant clear cytoplasm that some of the nuclei are crowded aside and can be distinguished only with difficulty. Proliferation of these tall clear cells may occur, with groups of cells scattered throughout the tumor separated only by sparse growth of the connective tissue stroma (Fig. 54–5, *B*).

The histologic pattern is not uniform, and the two forms may be found in the same tumor. In fact, many of the characteristics of dysgerminoma, teratoma, papillary cystadenoma, hypernephroma or any other ovarian neoplasm may be present. The two major types (*a*) and (*c*) outlined above are the two principal patterns for which to look.

Treatment

Since these tumors are highly malignant, the treatment regardless of age or parity should be total hysterectomy with bilateral salpingo-oophorectomy. Any attempt at conservation of ovarian tissue will usually fail whether the tumor appears to be encapsulated or not. Pathologists have been unable to correlate particular microscopic pictures with a better or worse clinical prognosis. Unlike the mesonephromas that appear in other areas of the female genital tract, such as cervix, vagina or uterus, where they are benign, mesonephroma of the ovary is clinically malignant whether the tumor is confined to the ovary or not.

SARCOMA OF THE OVARY

The malignant solid connective tissue neoplasms of the ovary are far less common than carcinoma, with the ratio placed at approximately one in forty. Sarcomas are said to represent about 6 per cent of all ovarian tumors. Contrary to the common belief that these are predominantly tumors of childhood and puberty, primary ovarian sarcoma may occur at any age. The majority occur either about the time of puberty or after the menopause. Some ovarian sarcomas appear to arise secondarily as malignant transformations of a pre-existing fibroma or teratoma.

Grossly, the masses lie relatively free in the abdominal cavity, because the tumor is mainly confined by the ovarian stroma and capsule. Only late in its course does it break through and implant on the peritoneal surfaces in the abdomen. Unlike fibromas, sarcomas tend to be bilateral, with the tumor in one ovary frequently much larger than the other. The similarity to fibroma appears in that the tumors tend to maintain the shape of the ovary and grow to large size on a pedicle. The surface is typically nodular and lobulated. Beneath the surface large dilated veins can be seen.

On cut section sarcomas have the same hard consistency as fibromas, particularly when they are composed of spindle cells. They do have a tendency like sarcomas elsewhere to necrose and leave cystic cavities full of broken-down tumor cells and blood. The "round cell" undifferentiated sarcomas are softer and have a mushy appearance when transected. Not infrequently mixed types of sarcoma are encountered.

The microscopic picture varies, depending on the predominance of the particular cell types. Sarcomas usually are composed of spindly cells. Many have considerable quantities of normal-appearing columns of collagenous fibrous tissue that surround accumulations of spindle cells with large nuclei and numerous mitoses. The cells are often undifferentiated, anaplastic and closely packed together.

Some of these firm spindle cell fibrosarcomas look much like a cellular fibroma

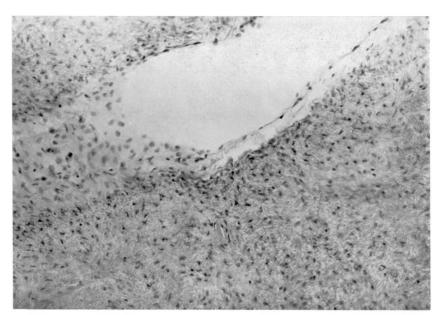

Fig. 54-6. An undifferentiated ovarian sarcoma of slight anaplasia. It is evidently invading the wall of the blood vessels shown, however, and is likely to metastasize via the blood stream to the lungs. Blood vessel invasion characterizes ovarian sarcomas, like other malignant connective tissue tumors that arise elsewhere.

The final differentiation will be based on the anaplastic disparity in size and shape of the cells, the mitoses and nuclear hyperchromatism of fibrosarcoma. The presence of collagen, demonstrated by green coloration after the Masson trichrome stain, or a red color when Van Gieson's stain is used, is helpful in proving the tumor to be a fibrosarcoma. Leiomyosarcoma cells are wider and have cytoplasm containing longitudinal myoglia fibrils that stain reddish with the Masson method.

The "round cell sarcomas" are the most dangerous, but fortunately are found even less often. They are particularly prone to appear in the young girl at puberty. It has been pointed out that many of the old group of so-called round cell sarcomas at this age are actually granulosa cell carcinomas or dysgerminomas. The differentiation is important, for the surgeon should be conservative and remove only the involved ovary if the tumor is a granulosa cell tumor or dysgerminoma, but should be radical in his approach if the neoplasm is a round cell embryonic sarcoma.

Grossly, these tumors are softer in consistency than their fibrosarcomatous counterparts. On cut section the mushy surface contains many cystic areas full of foul-smelling degenerating tumor and hemorrhage.

On microscopic section the small round embryonic types of cells are everywhere in evidence. They have large nuclei in proportion to the cell size that tend to be located centrally. The cells vary in size and shape and are hyperchromatic. Tumor giant cells with many nuclei are mixed in, freely covering the small rounded sarcoma cells. Immature blood vessels are seen with their lumens often packed with tumor cells.

Today pathologists would class such sarcomas as (1) malignant lymphomas, either primary or metastatic, including reticulum cell sarcoma and lymphosarcoma; (2) mixed mesodermal sarcomas, of Wilms type; and (3) undifferentiated sarcomas, including embryonic sarcomas and gonadoblastomas (Fig. 54-6).

What Are the Clinical Characteristics?

Unfortunately there is little to distinguish sarcomas from any other solid tumor of the ovary, either from a recounting of the history or a recording of the physical findings. They mostly lie rather free in the abdomen, grow on a pedicle and reach an appreciable size. The growth is so rapid, however, that the patient experiences weakness, cachexia and weight loss rather early in the course of the disease. Abdominal pain also occurs early because of torsion of the tumor pedicle and the rapid expansion in the size of the tumor. The abdomen enlarges, owing to the ascites that appears in nearly half of the patients.

Most types of sarcoma are highly malignant. Spread occurs by direct invasion as well as penetration of sarcomatous cells, particularly by blood vessel invasion and also along lymphatic channels. Metastases occur to lung and liver, while the tumor implants freely on the peritoneal surface. The regional lymph nodes may be involved.

Treatment

The surgical treatment, at whatever age sarcoma is encountered, is total hysterectomy with removal of both adnexa.

REFERENCES

Benirschke, K., Easterday, C., and Abramson, D.: Malignant Solid Teratoma of the Ovary. Report of Three Cases. *Obst. & Gynec.*, 15: 512, 1960.

Diddle, A. W., and Devereux, W. P.: Ovarian Mesenchymoma. A Five Year Followup Study. *Obst. & Gynec.*, 13: 294, 1959.

Gardner, G. H., Greene, R. R., and Peckham, B. M.: Normal and Cystic Structures of the Broad Ligament. *Am. J. Obst. & Gynec.*, 55: 917, 1948.

Idem: Tumors of the Broad Ligament. *Am. J. Obst. & Gynec.*, 73: 536, 1957.

Green, G. H.: Solid Malignant Teratoma of the Ovary. *Am. J. Obst. & Gynec.*, 79: 999, 1960.

Horn, R. C., Jr., and Lewis, G. C., Jr.: Mesothelioma of the Female Genital Tract. *Am. J. Clin. Path.*, 21: 251, 1951.

Jackson, R. L.: Ovarian Dysgerminoma. Report of 8 Cases. *Am. J. Obst. & Gynec.*, 80: 442, 1960.

Merrill, J. A.: Carcinoma of the Broad Ligament. *Obst. & Gynec.*, 13: 472, 1959.

Novak, E., Woodruff, J. D., and Novak, E. R.: Probable Mesonephric Origin of Certain Female Genital Tumors. *Am. J. Obst. & Gynec.*, 68: 1222, 1954.

Novak, E. R., and Woodruff, J. D.: Mesonephroma of the Ovary. Thirty-Five Cases from the Ovarian Tumor Registry of the American Gynecological Society. *Am. J. Obst. & Gynec.*, 77: 632, 1959.

Parker, T. M., Dockerty, M. B., and Randall, L. M.: Mesonephric Clear Cell Carcinoma of the Ovary. A Clinical and Pathologic Study. *Am. J. Obst. & Gynec.*, 80: 417, 1960.

Schiller, W.: Mesonephroma Ovarii. *Am. J. Cancer*, 35: 1, 1939.

Stowe, L. M.: On the Genesis of the So-Called Mesonephroma Ovarii. *Cancer*, 8: 446, 1955.

Thurlbeck, W. M., and Scully, R. E.: Solid Teratoma of the Ovary. A Clinicopathological Analysis of 9 Cases. *Cancer*, 13: 804, 1960.

Chapter 55

Functioning Tumors of the Ovary

THE SOLID tumors of the ovary that have an associated endocrine function, or so-called functioning tumors, occur relatively infrequently. Despite their rarity they continue to fascinate the clinician, the pathologist and the student. Some, such as the granulosa cell and theca cell tumors, are associated with feminization, owing largely to their inherent propensity to secrete estrin, while others, such as the arrhenoblastoma, Sertoli, Leydig and lipoid cell tumors, tend to produce masculinization, virilization or defeminization through their ability to produce androgen. In rare instances specific tumors may secrete an excess of corticosteroids and present some of the features of Cushing's syndrome. An unquestionable case of Cushing's syndrome would suggest adrenal disease rather than ovarian tumor, but the lipoid tumors, and perhaps the arrhenoblastomas, have the power to produce conditions that closely simulate it.

There is a strong tendency to attribute specific endocrine activity to tumors that bear a definite cell type. Although the granulosa and theca cell tumors are in most instances associated with feminizing phenomena, some of them are hormonally inactive, but others have been known to produce virilization. Conversely, a few Sertoli or Leydig cell tumors, which normally produce androgen and masculinization, have been known to induce feminization.

What Are the Cell Types Normally Responsible for Estrin Production?

It is not surprising that the granulosa cell, which is intimately concerned with the development of the follicle, should be considered partly responsible for the increased production of estrin when a tumor with this type of cell is discovered. Such tumors do secrete estrin in excess, as witnessed by the fact that clinically they produce precocious uterine bleeding in the prepuberal child or rhythmic reappearance of menstrual cycles after the menopause. The bleeding is due to hyperplasia of the endometrium secondary to estrin stimulation. Although there is incomplete evidence that endometrial hyperplasia leads to carcinoma, the association of a granulosa cell tumor with endometrial carcinoma is noted more often than one would expect from mere chance.

The granulosa cell, however, is not the only or even principal cell in the human ovary that secretes estrin. There is increasing belief that the theca cell actually produces most of the estrin in the granulosa cell tumor. We are aware that the supporting ovarian stroma responds to the growth of the follicle under normal conditions. The stromal elements are therefore normally implicated, and one may then expect some increase in feminine hormones in the presence of other types of ovarian tumor, such as the cystadenoma and adenocarcinoma, when a theca cell stromal response is present.

What Is the Origin of the Theca, Granulosa and Luteal Cell Tumors?

Since the thecoma, granulosa cell tumor and luteoma are all variants of the same "gonadal stromal" tumor, the discussion of their origin will be considered together.

The term "sex-cord mesenchyme tumor" has been suggested, since these neoplasms take their origin from either (a) the embryonic sex cords, in which case it is a more likely granulosa cell tumor, or (b) the stromal mesenchyma of the embryonic gonad. In the past there was much discussion of the origin of granulosa cell tumors from either ovarian follicles, perhaps atretic, or granulosa cell rests in the ovarian cortex which were left over from the development of the primary follicles. There can be no doubt that such rests actually exist, but there is considerable question that the granulosa cell tumors arise from them.

There is more general agreement now that these tumors arise from the undifferentiated ovarian stromal mesenchyma, termed the feminizing mesenchyma by Novak. Experimentally, both granulosa cell and the theca cell tumors have been produced by irradiating young or mature mice with x-ray. The tumors seem to arise from a primitive type of mesodermal tissue and appear either in mixed or pure form, with occasional types that show luteinization besides the granulosa cell variety. There is further suggestion that stimulation from the anterior pituitary may play a role in the development of these tumors. This stems from experiments whereby ovarian tissue was transplanted into the spleens of mice which had previously been castrated. The estrin elaborated by the ovarian graft in its new position filtered through the liver, where it was destroyed. The stimulating action of pituitary gonadotropic hormones on the transplant was therefore not checked by the feedback-control effect of estrin. Such transplants tended to develop granulosa cell tumors. Also animals joined in surgical parabiosis, like Siamese twins, grew similar tumors after the ovaries had been removed from one partner. If a chemical irritant was fed to the intact partner, whose ovaries were concurrently being stimulated by both pituitary glands, granulosa cell tumors developed.

A few human cases of granulosa cell tumor or thecoma have followed pelvic irradiation for some other condition, and radiation may have had some etiologic effect. Otherwise, in human cases there is no indication of their cause.

GRANULOSA CELL TUMOR

This tumor can appear in any age group. Somewhere between 5 and 10 per cent occur before the onset of puberty. The remainder are about equally divided between the reproductive and the postmenopausal years. There is no problem in either diagnosis or treatment when the tumors are encountered before puberty or after the menopause. The obvious physiologic manifestations, such as the appearance of cyclic uterine bleeding when none is expected, are enough to arouse a suspicion of their presence and to indicate the proper diagnosis. Likewise, there is no uncertainty in instituting proper therapy in the prepuberal or postmenopausal age group. One wishes to be conservative in the young and should be radical in the older age group, because there is a definite malignant tendency in this tumor which may be clinically obvious in as high as 30 per cent. They are rarely as malignant in the younger age group, however.

There is little to distinguish the granulosa cell tumor from any other tumor of the ovary in the reproductive age group. It may be a cause of amenorrhea due to its constant estrogenic activity. There are many causes of the excessive menstrual bleeding that may accompany it. In patients in the twenties and thirties one is faced with the problem of wanting to conserve the reproductive function, yet avoid the risk of late recurrences in the granulosa cell tumors that are more malignant.

Since this is the chief clinical problem, and the histogenesis and endocrine factors are the same for all age groups, the granulosa cell tumor and its variants, the thecoma and luteoma, will be discussed here in the thirty- to forty-year age group. The clinical elements will be outlined first.

What Symptoms and Signs Do Granulosa Cell Tumors Exhibit?

There are actually no symptoms in granulosa cell tumors which, in the thirty- to forty-year age group, can be considered pathognomonic. The tumors vary in size, but are usually readily palpable and average between 5 and 10 cm. in diameter. They may, however, be very small and escape detection on physical examination. Apparently there is no relation between the size of the tumor and the degree of hormonal response. A small tumor may produce large amounts of estrin and provide the explanation of excessive menstrual bleeding or amenorrhea.

The tumors can become so large that they fill the whole pelvic cavity. Many large tumors are hormonally inactive. The symptoms produced then are those attributable to any large pelvic mass and are usually pain and discomfort in the lower portion of the abdomen and the back. For the most part the tumors are unilateral and are rarely ever fixed to adjacent structures. Approximately 25 per cent of all granulosa cell tumors appear bilaterally. Since the granulosa cell tumors may resemble fibromas in many ways, it is not surprising that some of the patients will have both ascites and hydrothorax, such as one finds in Meigs's syndrome. The ascites is occasionally bloody.

The granulosa cell tumor, since it frequently produces estrin in excess, often manifests itself in this age group by abnormalities in the vaginal bleeding pattern.

The change in the nature and type of the menstrual flow varies with the amount of estrin being produced. It customarily manifests itself in one of two ways: (a) The patient may have a preliminary phase of amenorrhea, which may be either long or short, followed by excessive, prolonged vaginal bleeding. This type of bleeding is similar to that seen in metropathia hemorrhagica, in which endometrium is stimulated by estrin, unbalanced by adequate progestin. The probable explanation of the amenorrheic phase lies in the excessive estrin circulating in the blood. Vaginal bleeding follows perhaps when the estrin level drops, on account of secondary pathologic changes that may occur within the tumor. (b) The menstrual bleeding may appear at irregular intervals and be excessive for prolonged periods. In most instances menstruation occurs from a proliferative or anovulatory type of hyperplastic endometrium. In rare instances, particularly when considerable luteinization of the granulosa cells has taken place, the endometrium may be partly in the secretory phase. Pregnancy has been known to occur with small granulosa cell tumors, but the cycles of most patients will be anovulatory.

The uterus is usually enlarged to about twice its normal size. In part this is due to the estrin stimulation from the tumor, and in part to the presence of fibroids. Approximately 70 per cent of patients with granulosa cell tumors will also have fibroids. Owing in part to this same estrin stimulation, unbalanced by progestin, these patients are prone to have endometrial hyperplasia and also carcinoma. The association of endometrial carcinoma is noted in up to 20 per cent of women with this type of tumor. The coexistence of granulosa cell tumors and endometrial carcinoma is found less often in the twenty- to thirty-year age group than in the premenopausal and postmenopausal ages. Nevertheless the possibility should be constantly kept in mind when dealing with these tumors.

What Do They Look Like at the Time of Abdominal Exploration?

The gross appearance of the granulosa cell tumor is often not much different from that of any other solid tumor, such as a fibroma. It cannot be clearly distinguished grossly from the thecoma or luteoma, since they are probably variants of the same tumor. They are usually large, encapsulated tumors, smooth, round and occasionally lobulated. They vary in size, however, and may be either very small or so large that they fill the abdomen. Since they contain large amounts of fibrous tissue, the tumors are usually solid. Some contain smooth-walled clear fluid-filled cysts. The

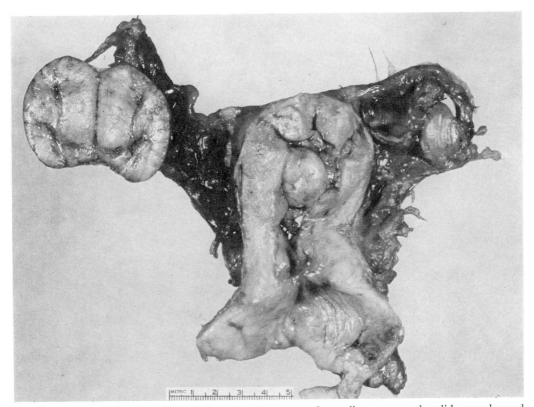

Fig. 55-1. The bisected ovary is replaced by a granulosa cell tumor, mostly solid, granular and yellow. The endometrium shows polyps and hyperplasia as evidence of estrogenic stimulation in a postmenopausal woman.

larger tumors also tend to undergo cystic degeneration within the substance of the tumor. On cut section there is a definite yellow to orange tinge, due to the high lipoid content of the tumor. It is more pronounced in those tumors that are endocrinologically active (Fig. 55–1).

What Is the Microscopic Appearance of the Granulosa Cell Tumor?

The cells one encounters in a granulosa cell carcinoma closely resemble the granulosa cells of a maturing graafian follicle. They are small round cells with scanty cytoplasm, relatively large nuclei and infrequent mitoses. The histologic arrangement of the cells is varied, but they tend to fall into one of three patterns:

1. Folliculoma. For the most part the cells arrange themselves in sheets that contain glandlike patterns which resemble follicles. These spaces vary in size from that of an immature follicle to areas several times that size. Each of the follicular areas is surrounded by neoplastic granulosa cells. Small cystic areas were originally thought to be ova, but are now recognized as follicular areas of liquefaction. The gland spaces are filled with secretion from the granulosa cells which may take a homogenous acidophilic pink stain (Fig. 55–2, *A*). These cystic spaces are termed Call-Exner bodies, and when seen are characteristic enough to make the diagnosis of granulosa cell tumor. This is the folliculomatous growth pattern. (2) Cylindroma. The cells may arrange themselves in strands or hollow columns, and a cylindrical pattern results. This is due to the increased amounts of fibrous tissue present. These isolated columns often seem to branch and anastomose with one another. This constitutes the cylindromatous growth pattern (Fig. 55–2, *B*). (3) Sarcoma-like. The cells may grow in a diffuse spread, at times showing evidence of trabeculation, while in

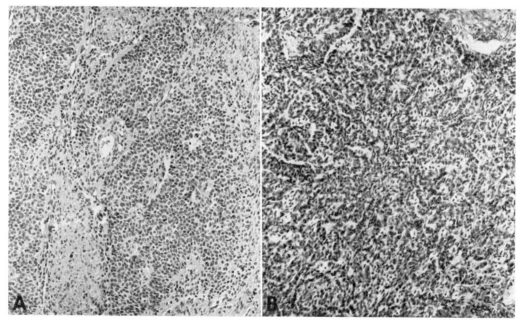

Fig. 55-2.   *A*, Granulosa cell tumors of the well differentiated folliculoma type in part form rosettes around empty spaces, the Call-Exner bodies, as seen on the right. Some thecomatous stroma is also evident. *B*, Cylindromatous growth pattern of a more anaplastic type is not so easily recognizable as a granulosa cell carcinoma. It is a more common histologic type than the folliculoma.

others a pseudoadenomatous appearance is noted. This has been called the mosaic type, or the sarcomatous pattern.

Most granulosa cell tumors will have a thecomatous stroma mixed with the granulosa cell elements. The differentiation between luteinized theca cells and granulosa cells can occasionally be difficult. The more theca cells there are, the more active the tumors are endocrinologically and the greater the chance of malignancy in both the breast tissue and the endometrium. Pure granulosa cell tumors are said to be nonfunctioning.

What Is the Relation to Endometrial Carcinoma?

There appears to be a definite association of granulosa cell tumors of the ovary and endometrial carcinoma. They are found concomitantly in a much higher percentage than one would expect from mere chance. Not all granulosa cell tumors secrete estrin, for some are hormonally inactive. The prolonged and excessive stimulation of the endometrium, unbalanced by progestin, may explain the fact that four fifths of the active granulosa cell tumors will be associated with cystic and adenomatous endometrial hyperplasia, while as many as 20 per cent will also have endometrial carcinoma. If the nonfunctioning granulosa cell tumors are excluded, the percentage of endometrial carcinoma will be appreciably higher. The association is not absolute, but it occurs often enough for the gynecologist to be on the alert for the two associated forms of malignancy—one in the ovary, the other in the endometrium.

What Is the Malignant Potential in the Ovary?

The more granulosa cell tumors are reported, the higher becomes the incidence of metastasis and recurrence. The tumor is obviously often slowly growing. It is an interesting clinical observation that recurrences may appear five, ten, and even twenty-five years after the primary tumors have been removed surgically.

The incidence of malignancy in granulosa cell tumors is generally recorded as ranging between 20 and 30 per cent. Pathologists are prone to consider a large majority to represent creeping forms of cancer. The variation in clinicopathologic opinion reflects the histologic nature of the tumor and the age at which it appears. The greater the theca cell component, the less the chance of malignant transformation. The younger the patient generally, the less likely the tumor will have clinically malignant behavior.

How Is the Diagnosis Made?

The index of suspicion is high when the tumor occurs before the menarche and after the menopause, but the clinical diagnosis of granulosa or theca cell tumors cannot be made with any certainty on the basis of the palpation of a solid tumor and a history of abnormal uterine bleeding during the active menstrual age. During this age span any adnexal tumor may produce the same physical findings and symptoms. It must also be kept in mind that some of the granulosa cell tumors are so small that they are unlikely to be felt. Such tumors may have more endocrine activity than the larger tumors that are frequently relatively quiescent hormonally.

Before the menarche practically any tumor capable of producing an endocrine effect is large enough to be felt on rectal examination.

How Does One Treat a Granulosa Cell Tumor?

The therapy of granulosa cell tumors is linked to their malignant potential, but should be modified by the age of the patient and the extent of the tumor.

Most granulosa cell tumors, at whatever age, are either malignant or potentially so. The rate of growth is apt to be slow, however, when histologic evidence of invasion is found. The tumor is rarely extensive in the younger age group. Thus the surgeon can afford to be conservative and to remove only the involved ovary when the tumor is discovered in infancy or the early reproductive years, provided there is no clinical evidence that the capsule is invaded or that disease has spread beyond the confines of the ovary. Should the pathologist on subsequent histologic study raise the question of malignancy in such a tumor, the gynecologist must rely on his own judgment as to whether to reoperate and remove the uterus and other ovary. He must make this decision, which is actually a calculated risk, for the pathologic description cannot accurately predict the clinical course in most of these tumors. If the decision is made to do nothing more, the patient should be followed up at regular yearly intervals for a considerable time, because metastases and recurrences may appear very late.

When the woman's family is complete or the tumor is discovered after the age of forty years, regardless of whether the cancer is confined to the ovary or not, the uterus and both adnexa must be sacrificed. The malignant potential in granulosa cell tumors in the older age group may run high. The late recurrences reported are usually found when the tumor has occurred in the late reproductive years, and have been known to appear from ten to over twenty years after primary surgery. Later recurrences seem to be more common than those noted within five years of the definitive treatment. There is a discrepancy in the figures reported for late recurrence; the percentage varies with the histologic pattern and ranges from 10 to 70 per cent.

THECA CELL TUMOR

The borderline between granulosa cell and theca cell tumors is not very clear-cut histologically. The clinical manifestations as well as the endocrinologic activities are also similar. Unlike the former tumor, the theca cell tumor, or thecoma, rarely appears before the age of thirty years and is less common after the menopause. Approximately 65 per cent appear in the mature reproductive years. Thecoma is the most common functioning ovarian tumor seen in general practice.

The extent of hormonal activity depends on the abundance of the theca cell elements that are found on histologic examination. Approximately two thirds are thought to be nearly pure theca cell tumors, and the remainder show variable quantities of granulosa cells in association. The tumors that present a more equal mixture of theca cell and granulosa cell elements appear to have the greatest functional activity. The pure types of either granulosa cell or theca cell tumors appear likely to produce less estrin and cause fewer menstrual disturbances.

What Do Thecomas Look Like Grossly?

The symptoms and physical signs produced by the theca cell tumors are identical with those of the granulosa cell tumor. Identification can be made only on histologic examination.

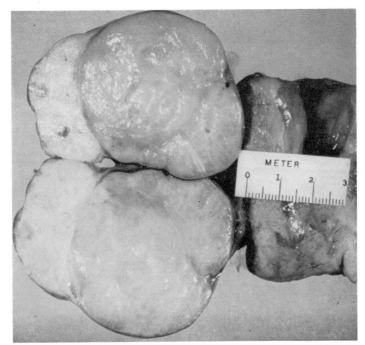

Fig. 55-3.   The ovary is spherically enlarged by a rounded tumor, solid and originally yellow-tan, in contrast to the paler, marginal, uninvolved ovarian tissue. The endometrium is hyperplastic and measures 5 mm. in thickness.

At the time of operation they appear as solid tumors varying in size from 5 to 10 cm. and covered by a smooth capsule. The tumor tends to be unilateral, and the opposite ovary is frequently atrophic. The uterus is large and appears healthy, but no corpora lutea are found in the contralateral ovary. On cut section the tumor surface appears fibrous and yellow to deep orange, depending on the lipid content, which in turn reflects the degree of physiologic activity produced by theca cells (Fig. 55–3). At times the cut surface has the same whorled appearance that one sees in a fibroma. It has been said that some fibromas are simply burned-out thecomas. The tumor characteristically is firm and hard for the most part, but may have areas of cystic degeneration in its substance.

How Do They Appear Histologically?

The pathologic criteria for the diagnosis of theca cell tumors are not as well defined as for granulosa cell tumors, since thecomas are apt to contain varying quantities of granulosa cells as well.

Microscopically, one finds bands of spindle or epithelioid stromal cells that are irregularly and either tightly or loosely arranged. The theca cells tend to blend marginally into the stroma of the normal portions of the ovary. The epithelioid cells that sometimes occur focally have clear cytoplasms, and represent the more fully luteinized theca cells. Mitoses are rarely found. Anaplasia or cancer in a thecoma is of great rarity. Localized bands of hyaline degeneration are characteristically present (Fig. 55–4, *A*). It is often difficult histologically to determine whether the plump spindle cells seen are actually theca cells or fibrocytes. It may hence be necessary to resort to special staining to distinguish between the fibroma and the thecoma. Fat

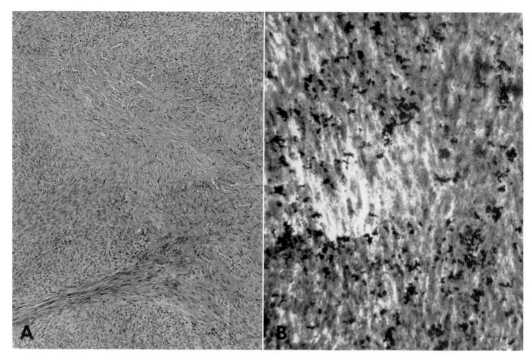

Fig. 55-4.   The cellular strands of thecomatous stroma are interspersed with hyalinized foci such as those in the upper part of the illustration. No cellular atypism or invasive behavior is ordinarily evident in thecomas. *B*, Abundant droplets of sudanophilic lipoid demonstrated in a frozen section of a spindle-celled solid ovarian neoplasm usually indicate it to be a thecoma.

stains bring out both intracellular and extracellular evidence of the presence of fat in abundance, which ovarian fibromas lack (Fig. 55–4, *B*). More elaborate staining techniques, such as silver procedures to detect the arrangement of the reticulum, are sometimes helpful in distinguishing the thecoma from the granulosa cell tumor. In the thecoma the reticulum appears to surround individual cells rather than groups of cells as in granulosa cell tumors. As noted, the two diagnoses are not mutually exclusive.

How Do You Treat a Theca Cell Tumor?

The pure thecoma, although endocrinologically active and capable of producing endometrial hyperplasia, uterine bleeding and perhaps endometrial carcinoma, is fundamentally a benign tumor. On extremely rare occasions evidence of invasion may be found together with anaplastic cells showing mitoses. The mixed types of thecoma are potentially malignant, with the degree dependent upon the amount of the granulosa cell component.

The same plan of therapy one uses for the granulosa cell tumor applies also to the treatment of thecoma. The problem is less difficult because the tumors rarely appear in adolescence or the most active reproductive years. Patients with large tumors or smaller ones that show invasion of the capsule should be subjected to total hysterectomy and bilateral salpingo-oophorectomy. The same procedure should be carried out if the tumor is found on both sides. Actually, the thecoma tends to be both benign and unilateral. In a woman in the early thirties the surgeon may safely excise the involved ovary and leave the uterus and opposite ovary.

LUTEOMAS (LUTEINIZED GRANULOSA-THECA CELL TUMORS)

This tumor has the same physical characteristics and produces the same symptoms as those of the granulosa and theca cell, for it is actually a variant of these tumors. The only essential differences other than their gross appearance and those observed histologically are that (1) they sometimes produce a secretory endometrium rather than a proliferative one, and (2) they are said to be more likely to undergo malignant transformation. A few luteomas have been reported that seem to have produced virilizing rather than feminizing effects. It is possible, however, that the masculinization may have been due to the failure to distinguish luteinization within granulosa cell tumor from possible adrenal rests or adrenocortical types of ovarian tumor. These adrenal tumors of the ovary have been called masculinovoblastomas.

How Do Luteomas Appear Grossly?

Like the theca and granulosa cell tumors, they are solid tumors which are often lobulated, and like the others they may contain areas of cystic degeneration in their substance. Since they contain large quantities of fat, the color of the tumor on cut section has a distinctly orange hue. Because of this they have been called xantho-fibroma-theca-cellulare.

What Is the Histologic Pattern?

The luteoma cells closely resemble miniature cells of a normal corpus luteum. There are usually large sheets of cuboidal or polygonal cells that blend into areas containing plump spindle cells like those of a thecoma. The cytoplasm takes an even pale acidophilic stain and may appear somewhat granular or vacuolated.

It is important to differentiate this fat-laden tumor from other tumors in this lipoid-rich category, such as those arising from adrenal cortical rests, Leydig cells or possibly from inclusions of embryonic kidney (Grawitz tumor of ovary). Some of the luteomas appear to be feminizing, and others are either nonfunctional or even reportedly androgenic. The mixed theca, granulosa and luteal cell tumors are said to be more active hormonologically. There is a greater chance of (*a*) finding associated endometrial carcinoma or (*b*) having the tumor undergo malignant change.

Treatment

In general, treatment is the same for luteoma as for a thecoma with granulosa-cell components. Conservative surgical removal is indicated in the absence of positive evidence of cancer.

TUMORS OF THE OVARY ASSOCIATED WITH MASCULINIZATION

The masculinizing ovarian neoplasms are always fascinating because of their bizarre endocrine manifestations. In actual practice they are suspected far more often than they are found. Any sign of virilism in the female, from whatever cause, is apt to be ascribed to some type of tumor which has androgenic properties, regardless of whether or not a pelvic mass can be felt. If no adnexal mass is palpable, the gyne-

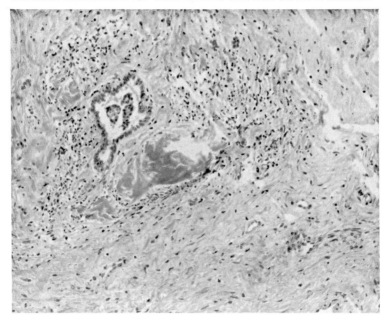

Fig. 55-5.   Portion of ovarian hilus of a postmenopausal woman showing the normal hilar structures. Between the foci of hyaline degeneration are wolffian type tubules of the rete ovarii. In a male they would have formed parts of the vas deferens. Around blood vessels are groups of small Leydig cells. These 2 ordinarily insignificant structures may form ovarian rete cysts and hilar masculinizing tumors, respectively.

cologist will do well to consider the adrenal or the nuclear sex chromatin pattern before he attributes the masculinizing effects to a nebulous ovarian tumor.

Nevertheless, rare masculinizing ovarian neoplasms of widely different origin do occur and provide great interest to the pathologist. Actually, there are many such tumors that never are reported, simply because the histologic pattern is either mixed or not distinct enough to make a definite diagnosis.

It should not be surprising that masculinizing neoplasms arise in the ovary. There are two main reasons for this: (1) In the course of normal development the embryonic ovary at its inception has a complete testicular scaffolding. The testicular elements atrophy as the differentiation toward the ovarian side progresses. The Sertoli cells, which arose from the sex cords in the embryonic testes, have their counterpart in the granulosa cells of the ovary. The stromal mesenchyma of testis contains the Leydig cells, which correspond to the ovarian theca cells. In many instances differentiation is not complete, and vestigia of the primitive testis normally persist in the hilus of the ovary (Fig. 55–5). These hilus cells are identical morphologically with the Leydig cells in the testis, which are androgen producers. Under certain conditions and in the presence of certain ovarian tumors such as the Sertoli-Leydig tubular adenoma (testicular-type adenoma of Pick), the less well differentiated arrhenoblastoma and the Leydig cell tumor, the ovary does secrete androgen and thus virilize the patient.

2. We have also noted that early in embryologic development the ovarian medulla and the adrenal cortex are intimately blended. In rare instances ovarian tumors appear which have the histologic appearance of the adrenal gland. The typical pattern shows cells resembling adrenocortical cells arranged in columns, sheets or clusters about blood vessels. Since these cells tend to produce corticoids, they have been thought to arise from adrenal rests, although no one has ever completely estab-

lished this. The cells more closely resemble the adrenal than the luteinized granulosa, or theca cells, with which they are often confused.

In summary, masculinizing tumors include: arrhenoblastoma, Sertoli-Leydig tumor, hilar cell tumor, adrenal rest tumor, gynandroblastoma.

The gynandroblastoma also is partly feminizing. So-called ovarian masculinization and the virilization that accompanies some metastatic cancers to the ovary are discussed in Chapter 56.

What about Masculinizing Ovarian Tumors with an Estrinizing Effect?

It is something of a paradox when certain tumors which have the histologic type of the known androgen producers are found to exert a feminizing influence. This same sort of phenomenon was observed in the discussion of testicular feminization in the section on adolescence.

There now appears to be evidence that cells formerly considered capable of producing only one kind of hormone may not do this consistently. The pathways of synthesis of the sex hormones tend to progress from cholesterol to progesterone to androgen to estrogen. It is reasonable and logical to postulate that in the presence of a functioning tumor of the ovary, for example, the synthesis may be incomplete or may be stimulated to progress further along the biosynthetic pathway than usually occurs. In this manner functional tumors with a cell type that would normally produce androgen may, under certain conditions, progress to the end-stage of estrin synthesis and manifest changes of a feminizing nature.

What Is the Clinical Behavior of a Masculinizing Tumor?

The clinical manifestations of these ovarian tumors are similar regardless of their pathologic conformation. A recounting of the clinical picture of the arrhenoblastoma will serve as a general background for all such masculinizing tumors.

Arrhenoblastoma

The virilizing effects of the arrhenoblastoma are well known to all medical students, despite the fact that most of their instructors have never encountered one in their own experience.

These tumors usually appear in the active reproductive period between twenty and thirty years in women who previously have had normal sex development and function. The departures from the normal may be listed as follows: (*a*) amenorrhea, (*b*) atrophy of the breasts, (*c*) a change to the male body type, (*d*) the appearance of the male hirsute pattern, (*e*) the development of an enlarged clitoris, and finally (*f*) deepening of the voice. The mere presence of amenorrhea, hirsutism and a unilateral pelvic tumor is not enough to make a diagnosis of arrhenoblastoma, but if the change appears abruptly in a young woman who has previously been normal, one may consider the possibility.

It is a fascinating observation that after the primary tumor has been removed all the physical characteristics regress toward the feminine side, except the voice, which continues to be harsh and deep. Most of the masculine signs have disappeared within a month of the surgical removal of the tumor. The menstrual periods return within

3 months, and approximately 10 per cent of the patients later become pregnant and deliver normal children.

Morphologic Appearance of Arrhenoblastoma

Grossly, these tumors have a rounded, smooth shape, and on section they are partly cystic and partly composed of brown or gray fibrous tissue. There are three principal histologic patterns:

1. TUBULAR ADENOMA OF PICK.   Tubules resembling an embryonic or child's testis are present. They lie in a fibrous stroma and appear to be lined by Sertoli cells. No interstitial cells of Leydig are identified. This type of arrhenoblastoma is least active functionally.

2. INTERMEDIATE TYPE.   Here there are cords somewhat like a poorly organized primitive testis, lying in a fibrous or loose areolar stroma. Usually some

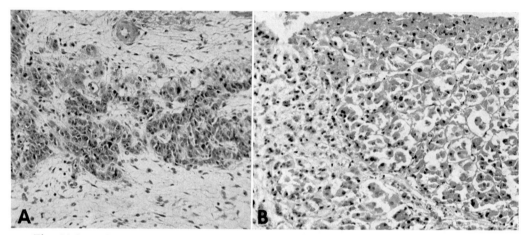

Fig. 55-6.   In arrhenoblastoma of the intermediate type it is possible to identify solid cell cords that resemble embryonic stages of testicular tubule formation. Nests of polygonal Leydig cells may occur in the tumor stroma, as seen in the upper part of the field. *B*, Part of an ovarian hilar cell tumor found incidentally at autopsy. The patient was moderately masculinized.

recognizable groups of polygonal eosinophilic Leydig cells are present. If one is fortunate, Reinke crystalloids of testosterone may be found in the cytoplasm of some Leydig cells (Fig. 55–6, *A*).

3. SARCOMATOUS TYPE.   This is a wild undifferentiated spindle cell sarcoma, unrecognizable as androgenic without other information. Curiously, this type is most apt to be functionally active.

Histologically, the intermediate and sarcomatous arrhenoblastomas appear malignant. Clinically, most of these tumors act like sluggishly invasive cancers. The Pick tubular adenoma is the rarest variant, clinically least active endocrinologically, and is usually benign.

SERTOLI-LEYDIG TUMOR

This rare entity may be differentiated histologically from the Pick adenoma by the presence of Leydig cells in the interstices between the testicular-type tubules. In some classifications it is regarded as synonymous with arrhenoblastoma, gynandro-blastoma or gonadoblastoma.

HILAR-CELL TUMOR

Clinically, these occur in older women, and produce more bitemporal alopecia, angularity of body contour and male facial appearance than clitoral hypertrophy or male aggressiveness. They are in a sense more masculinizing than virilizing.

Grossly, the tumors are sharply demarcated, solid, relatively small and soft and have a less dramatic gross appearance than other masculinizing tumors. On cut section they all have a brown or yellow tinge because of the high lipochrome pigment and lipoid content. Hilar cell tumors are composed microscopically of sheets of Leydig-type polygonal cells, without anaplasia or invasion (Fig. 55–6, *B*). Reinke crystalloids are present in about half the cases. No malignant hilar cell tumor has been reported yet.

ADRENAL REST TUMORS

Grossly, these are bright yellow, and either well or poorly demarcated. Micro-scopically, the cells are vacuolated with abundant lipoid, or eosinophilic. Their androgenic or estrogenic activities are not evident from pathologic scrutiny. The growth pattern may be that of either adrenocortical adenoma or carcinoma (Fig. 55–7).

The possibly related ovarian hypernephroma is grossly a bright yellow tumor that microscopically consists of sheets and cords of watery epithelial cells identical with those of the common renal cell carcinoma. Whether this so-called Grawitz tumor of the ovary is of renal or adrenal rest origin is not clear. These are more often nonfunctional than masculinizing.

Tumors either with adrenal-like cells, luteinized theca or Leydig cells present in

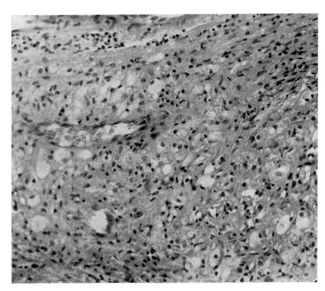

Fig. 55-7. An ovarian adre-nocortical rest tumor is characterized by cords of lipoid-rich vacuolated cells with intervening blood vessels that imitate the pattern of the adrenal zona fasciculata. This example is of the usual well differentiated benign appearance.

varying amounts are sometimes classified together under the name "lipoid cell tumors."

How Often Do These Tumors Occur, and What Is the Malignant Potential?

The so-called Sertoli-Leydig cell type of benign masculinizing tumor occurs for the most part in the active reproductive age group. These are extremely rare tumors.

The more differentiated and benign Leydig cell tumor has been reported in infancy and has been known to produce both masculinization and virilization. The undifferentiated arrhenoblastoma has not been seen before the age of fourteen years. When found in the reproductive age groups, they usually show either frank masculinization or changes away from the female characteristics. Occasionally Leydig-type tumors are found without clinical manifestations. Even in the presence of obvious virilization the urinary 17-ketosteroids show little variation from the normal.

A malignant potentiality exists in the undifferentiated arrhenoblastoma, in which the recurrence rate is in the range of 25 per cent.

The lipoid cell tumors are found even less frequently, since only fifty-odd cases have been reported. For the most part they are discovered in the active reproductive years. They appeared after the menopause in one third of the cases and only rarely produced virilization in the prepuberal child. It is unusual to find a lipoid cell tumor that does not show some masculinization. Because of the similarity of these cells to those of the adrenal cortex, it is not surprising that approximately 20 per cent will show some of the characteristics of Cushing's disease. Thus the patient may exhibit polycythemia, diabetes, weight gain and hypertension. Unlike in the Sertoli-Leydig tubular adenoma or the arrhenoblastoma, the urinary 17-ketosteroids tend to be elevated.

The malignant potential of adrenal rest tumors is somewhat less than that of the other masculinizing tumors.

Gynandroblastoma

In rare instances the pathologist encounters a form of arrhenoblastoma in which granulosa cell elements are also present. In most of them the masculinizing component predominates, and virilization occurs. Occasionally, however, estrogenic manifestations appear, the patient experiencing menorrhagia due to endometrial hyperplasia or carcinoma.

What Treatment Is Advised for Arrhenoblastoma, Gynandroblastoma, Hilar Cell or Adrenal Rest Tumor?

The malignant potential is approximately the same as that noted for the granulosa and theca cell tumors. There is about a 25 per cent chance of malignancy, and a recurrence rate of similar percentage.

In the late reproductive years or with the family complete this is enough to warrant total hysterectomy and bilateral removal of the adnexa. Except for the pure Sertoli or Leydig cell tumor, masculinizing tumors of the ovary are not found before puberty, and then they are virtually medical curiosities. The problem involving a choice of therapy therefore arises chiefly in the young woman. One can afford to be conservative in treatment, removing only the involved ovary, if the patient is young and the tumor encapsulated when there is no obvious evidence of metastasis.

Note that all hilar Leydig cell tumors so far reported have been benign, with one recent exception.

REFERENCES

Granulosa Cell Tumors

Biskind, M. S., and Biskind, G. S.: Development of Tumors in the Rat Ovary after Transplantation into the Spleen. *Proc. Soc. Exper. Biol. & Med.*, 55: 176, 1944.

Busby, T., and Anderson, G. W.: Feminizing Mesenchymomas of the Ovary—Includes 107 Cases of Granulosa-, Granulosa-Theca-Cell, and Theca-Cell Tumors. *Am. J. Obst. & Gynec.*, 68: 1391, 1954.

Diddle, A. W.: Granulosa- and Theca-Cell Ovarian Tumors: Prognosis. *Cancer*, 5: 215, 1952.

Duckett, H. C., Davis, C. D., and Fetter, B. F.: Granulosa Cell Carcinoma of Ovary; Clinical and Pathological Review of 17 Patients. *Obst. & Gynec.*, 2: 611, 1953.

Engle, R. B.: Roentgen Treatment of Granulosa Cell Carcinoma of the Ovary. *Am. J. Roentgenol.*, 80: 793, 1958.

Flick, F. H., and Banfield, R. S., Jr.: Theca- and Granulosa-Cell Tumors—A Review of 55 Cases. *Bull. Sloane Hosp. for Women*, 2: 31, 1956.

McKay, D. G., Robinson, D., and Hertig, A. T.: Histochemical Observations on Granulosa-Cell Tumors, Thecomas, and Fibromas of the Ovary. *Am. J. Obst. & Gynec.*, 58: 625, 1949.

Mackinlay, C. J.: Male Cells in Granulosa Cell Tumours. *J. Obst. & Gynaec. Brit. Emp.*, 64: 512, 1957.

Meigs, J. V.: Ovarian Tumors with Endocrine Significance. *Ann. Surg.*, 102: 834, 1935.

Morris, J. McL.: Functional Tumors of the Ovary. *Clin. Obst. & Gynec.*, 4: 821, 1961.

Morris, J. McL., and Scully, R. E.: *Endocrine Pathology of the Ovary*. St. Louis, C. V. Mosby Company, 1958.

Novak, E., and Brawner, J. N., Jr.: Granulosa Cell Tumors of the Ovary. A Clinical and Pathological Study of 36 Cases. *Am. J. Obst. & Gynec.*, 28: 637, 1934.

Sommers, S. C., Gates, O., and Goodof, I. I.: Late Recurrence of Granulosa Cell Tumors. *Obst. & Gynec.*, 6: 395, 1955.

Varangot, J.: *Les Tumeurs de la Granulosa*. Folliculomes de l'oveire. Paris, L. Arnette, 1937.

Functioning Tumors and Endometrial Carcinoma

Corbet, R. M., Miller, A. A., and Tod, W. H.: Endometrial Carcinoma Associated with Feminizing Tumours of the Ovary. Report of Two Cases. *J. Obst. & Gynaec. Brit. Emp.*, 59: 368, 1952.

Emge, L. A.: Endometrial Cancer and Feminizing Tumor of Ovaries. Significance of Their Coexistence. *Obst. & Gynec.*, 1: 511, 1953.

Hertig, A. T.: Endocrine Ovarian-Cancer Relationships. *Cancer*, 10: 838, 1957.

Ingram, J. M., Jr., and Novak, E.: Endometrial Carcinoma Associated with Feminizing Ovarian Tumors. *Am. J. Obst. & Gynec.*, 61: 774, 1951.

Larsson, E., and Olson, A. W.: Thecoma Associated with Adenocarcinoma of the Endometrium. *Am. J. Obst. & Gynec.*, 66: 432, 1952.

Theca Cell Tumors

Diddle, A. W., and Devereux, W. P.: Ovarian Mesenchymomas; Five-Year Follow-up Study. *Obst. & Gynec.*, 13: 294, 1959.

Flick, F. H., and Banfield, R. S., Jr.: Malignant Theca-Cell Tumors. Two New Case Reports and Review of the Eight Published Cases. *Cancer*, 9: 731, 1956.

Henderson, D. N.: The Malignancy of Special Ovarian Tumors. *Am. J. Obst. & Gynec.*, 62: 816, 1951.

Israel, S. L., and Mutch, J. C.: Endocrinologic Effects of Certain Ovarian Tumors. *Surg., Gynec. & Obst.,* 105: 166, 1957.

Jew, E. W., Jr., and Gross, P.: Malignant Thecoma with Metastases. *Am. J. Obst. & Gynec.,* 69: 857, 1955.

Novak, E., and Novak, E. R.: *Gynecologic and Obstetric Pathology.* 4th Ed. Philadelphia, W. B. Saunders Company, 1958.

Pedowitz, P., Felmus, L. B., and Grayzel, D. M.: Criteria for the Diagnosis of Malignancy in Theca-Cell Tumors. *Am. J. Obst. & Gynec.,* 68: 1519, 1954.

Poshyachinda, D., Kahana, L., Del Corral, F., and Hamblen, E. C.: Bilateral Functioning Cystadenofibromas of the Ovaries. Report of a Case. *Am. J. Obst. & Gynec.,* 79: 995, 1960.

Richardson, G. S., and Ulfelder, H.: Problems Presented by Benign Solid Ovarian Tumors. *Clin. Obst. & Gynec.,* 4: 834, 1961.

Rogers, W. S., Gordon, R. E., and Marsh, M. R.: The Incidence of Malignancy in Theca-Cell Tumors. *Am. J. Obst. & Gynec.,* 64: 1289, 1952.

Rubin, I. C., Novak, J., and Squire, J. J.: Ovarian Fibromas and Theca-Cell Tumors: Report of 78 Cases, with Special Reference to Production of Ascites and Hydrothorax (Meigs' Syndrome). *Am. J. Obst. & Gynec.,* 48: 601, 1944.

Schneider, G. T.: "Functioning" Ovarian Tumors. *Am. J. Obst. & Gynec.,* 79: 921, 1960.

Scully, R. E., and Morris, J. McL.: Functioning Ovarian Tumors; in J. V. Meigs and S. H. Sturgis, eds.: *Progress in Gynecology.* New York, Grune & Stratton, Inc., 1957, Vol. III, p. 20.

Masculinizing Tumors and Gynandroblastomas

Amromin, G. D., and Haumeder, E. M.: Feminizing Ovarian Gynandroblastoma. *Am. J. Obst. & Gynec.,* 77: 645, 1959.

Emig, O. R., Hertig, A. T., and Rowe, F. J.: Gynandroblastoma of the Ovary. Review and Report of a Case. *Obst. & Gynec.,* 13: 135, 1959.

Hughesdon, P. E., and Fraser, I. T.: Arrhenoblastoma of Ovary. A Case Report and Histological Review. *Acta Obst. et Gynec. Scand.,* 32 (Supp. 4), 1953.

Iverson, L.: Masculinizing Tumors of the Ovary. A Clinicopathologic Survey with Discussion of Histogenesis and Report of Three Cases. *Surg., Gynec. & Obst.,* 84: 213, 1947.

Javert, C. T., and Finn, W. F.: Arrhenoblastoma. The Incidence of Malignancy and the Relationship to Pregnancy, to Sterility and to Treatment. *Cancer,* 4: 60, 1951.

Novak, E. R., and Mattingly, R. F.: Hilus Cell Tumor of the Ovary. *Obst. & Gynec.,* 15: 425, 1960.

Sternberg, W. H.: The Morphology, Androgenic Function, Hyperplasia, and Tumors of the Human Ovarian Hilus Cells. *Am. J. Path.,* 25: 493, 1949.

Teilum, G.: Arrhenoblastoma—Androblastoma. Homologous Ovarian and Testicular Tumors, Including So-Called Luteomas and "Adrenal Tumors" of Ovary and Interstitial Tumors of Testes. *Acta path. et microbiol. Scand.,* 23: 252, 1946.

Idem: Classification of Ovarian Tumours. *Acta obst. et gynec. Scand.,* 31: 292, 1952.

Welch, J. W., and Hellwig, C. A.: Hypernephroid Carcinoma of the Ovary. Case Report. *Am. J. Obst. & Gynec.,* 80: 426, 1960.

Zuspan, F. P.: Testicular Feminizing Syndrome in Male Pseudohermaphroditism. A Report of Its Occurrence in Successive Siblings. *Am. J. Obst. & Gynec.,* 80: 454, 1960.

Chapter 56

Metastatic (Secondary) Ovarian Neoplasms

SOLID tumors of the ovary may not be primary neoplasms at all, but secondary metastases from malignant disease elsewhere. The ovary is a frequent site of metastases from an initial focus in the stomach, sigmoid colon, endometrium and breast. These occur far more frequently than we are accustomed to think, for small nests of cells are unlikely to be detected. Unless the ovary enlarges to appreciable size, the metastatic tumor of the ovary may not be recognized in life. The symptoms and physical findings are in no way different from those noted with any solid tumor of the ovary.

BREAST CANCER

We are accustomed to the logic of removing ovaries because of their hormonal influence on metastatic carcinoma from a primary lesion in the breast. We are less adjusted to the concept that the ovaries should be removed because they are a likely site of metastases. It is amazing how many ovaries of young women who have had bilateral oophorectomy to control metastases from breast cancer also will reveal malignant cell deposits (Fig. 56–1). The incidence has been placed at 20 per cent. When breast cancer metastases are seen in bone, secondary malignant involvement of the ovary reaches 60 per cent.

SIGMOID COLON CANCER

The first indication of malignant disease in the sigmoid may be the physical finding by palpation of a tumor in the region of the left ovary. Frequently there are no symptoms referable to the gastrointestinal tract, despite the fact that at operation an annular constricting lesion is found that is appreciable in size. We have encountered four such cases within the past year. Metastases to the ovary are so common in sigmoid carcinoma that the ovaries must always be suspected whether they show obvious metastases or not (Fig. 56–2). The cancer cell deposits may be microscopic. This is such a common association that some surgeons advocate total hysterectomy

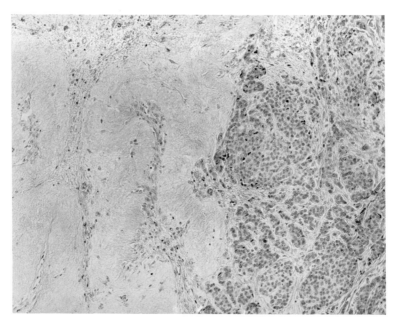

Fig. 56-1.   Metastatic carcinoma simplex of the breast, as found in surgical pathologic material after oophorectomy. Cords of carcinoma cells are infiltrating a corpus albicans.

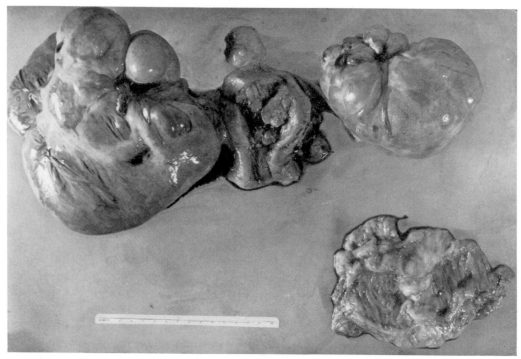

Fig. 56-2.   Large, bilateral ovarian metastases are present that arose from the primary annular carcinoma of the sigmoid colon shown at the lower right. Endometrial polyps and a fibroid were also found.

and bilateral oophorectomy as a regular part of the operation for resection of a sigmoid adenocarcinoma.

ENDOMETRIAL CARCINOMA

Metastases to the ovary from primary adenocarcinoma in the endometrium occur so frequently, in 12 per cent of cases, that it is standard procedure to remove the adnexa when performing a hysterectomy for endometrial cancer.

STOMACH CANCER

Though the stomach and sigmoid colon are the most common primary sites within the gastrointestinal tract that send metastatic deposits to the ovary, metastases may appear from lesions present anywhere along its course, including the gallbladder. In the past the stomach was always suspected when secondary tumors were found in the ovary. Actually, the other sites previously listed are more likely primary sources. Ovarian metastases from adenocarcinomas of the stomach microscopically may contain characteristic signet ring cells, similar to those seen invading the gastric wall.

Krukenberg originally described this type of ovarian tumor and pointed out the association of abnormalities in the stomach and ovary, though he actually believed it to be a primary ovarian sarcoma rather than metastatic ovarian carcinoma of gastric epithelial origin. There has been a tendency to apply the term "Krukenberg tumors" to all metastatic carcinomas of the ovary. This is obviously an error, for metastatic tumors to the ovary usually tend to have the same microscopic appearance as at the primary source. Metastatic tumors to the ovary from the stomach are most often bilateral and frequently large and lumpy, though the initial adenocarcinoma

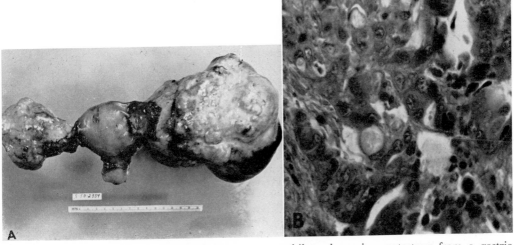

Fig. 56-3. *A,* Genuine Krukenberg tumors are bilateral ovarian metastases from a gastric carcinoma, shown here as large nodular masses. *B,* Mucous signet-ring cells of metastatic carcinoma simplex are the histologically characteristic finding in Krukenberg tumors. Such cells may be from a colonic carcinoma, and may fall within the definition of the Krukenberg type of ovarian metastasis.

in the stomach may be small (Fig. 56–3, *A*). It is not a genuine Krukenberg tumor unless it contains the characteristic signet ring cells containing mucous droplets, and usually lying in abundant fibrous stroma (Fig. 56–3, *B*).

HOW DO THE SECONDARY DEPOSITS GET TO THE OVARY?

The route of spread of metastatic cancer cells from primary sources to the ovary varies widely, depending on the location of the initial tumor. From the immediately adjacent sigmoid colon or endometrium metastases may occur by contiguous spread along lymphatic channels, or as in the case of endometrium by implantation through the open fallopian tubal lumen. In most instances, however, the metastatic deposits are found within the interior rather than on the surface of the ovary. This fact is a strong argument against the theory that cells were disseminated freely throughout the peritoneal cavity from primary gastric carcinomas. The probable method of spread from the stomach is retrograde through lymphatic channels, although dissemination via the blood stream is possible. The latter route would be most logical in explaining how metastases occurred from breast cancer.

The opposite ovary becomes involved from a primary contralateral carcinoma by lymphatic extension to the uterus and then to the hilus of the opposite ovary. Though the initial carcinoma in the ovary may be of unilateral origin, the spread to the opposite ovary occurs so frequently that the uterus and both adnexa should be removed as standard therapy in ovarian cancer.

WHAT DO THESE SECONDARY METASTATIC TUMORS LOOK LIKE?

Gross Appearance.   Metastatic carcinomas to the ovary are invariably solid and frequently bilateral. They are almost invariably free of any attachments. Within the smooth-surfaced solid tumors nodular areas and soft cystic spots are common findings. They vary in size, but for the most part are approximately spheroidal and about 15 cm. across. On rare occasions they may grow rapidly and produce a noticeable abdominal enlargement.

The Krukenberg tumor, alone among metastatic ovarian cancers, has typical gross characteristics. Such tumors tend to maintain the original shape of the ovary, regardless of the size they may achieve. These bilateral kidney-shaped tumors have the wrinkled surface convolutions that one is accustomed to see in the normal ovary.

On cut section one encounters solid fibrous and granular, nearly white accumulations of tumor cells scattered through what appears to be normal ovarian tissue. The Krukenberg tumors tend to be both fibrous and slightly gelatinous.

Microscopic Appearance.   In many instances metastatic foci in the ovary maintain the histologic picture of the primary cancer. It is unwise to try to determine the site of origin of a primary tumor, however, based simply on an ovarian biopsy. If the tumor originally arose from the stomach or large intestine, the metastatic carcinoma will tend to produce mucin, which varies in amount. There may be enough mucus to obscure the details of the cellular pattern.

The signet ring cells of the typical Krukenberg type of carcinoma metastasis are striking. The signet ring connotation is due to the ringlike appearance of the cell, which contains so much mucin that the nucleus is flattened and pushed to one side, while the remainder of the cell remains clear and basophilic, surrounded by a ring of cell wall. The microscopic appearance of Krukenberg tumors varies greatly. Not infrequently the reactive stroma is so abundant that the signet ring epithelial cells are few and far between, while the tumor takes on the misleading microscopic appearance of a fibroma or sarcoma. Mucus stained by PAS technique aids in making the correct diagnosis.

DOES THE TREATMENT OF SECONDARY TUMORS DIFFER FROM THAT GIVEN FOR PRIMARY OVARIAN CARCINOMA?

The only added factor in the treatment of cancer metastatic to the ovary is the necessity of determining the primary source. The stomach and remainder of the gastrointestinal tract should be scrutinized closely, for primary carcinomas arising here may metastasize without producing any local symptoms. Total hysterectomy and bilateral oophorectomy are indicated, even when the metastases seem grossly limited to one ovary.

REFERENCES

Karsh, J.: Secondary Malignant Disease of the Ovaries. A Study of 72 Autopsies. *Am. J. Obst. & Gynec.* 61: 154, 1951.

Rendleman, D. F., and Gilchrist, R. K.: Indications for Oophorectomy in Carcinoma of the Gastrointestinal Tract. *Surg., Gynec. & Obst.*, 109: 364, 1959.

Shaw, W.: Krukenberg Tumour of the Ovaries. *Proc. Roy. Soc. Med.*, 19: 49, 1925.

Soloway, I., Latour, J. P. A., and Young, M. H. V.: Krukenberg Tumors of the Ovary. *Obst. & Gynec.* 8: 636, 1956.

Wheelock, M. C., and Putong, P.: Ovarian Metastases from Adenocarcinoma of Colon and Rectum. *Obst. & Gynec.*, 14: 291, 1959.

Woodruff, J. D., and Novak, E. R.: The Krukenberg Tumor: Study of 48 Cases from the Ovarian Tumor Registry. *Obst. & Gynec.*, 15: 351, 1960.

Chapter 57

Diagnosis and Treatment
of Common Lesions of the Breast

SINCE the general physical examination is a fundamental step in the investigation of any patient who is suspected of gynecologic disease or malfunction, it is obvious that the physician who concentrates his interests on these problems will of necessity examine many more breasts than will the average physician. For this reason it is important to discuss some of the more common disease entities that are likely to be encountered. It is manifestly impossible to consider all the variations of tumor formation that can and occasionally do appear. Since the breast is an external organ which can readily be seen and felt, there is small reason for overlooking a tumor. In most instances the patient will have discovered it herself. Although the breast may change in size and contour because of the presence of a deep-seated tumor, the patient is usually unaware of it or fails to recognize its significance. In most instances the tumor, whether benign or malignant, is discovered accidentally while running the hand across the breast in the course of bathing.

Is the History of Any Help in Detecting Breast Neoplasms?

Although the patient frequently gives a history of injury to the breast and dates the discovery of a lump from the moment of trauma, in all probability the actual blow had nothing to do with the development of the tumor. One can so traumatize the fatty portion of the breast that a fat necrosis appears which is often indistinguishable clinically from malignant disease, but in most instances the trauma simply calls attention to a pre-existing tumor, as the patient explores the injured area.

THE SIGNIFICANCE OF PAIN.   Although it is not invariably true, there is a general rule of thumb in diagnosis of breast lesions that painful or tender lumps are unlikely to be malignant. In most instances pain suggests some physiologic alterations in the breast epithelium that result from hormonal imbalance. The symptoms tend to appear in the ten-day period preceding menstruation and to subside with its onset. The severity of the symptoms varies widely in the same patient, and the typical history of mastodynia (painful breasts) is marked by exacerbations interspersed with longer or shorter intervals of regression and quiescence. The patient is extremely concerned about the possibility of cancer, particularly when she can feel some irregular, tender masses. In most instances the patient can be reassured that her fears are unfounded.

If the symptoms are persistent and incapacitating, or if the physician entertains any doubt about the underlying situation, the breast should be biopsied and the offending lesion excised.

The Significance of Nipple Drainage.   One may have a serious lesion of the breast without discharge from the nipple, but when the patient observes it (a rare occasion) and tells the physician about it, both become much concerned. In many instances, in fact in the majority of cases, such discharge is entirely physiological, or it may represent an underlying inflammatory process. Discharge does not mean that the patient has breast carcinoma. This is particularly true if the physician or patient has to squeeze the breast to demonstrate the discharge. One should become more concerned if it appears spontaneously, particularly if it is bloody or thin and watery.

Several types of discharge are described by patients, and offer important clues in the differential diagnosis. The two most common are (*a*) the serous and (*b*) the bloody type of discharge.

The *serous discharge* usually stems from proliferative intraductal lesions such as the intraductal papilloma. Rarely it is associated with carcinoma. The discharge is usually thin, proteinaceous and yellowish when seen by the physician and appears as a yellowish stain on the brassière or night clothing when noted by the patient. Such duct epithelial proliferations are usually located superficially in the areolar area where they are easily traumatized. This probably explains the appearance of the serous type of discharge.

The *bloody discharge* varies in its appearance and consistency, depending on the concentration of red blood cells. In most instances it will be brownish. Occasionally it resembles true blood, and rarely it may be dark red or black. This type of discharge also springs from intraductal epithelial proliferations, and although in most instances they are benign, it is more alarming to the patient and physician. By and large the intraductal papillomas that produce it are due to irritation hormonal stimulation or form a part of cystic mastitis. It can be due to deep-seated intraductal carcinomas, but the physician usually need not become overexercised about the malignant possibilities.

The Milky Type of Discharge.   It is not an uncommon experience for women to observe a milky type of secretion for some months or even years after the termination of a pregnancy. The quantity is minimal and frequently is noted only upon pressure or on squeezing of the breasts. Occasionally it appears spontaneously, but this should not cause alarm, for the milky secretion has no pathologic basis. Prolactin secretion studies of the pituitary have never been perfected to the point at which they have any practical significance, and the cause of the continued production of milk is as yet unknown. It may be a hormonal imbalance, but to date attempts to suppress it by administering either androgen or estrin have usually been unrewarding.

The Thick, Yellowish-Green Type of Discharge.   As the descrption applies equally well to pus wherever it is seen, it is not surprising that such a discharge is usually associated with low-grade inflammatory processes located in and around the areola or within the superficial ducts of the breast. It is not an uncommon experience with women of middle age who have borne children to say that they can frequently express a drop of thick gray material from the nipple. Although this may sometimes be found in women who have epithelial proliferation in the ducts, it has no pathologic significance other than a mild degree of inflammation and duct ectasia.

The Thin, Watery Type of Discharge.   When this type of discharge appears spontaneously, it is far more likely to have an association with malignant disease than any of the other types of discharge.

How Valuable Are Cytologic Examinations of the Nipple Discharge?

In view of the amount of publicity given to early detection of cancer, it is not surprising that both patient and physician are interested in the observations that may be made on the nipple discharge when it is smeared and subjected to cytologic study after staining by the Papanicolaou technique.

The method has been both enthusiastically received and discounted. The chief disadvantage lies in the number of false positives that may lead to errors in diagnosis and treatment. There is no question that intraductal papillomas as well as carcinomas shed tumor cells that appear in the secretion. In many instances, however, it is practically impossible even for a trained cytologist to tell whether they are benign or malignant. Of more practical significance perhaps than the number of false positives, which will in all probability be followed by tissue biopsy, are the false negatives, which simply give an unwarranted sense of security.

It would appear, then, that the physician will be on safer ground to explore the areolar area and biopsy any suspicious lesion if there is reasonable doubt in his mind that the nipple discharge may have a malignant connotation.

What Can We Learn from Inspection of the Breast?

A considerable amount of information can be obtained simply by looking at the breast under adequate illumination. The inspection should begin with the patient lying on her back with her arms at her sides. The first thing that strikes your eye is the size, shape and contour of the breasts. If a physician trains himself to look at the breasts critically, it is amazing how quickly he learns to recognize departures from the normal. Only then does he realize that although the two breasts are similar in appearance, one breast may be larger than the other. This has no pathologic significance, but if he has noted this, he will also be quick to discover a depressed or bulging area in the skin overlying the breast tissue due to either a deep seated carcinoma that causes

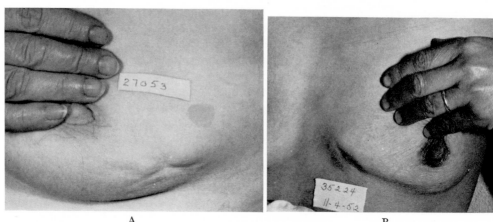

A   B

Fig. 57-1. *A,* Small area of skin retraction, typically caused by breast carcinoma. *B,* An indurated localized nodularity of the breast, due to either a benign or a malignant neoplasm. In this instance it was carcinoma.

skin retraction (Fig. 57–1, *A*) or an enlarging benign or malignant tumor that pushes the skin outward (Fig. 57–1, *B*).

He will note the color of the skin and the presence of dilated veins running over the breast surface. Thickening of the skin, which feels warm to the touch, may be an indication of an underlying inflammatory process that may be either benign or malignant. In most instances it will be a secondary manifestation of some acute or chronic infection in either the duct or the cystic lobular portions of the breast. On the other hand, a true, inflammatory, rapidly growing carcinoma of the breast, or one undergoing necrosis also will produce redness and increased superficial heat over the entire breast or perhaps in a localized segment.

Dilated veins running in the superficial skin often herald the rapid growth of tumor in the breast tissue beneath. This is particularly true of sarcoma, but it may also be found in expanding tumors which may be either benign or malignant In addition to the color, the *texture of the skin* may give important information. This is particularly true when the skin appears thickened and edematous. The so-called *peau d'orange*, in which the thick, pitted skin resembles that of an orange, is a typical finding in extensive or inflammatory carcinoma and is due to the blocking of the superficial skin lymphatics by tumor cells (Figs. 57–2, 57–3, *A*). The greater portion of the skin surface is implicated, but obvious thickening of the skin without the pockmarks may occur in localized areas, particularly in the more dependent portions of breast below the areola. This may be due to infection, but of greater significance is the fact that it may be the first indication of carcinoma arising deep in the substance of the

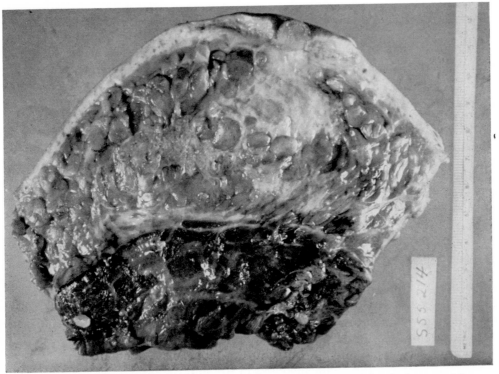

Fig. 57-2. Breast carcinoma has developed below and to the left of the nipple area, with upward spread. The results of invasion of the areolar area include thickening of the dermis, *peau d'orange* appearance and retraction of the nipple.

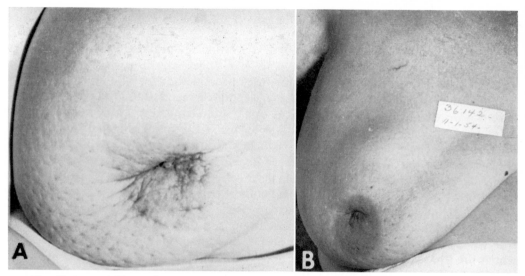

Fig. 57-3.   *A,* External appearance of nipple retraction and *peau d'orange* abnormality characteristic of breast carcinoma with skin involvement. *B,* A retracted nipple that points upward toward the bulging tumor mass indicates carcinoma in the upper breast quadrant.

breast. Actually, the point of origin of the mammary cancer may be remote from the area of dependent edema, such as in the upper outer quadrant. If the cancer arises in a more superficial portion of the breast, you may note a localized edema and thickening of the skin with perhaps some suggestion of skin retraction in this area.

Finally the *condition of the nipple* should be considered. The two things to look for are (*a*) the size and shape of the nipples and the direction in which they point, and (*b*) the nature of the epithelium that covers the areolae and nipples.

What Is the Significance of Nipple Retraction?

Retraction of the nipple may be normal in any woman, but it can have serious import. Many women have experienced trouble with an inverted nipple that they have noted for years, and it may have interfered with their desire to nurse their children. The inversion may be present on one or both sides, but whenever it is found to be insignificant, the size and shape of the nipple are in all other respects normal. It is also possible to find a retraction of the nipple secondary to an old breast abscess which drained spontaneously or had to be incised, but here too it is only the position of the nipple that has changed, not its contour.

When mammary carcinoma is present, however, definite changes are frequently noted in both the areola and the nipple. For example, a centrally placed cancer of the breast will in many instances cause the nipple to retract below the level of the skin. If the cancer is laterally placed or is in the upper quadrant of the breast, the nipple will tend to point in the direction of the tumor. This is due to the contracting effect of the fibrosis that always surrounds such malignant lesions. Not only is the direction of the nipple altered, but also the nipple itself tends to become larger, broader and flatter as the tumor increases in size and the productive fibrosis becomes more prominent (Fig. 57–3, *B*).

Not all malignant lesions behave in this fashion, and it is possible for benign masses to produce nipple retraction that closely simulates alterations due to malignant disease. Such cases, however, are the exception, not the rule.

What Is the Significance of Skin Retraction?

The mechanism involved in skin and nipple retraction is the same whether the lesion is benign or malignant. The extent of the retraction is due to the amount of fibrosis set up by the causative agent. Thus we may have fibrosis due to fat necrosis or an inflammatory process in the duct or lobular system. As the fibroblastic response becomes more mature, there is a natural tendency for the skin to retract, drawing everything toward the site of the original lesion. The normal anatomy of the breasts contributes, for the breast is anatomically situated between the deep layer of fascia that is attached to the pectoral muscle and the superficial fascia that is attached to the skin. The breast substance itself is separated into compartments by the fibrous tissue septa which in turn attach both to the skin and the deep pectoral fascia. Thus when carcinoma activates a fibroblastic response, there is a natural tendency for the skin to retract and for the tumor to become fixed to the underlying pectoral muscles. This is why dimpling of the skin in certain instances becomes apparent only when the patient puts her arms over her head, thereby putting the pectoral muscles on tension.

Most carcinomas of the breast will present some suggestion of retraction of either the nipple or skin. A few well differentiated, well circumscribed cancers will show little or no retraction simply because they progress at a more leisurely pace and set up less of a protective fibrotic response in the rest of the breast tissue. Conversely, some of the larger benign lesions, small intraductal papillomas or areas of fat necrosis may occasionally, when there has been a history of nipple discharge, be accompanied by superficial ulcerations in the epithelium of the skin overlying the nipple or areola. The discharge is usually attributed to these ulcerations, and the process is considered to be a simple eczema. It may well be, but even the most experienced observers cannot distinguish between a benign eczematoid lesion and the Pagetoid type of carcinoma that is common in this area. The differentiation can be made only by a biopsy of the lesion.

EXAMINATION OF THE BREAST

After a thorough inspection of the breasts a systematic further examination is indicated. It is well to keep in mind that the breast covers a wide area on the chest wall extending upward to the clavicle, to the sternum in the midline, well out laterally to the latissimus dorsi and into the axilla. If a malignant tumor is present in the breast tissue, it may metastasize to the lymph nodes in the supraclavicular region as well as the axilla.

Supraclavicular Examination

The examination should begin with palpation of the supraclavicular area with the patient in the sitting position. If the malignant process has metastasized to the neck lymph nodes, it may be felt at the border of the sternocleidomastoid muscle, where it attaches to the inner end of the clavicle and the sternum. The lymph nodes lie in the angle between the internal jugular and subclavicular veins and are often deeply placed. Therefore, when these nodes can be felt, it is usually an indication of rather widespread disease. The more superficial lymph nodes palpated laterally become involved in most instances only after the more centrally placed nodes (the so-called sentinel nodes) have become implicated.

Nodes found to contain tumor in this region augur a poor prognosis for the future and influence the nature of the therapy. There is little point in performing a radical mastectomy for the carcinoma, and one may choose to use radiation or some form of chemotherapy rather than surgery. Attempts to carry out more extensive dissections, which included a complete neck dissection, removal of the clavicle and breast tissue en bloc, have proved to be too destructive and completely valueless for cure of cancer.

Axillary Palpation

It is much easier to examine the axilla with a patient in the sitting position than it is with her lying down. The palpation is done with the tips of the fingers while the flat of the hand lies on the lateral wall of the chest. Little will be accomplished by digging the finger tips into the axillary space, and the gentler the palpation, the greater the degree of accuracy. Lymph nodes tend to lie along the distribution of the veins high up in the axilla or beneath the pectoral border (Fig. 57–4). By gently pressing the tips of the fingers into the uppermost part of the axillary space the nodes can be felt and sometimes can be pressed against the chest wall. If the patient is obese or the lymph nodes are situated high in the axilla, it may be impossible to be sure whether they are present or not. Haagensen stresses the fact that much more information can be obtained about the nodes that lie under the pectoral muscle if the muscle is permitted to relax. To ensure this he recommends that the patient rest her forearm on the left forearm of the examiner while he palpates the axilla with the right hand.

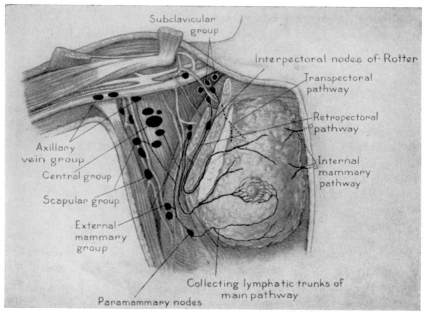

Fig. 57-4.   Location of regional lymph nodes and lymphatics of the mammary region. (C. D. Haagensen: *Diseases of the Breast.*)

WHAT INFORMATION DO YOU SEEK, AND HOW DO YOU INTERPRET THE FINDINGS OF AXILLARY PALPATION? If there is an obvious lump in the breast or the skin retraction sign is seen in the breast substance or nipple on inspection, the examiner is interested in whether the process is localized or has extended to the regional lymph nodes. He cannot feel them if the carcinoma is centrally placed and has metastasized directly to the lymph nodes of the internal mammary chain, but axillary metastases are far more common whenever the tumor is felt. Primarily, then, he is interested in how many nodes are present, their size and their degree of fixation to underlying structures such as the axillary veins or the overlying skin. By and large the bigger the lymph node, the greater the chances of metastases if the tumor in the breast is malignant. When a single node or a mass of nodes is felt, any individual masses that are greater than 1.5 to 2 cm. in size are almost certainly malignant. It would be a serious error, on the other hand, to regard an axilla as free of metastasis simply because no lymph nodes are palpated. The inaccuracy of preoperative estimation runs as high as 50 per cent. When masses are felt, the examiner will be correct if he assumes that they contain cancer about 80 per cent of the time. If large lymph nodes are present and seem to be fixed, it will be well for the physician to inspect the arm and hand on the same side to see whether there is any suggestion of blockage in either the lymphatic or venous return. Dilated veins on the back of the hand or edema of the arm would provide presumptive evidence of such obstruction.

Examination of the Breast Itself

A systematic examination of the breast itself can best be done with the patient lying on her back with her arms at her sides. If the breast is large and pendulous and does not lie flat on the chest wall naturally, Haagensen recommends that a small pillow be placed under the lower chest wall. The position mentioned is far better than if one tries to examine the patient's breast in the sitting position, for the simple reason that it is more accessible and the breast folds are much less thick when the patient is supine. The examination begins with the flat of the hand lying on the contour of the breast with the fingers extended. The entire region of possible distribution of breast tissue is then gently palpated, beginning at the periphery of the circle and systematically narrowing the examination down to the nipple area.

Particular attention should be paid to the lateral portions of the breasts, for the majority of lesions, both benign and malignant, are found in these regions. The cardinal sin in breast palpation is to pick up the breast tissue between the fingers and carry out the examination in this manner. Far more accurate examination will follow gentle pressure from the extended fingers with the hand flat against the breast. It is also essential that the opposite breast be felt, because benign disease is sometimes bilateral. Carcinoma is known to appear simultaneously in both breasts, and if no contralateral masses are felt, the change in the consistency of the suspicious region in the breast first examined will be much more apparent.

There is one part of the breast where palpation is somewhat unsatisfactory, namely, the area below the nipple in the so-called mammary fold. This is particularly true of the large, pendulous, flabby breast. Because this is the most dependent portion, the actual weight of the upper portion presses down on the breast tissue in this zone, producing an area of stasis and congestion. Since fibrosis is an invariable histologic sequence to the presence of chronic edema, this fold often feels firm, hard and ridgelike and gives an impression that tumor is present. If this situation exists, the patient should be asked to sit up and have this area of the breast examined again. It is now permissible to palpate the breast tissue under suspicion and examine it for tumor, which will be much more in evidence than if the patient remains supine.

The wise examiner on completion of his palpation will not fail to ask the patient where she thought she felt the lump that brought her to the physician. Women have an uncanny way of detecting the smallest mass in the breast, probably because their palpation is far more gentle than the surgeon's. On rechecking he may find something that he had missed previously or can concentrate on some other region than the one originally thought to be important. With moving pictures on breast self-examination being shown, we may expect more women to have an intelligent interest in their breasts than previously.

How Do You Interpret What You Feel?   The main problem in palpation of the breast is the decision that must be made as to whether a departure from normal represents (*a*) physiologic alteration in breast tissue, (*b*) inflammatory reaction or (*c*) a neoplasm, either benign or malignant. Obviously, if the breast changes are due to the physiologic action of hormones, nothing need be done, but sepsis may require drainage, and any tumor found must be biopsied or excised to determine whether or not a cancer is present.

Except for fat necrosis in the breast, which in many instances cannot be differentiated from a cancer by palpation, most inflammatory lesions in the breast will manifest themselves by increased heat, redness and tender tumor formation. It must be always kept in mind that a malignant tumor may break down and become infected, and such a process should not be considered benign solely on the basis of the factors mentioned above. If there is any suspicion of cancer, the region should be explored, biopsied and drained. In far too many instances of breast carcinoma this step has been too long postponed.

Irregular nodularity throughout the breast, but particularly in the upper outer quadrant, is a common finding in many women. The breast tissue in this area becomes heavy, nodular and exquisitely tender to the lightest pressure, even clothing. The discomfort and physical changes in the breast tend to become more pronounced in the ten-day period immediately preceding the onset of menstruation, largely owing to hormonal stimulation of the duct and lobular epithelium. This process may be regarded as entirely normal, and treatment should concentrate on making the patient more comfortable. Although it may be extremely difficult at times to decide whether the nodularity is benign or malignant, the timing of the physical signs and symptoms, together with the accompanying tenderness, does suggest physiologic changes rather than tumor formation. By and large, pathologic processes tend to localize to a single region or segment of the breast with the exception of chronic cystic disease and particularly blunt duct adenosis.

What Observations Should Be Made If Tumor Is Detected?   There are several observations that should be made when a tumor is felt in the breast. The size and location, shape and degree of demarcation, consistency and mobility of the tumor are all very important. They are of value both in differential diagnosis and in outlining proper therapy.

The Size and Location of the Tumor.   It is important to record the size of the original tumor in centimeters, as well as its location in the breast. For example, a medial quadrant tumor may metastasize to the internal mammary lymph nodes, and a lower quadrant neoplasm may involve the lymphatics of the rectus sheath. Both observations will influence therapy. If the internal mammary chain is involved, the surgeon may elect to attack it surgically or may give x-ray treatment to such a patient. Lower quadrant breast tumors should have the upper rectus fascia excised. Size is important in prognosis if the tumor is malignant. Prognosis is more dependent on the size of the initial primary cancer than any other single factor in the breast, as in other parts of the body.

The Shape of the Tumor.   Tumors of the breast assume many forms. The characteristic terms used to describe such tumors are irregular, nodular, rounded. Carcinoma, for example, is apt to be irregular in outline, and benign conditions such as adenofibrosis and cysts tend to have a rounded or discoid contour. Such masses are also apt to be discrete and distinct from the rest of the breast tissue. Other pathologic processes, both benign and malignant, grade off gradually into the uninvolved breast and do not appear to be as sharply demarcated. This is especially true of cystic disease, blunt duct adenosis and carcinoma.

There are many variables in these observations, and no hard and fast statements can be made. For example, we know very well that certain types of carcinoma, particularly those that grow slowly and are well differentiated frequently are manifested as discrete tumors. On the other hand, it is obvious that multiple small cysts can occur as a result of physiologic change, or blunt duct adenosis as well. These lesions may be found through the entire breast.

The Consistency and Mobility of the Tumor.   Because the malignant processes in the breast tend to set up a fibrotic response, such lesions are apt to be fixed either to the skin or to the underlying fascia. The degree to which they are fixed will depend in large part on the size of the tumor. It may become so extensive that the entire mass is fixed and the breast is contracted. Malignant lesions then are less likely to move about in the breast tissue on examination than adenofibrosis and cysts, which can be displaced readily.

When a tumor appears to retract the skin or be fixed to the underlying tissue, several other diagnostic maneuvers should be used to test the extent of its fixation: (1) Raising the arms above the head places the patient's pectoral fascia on stretch. If there is a suggestion of dimpling of the skin or if the tumor seems to be fixed to the pectoral muscles, the observations will now become much more apparent when the pectorals contract, as they do in this position. (2) Another method of accomplishing the same thing is to have the patient place her hands on her hips and then contract the pectoral muscles. This may be done either in the supine or sitting positions. (3) Lifting the breast tissue and cupping it around the tumor may bring out latent skin fixation. This maneuver, combined with pectoral contraction, will frequently bring out any fixation to the underlying fascia. The degree of motion will depend on the extent to which the tumor adheres to the fascia.

If it is only moderately fixed, the tumor may be moved over the underlying muscles without pectoral contraction, but a more pronounced excursion will be noted if the examiner holds the tumor and the patient puts the muscle on tension. With greater fixation not only will the tumor fail to move when it is pushed from side to side, but also no further movement is noted when the muscles contract. (4) If the breasts are relatively small, much useful information as to possible skin retraction or muscle fixation can be obtained by having the patient lean forward from the hips with chin upward and the extended hands placed on those of the examiner (Fig. 57–5). This is a favorite test of Haagensen. Normally the breasts would fall away from the chest wall, but with a tumor fixed to either skin or chest wall the retraction of the nipple

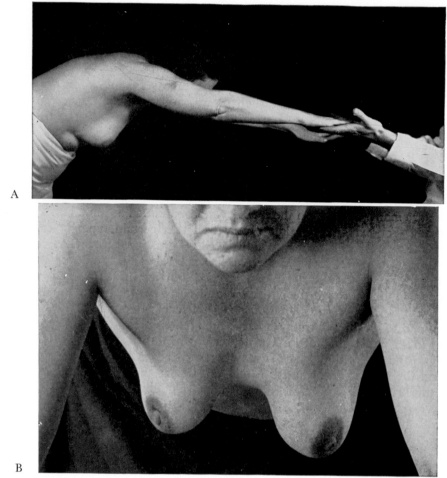

Fig. 57-5. *A*, The Haagensen forward-bending test. *B*, Asymmetry shown by bending forward, with fixation of the right breast and lateral deviation of its nipple, indicative of an upper quadrant carcinoma. (C. D. Haagensen: *Diseases of the Breast.*)

or breast tumor becomes obvious and the breast remains abnormally fixed to the chest wall. A tendency is noted for the nipple to deviate toward the site of the tumor.

In the face of these findings the physician should no longer entertain the wishful thought that the changes are due to benign physiologic alterations. The more experienced surgeon will biopsy such lesions, for the simple reason that he knows there are too many variables to permit him to rely solely on his clinical estimate.

WHAT OTHER DIAGNOSTIC MEASURES MAY BE USED SHORT OF INCISIONAL BIOPSY?

Although there are many enthusiasts for a variety of methods designed to differentiate benign from malignant lesions in the breast, the best and most accurate procedure is actual tissue examination under the microscope. The following procedures have their advocates.

Transillumination

In the past the method of shining a light through the breast tissue in a darkened room was widely practiced. It is true that when the patient leans forward, allowing the breast to fall away from the chest wall, opaque areas may appear which suggest that this area of the breast differs from others that transmit light more freely. It does not mean very much, however, for one still does not know whether the lesion is benign or malignant. There is little enthusiasm for this procedure today.

X-ray Examination of the Breast

Roentgenographic examination of the breasts continues to have its sponsors, although there is no general acceptance. The procedure may be carried out (1) after injection of the mammary duct system with a wide variety of media designed to produce a contrast with the rest of the breast tissue, or (2) by direct x-ray study of the breast with a technique intended to bring out soft tissue shadows. There is no doubt that soft tissue tumors can be delineated in this manner, particularly when the breast is purposefully allowed to fall away from the chest wall. Only the most enthusiastic disciples, however, are willing to declare that observations such as the finding of minute, granular opaque areas in the suspected tumor region, like psammoma bodies in ovarian tumors, are actually due to minute calcium deposits in a malignant tumor, or that any tumor seen is a cancer.

Just as the physical findings are suspicious rather than pathognomonic, so the diagnostic tests mentioned above are open to question, and the physician is forced to fall back on the microscopic study of tissue removed for biopsy.

What Biopsy Methods Are Available?

Although it has never been demonstrated in breast carcinoma that any actual harm has come from a delay in performing operation after the taking of a biopsy, nevertheless the ideal method of management is to perform an incisional biopsy under adequate anesthesia in the operating room, where preparations have been made to carry out a radical mastectomy if the frozen section is reported as cancer.

There are one or two office procedures that can be done if one so desires and is sufficiently well trained in interpreting the findings.

Aspiration Biopsy.   This is practiced under local anesthesia by some enthusiastic advocates. A syringe with a large-gauge needle is inserted in what is believed to be the most suspicious area of the breast. By suction, cells are aspirated into the lumen of the needle and are extruded onto a glass slide which is then immersed in fixative and stained. Again, there is no question if the needle is inserted in the proper region of the breast that tumor cells can be recovered, but the method has the definite disadvantage that there is no chance to study the arrangement of the cells in relation to the rest of the architecture of the breast tissue, either benign or malignant. In tumor diagnosis the arrangement of the cells is perhaps more important than the interpretation of the nature of individual cells. The method then becomes a cytologic study, and the pathologist is asked to interpret dispersed cells alone, many of which may have been poorly fixed or stained.

The method at best is only as good as the ability of the surgeon to select the proper area to aspirate. If a negative report is forthcoming, it means only that no

malignant cells were obtained from the material aspirated. Particularly in the pathologic entity, cystic disease, carcinoma may coexist with a tense palpable cyst, yet be
totally unrecognizable. Unless the tumor is large enough to be felt, aspiration has no
value, and in the smaller lesions located deep within the breast accurate aspiration
biopsy of this type is practically impossible.

TROCAR BIOPSY.   Some of the objections to aspiration biopsy are overcome
by using larger-bore trocars or trephines. Adequate tissue may be obtained in this
manner, but only a false sense of security will result if the biopsy site is incorrect.
Thus, although the material obtained may be adequately interpreted by the pathologist, in contrast to that obtained by aspiration, nevertheless the basic objection to the
method still holds, namely, that small carcinomas may be missed.

INCISIONAL BIOPSY.   By all odds the method of choice when the physical signs
indicate a breast lesion whose nature is uncertain is a surgical biopsy of the lesion
under suitable anesthesia. The only controversial point is whether the entire region
under suspicion should be excised or whether the surgeon should take his specimen
directly from the part he thinks most likely to be malignant. In general practice the
surgeon is apt to take a small wedge directly from the suspected malignant site when
all presumptive signs (e.g. retraction) are present. If the lesion is not circumscribed
and not stony hard, and the outlines are not definite, excision of the entire region
under suspicion should be carried out at a point well away from it.

There is a theoretical objection to both methods, for unquestionably tumor cells
are spread in the process. The important point, however, is that a biopsy must truly
represent the pathologic condition. This presupposes that the surgeon knows enough
gross pathology to take the specimen from the proper place. No surgeon wishes to
disseminate tumor cells unnecessarily, but it is of far greater importance that he
secure an adequate representative biopsy.

In most instances the pathologic interpretation can be made on frozen section
material, and it is axiomatic in surgery for malignant disease that radical surgery
should be done only after receiving a positive report of cancer. If there is doubt about
the microscopic findings or if the excisional biopsy is performed in a hospital with no
pathologist available, it is better to terminate the operation and await the final
microscopic diagnosis. This is far better than proceeding with surgery that may be
unnecessarily mutilating, unnecessary if the lesion is benign, or totally inadequate
if a simple amputation has been performed for a malignant lesion. The dictum that
definitive surgery should follow immediately upon receipt of a pathologic confirmation
is basically correct, but ill-advised operations without a proper diagnosis can never
be condoned despite the fact that the delay factor is minimized by the act. Collected
statistics would seem to indicate that the end-results are no worse when the final
surgical extirpation has been delayed even as long as two weeks. The surgeon can
therefore afford to be sure of the diagnosis, but should then act at once.

The pathologic and therapeutic aspects of breast cancer are discussed in problems
of the forty- to fifty-year age group (Chap. 62).

COMMON PATHOLOGIC ENTITIES ENCOUNTERED IN THE ADULT BREAST

A wide variety of dysplasias and tumors may appear in the female breast. Many
are benign, but with enough of the characteristics of malignant disease to make them
a problem in diagnosis and management. It is manifestly impossible to discuss here

all the rare inflammations, hyperplasias and tumors such as tuberculosis, sarcoidosis, panniculitis, adenoma, liposarcoma, rhabdomyosarcoma and others. They occur so infrequently and are so bizarre in their manifestations that a biopsy for diagnosis is obviously indicated. We shall therefore confine our discussion mostly to the more common disease entities, including adenofibrosis, cystic disease of the breast, intraductal papilloma, fat necrosis and breast abscess.

ADENOFIBROSIS

This condition was mentioned in breast problems of adolescence (Chap. 23). It is a diffuse process, usually in both breasts, characterized by fibrous tissue replacement of the normal mammary fat. Care should be taken not to confuse adenofibrosis with the common benign tumor of young women that is called either fibroadenoma or adenofibroma.

When Does Adenofibrosis Occur?

Adenofibrosis is often seen in young adult women in their thirties and forties. According to Nathanson, it has occurred in small, well formed, feminine, attractive infertile women more frequently than in other patients. Actually, the condition may develop at any time between the menarche and the menopause, and many patients do not fit the foregoing description.

What Are the Symptoms?

Typically, as the menstrual period approaches, the breast becomes diffusely tender and firm, producing a movable mass the size and shape of a thick pancake. This disappears with the menses. Edema and congestion of hormonal origin appear responsible, and the chronicity of these processes may stimulate fibrosis.

What Gross and Microscopic Features Identify Adenofibrosis?

Replacement of the normal, soft, yellow, fatty breast stroma by dense gray-white rubbery fibrous tissue is the main finding. Before excision and sectioning the mass may be hard, but slicing reduces it to a soft, resilient rubbery consistency. The process is not demarcated or sharply delimited, and some fat may remain intermingled.

Microscopically, adenofibrosis consists of a sheetlike interposition of collagenous fibrous tissue, rather poor in nuclei, among the breast lobules. Where fat should occur, fibrosis is found. The epithelial structures may show pressure atrophy, appear normal or develop small cysts.

What Is the Relation of Adenofibrosis to Cystic Disease?

Many authorities have considered that adenofibrosis is the initial stage in the development of cystic disease of the breast. Actually, if any cysts are found in a fibrous breast specimen, it will likely be diagnosed as cystic mastitis; otherwise it will be designated as adenofibrosis.

What Is the Therapy?

If a reliable diagnosis of adenofibrosis could be established without biopsy, probably few cases would receive any surgical treatment. But since firm, poorly demarcated and outlined breast masses that persist do properly disturb many patients and their physicians, excision often proves the diagnostic and therapeutic method of choice.

Medical treatments for adenofibrosis, as for cystic disease, have not proved generally successful.

CYSTIC DISEASE OF THE BREAST

Cystic disease, often called fibrocystic disease and chronic cystic mastitis, though there is rarely any inflammation present, is by all odds the most common benign lesion of the female breast. The true incidence is hard to come by, since statistical reports are usually based on the presence of cysts large enough to be palpated. A far larger group of women will be found to have minute cysts. According to autopsy studies, approximately half the women who show no palpable evidence of cystic disease will have cysts larger than 1 to 2 cm. in 20 per cent, or microscopic evidence of smaller cysts in 20 to 30 per cent.

From a practical point of view we are primarily interested in the number of women who have clinically obvious cystic disease. It has been estimated that one woman in twenty will have palpable evidence of cystic disease some time in the span of her menstrual life. Cystic disease is seen far less often in the postmenopausal years. When one considers the etiologic relation that appears to exist between cystic disease and carcinoma, however, the minute and microscopic cysts become important.

When Are We Most Likely to Encounter Cystic Disease?

Since cystic disease is a direct aftermath of duct and ductular epithelial proliferations caused by hormonal activity, particularly estrogenic, active benign cystic disease may be found throughout the reproductive years up to, but not far beyond, the menopause. It is most often seen and causes the biggest problems in differential diagnosis in the thirty- to forty-year age group.

What Symptoms Are Produced by Cystic Disease in the Breast?

Whether or not the patient complains of symptoms from her cystic disease depends largely on how many cysts she has, their size, location and how rapidly they enlarge. Thus a patient may have widely dispersed small cysts that are palpable as shotty nodules without being aware of their presence until an inadvertent blow causes the patient to feel her breast. On the other hand, an accumulation of relatively small cysts in the upper outer quadrant of the breast may cause considerable discomfort and pain in the days preceding the onset of the menstrual period when hormonal alterations are the greatest. A larger cyst, responding to the same stimulation, may become exceedingly painful as the fluid contents distend the restricting capsule, only to shrink or regress as the period comes on. The patient may actually observe a diminution in the size of the tender lump with the onset of each menstruation. This is an important observation, for tumors that respond in this fashion are rarely cancer. Pain and tenderness are frequently noted in benign cystic disease, but they are rare in solid tumors of the breast such as adenofibroma or carcinoma.

What Do Benign Cysts of the Breast Feel Like?

The physical findings in benign cystic disease of the breast vary with the size of the cyst, its location and the length of time it has been present. It was previously noted that the physical characteristics, as well as the symptoms, vary with the phases of the menstrual cycle.

In most instances the cyst stands out from the rest of the breast tissue as a well demarcated, rounded tumor. If it is a solitary tumor, the examiner can move it freely within the breast substance, but if there is an accumulation of multiple small cysts, particularly involving the lateral segments, it may tend to shade off into the rest of the breast tissue, and the mass is neither clearly delineated nor movable. A solitary cyst may be firm or hard, depending on how much fluid it contains and the phase of the menstrual cycle in which it is noted. When it is full of compressed fluid or if the cyst is of long standing, there is a resistance to palpation approaching hardness.

The main elements on palpation that distinguish the benign cyst from malignant neoplasm are (*a*) its mobility, (*b*) the absence of any suggestion of skin retraction, and (*c*) the presence of tenderness over the cyst.

It is a great temptation to confirm the cystic nature of the tumor by aspirating with a syringe and needle under a procaine infiltration of the overlying skin. This is particularly true if the patient complains of acute tenderness in the region, since aspiration of the contents will relieve the pain. If one chooses, the fluid obtained may be spun down in the centrifuge and the sediment subjected to microscopic examination after properly fixing and staining the smears. The results are not very rewarding, and a false sense of security may result.

In all probability the aspiration of cloudy gray or brownish fluid is good evidence of the benignity of a cyst, but occasionally carcinoma may appear on the external surface of the cyst or in a small focus adjacent to it. In the past, aspiration was frowned upon, but in recent years it has become a more common procedure. It is far safer, however, to explore the breast surgically, excise the offending or suspicious segment and submit the tissue to microscopic examination. There will be fewer hazards from aspiration if a cyst develops after a previous exploration in which benign cystic disease was encountered.

What Does Cystic Disease Look Like Microscopically?

Just as cysts of the breast vary grossly from pinhead-sized, yellow, gray or blue nodules to the large, solitary bluish cysts traditionally called blue dome cysts of Bloodgood, microscopically, cystic disease has a variable appearance (Fig. 57–6). By definition the old-fashioned entity "chronic cystic mastitis" includes either gross or microscopic cysts, or both.

The most common cysts are the largest, both grossly and microscopically. They arise by blunt outgrowths of branches of medium-sized ducts, which later apparently become pinched off. Such blunt duct cysts are lined by ordinary mammary duct epithelium, outside which is a layer of contractile myoepithelium, with the specialized hormone-responsive intrinsic breast stroma around the periphery. When these cysts are multiple, the condition is called *blunt duct adenosis*.

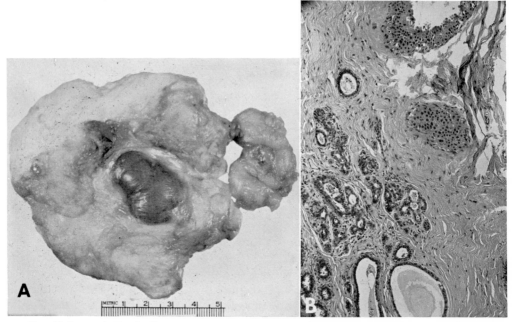

Fig. 57-6.   *A*, Cystic disease of the breast is grossly a variable intermingling of yellow fat, white fibrous tissue and cysts of different sizes. Large cysts containing yellowish fluid that appears blue, owing to reflected light, are traditionally referred to as blue-dome or Bloodgood cysts. *B*, Microscopically, cystic disease also is variegated in appearance, with stromal fibrosis, blunt duct cysts like those shown at the bottom, and apocrine metaplastic cysts such as the one at the top.

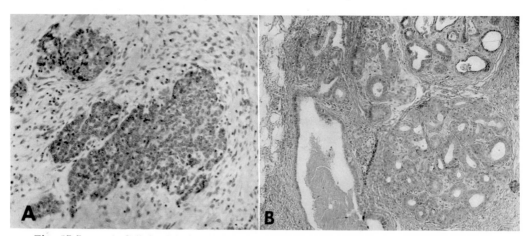

Fig. 57-7.   *A*, Cellular lobular proliferations engulfed in stroma are called sclerosing adenosis of the breast. They are not considered precancerous, despite their cellularity. *B*, Lobular and ductular epithelial hyperplasia may occur. This has a statistical relation to breast cancer development.

Some large microscopic cysts are lined by a tall, brightly eosinophilic, rather ominous-looking epithelium identical with that of the apocrine sweat glands found in the axilla and elsewhere. This was once called Schimmelbusch epithelium, but now it is referred to as *apocrine metaplasia*.

Lobular ductules mingled with their intrinsic stroma may form small masses in the breast that on section are granular, tan and slightly elevated. Microscopically, the small ducts and close-packed stromal cells produce localized cellular proliferations, and together they form small rounded knots of benign hyperplastic ductular and stromal cells. This process is called *sclerosing adenosis* (Fig. 57–7, *A*).

Around the ducts and ductules there may be a leukocytic infiltrate, predominantly lymphocytes and macrophages. Originally this was the reason for calling the condition mastitis, but it is now evident that this is not an inflammation, but a reaction to degeneration or leakage of the duct secretions.

Finally, varying degrees of microscopic piling up of the epithelial linings of ducts and ductules occur. When localized, these may produce papillomas and, when diffuse, a crowding of parts of ducts with solid masses of epithelial hyperplasia (Fig. 57–7, *B*). Foote and Stewart concluded that this hyperplastic process was the only part of chronic cystic mastitis that bore a definite relation to the development of mammary carcinoma.

What Is the Likelihood That Cancer Will Develop in a Breast Containing Cystic Disease?

There are two questions of great concern to both the patient and the physician in dealing with cystic disease of the breast: (1) Is cancer likely to develop later in such a breast? (2) Is there much chance that cancer may already be present in an otherwise benign cystic breast?

FREQUENCY OF CANCER APPEARING IN A BREAST THAT PREVIOUSLY CONTAINED GROSS CYSTIC DISEASE. If one can be sure that no cancer was present in the breasts at the time of exploration for benign cysts, and patients have been followed up for a sufficiently long time, e.g. five to twenty-five years, it is possible to get a fair idea of the

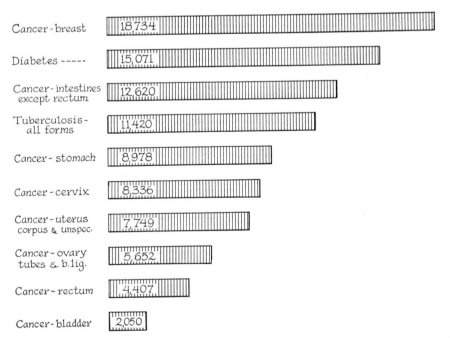

DEATHS IN 1950 FROM VARIOUS DISEASES AMONG WOMEN IN THE U.S.

Cancer-breast	18,734
Diabetes -----	15,071
Cancer-intestines except rectum	12,620
Tuberculosis- all forms	11,420
Cancer-stomach	8,978
Cancer-cervix	8,336
Cancer-uterus corpus & unspec.	7,749
Cancer-ovary tubes & b.lig.	5,652
Cancer-rectum	4,407
Cancer-bladder	2,050

Fig. 57-8. Comparison of breast carcinoma mortality with deaths from other diseases. (C. D. Haagensen: *Diseases of the Breast.*)

likelihood of carcinoma developing in a breast that contains cystic disease. One must also be sure that true cystic disease was present and that microscopic evidences of epithelial proliferation of either the duct or lobular portions are included, as well as cases with large, visibly evident blue-dome cysts. Too frequently in the reported series there were many patients lost in the follow-up study. Thus the residual evidence is heavily weighted on the side of an increased incidence of carcinoma when such an article appears. These factors must be taken into consideration when evaluating such reports.

It would appear that, when consideration is given to the estimated attack rate for breast carcinoma in the general population, a patient with cystic disease is approximately three and one half to four times more likely to have cancer in one breast than a woman not so afflicted. Since approximately 4 per cent of mature women may be expected to have carcinoma of the breast, this is a significant figure. When the information is based solely on follow-up studies, the reported incidence runs from 1 to 6 per cent. Haagensen, who had better than a 70 per cent follow-up on approximately 150 patients after 10 years, found 8 cases of carcinoma, 4 of which appeared in the same breast and 4 in the opposite breast, or roughly 5 per cent. Applied to the estimated breast cancer death rate for the United States, there were four times as many cancers as one would normally expect (Fig. 57–8).

What Is the Chance That Cancer May Coexist in the Breast That Contains Cystic Disease?

Obviously this kind of information can be obtained only by several studies of breast tissue taken from patients who have had their breasts removed for carcinoma. Pathologists, after thorough search of breasts removed for carcinoma, are able to find microscopic evidence of multiple cysts as well in approximately 60 per cent. There is less evidence that the larger cysts (those over 1 to 2 cm.) that can be seen grossly bear any particular relation to carcinoma, since they are seen about as frequently (25 per cent) in the noncancerous as in the malignant breast. It would appear, then, that the minute cyst has importance in the etiology of breast carcinoma.

From a practical point of view the 1- to 2-cm. cysts cannot be felt, but they can be seen at the time of surgical breast exploration. Clinically, it is a comparatively rare occurrence when the surgeon encounters both carcinoma and obvious cystic disease in the same breast. If the surgeon excises the area in the breast that is under suspicion with sufficiently wide margins and receives a report of benign cystic disease, it is unlikely that he will have missed a focus of carcinoma. This occurred once in the practice of each of two famous surgeons in a ten-year period.

If the cystic disease occupies a large portion of the breast tissue, the surgeon should try to excise as much as possible without producing an emotionally disturbing deformity. Simple mastectomy has been recommended for these patients, but it is justified only in the exceptional case. Before advocating such a radical procedure the surgeon would be wise to consider the facts that (a) cystic disease tends to appear in both breasts, and (b) the process usually subsides with the onset of the menopause. The recurrence of a cyst or the appearance of carcinoma is just as likely to occur in the opposite breast. The surgeon then can afford to procrastinate, since the basic pathologic process commonly regresses in time. Bilateral or even a single simple mastectomy is a frightful price for a woman to pay as prophylaxis for a carcinoma that has a limited chance of developing. Women hate to have any operation that they believe lessens their attractiveness to the male sex and will tolerate a hysterectomy, since the manifestations are not obvious, far more readily than they will a mastectomy. Unless the index of suspicion of malignant disease is high, there seems to be little rationale for either single or bilateral mastectomy for cystic disease.

What Treatment Is Recommended for Cystic Disease of the Breast?

In the discussion above we have suggested that the optimum treatment for cystic disease of the breast is surgical excision of the area under suspicion, performed in a hospital under suitable anesthesia. The tissue is then submitted for frozen section if a pathologist is available, but if not, the material is preserved for subsequent pathologic evaluation. The type and extent of the excision will be dictated by the location of the mass and the degree of deformity that may result. To determine adequately the dispersion of the cystic disease, a dry operative field is essential. After removing the cystic area the surgeon should inspect the specimen, paying particular attention to the interior walls of the cysts as well as their exterior and the possible presence of papillary excrescences.

ASPIRATION.   In the discussion of diagnostic measures mention was made of the practice of aspirating obvious cysts of the breasts. It was suggested that this method of therapy be confined to the group of patients who have recurrence of the cysts after a previous biopsy excision. The chance of subsequent malignancy is naturally reduced under these conditions. It is amazing how few of these cysts reappear after they have once been aspirated. The explanation of this is unknown. The fact that the previous excision revealed only benign disease does not guarantee, however, that carcinoma of the breast will not appear subsequently. If the physical findings suggest a cyst, it is probably just that, and aspiration of cystic fluid will confirm it, but if the mass is solid and no contents are aspirated, the breast should be re-explored, for it is probably malignant.

HORMONE THERAPY.   Since the morphology of the breast varies with phases of the menstrual cycle, cystic mastitis has been linked to fluctuations in the levels of the ovarian hormones. The epithelial changes in ducts and lobules might be expected to be due to excessive stimulation by estrogen, but laboratory evidence suggests that the patients who have cystic disease actually show no fluctuation in estrogen secretion and that the peaks of secretion normally found in the menstrual cycle are lacking. Thus it is the constant estrogenic stimulation that is apparently most important. There is little excuse, then, for giving androgen to balance the hypersecretion of estrogen, for none exists.

On the other hand, it is both meddlesome and useless to give estrogen to make up the apparent deficit. There is a tendency for cystic disease to regress spontaneously. The part of wisdom would suggest that the patient will do better if (*a*) the breasts are supported by an uplift type of brassière that may be worn at night when the symptoms are severe, (*b*) cold ice packs are applied to tender areas of the breast, and (*c*) some form of diuretic is given coupled with a restriction of salt intake.

BLUNT DUCT ADENOSIS AND SCLEROSING ADENOSIS

There are two subdivisions of cystic mastitis that bring about more than the usual amount of confusion in establishing a clear-cut differential diagnosis between benign and malignant disease in the breast. In nearly every case of cystic disease the clinician will feel small lumps, and the pathologist will find corresponding areas of small ducts and larger lobules that extend out into the breast stroma and set up a reactive fibrosis around foci of blunt duct adenosis. This has no particular clinical significance, except occasionally when the focal areas of epithelial proliferation are so marked that one might suspect a neoplasm, and particularly carcinoma.

In What Particular Way Does Blunt Duct Adenosis Resemble Carcinoma?

Clinically, there is little to distinguish blunt duct adenosis from carcinoma, except that adenosis shows little tendency to produce skin retraction and by and large does not occupy as much breast tissue as a carcinoma does. The confusion lies in the fact that both feel firm, hard and irregular to a light touch and seem to diffuse into the surrounding breast tissue with little tendency to demarcate. Since some smaller carcinomas may exist without evidence of any skin retraction, there is little on palpation to distinguish the two. If definite cysts can be felt, the examiner leans to the side of cystic disease, because blunt duct adenosis often is a part of it, but if no cysts are felt, a suspicion of carcinoma should arise. The best way to establish the diagnosis is to explore and biopsy the area of breast tissue that has set up the doubt.

What Are the Gross Pathologic Characteristics?

The operator should not try to make a differential diagnosis on the basis of the gross appearance of the cut surface of the mass. In general, blunt duct adenosis is less firm and gritty than carcinoma, but this is all relative, and it is unwise to rely on the observation. Actually, the tissue, once excised, often feels less stony hard than it did before. This is probably due to the release of tension in the fibrous tissue strands.

On gross inspection we look for the telltale white streaks spreading out into the breast stroma from a focus that is frankly cancer. Streaks are usually absent with blunt duct adenosis. Here again it is unwise to rely entirely on such observations. The final diagnosis depends on the microscopic picture.

Since there is little about blunt duct adenosis that distinguishes it absolutely from carcinoma either clinically or upon gross inspection of the biopsy specimen, the final diagnosis must rest with the pathologist's interpretation of the microscopic picture. This may also offer some points of difficulty unless the slides are thoroughly studied. In blunt duct adenosis it is the occasional lack of orderly arrangement coupled with epithelial proliferation that might cause confusion with carcinoma. This could lead to a serious error, particularly by someone not used to interpreting frozen section biopsy material. If there is the least doubt, definitive surgery should be deferred until the pathologist has a chance to review the permanent microscopic sections.

PATHOLOGIC CHARACTERISTICS OF SCLEROSING ADENOSIS.   The brown or tan granular foci that protrude from the sectioned breast specimen in localized areas may also be confused with carcinoma. The same factors are at work to provide problems, namely, excessive amounts of epithelial proliferation with many ductules expanding out into the breast stroma. Microscopically, the cells may be seen in mitosis and may vary in size and shape. In early stages of this lobular proliferation it is easy on frozen section to confuse the picture with carcinoma. In later stages of the process, fibrosis in the stroma of the breast gives the clinical sense of firmness to the tissue. Increasing

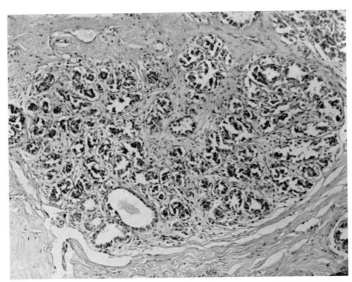

Fig. 57-9. A lobule with sclerosing adenosis is peripherally demarcated. Despite the cellularity of the ductules, there is no anaplasia or invasion, and the process is benign.

fibrosis may tend to break up the normal pattern of ductular development and regression. Thus we see a histologic variation in the size and shape of cells and a disorderly pattern of growth, both of which are found in carcinoma. Nevertheless neither anaplasia nor invasion, the two hallmarks of cancer, are found, and sclerosing adenosis is properly regarded as neither a neoplastic nor precancerous condition (Fig. 57–9).

What Is the Best Treatment of Sclerosing and Blunt Duct Adenoses?

If one is sure of the diagnosis, simple excision of the involved regions will suffice, and any recurrence or subsequent appearance of carcinoma in such a breast is extremely unlikely. The chief point in therapy is to be sure what you are dealing with. If doubt of the true nature of the biopsy specimen should arise on frozen section diagnosis, it is far better to wait on the report of the permanent sections. If it is a sclerosing or blunt duct adenosis, local excision is adequate therapy, and you have avoided unnecessarily mutilating your patient. In the rare instance in which the final diagnosis is carcinoma you have done your patient no great disservice, for although you prefer to follow biopsy with definitive surgery if the diagnosis is cancer, there is no convincing statistical evidence to date that the patient is damaged irreparably if the final excision is completed within the first few days after the biopsy.

Intraductal Papilloma

Epithelial proliferations in the form of papillary excrescences that occur within the duct system of the breast are called intraductal papillomas. In most instances they are benign, but since, like carcinoma, they tend to produce a nipple discharge that may be either serous or bloody, the possibility of malignant disease must constantly be kept in mind. Papillomas do not appear as often as carcinoma and have no particular predilection for any age group. One would normally expect to find the greatest concentration of these lesions at the age when hormonal stimulation is at its height. Intraductal papillomas, however, actually occur in all age groups from the early twenties into the eighties.

Before the true incidence of intraductal papilloma can be determined it is necessary to agree on what actually constitutes a papillary growth within the duct. If, for example, one includes papillomas that are evident only on microscopic examination, the incidence will be high, because they are common in cystic disease of the breast. Since such proliferations are unlikely to produce palpable tumor formations or nipple discharge, they will not be recognized clinically. We are primarily concerned here with the papillomatous lesions that do produce symptoms and a sufficient growth to be seen and felt. The principal clinical problem is whether these changes are due to a benign intraductal papilloma or malignant disease.

What about Nipple Discharge?

A spontaneous discharge from the nipple is virtually the only symptom of any consequence produced by an intraductal papilloma. When a discharge does appear, it is often sporadic, persisting for several days or weeks, only to disappear for long periods of time before it is seen again. This well recognized pattern is of considerable help in establishing the differential diagnosis between benign and malignant breast disease, for in malignant growth the discharge usually is of recent origin.

It makes some difference where the papilloma is located within the duct system and how it grows as to whether or not the patient has a nipple discharge. For example, if the epithelial proliferation takes the form of a papillary growth that tends to grow out into the lumen of a major duct on a stalk, one might expect to note nipple discharge, for such lesions are fragile and easily traumatized. If the growth happens to be near the areola, in the central portion of the breast, the chances of nipple discharge increase materially. On the other hand, intraductal papillomas sometimes grow as almost solid glandular structures. Such lesions are less likely to produce a discharge that can be seen, from the very nature of their growth pattern and the fact that they tend to appear in the more peripheral areas of the breast.

What Are the Gross and Microscopic Pictures of Intraductal Papilloma?

Some surgeons palpate all quadrants of the breast under anesthesia until the segment responsible for the nipple discharge is located, and then open the responsible duct along a grooved director. When this technique is used, the papilloma typically appears as a soft, tan, microcystic, pedunculated nodule arising from the smooth, pale gray duct lining. Most are from 0.3 to 1.0 cm. in diameter and lack a definite stalk. Ordinarily they are more commonly multiple in different ducts than single.

If a segment of breast is excised for frozen section without prior identification of the ducts, one feels fortunate to identify a papilloma on sectioning the tissue, because grossly it is often indistinguishable from sclerosing adenosis and is easily missed.

Microscopically, most papillomas are cellular aggregations of epithelium piled up in layers on a delicate fernlike stroma (Fig. 57–10). The stalk is short or not identifiable. Cytologic variations in the epithelium are unusual. Papillomas vary in

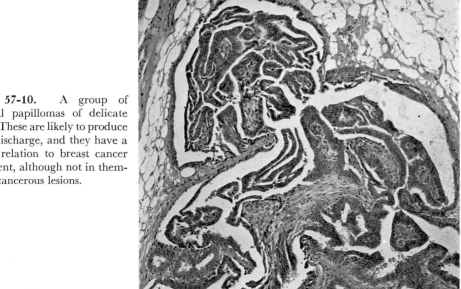

Fig. 57-10. A group of intraductal papillomas of delicate structure. These are likely to produce a nipple discharge, and they have a statistical relation to breast cancer development, although not in themselves precancerous lesions.

the amount of stroma they have, and a few are mostly polyps of fibrous connective tissue covered by little or no epithelium.

The first type, or predominently epithelial papilloma, is what Foote and Stewart related statistically to an increased frequency of carcinoma developing in the same breast. The second type, or fibrous polyp variant of papilloma, is without any such significance.

What Is the Significance of Tumor Formation in Association with a Spontaneous Nipple Discharge?

In most instances the patient comes to her physician because she is concerned about the cause of her nipple discharge. She may have had it on and off for years. Rarely does she ever note any tumor. On rare occasions she may have discovered a slowly enlarging small lump in the region of the areola when the nipple discharge had disappeared, only to have the lump regress when discharge again appeared.

By gentle, painstaking palpation the physician will occasionally be able to demonstrate either a tumor or a particular area within the areola of the breast where gentle pressure produces a discharge. Occasionally a 2- or 3-centimeter mass can be felt in the subareolar region, but in most instances about all the physician can feel is a sense of resistance or thickening on light pressure of the extended finger tips. This thickening can often be traced back along the duct into the deeper breast tissue for a distance of 2 or 3 cm. Rarely is there ever enough tumor present to produce a nipple retraction.

The association, however, of palpable tumor and a history of spontaneous discharge of serous or bloody fluid from the nipple should heighten one's index of suspicion that malignant disease may be present within the breast. Rarely this combination can be produced by cystic disease, blunt duct adenosis, mammary duct ectasia or even pregnancy, but by and large, when tumor and discharge coexist, either an intraductal papilloma or carcinoma provides the explanation.

How Is the Differential Diagnosis Established?

Since there may be few localizing signs, the differential diagnosis between a benign and malignant cause is not easy.

If localizing signs are present, the diagnosis can be made only by exploration and biopsy.

There are a few observations that may help in localizing the area in the breast that should be explored. We have mentioned the presence of palpable tumor and a pressure point that produces nipple discharge. These are important localizing signs, for intraductal papillomas are clinically in most instances single lesions. They may occur histologically in several regions within the same breast or in the opposite breast, but in general they tend to appear to the surgeon as single lesions.

The problem of determining the true cause of the nipple discharge becomes more complex when no tumor of any sort can be felt. It may be wise to advise a surgical exploration in these patients, but if you do not know where to begin the exploration, you have a considerable reluctance in advising the patient to submit to it. There is a good practical point already touched on which may prove of considerable value in selecting the area to be biopsied when no tumor can be felt. In gentle palpation around the areolar area there often appears to be one single point which is invariably followed by nipple discharge, even though no tumor can be felt. This discharge always seems to appear at the same point on the surface of the nipple. This is probably due to the anatomic arrangement of the duct outlets as they appear on the nipple surface. Discharge noted at the twelve o'clock position on the nipple when pressure is made in the corresponding segment of the areola simply means that the duct papilloma is located in the duct that drains that region. This, then, is the area to explore.

If no tumor, pressure point or other localizing signs such as the ones we have just mentioned are present, the patient should be examined at regular intervals and exploration be deferred until localizing signs do appear. Concern about the possibility of missing a rare carcinoma or the patient's apprehensions, increased by the need for repeated examination, may force the surgeon into exploration of the entire areolar area in the absence of localizing signs.

What Is the Proper Treatment of Intraductal Papilloma?

If the diagnosis can be accurately established by competent microscopic study, simple excision of the involved area is all that need be done. There is little reason for simple mastectomy and less for more radical procedures. Although some pathologists feel that intraductal papillomas have varying degrees of malignant potentiality, there is little good evidence that any one clinically evident benign papilloma becomes a malignant one. Pathologically, greatest suspicion is directed toward the papillomas that are more solid, sessile and glandular.

Where the microscopic interpretation is so important, the initial step in therapy should be adequate biopsy of the area under suspicion and not a mastectomy based on the observations made from frozen section material. Permanent paraffin sections are much easier to evaluate, and the patient loses nothing if subsequent reports point out the need for more extensive surgery.

The greatest point of diagnostic confusion, based on frozen section interpretation, arises in trying to differentiate between a benign papilloma and papillary carcinoma.

The latter, however, are rare, and when they do exist are usually well differentiated. There is no great need for speed in carrying out any definitive surgery. One can afford to establish an accurate diagnosis without any concern about jeopardizing the future health of the patient.

Since localizing signs are at best somewhat nebulous, the burden of proof of whether or not the patient has papilloma or malignant disease is placed squarely in the hands of the surgeon. He must be sure that he has provided the pathologist adequate material taken from the proper area within the breast in order that the pathologic interpretations mean anything. If he has done so and the diagnosis of intraductal papilloma is correct, simple local excision is adequate therapy. Clinically, the two conditions coexist uncommonly, intraductal papillomas with discharge are usually single entities, and the patients who have had adequate excision practically never have carcinoma subsequently, though they may on rare occasions have another papilloma in the same or opposite breast.

The technique for thorough exploration of the areolar area of the breast in a patient who has spontaneous discharge from the nipple is well described by Haagensen.

Fat Necrosis

Since the breast occupies such an exposed position, it is not surprising that trauma to it may occur. Since the breast has a high component of fat, any blow may create a subcutaneous hemorrhage within the fatty tissue of the breast. Rake handles, broom handles and being pawed by a dog are common sources of injury.

Traumatized fat responds in much the same way wherever it is encountered in the body. The mechanism is not entirely clear, for the inflammatory response may be due to (*a*) actual destruction of the fat by crushing or (*b*) ischemic necrosis within it due to the hemorrhage caused by the blow. A similar response to lipid is noted in mammary duct ectasia in which irritating material escapes from the duct lumens and permeates the fatty periductal tissue. Here, too, a firm or hard fibrotic tumor develops. The important point to remember is that in many instances the physical findings in the breast are practically indistinguishable from those of carcinoma.

In general, fat necrosis tends to be more sharply circumscribed than carcinoma, but the stony hardness of the tumor and the fact that the fibrosis in and around the area of fat necrosis not only fixes the tumor to the underlying tissue, but actually causes skin retraction over it, make the area truly suspect for malignant disease. In most instances fat necrosis occurs primarily in the tissue just beneath the skin, spreading deeper as hemorrhage causes more necrosis. The superficiality of the necrotizing process further contributes to the element of skin retraction that is also so characteristic of carcinoma.

After trauma the area of fat necrosis gradually enlarges in much the same way that a carcinoma develops. If no ecchymosis ever appeared at the site of the trauma or subsided before the tumor was noted, such a history of slow growth in a firm hard tumor strongly suggests neoplastic cause. If there never had been a tumor in this area, the presence of ecchymosis would point to traumatic fat necrosis.

Areas of fat necrosis may break down and set up an inflammatory process first manifested by increased heat and redness in the skin overlying the tumor. This is undoubtedly due to the superficial position of the tumor. The skin changes simply reflect the underlying lesion. Unfortunately carcinoma occasionally behaves in a similar manner.

The final diagnosis must depend on exploration and biopsy. One does not like to incise an inflammatory carcinoma, but the chance of spreading carcinoma must be balanced against the obvious mistake of performing a radical mastectomy for a process that should require only local excision or perhaps incision and drainage. Biopsy is indicated in the presence of a lesion with these characteristics whether there is any history of tumor or not. The clinical differential diagnosis is too obscure to follow a policy of observation.

What Is the Pathologic Picture of Fat Necrosis?

The fresh specimen of fat necrosis may look exactly like a scirrhous carcinoma, with radiating bands of hard white tissue spreading from a central focus into the breast. Some specimens are abnormally dark yellow, oily and soft. Few specialists, however, would base any therapeutic decision upon being able to distinguish between fat necrosis and cancer without the aid of the microscope.

On frozen section there is usually clear histologic evidence of ruptured fat cells with pools of extracellular lipid surrounded by abundant lymphocytes, macrophages and sometimes giant cells. Fibroblastic reaction is evident. Occasionally the cellularity of the leukocytic exudate may make for some difficulty in excluding cancer. Permanent sections demonstrate the severe macrophage and foreign body giant cell reactions with fibrosis that typify fat necrosis anywhere in the body (Fig. 57–11).

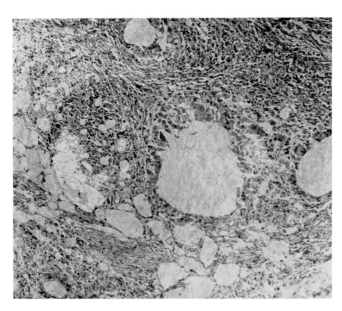

Fig. 57-11.   Fat necrosis of the breast involves rupture of fat cells, pooling of their lipoid contents, considerable macrophage reaction and inflammation. Later, foreign body giant cells and fibrosis are prominent.

Treatment of Fat Necrosis

As indicated above, the important point in therapy is an accurate pathologic diagnosis. When the diagnosis of fat necrosis has been established, local excision of all the involved tissue, in much the same fashion that a carbuncle is treated, will suffice. In all probability the wound should be drained, because it is difficult to maintain a dry operative field however hard you try.

COMMON INFECTIOUS PROCESSES OCCURRING IN THE BREAST

In addition to the exudative inflammation that accompanies fat necrosis, mammary duct ectasia and inflammatory carcinoma, there are a few infections which are primary in the breast. Because of the large fatty component of breast tissue and the rather widely dispersed blood supply, infection here is rarely fulminating, but tends to progress slowly and to give rise to varying degrees of induration. There is small likelihood that an abscess and the surrounding connective tissue fibrosis will be confused with carcinoma, but the possibility should still be kept in mind, particularly when redness is accompanied by edema and infiltration of the skin. If any doubts exist, the lesion should be biopsied.

Abscess in a Lactating Breast

It is not uncommon for infection to develop in the breast tissue of a woman while she is nursing a newborn infant. The source of the infection is usually through an abrasion or crack in the epithelium covering the nipple. It may be mild and simply represent an area of tenderness accompanied by redness of the overlying skin. Common obstetrical practice calls for discontinuance of nursing when these signs appear. The infection then usually follows one of two courses: (1) It may subside completely under a regimen of rest, supplemented by the administration of broad-spectrum antibiotics, in a matter of a few days. If this be the case, the patient can continue nursing when the signs of infection have disappeared. (2) The infection may progress into a full-blown abscess associated with a protective ring of fibrosis which tends to wall it off from the surrounding breast tissue.

From time immemorial we have always associated infection, wherever it occurs, with tumor, rubor, calor and dolor. Infections in the breast are no exception. In addition, the overlying skin tends to become edematous, and if infection has been present for any length of time, induration follows. Since all these factors may be present in either carcinomas of the inflammatory type or those undergoing central degeneration, the obstetrician should not forget the remote possibility that carcinoma may be present. If the patient is now nursing or has recently abandoned it, the chances are more in favor of a true abscess, for breast abscess is uncommon in the nonlactating woman.

Treatment of a breast abscess calls for adequate incision and drainage if the process does not subside promptly under antibiotic therapy. The architecture of the breast is such that infection tends to pocket in fatty tissue walled off by fibrous compartments. Antibiotic therapy is therefore frequently inadequate. For the same reason the incision and drainage must be sufficiently wide in scope to enter all the potential compartments where infection may be present. It is always a good policy to biopsy any indurated tissue and to send it to the laboratory for pathologic review.

The Subareolar Abscess

Until recently the treatment of small localized abscesses occurring in the areolar area has been most unsatisfactory, for they were prone to recur. The reason for the recurrence lies in the fact that the sinus tracts that form and lead down to the collecting ducts at the base of the nipple become lined with epithelium. Antibiotic therapy and simple incision and drainage are ineffective. Cure takes place only after the entire sinus tract and associated collecting ducts have been excised in toto.

OTHER TYPES OF BREAST MASSES

In rare instances such entities as tuberculosis, syphilis or sarcoid may appear in the breast tissue. They occur so infrequently that their clinical characteristics, differential diagnosis and treatment will not be discussed here. For the same reason we have elected to exclude such neoplastic entities as Hodgkin's disease, myelogenous leukemia, lymphoblastoma or leukemia, which can, but rarely do, appear in the breast

PLASMA CELL MASTITIS

One of the most interesting inflammatory lesions of the breast is an unusual entity called plasma cell mastitis. It derives its name from the preponderance of plasma cells seen in histologic sections of the tumor. Ordinarily plasma cells are not found in any great concentration on pathologic review of any abnormal breast tissue. In plasma cell mastitis, however, they are present in abundance, frequently appearing as sheets of cells. Though rare, we have elected to discuss its clinical manifestations, for when discovered, it is almost invariably confused with and treated as extensive carcinoma of the breast. Actually, it is a benign process not of precancerous nature. There is little tendency even for it to recur locally, much less metastasize, if the pathologic diagn sis is correctly made.

What Is the Background of Plasma Cell Mastitis?

The mechanism by which plasma cell mastitis appears in the breast is similar to that of ordinary mastitis, traumatic fat necrosis and mammary duct ectasia. Haagensen feels strongly that plasma cell mastitis is simply the end-stage in the natural history of mammary duct ectasia. Still, there does seem to be some difference in the age groups at which the two conditions are discovered. Mammary duct ectasia tends to occur in the atrophic breast of the older woman, but the great majority of women who have plasma cell mastitis are in their thirties. Owing to the associated nipple discharge, there is a tendency to attribute the pathologic changes to disturbances within a lactating breast, but the majority of these patients have plasma cell mastitis years later. It is true, however, that there is usually a history of multiple pregnancies. Possibly one might postulate that alterations within the architecture of the breast may have caused a mechanical interference with free drainage along the mammary ducts, as suggested by Adair.

The underlying defect is in all probability a distention of and leakage around the terminal ducts in the areola and nipple involving fatty debris of cellular origin. Plugged at the outlet in the areola, the duct distention extends back into the collecting ducts within the breast substance. The material contained within them is irritating and destructive to the epithelium lining the ducts, which become thickened and fibrosed as their walls become infiltrated with lymphocytes. As Haagensen suggests' the ducts become not only thicker, but also foreshortened. For this reason retraction of the nipple takes place.

Up to this point there may be nothing in the way of symptoms, and only nipple discharge and retraction as physical findings. Eventually, however, the ducts weaken in spots, and the irritating fat-containing contents escape into the stroma. Since they are poorly tolerated by the supporting tissues, they set up a chronic inflammatory reaction within the breast stroma which becomes clinically obvious as a tumor that develops beneath the areola deep in the substance of the breast. The patient now becomes aware of discomfort and pain, as well as redness of the skin overlying the tumor. Probably because of the central, deep location of the tumor within the breast, the swelling may not be particularly tender. In most instances the pain subsides and evidence of inflammation gradually disappears under a regimen of cold applications. The patient who subsequently is proved to have plasma cell mastitis almost invariably has such a history. Unfortunately, the physician rarely sees the patient until after the inflammatory element has gone. It is the lack of pain, together with the presence of a mass, nipple retraction, discharge and skin fixation that gives the impression that the process is malignant.

Although the initial evidence of inflammation may subside, the inflammatory tumor does not necessarily regress. It may, in fact, gradually involve the entire breast. The axillary lymph nodes become implicated, and in most instances they are enlarged, firm and hard. The entire nodal chain may be traced from the breast into the axilla.

In most instances the correct diagnosis is not made preoperatively. The developmental phases, however, are so constant that the physician should question the diagnosis of carcinoma when these factors appear in the history of a woman in her thirties or forties who presents herself with a mass in a nonlactating breast.

The physical findings are so characteristic of malignant disease that observation of the points brought out in the history is very important. Characteristically, the following findings are noted on physical examination: (1) There is a mass of varying size deep in the substance of the breast on one side. (2) There is little tenderness on palpation of the mass. (3) It is firm, stony hard, usually sharply localized, but sometimes diffuse. (4) A creamy, often watery, discharge can be expressed from the retracted nipple of the breast. If it is examined cytologically, cellular detritus, mucus and desquamated cells are seen. (5) Occasionally there is enough edema of the dependent skin overlying the defect to give the *peau d'orange* effect so characteristic of carcinoma. (6) In many instances the overlying skin is fixed to the tumor. (7) The axillary lymph nodes are enlarged, firm or hard.

What Is the Microscopic Appearance?

The danger in this sort of a case lies in the fact that the criteria of malignant disease appear so obvious that the surgeon often elects to perform a radical mastectomy without a previous pathologic confirmation obtained by biopsy and frozen section.

The principal histologic factors that appear on microscopic review of sections obtained by biopsy, according to Adair and Ewing, are (1) infiltration of the breast stroma with plasma cells. This seems to be the main pathologic consideration in establishing the diagnosis, because mature plasma cells are infrequently noted in any quantity in other breast lesions. (2) There is proliferation of cells lining the ducts. As many as "six to eight rows of hyperchromatic epithelial cells" are sometimes seen. This would appear to be a point of difference between plasma cell mastitis and mammary duct ectasia. The latter, which occurs in the atrophic breast, shows atrophy rather than proliferation of the epithelial lining. The proliferation of the ductal epithelium in plasma cell mastitis is often so extensive that a comedocarcinoma is suspected. (3) Collections of giant cells are seen in the proliferating epithelium which may cause the pathologist to wonder about the possibility of tuberculosis as a diagnosis.

How Should Plasma Cell Mastitis Be Treated?

The primary consideration in therapy revolves around the establishment of the true diagnosis. With suspicion aroused and the diagnosis in doubt, a biopsy of the mass is indicated.

In all probability local removal of the tumor is all that is necessary. If the mass is large enough, a simple mastectomy may have to be performed. There is little evidence that a true plasma cell mastitis, despite the proliferation of the duct epithelium, goes on to cancer if left undisturbed. Adair followed up two cases for two years without any appreciable change noted in the tumor. There have been a few cases reported, however, that apparently recurred locally after a simple excision of the tumor. In addition, a breast neoplasm has been found in a few cases in which the predominant cells were plasma cells—plasmacytoma of breast, either malignant or less often benign.

To avoid local recurrence of the tumor, all of it must be excised, including the entire breast if necessary. If subsequent pathologic study reveals the presence of carcinoma, x-ray treatment might be given in the manner advocated by McWhirter.

REFERENCES

Nipple Discharge

Adair, F. E.: Sanguineous Discharge from the Nipple and Its Significance in Relation to Cancer of the Breast. *Ann. Surg.*, 91: 197, 1930.

Bloodgood, J. C.: Benign Lesions of the Female Breast for Which Operation Is Not Indicated. *J.A.M.A.*, 78: 859, 1922.

Campbell, O. J.: The Bleeding Nipple. *Surgery*, 19: 40, 1946.

Copeland, M. M., and Higgins, T. G.: Significance of Discharge from the Nipple in Nonpuerperal Mammary Conditions. *Ann. Surg.*, 151: 638, 1960.

Donnelly, B. A.: Nipple Discharge; Its Clinical and Pathologic Significance. *Ann. Surg.*, 131: 342, 1950.

Fitts, W. T., Jr., Maxwell, J. D., and Horn, R. C., Jr.: The Significance of Nipple Discharge. *Ann. Surg.*, 134: 29, 1951.

Kilgore, A. R., Fleming, R., and Ramos, M. M.: The Incidence of Cancer with Nipple Discharge and the Risk of Cancer in the Presence of Papillary Disease of the Breast. *Surg., Gynec., & Obst.*, 96: 649, 1953.

Madalin, H. E., Clagett, O. T., and McDonald, J. R.: Lesions of the Breast Associated with Discharge from the Nipple. *Ann. Surg.*, 146: 751, 1957.

Papanicolaou, G. N., Holmquist, D. G., Bader, G. M., and Falk, E. A.: Exfoliative Cytology of the Human Mammary Gland and Its Value in the Diagnosis of Cancer and Other Diseases of the Breast. *Cancer*, 11: 377, 1958.

Saphir, O.: Cytologic Examination of Breast Secretions. *Proc. Second Nat. Cancer Conf.*, 2: 1238, 1952.

Dysplasia and Cystic Disease of Breast

Bloodgood, J. C.: The Pathology of Chronic Cystic Mastitis of the Female Breast, with Special Consideration of the Blue Domed Cyst. *Arch Surg.*, 3: 445, 1921.

Idem: Borderline Breast Tumors. Encapsulated and Nonencapsulated Adenomata Observed from 1890 to 1931. *Am. J. Cancer*, 16: 103, 1932.

Copeland, M. M.: Mammary Dysplasia: Diagnosis and Treatment. *Texas J. Med.*, 55: 801, 1959.

Fanger, H., and Barker, B. E.: Histochemistry of Breast Diseases. A.M.A. *Arch. Path.*, 67: 293, 1959.

Franz, V. K., Pickren, J. W., Melcher, G. W., and Auchincloss, H., Jr.: Incidence of Chronic Cystic Disease in So-Called "Normal Breasts," a Study Based on 225 Post Mortem Examinations. *Cancer*, 4: 762, 1951.

Gershon-Cohen, J., and Ingleby, H.: Mazoplasia. *Am. J. Path.*, 27: 732, 1951.

Haagensen, C. D.: *Diseases of the Breast*. Philadelphia, W. B. Saunders Company, 1955.

Ingleby, H.: Normal and Pathological Proliferation in the Breast, with Special Reference to Cystic Disease. *Arch. Path.*, 33: 573, 1942.

Kistner, R. W.: Observations on the Use of a Nonsteroidal Estrogen Antagonist. I. Cystic Disease of Breast. *Am. J. Obst. & Gynec.*, 81: 233, 1961.

Lewison, E. F.: Relationship between Benign and Malignant Breast Disease. *Ca.*, 9: 155, 1959.

Idem: Value of Periodic Examination in Early Cancer of the Breast. *Postgrad. Med.*, 27: 297, 1960.

Linden, G., Cline, J. W., Wood, D. A., Guiss, L. W., and Breslow, L.: Validity of Pathological Diagnosis of Breast Cancer. *J.A.M.A.*, 173: 143, 1960.

Massie, F. M., and McClellan, J. T.: An Analysis of 1500 Breast Biopsies. *Am. Surg.*, 26: 509, 1960.

Nathanson, I. T.: Present Concepts of Benign Breast Disease. *New England J. Med.*, 235: 516, 548, 1946.

Oberman, H. A., and French, J.: Chronic Fibrocystic Disease of the Breast. *Surg., Gynec., & Obst.*, 112: 647, 1961.

Oliver, R. L., and Major, R. C.: Cyclomastopathy: Physiopathological Conception of Some Benign Breast Tumors, with an Analysis of Four Hundred Cases. *Am. J. Cancer*, 21:1, 1934.

Pessagno, D. J.: Cystic Disease of the Breast. *Am. Surgeon*, 23: 65, 1957.

Rivers, L., and others: Carcinoma of the Breast. The Diagnostic Significance of Pain. *Am. J. Surg.*, 82: 733, 1951.

Saltzstein, S. L.: Histologic Diagnosis of Breast Carcinoma with Silverman Needle Biopsy. *Surgery*, 48: 366, 1960.

Simmons, C. C., Daland, E. M., and Wallace, R. H.: Delay in the Treatment of Cancer. *New England J. Med.*, 208: 1097, 1933.

Sloss, P. T., Bennett, W. A., and Clagett, O. T.: Incidence in Normal Breasts of Features Associated with Chronic Cystic Mastitis. *Am. J. Path.*, 33: 1181, 1957.

Urban, J. A.: Early Diagnosis of Breast Cancer. Salvage Data with Lesions Considered Clinically Benign or Doubtful Prior to Operation. *Cancer*, 9: 1173, 1956.

Vassar, P. S., and Culling, C. F. A.: Fibrosis of Breast. A.M.A. *Arch. Path.*, 67: 128, 1959.

Warren, S.: The Prognosis of Benign Lesions of the Female Breast. *Surgery*, 19: 32, 1946.

Womack, N. S.: Endocrine Relationships between Chronic Cystic Mastitis and Cancer of Breast. *Am. Surgeon*, 24: 618, 1958.

Blunt Duct and Sclerosing Adenoses

Foote, F. W., Jr., and Stewart, F. W.: Comparative Studies of Cancerous versus Non-cancerous Breasts, *Ann. Surg.*, 121: 6, 197, 1945.

Heller, E. L., and Fleming, J. C.: Fibrosing Adenomatosis of the Breast. *Am. J. Clin. Path.*, 20: 141, 1950.

Hill, R. P., and Miller, F. N., Jr.: Adenomas of the Breast, with Case Report of Carcinomatous Transformation in an Adenoma. *Cancer*, 7: 318, 1954.

Marx, R.: Significance of Ductal Sclerosis in Paget's Disease—Regression of Intraductal Carcinoma. *Arch. Path.*, 47: 404, 1949.

Sandison, A. T.: A Study of Surgically Removed Specimens of Breast, with Special Reference to Sclerosing Adenosis. *J. Clin. Path.*, 11:101, 1958.

Urban, J. A., and Adair, F. E.: Sclerosing Adenosis. *Cancer*, 2: 625, 1949.

Intraductal Papilloma

Congdon, G. H., and Dockerty, M. B.: Malignant Lesions of Nipple Exclusion of Paget's Disease. *Surg., Gynec., & Obst.*, 103: 185, 1956.

Gillis, D. A., Dockerty, M. B., and Clagett, O. T.: Preinvasive Intraductal Carcinoma of the Breast. *Surg., Gynec. & Obst.*, 110: 555, 1960.

Haagensen, C. D., Stout, A. P., and Phillips, J. S.: The Papillary Neoplasms of the Breast. I. Benign Intraductal Papilloma. *Ann. Surg.*, 133: 18, 1951.
Hendrick, J. W.: Intraductal Papilloma of the Breast. *Surg., Gynec. & Obst.*, 105: 215, 1957.
Howard, M. A., and Rosenblatt, M. S.: Management of Intraductal Papilloma. Its Relationship to Cancer of the Breast. *Am. J. Surg.*, 92: 142, 1956.
Moore, S. W., Pearce, J., and Ring, E.: Intraductal Papilloma of the Breast. *Surg., Gynec. & Obst.*, 112: 153, 1961.
Saphir, O., and Parker, M. L.: Intracystic Papilloma of the Breast. *Am. J. Path.*, 16: 189, 1940.
Snyder, W. H., Jr., and Chaffin, L.: Main Duct Papilloma of the Breast. *Arch. Surg.*, 70: 680, 1955.
Stapley, L. A., Dockerty, M. B., and Harrington, S. W.: Comedocarcinoma of the Breast. *Surg., Gynec. & Obst.*, 100: 707, 1955.
Stewart, F. W.: *Tumors of the Breast.* Washington, D.C., Armed Forces Institute of Pathology, 1950.

Fat Necrosis

Adair, F. E., and Munzer, J. T.: Fat Necrosis of the Female Breast. Report of 110 Cases. *Am. J. Surg.*, 74: 117, 1947.
Cohn, L. C., and Bloodgood, J. C.: Chronic Lactation Mastitis, Suppurative and Non-suppurative. *Am. J. Cancer*, 16: 487, 1932.
Dunphy, J. E.: Surgical Importance of Mammary and Subcutaneous Fat Necrosis. *Arch. Surg.*, 38: 1, 1939.
Lee, B. J., and Adair, F. E.: Traumatic Fat Necrosis of the Female Breast and Its Differentiation from Carcinoma. *Ann. Surg.*, 80: 670, 1924.
Menville, J. G.: Fatty Tissue Tumors of the Breast. *Am. J. Cancer*, 24: 797, 1935.

Breast Infections and Cancers Simulating Infections

Barber, K. W. Jr., Dockerty, M. B., and Clagett, O. T.: Inflammatory Carcinoma of the Breast. *Surg., Gynec. & Obst.*, 112: 406, 1961.
Case, T. C.: Tuberculosis of the Mammary Gland. *New York State J. Med.*, 59: 3789, 1959.
Knight, I. C., and Nolan, B.: Breast Abscess. *Brit. M.J.*, No. 5131, 1224, 1959.
McGregor, J. K.: Hodgkin's Disease of Breast. *Am. J. Surg.*, 99: 348, 1960.
Rogers, C. S., and Fitts, W. T., Jr.: Inflammatory Carcinoma of Breast; Critique of Therapy. *Surgery*, 39: 367, 1956.
Schmitz, R. L.: Breast Disorders Complicating Pregnancy and Lactation. *M. Clin. N. Amer.*, 45: 107, 1961.
Soltau, D. H., and Hatcher, G. W.: Some Observations on the Aetiology of Breast Abscess in the Puerperium. *Brit. M.J.*, 1: 1603, 1960.

Plasma Cell Mastitis

Adair, F. E.: Plasma Cell Mastitis—A Lesion Simulating Mammary Carcinoma. *Arch. Surg.*, 26: 735, 1933.
Cheatle, G. L., and Cutler, M.: *Tumors of the Breast.* New York, Edward Arnold & Co., 1931, p. 298.
Cromar, C. D. L., and Dockerty, M. B.: Plasma Cell Mastitis. *Proc. Staff Meet., Mayo Clin.*, 16: 775, 1941.
Gaston, E. A.: Plasma Cell Mastitis. *Surgery*, 21: 208, 1947.
Halpert, B., Parker, J. M., and Thuringer, J. M.: Plasma Cell Mastitis. *Arch. Path.*, 46: 313, 1948.
Lepper, E. H., and Weaver, M. O.: Generalized Distention of Ducts of Breast by Fatty Secretion. *J. Path. & Bact.*, 45: 465, 1937.
Manoil, L.: Plasma Cell Mastitis. *Am. J. Surg.*, 83: 711, 1952.
Parsons, W. H., Henthorne, J. C., and Clark, R. L., Jr.: Plasma Cell Mastitis; Report of 5 Additional Cases. *Arch. Surg.*, 49: 86, 1944.
Payne, R. L., Strauss, A. F., and Glasser, R. D.: Mastitis Obliterans. *Surgery*, 14: 719, 1943.
Tice, G. I., Dockerty, M. B., and Harrington, S. W.: Comedomastitis. *Surg., Gynec. & Obst.*, 87: 525, 1948.

PART V

Disorders Common to the Premenopausal and Menopausal Periods (Ages 40 to 50 Years)

Chapter 58

Abnormal Uterine Bleeding

THE EMPHASIS on the interpretation of the causes of abnormal uterine bleeding shifts sharply in the direction of malignant disease in the span of years between forty and the menopause. Cancer of the uterus, primary in either the cervix or endometrium, may appear in younger age groups, but the likelihood of its occurrence rises abruptly after the age of forty years. The most probable explanation of vaginal bleeding is still dysfunctional, but the most important cause will be cancer.

By far the highest percentage of patients who bleed abnormally at this age will show histologic evidences of persistent proliferation or hyperplasia of the endometrium, with an occasional case that presents irregular ripening or shedding. These are the so-called functional bleeders. This appears to be true whether there is palpable pelvic disease or not. Approximately 10 per cent of patients in this age group will have vaginal bleeding due to cancer. For this reason any abnormal bleeding pattern in a woman over forty years of age should be regarded with a suspicion that increases as she approaches the menopause.

The most perplexing problems arise during the climacteric, which may be defined as the period in a woman's menstrual life that precedes the actual cessation of flow (menopause). During this span of years (roughly at age forty-five to forty-eight years) the menstrual periods are apt to be irregular. It is common to have prolonged stretches of amenorrhea followed by continuous and sometimes excessive bleeding. Psychic unrest, emotional instability, inability to concentrate, and at times vasomotor phenomena (hot flashes), are common at this time in a woman's life.

Both the physician and the patient prefer to attribute any departure from the established bleeding pattern as normal for her because she is in this climacteric period. It must be kept in mind, however, that malignant disease as well as dysfunctional bleeding is common in this age group and manifests itself by abnormal uterine bleeding. Unfortunately, owing to the defeatist attitude of a large segment of the medical profession toward cancer, the diagnosis of malignant disease is not entertained, either because the physician does not want to believe that his patient might have cancer, or because a cancer diagnosis is reached only by the exclusion of all benign causes. In too many instances the physician prefers to explain away the symptoms, prescribing hormone therapy for benign functional bleeding rather than investigating the cause. Since malignant disease is by far the most important source of abnormal bleeding shortly before the menopause, the physician will do well to rule out cancer before accepting a diagnosis of benign functional bleeding.

History

The accurate taking of the history, as it concerns the nature of the vaginal bleeding, is of the utmost importance, particularly as to the degree, duration and timing of flow in relation to the cycle. The physician should ask the patient: (1) When did she first note a change from her normal menstrual pattern? Any change should be regarded with a careful appraising eye in this age group. (2) Have there been similar deviations from the normal in the past? This may be an indication of a functional cause that has righted itself spontaneously or after therapy, or it may point the finger of suspicion to possible cancer of the endometrium. Many patients give a history of disturbed menstrual patterns for some years preceding the final diagnosis of cancer. (3) Has the interval between the periods varied, and in which direction (shorter or longer)? Shortening of the interval causes no great concern, unless it is associated with some constitutional disorder. Such a history suggests a functional explanation of the bleeding. An increasing tendency to prolongation of the flow beyond eight days, especially when the amount tends to increase, suggests an organic cause. (4) Has the patient noted intermenstrual spotting or flowing, and in what amounts? This may point to a functional cause such as overstimulation of the endometrium by estrin in the absence of progestin. On the other hand, cancer of the cervix may cause periodic vaginal spotting, though the menstrual period is in no way altered.

5. Has she ever noted postcoital staining or bleeding following the use of instruments such as a douche nozzle? The explanation may lie in the presence of a cervical or endometrial polyp, but this also is the most common single symptom of cancer of the cervix. (6) Has the amount of flow diminished or increased? A decreasing quantity may point to a gradual diminution in ovarian stimulation, suggesting the onset of the climacteric. An increasing amount of flow, particularly when the duration is prolonged, suggests the possibility of cancer. If so, does the increased amount vary from day to day? (7) What is the nature of the vaginal flow? Is it spotting, flooding or gushing? Spotting may be more significant than flooding or gushing spells, which are common with submucous uterine fibroids or hypothyroidism.

8. Does the patient have symptoms of any constitutional disease? The hypothyroid patient may bleed profusely. As she approaches the menopause, thyroid hormone output diminishes. Chronic iron deficiency due to blood loss may cause an anemia which in turn produces bleeding. Thrombocytopenic purpura may be secondary to leukemia. Hypertensive patients may have uterine bleeding. (9) Has the patient been taking estrogen or any other hormone, and on what dose schedule? The patient may bleed from an endometrium overstimulated by estrin or from the sudden withdrawal of estrin, as the medication is discontinued. If a carcinogenic factor is associated with the hormones, it is in all probability due to the continuity of the dosage rather than the amount. The patient may likewise bleed after the withdrawal of progestin therapy. (10) Has the patient ever had radiation therapy for the control of uterine bleeding? This is another by-product of an abnormal vaginal bleeding pattern common in the history of patients who have carcinoma of the endometrium. Patients who have received radium or x-ray treatment for uterine bleeding may later have cancer of the endometrium more often than unirradiated women.

What Is the Relation of Abnormal Vaginal Bleeding to the Physical Findings?

Bleeding may arise from a variety of pathologic entities that commonly manifest themselves in this age group.

When no gross pelvic disease can be felt, many of the patients who bleed abnormally will present histologic evidence of either chronic endometritis, a persistently proliferative endometrium or irregular ripening or shedding after endometrial biopsy sampling or curettage. Nearly 25 per cent, however, will have hyperplasia of the endometrium. The relation of this form of endometrium to endometrial cancer is not an invariable one, but it occurs often enough to make such a patient a cancer suspect in this age group.

The benign pathologic entities that give physical evidence of their presence and are often associated with abnormal bleeding are uterine fibroids, adenomyosis, polyps, external endometriosis and pelvic inflammatory disease. The common uterine neoplasms which alter the menstrual pattern and produce an abnormal bleeding picture are cancers of the cervix and endometrium. Cancer of the ovary is associated with uterine bleeding in less than 10 per cent of cases.

In the presence of grossly palpable pelvic disease a uterine fibroid will appear about six times as frequently as pelvic inflammation and nearly ten times as often as endometriosis or adenomyosis. There appears to be little difference in the frequency of polyps whether there is palpable disease or not. Approximately 3 per cent of patients with uterine fibroids will have malignant disease in association.

It is a common misunderstanding that a fibroid is the cause of the bleeding. Except for a submucous fibroid, which cannot be felt on vaginal or rectal examination, the patient bleeds not because she has a fibroid, but from the ovarian dysfunction accompanying it. A large fibroid rising to the umbilicus may be completely asymptomatic. Inspection of the ovary at the time of operation for removal of a fibroid uterus that bleeds will, in most instances, reveal single or multiple large follicular cysts of the ovary without evidence of a recent corpus luteum. The endometrium will be proliferative or hyperplastic, regardless of the time of the cycle. The same observations hold true for pelvic inflammatory disease and endometriosis. It is important, therefore, not to be disturbed by the finding of a pelvic tumor when you are in search of the cause of uterine bleeding. The same thing is true of small lesions that can be seen externally, such as urethral caruncles or polyps. They can cause vaginal spotting or even bleeding, but they can also be a misleading "red herring." The patient may still have a cervical or endometrial cancer.

How Do We Rule out Cancer as a Cause of Abnormal Vaginal Bleeding?

Any departure from the type of bleeding the woman is accustomed to experience calls for an investigation, regardless of the extent of the variation in the years past forty. It is imperative in the woman in the climacteric period when cessation of the menstrual periods is imminent.

DIRECT INSPECTION AND PALPATION.   Naturally attention should be focused on the genital tract only after one is sure that the bleeding is not coming from the urinary bladder or rectum. If the bleeding is in small quantity and appears only sporadically, the patient is often confused as to its source. Careful questioning, accompanied by examination of the sediment of a catheterized specimen of urine, will usually rule out the bladder. Inspection and digital examination of the anus and lower portion of the rectum will eliminate obvious sources in this area.

Direct inspection of the external genitalia and vagina should be done routinely. The patient may have vaginal spotting from atrophic changes in the vaginal epithelium, *Trichomonas vaginalis* or cervical polyps. The external portion of the cervix should be thoroughly inspected and any suspicious areas biopsied. Unfortunately many cervices appear entirely normal on direct inspection and palpation, yet harbor carcinoma in the endocervix. To eliminate the vagina and cervix completely as the site of abnormal bleeding, one must not only see and feel but also biopsy any suspicious areas that can be seen, as well as those not visible externally in which cancer may be hidden.

The size or contour of the uterus is not very helpful in establishing the cause, for the abnormal bleeding from a cancer may arise within a small area in the endometrial cavity of a uterus distorted by the presence of fibroids or in a large symmetrical uterus that contains a single tumor. If the mass is eccentrically placed, one must be sure that the tumor is a subserous fibroid and not a solid neoplasm of the ovary. Since it is impossible to make this differentiation with any surety, these patients should be surgically explored.

Fixation of the uterus and induration in the vaginal vaults may be due to a variety of causes, some of them recent, others of long standing. It may be due to residual endometriosis, pelvic inflammation, chronic pelvic peritonitis or lymphatic spread from cancer of either the endocervix or endometrium. The abnormal vaginal bleeding in association with these causes and with these physical findings may well be functional, but can also be due to a malignant disease.

VAGINAL SMEAR.   The vaginal cytology smear is most useful in this age group. The appearance of tumor cells at this time, when genital cancer is at its peak, means that cancer is most likely present somewhere in the genital tract. Rarely urethra, bladder or rectum may be the source of the tumor cells. The abnormal bleeding then must be considered due to cancer, until thorough investigative procedures have ruled it out.

Cancer of the cervix is at its peak incidence at forty-five years of age in parous women. In most instances some suspicious area appears on the external cervix, but, as noted previously, carcinoma may arise within the canal of a cervix whose outward appearance is completely normal. A positive Papanicolaou smear then would call for endocervical biopsy or curettage. Less than 2 per cent of positive vaginal smears are in error when a cancer of the cervix is suspected. The error is far greater in endometrial cancer, in which smears are reported as negative in 25 per cent of patients who prove to have a cancer of the uterine fundus. If there is any doubt about the interpretation of the smears, or if the Papanicolaou smears add nothing to help diagnose the cause for the abnormal bleeding, curettage is indicated. Vaginal smears are helpful, but the final diagnosis and outline of subsequent therapy depend on pathologic examination of tissue obtained by biopsy or curettage.

CERVICAL BIOPSY AND CONIZATION.   Any area of the external portion of the cervix that appears abnormal should have a biopsy. If no such areas are visible to the naked eye, but the symptoms suggest and vaginal smears confirm the possible presence of cancer, the squamocolumnar junction should be biopsied in all four quadrants. The preliminary use of Lugol's or Schiller's solution to delineate the proper areas from which to take the biopsy is a helpful adjunct (see Chap. 48).

Under similar conditions the endocervical canal should be scraped with an endometrial biopsy curet, or random four-quadrant biopsies should be taken blindly within the canal. Specimens of this sort can be taken as an office procedure. If the diagnosis is still in doubt, the patient should be hospitalized and a cone of tissue containing the entire endocervical canal should be removed with a cold surgical knife.

ENDOMETRIAL BIOPSY.   This is a simple office procedure readily accomplished with minimal discomfort to the patient. Although it is not 100 per cent accurate, it does provide a working background upon which to base therapy. If the explanation of the bleeding is entirely functional, histologic examination will show changes that reflect the hormonal activity. In most instances the sample obtained is representative of the entire endometrium (Fig. 58–1). It must be constantly kept in mind, however, that you are only dealing with a sample. For example, carcinoma of the endometrium is usually found in association with endometrial hyperplasia and anovulatory cycles. It is possible to have a normal secretory endometrium in the greater portion of the uterine cavity, but a small focus of carcinoma in a localized area. Adenomatous hyperplasia has been noted accompanying an otherwise normal secretory pattern, probably because a series of anovulatory cycles has been followed by ovulation.

Despite these obvious objections the endometrial biopsy does provide a reasonable estimate of what is going on within the endometrium. When suspicions of malignant disease arise, the most logical diagnostic procedure is a curettage. Unfortunately, not all patients take kindly to this suggestion and may refuse to have it done, despite serious efforts to convince them of its importance. An endometrial sample obtained by biopsy curet is better than no specimen at all. If the histology shows a persistent proliferative phase at a time when it should be secretory, one may safely resort to progesterone therapy, for in most instances the bleeding will be functional. If bleeding persists despite hormonal substitution therapy, a curettage, often with a subsequent hysterectomy, is indicated.

CURETTAGE.   Since the suspicion of malignant disease should always arise in the doctor's mind when abnormal vaginal bleeding occurs in this age group, and particularly at the climacteric, generally curettage should be advised. In too many instances we speak of *diagnostic* curettage. It is, to be sure, a diagnostic procedure, but patients for some reason feel that there is doubt of its value in the surgeon's mind and that perhaps after all they do not need it. For this reason they may postpone having a curettage done or even refuse it. Since much of the vaginal bleeding is functional, curettage actually may be curative as well as diagnostic. This element should be stressed.

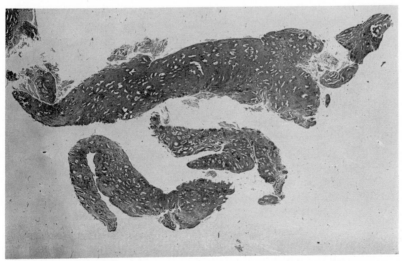

Fig. 58-1.   Endometrial biopsy expertly performed will provide strips of endometrium adequate for the analysis of diffuse processes that may cause abnormal vaginal bleeding.

Curettage is preferable to endometrial biopsy, for all of the endometrium then is available for histologic review, not just a sample. Every piece of tissue, however small, should be sent to the laboratory. Rubber dam is preferable to gauze for collecting the small fragments of curetted material.

Curettage is not 100 per cent accurate, for a small focus of carcinoma may exist at the upper corners of the endometrial cavity, or cancer may arise and be hidden behind a submucous fibroid or a polyp. In both instances the curettement may fail to reveal the most significant lesion. A continuation of the symptoms should call for a repeat curettage or hysterectomy. This occurs infrequently, but often enough so that it has become an invariable rule to have the entire interior of the specimen uterus inspected before the abdomen is closed after a hysterectomy.

Fractional Curettage. Since the source of the bleeding from within the cavity is not known, the endocervical canal should be curetted independently of the endometrial cavity. Carcinoma arising in the endocervix is much more vicious than superficial cancer within the endometrium and must be treated more drastically. This should be known before, not after, a hysterectomy is done. The fractional curettings from the two areas should be kept separate. After thorough scraping of the endocervical canal the endometrial cavity is then subsequently investigated.

Treatment of Abnormal Bleeding

ESTROGENIC THERAPY. Many patients in this age group are in the habit of taking estrogen, not always under the direction of a physician. The dosage schedules vary widely. In many instances the patient will have taken the hormone continuously over a long time. Bleeding varying from the normal menstrual pattern may occur in a patient receiving estrin therapy in one of two ways: (1) the continued stimulation of the endometrium by the estrin supplement produces an overabundant, proliferative type of endometrium. For much of the time the patient is amenorrheic, but when the growth of endometrium exceeds its local blood supply, a "break through" bleeding occurs as localized portions of the endometrium slough. (2) Sudden discontinuance of estrin therapy will also produce prolonged and sometimes excessive bleeding. Such vaginal bleeding may be expected to persist for as long as three weeks without raising any suspicion of a possible organic cause. Any bleeding beyond that time should be regarded with concern and lead to a more intense diagnostic maneuver.

If the patient is bleeding abnormally, but is known to be taking estrin, a vaginal smear and endometrial biopsy should be taken. Too often the bleeding is attributed to estrin therapy without investigating the cause. If these tests provide no suspicion of cancer, one is justified in omitting the estrin, and waiting to see whether the vaginal bleeding ceases. If it is excessive, progesterone substitution therapy should supply the deficiency that is commonly inherent in dysfunctional bleeding and stop the uterine bleeding.

HOW DO WE TREAT RECOGNIZABLE BENIGN PATHOLOGIC ENTITIES THAT PRODUCE ABNORMAL BLEEDING?

We have noted that such pathologic entities as fibroids, pelvic inflammation, endometriosis and adenomyosis may be present in patients who have abnormal uterine bleeding.

In treatment the decision for or against therapy and the choice of the procedure for correction depend on the sum total of the symptoms presented and the clinical judgment of the surgeon. Vaginal bleeding is only one factor in the final decision. The majority of the pathologic conditions mentioned bleed because of ovarian dysfunction. The exceptions are polyps and submucous fibroids. Endometriosis or adenomyosis, for example, may produce such dyspareunia, pelvic pain and dysmenorrhea that hysterectomy might be indicated for these reasons alone. Excessive or prolonged vaginal bleeding would simply provide an added reason for the procedure. It must be remembered that cancer of the cervix or endometrium can occur in patients who have a fibroid uterus or the other pathologic entities mentioned.

CERVICAL POLYPS

Polyps projecting through or presenting at the cervical os may be a cause of prolonged, often intermittent, spotting or excessive vaginal bleeding, since they are in a location where they are readily traumatized (Fig. 58–2). Cancer rarely occurs in a cervical polyp or in an endometrial polyp occurring at this age. When it does, malignant changes are usually noted at the base of the polyp. This fact must be taken into consideration when deciding how the polyp had best be removed. If it is possible to excise the polyp in its entirety, including the base, it may be done as an office procedure. On the other hand, a polyp on a long stalk which takes origin high in the uterine fundus should be removed under anesthesia in order to be sure that the base has been removed. The same may be said of large or multiple polyps. At times the cervical canal may be so strictured that it is impossible to get at the base in an office maneuver.

The decision as to whether the patient should be hospitalized also hinges on a number of other factors. Before one can be satisfied that the polyp should be removed as an office procedure one should have other evidence that cancer does not exist, such

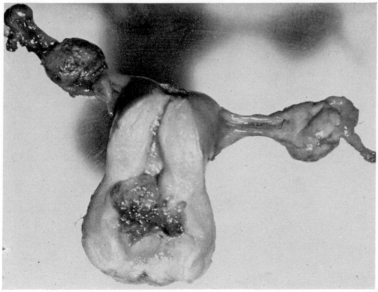

Fig. 58-2.   A cervical polyp with an eroded and necrotic tip, traumatized by pressure and friction in the cervical canal, may be a cause of excessive vaginal hemorrhage.

as is provided by a smear and an endometrial biopsy. If there is any question, the patient should be hospitalized and the polyp removed as part of a general cleansing of the entire uterine cavity. Some polyps have too broad a pedicle to make it safe to remove them in the office, for brisk hemorrhage is possible. If significant bleeding or another polyp appears after the initial excision, the patient should be sent to the hospital for curettage. This happens not infrequently.

FIBROIDS

We have noted that excessive and abnormal vaginal bleeding may occur in patients who have a fibroid uterus. In most instances the combination is enough to influence the physician to advocate hysterectomy. The bleeding factor again is simply one element in the decision. For various reasons the patient may not wish to have the uterus removed, particularly if bleeding is the only symptom and there are other means to correct it. If the surgeon can be assured through smear, biopsy or curettage that no cancer exists, he may treat the bleeding factor with progesterone out of respect for the patient's intense desire to preserve the uterus. It must be remembered, however, that uterine fibroids and carcinoma of the endometrium are frequently associated. The surgeon will do better if he advocates hysterectomy. Intrauterine and external radiation given after curettage are poor choices as alternate therapy, for they accomplish their purpose partly at the price of radiation castration and do not remove the site susceptible to develop a subsequent cancer (Fig. 58–3).

When the vaginal bleeding is excessive or gushing and the blood loss so extreme

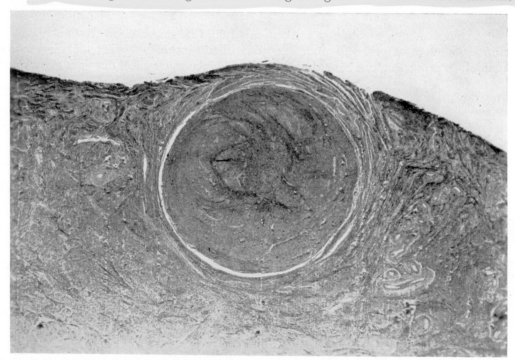

Fig. 58-3.   A small, strategically located submucous fibroid tumor may stretch the overlying endometrium and be responsible for uterine bleeding that is unresponsive to curettage.

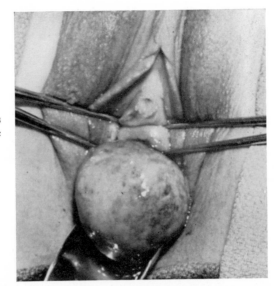

Fig. 58-4. Sometimes a large submucous fibroid may become pedunculated and prolapse outside the vulva, with associated hemorrhage.

that the hemoglobin level drops below 10 gm. per 100 ml., the patient is likely to have a submucous fibroid or fibroid polyp with a broad base (Fig. 58-4). They cannot be excised without taking out the uterus, and no amount of hormone substitution therapy will correct the bleeding problem.

FUNCTIONAL BLEEDING

Abnormal uterine bleeding due to endocrine factors or a lack of responsiveness on the part of the endometrium to normal hormonal stimulation is common in the forty- to fifty-year age group, and particularly in the years immediately preceding the cessation of menstrual periods. The same type of ovarian dysfunction is noted at the other end of the menstrual spectrum, during puberty and adolescence. There it is due to the immaturity of the ovary, in contrast to the older age group, in which either the aging ovary fails to respond in the usual way to normal or abnormal pituitary stimulation, or the target organ endometrium does not react consistently to the varying quantities of ovarian hormones. The defect is usually on the progestin side, and the cycles tend to be anovulatory. Before the bleeding can be considered functional the physician must be convinced that no organic cause for the bleeding is present.

When Is the Bleeding Pattern Abnormal?

At times it may be difficult to decide when the bleeding is actually abnormal. Alterations in the customary menstrual pattern frighten women at this age, not because of the fear of cancer, but rather the dread of the approaching menopause. Disturbances in menstrual rhythm are not uncommon during this age span. One may then expect an occasional period which is longer and associated with greater blood loss than normally expected. Such bleeding should not be considered abnormal unless the pattern repeats itself. The sporadic menorrhagic outbursts frequently correct themselves without medical help.

Abnormality here is an individual thing. For it to mean anything the present vaginal bleeding problem must be compared with the patient's previous menstrual history. Some patients without endocrine abnormality or disturbed thyroid function bleed heavily with every period. The interval between menstrual cycles varies between women, and in some women it is not always the same. Similar observations may be made about the duration and nature of the flow. Clots are not always a symbol of menstrual bleeding abnormality.

At this time of life the periods may be too short or too prolonged in duration, or too frequent or too delayed in interval. Dysfunctional vaginal bleeding is far more apt to be associated with shortened intervals. Abnormal bleeding is usually prolonged or associated with intermenstrual or postcoital spotting.

Curettage and Hysterectomy

In this particular age group there is far less indication for hormone therapy than in the earlier reproductive years, when one should and can be conservative, since the likelihood of cancer as the explanation of bleeding is more remote. When no visible or palpable pathologic change is evident, yet the patient bleeds abnormally, a curettage is the best form of therapy. If the uterine bleeding is purely functional, this frequently provides a cure. Whether or not a hysterectomy is performed at the time of curettage will depend on the physical findings, the interpretation of the histologic picture seen on frozen section of the endometrial tissue removed, and the extent of the uterine bleeding, as indicated by the type and amount of flow and the degree of anemia produced. In many instances other factors, unrelated to the vaginal bleeding, influence the surgeon in the direction of hysterectomy, such as pelvic relaxation or associated abnormalities like fibroids or endometriosis, unsuspected until the patient was under anesthesia.

Hormone Therapy

If the surgeon has carried out extensive diagnostic measures and has good reason to believe that no cancer is present, he may take a calculated risk and give the patient progesterone therapy. Since much of the time functional bleeding is anovulatory, the hormone deficiency likely is on the progestin side and is due to the unbalanced stimulation of estrin upon the endometrium. The basic aim in such therapy is to provide a medical curettage that produces a complete sloughing of the endometrium, rather than the patchy desquamation that occurs with anovulatory periods.

The dosage schedule varies with the individual uterine bleeding problem. If the bleeding is excessive and continues, an injection should be given immediately. Fifty milligrams of Proluton, intramuscularly, for three days should stop the bleeding and produce complete withdrawal bleeding three days later. This period of flow may be profuse, but it should terminate in about four days. If the patient still has a recognizable cycle, but simply bleeds excessively at the time of her period, Delalutin, 2 cc., should be given as one injection beginning on the eighteenth day of a 28-day cycle, or Proluton, 20 mg., given as an intramuscular injection daily for 5 days. Withdrawal bleeding should occur approximately ten days after the Delalutin or four days after the last Proluton injection.

If the patient continues to bleed, or the same excessive bleeding occurs in subsequent cycles, hormone therapy should be abandoned and hysterectomy performed after a preliminary curettage.

THE PATHOLOGIC PICTURE OF THE ENDOMETRIUM IN PATIENTS WHO BLEED ABNORMALLY AT THE CLIMACTERIĆ

METROPATHIA HEMORRHAGICA

A large number of patients who have an abnormal bleeding pattern in this age group have so-called metropathia hemorrhagica. It is true functional bleeding, for there are rarely other pathologic conditions found with it. The history is usually that of prolonged periods of amenorrhea followed by excessive, and often prolonged, uterine bleeding. The patient experiences nothing except the symptoms of anemia, which are noticeable only after the bleeding has continued for some days or weeks.

Estrogen production is primarily due to the persistent activity of one large graafian follicle, several follicle cysts or hyperplastic ovarian cortical stroma. There are no corpora lutea. The estrin stimulation of the endometrium is therefore not adequately balanced by progestin, and a persistent proliferative type of endometrium results. The endometrial picture varies, depending on the duration of the stimulus and the responsiveness of the individual endometrium to estrin stimulation. In many the pathologic picture is that of a well established endometrial hyperplasia. Others seem to bleed excessively from a proliferative endometrium that shows little tendency to become hyperplastic. Regardless of the degree of proliferation, the majority show no secretory changes.

PERSISTENT PROLIFERATIVE ENDOMETRIUM

Under estrogenic stimulation the endometrial glands and stroma tend to grow progressively. The glandular epithelium grows faster, so that the glands become more tortuous and irregular in the absence of ovulation and subsequent menstruation. Grossly, the endometrial layer is abnormally thickened, with or without polypoid changes. Microscopically, there are mitotic figures in the glands, which are lined by crowded palisaded nuclei that may form several layers (Fig. 58–5, *A*). Eventually, after the equivalent of two or three successive anovulatory cycles, the glands are seen to bulge irregularly and take on locally cystic or glove-finger abnormalities of shape. Beyond about four successive months of anovulatory proliferation such architectural alterations become sufficiently widespread to constitute a slight endometrial hyperplasia, and if this process continues uninterrupted for one or two more cycles, the changes merge into the typical histologic picture of endometrial hyperplasia. The pathologic diagnosis of proliferative endometrium consistent with anovulatory cycles is equivalent to a clinical impression of metropathia hemorrhagica in many instances.

HYPERPLASIA OF THE ENDOMETRIUM

GROSS APPEARANCE. The endometrium obtained by endometrial biopsy or curettage is fairly characteristic when hyperplasia is present. The material is found in abundance, and large quantities are obtained with ease. It usually retains its smooth sheen and hangs together well, in contrast to carcinoma, in which the tissue is granular and very friable when the examining finger is passed over it. The more yellow or white and dry the biopsy specimens are, the more suspicious one becomes that cancer is present.

MICROSCOPIC APPEARANCE. A true hyperplastic endometrium can sometimes

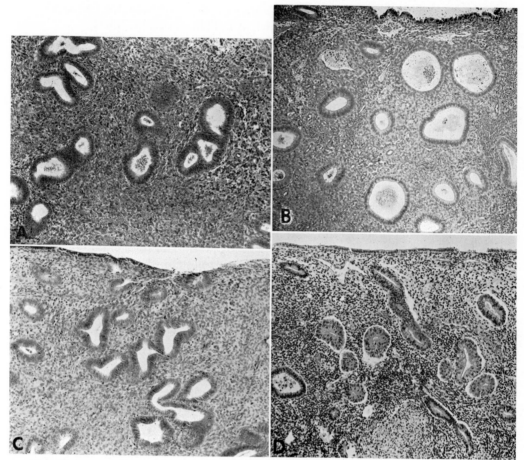

Fig. 58-5.   *A*, Persistent proliferative endometrium that follows several anovulatory cycles is recognized by the tortuous glands lined by crowded and abnormally palisaded epithelial nuclei. Mitoses are found at higher magnification. The stroma is compact. *B*, Cystic endometrial hyperplasia is evident when the glands are spherically dilated and lined by a crowded columnar epithelium. Pus in some gland lumens indicates pyometra, a commonly associated abnormality. *C*, Adenomatous endometrial hyperplasia has irregular out-pouchings of the glandular epithelium into the stroma, and usually a notable palisading of the epithelial linings. *D*, Anaplasia involves irregular sizes, shapes and arrangements of the glandular epithelial cells, frequently with hyperchromatic nuclear staining. Leukocytes, chiefly lymphocytes, are commonly present in the endometrial stroma in adenomatous hyperplasia and anaplasia.

be diagnosed by holding the slide up to a strong light without the benefit of a microscope. This is due to one characteristic gland pattern which has been called *swiss cheese* endometrium, a colorful, not particularly accurate or appealing bit of medical slang. Throughout the specimen there are many cystic spaces, both large and small. The normal cylindrical glandular pattern seen in the early proliferation of the epithelium has been lost. Tall columnar crowded epithelium lines the cystic hyperplastic glands, which have proliferated equally rapidly in all directions (Fig. 55–5, *B*). There is proliferation also of the stromal elements. Mitoses may be evident in both stromal and epithelial cells. Lymph follicles also are present.

Degenerative areas are seen at times and are said to be due to local vascular changes in the endometrium, secondary to hormonal imbalance. Although these infarct-like areas of necrobiosis are believed to be one explanation for the excessive bleeding, the patient may bleed profusely without their occurrence being noted at all. Venous thrombi of clotted blood also may be present. The obsolete term "hyperplastic endometritis" referred to the triad of cystic glands, lymphatic follicles and venous thromboses. Nowdays this would be called cystic hyperplasia of the endometrium.

Though the patient with hyperplasia of the endometrium may bleed heavily, she does not do so merely because the endometrium has proliferated. If the stimulating force, in this case estrin unbalanced by sufficient progestin, were constant, the endometrium would simply build up without any bleeding episodes. Bleeding follows when the estrin level fluctuates because of the irregular stimulating action of the pituitary, with "teetering of the titer" of estrogen.

Endometrial hyperplasia presenting the typical cystic swiss cheese pattern is benign, both pathologically and clinically. There is no evidence that such an endometrium becomes carcinomatous, unless subsequent more sinister alterations ensue.

ADENOMATOUS HYPERPLASIA

More extreme degrees of proliferation lead to an increase in the number of glands as well as a more atypical pattern within them. Grossly, the material is not distinctive. Microscopically, the glands have unusual shapes, like figures of eight and clover leaves, due to finger-like outpouchings from the main glands (Fig. 58–5, *C*). Unlike in cystic hyperplasia, the adenomatous glandular epithelium thus grows irregularly and tends to invaginate locally into the stroma. The glands may be in such profusion that they appear nearly "back to back" with only a little stroma between them. The stroma itself is not remarkable, but the epithelium of many of the glands is crowded, and there is ample evidence of epithelial hyperactivity.

Within the glands the cellular pattern changes from one layer of cuboidal or columnar cells to an irregular palisading in localized areas within the glands. This may lead to local papillary buddings or infoldings. The cells themselves are slightly hyperchromatic. Some mitotic activity is evident, but atypical mitoses and tumor giant cells are absent. The basement membrane is everywhere intact, and there is no evidence of stromal invasion.

It is the epithelial hyperactivity, atypicality of the glandular pattern, and the piling up of the endometrial glands that may make the frozen section diagnosis difficult. Grossly, however, the moist, soft hyperplastic endometrium usually is distinguishable from the drier, friable carcinomatous curettings.

ENDOMETRIAL ANAPLASIA

Beyond the structural changes that result in cystic or adenomatous glandular alterations, the individual epithelial cells may show cytologic abnormalities. When neighboring glandular cells vary noticeably in arrangement, cell size and staining, and when the nuceli particularly have a wide range in size, orientation toward each other and staining, this is termed "atypical hyperplasia" or anaplasia (Fig. 58–5, *D*). Some cells may be dying or have pyknotic nuclei, which of course needs to be distinguished from anaplasia. Although anaplasia is one facet of cancer, alone it is not convincing evidence either of an actual or potential neoplasm, and may regress completely. Alone, anaplasia does not justify a hysterectomy, but it may when other information also favors removal of the uterus. In any case a patient with either endometrial adenomatous hyperplasia or anaplasia should be followed up with care by smears and repeated curettage.

The logic of such treatment becomes evident when one considers that as many as two thirds of the patients who subsequently had carcinoma of the endometrium have been found to have had adenomatous hyperplasia as a precursor in curettings in the years before the final diagnosis of cancer was made.

CARCINOMA IN SITU OF ENDOMETRIUM

This is a microscopic diagnosis that requires strict adherence to certain criteria and prior opportunities to see similar cases. The glands with carcinoma in situ are distinguished by an eosinophilic-staining cytoplasm. Usually they have an adenomatous arrangement, and they must be sharp, clean-cut and healthy in cytologic appearance. The epithelial nuclei are large and abnormally pale, and they have folded or notched nuclear membranes in some cells. No invasion is evident, the carcinomatous cells are not degenerated, and adjacent stroma is not infiltrated with leukocytes (Fig. 58–6, *A*). Endometrial carcinoma in situ occurs in the same uterus as invasive endometrial cancer, or alone as part of a localized or diffuse hyperplasia, or in a polyp.

In the endometrium carcinoma in situ is considered an irreversible neoplastic change that will proceed to invasion unless it is removed or destroyed. Nevertheless it may average as much as five years or more, in retrospective studies, between the recognition of endometrial cancer in situ and invasive carcinoma. Further, carcinomas in situ in younger women in some cases are thought to have regressed after pregnancy. Thus the diagnosis need not constitute a surgical emergency.

Carcinoma in situ of endometrium, under various names, has been known or rediscovered at intervals for at least sixty years. It is uncommon, and occurs in a general hospital perhaps once in two or three years. Unlike the endometrial hyper-

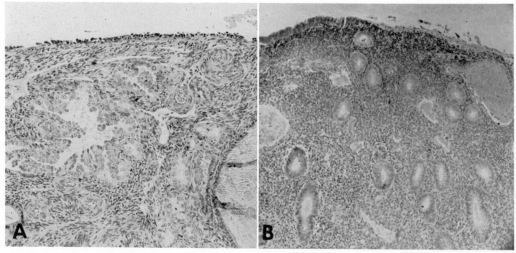

Fig. 58-6. *A*, Endometrial carcinoma in situ is characterized by localized noninvasive proliferations of glands with unusually pale, prominent nuclei and acidophilic cytoplasm. Necrobiosis, degeneration and leukocytic infiltration are absent, and their presence casts doubt on the diagnosis of carcinoma in situ. *B*, Atypical epithelial changes in parts of an endometrial polyp lack the clear-cut criteria of anaplasia or carcinoma in situ, and are ordinarily not of clinical significance.

plasias, which are classified with considerable accuracy, a tendency exists to confuse endometrial carcinoma in situ with secretory exhaustion, decidual reaction, glandular degeneration, squamous metaplasia and changes accompanying chronic endometritis, all of which lack any neoplastic significance. On this account it is well to maintain a conservative attitude toward the diagnosis of this condition.

ENDOMETRIAL POLYPS

Polyps are frequent findings and may provide the only explanation for excessive uterine bleeding at the climacteric. They may be single or multiple, grow on a long pedicle or simply have a wide, flat base. The size varies from about 0.5 to 3 cm. Grossly, polyps have a smooth surface, and microscopically they are like peninsulas covered by surface epithelium on three sides. Usually the stroma appears edematous or fibrous, and the glandular pattern most often resembles that seen in cystic hyperplasia. Old polyps may show epithelial degeneration.

When polyps arise out of a background of actively proliferating hyperplastic endometrium, cellular changes may be seen within the polyp that simulate the appearance of malignancy. The glands may be closely packed, and the epithelial activity is so extreme that malignancy in the polyps is occasionally reported. Strict criteria of anaplasia may not actually be met. Since carcinoma of the endometrium sometimes grows in a polypoid fashion, it is important to distinguish between mere atypical change within a circumscribed polyp (Fig. 58–6, B) and true carcinoma of the endometrium. The atypical changes in the polyp have little clinical significance, except that they contribute to the bleeding picture. In order that the distinction be thoroughly established, the base of the polyp and adjacent endometrium should be sharply scrutinized histologically.

Endometrial carcinomas that arise in polyps are more common in an older age group, particularly in women over sixty years old. In younger women polyps are no more sinister than cystic hyperplasia in most instances. Of course this does not apply to a carcinoma that grossly may resemble a polyp.

REFERENCES

Diagnosis and Management

Adamson, T. L., Brown, R., and Myerscough, P. R.: Post-menopausal Bleeding. *J. Obst. & Gynaec. Brit. Emp.*, 64: 566, 1957.

Albright, F.: Metropathia Hemorrhagica. *Maine M.J.*, 29: 235, 1938.

Benson, R. C., and Miller, J. N.: Surgical Curettage; Its Value in Abnormal Uterine Bleeding. *Obst. & Gynec.*, 8: 523, 1956.

Brewer, J. I., and Miller, W. H.: Postmenopuasal Uterine Bleeding. *Am. J. Obst. & Gynec.*, 67: 988, 1954.

Buldain, M., and Jacobs, W. M.: Postmenopausal Uterine Bleeding. *Obst. & Gynec.*, 6: 671, 1955.

Cope, T. I.: Some Aspects of Postmenopausal Bleeding. *Obst. & Gynec.*, 7: 153, 1956.

Diamond, L. K., and Porter, F. S.: The Inadequacies of Routine Bleeding and Clotting Times. *New England J. Med.*, 259: 1025, 1958.

Israel, S. L., and Weber, L. L.: Postmenopausal Bleeding. *West. J. Surg., Obst. & Gynec.*, 64: 515, 1956.

McLane, C., Miller, N. F., TeLinde, R. W., and Aldridge, A. H.: Indications for Hysterectomy. *Am. J. Obst. & Gynec.*, 72: 534, 1956.

Payne, W. R.: Hysterectomy—A Problem in Public Relations. *Am. J. Obst. & Gynec.*, 72: 1165, 1956.

Rodman, N. F., Jr., Barrow, E. M., and Graham, J. B.: Diagnosis and Control of the Hemophilioid States with the Partial Thromboplastin Time (PTT) Test. *Am. J. Clin. Path.*, 29: 525, 1958.
Seaman, A. J., and Benson, R. C.: Coagulation Studies of Patients with Abnormal Uterine Bleeding. *Am. J. Obst. & Gynec.*, 79: 5, 1960.
Speert, H.: The Endometrium in Old Age. *Surg., Gynec., & Obst.* 89: 551, 1949.

Cervical and Myometrial Abnormalities

Counseller, V. S., and Collins, D. C.: Fibromyoma of the Cervix Uteri. Report of a Case. *Am. J. Obst. & Gynec.*, 30: 108, 1935.
Fluhmann, C. F.: *The Cervix Uteri and Its Diseases.* Philadelphia, W. B. Saunders Company, 1961.
Kelly, H. A., and Cullen, T. S.: *Myomata of the Uterus.* Philadelphia, W. B. Saunders Company, 1909.
Mezer, J.: Metaplasia and Carcinoma in Cervical Polyps. *Surg., Gynec. & Obst.*, 75: 239, 1942.
Miller, N. F., and Ludovici, P. P.: On the Origin and Development of Uterine Fibroids. *Am. J. Obst. & Gynec.*, 70: 720, 1955.

Endometrial Abnormalities

Gusberg, S. B.: Precursors of Corpus Carcinoma. Estrogens and Adenomatous Hyperplasia. *Am. J. Obst. & Gynec.*, 54: 905, 1947.
Hertig, A. T., Sommers, S. C., and Bengloff, H.: Genesis of Endometrial Carcinoma. III. Carcinoma in Situ. *Cancer*, 2: 964, 1949.
Novak, E., and Rutledge, F.: Atypical Endometrial Hyperplasia Simulating Adenocarcinoma. *Am. J. Obst. & Gynec.*, 55: 46, 1948.
Overstreet, E. W.: Endometrial Polyps. II. Their Diagnosis at Curettage. *Obst. & Gynec.*, 14: 394, 1959.
Peterson, W. F., and Novak, E. R.: Endometrial Polyps. *Obst. & Gynec.*, 8:40, 1956.
Schröder, R.: Endometrial Hyperplasia in Relation to Genital Function. *Am. J. Obst. & Gynec.*, 68: 294, 1954.
Scott, R. B.: The Elusive Endometrial Polyp. *Obst. & Gynec.*, 1: 212, 1953.
Speert, H.: The Premalignant Phase of Endometrial Carcinoma. *Cancer*, 5: 927, 1952.
TeLinde, R. W., Jones, H. W., and Galvin, G. A.: What Are the Earliest Endometrial Changes to Justify a Diagnosis of Endometrial Cancer? *Am. J. Obst. & Gynec.*, 66: 953, 1953.

Chapter 59

Adenomyosis

THE PRESENCE of endometrial tissue in islands scattered through the muscle wall of the uterus has been called adenomyosis, or internal endometriosis. The response on the part of the myometrium to this benign invasion is a nodular or diffuse overgrowth that may produce a grossly enlarged uterus. The diffuse form of uterine enlargement should be distinguished from the localized form, which has been called an *adenomyoma*. The two are actually different, though endometrial gland structures are found in both. The adenomyoma is much like a fibroid and is diagnosed and treated as such. Adenomyosis in the diffuse form so infiltrates the muscle that it is impossible to find any line of demarcation between the process and the rest of the uterine wall.

How Does Adenomyosis Arise?

There are many theories as to how the glandular epithelium of the endometrial cavity gets into the uterine muscle. The actual mechanism is not known. Cullen, who originally described adenomyosis, believed that gland epithelium directly invaded the myometrium during involution of the uterus after repeated pregnancies to become partially pinched off and left there (Fig. 59–1). Under the stimulation of the ovarian hormones it often continues to respond as though the endometrium were normally placed. Cullen's suggestion gains some support from the observation that adenomyosis is three to four times more common in multiparous women than in the nulliparous. Actually, it may be thought of as endometrial herniations into weak spots of the myometrium in a physiologically overactive uterus. Other less likely theories mention misplaced remnants of müllerian duct epithelium, origin from the mesonephric tissue of the wolffian duct, celomic metaplasia and lymphatic or hematogenous spread of the endometrial glands into the muscle.

In all probability external endometriosis and adenomyosis are two distinct pathologic entities, with little in common, although they both manifest themselves by ectopic endometrium and are frequently observed together.

How Frequently Is Adenomyosis Found and in What Age Group?

A moderate degree of adenomyosis is to be expected in the uterus of an occasional multiparous woman beyond the age of forty years. Approximately 10 per cent of uteri removed for all causes will show some evidence of it. When external endometriosis is also present, the incidence of ectopic epithelium within the uterus rises sharply.

865

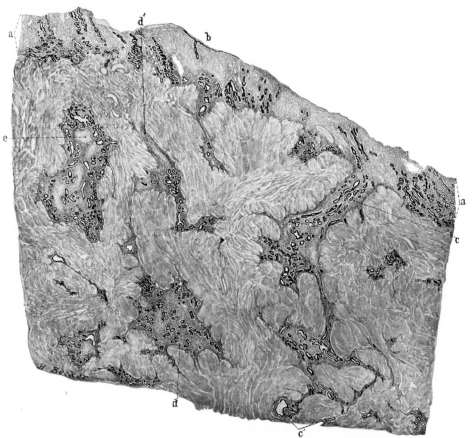

Fig. 59-1.　　Drawing of the uterine wall in adenomyosis to show the islands of endometrial glands and stroma within the myometrium. Although many are apparently isolated foci, reconstructions of serial sections demonstrate that most of the adenomyotic tissue is in continuity with the uterine lining endometrium, as shown at *c*. (From T. S. Cullen: *Adenomyoma of the Uterus*. New York, Appleton & Co.)

The actual incidence is hard to determine, because discrepancies occur in interpretation of the dipping down to various depths of the endometrium into the myometrium. Marginal involvement is called adenomyosis by some pathologists and not by others. This explains the variations in the reported incidence, which vary from 5 to 50 per cent.

There is general agreement that the incidence increases as the patient passes into the forty- to fifty-year age group. This is in contrast to external endometriosis, which is most commonly associated with the thirties.

What Symptoms Are Produced by Adenomyosis?

The chief symptoms produced by the presence of adenomyosis within the uterus are abnormal uterine bleeding and severe dysmenorrhea. Clinically, adenomyosis of the uterus is practically indistinguishable from a fibroid uterus on palpation and superficial appearance. The differentiation may be difficult even at the time of operation with the abdomen open and the uterus in hand. The true nature may not be disclosed until the uterus is transected after its removal. Both adenomyosis and fibroids produce uterine enlargement and are associated with excessive bleeding.

Abnormal uterine bleeding is usually the rule with adenomyosis. Frequently it takes the form of a prolonged menstrual flow, which is sometimes so excessive that it reaches hemorrhagic proportions. In some instances it is not unlike the flow seen with the submucous fibroid, though there is less of the sudden gushing element. As with the submucous fibroid, the bleeding does not respond to hormone therapy and is not relieved by curettage.

The chief point of differentiation between adenomyosis and fibroid is pain. The fibroid for the most part is a painless tumor. One should expect adenomyosis when a patient has a diffusely enlarged uterus with symptoms of a cramplike dysmenorrhea that persists through the entire period rather than the first few hours. The dysmenorrhea becomes progressively more severe and disabling as the patient approaches the climacteric. During the rest of the menstrual cycle the adenomyosis is relatively asymptomatic. This tends to distinguish it from genuine endometriosis, which sometimes produces pelvic discomfort throughout the month.

The explanation of the pain probably lies in the observation that the ectopically placed endometrium continues to respond to hormonal stimulation just like the normal endometrium. The areas of glandular epithelium within the muscle are commonly thought to menstruate each month under the influence of the hormones. This is debatable, for frequently the endometrial tissue is found to be proliferative when a secretory endometrium would be expected, but certainly changes do take place accompanied by stromal edema. Since the muscle walls are unyielding and do not permit any expansion, pain results. It is also possible that the increase in the vascularity of the uterus, which is a common observation with adenomyosis, may contribute to the pain as the uterine wall becomes engorged. This element, plus the scarring within the wall, interferes with the normal contractility of the muscle wall.

What Is Found on Physical Examination?

An accurate diagnosis of adenomyosis is hard to make on the basis of the physical findings alone. It is suspected when a diffusely large uterus is found in a patient who has increasingly severe cramplike pain at the time of, and through, the menstrual period. There is so much associated disease in the form of external endometriosis and fibroids that a primary diagnosis of adenomyosis is rarely made preoperatively. In the absence of fibroids or endometriosis the uterus is usually diffusely enlarged and firm. It rarely exceeds three times normal size, however. With lesser degrees of enlargement the patient is frequently thought to have functional bleeding and is treated unsuccessfully by curettage or hormone therapy.

The process typically extends diffusely through parts of the fundal portion of the uterus, rarely involves the cervix and is most frequently encountered in the posterior wall.

What Does the Uterus Look Like Grossly on Cut Section?

Because it closely resembles a uterus symmetrically enlarged by a large single fibroid, the final diagnosis may await transection after removal of the uterus. The most striking finding, other than its rather constant location in the posterior wall, is the total lack of any capsule demarcating the thickening from the rest of the musculature. Encapsulation is a common observation in a fibroid uterus. In adenomyosis there is no delineation, and the walls are diffusely thickened.

On cross section the surface has a coarse, trabeculated appearance with scattered

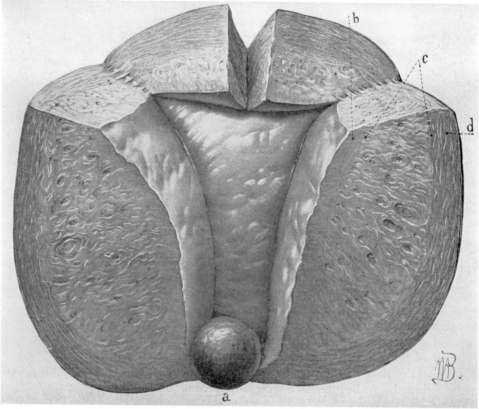

Fig. 59-2.   Drawing of the thickened uterine wall, with a coarse, trabeculated appearance of the inner half to four fifths of the myometrium that is typical of adenomyosis. The outermost part of the myometrium seems to be uninvolved (*d*). A submucous adenomyoma is present. (*a*). (Max Brödel in T. S. Cullen: *Adenomyoma of the Uterus.* New York, Appleton & Co.)

dark hemorrhagic or chocolate-colored areas, varying in size from a few millimeters to large cystic spaces several centimeters in diameter. In the majority of cases the ectopic endometrial foci are situated in the inner half of the uterine wall near the junction of the endometrium and myometrium. The process often seems to communicate with the mucosal layer. There appears to be an increase in vascularity throughout the fundal portion of the uterus (Fig. 59–2).

What Is the Microscopic Appearance?

The final diagnosis awaits review of the pathologic sections. The histology of adenomyosis and the diagnosis are based on the microscopic finding of endometrial glands and stroma, arranged in relatively orderly fashion, within the uterine musculature. They may be in abundance, or only a few may be encountered.

To establish the diagnosis, the ectopically placed glands must be found sufficiently deep in the muscle wall and usually are not in obvious continuity with the surface epithelium in the endometrial cavity. An arbitrary point of separation of adenomyotic glands from the base of the endometrium by one low-power microscopic field is commonly required (Fig. 59–3, *A*). In addition to presence of endometrial glands within the muscle, there is generally a proliferation of intermuscular fibrous tissue elements. This varies in extent in different specimens, but it is diffusely

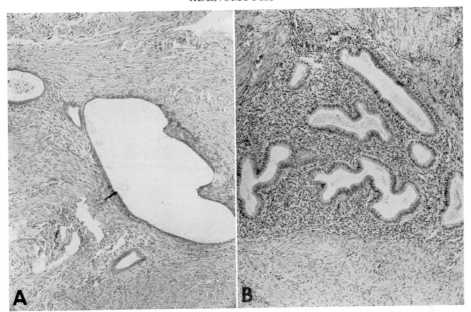

Fig. 59-3. *A,* The basal layer of normal endometrium is just along the top of the figure, and both endometrial glands and stroma are penetrating sufficiently deeply into the myometrium to justify a diagnosis of adenomyosis. Some glands here are cystic and atrophic; others are of normal appearance. *B,* Sometimes adenomatous hyperplasia or secretory activity, or both, occur in adenomyosis in a uterus with atrophy of the endometrial lining after the menopause or bilateral oophorectomy.

distributed and not localized as in a fibroid. Fibrosis in part accounts for the firmness of the process.

The consistency of the thickening is not uniform, though the general impression on palpation is that the uterus with adenomyosis is firmer than one that contains a fibroid. In part this is due to the amount of fibrous tissue it contains, and in part to the extent of degenerative changes that may take place in both muscle and connective tissue.

There are wide variations in the functional response of the ectopic glandular implants to hormonal stimulation. Complete cystic hyperplastic changes may be evident in all or only in a few isolated glands, but for the most part the ectopic areas respond only to estrogenic stimulation.

The Response of the Endometrium Itself

There seems to be little doubt that adenomyosis is in some way related to hormonal imbalance. The bleeding factor and the frequent anovulatory cycles suggest a continuous stimulation of estrin unbalanced by adequate progestin. Approximately 70 per cent of the menstrual cycles in patients with adenomyosis will be anovulatory. One may then expect to find either hyperplasia of the endometrium or persistent proliferative endometrium most of the time. Some pathologists feel, however, that the timing of the endometrial sampling, or hysterectomy, may account for the preponderance of proliferative endometrium, since both are usually carried out after long periods of bleeding. The endometrium in such a case might be expected to be in the reparative or proliferative phase. The majority feel that overstimulation by estrin is responsible for the development of hyperplasia and adenomyosis, though the causal relation cannot readily be established.

If the implant is under hormonal control, it is usually subject to regressive changes, particularly in this age group, when hormonal activity fluctuates and may be on the wane. Rarely, however, does one find carcinoma arising in an ectopic implant within the muscle wall. Some implants, nevertheless, continue to grow actively after the ovaries have been sacrificed (Fig. 59–3, *B*).

How Had Adenomyosis Best Be Treated?

Since the diagnosis frequently cannot be made until pathologic sections are studied, the patient is often treated for what is believed to be functional bleeding. As previously noted, curettage and hormone therapy alone or in combination rarely control the bleeding.

The common association of a firm, enlarged uterus with a history of increasing dysmenorrhea and frequently some abnormal bleeding is enough in this age group to warrant definitive therapy by hysterectomy. Since the differentiation between adenomyosis and a sarcoma of the uterus may be hard to make, the ovaries should probably be removed at the time the uterus is totally excised.

FIBROSIS UTERI (MYOMETRIAL HYPERTROPHY)

This is a less common condition clinically and grossly usually indistinguishable from adenomyosis. Microscopically, however, there is simply an obvious overgrowth of myometrial smooth muscle intertwined with increased collagenous fibrous tissue

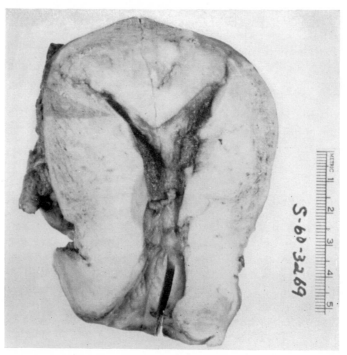

Fig. 59-4. A uterus with myometrial hypertrophy (fibrosis uteri) characteristically has a rather coarse muscular wall, over 2.5 mm. in thickness. Microscopically, both the smooth muscle and fibrous components are increased.

The basis of fibrosis uteri, manifested by a thickened, coarse, tough myometrium, is not known, but the condition usually affects multiparous women, and it is thought to be related to incomplete postpartum involution of the uterus.

Usually a clear-cut case of myometrial hypertrophy has a uterine wall diffusely thickened, measuring more than 2.5 cm. (1 inch) from the endometrial cavity to the serosal surface (Fig. 59–4). The diagnosis is usually first made pathologically after a hysterectomy performed for dysmenorrhea or excessive menstrual flow in a woman over forty years old.

REFERENCES

Benson, R. C., and Sneedem, V. D.: Adenomyosis: A Reappraisal of Symptomatology. *Am. J. Obst. & Gynec.*, 76: 1044, 1958.

Brines, O. A., and Blain, J. H.: Adenomyosis of the Uterus. *Surg., Gynec. & Obst.*, 76: 197, 1943.

Colman, H. I., and Rosenthal, A. H.: Carcinoma Developing in Areas of Adenomyosis. *Obst. & Gynec.*, 14: 342, 1959.

Cullen, T. S.: Adenomyoma Uteri Diffusum Benignum. *Johns Hopkins Hosp. Rep.*, 6: 133, 1897.

Idem: *Adenomyoma of the Uterus*. Philadelphia, W. B. Saunders Company, 1908.

Dockerty, M. B., Pratt, J. H., and Decker, D. G.: Primary Adenocarcinoma of the Recto-vaginal Septum Probably Arising from Endometriosis. *Cancer*, 7: 893, 1954.

Emge, L. A.: Problems in the Diagnosis of Adenomyosis Uteri, with Special Reference to Dysfunctional Bleeding. *West. J. Surg., Obst. & Gynec.*, 64: 291, 1956.

Hyams, L. L.: Adenomyosis—Its Conservative Surgical treatment (Hysteroplasty) in Young Women. *New York State J. Med.*, 52: 2778, 1952.

Johnson, R. V., and Roddick, J. W., Jr.: Incidence of Adenomyosis in Patients with Endometrial Adenocarcinoma. A Study of 100 Patients. *Am. J. Obst. & Gynec.*, 81: 268, 1961.

Kovar, W. R., Russum, B. C., and Grier, M. E.: What is Fibrosis Uteri? A Clinicopathologic Investigation of Fifty Cases. *Obst. & Gynec.*, 4: 311, 1954.

Kumar, D., and Anderson, W.: Malignancy in Endometriosis Interna. *J. Obst. & Gynaec. Brit. Emp.*, 65: 435, 1958.

Novak, E., and DeLima, O. A.: A Correlative Study of Adenomyosis and Pelvic Endometriosis, with Special Reference to the Hormonal Reaction of Ectopic Endometrium. *Am. J. Obst. & Gynec.*, 56: 634, 1948.

Scott, R. B.: Uterine Adenomyosis and Adenomyoma. *Clin. Obst. & Gynec.*, 1: 413, 1958

Chapter 60

Sarcoma of the Uterus

THIS RARE form of malignant disease is most frequently encountered in the forty- to fifty-year age group. Sarcomas constitute only about 3 per cent of all malignant tumors of the uterus. The ratio of the occurrence of sarcoma to carcinoma within the uterus is roughly one to forty. It is said that approximately 0.5 per cent of fibroids undergo sarcomatous degeneration.

The classification of sarcomas is a broad one, since they may take origin from (1) the smooth muscle cells of the uterine wall or a fibroid; (2) the connective tissue of the uterine wall or that of a fibroid; (3) stromal cells in the endometrium or cervix; (4) the blood vessels within the endometrium; and (5) embryonic rests or misplaced tissue elements. The general consensus is that sarcoma arises from poorly differentiated mesodermal cells and not from normal adult muscle or normal connective tissue cells. The classification based on cellular origin is not very practical for the following reasons: (*a*) The tumors are so anaplastic, grow so rapidly and invade so extensively that the actual site of origin can rarely be traced with any certainty; (*b*) representative cells of various histologic types may appear in the same tumor.

Once it was satisfactory to classify sarcomas into the predominant cell shapes, such as round cell, spindle cell or mixed cell. Of the three, the round cell was least common. Modern classifications involve identification of the basic cell type from which a sarcoma develops. The sarcoma is then named for the cell type of origin. Some classifications are complex. In this chapter sarcomas will be dealt with under categories of undifferentiated, leiomyosarcomatous, endometrial, mixed, rhabdomyosarcomatous and carcinosarcomatous subtypes.

What Are the Gross Characteristics of Sarcoma Arising in the Myometrium?

There are three different macroscopic types of sarcoma that arise in the uterine wall: (*a*) the diffuse type, (*b*) circumscribed tumors, and (*c*) sarcoma arising in a fibroid.

THE DIFFUSE FORM OF SARCOMA OF THE MYOMETRIUM.   Since this tumor is diffuse in its growth process, it produces symmetrical enlargement of the uterus not unlike that seen in a normal pregnancy, with which it is sometimes confused. The differentiation between sarcoma and a degenerating cellular fibroid that occupies the whole fundus of the uterus may not be easy to make. The presence of moist edematous tissue suggests sarcomatous proliferation and there is no restraining capsule (Fig. 60–1). This type is least common.

THE CIRCUMSCRIBED SARCOMA OF THE UTERINE WALL.   Sometimes a sarcoma does arise within the uterine wall as a solitary globular or pedunculated tumor that has some parts of a capsule when discovered early in its development. As growth progresses the encapsulation disappears, and there is little gross difference between its appearance and that of the diffuse type.

WHAT DO THESE TWO TYPES LOOK LIKE ON CUT SECTION?   When the tumor is transected, it presents a characteristic appearance that has been described as looking like "fish flesh" or "raw pork." The sarcomatous tissue that goes to make up the tumor has a smooth, slick cut surface with a yellowish tinge, and it is relatively soft and friable. Within its substance one may see cystic areas of degeneration with hemorrhagic contents. There is also straw-colored fluid, suggesting edema as the result of lymph stasis. Large dilated blood vessels with venous sinuses are present occasionally over the surface. Though the sarcoma arises in the uterine wall, it frequently juts into the endometrial cavity or out into the peritoneal cavity or the broad ligament. It is not uncommon to note a polypoid sarcoma within the cavity of the uterus that has arisen from a primary site within the wall (Fig. 60–2).

MICROSCOPIC PICTURE.   The appearance of undifferentiated uterine sarcomas is histologically somewhat reminiscent of umbilical cord. As in the Wharton's jelly, the cells are lying in a faintly stained, slightly gelatinous or myxomatous matrix. Individual cells are stellate, with large irregular nuclei, prominent nucleoli and considerable anaplastic variation. Mitoses and evidences of invasion are easily demonstrated. Recognition that a malignant neoplasm of sarcomatous type is present is not difficult. Nevertheless no differentiated elements are recognized with certainty in many cases.

Traditionally, if the sarcoma forms polypoid smooth masses and hangs down into the uterus or vagina like a bunch of grapes, it is called *sarcoma botryoides*, from the gross appearance. Microscopically, sarcoma botryoides may prove to be an undifferentiated sarcoma, as described above. Or more characteristically, there may be identifiable foci of fibroblastic, chondroblastic, myoblastic or other types of differentiated sarcoma cells, as described later (Fig. 60–3).

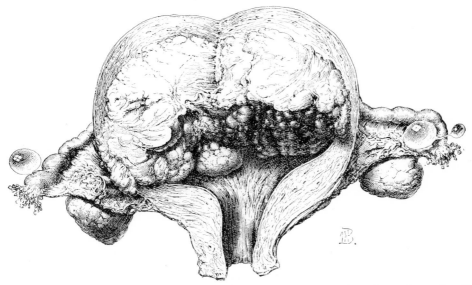

Fig. 60-1.   A diffuse uterine sarcoma protruding in a botryoid manner into the uterine cavity. (From a drawing by Max Brödel in T. S. Cullen: *Cancer of the Uterus.* New York, Appleton & Co., 1900.)

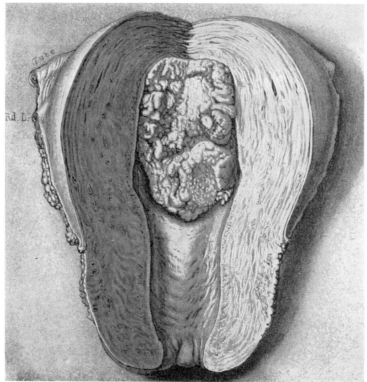

Fig. 60-2.   Drawing of a polypoid sarcoma protruding into the endometrial cavity. A carcinoma would usually appear more granular and friable.

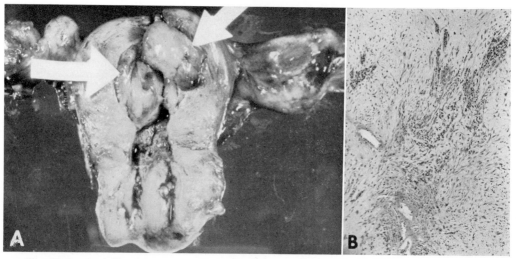

Fig. 60-3.   *A*, Uterine sarcoma botryoides has rounded tumor masses that bulge into the endometrial cavity, either from the fundus as in this case, or from the lower uterine segments. Note the smooth surfaces of the sarcomatous nodules. *B*, Variegated histologic features of the sarcoma botryoides include undifferentiated sarcoma, foci of malignant smooth or striated muscle and other connective tissue types.

Many uterine sarcomas characteristically invade blood vessels and embolize to the lungs and other distant sites, a fact which accounts in large part for their over-all poor prognosis. One should search for blood vessel invasion, in doubtful cases with the aid of special histologic stains for elastic tissue, which make identification of arteries and veins considerably easier.

LEIOMYOSARCOMA ARISING IN A FIBROID

This is by all odds the most common form of sarcoma found in the uterus. When one considers all the fibroids that occur, the chance of sarcomatous degeneration occurring within any one is not great, and collected statistics place the incidence at approximately 0.5 per cent.

It is often difficult to decide whether one is dealing with a cellular myoma or sarcomatous change in a pre-existing fibroid. Further difficulties are encountered when the pathologist attempts to differentiate between a circumscribed sarcoma within the uterine wall and sarcoma that has arisen within a fibroid. There can be no doubt about recognizing the sarcoma that develops in the center of a large fibroid, which is not unlikely to occur. It is interesting to note that there may be several fibroids within the uterus, only one of which may show sarcomatous alteration.

The gross appearance of the sarcomatous fibroid is recognizably different from one that is not malignant. Such tumors tend to be externally softer and often show gross evidence of edema. On cut section the leiomyosarcomatous tissue has a smooth yellow, tan or maple-colored bulging surface, at times with areas of necrosis and hemorrhage (Fig. 60–4, *A*). It is not white, whorled and fibrous like an ordinary leiomyoma. Some pathologists believe that the smooth, pale tan appearance reflects hypercellularity. These changes may appear within the center of the fibroid. The sarcomatous area may be small and surrounded by benign leiomyomatous tissue or a capsule. Sometimes this is called *leiomyosarcoma in situ.* In other instances the entire fibroid may be so involved that the protective capsule is lost and the myometrium or serosa is invaded. The prognosis may depend on the degree to which the tumor is encapsulated.

Microscopic Picture

It will be recalled that benign leiomyomas are cellular when they are small and relatively rapidly growing; an active growth also occurs during pregnancy. Most gross fibroid tumors thus have already passed through their growth phase and when removed are less cellular histologically, with abundant fibrosis and degeneration. Leiomyosarcomas are usually either just as cellular or contain even more closely packed smooth-muscle elements than the average benign leiomyoma in its growth phase. Thus the first criterion of leiomyosarcoma is an abnormal hypercellularity (Fig. 60–4, *B*). To be certain of this requires experience and judgment. In the days when celloidin sections were used, five or six times thicker than the paraffin sections now available, histologically many benign leiomyomas appeared abnormally cellular because of the layers of nuclei observed. This was one reason why the undesirable term "leiomyosarcoma, clinically benign" arose.

Leiomyosarcoma cells histologically vary in size, shape, arrangement and staining, and show nuclear hyperchromatism. Giant or double nuclear forms occur. Some

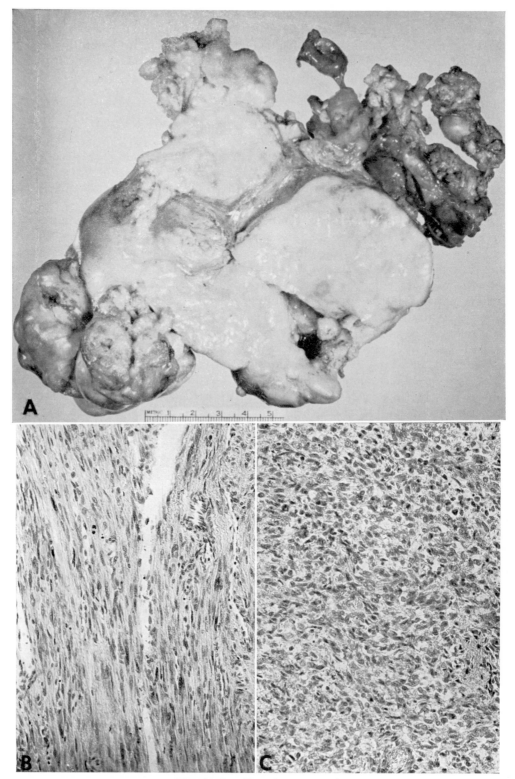

Fig. 60-4. (*Legend on page 877.*)

cells lie at right angles to the main axis of the tumor growth. Anaplasia of this sort is an essential part of leiomyosarcoma, and it must be present if this diagnosis is to be made accurately. Ischemic changes in a benign fibroid may lead to some irregular swelling, shrinkage and altered cellular and nuclear shapes, and these should not be confused with anaplasia. Nuclear pyknosis due to vascular insufficiency likewise must be distinguished from hyperchromatism.

Provided that hypercellularity and anaplasia are both present, the diagnosis still rests between a benign leiomyoma with atypical growth behavior and a leiomyosarcoma. Once the two criteria are met, a search for mitotic figures is made. If mitoses are present in a hypercellular leiomyomatous tumor with anaplasia, this is usually considered to indicate that it is a leiomyosarcoma of low-grade malignancy. In such cases the prognosis will depend upon the size, encapsulation and location of the leiomyosarcoma, the presence or absence of blood vessel invasion and the type of operation performed. Many cases are cured by a simple hysterectomy before the pathologic diagnosis is made. But these are real sarcomas, potentially lethal, and not to be stigmatized as "leiomyosarcoma, clinically benign." In modern practice there is no need for such a confusing diagnosis.

Other, more undifferentiated leiomyosarcomas are microscopically wildly anaplastic and obviously malignant, with many normal and abnormal mitoses and tumor giant cells (Fig. 60-4, *C*). One problem, aside from assaying the invasion of adjacent tissues and blood vessels, is to identify the sarcoma cells as leiomyoblasts. Special staining by the Masson method will color smooth-muscle cells red and distinguish them from the fibrocollagen, which stains green. Also phosphotungstic acid hematoxylin (PTAH) will show the cell walls and longitudinal cytoplasmic myofibrils that characterize smooth-muscle cells. In this way an anaplastic sarcoma can sometimes be identified as leiomyosarcomatous. Tissue cultures may help.

In view of the number of uteri that contain multiple fibroid tumors, in most laboratories it is not practicable to sample every fibroid for histologic study. The usual practice is to bisect every nodule and examine every fibroid grossly on cut section. Should any of them be soft or smooth on cut surface, or yellow or tan in color, or resemble "fish flesh," a portion of such a tumor is submitted for microscopic examination. The uterine specimen is saved, pending final diagnosis.

As with all sampling techniques, there is a possibility of overlooking a focus of sarcoma or of submitting an unrepresentative specimen. Careful gross and microscopic study usually results in recognizing a leiomyosarcoma in one of multiple fibroids, but on occasion a primary sarcoma is overlooked.

What Is the Malignant Potentiality of a Sarcoma Arising in a Fibroid or within the Wall of the Uterus?

In general it may be said that uterine sarcoma is a lethal form of cancer. The prognosis is better if the sarcoma arises in a fibroid, provided the tumor remains

Fig. 60-4. *A*, This large leiomyosarcoma arising in a fibroid uterus is poorly demarcated and invading through the uterine wall into the parametrial regions. The pale, slick, moist "fish flesh" appearance of the cut surface is typical of sarcoma. *B*, Well differentiated leiomyosarcoma has evident anaplastic variations of the smooth muscle cells, with abnormally large and hyperchromatic nuclei. Mitoses are present in the left central part of the field. *C*, Anaplastic leiomyosarcoma is not easily identified as of smooth muscle origin without special staining. The arrangement of the cells is irregular, with great variation in their size and staining qualities.

encapsulated. Sarcoma of either the nonmyomatous myometrium or endometrium is less amenable to therapy. Metastases are far more likely to occur from embolic spread via blood vessels than by direct contiguity or dissemination by lymphatic channels. The favorite sites for metastatic lesions to appear in are the lungs and liver. The regional lymph nodes are rarely involved.

It once was customary to evaluate the prognosis on the basis of the relative number of mitoses seen on the histologic sections. A rough parallelism appears to exist between the number of mitoses and the clinical estimation of malignancy, corresponding to sarcomas of either low-grade or high-grade malignant behavior. The patients who seem to do well after therapy for sarcoma tend to have either tumors with few mitoses or sarcomas that arise within the confines of leiomyomas. This rule of thumb may have some statistical accuracy, but it cannot be relied upon. For example, the diagnosis of "leiomyosarcoma, clinically benign," in two women known to us was made in the past by pathologists who based their estimation of the prognosis on the number of mitoses seen in pathologic sections. A hindsight review of the pathologic slides produced the same diagnosis and a favorable prophecy as to the prognosis. In both instances the patients died within six months of widespread metastases to lung, liver and, in one case, to buccal mucosa and soft parts of the shoulder. Similar unpredictable factors may be operative in explaining why the so-called malignant myomas recur or metastasize after their removal. Frequently the pathologic interpretation and the clinical behavior of the tumor do not correspond.

It is evident that there are many factors that influence the malignant potential other than the degree of mitotic activity and the histologic pattern of the tumor. The prognosis does warrant more optimism if the leiomyosarcoma is confined to a fibroid.

SARCOMA OF THE ENDOMETRIUM

Tumors that take origin from the endometrium may be either diffuse or circumscribed. Both are relatively rare. The *diffuse* type arises in the fundus and may gradually spread within the endometrium of the entire cavity, where it remains relatively confined. Occasionally the cervical epithelium is involved. Eventually the sarcoma invades the myometrium and implicates both the lymphatic and venous channels. The uterus then becomes soft and symmetrically enlarged, simulating pregnancy. The *circumscribed* type is seen more frequently. The sarcoma arises as a solitary endometrial nodule of the uterine cavity. It then spreads in one of two ways: (1) extension may take place into the myometrium, or (2) the sarcoma may assume the general appearance of a polyp that protrudes into the cavity.

Endometrial sarcoma frequently appears as a polypoid tumor. Sarcomatous polyps are softer, bulkier, and more friable than the benign endometrial polyp, with which they may be confused. They frequently become necrotic and present themselves with an ulcerated surface. The ulceration is particularly likely to appear when the sarcoma arises near the cervical epithelium. Not infrequently the gross appearance is of a malignant neoplasm practically indistinguishable from epidermoid carcinoma of the cervix (Fig. 60–5).

Grossly, endometrial sarcomas are not usually distinctive enough to be recognized, since they resemble polyps, fibroids or carcinomas. Microscopically, most are rather wildly anaplastic and composed of small, close-packed cells of various sizes and shapes, with mitoses and occasional tumor giant cells. From the intimate intermingling

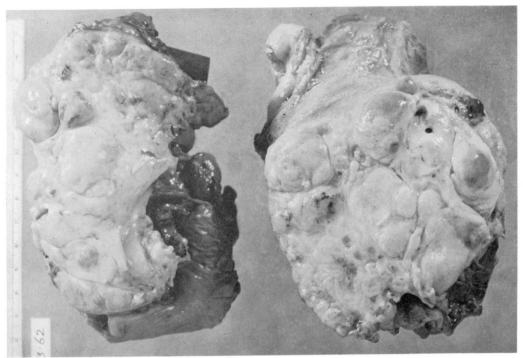

Fig. 60-5.   A bulky tumor of endometrial stromal sarcoma type. The smooth appearance typical of sarcomatous tissue is evident, as well as the bulging nodularity of its growth.

of the sarcoma with endometrial glands and noncancerous endometrial stroma, and by the general structure of the tumor cells, it is possible to classify them as of endometrial stromal origin.

Like other uterine sarcomas, endometrial sarcoma invades the myometrium and metastasizes characteristically via blood vessel embolism, so that these aspects must be looked for as part of the pathologic study.

Endolymphatic Stromal Myosis

This extremely rare form of endometrial sarcoma has been described under a variety of names such as stromal endometriosis, stromal adenomyosis, stromal myosis and stromatous endometriosis. Originally it was believed to be a form of adenomyosis, but in all probability there is little relation to either adenomyosis or endometriosis. There does appear to be a clinically benign form of adenomyosis in which the stroma is the predominant but not the sole element in the myometrial involvement. Unfortunately cases of genuine stromal myosis are not so benign. Occasionally, seemingly innocuous tumors recur years later, and they also invade the myometrium. Such behavior on the part of some of these tumors, coupled with their microscopic picture, has led many pathologists to the belief that stromal myosis is actually a form of endometrial sarcoma of low malignancy and not a variant of adenomyosis.

The lesion may arise in the endometrium or within the uterine wall. The condition may be diffuse or localized, although the uterus is usually symmetrically enlarged. On cut section sometimes cordlike strands can be seen extending macroscopically through the myometrium. The gross appearance is not unlike that of

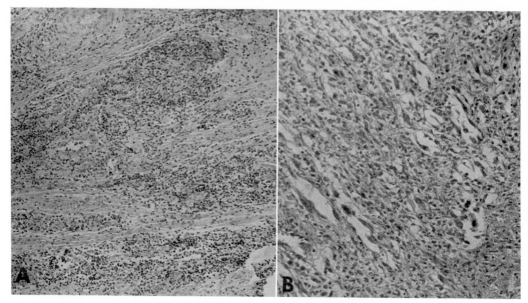

Fig. 60-6. *A,* In endometrial stromal sarcoma of the stromal myosis type the myometrium is permeated by cords of small dark cells that resemble the endometrial stroma. These lie in and around the myometrial lymphatics and spread toward the serosal surface. *B,* Part of a mixed sarcoma of botryoid type shows a variable intermingling of undifferentiated malignant stromal cells with straplike cells of rhabdomyosarcoma.

adenomyosis, except for this. Under the microscope the cords of tissue that were perhaps seen grossly appear as close-packed, spindly endometrial stromal cells growing between muscle bundles and also in channels or lymphatic spaces that are separated from the normal connective tissue and myometrium by a single layer of endothelial cells. Throughout the tumor solid masses of small, elongated cells are seen that closely resemble stromal cells of the endometrium (Fig. 60–6, *A*). Mitoses may be few or numerous, but there is little alteration in cell size or staining quality. The entire picture closely matches the microscopic appearance of a small cell spindle sarcoma. Endometrial glands are absent. The suggestion has been made that the malignant stromal cells seen may have overrun and outgrown the glandular elements of adenomyosis. This is the exact reverse of the microscopic picture of adenocarcinoma of the endometrium, in which the glands proliferate at the expense of the stroma.

The *treatment* is obviously removal of the uterus and adnexa. Most cases are controlled by local surgery, even when there is a pelvic recurrence. We have encountered metastases to regional lymph nodes and the lateral pelvic wall lymphatic channels, where finger-like processes, seemingly encapsulated and covered with smooth endothelium, have infiltrated widely. Only the most radical surgery could hope to encompass such a tumor.

RARER FORMS OF UTERINE SARCOMA

On rare occasions uterine sarcomas are associated with other tissue elements that are more fully differentiated, such as cartilage, bone and muscle. Grossly, they often resemble leiomyosarcomas.

SARCOMA BOTRYOIDES

This multifarious type of mixed mesodermal uterine sarcoma is most frequently seen in very early infancy but is occasionally encountered at other times, such as after the menopause. The gross appearance is characteristic. It has been called a "grape-like" sarcoma of the cervix. Multiple vesicular, globular masses of tumor on long stalks, looking like a bunch of grapes, may arise from the uterine fundus, cervix or upper part of the vagina. The multiple, pinkish, individual small masses are in all probability due to the rapid development of the sarcoma and the edema that is usually associated with such a growth pattern. In a relatively short time the entire vagina may be found to be full of tumor which eventually pouts out through the introitus. The lateral vaginal walls rapidly become involved in the spread of the tumor.

On microscopic section of the sarcoma a wide variety of embryonic connective tissues may be found. Much of the sarcoma may be undifferentiated, as already described. Among the recognizable mesodermal elements present at times are embryonic and cross-striated muscle and hyaline cartilage (Fig. 60–6, *B*). Microscopically, one finds an epithelial covering of normal glandular or squamous cells overlying the multiform stroma described.

This form of sarcoma, whether it occurs in infancy or after the menopause, ordinarily is rapidly fatal. The tumor recurs rapidly unless extensive procedures are performed, embracing total exenteration of the pelvic viscera. Several successful surgical cases of this sort have been reported.

MIXED MESODERMAL TUMORS

These are unusual types of sarcoma which may appear in the older age groups. They have been reported at both ends of the reproductive age spectrum and are not unlike sarcoma botryoides except that they do not form polypoid grapelike masses or bulge into the vagina. These tumors contain a wide variety of mesenchymal elements. Analogous mixed sarcomas elsewhere are called *malignant mesenchymomas* or *mixed mesenchymal sarcomas*. In addition to neoplastic cartilage and bone, smooth and striated muscle are frequently seen. Tumors with striated muscle components have been called *rhabdomyosarcomas*, but this term is best reserved for a relatively pure sarcoma made up of striated rhabdomyoblasts (Fig. 60–7). Like many other sarcomas, they are highly malignant. Recurrences and metastases appear in areas remote from the primary source fairly promptly after what should be adequate therapy.

Other tumors of mesenchymal origin are even more rarely encountered. Since they produce the same sort of symptoms and behave in essentially the same way, they need only be recorded. Pure myxosarcoma, lipomyxosarcoma, melanosarcoma, lymphosarcoma, angiosarcoma and chondrosarcoma have all been reported to arise primarily in the uterus.

CARCINOSARCOMA

This is a rare form of endometrial sarcoma in which both carcinoma and sarcoma appear in the same uterus. In any one case there is considerable doubt as to whether there is transition from one to the other or whether both arise independently and

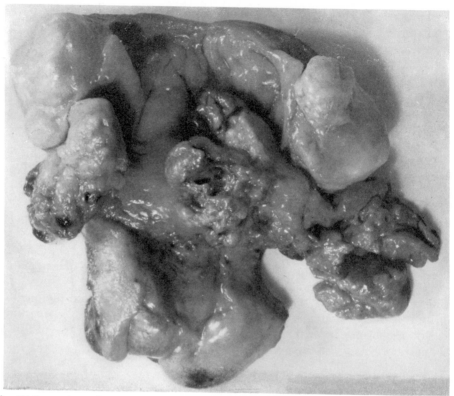

Fig. 60-7.   A uterine sarcoma of a relatively pure striated muscle type, or rhabdomyosarcoma. It is somewhat botryoid and friable, with the gross appearance of partially hemorrhagic and necrotic sarcoma invading the uterine wall.

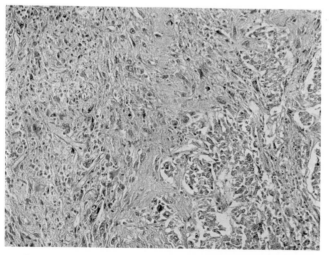

Fig. 60-8.   Carcinosarcoma is a distinctive neoplasm, since the appearance is partially that of an anaplastic sarcoma, as shown on the left, which merges locally with a carcinomatous growth, as seen on the right. Both structural patterns reminiscent of the endometrial glands and stroma may be recognized.

produce a collision tumor. The sarcoma is supposed most likely to have developed from the stromal elements of an adenocarcinoma. It is possible that the stromal cells have changed their morphologic pattern from a type originally carcinomatous.

Gross examination of a carcinosarcoma shows friable cancerous tissue, perhaps polypoid like an endometrial carcinoma. Microscopically, there is some highly undifferentiated carcinomatous growth, some intermingled spindle cells of sarcomatous appearance and other cells that are unclassifiable as either carcinoma or sarcoma (Fig. 60–8).

About half of such cases have a history of previous pelvic irradiation, which is believed to increase the chance of carcinosarcoma developing. The prognosis of uterine carcinosarcoma is poor.

DIAGNOSIS AND TREATMENT OF UTERINE SARCOMAS

What Is the Clinical Course of Most Uterine Sarcomas?

There are so many large dilated vessels in these tumors that it is not surprising to find metastatic deposits in lung, liver and bone appearing early in the course of the disease, brought there by hematogenous routes. Not infrequently the sarcomatous cells can actually be seen in the vessels on microscopic investigation. Since the tumor invades vigorously and rapidly in all directions, lymphatic pathways in the uterine wall may carry tumor cells to the intestine, spleen and kidney. Blood vessel dissemination is far more common, and regional lymph nodes are infrequently involved.

Sarcoma primarily involves the fundal portion of the uterus rather than the cervix. Because of its growth pattern the uterus increases in size rapidly and more dramatically than in other forms of cancer. The cervix can become involved. The most striking form of cervical sarcoma is the sarcoma botryoides. This tumor has been discussed above and in the section on infant problems (Chap. 9). There is another form of cervical sarcoma rarely seen that resembles in many ways a fibroid polyp. A smooth surface with areas of ulceration may give it somewhat the appearance of a cervical carcinoma.

What Are the Physical Signs and Symptoms?

The physical findings are more suggestive in the diagnosis of sarcoma of the uterus than the symptoms. Abnormal vaginal bleeding and discharge, the chief symptoms, are common to a wide spectrum of pathologic conditions within the uterus.

The most significant finding is a rapid increase in the size of a uterus which was believed to contain a harmless fibroid. The enlargement is frequently symmetrical, and since the uterus feels soft, the patient of proper age may be suspected of being pregnant. There may well be amenorrhea, unless the endometrium is involved either primarily or secondarily. The enlargement need not be symmetrical, for sarcoma may occur within the interior of one of many fibroids in the uterus.

Abnormal bleeding occurs when the endometrium is invaded or the tumor arises as a primary endometrial sarcoma. It may reach hemorrhagic proportions, but uterine bleeding is far more likely to be irregular or continuous in lesser amounts. Vaginal discharge is common when sarcoma is present. Early in the course of the disease it may be thin and watery, but as the process within the endometrial cavity continues the nature of discharge changes, and one may expect it to become serosanguineous with a rather offensive odor. In the late stages the patient frequently passes necrotic tumor particles if there is a tendency on the part of the sarcomatous lesions to degenerate and become infected.

Pain is rarely an early symptom. When it occurs in a patient who is known to have a fibroid, it is probably due to an accident within the fibroid itself and not to a malignant alteration. Unfortunately the tumor grows so fast that pain soon follows as the tumor invades. Pain may be intense and continuous later on in the disease.

Constitutional symptoms, such as anemia, weakness, cachexia, sleeplessness and weight loss out of proportion to the amount of bleeding or discharge, are commonly found in the later stages of the disease. Because of the frequency with which the sarcoma becomes infected, the patient may have an elevated temperature.

In many instances the first indication of disease within the uterus is its rapid increase in size, but the symptoms mentioned above should arouse suspicion regardless of the size of the uterus. The diagnosis of sarcoma is frequently made only after the abdomen has been opened for conditions believed to be benign.

What Are the Problems in Therapy?

If sarcoma is suspected and there is no x-ray evidence of metastatic deposits in the lungs or suggestion of spread of the disease beyond the uterus, a total hysterectomy and bilateral salpingo-oophorectomy should be done.

When gross pathologic changes are noted, such as a softer consistency and edema in one of many fibroids, when the operation is a myomectomy, the operation should be changed to a total hysterectomy with removal of the ovaries. If the fibroid has already been enucleated, the pathologist may be helpful in deciding whether it is a sarcoma or simply a degenerating cellular myoma. If anaplasia or the number of mitotic figures is excessive, the uterus should come out. This is a difficult decision to make based on frozen section diagnosis. The surgeon's judgment must dictate the subsequent operative course. If there is an overpowering reason to save the uterus, he and the patient may take a calculated risk. In the forty- to fifty-year age group the uterus and adnexa should be removed.

Is RADIATION THERAPY ADVISABLE?   Radiation treatment in the form of external irradiation may be given in a dosage up to 3000 gammas of tumor dose as an adjunct to surgery if the sarcoma involves the uterine wall in either a diffuse or circumscribed fashion. There would be little advantage and some contraindication to giving radiation therapy if the sarcoma is found only within the central portion of a well encapsulated fibroid tumor. If the sarcoma recurs locally after adequate primary treatment in an area where surgical excision would jeopardize the function of normal organs such as the bladder and rectum, external irradiation may be tried. The tumor response to irradiation treatment for sarcomatous lesions is variable.

WHAT TREATMENT SHOULD BE GIVEN IF SARCOMA IS DISCOVERED UNEXPECTEDLY? In a fair number of instances the surgeon becomes aware of the presence of sarcoma within the uterus or myoma that he has removed only when he is told later by the pathologist. The operation may be less than ideal for such a lesion. For example, the surgeon might have done a supravaginal hysterectomy, leaving the cervical stump. This poses a problem in further therapy as to what should be done. In general, if the sarcoma has been found within a fibroid located in the fundal portion of the uterus, nothing more need be done. The malignant potential of these tumors is so variable that in all probability either the patient was cured by the first operation or total hysterectomy originally or cervicectomy now will not prevent a recurrence or metastasis. This is not to be construed as an argument for doing a supravaginal rather than a total hysterectomy.

The ovaries may be spared in a young patient who has a sharply localized sarcoma within a fibroid, but otherwise the primary operation is total hysterectomy with removal of the adnexa. The further question is whether a second operation will improve the prognosis. When the fibroid containing the sarcoma is located close to the amputated cervix, the cervical stump should also be removed.

At times, but rarely in the forty- to fifty-year age group, sarcoma is found in a uterine fibroid after a myomectomy. The decision as to whether to do a second operation and remove the uterus will depend on the extent to which the sarcoma is encapsulated and the degree of mitotic activity in the tumor. If it is a low-grade leiomyosarcoma and well protected by normal fibroid tissue, the surgeon may elect to do nothing. The prognosis is supposed to parallel the degree of mitotic activity in the sarcoma, but this is not invariable, and one may be disappointed if this is the only basis for the decision in favor of or against further treatment.

REFERENCES

Leiomyosarcoma

Corscaden, J. A.: *Gynecologic Cancer*. Baltimore, Williams & Wilkins Company, 1956.

Corscaden, J. A., and Singh, B. P.: Leiomyosarcoma of the Uterus. *Am. J. Obst. & Gynec.*, 75: 149, 1958.

Davis, G. H., Howe, J. S., and French, W. G.: Leiomyosarcoma of the Uterus; Report of 16 Cases. *Am. J. Obst. & Gynec.*, 56: 1048, 1948.

Hertig, A. T.: Seminar on Tumors of the Gynecologic System. Proc. 18th Seminar of Am. Soc. Clin. Path., Chicago, 34, 1953.

Novak, E., and Anderson, D. F.: Sarcoma of the Uterus. Clinical and Pathologic Study of 59 Cases. *Am. J. Obst. & Gynec.*, 34: 740, 1937.

Steiner, P. E.: Metastasizing Fibroleiomyoma of the Uterus. Report of a Case and Review of the Literature. *Am. J. Path.*, 15: 89, 1939.

Thornton, W. N., and Carter, J. P.: Sarcoma of the Uterus; A Clinical Study. *Am. J. Obst. & Gynec.*, 62: 294, 1951.

Webb, G. A.: Uterine Sarcomas. *Obst. & Gynec.*, 6: 38, 1955.

Endometrial Sarcomas

Corscaden, J. A.: Sarcoma of the Endometrium. *Am. J. Obst. & Gynec.*, 61: 743, 1951.

Ginzler, A. M., and Herrera, N. E.: Sarcoma Arising in an Omental Endometrial Cyst. *J. Mt. Sinai Hosp.*, 24: 869, 1957.

McDonald, J. R., Broders, A. C., and Counseller, V. S.: Sarcoma of the Endometrial Stroma. *Surg., Gynec. & Obst.*, 70: 223, 1940.

Ober, W. B., and Jason, R. S.: Sarcoma of the Endometrial Stroma. *Arch. Path.*, 56: 301, 1953.

Tudhope, G. R., and Chisholm, A. E.: On the So-Called Sarcoma of the Endometrium. *J. Obst. & Gynaec. Brit. Emp.*, 41: 708, 1934.

Endolymphatic Stromal Myosis

Benjamin, F., and Campbell, J. A. H.: Stromal "Endometriosis" with Possible Ovarian Origin. *Am. J. Obst. & Gynec.*, 80: 449, 1960.

Hunter, W. C.: Benign and Malignant (Sarcoma) Stromal Endometriosis. Eleven Year Progress Report of Previously Reported Cases. Ten New Examples, Including One Followed for Twenty-Four Years. *Surgery*, 34: 258, 1953.

Hunter, W. C., Nohlgren, J. E., and Lancefield, S. M.: Stromal Endometriosis or Endometrial Sarcoma. A Re-evaluation of Old and New Cases, with Especial Reference to Duration, Recurrences and Metastases. *Am. J. Obst. & Gynec.*, 72: 1072, 1956.

Park, W. W.: Nature of Stromatous Endometriosis. *J. Obst. & Gynaec. Brit. Emp.*, 56: 759, 1959.

Robertson, T. D., and others: Benign and Malignant Stromal Endometriosis. *Am. J. Clin. Path.*, 12: 1, 1942.

Symmonds, R. E., and Dockerty, M. B.: Sarcoma and Sarcoma-Like Proliferations of Endometrial Stroma. A Clinicopathologic Study of 19 Mesodermal Mixed Tumors. *Surg., Gynec. & Obst.*, 100: 232, 1955.

Welling, S. K., Mikuta, J. J., and Greene, J. W., Jr.: Stromal Endometriosis—Report of a Case. *Obst. & Gynec.*, 16: 610, 1960.

Wheelock, M. C., and Strand, C. M.: Endometrial Sarcoma; Relationship to Certain Instances of Stromal Endometriosis. *Obst. & Gynec.*, 2: 384, 1953.

Rarer Uterine Sarcomas

Alznauer, R. L.: Mixed Mesenchymal Sarcoma of the Corpus Uteri. *Arch. Path.*, 60: 329, 1955.

Bickel, D. A., and Bennett, J. R.: Rare Mesodermal Tumors of the Uterus and Vagina. *Am. J. Obst. & Gynec.*, 67: 1257, 1954.

Greene, R. R., and Gerbie, A. B.: Hemangiopericytoma of the Uterus. *Obst. & Gynec.*, 3: 150, 1954.

Hertig, A. T., and Gore, H.: *Atlas of Tumor Pathology: Tumors of the Female Pelvis.* Washington, D.C., Armed Forces Institute of Pathology, 1960, Part II.

Kulka, W., and Douglas, G. W.: Rhabdomyosarcoma of the Corpus Uteri. Report of a Case Associated with Adenocarcinoma of the Cervix, with Review of the Literature. *Cancer*, 5: 727, 1952.

McFarlane, K. T.: Sarcoma of the Uterus. An Analysis of 42 Cases. *Am. J. Obst. & Gynec.*, 59: 1304, 1950.

Ober, W. B.: Uterine Sarcomas: Histogenesis and Toxonomy. *Ann. New York Acad. Sc.*, 75: 568, 1959.

Pena, E. F.: Primary Chondrosarcoma of the Uterus. *Am. J. Obst. & Gynec.*, 61: 461, 1951.

Scheffey, L. C., Levinson, J., Herbut, P. A., Hepler, T. K., and Gilmore, G. H.: Osteosarcoma of the Uterus. Report of a Case. *Obst. & Gynec.*, 8: 444, 1956.

Sternberg, W. H., Clark, W. H., and Smith, R. C.: Malignant Mixed Müllerian Tumor (Mixed Mesodermal Tumor of the Uterus). A Study of Twenty-One Cases. *Cancer*, 7: 724, 1954.

Walton, L. L.: Lymphosarcoma of the Uterus. *Connecticut State M.J.*, 17: 819, 1953.

Carcinosarcomas

Goodfriend, M. J., and Lapan, B.: Carcinosarcoma of the Uterus. *New York State J.M.:* 50: 1139, 1950.

Hill, R. P., and Miller, F. N., Jr.: Combined Mesenchymal Sarcoma and Carcinoma (Carcinosarcoma) of the Uterus. *Cancer*, 4: 803, 1951.

Klein, J.: Carcinosarcoma of the Endometrium. *Am. J. Obst. & Gynec.*, 65: 1212, 1953.

Peery, T. M., and Miller, F. N.: *Pathology: A Dynamic Introduction to Medicine and Surgery.* Boston, Little, Brown & Company, 1961, p. 437.

Chapter 61

Cancer of the Cervix

CARCINOMA arising in the cervical portion of the uterus is the commonest form of cancer occurring in the female genital tract and in the United States is now exceeded only by cancer of the breast as the most frequent form of malignant disease in women. It is estimated that approximately 25,000 women die yearly from malignant disease of the female reproductive organs, of whom 16,000 have cancer in the uterine cervix. Statistics available from upper New York state indicate that 23 women per every 1000 now have cancer of the cervix while 17 more per 1000 will have cancer of the endometrium. Thus 4 out of every 100 women over the age of 35 years, regardless of their marital state, will have uterine malignancy.

Despite the fact that we are dealing with a form of cancer that produces a definite train of symptoms and arises in an area that can be seen and felt, the 5-year salvage figure reported for cancer of the cervix in the world literature is at best no better than 50 per cent. Such reports provide a definite challenge to the medical profession to improve our techniques in both diagnosis and therapy. As we shall try to show later in the discussion, carcinoma of the cervix tends to remain localized in the pelvis. If the method of treatment is sufficiently all-encompassing, we should be able to improve on our existing salvage rates. Unlike carcinoma in other regions of the body, a treated patient alive without evidence of disease at five years is likely to remain so. The chances of achieving permanent success improve tremendously if treatment is carried out in the early stages of the disease.

What Factors Bear on the Incidence of Cervical Cancer?

There have been some recent signs that both patient and physician are becoming aware of the fact that cancer of the cervix can be detected early in its development, when the prognosis from adequate treatment is maximal. Not only do life insurance statistics suggest that the incidence of cancer of the cervix is declining, but also those that are seen now tend to be in the form of localized disease (League of Nations stage 0, I or II). Approximately 70 per cent of the patients seen today appear in these classifications, whereas the reverse was true as recently as 15 years ago. The improvement may be traced to the intensive efforts made to educate both the public and the physician. Much credit should go to widespread use of the vaginal smear, since nearly one third of the cases are not clinically obvious.

In addition to early detection, there are a number of factors that bear on the incidence of cervical carcinoma.

AGE.   In an earlier discussion of the preinvasive phase of carcinoma of the cervix (carcinoma in situ) (Chap. 48) we noted that the greatest concentration of cases occurred in the mid-thirties. The peak incidence of invasive carcinoma appears some ten years later, around the age of forty-five years. Although it is possible for a girl to have cervical carcinoma before the age of thirty years, the chances are somewhat less than 2 per cent. There are reports of accredited cases occurring in infancy, but almost invariably they are undifferentiated or adenocarcinomas rather than epidermoid carcinomas. Squamous carcinoma of the cervix can also appear in extreme old age, but the incidence declines sharply after the age of sixty.

This is the reverse of carcinoma of the endometrium, another type of malignancy that arises in the same organ. Here the majority of cases are concentrated around the age of fifty-seven, but 25 per cent of all endometrial cancer still appear before the menopause.

There is an old medical school axiom that any type of postmenopausal bleeding should be regarded as evidence of cancer of the endometrium until proved otherwise. This observation is correct, but, for practical reasons, the old proverb should be revised to include carcinoma of the cervix as well as endometrium. Carcinoma of the cervix at present occurs about three times as often as cancer of the endometrium. Until recently the relative incidence was about eight to one. Since carcinoma of the cervix is more common and does occur after the menopause, it may well cause the symptoms. The important fact is that therapy designed to cure cancer of the endometrium will prove totally inadequate for cancer of the cervix.

Epidemiologic Factors

There are many interesting epidemiologic factors concerned with the etiology of cervical carcinoma. Some of them are racial; others are concerned with religious practices, while the majority relate to marriage and parity.

RACIAL FACTORS.   There seems to be good statistical evidence that the white population has a lower incidence of cancer of the cervix than the nonwhite. This may not be due entirely to racial predisposition, for other epidemiologic factors must be considered, such as economics, obstetrical practices and personal hygiene, to name a few.

RELIGIOUS PRACTICES.   It is a striking observation that carcinoma of the cervix is rare among the religious groups in whom circumcision of the male is common practice. It is possible for a Jewish woman married to a circumcised man to have cancer of the cervix, but the ratio is about one Jewish woman to nine non-Jewish. The same discrepancy is noted between the Mohammedan peoples, who practice circumcision, and the Hindus, who do not, despite the fact that other factors in the environment are comparable.

PARITY AND CARCINOMA OF THE CERVIX.   There appears to be a definite relation between successful pregnancy and the subsequent development of carcinoma. For example, only 10 per cent of nulliparous women have cancer of the cervix regardless of their marital status. Cancer of the cervix is also rare in nuns within religious orders, although other forms of cancer in other organs occur about as frequently as in the general population. The more children the woman has, the greater the chances of cervical cancer.

MARRIAGE AND CERVICAL CANCER.   One may jump to the conclusion that mechanical trauma incident to repeated pregnancy is the obvious explanation, but such an assumption is not entirely warranted. Some observers believe that the important factor is marriage itself, not parity, and point to the statistical fact that married women are twice as likely to have cervical cancer as single women, irrespective of parity. Lombard and Potter, after careful review of the histories of patients with cervical malignancy in the state of Massachusetts, go one step farther. They believe that marriage, not childbearing, is the important factor, but add that the age at which marriage took place is also important. Over 50 per cent of the patients with cervical cancer married before the age of twenty. One can only speculate on why this is so.

The unknown factor could possibly be hormonal or a number of other different matters, but in all probability it is not a hereditary one. It is true that in experimental animals, chiefly mice, heredity does seem to be operative, but this experience cannot be transposed to the human being. Cancer may appear in the same family, and indeed multiple cases of cervical carcinoma occurring through several generations have been documented, but at most one may only postulate that a faulty tissue substrate may be present that will permit cancer to develop if it is abnormally stimulated by an activating force as yet unknown.

What Is the Role Played by Chronic Irritation?

One of the predisposing factors in the etiology of cervical carcinoma could be chronic irritation resulting in cervical infection (cervicitis). Trauma to the exposed squamous epithelium covering the exocervix and to the columnar epithelium of the endocervix frequently leads to inflammation. The invariable histologic sequence in the repair process results in scar tissue. Wherever found in the cervix, chronic infection and subsequent scar tissue formation appear to be linked to carcinogenesis.

EVIDENCE AGAINST THE ETIOLOGIC ROLE OF CHRONIC IRRITATION. Not all pathologists are in agreement and point out that many severely infected cervices show no epithelial variation from normal. Also cancer may arise here in the absence of any irritating signs, past or present. For example, carcinoma of the cervix does appear in the nulliparous woman, though the frequency is far less than in her parous sister. Conversely, not every ulcerated cervix becomes carcinomatous. It is a rare finding, for example, in procidentia, in which the cervix prolapses beyond the introitus and becomes subject to repeated trauma. In the past gynecologists frequently made the statement that cervical cancer and procidentia never went together. This is not true, for approximately 1 per cent of all procidentias will develop malignancy in the cervix. In San Salvador, for instance, where the incidence of cancer of the cervix is high in a mixed population, Diaz-Bazan has reported twenty-five proved cases in which cervical cancer was found in association with procidentia.

We have noted that carcinoma of the cervix occurs far less frequently than with normal expectancy in the Jewish and Mohammedan peoples among whom male circumcision is a routine practice. Cancer of the penis is equally rare among circumcised men. Inconclusive but interesting attempts have been made to implicate penile smegma as the carcinogenic agent in both cases.

Chronic irritative processes alone are not enough to incite the cervical epithelium to undergo malignant change. Some stimulating force must be added. There is experimental evidence to suggest that this element may be estrin unopposed by adequate progesterone. Clinical observations are against this. For example, we recently encountered a carcinoma of the cervical stump in a woman who had had her ovaries removed forty years before. Perhaps the adrenal gland provided the estrin source, but this assumption is pure conjecture. Some idea of how little most clinicians believe estrin to be the stimulating agent can be gathered from the present tendency to recommend that ovaries be left in situ in the younger woman when radical surgical extirpation of the uterus is done for carcinoma of the cervix.

Actually, the stimulating force that causes a cervix to change from a benign to a malignant epithelium has not been determined. It is obvious that many factors, alone or in combination, are implicated and that chronic irritation is not the only element involved.

EVIDENCE FOR CHRONIC IRRITATION AS AN ETIOLOGIC FACTOR.   Despite the fact that cancer of the cervix may appear in the absence of chronic irritation, the clinical evidence supporting the importance of its role in carcinogenesis is strong. It derives from the observations that:

1. Carcinoma of the cervix appears most often in patients who have had multiple pregnancies.

2. Cervical erosions and unrepaired lacerations are the common sites where carcinoma appears.

3. The repaired cervix rarely becomes cancerous.

4. Venereal disease, usually gonorrhea or syphilis, increases the incidence of carcinoma of the cervix, according to several studies. Presumably this is another type of chronic irritation affecting the cervix, so far as the relation to cancer is concerned. It is interesting that there is also a statistically demonstrable effect of syphilis in connection with development of carcinomas of the oral region and tongue.

Cancer of the Cervix and Repeated Pregnancy

Where obstetrical care is at a low ebb or economic conditions are unfavorable, the relative frequency of carcinoma of the cervix will increase, though breast cancer is less often encountered. The patient cannot afford good obstetrical care, nor can she do other than breast-feed the baby. Cancer of the cervix appears in the poorer economic groups. Repeated pregnancies are the rule. Nearly all marry early and have their children before the age of twenty, and parity before twenty years of age has some important unexplained effect that increases the risk of carcinoma. A lacerated cervix unrepaired surgically after repeated pregnancies typically becomes chronically infected. Chronic infection and resultant scar tissue appear to be intimately concerned in the development of cervical carcinoma.

CERVICAL EROSIONS AND UNREPAIRED LACERATIONS.   The unrepaired cervical laceration that results in eversion of the cervical epithelium and the ordinary cervical erosion are two benign conditions that may be considered predisposing to the development of malignant disease. Trauma to the exposed epithelium of the endocervical lining of the cervix invariably leads to chronic inflammatory changes. Carcinoma tends to arise at the border of a cervical erosion. Most cervical carcinoma in situ appears in lesions that were regarded clinically as benign erosions. Carcinoma first makes its appearance at the point where the endocervical epithelium of the cervical canal joins the squamous epithelium covering the external cervix. Because of the lacerations and accompanying erosions, this area may be at some distance from the external os. This is the area which must be biopsied.

CANCER OF THE CERVIX RARELY APPEARS IN THE REPAIRED CERVIX.   The concept that carcinoma is more likely to develop when a stimulating force, as yet unknown, acts upon a cervix already irritated by chronic infection derives its best support from this observation. The reports of thousands of cases indicate that patients who have had adequate treatment for their chronic cervicitis rarely (0.001 per cent) have carcinoma.

PRECANCEROUS LESIONS

In oncologic discussions the term "precancerous" is used rather freely. There are some authorities, however, who question whether there is such a thing, for when the word "precancerous" is used, you assume that (*a*) such a lesion represents the connecting link between benign conditions and true carcinoma and that (*b*) it will invariably progress to cancer unless something to prevent it is done. This is not necessarily so. The same reservations hold for the two main conditions that appear in the cervix and have often been called precancerous: (1) carcinoma in situ and (2) leukoplakia. The former has been discussed in detail in the section devoted to the problems of the thirty- to forty-year age group (Chap. 48), because this is the time when most of the controversial problems arise both in diagnosis and in therapy (Fig. 61–1, *A*, *B*).

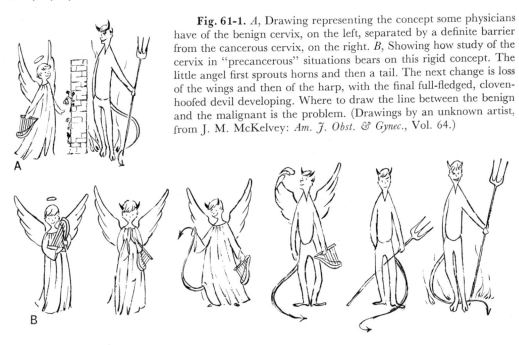

Fig. 61-1. *A*, Drawing representing the concept some physicians have of the benign cervix, on the left, separated by a definite barrier from the cancerous cervix, on the right. *B*, Showing how study of the cervix in "precancerous" situations bears on this rigid concept. The little angel first sprouts horns and then a tail. The next change is loss of the wings and then of the harp, with the final full-fledged, cloven-hoofed devil developing. Where to draw the line between the benign and the malignant is the problem. (Drawings by an unknown artist, from J. M. McKelvey: *Am. J. Obst. & Gynec.*, Vol. 64.)

LEUKOPLAKIA

Clinically, leukoplakia is readily recognized as a small to large whitish plaque, either single or multiple, appearing usually on the anterior lip of the cervix and the portio vaginalis. These areas may give rise to symptoms of bleeding and discharge. When Lugol's or Schiller's solution is applied to the cervix, white plaques of leukoplakia stand out against the mahogany brown background of the normal cervical and vaginal epithelium. They cannot be displaced by vigorous rubbing, but are readily accessible to biopsy.

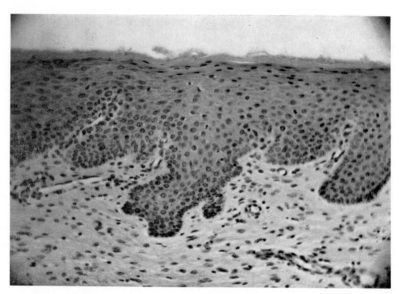

Fig. 61-2.   Leukoplakia of the cervical pars vaginalis is histologically characterized by a superficial hyperkeratotic and parakeratotic scale, irregular maturation of the intermediate epithelial layers and some basal cell hyperplasia. Stromal perivascular leukocytes may be sparse or abundant.

Microscopic Examination

Microscopic examination of the biopsy specimen reveals a varied pattern, depending on the extent of the process. Criteria of leukoplakia vary between different laboratories, and most texts give a rather vague description of the pathologic changes or assert that there is no way of recognizing leukoplakia histologically. Actually, the white appearance of the patch is due to a reflection of light from abnormally thick surface layers of hyperkeratotic scale that contain keratinized cells, some of which retain their pyknotic nuclei all the way to the most superficial strata. This latter abnormality of epithelial keratinization is called "parakeratosis."

The essence of leukoplakia microscopically is a laggardly and irregular maturation of a keratinizing epithelium. Thus there may locally be three or more layers of basal cells rather than the normal single stratum. Precornified, immature and unkeratinized cells are mixed in the upper layers with some completely mature keratinized cells that may be found singly or in nests. Mitotic activity is usually increased, and fingers of hyperplastic epithelium extend down in places into the connective tissue. The underlying stromal tissue typically has an inflammatory infiltrate of lymphocytes, macrophages and plasma cells (Fig. 61-2).

Sometimes the downgrowth of epithelial pegs is called pseudoepitheliomatous hyperplasia. This is a poor term, in that it sounds ominous, but actually means only that the process imitates a cancer. True anaplasia is not an integral part of leukoplakia, although it may appear as a complication. Carcinoma also may complicate leukoplakia, but there is no definite pathogenetic relation in any one biopsied case that justifies regarding ordinary leukoplakia as an obvious precancerous condition.

As in carcinoma in situ, with which leukoplakia is often associated, there are two common observations in the microscopic picture: (1) The abnormal cell changes are confined to the epithelium and do not penetrate the basement membrane. (2) The transition between pathologic and normal epithelium is abrupt.

Clinicopathologic Correlations

Leukoplakia is a reversible histologic process. Statistically, it is related to the development of carcinoma beyond doubt, but not to the extent that requires any drastic therapy, unless it is accompanied by anaplastic or neoplastic changes.

Because of the vague definition of the process there is doubt in the minds of many pathologists as to whether leukoplakia is an early phase of malignant disease in the cervix. Hinselman, on the basis of exhaustive studies with the colposcope, which provides direct vision of the cervix at ten to fifteen times magnification, and Antoine with the more elaborate colpomicroscope, believe that leukoplakia is precancerous. Novak and Meyer find no more reason to believe that carcinoma will develop from a background of leukoplakia than to conclude that the rare finding of malignant change in a cervical polyp proves that polyps are precancerous.

Nevertheless there are some cases that appear to have progressed from leuko- plakia to frank carcinoma. There can be little doubt that the two conditions may coexist. If leukoplakia does not actually become malignant, it may mask a carcinoma growing beneath. Therefore, in the interest of complete diagnosis as well as prophy- laxis, leukoplakic lesions should be excised. In most instances this can be simple excision. More extensive processes may call for shallow conizing or amputation of the cervix.

Carcinoma in Situ

The problems involved in the recognition and treatment of carcinoma in situ, together with the diagnostic procedures essential to establish a final diagnosis, have been discussed previously. It was mentioned then and is repeated now that the appearance of the cervix may give little or no indication of harboring malignant disease. Most cases of early carcinoma occur in lesions that were thought to be benign erosions. Suspicions aroused by the history and heightened by the findings in vaginal smears are confirmed by either multiple punch biopsies or cervical conization. Too frequently cancer is found on routine examination of a uterus removed for other reasons.

ESTABLISHED CERVICAL CANCER

What Are the Symptoms of Invasive Cancer of the Cervix?

In the discussion of the preclinical phase of cancer of the cervix the comment was made that there were no pathognomonic symptoms. The same may be said for invasive cervical cancer. The three principal symptoms of bleeding, discharge and pain are present, but all may be due to a cause other than cancer. Because uterine carcinoma is by all odds the most important cause, and since it appears so frequently in this age group, it must be ruled out before a benign explanation can be accepted. Of the three symptoms, only bleeding and discharge can be considered indications of early growth. Pain is present only when the disease has progressed beyond the confines of the cervix.

It is practically impossible to determine the duration of the disease or the rate of growth on the basis of the symptoms. In established cancer the symptoms may be

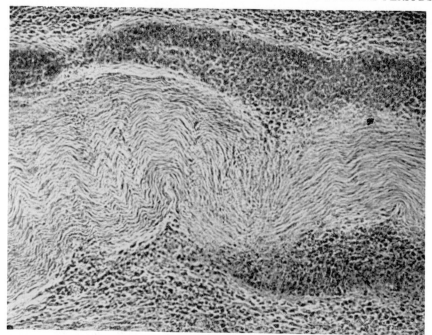

Fig. 61-3.   Cords of cervical cancer cells are invading the lymphatics and tissue spaces both above and below a large pelvic nerve. From a giant histologic section made of an exenteration specimen. (Courtesy of Dr. G. H. Friedell, Massachusetts Memorial Hospitals, Boston.)

long delayed, and all too frequently the growth is discovered late on routine examination of the patient.

Bleeding is by far the most common symptom. Since the menstrual cycle is not changed in rhythm or amount of flow, it is the intermenstrual bleeding that carries the greatest significance. The patient may note slight spotting on straining at stool or exercise, or perhaps after riding in an automobile. In most instances bleeding is noted after intercourse or taking a douche. As the cervical growth is traumatized, the bleeding usually is slight in amount and may be described as "spotting." It is frequently not enough to require wearing a pad and may not appear regularly. Several days may go by without any evidence at all. Except in the more advanced stages the bleeding rarely comes in gushes or assumes hemorrhagic proportions.

Unfortunately the bleeding is insufficient to alarm the patient. Cancer of the cervix tends to appear in women approaching the menopause. They attach little importance and pay no attention to small amounts of bleeding, particularly when not associated with pain. The symptoms are attributed to the menopause. After the menopause the vaginal staining receives even less attention. The cancer is thus firmly entrenched before the patient seeks an explanation of the cause. This is the reason why so few carcinomas of the cervix are discovered early enough to expect the best result from therapy. Postcoital bleeding or intermenstrual staining may be due to cervical polyps or erosion, but the most important cause is carcinoma. A real hemorrhage occurring intermenstrually may mean necrosis in a large, friable growth. However small the amount of bleeding, the symptoms demand an explanation.

Discharge is such a common symptom among women of all ages that it rarely induces the patient to seek medical advice until it becomes a nuisance. In the early phases it is slight in amount though constant, unless there is a large proliferative

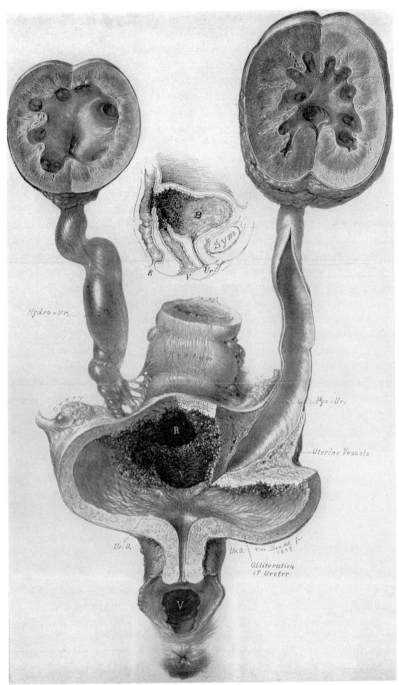

Fig. 61-4. The typical end-stage of advanced cancer of the cervix. The carcinoma has invaded the bladder and rectum, producing a cloaca, as shown also in the insert. The ureters are obstructed at their lower ends by cancer growth, with secondary bilateral hydroureter, hydronephrosis, kidney infections, and death in uremia. (From T. S. Cullen: *Cancer of the Uterus*. New York, Appleton & Co., 1900.)

growth. Despite the fact that discharge may come from a necrotic tumor, it rarely has an offensive odor unless saprophytic organisms are present. The discharge is thin and watery, and the color varies from yellow to brown, depending on the amount of associated bleeding. In most instances it can be described as serosanguineous. Rarely does the discharge precede the bleeding, and they often coexist. Two thirds of patients seen will have bleeding and discharge either alone or in combination.

These symptoms are all that occur in the early stages of cancer of the cervix. It is unfortunate that the disease does not affect the well-being of the patient or produce pain. Were it so, the patient would consult the physician earlier in the course of the disease.

SYMPTOMS OF ADVANCED DISEASE.   As the growth progresses, *bleeding* appears more frequently and increases in amount, though it may never be excessive, particularly in the postmenopausal age groups. Bleeding, however, is one cause of death in the terminal phases of cervical carcinoma. The nature and amount of discharge change as the growth process continues. It now becomes both profuse in amount and malodorous.

Pain, combined with discharge and hemorrhage, is the most common symptom in patients with advanced disease. It is due to blocking of the lymphatics and impingement on nerve ganglia by progressive infiltration of malignant disease (Fig. 61–3). Some part of the pain may be secondary to the inflammatory reaction produced by septic necrosis within an ulcerating tumor.

The constant boring type of pain localizes in the lower back and sacrum as the disease spreads posteriorly along the uterosacral ligaments. It tends to vary in its severity, is usually worse at night and is unrelieved by lying down. When the sacral nerve plexus becomes involved, the pain radiates down the back of the leg like a true sciatica. Increased doses of morphine are now required for relief. Regional lymph node metastases encasing the obturator nerves may cause pain down the inner sides of the legs. Advancing disease commonly blocks the ureters, resulting in a hydronephrosis that gives rise to flank and costovertebral pain. Encroachment of the disease upon the bladder or the rectum often produces pain on voiding or defecation. Eight per cent of untreated cancers of the cervix will develop either vesicovaginal or rectovaginal fistulas. Death is predominantly due to uremia as the ureters become obstructed and pyelonephritis develops (Fig. 61–4).

What Is the Gross Appearance of Invasive Cervical Cancer?

To establish the diagnosis of invasive cancer of the cervix the physician must (*a*) palpate the cervix, (*b*) subject it to direct inspection, and (*c*) biopsy it.

The gross appearance of the cervix is subject to many variations. Occasionally the lesion cannot be distinguished clinically from a simple erosion. Approximately one third of all carcinomas of the cervix are not evident on gross examination. The only clinical evidence may be the palpation of a firm, hard, slightly enlarged cervix that bleeds easily when the reddish granulation tissue around the external os is traumatized by the examining finger. It need not be firm and hard. The younger the subject, the softer the lesion.

When a questionable or positive vaginal smear is obtained from a patient who gives a history of intermenstrual bleeding or postcoital spotting, but who shows nothing abnormal on gross inspection or palpation of the cervix, the examiner should take particular pains to investigate the endocervical canal. Excavating cancer may be present without obvious external manifestations. The suspicion is heightened, however, when the total bulk of the cervix is increased, and it assumes a barrel-like contour.

What Does Early Carcinoma of the Cervix Look Like?

After taking the vaginal smear and palpating the cervix, and areas adjacent to it, the cervix and vagina must be inspected, using a speculum and a strong light. Before the actual development of a papillary fungating growth or frank ulceration, the cervix may simply give the impression that it is not quite normal. Actually, there is no gross picture that characterizes carcinoma of the cervix before the time when there is no longer any question of the diagnosis. A fine granular surface overlying an erosion or an eversion of the endocervical epithelium of a lacerated cervix that bleeds to the slightest touch are suggestive (see Frontispiece). This is an important observation, but it does not make the diagnosis, because red raised papillary growths are often seen with inflammatory lesions. The index of suspicion is raised, however, for we know that cervical carcinoma typically tends to arise at the border of what may appear to be a benign erosion. It will be strengthened further if the cervix has a worm-eaten appearance or if actual ulceration has taken place (Fig. 61–5).

In many instances the part of the cervix that has undergone malignant change will appear redder, darker and less shiny than the uninvolved portions. It is said to have a "tomato blush." Unfortunately, however, the variables in the appearance of early carcinoma are so great that the more experience one has had with cervical cancer, the less one relies on clinical impressions and the more one biopsies any suspicious-looking area that fails to take the Schiller stain (see Frontispiece).

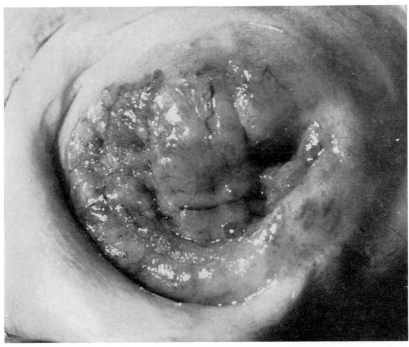

Fig. 61-5.   Ulcerated carcinoma of the cervix, one of the most easily recognizable types of advanced cervical cancer.

The diagnostic aids, the method of taking a biopsy and the variables in the interpretation of the histology have been discussed in Chapter 48.

What Is the Usual Pattern of Growth?

By and large, clinically recognizable invasive cancer of the cervix (*a*) grows as an exophytic lesion (Fig. 61–6), or (*b*) appears as an ulceration (Fig. 61–7, *A*). On occasion the carcinoma may begin as a cauliflower-like growth, but proliferates so rapidly that it outgrows its blood supply and sloughs, leaving an ulcerated granular base. The appearance then is much like that of the carcinoma that has begun as an ulcerating lesion. The pattern of growth has a bearing on the prognosis, since it must be obvious that a carcinoma expending its energy in an expansive proliferative manner will be less dangerous than one that begins as an infiltrative growth. An exophytic lesion, because of its exposed position, is more readily subject to trauma and will manifest itself sooner by bleeding than the more protected ulcerative form. It will, therefore, be diagnosed earlier.

THE PROLIFERATIVE, EXOPHYTIC OR CAULIFLOWER TYPE OF GROWTH.   This is the most common form of cervical cancer. It may arise from one or both lips of the cervix or from the endocervix. The principal growth effort goes into the production of a tumor that projects down into the vaginal canal. It varies in size, but may assume formidable proportions (Fig. 61–7, *B*). Its cauliflower-like appearance stems from the presence of multiple lobulations, furrows and crevices that make up the surface of the tumor. As we have previously noted, the expanding tumor may outgrow its blood supply. When it does, the proliferating cancer becomes necrotic, and the growth takes on a grayish-green, degenerated appearance. The bulk of the tumor may slough, leaving an undermined ulcer. Occasionally the proliferating type of cervical cancer spreads over the surface of the cervix and extends onto the vaginal fornices. Eventually the deeper tissues are invaded, either from the point of its origin into the cervical stroma, or into the paravaginal tissues when the tumor has extended to the surface epithelium of the vaginal vaults.

When the exfoliative cancer arises from the endocervix, the same kind of exo-

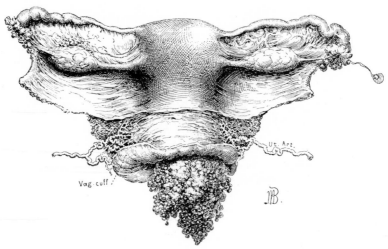

Fig. 61-6.   Drawing of a large protruding exophytic carcinoma of the cervix. (From T. S. Cullen: *Cancer of the Uterus.* New York, Appleton & Co., 1900.)

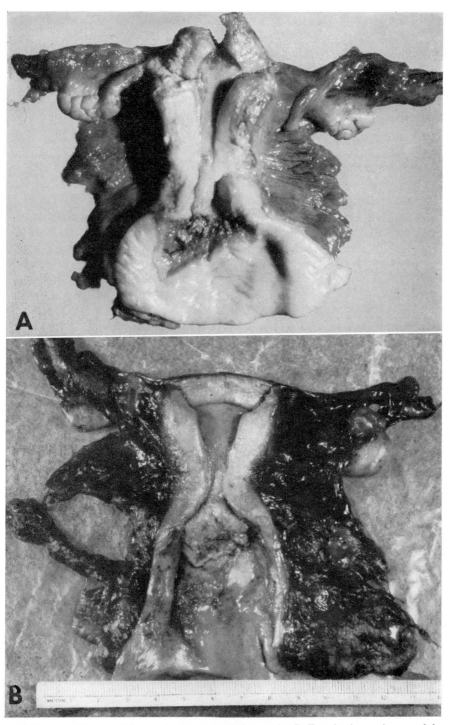

Fig. 61-7. *A*, Ulcerated form of carcinoma of the cervix. *B*, Exophytic carcinoma of the cervix and posterior vaginal fornix. Both specimens were removed by Wertheim hysterectomy. Note the parametrial tissues and vaginal cuffs included in the surgical excisions.

phytic growth may be encountered. Most cervical carcinomas will be epidermoid (95 per cent), but with an endocervical origin the same bulky type of tumor projecting into the vaginal lumen may be an adenocarcinoma. Outwardly they are indistinguishable. The final differentiation awaits histologic interpretation of the tissue provided by biopsy. It is important that the distinction be made, because cervical carcinoma of endocervical origin may respond less readily to irradiation. If the pathologic diagnosis is known, one may elect (*a*) to perform operation as the sole form of definitive therapy, or (*b*) to observe carefully the radiation response and be prepared to switch to surgery if the tumor does not regress satisfactorily during the initial phases of radiation therapy.

THE ULCERATIVE FORM OF CERVICAL CANCER is seen less often. In the older patient carcinomas of this sort have varying powers of invasion. In some a flat, irregularly shaped ulcer with a nodular edge appears in an eroded area on the cervix. To palpation the edge is hard and unyielding. The base of the ulcer is usually granular and bleeds easily from the slightest trauma. There is, however, a moderate degree of invasion. In some there seems to be more fibrous tissue than tumor.

For the most part, however, the excavating ulcerating type of tumor has a higher lethal potential than the exfoliating type, for the reasons previously mentioned. This is particularly true of the endocervical cancers that often infiltrate and destroy the deep cervical musculature, leaving only a shell of normal cervix, without giving any external manifestation of their presence. This is the type of cervical cancer that creates the "barrel-shaped" cervix.

As the ulcerating type of growth persists the entire cervix becomes implicated, whether the point of origin was external or within the canal. The ulcerating lesion with the firm, hard nodular edges and the moth-eaten base progresses to the point at which the anatomic landmarks vanish, to be replaced by a conical cloaca covered with sloughing, friable carcinomatous tissue in the area formerly occupied by the cervix. By this time the paracervical and paravaginal tissues are invaded (Fig. 61–4).

Occasionally there may be an extensive undermining of the cervical epithelium with little in the way of ulceration. Such a tumor is particularly dangerous, for the only indication of its presence may be cervical enlargement. The cervix feels firm and nodular, and the surgeon may be trapped into believing that he is dealing with a simple, benign cervical hypertrophy and proceed to treat it accordingly. The error is discovered only after the tissues have been examined pathologically.

Any ulcerating lesion of the cervix should be biopsied. If (1) the surrounding epithelium is dull red, (2) the undermining edges of the ulcer are firm and resistant to touch, and (3) the granulating base bleeds readily, there is an excellent chance that the lesion is cancer and not erosion.

Microscopic Pathology

The average case of cancer of the cervix presents no particular problem in pathologic diagnosis. The main problem is the case on the borderline between benign and malignant growth. The orderly arrangement of the normal cervical epithelium is so definite that important alterations can often be seen by low-power inspection. This is particularly true when specimens are taken from the advancing margin of the growth. The normal stratified cervical epithelium consists of three layers: (1) a superficial layer composed of partly flattened cornified cells with well marked cell outlines and pyknotic nuclei; (2) an intermediate precornified layer that contains smaller cells with less cytoplasm and larger nuclei; (3) a basal layer consisting of a single or double layer of small, deeply staining cells arranged at right angles to the surface layer. The hairline basement membrane sharply divides the epithelium from the underlying stroma.

Criteria of Malignancy

The two criteria necessary for the diagnosis of carcinoma in the cervical epithelium are (1) anaplastic atypicality of the epithelial cells and (2) evidence of invasion. As in carcinoma in situ, variations in the size, shape and staining qualities of the cells must be present. More important is the irregular increase in size and nucleoprotein content of the nuclei. Hyperchromatism is evident, since the nuclei stain more intensely. Mitoses may be few or abundant; some are normal, others perhaps atypical (Fig. 61–8).

In most instances epidermoid carcinoma arises from the deeper layers of the

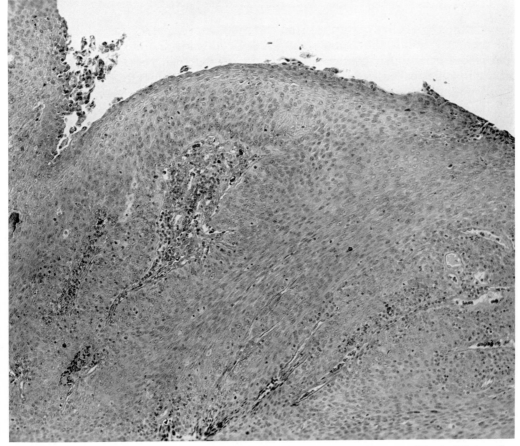

Fig. 61-8. Epidermoid carcinoma of a moderate grade of malignancy (Grade II) invading downward from the surface. Malignant tumor cells are desquamating from the surface at the upper left. In the body of the carcinoma there is keratinization of some individual cells; reasonably abundant mitotic figures and rare tumor giant cells are present.

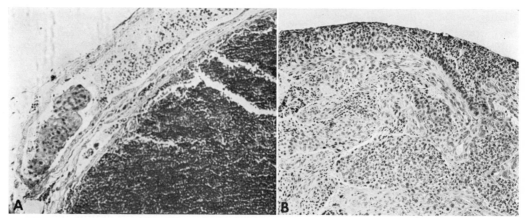

Fig. 61-9.   *A,* Lymphatic invasion by carcinoma of the cervix, even in small tumors, may result in tumor embolism to regional lymph nodes, with resulting metastasis. *B,* Spray pattern of epidermoid carcinoma of the cervix. The surface epithelium overlying the carcinoma is anaplastic, but with superficial differentiation.

epithelium. Occasionally it arises from the more superficial strata as a more highly differentiated tumor that shows less cytologic departure from the normal. Such epidermoid carcinomas contain small groups of flattened cells arranged in a concentric manner, called *epithelial pearls*. Pearls are less often found in the wilder, more undifferentiated tumors that may arise from the deeper layers.

To be clinically malignant a tumor must have evidence of invasion to accompany the anaplastic cellular changes. In carcinoma in situ of the cervix we noted that anaplastic cell changes were present, but that the basement membrane was intact. When this layer is broken, buds and columns of carcinoma cells push into the stroma like the growing roots of a plant. If these columns of cells with their varying sizes and shapes are sectioned transversely, they may appear as separate masses or nests of malignant cells bordered by a well defined fibromuscular stroma far below the surface. They may also be seen invading lymphatics of the cervix (Fig. 61–9, *A*). Nature's response to invasion of the stroma is an inflammatory reaction consisting of lymphocytes and sometimes polymorphonuclear leukocytes. The leukocytes are not usually evident in benign lesions that simulate invasive cancer. The more advanced the growth at times the greater the degree of lymphocytic infiltration into the loosened fibromuscular stroma.

"Spray Carcinoma"

Small, focal epidermoid carcinomas were described by Schiller that microscopically were seen to have arisen from the deeper epithelial layers of the cervix. These carcinomas had not invaded up to the surface of the cervical epithelium or laterally among the epithelial cells, but had "sprayed" downward locally into the stroma (Fig. 61–9, *B*). No associated carcinoma in situ was found. Schiller called this a "spray carcinoma."

It is important for two reasons: (1) as an indication that not all cervical cancers necessarily pass through a stage of carcinoma in situ; and (2) negative vaginal smears would accompany this type of invasive cancer, since it had not reached the epithelial surface anywhere.

Histologic Types

There are two main histologic types of cancer arising in the cervix. Carcinoma may arise from the stratified squamous epithelium covering the vaginal portion of the cervix or from the cylindrical, gland-forming epithelium of the endocervix. *Squamous, squamous cell* or *epidermoid carcinoma* is the type found in 95 per cent of cervical carcinomas, and adenocarcinoma accounts for the remainder. Novak observed that there have been a number of reports of adenocarcinoma appearing in young children, one being recorded in a seven-month infant, while epidermoid carcinoma has not been seen below the age of twelve years.

Adenocarcinoma of the Cervix

Adenocarcinoma arises either from the columnar epithelium lining the endocervical canal or from the gland tubules. Normally the cervical glands have a uniform appearance, lined by mucinous secretory goblet cells and evenly distributed through the stroma. In addition to anaplastic atypicality of the cells and stromal invasion, adenocarcinoma of the cervix is characterized by an increase in the number of glands found. Tubular or solid projections from the lumens of the endocervical glands are found invading the stroma.

Most adenocarcinomas of the cervix are well differentiated and secrete mucus into the gland lumens. The glands are irregular in size, shape and relation to each other. Some glands form back-to-back without any intervening stroma (Fig. 61–10). The individual cells are irregularly crowded and palisaded, with heavily stained nuclei. Usually invasion is by contiguity, and tumor cells do not break loose indi-

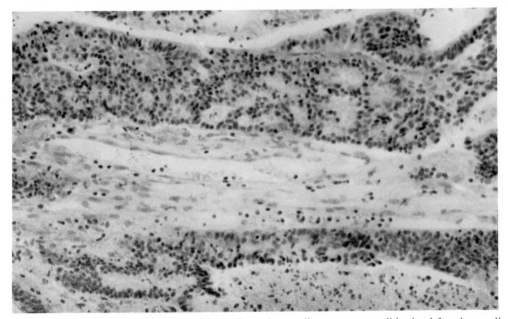

Fig. 61-10.   Adenocarcinoma of the endocervix usually grows as a solid, gland-forming malignant tumor, either with or without mucus secretion. The glands are back to back, but otherwise fairly well formed.

vidually. The over-all picture is often not unlike that seen in adenocarcinoma of the large intestine.

Relative Degree of Malignancy in Relation to Histologic Grading

In the past, treatment was outlined and prognosis evaluated on the basis of the histologic grade of the tumor. Today emphasis is placed on the extent of the disease rather than its histology. Confusion exists between the grade of the tumor, which depends on the individual cell characteristics, and the stage of the disease, which is simply a clinical estimate of the total amount of cancer present. The stage of disease far outweighs pathologic grading as the main factor in estimating prognosis in carcinoma of the cervix.

MARTZLOFF CLASSIFICATION.   There are three classifications in common usage by which attempts are made to evaluate the degree of malignancy on the basis of the histologic characteristics of the epidermoid carcinoma cells. Martzloff grades the tumor, depending upon the degree of cellular differentiation, into three groups—spinal cell, transitional cell and spindle cell. Supposedly the more differentiated the cell is, the less the degree of malignancy, and the more immature the cell is, the greater its growth activity and the wilder the cancer biologically.

A lower degree of anaplasia can be expected from the more highly differentiated spinal (prickle) cells that arise in the keratinized layer of the cervical epithelium in approximately 15 per cent of cancer cases. The cells are mature with large nuclei and abundant cytoplasm that takes a pale orange-red eosin stain. The cells are large and polyhedral. Epithelial pearl formation is often present.

The majority of carcinomas, approximately two thirds of the entire group, come from the transitional cell layer. Here the cells are rounded, contain small amounts of cytoplasm and have nuclei that stain deep purple with hematoxylin. They appear to arise from the precornified middle layers of the stratified squamous epithelium, but have little to suggest a squamous origin. Novak calls the transitional cell type a "sort of dumping ground" where the cells are neither spinal cell nor spindle cell.

The spindle cell type seems to come from the basal cell layer. Like the spinal cell, they appear far less frequently than the transitional cell tumors, roughly in 15 per cent of cervical cancers. The cells are small and spindle-shaped with deeply staining nuclei, not too unlike cells seen in certain sarcomas.

In the past the spinal cell tumors gave the best prognosis for surgical treatment, since they were the least malignant and the most likely to remain as localized tumors. Moreover, they did not appear to be as sensitive to radiation as the more immature transitional or spindle cell tumors. Recently, however, Day and Glucksmann noted that radiation sensitivity did not necessarily add up to a cure. Though the immediate response to radiation was satisfactory, many of the cells demonstrated persistent mitotic activity which later blossomed out as recurrences.

BRODERS CLASSIFICATION.   The classification devised by Broders of the Mayo Clinic uses four numerical grades (I, II, III and IV) for both epidermoid carcinoma and adenocarcinoma of the cervix. It is the classification most commonly used in this country. The basis for the classification is the well known observation that the degree of malignancy keeps pace with the degree of cell differentiation. The more highly differentiated carcinomas are classed as grade I, and relatively more immature, undifferentiated and anaplastic cells appear in grade II. It is the extent of cellular differentiation that determines the grade into which each tumor falls. For example, grade II will have between 25 and 50 per cent embryonic-type cells, and 50 to 70 per cent of cells in grade III tumors are undifferentiated.

The histologic classification, based as it is on biopsy specimens, has obvious limitations. Specimens taken from an area remote from the initial biopsy may vary in grade. The high preponderance of cases falls in the transitional cell group of Martzloff or the grade II grouping of Broders. Because of this, clinical staging of the extent of the disease has superseded grading as the crucial factor in determining prognosis and as a guide to treatment.

The original Broders grading method was cumbersome to apply, since as many as thirteen different cytologic characteristics had to be observed and evaluated. Most pathologists now use a simplified version.

In the northeastern area of the United States, influenced by teachings of Ewing, only three grades are used in some institutions. Actually, in reporting 5-year results, on over 2000 cases, one paper from the Mayo Clinic showed a difference in cure rate of epidermoid carcinoma grade III less than 2 per cent better than for grade IV. In the Ewing-inspired three grades, Broders grades III and IV are combined and called grade III.

A simple scheme for estimating the grade of an epidermoid carcinoma is as follows:

	GRADE		
	I	II	III
Epithelial pearls	Present	Absent	Absent
Individual keratinized cells	Many	Few	Rare
Intercellular bridges	Present	Absent	Absent
Tumor giant cells	Absent	Absent	Present
Mitoses per high-power field	Below 2	2 to 4	Over 4

Pathologists differ in the weight they assign to each of these factors. Counting mitoses is the easiest reproducible criterion, but these vary in number in different parts of a tumor. One axiom in use is that a neoplasm is named from its most differentiated portion and graded from its least differentiated parts.

There is so much subjective variation in grading cancers that it is doubtful whether any therapy should either be given or withheld on the basis of this type of grading information.

WENTZ AND REAGAN CLASSIFICATION. This is based on cytologic characteristics of epidermoid carcinoma cells in Papanicolaou smears, which are then applied to growth patterns as seen in biopsy and hysterectomy specimens. There are three groups: (1) *Keratinizing carcinoma,* with large pleomorphic cells, pearl formation and individual cellular keratinization. (2) *Large-cell nonkeratinizing carcinoma,* with large nucei, basophilic staining of cancer cells and a higher mitotic index. (3) *Small-cell carcinoma,* composed of uniform small basophilic cells, with the highest mitotic index of any of the three groups. The 5-year survivals for the three groups were 48, 79 and 20 per cent respectively.

How Does Cancer of the Cervix Spread?

Cancer of the cervix spreads from the primary site within the cervix in a number of different ways. It may extend (*a*) by direct infiltration of the adjacent supporting tissues, (*b*) by permeation along lymphatic channels, (*c*) by following the tissue planes

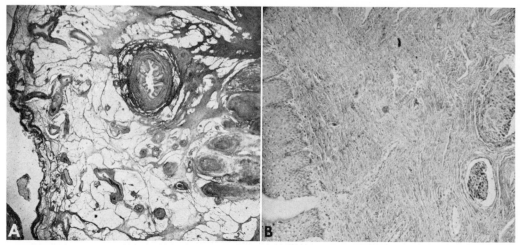

Fig. 61-11. *A,* Portion of a giant histologic section. Several distinct nests of carcinoma cells extend from the right-hand margin of the field and are invading the periureteral fibrous tissue. The ureter is present just above the center of the illustration. and carcinoma of the cervix typically spreads to involve it close to the bladder wall. *B,* Cervical carcinomatous emboli shown within lymphatics beneath the uninvolved vaginal epithelium, as a part of the spread of cancer downward in the pelvis.

of least resistance along parasympathetic nerves or blood vessels, (*d*) by lymphatic embolization directly to regional lymph nodes, or (*e*) by blood vessel invasion.

LYMPHATIC SPREAD. In the review of tissue sections of the local tumor the pathologist frequently observes cancer cells in lymphatic channels either within the tumor or in the connective tissue immediately adjacent to it. This is a microscopic discovery and will not be evident clinically. The overlying cervical or vaginal epithelium may be completely normal. Local invasion of the lymphatics is often seen in the earliest forms of invasive cancer.

Once the carcinoma has spread beyond the cervix, either by direct invasion of the paracervical tissues or by involvement of the neighboring vaginal epithelium as cancer cells enter the supporting tissue, they either propagate and form bulky local tumors or are picked up in the abundant network of deeper lymphatics common to this area. Many early, as well as advanced, cases will show lymphatic infiltration in the tissue adjacent to the primary tumor in the cervix.

WHAT HAPPENS WHEN THE CANCER REMAINS AS LOCAL TUMOR? If the carcinoma proliferates and grows locally, it tends to spread out laterally, but it also extends in a fore and aft direction to implicate the bladder or rectum, or both (Fig. 61–11, *A*). The bladder is reasonably well protected by the firm fascial envelope that surrounds it, so that the wall becomes infiltrated only when extensive growth is present. The chances of early bladder invasion increase when the carcinoma arises within the endocervical canal. The examiner may suspect bladder invasion when bullous edema of the bladder mucosa is seen by cystoscopy, even though there may be no actual evidence of tumor. Bullous edema in the absence of any past history of kidney infection and in the presence of proved cervical carcinoma is a fair indication that cancer is present in the bladder wall lymphatics. The posterior spread takes place along the uterosacral ligaments.

In addition to the anteroposterior extension of cervical cancer, the tumor also has a pronounced tendency to grow out laterally. It may do this on one or both sides and to different degrees. If it extends far enough out, the ureter may become occluded to such an extent that the patient has a hydroureter or hydronephrosis. Uremia is the most common cause of death from cancer of the cervix. As the disease becomes more advanced the growth may fix to the side wall of the pelvis.

WHAT HAPPENS WHEN TUMOR CELLS ENTER THE LYMPHATIC PATHWAYS? Permeation of cancer cells along lymphatic channels to reach remote areas in the vaginal canal and the regional lymph nodes in the pelvis is usually accepted as the most common method of spread of cervical cancer. It is interesting, however, that it is a difficult matter to discover tumor cells in transit on a histologic review of tumor sections. We know that tumor reaches the regional nodes, and it probably gets there through lymphatic pathways, but it is not always possible to prove this. Lymphatic extension may also occur in the deep tissue beneath a normal-appearing vaginal epithelium at a point distant from the primary focus in the cervix. This may explain some local recurrences of tumor noted after adequate therapy (Fig. 61–11, *B*).

What Lymph Nodes Are Involved? Once the nodes are involved, the tumor takes on a new growth pattern. The pattern of extension is fairly consistent. The nodes most often involved lie (*a*) in the chain beneath and lateral to the external iliac veins; (*b*) in the obturator spaces each bounded by the obturator nerve below, the side wall of the pelvis laterally and the external iliac vein above; (*c*) along the internal iliac or hypogastric arteries, particularly at the point of junction with the external iliac arteries; (*d*) in the sacral areas at the promontory and just medial to each common iliac artery and vein.

The cancer may lie dormant in these nodal areas, or may pass on through afferent lymphatic channels to the secondary chain of lymph nodes that lie lateral to the internal iliac arteries, vena cava and aorta. Further spread may take place to the mediastinal lymph nodes and is recognizable by x-ray, and to the left supraclavicular area, where it may be palpated.

There is no absolute rule about lymphatic spread of cervical carcinoma. Clinically, many variables appear in the usual pattern. Cervical cancer does, however, tend to remain localized to the pelvis. Metastases to liver, lung and bone occur, but far less often than one would normally expect from experience with cancer in other organs and sites.

How Often Are the Lymph Nodes Involved? One of the most striking things about cancer of the cervix is its tendency to remain localized to the cervix and the immediately adjacent paracervical and paravaginal tissues. Since the nodal areas cannot be palpated with accuracy, the true incidence of nodal involvement can only be surmised. For example, if radiation is chosen as the sole form of therapy, the extent of metastases to the regional lymph nodal area cannot be determined unless lymphadenectomy is done as a preliminary step. The information we do have comes from surgical experience. Since the Wertheim type of hysterectomy, combined with bilateral pelvic lymphadenectomy, is offered only to stage I and II cases, the data are again restricted. For the more advanced cases in stages III and IV the spread of cervical cancer to nodes can only be evaluated from the retroperitoneal or transabdominal lymphadenectomy performed before irradiation, or the exenteration procedures carried out as definitive therapy. The number of cases in these two categories is limited.

From the combined experience, however, it is obvious that nodal involvement occurs far less often than one would suppose. A sizable number of cases have been done for stages I and II, with a few cases in stage III. The incidence of positive lymph nodes ranges from 16 to 19 per cent. Broken down into stages, which reflect the clinical estimate of the amount of disease, a patient with stage I (cancer confined to the cervix) will demonstrate metastases to nodes in about 15 per cent. Approximately 25 per cent will have positive regional nodes in stage II.

It would be reasonable to expect that the incidence of regional metastatic disease would increase sharply as more intrapelvic malignant disease is encountered, but this is not the case. When exenteration procedures, which remove the entire soft-tissue contents of the pelvis, including the bladder and rectum, have been done as the sole definitive therapy for carcinomas too far advanced to hope that the Wertheim operation will be adequate (stages III and IV), the percentage of positive nodes recovered ranges between 25 and 30 per cent. Moreover, when exenteration operations are performed as the last recourse after irradiation failure, nodes are positive in only 42 per cent.

It is obvious, then, that the life history of carcinoma of the cervix differs from that of many other forms of cancer within the body. Cancer of the cervix is less likely to become a generalized disease, and it prefers to remain local. Autopsy studies on patients who died with their cervical cancer untreated indicate that 60 per cent succumb with the cancer confined to the pelvis. They died of uremia or hemorrhage through encroachment of the disease upon ureters and blood vessels. Although they do demonstrate distant spread to lung, liver, bone, mediastinal and supraclavicular nodes and do have metastases to regional lymph nodes, they have these less often than expected. There are several reasons why this may be true, the chief one being the tendency of cervical carcinoma to spread along tissue spaces.

SPREAD IN TISSUE SPACES.   The fact that cancer of the cervix tends to remain localized even in the face of extensive disease lends support to the more extended radical surgery designed to encompass it. It is interesting to speculate why cancer of the cervix often produces large masses of tumor in the tissues adjacent to its original site, but shows little in the way of nodal extension. In the past the explanation offered was that cancer cells in lymphatic channels were trapped in a protective fibrous barrier set up to restrict an invader. In more recent studies made on giant sections that include all the material removed by either the Wertheim or exenteration operations (discussed in detail later) another pattern of growth appears (see frontispiece). It would seem that cancer of the cervix, after it has left the primary site, may grow along tissue spaces following parasympathetic nerves rather than actually lying in lymphatic channels (Fig. 61–12, A). Serial sections allow the pathologist to trace the tumor back along the nerves to ganglion cells. The small lymph nodes found around the parasympathetic ganglia are often not involved in cancer, but accumulations of lymphocytes without the complete structure of nodes are frequently invaded. Further studies are in progress, but the work to date suggests a possible explanation of why cancer of the cervix is fundamentally a local disease. If this is so, there should be a reasonable chance of cure, provided the initial therapy is adequate. The same observations are now being collected for cancers of the breast and the prostate.

EMBOLIC SPREAD.   It is also evident on clinical grounds that permeation along lymphatic pathways is not the only method of spread. In general we expect to find fewer metastases to lymph nodes in early cases of cervical cancer. The statement is often made that a lesion less than 1 cm. in size will never show metastasis. Twenty per cent of carcinomas, however, that have disease confined to the cervix show cancer in the regional nodes without clinical or pathologic evidence of malignancy in the intervening tissue. The presence of cancer in the regional nodes of these patients suggests the possibility of an embolic spread.

It is a rare finding to note cancer cells in the lymphatics that intervene between primary tumor and regional node. Not infrequently tumor cells can be seen in afferent vessels at the periphery of a lymph node and can be traced into the node itself. One may infer that the cancer got there because of embolization from the primary tumor.

BLOOD VESSEL SPREAD.   In a further attempt to explain (*a*) why extensive carcinoma fails to metastasize to lymph nodes, and (*b*) why some patients with a relatively small tumor have recurrences locally or in distant regions despite adequate therapy, the giant tissue sections have been extended to include a study of possible blood vessel invasion. In the past, observations on blood vessel involvement were mostly made with hematoxylin and eosin stains. Special Verhoeff elastic tissue stains are necessary to bring out the details of blood vessel walls. Tumor that seems to be lying in the paracervical tissue, presumably in lymphatic spaces, can often be shown to be within a blood vessel when these stains are used (Fig. 61–12, *B*). We formerly believed that blood vessel invasion was a late manifestation of cancer spread which accounted for the metastases found in distant organs. Twenty-five per cent of terminal cases will show cervical carcinoma in liver, lung and occasionally spleen. This may occur without involvement of the regional lymph nodes, and there is increasing evidence that such spread may occur early as well as late.

SUMMARY.   Unlike carcinoma in other regions of the body, the life history of carcinoma of the cervix seems to suggest that the cancer is often confined to the pelvis,

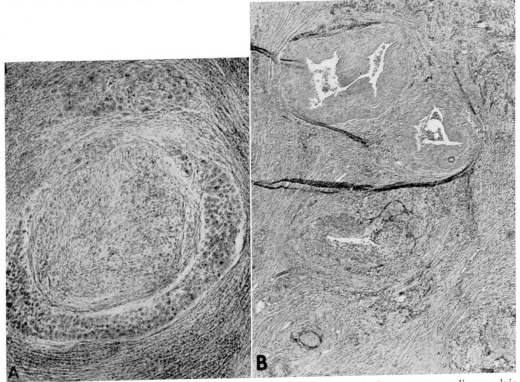

Fig. 61-12.   *A*, Field from a giant histologic section, to show cervical cancer surrounding a pelvic parasympathetic nerve. This may involve extension along tissue spaces rather than lymphatics. *B*, Just below the transverse artefactual wrinkle in the giant section is a vessel lined by cervical carcinoma. With the Verhoeff elastic tissue stain this was shown to be a vein, with blood vessel invasion by cancer. Cytologic detail in the giant celloidin sections is not present to the extent expected in paraffin sections.

since 40 per cent of patients dying of the disease show no cancer extension beyond. This fact provides encouragement for the success of adequate therapy.

How Much Carcinomatous Disease Does the Patient Have?

From the preceding discussion it is evident that the growth of cancer of the cervix produces a minimal number of symptoms so trivial that the patient fails to be impressed by their significance. They should not so deceive the physician that he prescribes for the symptoms without a thorough investigation. There can be no further delay in diagnosis, because the symptoms that finally induced the patient to consult her physician may already be late manifestations of the disease. It is the obligation of the physician to pay attention to the symptoms and to examine the patient, despite any reluctance on her part. Only in this manner can we increase the number of early diagnoses.

The appearance of preclinical carcinoma of the cervix has been reviewed. We are now primarily interested in how much cancer the patient has, not whether there is malignant disease present. The clinical estimate of the extent of the cancer determines the type of therapy and is the most important single factor in estimating prognosis. Estimation is done with the examining finger, with limited help from x-ray and cystoscopy.

The most important point to establish in evaluating the extent of the carcinoma is the mobility of the cervix and uterus. If the cancer is confined to the cervix, it may move freely, but any degree of fixation is suggestive evidence that cancer has extended beyond its confines into the surrounding tissue. Whether this has occurred is determined by a one-finger vaginal examination, followed by a digital exploration of the rectum. Rectal examination produces the greatest amount of information. The examiner should first feel the back of the cervix to determine how easily the uterus can be moved. When the uterus is fixed, the uterocervical segment should next be felt. Normally this narrows as the finger moves down from the fundus to the cervix. If it feels broad, this is the point where cancer most often extends into the paracervical tissues. A layer of induration palpated anteriorly in the upper vaginal wall may indicate bladder wall involvement. This should be checked by cystoscopy. Thickening of the uterosacral ligaments extending laterally and posteriorly is evidence of spread in these directions. The base of the broad ligaments is then felt. Unilateral or bilateral fixation may be due to disease. It is important to know whether the induration reaches to the side wall of the pelvis. If there is no sulcus or palpable edge to the lateral induration, the carcinomatous disease is probably fixed to the side wall.

One of the most difficult factors to evaluate accurately in determining the extent of the carcinoma is the firm induration that is a part of the picture of lateral extension. It may be cancerous infiltration or a fibrous barrier set up in response either to inflammatory breakdown in the primary tumor or as nature's response to a lethal invader. In either case the ureters may become occluded. Since the treatment and prognosis of cancer are directly dependent on the extent of disease, it is important to distinguish protective induration from malignant infiltration. To select proper therapy we must have some idea of how much disease actually exists.

Based on the evaluation of the extent of disease, an International Classification has been set up by the League of Nations. This is useful in comparing statistical reports of the results of different types of therapy for cervical carcinoma from the world's clinics. It is also useful as a guide to therapy.

INTERNATIONAL CLASSIFICATION OF CANCER OF THE CERVIX BY STAGES ON THE BASIS OF THE ANATOMIC EXTENT OF GROWTH (CLINICAL ESTIMATE).

Stage 0:   Carcinoma in situ. This is also known as intraepithelial or preinvasive or noninvasive cancer.

Stage I: The carcinoma is strictly limited to the cervix. It may arise from one or both lips and be either exophytic or ulcerative.

Stage II: The carcinoma has extended beyond the cervix.
   (a) To involve a small portion or all of the upper part of the vagina, but not the lower third.
   (b) To infiltrate the entire broad ligament on one or both sides, but not involve the side wall of the pelvis. The ureters may be occluded and the patient dying of disease and still be in stage II.
   (c) Into the endometrial cavity from a primary focus in the endocervix.

Stage III: (1) The disease has now invaded the side wall of the pelvis.
   (a) This may be by direct cancerous infiltration on one or both sides. No free space can be felt between the tumor and the pelvic wall.
   (b) The side wall may also be invaded by isolated pelvic metastases from a small growth in the cervix itself. This suggests embolic spread.
   (2) The carcinoma involves the lower third of the vagina.

Stage IV: The disease has now invaded adjacent viscera or has spread beyond the pelvis to distant organs or nodes. Carcinoma involves the bladder by direct extension. Vesicovaginal fistulas may be present.
   The spread may be posterior through the vaginal fornix or rectovaginal septum to involve the rectum.
   Rectovaginal fistulas may appear (Fig. 61-13).

This classification is useful, but it is only as good as the examination. The actual amount of disease is difficult to determine. The fixation may be due to pelvic inflammatory disease or endometriosis as well as elements of sepsis within a tumor, as previously mentioned. Independent of these elements, it is impossible to tell clinically whether the regional lymph nodes are involved or not. Therapy is based on the clinical appraisal of the extent of the disease. A stage I cancer may have metastases to lymph nodes impossible to detect before treatment. This case is really in stage III, but for comparison it must be regarded as stage I. The classification is also subject to human error in interpretation.

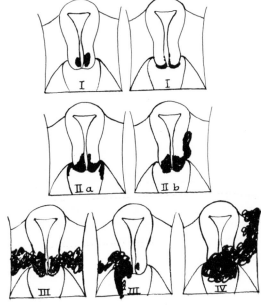

Fig. 61-13.   Diagrams to show examples of cancer of the cervix in stages I, IIa and IIb, III and IV. Sometimes these drawings are useful parts of the patient's clinical chart to help determine the best therapy.

SURGICAL-PATHOLOGIC CLASSIFICATION OF MEIGS AND BRUNSCHWIG. To circumvent the obvious deficiencies in the clinical classification and to provide a better correlation between the actual extent of disease and the type of therapy to be chosen for any given patient, Meigs and Brunschwig have devised a pathologic classification based on the amount of cervical cancer present in the operative specimen. By using this surgical-pathologic type of classification it is possible (a) to provide a better idea of the eventual prognosis, and (b) to compare the results of surgical therapy on a more realistic basis.

Class O: Carcinoma in situ. The disease is confined to the epithelium, and there is no histologic evidence of invasion. A variety of names are used which are synonymous with carcinoma in situ, such as intraepithelial carcinoma, preinvasive carcinoma and occasionally microcarcinoma.

Class A: The carcinoma is confined to the cervix. The tumor may be exophytic or ulcerative and involve one or both lips, but the cancer is still restricted to the cervix itself.

Class A₀: After a positive biopsy of infiltrating carcinoma no tumor is found in the cervix upon examination of the surgical specimen. These cases will be present in all irradiation series, but many surgeons exclude them in order that a true estimate be obtained of the results of surgery.

Class B: The cancer has spread from the cervix to involve the upper part of the vagina (the lower third is excluded) or the endometrial cavity, or both. The spread may be either direct or by permeation along lymphatic channels.

Class C: The carcinoma has now involved the entire thickness of the muscular walls of the cervix and extended into the paracervical and/or paravaginal tissues, as well as to any small lymph nodes that may be located in this region. There may be either direct or lymphatic spread to the tissues in the lower part of the vagina.

Class D: Cervical cancer has now spread beyond the immediately adjacent paracervical and paravaginal regions to involve the tube and ovary, as well as the regional lymphatics located along the iliac vessels or in the obturator areas.

Class E: Anterior-posterior spread has now taken place, and the serosa, musculature or mucosa of the bladder and rectum are now involved.

Class F: The carcinoma has involved the pelvic wall. The extension may be to fascia, muscle, bone or the sacral nerve plexus.

To facilitate further the comparison of methods of therapy the following additional prefixes precede the alphabetical classification: (1) If the patient has had preliminary radiation followed by surgery, the prefix "PR" appears. (2) "R" is used when the patient is operated upon after irradiation failure. (3) "S" is used when further surgery is done after the initial attempts to cure by operation have failed. (4) "RS" is added when both preliminary irradiation and surgery have been ineffective and more extensive surgery is indicated.

The classification has merit, and it is relatively simple so long as surgery has been both adequate and the sole definitive form of therapy. It becomes a little cumbersome when previous irradiation or surgery has been used for one reason or another.

TREATMENT OF INVASIVE CANCER OF THE CERVIX

The choice of treatment and the prognosis after therapy are directly dependent upon the extent of the cervical carcinoma. Other factors that influence the selection of therapy are the patient's age, general condition and associated diseases. The growth pattern, grade and the biological nature of the cancer also have a bearing on prognosis. By far the most important element, however, is the extent of the malignant disease. In selecting therapy for the patient with cancer confined to the cervix and/or the immediately adjacent vaginal and paracervical tissues, one may elect to treat with either surgery or radiation. In making this choice one must assume that the radiologist and the surgeon are equally competent in their respective fields and have both the equipment and the knowledge to carry out ideal cancer therapy. Approximately 33 per cent of cervical cancer cases have sufficiently localized disease to permit a choice. The remainder have too much disease to hope that surgery will encompass the entire malignant process and had best be treated by irradiation.

Why Do We Not Cure More Patients by Radiation or Surgery?

There are many factors concerned with the favorable response of the patient with cervical carcinoma to therapy, whether it be radiation or surgery. Although the histologic characteristics of the tumor and the extent of its spread have much to do with prognosis, it is obvious in any large experience that other elements are present, among them host resistance, which are equally important. All therapists are disappointed when the patient who has a relatively small amount of cancer of the cervix fails to respond to therapy and are equally surprised by the patient who has a bulky tumor and survives. Some patients will be cured, despite inadequate surgical excision or radiation given in insufficient quantity or of obsolescent type.

We should continue to offer the patient the best in therapy and individualize, as far as we know how, in the kind of treatment we give, but we must recognize that in a certain number failure in cancer therapy seems to be foreordained. Certain carcinomas appear to grow like a fungus and can be destroyed, provided the therapy is sufficiently powerful, but others seem to be part of the individual and cannot be eradicated by any means yet available without destroying the patient at the same time. It is interesting to speculate on why this is so, and to consider the methods now in use which are designed to sift out the patient who is curable from the one who is not.

What Are the Methods Used to Select the Proper Patient for the Proper Type of Therapy?

Before we can attribute the cause of therapeutic failure to the method used we must be sure that the treatment given was adequate for the amount of cancer the patient had. We have previously noted that there is a 30 per cent error in the clinical estimation of the extent of disease, as well as the fact that it may be present in (*a*) areas inaccessible to palpation, or (*b*) in embolic form, where it cannot be felt in regions that can be readily approached. It is unrealistic if the initial therapy has been inadequate to trace the cause of failure to (1) lack of radiation sensitivity, (2) acquired radiation resistance, (3) biological nature of tumor growth, (4) host resistance or (5) immunologic variables. With the fact of adequate therapy established, methods now being used in a variety of clinics are of the utmost importance to assess the nature of cancer growth and to provide guidance in the selection of therapy. This is a necessity if prognosis of therapy for this localized form of cancer is to improve.

Since the fundamental treatment for the majority of cases of cancer of the cervix, as we now know it, seems to be irradiation, the principal problems seem to revolve around radiation sensitivity and radiation resistance. If certain tumors are primarily resistant to radiation and it is possible to establish this as a fact, it would be foolish to persist in a form of therapy that was doomed to fail. These patients had best be offered surgery. A yardstick is badly needed to help in selecting the proper therapy for the proper patient.

What Methods Are Used to Measure Radiation Sensitivity and Resistance?

In any intensive study of the problems concerned with radiation sensitivity it soon becomes obvious that the response to ionizing radiation varies widely, even in the same patient. There appears to be a difference in sensitivity, for example, in various parts of the same tumor, the periphery being more amenable to treatment than the central portion. Moreover, epidermoid carcinoma of the cervix, metastatic to a regional lymph node, appears to be harder to cure than cancer at the primary site. One may postulate that the tumor takes on a different pattern after it has left the primary site. The difference may well be due to the nature of the more normal tissue that surrounds the tumor, in other words, the tumor bed or stroma. The radiologist counts on the preservation of this supporting tissue both in planning to achieve recovery and in palliative tumor control. By balancing the effect of radiation on the tumor as well as on the tissue bed the therapist has had far more success, in recent years, in treating cases that previously had been regarded as radiation-resistant. It is well known that some cancer foci within the field of ionizing radiation are destroyed by less than the usual amount, while others may require more. The main factor that appears decisive in tumor control is more the ability of the supporting tissue to restrict the rate and dispersion of cancer growth than the effect of irradiation on the tumor cells.

The term "radioresistant" is used loosely to apply to such tumors as adenocarcinoma that are believed generally to respond less readily and in a more unpredictable fashion to radiation than do epidermo d cancers. In individual instances, however, the glandular tumors may do as well as if not better than the squamous carcinomas. We know, for example, that a cancer of the endometrium can be destroyed by radiation. We prefer to operate on such patients, not because the tumor is resistant to radiation, but largely because the uterus is in an accessible location. Actually, the only true way of knowing how an individual tumor will respond is to give a trial dose of radiation. A variety of laboratory procedures are available to measure the radiation effect.

THE HISTOLOGIC APPROACH.   When the pathologist attempts to pinpoint a parallel relation between the degree of histologic differentiation and radiation sensitivity or resistance without exposing the patient to prior x-radiation, it becomes obvious that the terms "sensitivity" and "resistance" are purely relative. For example, a proliferative protrusive type of growth will have the same histologic architecture as the ulcerating infiltrating tumor that has an entirely different tumor bed. The latter has far more prognostic significance than the morphologic picture (Table 8).

Table 8.   Five-Year Survival Rate of 259 Patients with Anaplastic Tumors for Comparison with That of 87 Patients with Differentiated Tumors

CLINICAL STAGE	ANAPLASTIC CARCINOMA		DIFFERENTIATED, SQUAMOUS CARCINOMA	
	NO. CASES	5-YEAR SURVIVORS %	NO. CASES	5-YEAR SURVIVORS %
I	15	6	40	15	7	46
II	48	11	23	27	9	33
III	107	18	16	32	11	34
IV	89	5	5	13	1	7

For many years investigators have attempted to forecast cancer prognosis from therapy by histologic study of the actual tumor cell and its response to radiation. They looked for evidence of postirradiation nuclear and cytoplasmic changes, together with the amount of swelling or vacuolation in both cell and nuclei. Although this approach reflected prognosis to a degree, it was soon evident that radiation sensitivity was as much concerned with the response of the normal cells and supporting stroma as it was with the tumor cell itself.

Subsequently Glucksmann took a series of tumor biopsies from the growing edge of the carcinoma weekly during the course of radium treatment. A favorable response to radiation could be expected when the tumor cells showed (*a*) an increase in the number of cancer cells that showed differentiation, and (*b*) a disappearance of mitoses and more resting cells (Table 9). These observations have cast doubt on the generally accepted theory that the more highly anaplastic cells are the most radiosensitive. They add support to the contention that radiosensitivity and radiocurability do not necessarily go hand in hand. The chief disadvantage in this approach lies in the fact that repeated biopsies tend to negate the effect of radiation, for the treated tumor is believed not to heal as well.

Table 9. Correlation between the Histologic Prognosis and Response to a Trial Dose of Radiation with End-Results of Full Radiation Therapy in 1039 Cases of Cancer of the Cervix

CLINICAL STAGE	FAVORABLE PROGNOSIS		UNFAVORABLE PROGNOSIS		TOTAL	
	NO. CASES	% CORRECT	NO. CASES	% CORRECT	NO. CASES	% CORRECT
I.............	83	80	96	80	179	80
II.............	124	68	396	87	520	82
III.............	29	76	256	88	285	87
IV.............	2	100	53	84	55	94
Total..........	238	73	801	87	1039	84

From the Strangeways Research Laboratory Report 1954 by Courtesy of Dr. A. Glucksmann. Quoted in Recent Advances in Obstetrics & Gynecology, by Bourne and Williams. 9th Ed. Little Brown & Co., Boston, 1958, p. 298.

THE CYTOCHEMICAL TEST. Gusberg and other investigators have studied and have expressed interest in the concentration of nucleoproteins in the irradiated cell. It has been shown that cancer cells dying in the course of radiation treatment alter their nucleic acid composition before any change can be noted in the histologic pattern.

Two types of cells are noted. The so-called A cell is frequently noted in the proximity of blood vessels near the growing edge of the tumor. These cells are extremely viable and are aggressive in their growth pattern. Chemically, the heavy chromatin network within the nucleus has a high concentration of deoxyribonucleic acid (DNA). The accompanying nucleolus tends to be obscure in contrast to the B cell, in which the chromatin pattern is diminished and the nucleolus is enlarged. The DNA content is lowered, but the concentration of ribonucleic acid (RNA) is increased. These cells are prenecrotic and tend to be either inactive or devitalized. The differentiation between the two is made by ultraviolet spectrophotometry. In a case that shows a favorable radiation response the A cells change into the B category.

THE VAGINAL SMEAR METHOD. Ruth and John Graham believe that successful radiation depends as much on the response of the normal supporting tissue as on the radiation sensitivity of the tumor cell. They have studied by cytologic techniques the normal cells in vaginal secretions both before and after irradiation. This concept involves the role of the host response to radiation in cancer therapy. The normal cells in vaginal secretion are reviewed with greater facility, because there are always more normal than tumor cells present.

The so-called RR or radiation response is determined after a trial dose of radium, totaling 1000 mg.-hours. The following changes are sought: (*a*) a yellowish brown staining of the cytoplasm, (*b*) enlargement of the cells and nuclei, (*c*) vacuolization of the cytoplasm, (*d*) increase in the number of nuclei, (*e*) derangement of the chromatin.

A favorable response may be anticipated if more than 75 per cent of the cells show a good RR, while the converse is true when the percentage drops below this figure. The findings check well when they are applied to the five-year end-result statistics. Thus one may expect a survival figure after radiation therapy in the range of 65 to 90 per cent when the RR was recorded as good, but only 10 to 35 per cent when a poor RR was observed.

One of the most interesting and promising offshoots of this attempt to measure radiation sensitivity or perhaps host resistance is the application of the method to the patient before any treatment is given. To test the sensitization response (SR), the cytologist seeks characteristic changes which appear in the basal and parabasal cells that normally desquamate from benign squamous vaginal epithelium. The basal cells appear in round or oval forms and have no "squared-off" corners characteristic of the polygonal cells from the intermediate or superficial cells. The distinguishing factors by which the SR is determined are (1) the lavender tinge that is seen in the cytoplasm, (2) vacuolization, and (3) increased density in the cytoplasm.

By correlating these observations clinically, a favorable result from radiation therapy may be expected when more than 10 per cent of SR-type cells are present in the vaginal smear. The 10 per cent end-point is chosen because the greatest differences in the survival rates were noted at this level. A 69 per cent 5-year survival could be expected from radiation if more than 10 per cent basal SR cells were present as against 18 per cent survival when the number was 10 per cent or less.

Although the correlation is not as close in patients with stage I carcinoma as it is in stages II and III, the fact that the patient with poor SR does so badly with radiation suggests that these patients might be better served by offering them surgery rather than radiation. The survival statistics reported by the Grahams support this contention. If the SR truly reflects a protective role assumed by all benign epithelial cells of the body, it should serve as an index of host resistance. In this regard it is interesting that the patients who have a poor SR tend to have fewer metastases to lymph nodes. This may be the reason why the surgical results are strikingly better in patients with poor SR than those achieved by radiation. We have recently encountered a patient with a poor SR and enough bulky tumor to place her in the clinical classification of stage IV. Fifty-one negative lymph nodes were found when a pelvic exenteration was performed as the sole form of treatment. This patient gained 70 pounds and is alive and active without disease after 3 years.

Many observers have criticized this approach based on the fact that the changes observed are so subtle that the technique cannot be easily mastered, and the interpretation is too refined for most observers to make clear-cut observations. Too many cases are borderline. It is an interesting and important suggestion, however, and if enough laboratories confirm the findings, it could provide the yardstick needed to allow the physician to choose between surgery and radiation as the best mode of therapy. Unfortunately, some nonconfirmatory studies have already been published.

THE BUCCAL SMEAR.   Recognizing the difficulties inherent in interpreting accurately the epithelial changes within the vaginal epithelium after irradiation and desiring to make the same postirradiation cytologic observations in an area thought free of hormonal influence, Jones has elected to take smears from the buccal cavity after 1000 roentgens of radiation to this region.

In general the clinical end-results did not correlate too well with the cytologic findings, except as they applied to the degree of macrocytosis and the number of multinucleated cells noted. When more than 10 per cent showed these responses the clinical results were excellent.

TISSUE CULTURES AND TUMOR TRANSPLANTS.   There are two reasons why the end-result responses are not more uniform for any given amount of disease: (1) The clinical course in the untreated patient varies widely. (2) The response to radiation therapy is not uniform. Both observations can be confirmed not only clinically, but also in tissue cultures and tumor transplant experiments.

Clinically, we are aware of the patient who has a small carcinoma that has been well treated, yet dies in a relatively short time with extensive metastatic disease. The best known case was associated with the so-called HeLa cell strain used in tissue culture experiments. This patient had such minimal tumor that it was barely looked on as suspicious, yet she died in less than three months. Biopsy material in tissue culture grew with abandon. In contrast, we all know of patients that had pathologic confirmation of invasive cancer, but remained well five or more years without treatment of any sort. There are some statistics from the California Tumor Registry that indicate that 13 per cent of patients with cancer of the cervix, diagnosed but untreated, live 5 years.

Carcinoma of the cervix has a good transplantability rate when introduced into the hamster cheek pouch, but it is also true that not all cases grow equally well. The same individual variability is noted in tissue culture experiments, when any human cancer is utilized.

When subjected to radiation, the growth of cancer cells in tissue culture may prove either very sensitive or resistant to radiation. In certain instances new growth is noted after an initial period of destruction, just as we see in some irradiated patients. The effect here, of course, is evidently directly on the tumor cells. The same observations, however, are made in irradiated tumor transplants where the tumor bed and its vascularity also play a role. There does seem to be a definite relation between the size of the x-radiation dose and its lethal effect on the tumor. Nevertheless the same difference in radiosensitivity appears in different tumor transplants that we noted in patients.

There is much that we do not know about the biology of tumor growth, and the response of tissues of the host. There does appear to be such a thing as tissue immunity not unlike that encountered in virus infections. Patients with the same amounts of tumor and identical microscopic patterns may either go rapidly downhill and die or survive without any treatment. The methods briefly discussed above are basically attempts to differentiate between the two.

Can Cancer of the Cervix Metastatic to Regional Lymph Nodes Be Cured?

There is another factor with a bearing on the explanation of why we are unable to cure more patients with cancer of the cervix despite its tendency to grow as a local disease. The prognosis after therapy is intimately linked to the extent of cancer spread to the regional lymph nodes. The presence of even a single positive node will affect the prognosis adversely. Approximately 15 per cent of patients classified as stage I and 25 per cent of stage II cases will have positive lymph nodes in the iliac and obturator regions.

Surgeons primarily, but many radiologists and pathologists as well, express doubt about the efficacy of ionizing radiation to destroy cancer in lymph nodes. Of course cancer can be localized or neutralized by irradiation without killing all the tumor cells. Similar observations have been made about the curative effects of radiation when lymph nodes are found in other parts of the body such as the neck and inguinal regions and where the nodes are more superficially placed than those in the pelvis. It is possible, of course, that cancer may have spread over such a wide area that not all the lymph nodes were included in the field of radiation, but there is sufficient evidence to question the ability of irradiation to destroy cancer in involved nodes wherever they are placed. Metastatic cancer is more resistant to irradiation than the primary growth. The failure to salvage more patients by radiation therapy in stage I may be due to the fact that between 15 and 20 per cent will have undetectable nodal cancer spread (Table 10).

Undoubtedly the biological nature of the tumor enters into the explanation. As we shall show later, surgical removal of the regional lymph nodes at the time of radical excision of the uterus and the intervening lymphatics will result in a 30 per

Table 10. **Five- and Ten-Year Survival in Cases Submitted to Surgery and Found to Have Lymph Node Involvement**

	5 YEARS	10 YEARS
Number of patients submitted to surgery	284	190
Number found without node involvement	225	151
Number found with node involvement	59	39
Percentage of patients with node involvement	20.8%	20.5%
Number alive without node involvement	138	85
Number alive with node involvement	19	9
Survival rate in patients without node involvement	61.3%	56.3%
Survival rate in patients with node involvement	32.2%	23.1%

Plan of radiation treatment:
(a) 30 mg. in cavity   } for 100 hours
    20 mg. in vaginal fornices } Total dose, 5000 milligram-hours of radium
(b) x-ray therapy
    Operability rate: 50%

RESULTS, 1946–51 (299 PATIENTS TREATED)

	NO. CASES	ALIVE WITH NO DISEASE	RELATIVE APPARENT RECOVERY RATE
Stage I	51	36	70.6%
Stage II	131	66	50.0%
Stage III	100	27	27.0%
Stage IV	17	1	5.9%
SURGERY			
Stage I	46	33	70.0%
Stage II	105	64	60.0%
Stage III	32	17	50.0%

Carcinoma cervicis uteri, 1930–46, with lymph node involvement, Royal Prince Alfred Hospital, Sydney, N.S.W., Australia.

cent salvage of patients who have cancer in these areas. The chance of achieving a five-year cure, which is tantamount to permanent survival in cancer of the cervix, is dependent on the extent of the disease present. Approximately 50 per cent of patients with a stage I cancer and positive nodes will be alive at 5 years, but only 20 per cent of those who have enough disease to be placed in the stage II category. Rarely will there be a significant salvage when the patient has more extensive disease. Most cured patients had only local carcinomas present in varying amounts.

Factors Complicating the Choice and Management of Therapy

There are certain pathologic conditions in the pelvis that are not infrequently associated with carcinoma of the cervix. They complicate the clinical evaluation of the extent of the disease, as well as provide definite problems in treatment simply by their presence. The common pelvic lesions that influence and complicate radiation therapy are pelvic inflammation, fibroids, ovarian tumors and pregnancy. For all but pelvic inflammation, the history and physical examination will be sufficient to distinguish between coexisting diseases and dissemination from a primary cervical cancer. For example, these data should be adequate to establish a diagnosis of pregnancy when combined with a rabbit or a frog test. The presence of the pregnancy, however, makes planned radiation a problem.

PELVIC INFLAMMATION. It is not always easy to distinguish between pelvic inflammatory disease and cancer spread. Rectal examination gives identical findings in both. If one encounters fixed bilateral sausage-shaped masses in the pelvis and perhaps distended Bartholin's glands, one is justified in assuming that there are two disease entities to explain the findings. At the same time we are also aware of the fact that inflammatory reactions in the broad ligament go hand-in-hand with malignant extension. We are alert to the fact that radiation given to a patient with clinical evidence of a past history of pelvic cellulitis may light up a pre-existing infection and produce peritonitis. Also there is a real danger that bowel may be adherent to the uterus, thereby increasing the danger of irradiation damage to either the small intestine or rectum. Nevertheless we cannot neglect to institute a therapy designed to cure. Only in the presence of distant metastases should treatment be undertaken only for palliation.

Whether the treatment for cervical carcinoma be radiation or surgery, the patient should be hospitalized. Supportive measures are an essential part of the treatment if complications are to be avoided. Diet rich in protein and vitamin content should be given. The anemia must be corrected by iron and blood transfusions Broad-spectrum antibiotics should be instituted to control sepsis, either active or latent. Any obvious pelvic abscess should be drained surgically. With extensive necrosis of the cervical tumor and cervical stenosis a pyometra is often present. The cervical canal must be dilated, the endometrial cavity explored and drainage maintained by the insertion of a T-tube similar to that used in biliary surgery for drainage of the common duct.

With the patient adequately prepared, therapy may then be started. If the cancer is confined to the cervix and the surgeon is convinced that the broad ligament induration present is associated with pelvic inflammation and not an extension of cancer, he may elect to do a Wertheim hysterectomy with lymph node dissection. This eliminates the dangers of irradiating adherent bowel. If he has underestimated the extent of the disease preoperatively, he may free up the bowel, remove the ovaries, mark the gross outlines of the cancer with dura clips as a guide to radiation therapy and abandon the idea of further surgery.

If the surgeon prefers, or the cancer is too extensive for surgery, external radiation should be begun in reduced dosage under the protection of chemotherapy. Radium is much more apt to make a pelvic peritonitis flare up. Approximately 200 roentgens of external radiation are therefore given daily, with rotation of the entry portals. When it is evident that the therapy will be tolerated, as noted by the lack of temperature elevation, leukocytosis, chills, fever and malaise, the dosage may be increased.

FIBROIDS.   Cancer of the cervix is common in the fibroid uterus. Too infrequently it is first discovered by the pathologist after total hysterectomy for the fibroids. This can be avoided by (1) keeping in mind that a fibroid other than a submucous fibroid does not usually bleed and (2) by doing a preliminary cervical biopsy and curettage to determine the cause of vaginal bleeding before proceding with the removal of the uterus.

When the diagnosis of cancer has been established, the presence of a fibroid in the uterus complicates the planned radiation only if the leiomyoma is pedunculated, either outside or inside the uterus. Radiation in either case may so destroy the blood supply of the pedicle that necrosis of the leiomyoma can lead to infection and cellulitis if within the uterus, or peritonitis if the tumor arises from the fundus within the abdominal cavity. A large uterus does not make radiation therapy any easier, but a calculated risk may be taken without too much danger.

When there is a large pedunculated tumor present with extensive malignant disease in the cervix, complications in therapy may be prevented by surgical removal of the tumor at the same time radium is applied to the cervix. At exploration a bilateral lymphadenectomy may be performed, or if this proves undesirable, the gross extension of the tumor may be palpated and outlined by dura clips as a guide for subsequent external radiation.

If the disease is confined to the cervix, the senior author would prefer to carry out definitive treatment by surgery, doing a Wertheim hysterectomy and bilateral pelvic lymphadenectomy.

The same course of action would be the treatment of choice for a pedunculated intrauterine fibroid polyp or submucous fibroid tumor mass. If the malignant disease has extended beyond the cervix, the polyp should be removed and radium applied at the same time.

OVARIAN CYST.   The same problems in therapy are presented by the finding of a coexisting ovarian cyst. Here the indications for intra-abdominal intervention are increased. In most instances ovarian cysts lie relatively free in the abdominal cavity and obtain their blood supply from a pedicle. Radiation may destroy the blood supply with resultant necrosis of the tumor and peritonitis. Moreover, there is always the chance that the cyst may contain an independent cancer.

If the primary carcinoma of the cervix is in stage I or early stage II, the senior author would prefer to perform a Wertheim hysterectomy and bilateral pelvic lymphadenectomy. If the disease is more widespread, abdominal exploration, bilateral salpingo-oophorectomy and demarcation of the gross tumor by dura clips with or without lymphadenectomy are indicated.

PREGNANCY.   The presence of cancer of the cervix with pregnancy always sets up a problem in therapy. The fact that the cancer is usually discovered by accident points out the need of a periodic inspection of the cervix combined with vaginal smear examinations throughout the course of pregnancy, whether the patient has symptoms or not. Any suspicious lesion may be biopsied without fear of producing abortion or inducing labor.

The treatment will depend upon the extent of the disease and the duration of the pregnancy.

In the first trimester of pregnancy definitive treatment may be carried out by the Wertheim operation, combined with bilateral pelvic lymphadenectomy, provided the disease is in stage I or early stage II.

If the obstetrician prefers radiation as definitive therapy, or if the disease is too advanced for surgery, the uterus must be emptied by curettage or abdominal *hysterotomy* before the application of radium or the administration of x-ray therapy. It is unwise to give radiation with the pregnancy in utero, owing to the risks both of sepsis and of further dissemination of carcinoma as the products of conception are expelled through an ulcerating cervical os.

In the last trimester one gives greater consideration to the problem of obtaining a viable infant, while at the same time adequate therapy is given to the cancer. In this instance it may be wise to defer all treatment for two or three weeks until there is a reasonable chance of obtaining a live baby that will survive. An abdominal cesarean section is then performed, and the full course of radiation is begun approximately two weeks thereafter.

When a cancer of the cervix is encountered at the fifth or sixth month of pregnancy, the obstetrician is forced to disregard the gestation and to concentrate on the treatment of malignancy. The period of delay is too great, if we are to wait for a viable infant. The pregnancy should be immediately terminated by abdominal cesarean section and radiation therapy begun after approximately two weeks. Religious doctrine of Catholics may modify this decision, and this factor requires due consideration.

Radiation Therapy

Radiation is the treatment of choice for the majority of patients with cancer of the cervix and for all but the most accomplished of pelvic cancer surgeons. This is largely due to the extent of the neoplastic disease. At best only 30 per cent of patients with cervical cancer will be in stages I and IIa, in which the radical Wertheim operation with bilateral pelvic lymphadenectomy can be performed with results equal to or better than those obtained after irradiation. Furthermore, not all patients with cancerous disease confined to the cervix or the immediately adjacent paracervical and paravaginal tissues are suitable candidates for an operation of this magnitude. Most patients have too much disease for the average surgeon to cope with. Nothing short of a total or partial exenteration of all pelvic viscera with diversion of the urinary tract to a newly constructed ileal bladder or colon will suffice. Until surgical training progresses to the point at which the radical surgical procedures for cancer of the cervix can be carried out adequately with a low morbidity and mortality rate, the fundamental treatment of cervical cancer will be ionizing radiation.

HISTORY.   Until the early years of the twentieth century surgery had been the sole method of therapy for cancer of the cervix. Without the present knowledge of electrolyte balance, postoperative care, anesthesia, antibiotics, blood and fluid replacement, the complications were many and lethal, and the results were poor indeed. With the appearance of clinically applied radium about 1918 surgery disappeared, because it soon became obvious that the use of intracavitary radium would

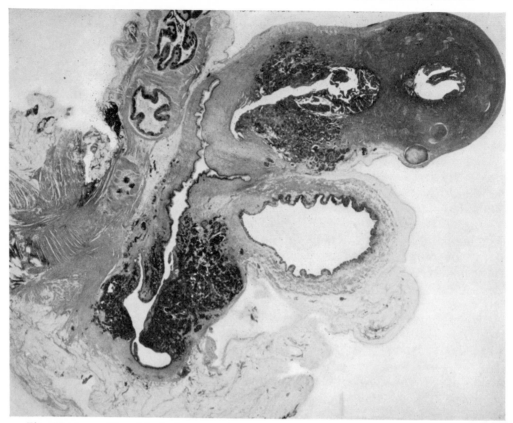

Fig. 61-14. Giant histologic paramedian section showing from left to right the rectum, vagina and a tangential section of uterus. The bladder is demonstrated below the uterus. The dark-stained nodules in the vaginal walls and lower uterine segment are cervical carcinoma, not susceptible to cure by radium therapy because of the depth of invasion. From an exenteration specimen.

produce an increasing number of five-year cures without the mortality and morbidity that accompanied the surgical procedures. The improvement in the five-year results, however, was noted largely in the group in which the cancer was confined to the cervix and the regions immediately adjacent to it. Most patients had more extensive disease. It was logical then to try to increase the dose of radium applied to the cervical canal and upper part of the vagina, with the idea of destroying cancer growth at a distance from the cervix. This experiment failed for the simple reason that the effect of radium decreases in geometric proportion as the square of the distance from the central point of application. To increase the dosage is to cause more extensive destruction of tissue in the immediate vicinity of the cervix without appreciably influencing the amount of radiation delivered to tumor situated farther out laterally (Fig. 61–14). After approximately twenty years it became obvious that if lateral extensions of tumor and the regional lymph nodes were to be properly irradiated, external radiation in the form of x-ray would have to be added to the local application of radium to the cervix. In the past twenty-five years accepted therapy for cancer of the cervix has been the combined use of x-ray and radium. The five-year salvage has shown a steady improvement over this period.

PROGNOSIS. The eleventh volume, annual report of the Radiumhemmet in Stockholm on the results of treatment of cancer of the uterus, presents the relative

5-year recovery rates in over 42,000 cases treated in 84 centers throughout the world for the years 1947–1951. The mean average salvage for stages I through IV was approximately 43 per cent. This is a considerable improvement from the 25 per cent achieved from the use of radium alone, as reported in the past. By individual stages the 5-year salvage rate was as follows: stage I, 70 per cent; stage II, 49 per cent; stage III, 27 per cent; and stage IV, 7 per cent. It is still unfortunate that only 20 per cent of the total number of cases treated are in stage I. The experience expressed in these combined statistics is approximately the same as that reported in different centers in this country over the same period of time. For example, the results from the Los Angeles Tumor Institute for stages I through IV treated by radiation are 74, 53, 28 and zero per cent. The improved salvage noted from the combined use of radium and x-ray gives cause for encouragement, but none for complacency. Too few early cases are seen, and too many women die after the best of treatment.

WHAT ARE THE PROBLEMS THE RADIOTHERAPIST MUST FACE?   The basic aim in irradiation is to destroy cancer at the primary site within the cervix, as well as in all areas within the pelvis to which it may have spread. Unfortunately the actual amount of disease can be determined only by the examining finger with some help from the intravenous pyelogram that allows you to form an opinion of the degree of encroachment of tumor upon the ureters and bladder (Fig. 61–15). The actual direction and extent of spread are open to question. There may prove to be more or less cancer, or it may be found in regions that we do not become aware of by clinical appraisal. For example, some stage I lesions have regional lymph node involvement, which cannot be felt, in 20 per cent of the cases.

Since judging the amount of malignant disease present is only a clinical estimate,

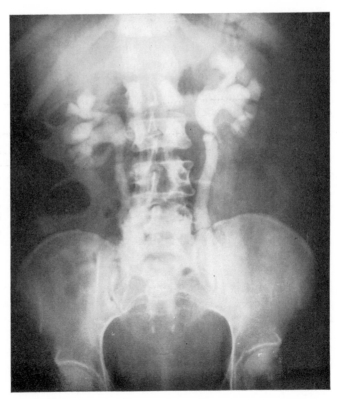

Fig. 61-15.   When an intravenous pyelogram in a patient with cancer of the cervix shows advanced bilateral hydronephrosis and hydro-ureter, the tumor has evidently involved the ureterovesical region extensively. Hope for adequate palliation by irradiation in such a situation is scant.

the combined dose of radium and x-ray must be uniform for cancer throughout the pelvis and lethal for cancer cells wherever encountered. This presents a real problem for the radiotherapist, because the region of potential spread is extensive. The field to be included extends from the anterior superior iliac spine to the anterior superior iliac spine, from the bifurcation of the aorta to the symphysis pubis and at varying depths from the skin, depending on the general body build and adiposity of the patient.

The dosage must also be delivered at the tumor site without damaging adjacent organs, such as the bladder, small intestine, and rectum. It is not inconceivable, since there is such a wide area to cover, that some spots may receive inadequate irradiation and others too much. To prevent overconcentration of ionizing radiation at any one point the amount of external irradiation must be carefully balanced with that from the intrauterine source. The principal effect of radiation may well be the destruction of cancer cells, but the effect on the supporting tissues must be considered, for if they are devitalized by too intensive irradiation, some of the actual resistance to cancer invasion may be lost. The optimal dose of irradiation to cure cancer of the cervix is not far below the tolerance level for normal tissue. There is a tendency to overtreat the early case with limited amounts of cancer and to undertreat the patient with more advanced disease. The dosage for the combined use of radium and x-ray must be planned with precision, giving proper emphasis to each element to avoid undesirable damage to normal tissue as well as to the tumor bed.

How Does the Radiologist Meet the Problem?   These are practical matters that are well known to the therapeutic radiologist. Tremendous strides have been made to overcome these barriers to successful therapy. Physical tables now correlate the amount of radiation given by x-ray with that administered by intrauterine radium application. The dose is calculated for its effect at the tumor site and the most likely areas of tumor extension. The dosage therefore becomes more precise.

Attempts are now being made actually to measure the amount of radiation in tissue through the use of ionization chambers placed in the bladder and rectum and dosimeters implanted interstitially. More attention is being paid to the time, spacing and rate of administration of the radiation as well as the recovery rate in different tissues. This probably is more important than the voltage of the machine that delivers the radiation. The majority of cases of cervical cancer in this country today are being treated by the 250-KV x-ray machines. The dosage that can be delivered is limited by the tolerance of the skin of the abdominal wall and back. In recent years higher voltage machines such as the 2000-KV machine and high-energy units like the linear accelerator, betatron (22.5 million volts) and isotopic cobalt machines have been developed and are now in use. All are designed to deliver the optimum dose to the cancer without (*a*) producing tissue necrosis in normal structures, (*b*) interfering with the protective mechanism in normal tissue, (*c*) instituting adverse constitutional effects.

Just what the actual dose should be in an individual cancer patient is another problem. In the past there was altogether too much standardization in therapy. Actually, there is no standard radiation dose that can be expected to produce predictable results in every instance. Because we know the approximate amount of radiation that will destroy tumor cells and can be tolerated by the supporting tissue, we speak of a cancericidal dose, placed roughly at 6000 roentgens delivered at the tumor site, not as measured in air. Clinically, however, we are aware that any given patient may be cured by less than that amount, while in others 6000 roentgens may be inadequate for a carcinoma of comparable size and histologic appearance.

In the present trend toward individualization in cancer therapy we should strive to give the patient the amount of radiation that she needs for cure and not expose her to the maximum dosage simply because she has cancer of the cervix. It is of the utmost importance that the dosage at the tumor site be measured physically, but successful radiation therapy in the future will probably depend more upon the ability of the radiologist to estimate the response of the tumor than upon the total dose or the voltage of the apparatus that delivers it. The explanation of why cancers of equal size, clinical stage and histologic nature respond in different fashion will await a better understanding of the biological nature of the tumor itself.

How Is the Radium Given?   To give radium effectively there must be flexibility of method. To the uninitiated the technique of the radium application seems amazingly simple. Radium with accompanying instructions for its use can be obtained from commercial companies. The patient and her tumor, therefore, must conform to the type of radium and applicator available.

The trained radiotherapist, however, recognizes that special problems presented by anatomic variations in the uterus and vagina, as well as the irregular spread of the local cancer growth, may not lend themselves to one standard method of radium application. The treatment must be individualized, and the dosage given, as well as the type of applicator used, must be adjusted to the situation that presents itself. For example, a patient may have a cervical cancer develop in a uterus which is fixed in retroversion. Great care must be taken then that the large bowel mucosa be not too heavily radiated. Blakey has pointed out that the average diameter of the cervix is approximately 3 cm., and the combined thickness of the posterior vaginal and bowel walls is roughly 0.5 cm. Most radium applicators in general use have a minimum diameter of 0.6 cm. This places the bowel mucosa, which is extremely sensitive to the effects of irradiation, not over 2 cm. away. With the uterus held in retroversion the chances of getting radiation proctitis and subsequent fistula are better than average. The method of administering radium in a case like this is most important.

The most common techniques for intrauterine and vaginal application of radium today are (1) the Stockholm box method, (2) the Manchester ovoid method, and (3) the Ernst type of applicator. They are basically the same, varying in the amounts of radium used in the different units, the duration of application, the time-spacing of the treatments, and the total amount of ionizing radiation to be given (Fig. 61–16). In most instances the radium is inserted in 10-mg. units for a total amount of 50 to 60 mg. and remains in position long enough to give a total dose of 5000 mg.-hours. In addition to the intrauterine and vaginal types of applicator, local radium treatment can be given by implanting platinum needles containing radon directly into the tissues at approximately 1 cm. intervals (method of Pitts and Waterman.) Whatever the method, success will be heavily influenced by the attention paid to the details of administering it.

We have noted that the total dose to be given must be balanced with the amount of radiation administered by external x-radiation. The radium is expected to destroy cancer in the cervix and the immediately adjacent region, while the external x-ray sources are counted on to destroy tumor more laterally placed. Arbitrary points are set up by which the total tumor dose may be estimated. Point A is located 2 cm. lateral to the cervix at about the level of the internal os. Point B is located on the side wall of the pelvis. Theoretically, the external x-radiation sources concentrate on

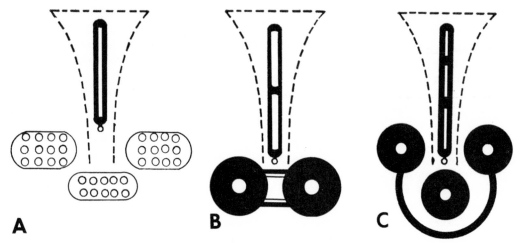

Fig. 61-16.   Diagrams of techniques of radium application to the cervix. *A*, Stockholm method; *B*, Manchester method; *C*, Paris method. (Fluhmann: *The Cervix Uteri and Its Diseases.*)

this latter area with the idea of destroying tumor in the lymphatic channels intervening between the primary cancer and the possible lymph nodal extension. In most instances a total dose of 5000 mg.-hours of radium will be delivered by the intra-uterine and vaginal applicator. The tumor dose at point A will be approximately 3000 roentgens.

The shape of the cervix, the position of the uterus and the direction of tumor spread all will influence the calculated dose. The time elements and the spacing of treatments are extremely important. Most radiotherapists prefer to give a lower dose over a longer time, rather than a high concentration for a shorter interval, although the total dose is the same. It is never given in a single application. The plan of treatment varies in different clinics, but many now give external x-radiation for two weeks, a radium application, two more weeks of external radiation and a final radium treatment.

How Is External Radiation Given?   External radiation delivered by an x-ray machine is directed toward point B on the lateral pelvic wall with the avowed purpose of introducing a lethal dose of radiation into the regions of potential spread, namely, the lymphatic channels intervening between the primary growth and the regional nodes.

When the conventional 250- and 450-KV x-ray units are used, 4 portals of entry, measuring roughly 10 by 10 cm. or 10 by 15 cm. are used. A central portion between the two anterior abdominal wall fields is protected from the external radiation by lead strips, since this area has been covered by the intrauterine radium. Similar portals are outlined on the back. In addition a transvaginal field is sometimes utilized, in combination with the usual portals. In this case the amount of intrauterine radiation is either sharply curtailed or omitted entirely. There is a temptation to use lateral fields, but there is great danger of producing aseptic necrosis of the femoral heads by this approach.

Daily treatments are given on an outpatient basis in most instances, with a daily dose not in excess of 300 roentgens. The total tumor dose of 4000 roentgens is given in about 4 weeks. When combined with the radiation given in the uterine canal, in the form of radium, the total tumor dose will be in excess of 7000 roentgens. To give more is to run the risk of severe complications from overirradiation.

The supervoltage units such as the 2000-KV machine, the cobalt-60 unit and the 22,500-KV betatron radiation sources can deliver much higher doses of radiation to the pelvis without causing troublesome skin damage or constitutional reactions. In addition to the 5000 mg.-hours of intrauterine radium the patient also receives 4000 to 5000 tumor dose roentgens from these external sources, delivered in daily doses over a 4- to 6-week period. Lead shields are used in the center of the fields to protect the area to be irradiated by the intrauterine and vaginal sources. It is possible to give much higher doses with the supervoltage units, but an increasing number of complications may be expected when this is done. If the radiation given by external sources is increased, the amount of x-radiation given in the form of radium must be reduced. This is unwise in carcinoma patients who are in stage I and II, but can be done when patients have more extensive disease. When the cobalt-60 unit is used for more extensive disease in stages III and IV, a total tumor dose of 6000 r may be given if the radium is omitted.

The effectiveness of radiation therapy will be modified by the patient's general health. Much greater attention is now given to getting the patient in better general condition before attempting to carry out an intensive irradiation program. Liver, iron and blood transfusions may be given to correct any anemia, antibiotics are given to reduce the element of sepsis, and a general supportive regimen is carried out in an attempt to improve the patient's own resistance to her tumor. In the past some have been more interested in the mechanics of treating the patient's cancer than in the patient herself.

WHAT DOES RADIOACTIVE GOLD HAVE TO OFFER? In keeping with the constant desire of the radiotherapist to find some method of therapy that will deliver a uniform cancericidal radiation to the more remote foci of carcinomatous spread within the pelvis, radioactive gold has been tried with varying degrees of success. It is given in one of two ways: (a) direct injection of gold transvaginally into each paracervical and paravaginal region in total doses ranging from 70 to 150 microcuries; (b) 150 microcuries of gold are implanted under direct vision into the tumor-bearing area after abdominal exploration, pelvic lymphadenectomy and biopsy. Intracavitary radiation in the usual amount is given in two applications one week apart in both instances.

Although there has been some initial enthusiasm for this sort of therapy, it has cooled appreciably in the face of the high rate of complications that have followed its use. Several deaths have been directly traced to tissue necrosis after treatment. The incidence of radiation proctitis, both early and late, leading to fistulas and intestinal obstruction, is much too high. Many of the patients have complained of persistent pain with a sciatic distribution, and a few have had ureteral strictures. The complications after abdominal exploration and lymphadenectomy have been more numerous and severe, and the number of survivors is appreciably less than one has come to expect from traditional radiation therapy.

To be effective the gold must circulate rapidly and be dispersed to all potential tumor-bearing areas, for it has a half-life of only two and one-half days. It does this very well in animal experiments, and the effect on regional lymph nodes is dramatic. In the patient with cancer, however, this rapid rate of dispersion seems to be lost. As a result of pooling and delayed absorption of the gold, "hot spots" occur, and local tissue necrosis follows. This probably is the reason why the complications are more frequent when gold is implanted after pelvic lymph node dissection. Not only are the lymphatic pathways perhaps obstructed by tumor, but also the surgery in all probability further disturbs the tumor bed and interferes with the dissemination of the radioactive gold.

COMPLICATIONS OF RADIATION THERAPY.   There are serious dangers inherent in ionizing radiation. The immediate mortality associated with its use is minimal, but morbidity both at the time the radiation is given and later is frequently encountered despite every effort at avoidance. The structures chiefly damaged are the bladder and the rectum. Progressive small bowel necrosis may take place if radiation has been given to a patient with chronic pelvic inflammatory disease or one who has had a previous laparotomy. Extensive radiation destroys the blood supply in the small bowel mesentery. The effect on bladder and rectum is more direct, since the epithelium of both structures is sensitive to the effects of radiation. Furthermore, the rectum may also be adherent to the uterus as a result of pre-existing disease process or pelvic surgery.

In addition to the above-mentioned elements that produce serious sequelae, other factors complicate the normal course of radiation therapy. They are (1) the reactions of the skin to external therapy, (2) radiation sickness.

In recent years both the radiologist and the surgeon have increased the scope of their particular form of therapy in the hope that the cure rate for what is fundamentally a local form of cancer will improve with more intensive therapy. Inevitably there has been a pronounced increase in the number of unpleasant complications after both methods of therapy. This is particularly true of radiation.

The amount of radiation must be calculated and administered so that the dosage is lethal for the cancer, while normal tissue is undamaged. Since there are two sources of radiation utilized, the excessive radiation reaction may be due to either local application of radium or external x-ray therapy. Cystitis or proctitis may occur during the course of therapy which can lead to bladder or bowel ulceration and to rectovaginal or vesicovaginal fistulas at a later date. The incidence of rectovaginal or vesicovaginal fistulas ranges from 4 to 8 per cent, with the higher incidence in the group treated for more extensive disease. It is unfair to blame radiation entirely for these unfortunate results, because 8 per cent of untreated patients will also suffer vesical and rectal fistulas. Nevertheless the hazard remains.

A sustained temperature elevation during the application of radium is a suggestive sign of overirradiation. It may be advisable to remove the radium before completing the treatment. If extensive instances of cystitis or proctitis develop during external x-radiation, the treatment may have to be abandoned temporarily or the daily dosage be materially reduced.

What about Radiation Injuries of the Intestine?   Rectal injuries are most distressing to the patient and occur much more often than bladder complications, roughly in the ratio of three to one. There is a good reason for this, since there is experimental evidence to show that intestinal epithelium is far more sensitive to the effects of radiation than that of the bladder. In most instances the damage is caused by external roentgen-ray therapy, but injuries can also be produced by (a) malposition of the radium applicator in the uterine canal, (b) overloading of radium in the vaginal containers, or (c) a change in the position of the applicators in the course of treatment. It is important that the position of the applicators be checked by x-ray. The danger from radiation sources within the uterus increases if the uterus is fixed in retroversion or if the disease extends to the posterolateral fornix of the vagina.

Rectal irritation is far more common during external x-radiation than bladder damage. Diarrhea, tenesmus and bloody stools are the most common symptoms.

Fortunately they appear late in the course of treatment, usually in the third week. The complaints can be so severe that the treatments may have to be discontinued for a week or more, or the normal daily tumor dose of 200 roentgens may have to be reduced to 100 to 150 roentgens when the treatments are resumed. The frequency of severe rectal irritation is about the same whether the 250-KV or 2000-KV machine is used. The symptoms are probably due to the direct necrotizing effect of the radiation on the sensitive intestinal mucosa.

Late bowel complications take the form of (1) ulceration, (2) stricture, (3) fistulas, (4) malnutrition, or (5) intestinal obstruction.

If the rectum is examined by proctoscope, an edematous area can be seen surrounded by an indurated border on the anterior rectal wall. This bleeds easily at the touch. Subsequently this portion of the wall may ulcerate and lead to fistula formation. The patient complains bitterly of cramplike tenesmus and bloody discharge over a long period of time. Rectal stricture is common, appearing from one to several years after an early radiation proctitis. It may, however, appear without any preceding history of rectal injury or may follow a long quiescent period. If the stricture is extreme enough to produce intestinal obstruction or a rectovaginal fistula, it may be necessary to do a colostomy to divert the fecal stream.

The intestinal complications do not end here. Owing largely to the progressive endarteritis and thrombosis of the vessels that supply the rectum or small bowel, two things may happen years after the course of pelvic irradiation: (a) the small bowel either obstructs or perforates, or (b) the motility and hence the function of the intestine become so altered that the patient suffers from chronic malnutrition (Fig. 61–17).

How Does Radiation Affect the Bladder? The bladder epithelium is much more resistant to the effects of radiation than that of the rectum. Nevertheless the urinary tract is often severely damaged by it. It is a rare thing not to have some degree of dysuria or mild hematuria during the course of the radiation treatment.

Bladder injuries are most often due to the local intracavitary application of radium. External radiation rarely is a contributing cause. Occasionally, when large doses are given, ureteral obstruction may result from the fibrosis that follows the initial destructive effect of x-ray therapy.

Radiation reaction in the bladder can be distressing, with extensive dysuria as the chief symptom. On cystoscopic examination erythema, edema and petechial hemorrhages are seen in the bladder mucosa. The emphasis in treatment should be on preventing the occurrence of such radiation damage. Antibiotics should be given and

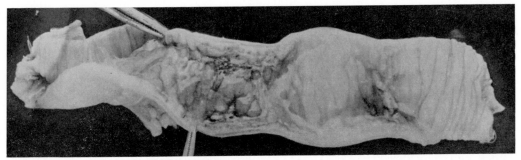

Fig. 61-17. Severe radiation reaction of the intestine characterized by chronic edema with ulceration and granulation tissue replacement of the mucous membrane locally, as shown near the clamps, and sometimes localized damage to the deeper structures that may produce penetrating ulcers or perforation, as shown at the right.

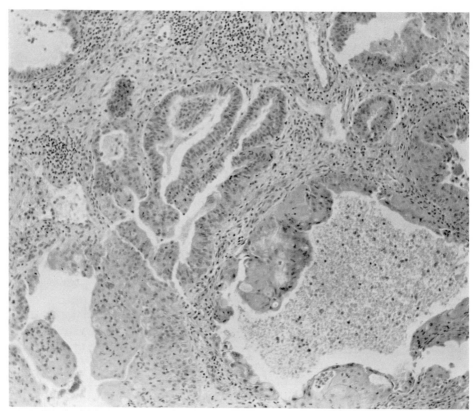

Fig. 61-18.   Biopsy of the urinary bladder after radiation therapy. The glandular and squamous metaplasia, degenerative epithelial changes and apparent anaplasia are attributed to radiation reaction, and not considered to represent carcinomatous involvement.

the radium applicators should be removed before the treatment is completed if an elevation of temperature occurs.

The late results of radiation damage to the bladder are extremely unpleasant. Frequency, extreme dysuria and occasionally bloody urine are the most frequent symptoms. They are due to small ulcerations on the floor of the bladder and a decreased bladder capacity. Unless the urologist has had considerable experience, the differential diagnosis between radiation reaction and recurrence of cancer may be difficult to make, for both produce indurated ulcers. The pathologic diagnosis also may be difficult, because in small biopsies radiation reaction of bladder epithelium can closely simulate the anaplasia of epidermoid carcinoma (Fig. 61–18).

Reaction of the Skin to Radiation Therapy.   The amount of external irradiation that can be given to a patient is sharply limited by the tolerance of the skin. Rarely is it possible to deliver more than 3000 roentgens in air to each of the 4 skin portals commonly utilized in therapy from a 250-KV machine. With the higher-voltage machines less of the radiation is dissipated in the skin, and larger tumor doses may be given. When the external radiation is given transvaginally, the amount is determined by the local response of the skin. The perineal skin does not tolerate radiation as well as the skin of the abdominal wall and back.

Radiation sensitivity of the skin is shown by severe degrees of erythema, to the point of blistering. By applying some preparation such as Aloe Vera ointment two or three times daily skin irritation is ameliorated so that it is rarely necessary to discontinue treatment. The ointment includes an extract of cactus leaf similar in its healing properties to chlorophyll. In overcoming this handicap to treatment it is more important to know what to avoid than what to put on. The skin areas should be kept dry. Water should be avoided. White Vaseline, Aloe Vera or Alphagel ointment helps, but other kinds of ointment should not be used. Erythema and blistering are immediate reactions. Years later the skin shows telangiectasis, pigmentation and induration over the portals of entry. Irradiated skin may break down, leaving painful indurated ulcers that can be cured only by excision and grafting.

The same reaction to radiation is noted in the vaginal epithelium at the apex of the vagina. This leads to obliteration of the upper portion and foreshortening of its length. The adhesions here should be broken up to make it possible to examine the patient later for evidence of cancer recurrence.

Radiation Sickness. In certain patients nausea and vomiting may become so intense and persistent during x-radiation that the plan of therapy has to be modified. The important thing to remember is that these symptoms provide a warning signal that the radiotherapist is approaching the maximum point of tissue tolerance. Bone marrow and peripheral blood studies will usually show a leukopenia that persists for several weeks after radiation therapy. The bone marrow depression leads to both a leukopenia and an anemia that should be corrected by transfusion.

By varying the dosage and spacing the treatments radiation sickness can be avoided, and the therapy can be allowed to proceed. At times it may be necessary to interrupt the treatment program. This is far better than persisting in carrying out the planned course and trying to overcome the nausea and vomiting with tranquilizing drugs such as chlorpromazine (Thorazine) or drugs that are effective for motion sickness such as Dramamine or Bonamine. If the therapist recognizes the fact that the symptoms of radiation sickness do give indications that maximal tissue tolerance is nearly reached, and the dosage schedule is modified, then chlorpromazine in 10-mg. doses 3 times daily, or Bonamine and Dramamine, 25 mg. 3 times a day, combined with Cortate will be helpful adjuncts to therapy.

Has Supervoltage Therapy Reduced the Number and Severity of the Complications? The advent of the supervoltage x-ray units and high-energy sources such as the betatrons and cobalt units was hailed with great enthusiasm, since the radiologist hoped that increasingly large cancericidal doses of radiation could be delivered to the tumor without producing damage to normal structures in the same area. Until this time the amount of external radiation that could be given was sharply limited by the tolerance of the skin. Any attempt to give more than 3000 roentgens tumor dose in the usual period of a month with the older type of 250-KV x-ray machine was apt to bring unwanted skin damage. The main factor in therapy, by necessity, had to be intra-uterine and intravaginal radium. Radium given in this manner produced its own series of complications, as attested by the number of bladder and rectal sequelae. The amount of radiation from both sources, external and internal, had to be carefully gauged.

By use of supervoltage therapy increasingly large cancericidal tumor doses have been given, and it is now well documented that this can be done without damaging the skin. As the amount of radiation from external sources has been stepped up, however, there has been a corresponding increase in the number of complications. These are serious and not readily corrected. Since the object of therapy is to cure the patient, not destroy her by your attempts to do so, the amount of radiation any patient can be given is bound to be limited by tissue tolerance, as measured by the number and degree of severity of the complications produced.

Most of the complications, when intracavitary and intravaginal radium was given in combination with external radiation delivered by the 250-KV x-ray machine, were traceable to radium. The usual plan of treatment called for the application of radium in 10-mg. units, using a variety of types of applicators to the uterine cavity, external cervix and upper part of the vagina. The total number of milligram-hours ranged from 4500 to 6000. The local radium was calculated to deliver at an arbitrary point A, 2 cm. lateral to the cervix at the level of the internal os, a tumor dose of roughly 3000 roentgens. External x-radiation was then given over the period of a month in doses calculated to produce a tumor dose at point B, on the lateral pelvic wall, of another 4000 roentgens. Few complications resulted from the additional external irradiation.

In the past ten years, in keeping with the attitude of both surgeon and radiologist, a more vigorous attack has been made on cancer of the cervix. The radiologist with the supervoltage and high-energy units at his command has steadily increased the amount of external radiation apart from the intrauterine and vaginal sources.

No mass statistical information is available to permit an adequate evaluation of the effect of this accelerated program upon the over-all cure rate. It is becoming apparent, however, that serious complications are definitely increasing.

A number of reports have appeared recently that make it fairly obvious that one cannot hope to increase the dose of external radiation limitlessly without getting into difficulty, particularly if one continues to use the same amount of intrauterine and intravaginal radiation. The majority of serious complications seem to occur when the tumor dose delivered by external radiation exceeds 4000 roentgens, and they tend to concentrate on the rectum. The mortality rate is minimal, ranging from 0.5 to 2 per cent, but the morbidity from fistula formation, ureteral obstruction due to radiation fibrosis, and intestinal malfunction is increasingly high. Far fewer complications appear when the tumor dose of external radiation is kept below 3500 roentgens. The alternative is to reduce the amount of radiation supplied by local radium inserted at the tumor site. This is probably unwise.

It is apparent that we have much to learn about the tissue effects due to high-voltage therapy. When this type of therapy is used in combination with radium, the dose must be carefully worked out by physical tables. Some of the problems involved will tax the ingenuity of the best-trained radiation physicists.

Surgery as a Method of Treatment of Carcinoma of the Cervix

Surgery alone or in combination with radium has a definite place in the resources of treatment for cancer of the cervix. It holds its place by virtue of the trend toward individualization in therapy for cervical carcinoma. Surgery is not advocated as a substitute for radiation, nor is radiation the only form of treatment available. It is not a question of which is the better form of therapy, but which will provide a given patient the greatest chance of cure.

There are two operations that are commonly performed for early carcinomas in stage I and II, in which the disease is confined to the cervix or immediately adjacent paracervical and paravaginal tissues. Approximately 33 per cent are in this category. The types of operation are: (1) the Wertheim operation and pelvic lymphadenectomy. This is commonly called radical hysterectomy and node dissection. (2) The radical vaginal hysterectomy (Schauta), less commonly done in the United States, but popular in other countries. The regional lymph nodes are removed as a separate procedure. These operations may be used alone or in combination with radiation.

WHAT DOES SURGERY OFFER AS DEFINITIVE TREATMENT? All are agreed that the optimum treatment for most cervical carcinoma cases is radiation, since 70 per cent of patients either have too much disease or are too old, too fat or too debilitated for one to hope for a cure from surgery. In most instances extension of cancer beyond the cervix presents the average surgeon with more of a problem than he can cope with. Nevertheless there is a definite place for surgery in the treatment of cancer of the cervix.

The reasons why surgery is considered definitive treatment are based on the observed facts that: (1) There are too many local cancer recurrences after radiation therapy. (2) Clinical evaluation of the extent of the disease is often faulty. Undetected cancer extension to paracervical and paravaginal tissues, as well as to the regional lymph nodes, may be present. (3) There is a question of the effectiveness of x-ray to cure cancer in these nodes. (4) Some cancers are radiation-resistant. (5) Associated abnormalities may be present. Small intestine or rectum adherent to the uterus materially increases the risk of radiation therapy. Radiation of a pedunculated uterine tumor or ovarian cyst may produce necrosis and peritonitis.

In recent years there has been a strong revival of interest in surgery for the definitive treatment of cancer of the cervix. With the initial enthusiasm have come many misconceptions and much confusion about (1) which patients should be operated upon and (2) how much surgery is necessary to produce a cure. At present many women are being operated upon who might better have had radiation therapy, and many operations are inadequate. If one is to choose surgery as the method of choice in therapy, it must be adequate. Good radiation therapy is far superior to inadequate surgery. Moreover, inadequate radiation allows the patient to live longer and does not immediately cause the havoc that follows inadequate surgery.

WHICH PATIENTS SHOULD HAVE SURGERY AS DEFINITIVE TREATMENT? The Wertheim procedure and the Schauta operation fell into disrepute in the days before radium usage because of the high mortality rate. Modern surgery, chemotherapy, blood replacement and a better understanding of the physiology of the postoperative period have made it possible to adopt a more radical concept toward the surgical treatment of cervical carcinoma. The operative mortality rate now ranges between 1 and 3 per cent. It will be higher in the more inexperienced hands, for the operation has certain technical aspects which must be understood. There is nothing about the technique, however, that cannot be mastered by a well trained surgeon who is willing to take the trouble to learn the pitfalls. In this respect it is no different from radiation therapy.

The indications for the Wertheim procedure and lymph node dissection are sharply drawn. In the confusion as to the proper place of surgery the chief indications appear to have been overlooked:

1. The patient must be in good general condition.
2. She should not be elderly and preferably not obese.
3. The disease must be confined to the cervix and/or the immediately adjacent paracervical and paravaginal tissues.

The operation should be reserved for carcinomas in stage I and early stage II in the group of patients who are reasonable operative risks. The role of surgery is thus sharply limited by the extent of the cancer. This is not easily determined, since the examining finger is practically the sole arbiter. Some help may be had from the intravenous pyelogram. Mobility of the uterus and the degree of fixation of the paracervical and paravaginal tissues are the important factors. It is often difficult to tell whether we are dealing with a cancerous infiltration or a fibrosis secondary either to pre-existing disease such as pelvic inflammation or to endometriosis. In some instances it is simply an inflammatory reaction due to ulceration in the cancer or the mere presence of the tumor itself.

We must determine whether the cancer is confined to the cervix or the immediately adjacent areas, for the Wertheim and the Schauta operations are designed to excise safely this extent of disease, but no more. The presence of induration may swing the decision away from surgery. A mobile uterus, on the other hand, may influence a decision in favor, because the lymph nodes may be involved by cancer through embolic spread, despite the fact that the palpable tumor seems to be confined to the cervix on digital examination.

To extend the operative indications to the more obese patient or to one with more extensive cancer is to run the risk of increasing the number of ureterovaginal and vesicovaginal fistulas and, more important, the number of recurrences. The surgeon experienced in this kind of surgery can do the operation with less risk to the patient than the well trained surgeon who has had little experience with the problems of surgery for malignant disease in the pelvis, but the risk is still present.

How Much Surgery Is Needed?   If there is some confusion as to which patients should be offered surgery, there is more about what constitutes adequate surgery. To be successful the operation must encompass the malignant disease process. Since we cannot tell with accuracy how much cancer the patient has, the operation must remove the primary tumor, the intervening lymphatics and the regional lymph nodes. In a recent series of examinations of pathologic specimens removed by radical surgery for stage I carcinomas of the cervix, the patient had more extensive disease than the preoperative estimate in 25 per cent. Study of giant tissue sections obtained from Wertheim and exenteration specimens done for cervical cancer without any preliminary radiation indicates clearly that the spread, in either lymphatic or tissue spaces, tends to follow along the parasympathetic nerves and blood vessels. They may be traced back 3 or 4 cm. in serial sections to nerve ganglia. It is also evident that bulky tumor often extends in a fore-and-aft direction toward the bladder and rectum as much as it does laterally. Finally, nests of tumor cells can be detected lying in lymphatic or tissue spaces in foci remote from the primary tumor of the cervix in the paravesical area deep to the surface bladder epithelium (Fig. 61–19).

If operation is to be performed with the primary aim of curing the patient of her cancer, it must be sufficient in scope to encompass all the regions of potential spread. Many so-called radical surgical operations done today do not fulfill these criteria.

The term "radical hysterectomy and node dissection" is in common use. The word "radical" can be misinterpreted. It suggests that a satisfactory operation can be done by performing a hysterectomy which is a little more extensive than the surgeon is accustomed to perform for benign disease in the uterus and then adding a lymph node dissection. This is radical in terms of the surgeon's experience, but it is not adequate for the malignant disease present. The intervening lymphatics must be removed. Forty of 100 uteri removed by radical operations for cervical cancer had tumor in the paracervical or paravaginal area on at least one side. It was often found on the side that had the least induration. Clinically, palpable infiltration usually proved to be proliferation of connective tissue. These observations point up the difficulties encountered in making a true estimate of the extent of cancer by preoperative examination. The percentage error is not materially reduced by a palpation carried out under anesthesia.

In recent years there has been a tendency to place the emphasis in therapy upon dissection of the lymph nodes with less of a dissection around the bladder and paracervical and vaginal areas. We now know that this is the important area. It will do the patient no good to perform a beautiful regional node dissection if the excision of the tissue adjacent to the cervix has been less than adequate. To remove this area of paracervical and paravaginal tissue is to increase the danger of fistula formation, for this can be a vascular and bloody area. Not to remove it is to run the risk of recurrence. To leave cancer behind with the idea that the patient can then be subjected to radiation therapy is a fallacy. It is the rare case that can be salvaged by subsequent x-ray therapy. The primary extirpative attack is the only good chance the surgeon has to cure the patient, and it had best be adequate.

How Important Is It to Remove the Lymph Nodes? In the previous discussion we pointed out that the dissection of the paracervical and paravaginal areas is more important than the nodal excision, if we are to hope for a cure. This statement should not be construed as a condemnation of lymph node dissection. The regional nodes should be removed, for a 35 per cent salvage rate can be expected among those who have metastatic disease, provided the dissection around the cervix has been adequate.

One of the reasons why surgery has gained favor for the treatment of confined malignant disease is that the regional lymph nodes are found involved in at least 20

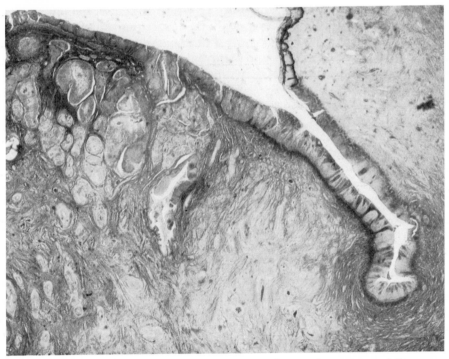

Fig. 61-19. In giant histologic sections of exenteration specimens removed for cancer of the cervix many nests of carcinoma cells, detached from the primary carcinoma, may be found growing beneath the vaginal epithelium.

per cent. There is some doubt that these women can be cured by external radiation. On the other hand, we know that 50 per cent of patients who have positive nodes with carcinomas in stage I, when the disease is confined to the cervix, and 20 per cent of those in stage II, when the disease has spread to the neighboring tissue, will be alive at 5 years. This is tantamount to a permanent salvage, for the 10-year survival rate is only 5 or 6 per cent less than that at 5 years, including patients who have died of intercurrent disease without any recurrence of their cancer.

Radiologists may question the observation that intensive x-ray therapy will not cure metastatic disease in lymph nodes. They point to the fact that 10 per cent fewer positive nodes than expected for the stage of carcinoma are recovered when nodal dissections are done after a complete therapeutic course of radiation. This has not been the general experience, however. The senior author's own experiences with extraperitoneal node dissection after complete radiation by radium and x-ray administered by 250-KV, 450-KV and 1200-KV machines tend to support the contention that radiation does not sterilize the nodes. It is true that the majority of cases were carcinomas in stage II, and therefore they had more extensive disease and possibly a different life history. Nevertheless 28 per cent of positive nodes were recovered after a complete course of radiation. This is about the same expectancy as without radiation therapy.

From the evidence at hand and accumulating as larger series of cases report wider surgical experience, it would appear that surgical excision will result in a reasonable percentage of cures when the cancer is confined to the cervix or the immediately adjacent areas. There is a decreasing incidence of cure when the cancer has spread more extensively.

It should be noted, however, that only 20 to 25 per cent of the patients seen are in the stage I classification, indicating confined disease, and that we cure at best 50 per cent of these. The emphasis in therapy should be placed, therefore, on a painstaking dissection of the paracervical and paravaginal areas rather than on the nodal areas alone, if we are to hope to increase the salvage of patients with cervical cancer.

How Does Lymph Nodal Involvement Relate to Prognosis?   Whether the patient has metastases to the regional nodes is the most important single factor in prognosis. We have pointed out that 50 per cent of patients with cancer confined to the cervix and immediately adjacent tissue will survive 5 or more years after their excision. The percentage of survival drops sharply, however, when the primary disease is more extensive. A 20 per cent 5-year cure rate is about the maximum when the extent of the patient's cancer places her in the category of stage II.

On the other hand, well over 80 per cent of patients in these classifications are salvaged when the lymph nodes are negative for cancer, and an adequate local dissection has been done. To emphasize further the importance of nodal involvement in relation to permanent cure, one can point to the facts that (*a*) 70 per cent of the patients with cancers in stage II who had negative lymph nodes after an extraperitoneal node dissection following complete radiation are alive and well 10 or more years after operations; and (*b*) 62 per cent of patients who had complete exenteration procedures for advanced disease are alive 5 or more years after operation when the lymph nodes were negative for cancer. None of the patients who had positive lymph nodes survived in this group. It is interesting to note that seven of the patients in the total exenteration group are alive without malignant disease ten or more years after operation.

THE RADICAL VAGINAL OPERATION FOR CANCER OF THE CERVIX (SCHAUTA). The radical operation commonly performed in the United States is an abdominal operation that permits extirpation of the entire uterus, intervening lymphatics and regional lymph nodes. The Schauta operation accomplishes the same thing through the vaginal approach, except that the regional lymph nodes are left untouched.

In many foreign clinics and in some treatment centers in this country radical removal of the uterus is carried out through the vagina. To the surgeon trained in this type of surgery it is possible to do a complete removal of the uterus and adjacent lymphatic tissue. It has two obvious disadvantages: (1) the regional lymph nodes are not removed, and (2) the problem of unsuspected cancer involvement of the bladder cannot be adequately dealt with through the vaginal approach. Retroperitoneal node dissections three or more weeks after operation are now being done in many clinics. The procedure has a real place in the obese patient who has cancer confined to the cervix of a mobile uterus.

WHAT ARE THE DISADVANTAGES OF SURGERY? The chief disadvantage of the surgical approach is the morbidity that follows extensive surgery in and around the bladder. This manifests itself chiefly in two ways: (1) the possibility of ureterovaginal and vesicovaginal fistulas, and (2) bladder atony and consequent dysfunction. These are serious drawbacks to the surgical approach. Both are definite possibilities if adequate surgery is to be done. The remaining complications are traceable to sepsis that may be present within the wound or deep in the pelvis. On rare occasions this may lead to wound disruption or to pelvic thrombophlebitis.

Fistula. Ureterovaginal or vesicovaginal fistulas are by far the most undesirable sequelae of radical surgical procedures for cervical cancer. Together with pyelitis and pyelonephritis they also are the most frequent complications to appear. The incidence is in the neighborhood of 10 to 12 per cent. The more extensive the cancer, the greater the chance that fistulas will develop.

Ureterovaginal Fistulas. Although the surgeon makes every attempt to avoid the subsequent development of a fistula by (a) delicate handling of the ureter in the course of its dissection, (b) leaving the ureter in contact with the peritoneum as far as possible, (c) making omental flaps to surround the ureter, (d) translocating the ureters from their usual retroperitoneal position, (e) providing catheter drainage of the retroperitoneal space after operation, and (f) using constant drainage through an inlying catheter for several months after the operation, ureterovaginal fistulas continue to plague the surgeon.

Unfortunately it is not entirely a question of familiarity with the technique of the operation. The percentage of fistulas seems to rise in inverse proportion to the experience of the operator. The surgeon who is well informed recognizes that the paracervical tissue through which the ureter runs must be removed if he is to do an adequate operation, realizing full well that he is running the risk of getting a fistula. The less experienced operator will avoid fistulas and bladder atony by doing an incomplete operation.

One might expect that the incidence of fistula formation would decline as surgical experience increased, but unfortunately the percentage (roughly 10) seems to remain fairly constant. In most instances it is not the damage produced at the time of operation that leads to the development of the fistula. The majority occur in the ten-day to two-week period following the operation, however careful the surgeon is with his technique. The fistulas appear because of tissue necrosis secondary to the loss of blood supply to the lower end of the ureter. The more cancer the patient has, the greater also the chance of making a false opening.

The ureterovaginal fistula will often heal spontaneously if full bladder drainage is constantly maintained by use of an inlying catheter that drains into a thigh urinal. It may repair itself in three weeks or take as long as three months. If the fistula does not close, the surgeon has the option of (*a*) trying to reimplant the ureter into the dome of the bladder, or (*b*) doing a nephrectomy. Nephrectomy is preferred if there is any element of obstruction or pyelonephritis.

Vesicovaginal Fistula. A fistula may also form between the bladder and the vagina. This is usually due to extensive dissection around the base of the bladder. Weak spots are set up in the bladder wall, and tissue necrosis produced through interruption of the blood supply also contributes. The vesicovaginal fistula, unlike the ureterovaginal type, rarely ever heals spontaneously, however small it may be. Almost invariably these will have to be closed surgically. Because of the inconvenience to the patient caused by the continual urine leakage through the vagina, the surgeon is often stampeded into attempting to close the fistula too soon after operation. The operator will make a foolish move if he attempts any kind of plastic repair before four to six months have passed. The tissues need time to recover, and a new blood supply is an essential requirement to successful repair. Done at the proper time, the fistula can be satisfactorily closed in most instances.

Cortisone Therapy. When the blood supply is not an important factor, the time between the appearance of the fistula and its repair may be reduced by giving cortisone, 100 mg. 3 times daily for 10 to 12 days. The induration of tissue in and about the fistula is thereby materially reduced. Operative attempts to cure the fistula may then be undertaken in four to six weeks. It is the general experience, however, that fistulas secondary to intensive radiation damage or extensive surgery have a large element of deficient blood supply. The results of cortisone therapy in this group are much less dramatic, and the surgeon faced with this problem will do better if he delays his attempts at surgical repair for several months.

Bladder Atony.   Because the nerve supply to the bladder is jeopardized in the course of the operation, and fibrosis around the neck of the bladder occurs as a natural part of the postoperative repair process, the patient frequently has bladder atony and occasionally a stress incontinence.

Bladder atony is unavoidable if an adequate operation has been done. The older the patient, the more trouble she has with this complication. A few patients have been able to void only in the standing position and with the assistance of hand pressure over the pubis. Recovery is usually complete after some months, although some patients are unable to tell when the bladder is full. Because of the lack of tone in the bladder wall in the weeks immediately following operation we have followed Meigs's plan of leaving an inlying catheter in place to drain freely into a thigh urinal. This is removed in two months. By this time the bladder musculature has had some return of function, although there is still enough impairment to have the patient follow a schedule of voiding every two hours by the clock, whether she has any urge to do so or not.

Stress Incontinence.   This is a late sequel which may prove so troublesome that a bladder neck suspension of the Marshall-Marchetti type is indicated. Why this occurs in certain patients is not entirely clear, but the cause is probably mechanical. A large part of the vaginal canal is removed in this operation. In the repair stage the anterior wall adheres to the posterior, forming a pointed, foreshortened vagina with the apex of the cone at the top. This tends to put the neck of the bladder on traction in such a manner that the posterior angle of bladder to urethra is lost, and stress incontinence follows. The muscle-setting exercises recommended in a later section (p. 1042) may be tried before recommending bladder neck suspension.

Other Complications. The Wertheim operation and lymph node removal call for a wide dissection of the pelvic contents. Despite drainage through the open vagina, hematomas are apt to form. Occasionally they become infected, producing cellulitis, abscess and rarely thrombophlebitis. Antibiotics coupled with transfusions usually correct the infection. Rarely is drainage necessary. Some authorities have recommended cortisone therapy for the firm, boardlike cellulitis that may on rare occasion produce enough fibrosis to obstruct the ureteral flow.

WHAT SALVAGE CAN BE EXPECTED FROM THE WERTHEIM AND SCHAUTA OPERATIONS? *Wertheim Operation.* We have noted that the choice of therapy and the prognosis depend on the extent of the disease. The Wertheim hysterectomy and bilateral lymphadenectomy and also the Schauta operation combined with extraperitoneal node dissection are designed to encompass the amount of cancer which places cases in the categories of stage I and early stage II. Technically, it is possible to extend the operation to cases with late stage II and III lesions, but the five-year salvage drops appreciably. The morbidity and the number of fistulas are increased, and more local cancer recurrences appear also.

Meigs, who is largely responsible for the return of the radical surgical therapy for cancer of the cervix, reports an 82 per cent survival rate for stage I lesions, but only a 62 per cent alive and well at 5 years for stage II. In stage I only 18 per cent have positive lymph nodes, of which he salvaged 42 per cent. There were more cases with metastases to regional lymph nodes in stage II (32 per cent), but only a 9 per cent salvage rate.

There has been some criticism about the reporting of surgical results, because in many series radiation therapy has also been used either before or after the operation. Recently we reported on a series of eighty patients in whom no radiation of any sort was used, and all patients with a positive invasive carcinoma biopsy in whom no disease was found in the postoperative Wertheim specimen were excluded. The operations were tailored to the amount of disease the patient had. The Wertheim operations were performed for carcinomas, stage I (confined to the cervix) and stage IIa (the disease had left the immediate confines of the cervix to involve the paracervical area and upper vaginal epithelium). A few Wertheim operations were done for patients who were classified as carcinomas, stage IIb. Patients in stages III and IV were subjected either to anterior exenteration (Wertheim dissection plus removal of the bladder) or total exenteration (Wertheim excision plus removal of both the bladder and the rectum).

The results are interesting, comparing favorably with those of Meigs, Brunschwig and others who subscribe to the more extensive pelvic dissections, and tend to support the contention that the Wertheim operation should be restricted largely to the cancers in stages I and early IIa. The salvage rate for the combined cases of stages of I and IIa was 79 per cent, with a 67 per cent survival in stage II. A casual glance would suggest that the Wertheim operation did very well for stage II, but when this is broken down into early IIa and more extensive disease IIb, it becomes obvious that the Wertheim procedure was satisfactory for the former (85 per cent salvage), but far from satisfactory for the latter (43 per cent). In cancers in stage I 50 per cent of patients with positive lymph nodes survived 5 years, but only 20 per cent of patients who had regional nodes containing cancer in stage II survived. All the cancer recurrences and most of the fistulas occurred when attempts were made to extend the indications for the Wertheim operation to patients with stage II disease. The improved salvage rate in cancers in stage IIa over IIb suggests that the operation satisfactorily encompasses the total extent of malignant disease in the former, but not in the latter. This is true regardless of the number of patients with lymph nodes involved by cancer.

The magnitude of the dissection for cancer of the cervix varies widely in this country and abroad. Table 11 lists some of the end-results as published by different centers in the recent literature.

The foreign experience can be scanned by reviewing the results reported in the above-mentioned *Annual Reports on the Results of Treatment in Carcinoma of the Uterus.* In the eleventh volume of this report it is noted that 5030 cervical carcinoma patients were treated by hysterectomy with or without preoperative irradiation in the years 1947–1951. The surgical cure rate for carcinomas in stage I was 74 per cent as compared to 65 per cent for radiation therapy. In stage II cancers surgery salvaged 56

Table 11.   Experience of 86 Institutions in Treatment of Carcinoma of the Cervix, 1947–1951

Total number of patients treated	42,130
Number of patients alive with no disease	18,031 (42.8%)

STAGE I

Total number of patients treated	9087 (21.3%)
Number of survivors without disease at 5 years	6120 (56.3%)
Total operations performed for stage I	2746 (30%)
Number of patients without disease at 5 years	2016 (74%)
Number of patients having radiation treatment	6323 (70%)
Number of patients without disease at 5 years	4104 (65%)
Mean average survival	68.5%

STAGE II

Total number of patients treated	16,046
Number of survivors without disease at 5 years	7,797 (48.6%)
Total operations performed for stage II	2,284 (14%)
Number of patients without disease at 5 years	1,268 (55.5%)
Number of patients having radiation treatment	13,762 (86%)
Number of patients without disease at 5 years	6,528 (47.8%)
Mean average survival	48%

STAGE III

Total number of patients treated	14,387
Number of survivors	3,914 (26.5%)
Total operations performed for stage III	262 (2%)
Number of patients surviving operation	81 (30%)
Mean average survival	23.5%

STAGE IV

Total number of patients	2986
Number of patients without disease at 5 years	201
Mean average survival	6.9%

per cent as against 48 per cent for radiation. When stages I and II were combined, the 5-year surgical survival rate was 65 per cent compared with 52 per cent for radiation. In comparing results obtained from the two methods of therapy we must keep in mind that three times as many stage I cancers and six times the number in stage II had radiation treatment. The surgical cases are obviously a selected group.

The disciples of radiation therapy see no reason to consider surgery when radiation does as well and carries less mortality and morbidity. The comparison of the best in surgery with the best in radiation, however, gives encouragement to those who prefer the operative approach. For example, Meigs cured 82 per cent of a large series when the malignant disease was confined to the cervix, and 62 per cent when the cancer had spread to the lymphatic areas around the cervix. In our series the total salvage rate for all stages of disease, including cancer cases in stages III and IV, was 65 per cent. In stage I the survival rate was 78 per cent, and 67 per cent for stage II.

Surgery as the sole definitive form of treatment has a rightful place in the treatment of cancer of the cervix. The dissection must be adequate, and to get the best results the extent of the surgical excision should be tailored to the amount of carcinoma the patient has.

Schauta Operation. It is difficult to evaluate the results of the Schauta operation, because in many large series preliminary radiation therapy has been given. Again, the operation is primarily designed for stage I and II carcinomatous lesions. The majority of cases in stage III and all patients in stage IV are treated by irradiation. Mitra, for example, reports a 50 per cent salvage rate for cancers in stages I and II, as against 75 per cent for Meigs. Some of the discrepancy may be traced to the fact that Mitra, operating in India, has not been able to trace all his patients. Some of the patients considered dead may well be alive. The operability rate is higher for the group treated by the Schauta operation (76 per cent), while only 60 per cent of Meigs's cases were in the operable group. It is also true that the Schauta operation, as originally performed, made no attempt to remove the regional lymph nodes. In the survival figures quoted by Meigs, six of twenty-three patients with nodes positive for cancer that were excised survived five or more years. The extra-peritoneal lymphadenectomy is too recent an addition to the Schauta operation to give any idea of the salvage rate that can be expected from the combined techniques.

The one conclusion that appears to be valid is that an adequate dissection for the primary cervical tumor and the areas immediately adjacent to it will produce a respectable number of five-year cures.

WHAT DO THE EXENTERATION OPERATIONS HAVE TO OFFER AS DEFINITIVE THERAPY? The partial or total removal of all the pelvic contents, coupled with a variety of methods of creating urinary diversion, is called partial or total exenteration. It was first proposed and performed by Brunschwig and is a relatively new approach to the surgical treatment of cervical cancer. The total exenteration operation calls for the excision en bloc of uterus, adnexa, bladder, rectum, vagina and vulva, together with a bilateral pelvic lymphadenectomy. The anterior exenteration removes all the organs mentioned above, but leaves the rectum intact. In both procedures it is necessary to divert the urinary stream by (a) creating a new bladder out of an isolated segment of ileum and transplanting the ureters into it, (b) performing a uretero-intestinal anastomosis into the sigmoid colon with or without an accompanying colostomy. If a tranverse colostomy is performed, the urinary drainage is no longer in contact with the fecal stream, and the chances of ascending infection, pyelonephritis and hyperchloremic acidosis due to electrolyte imbalance are minimized. Or (*c*) it is feasible to bring the ureters out to the skin as skin ureterostomies.

The rationale of these extensive procedures is based on the fact that cancer of the cervix is primarily a local disease. If the excision is extensive enough, it should be possible to remove all the malignant disease and to obtain some salvage in a group of patients who have little chance to survive by any other kind of treatment. For example, the anticipated salvage in stages III and IV carcinomas treated by radiation therapy is at best not much better than 20 per cent. In the majority of instances the radiologist treats such patients with the primary aim of palliation, not cure.

This sort of procedure was originally applied to patients who had had a full course of radiation and either were not responsive or later had a recurrence. When it was noted that (*a*) patients could survive such extensive surgery, (*b*) they could return to a happy useful life, and (*c*) survive for an appreciable time—a fair number have now lived 10 years or more, and 25 per cent survived 5 years—the operation was offered to those who had extensive disease in lieu of radiation therapy.

This is not an operation that should be undertaken lightly. It is a formidable surgical procedure which taxes the ability of all concerned with patient care both before, during and after operation. The problems in the convalescent period may be as troublesome as those encountered at the time of operation.

Despite these obvious disadvantages there is a logical place for this type of ultra-radical surgery in the treatment of extensive cervical cancer. In addition, sometimes the surgeon attempting to perform a Wertheim dissection for what was believed to be a stage I or IIa cancer may find that there is more malignant disease than he anticipated. There is little point in persisting in this type of excision if it is apparent that gross disease will be left behind. The choice must be made at the operating table (*a*) to abandon the dissection and mark the obvious extent of the tumor with dura clips so that the radiologist can have a better target for direction of the external radiation, or (*b*) to extend the operation to include either bladder or bladder and rectum, depending on the extent and direction of spread of the tumor.

An insufficient number of patients have had operations in the distant past to give more than indications of what can be accomplished in terms of long-time survival, but the results to date have been encouraging. A 33 per cent 5-year survival may be expected in the small group so far reported. It is surprising how many of these patients have negative lymph nodes despite their advanced stage of disease. When the nodes are negative, the long-term salvage rate is in the range of 62 per cent.

Combination of Radiation Therapy and Surgery

The initial attack on cancer of the cervix should be carefully planned. Taking all factors into consideration, the physician should choose either radiation or surgery and stick to it, giving the best treatment possible. It is unwise to embark on a course of therapy with the idea that if it fails, recourse can be had to its counterpart, whether radiation or surgery.

Nevertheless there is a place for the combination of radiation and surgery, as follows:

1. A trial dose of radiation may be undertaken with serial cervical biopsies and smears. This has been discussed (p. 915).

2. A partial dose of radiation is given as a preliminary step to definitive treatment by radical surgery.

3. In certain clinics radical surgery is being performed after full radiation treatment.

4. Surgical attacks on the regional lymph nodes are made either transabdominally or extraperitoneally before or after completion of full irradiation.

5. Appropriate surgery for the extent of the disease present is essential for the case already proved to be radiation-resistant.

6. Associated abnormalities may complicate therapy, making it necessary to carry out a combined surgical and radiation attack.

In specific situations surgery is often combined with radiation as follows:

1. Retroperitoneal or transabdominal dissection of the regional lymph nodes may be done either before or after a full course of radiation by radium and x-ray. The rationale for this approach is based upon the questionable value of x-rays to destroy cancer in regional nodes.

2. Full irradiation is followed by the Wertheim procedure and pelvic lymphadenectomy in certain clinics. This is done to eliminate a faulty substrate which may lead to reappearance of the tumor. It also minimizes the danger of implant metastasis through handling of the cancer at operation.

3. The *radiation-resistant* case is a problem. To test for radiation resistance a trial dose of radium may be given, followed by the Wertheim operation and pelvic lymphadenectomy or a pelvic exenteration, depending on the extent of the disease.

4. The recurrence of cancer in a local area may offer an opportunity for the Wertheim operation and pelvic lymphadenectomy in lieu of further radiation.

5. In selected patients with far-advanced cancer or recurrence after completed radiation therapy the pelvic exenteration operation may be tried.

RADICAL SURGERY FOLLOWING FULL RADIATION THERAPY.   The rationale of this approach is based on too many local recurrences that appear after full irradiation. To avoid cancer recurrence or the appearance of new growth, radical surgery is performed to remove the uterus and adjacent lymphatics as well as the lymph nodes.

It has obvious disadvantages. There are dangers in this form of therapy. It is not a question of technical facility or familiarity with the operative procedure. In many instances surgery in a previously irradiated field is surprisingly easy. The disappointments come in the higher percentage of complications, such as fistulas which appear not because of the technical difficulties encountered at the time of operation, but from the inadequacy of the blood supply when surgery follows full irradiation. It would seem more logical to direct more attention to the radiation techniques in order to reduce the incidence of local recurrence or to determine the sensitivity of the tumor.

RADICAL SURGERY FOLLOWING PARTIAL RADIATION THERAPY.   This procedure has merit where there is bulky tumor arising from the cervix, but confined to it with minimal spread to the adjacent tissue. A preliminary dose of local radium or a transvaginal course of x-ray therapy will reduce the bulk of the tumor and seal the lymphatics, so that cells will not seed in the operative site as the carcinoma is handled in the course of operation.

In many clinics a preliminary course of radiation is given, using half the usual amount of radium, as a preliminary step to the definitive radical surgery.

LYMPH NODE DISSECTION FOLLOWING A FULL COURSE OF RADIATION.   Based on the assumption that irradiation may not destroy malignant disease in lymph nodes, surgical removal is undertaken, either transabdominally or by the extraperitoneal approach. A sufficient period of time, usually three months, is allowed to pass to be certain that the local disease is controlled by radiation.

Taussig first advocated the transabdominal approach. The primary tumor and the intervening lymphatics are left undisturbed. Radiation is expected to take care of the disease in these areas. The node dissection is simply an adjunct to full radiation therapy. These lymph nodes can best be removed by using the extra-abdominal approach as advocated by Nathanson. The operation has a wider application, since it can be performed with less risk in the obese patient.

Recently a number of clinics have performed pelvic lymphadenectomy as a preliminary step to full radiation therapy. Again this may be done either trans-abdominally or extraperitoneally. The chief advantage of this mode of attack lies in the fact that radiation can be concentrated on the site of the primary tumor and the immediate pathways of extension from it. Theoretically, the complications should be fewer, for the lymph nodes are dissected from a nonirradiated field.

The combination of radiation therapy and surgery for the radiation-resistant case and for the patient who has associated abnormalities will be discussed under Treatment of Cancer Recurrences.

SUMMARY. The end-results from the combination of x-radiation and surgery bring forth the same observations that appear when either one is used as the sole definitive method of therapy. If the lymph nodes are negative, an 80 per cent salvage rate can be expected, in contrast to the 35 per cent survival in the group whose nodes are positive. The incidence of complications, however, tends to rise when radiation is used in conjunction with surgery, owing for the most part to the likelihood of tissue necrosis as the blood supply is jeopardized.

Cancer of the Cervical Stump

For many years and for adequate reasons total hysterectomy was considered the treatment of choice when there were indications for removal of the uterus. Many supra-vaginal operations are still done, however. Cancer arises in the cervical stump after this operation in about the same incidence that one may expect from the population at large. Some were obviously present at the time operation was performed, others develop later. The chance of cancer appearing in the remaining portion of the cervix increases if chronic infection existed at the time of the original subtotal operation.

The presence of cancer in the cervical stump complicates therapy, for there is no protection of normal tissue to shield the bladder and the rectum from the penetrating radiation. Proctitis and cystitis develop so frequently that the dosage of local radium to the cervix must be halved to prevent overirradiation and the possibility of vesico-vaginal or rectovaginal fistulas. Though external radiation may be given in full amounts, it must be administered cautiously, because both the small and the large bowel may be adherent to the cervical stump as the result of previous pelvic surgery. Radiation damage to the intestine is a danger. When the malignant disease is confined to the cervix, it may be best to resort to surgery. When it is more extensive, one must assume the risks inherent in irradiating this kind of case.

Treatment of Cancer Recurrences

Unfortunately the best in radiation therapy or surgery is not always greeted by a favorable response. Many of these cancer patients are relatively young women with growing families. If nothing further is done, they will live on the average of fourteen months. Since the cervical carcinoma tends to remain confined to the pelvis, there is a great temptation to attempt additional therapy.

There are two methods of therapy that may reasonably be considered. Radiation is the most readily available instrument and the method commonly used.

The dangers of x-radiation magnify when further radiation is added in the patient who has a cancer recurrence after a previous adequate course of radiation. In general the longevity is not increased, and the patient may be made more miserable. If the recurrence appears in an isolated area within the vagina, it is justifiable to give a surface radium application or to infiltrate the area with interstitial radon needles, provided only a small dose is given. This should not exceed 1000 mg.-hours. To give more intense local radiation or further x-ray therapy is to increase the danger of tissue necrosis.

If the previous radiation has been inadequate by common standards, which roughly are 5000 mg.-hours of radium and 4000 roentgens tumor dose by x-ray machine (7000 gamma roentgens total tumor dose), it is reasonable to attempt to give further radiation. Experience with this type of radiation is most disheartening and emphasizes the fact that the only good time to treat a patient is in the first course of x-irradiation.

The most recent addition to therapy for recurrent cancer is either the Wertheim procedure or the ultraradical pelvic exenteration operations suggested by Brunschwig for radiation failures. We recently completed a series of 100 cases of patients with cancer of the cervix who had a recurrence after radiation therapy. The magnitude of surgery was tailored to the amount of disease the patient had. It is interesting that the patients had more, rather than less, disease when the operative specimens were classified according to the tenets set up by Meigs and Brunschwig for evaluation of the extent of disease following surgery. The 5-year survival rate for 80 of the 100 patients (done over 5 years ago) was approximately 35 per cent.

WERTHEIM OPERATION. When the recurrent malignant disease appeared to be localized to the upper part of the vagina and cervix and did not encroach on the bladder or rectum, the Wertheim hysterectomy and a pelvic lymph node dissection were used instead of local radium application or external irradiation. The advantage of the surgical approach lies in the fact that it removes the entire vaginal canal and lymphatic pathways as well as the nodes, which may harbor trapped malignant cells. The obvious area of recurrence may represent only one site, while others are more remote or hidden from view and inaccessible to palpation. In the series of cases mentioned above the 5-year salvage rate for the Wertheim operation was better than 65 per cent. Eighty per cent of the patients with negative lymph nodes and four of nine patients with metastatic disease in nodes are alive and well without evidence of disease, five or more years after the operation.

PELVIC EXENTERATION. The ultraradical pelvic exenteration operation is reserved for extensive disease persistent or recurrent after radiation. The details of the different types of exenteration and the methods used to provide urinary diversion have been described (p. 941).

These are formidable surgical procedures which carry an operative mortality rate as high as 25 per cent. They should only be done by a surgeon with a wide experience with this sort of operation. A great strain is placed on the hospital, nursing and laboratory facilities to ensure a successful outcome. The problems of the postoperative period are as fraught with difficulty as the actual details of the operation.

Since lethal amounts of neoplastic disease may be present in the pelvis without any spread to remote areas, the operation is a rational approach for those cases previously regarded as hopeless. The operation has been performed in sufficient numbers for a long enough time to evaluate it in terms of end-results. We now know that these cancer patients can receive valuable palliation and have a 25 per cent chance of living 5 or more years, despite the high initial mortality rate from the operation. In the past all these patients would be dead. More important, perhaps, is the fact the patients can return to their former occupations and live useful, happy lives. Seven of thirty-seven patients in our own series are alive and active after ten years.

The likelihood of success increases if the cancer has spread anteriorly or posteriorly to involve bladder and rectum, rather than laterally. It is amazing how few of these patients with extensive disease have nodal involvement. In an experience totaling nearly 150 cases, metastases to regional lymph nodes have been found in only 42 per cent. When the nodes have been involved, we have obtained satisfactory palliation in many instances, but no five-year salvage. The 25 per cent salvage rate can be attributed to the fact that a complete excision of all tumor-bearing areas had been accomplished, together with the fact that these patients were free of regional lymph node metastases.

These operations have a restricted place in the treatment of cervical cancer and will be chiefly of value in the patients who have (*a*) radiation therapeutic failures, (*b*) vesicovaginal or rectovaginal fistulas, either as the result of cancer or irradiation, and (*c*) in a limited group whose cancers have recurred after inadequate surgery. Although there is palliation to be had from these operations, they should be undertaken with the idea of curing the patient, not palliating her. In too many instances the complications are so severe and prolonged that the patient has too little time to profit from her palliation before she succumbs to her disease.

How to Manage the Hopeless Cervical Cancer Case?

The majority of patients with extensive cancers are not suitable candidates for the pelvic exenteration operation. Uremia is the commonest cause of death from cancer of the cervix. Unless complicated by intractable pain or hemorrhage, it is an easy form of death. There is an axiom in surgery that it is well to let the patient pick her own way to die. If we cannot cure, and palliation can be accomplished only at the price of further trauma, we had best direct our energies toward the alleviation of the most distressing symptoms.

The most troublesome problem the cancer patient has to face is pain. Mental suffering also plays a part. Attractive surroundings and sympathetic care provide some relief. The patients are usually anemic, and high protein diets and occasional transfusions may be given to improve their condition. These should be given with the main purpose of making the patient more comfortable, rather than trying to prolong existence. Blood loss may reach hemorrhagic proportions frightening to the patient. Diethylstilbestrol has a hemostatic effect in moderate doses. If the bleeding is still excessive, one may consider ligation of the internal iliac arteries. When fistulas develop, constant nursing care is required to prevent distressing ulcerations of the skin produced by the discharges.

One may elect to try hormone therapy in the form of testosterone, given either orally or parenterally. Testosterone propionate, 75 mg. weekly by injection, or oral methyltestosterone, 25 mg. daily, is helpful largely because of the protein-sparing effect of testosterone. Cervical carcinoma is not hormone-dependent, and the hormones have only supportive action.

Relief of pain is the most urgent need. When the patient with advanced cancer of the cervix has pain, there is a real problem in management. Since the pain is severe and continuous, the tolerance to drugs increases rapidly, so that larger doses of opiates are necessary to obtain relief. Unless some vital structure becomes involved or hemorrhage occurs through invasion of a major vessel, the patient may live a year or more. Supportive treatment must be planned to ensure the patient's comfort over a long time. It is better at the outset to rely on the relief that can be obtained from analgesics supplemented by codeine or Demerol. These drugs will not suffice for long, but it is best to begin the long voyage in this way rather than rely too early in the terminal illness upon morphine. The morphine habit is quickly established. Heavier and heavier doses are required, and soon there is the problem of sufficient food intake and bowel elimination.

Cordotomy may be a great boon to the cancer patient who has intense pain that cannot be adequately controlled by morphine. In the past it was offered too late in the course of the disease to be of any lasting value. The operation carries with it the risk of excessive spinal cord damage as the spinothalamic tracts in the thoracic region are severed. Mobility, and bladder and bowel elimination may be altered as a result. To the patient who is likely to suffer intensely for many months, relief of pain is adequate compensation for the risks taken. Cordotomy should be performed more often and much earlier in the terminal phases of the incurable form of this disease.

REFERENCES

General Information

Arneson, A. N.: Presidential Address—Responsibilities of the Obstetrician-Gynecologist in the Treatment of Uterine Cancer. Am. J. Obst. & Gynec., 79: 833, 1960.
Ayer, J. E., Castillo, A., Rogers, W. S., and Jack, R.: Conservative Surgery for Early Cervical Cancer in Young Women. Obst. & Gynec., 10: 544, 1957.
Blaikley, J. B., Lederman, M., and Simmons, C. A.: Surgery or Radium for Cancer. Lancet, 1: 159, 1958.
Clayton, R. S. S.: Carcinoma of the Cervix Uteri—Ten Year Study with Comparison of Results of Irradiation and Radical Surgery. Radiology, 68: 74, 1957.
Decker, D. G.: The Management of Invasive Carcinoma of the Cervix. S. Clin. N. Amer., 39: 1061, 1959.
Del Regato, J. A.: Comparative Results of Surgery and Radiotherapy in Carcinoma of the Cervix. J. Lancet, 77: 454, 1957.
Fricke, R. E., and Decker, D. G.: Treatment and Prognosis in Elderly Patients with Cancer of the Cervix. J. Am. Geriat. Soc., 5: 183, 1957.
Graber, E. A., and O'Rourke, J. J.: Therapy in Gynecological Cancers: A Re-evaluation. Obst. & Gynec., 14: 714, 1959.
Holzaepfel, J. H., and Ezell, H. E.: Carcinoma of the Cervix: A Preventable Disease. West. J. Surg., Obst. & Gynec., 68: 378, 1960.
Horne, H. W., Jr.: Carcinoma of the Cervix Uteri. 1926-1948, Obst. & Gynec., 9: 167, 1957.
Kottmeier, H. L. (ed.): Annual Report on the Results of Treatment in Carcinoma of the Uterus. Stockholm, P. A. Norstedt & Sons, 1957, Vol. 11.
Idem: Current Treatment of Carcinoma of the Cervix. Am. J. Obst. & Gynec., 76: 243, 1958.
Lund, C. J.: An Epitaph for Cervical Carcinoma. J.A.M.A., 175: 98, 1961.
Meigs, J. V.: Editorial: Carcinoma of the Cervix. Surg., Gynec. & Obst., 108: 616, 1959.
Schlink, H.: Cancer of the Female Pelvis. J. Obst. & Gynaec. Brit. Emp., 67: 402, 1960.

Stallworthy, J.: Uterine Cancer—Advances and Unsolved Problems in Treatment. *Northwest. M.J.,* 57: 719, 1958.

Strand, C. M., and Wheelock, M. C.: Ratio of Cervical Carcinoma to Corpus Carcinoma. *Obst. & Gynec.,* 4: 380, 1954.

Twombly, G. H.: When Shall We Use Radical Hysterectomy and When Irradiation Therapy in the Treatment of Cancer of the Cervix?; in J. H. Mulholland, E. H. Ellison and S. R. Friesen, eds.: *Current Surgical Management.* Philadelphia, W. B. Saunders Company, 1957, p. 332.

Wall, J. A., Mastrovito, R., and Earl, D. M.: The Team Approach in Cervical Neoplasia. *Am. J. Obst. & Gynec.,* 75: 606, 1958.

Epidemiology

Christopherson, W. M., and Parker, J. E.: A Study of the Relative Frequency of Carcinoma of the Cervix in the Negro. *Cancer,* 13: 711, 1960.

Diaz-Bezan, N.: Cancer del cuello uterino associado con prolapso total en El Salvador. Revision de la literatura y reporte complementario de 25 casos. Extrait due Deuxième Congrès International de Gynecologie et d'Obstetrique de Montréal en 1958, 1:226, 1958.

Dorn, H. F., and Cutler, S. J.: Morbidity from Cancer in the United States. Washington, D.C., U.S. Department of Health, Education and Welfare, Public Health Monograph No. 29, 1955.

Dougherty, C. M.: Morbidity from Cancer of the Uterus in East Baton Rouge Parish. *Obst. & Gynec.,* 16: 535, 1960.

Dunn, J. E., Jr., and Buell, P.: Association of Cervical Cancer with Circumcision of Sexual Partner. *J. Nat. Cancer Inst.,* 22: 749, 1959.

Editorial: Epidemiology of Cancer of the Cervix. *J.A.M.A.,* 174: 1852, 1960.

Gagnon, F.: Contribution to the Study of the Etiology and Prevention of Cancer of the Cervix of the Uterus. *Am. J. Obst. & Gynec.,* 60: 516, 1950.

Idem: The Lack of Occurrence of Cervical Carcinoma in Nuns. *Proc. Second Nat. Cancer Conf.,* 1: 625, 1952.

Haenzel, W., and Hilhouse, M.: Uterine Cancer Morbidity in New York City and Its Relation to the Pattern of Regionlal Variation within the United States. *J. Nat. Cancer Inst.,* 22: 1157, 1959.

Heins, H. C., Jr., Dennis, E. J., and Pratt-Thomas, H. R.: Possible Role of Smegma in Carcinoma of the Cervix. *Am. J. Obst. & Gynec.,* 76: 726, 1958.

Hochman, A., Ratzkowski, E., and Schreiber, H.: Incidence of Carcinoma of the Cervix in Jewish Women in Israel. *Brit. J. Cancer,* 9: 358, 1955.

Jones, E. G., MacDonald, I., and Breslow, L.: Study of Epidemiologic Factors in Carcinoma of the Uterine Cervix. *Am. J. Obst. & Gynec.,* 76: 1, 1958.

Kaiser, R. F., and Gilliam, A. G.: Some Epidemiological Aspects of Cervical Cancer. *Pub. Health Rep.,* 73: 359, 1958.

Levin, M. L., Kress, L. C., and Goldstein, H.: Syphilis and Cancer: Reported Syphilis Prevalence among 7761 Cancer Patients. *New York State J.M.,* 42: 1737, 1942.

Lombard, H. L., and Potter, E. A.: Epidemiological Aspects of Cancer of the Cervix. II. Hereditary and Environmental Factors. *Cancer,* 3: 960, 1950.

Pereyra, A. J.: The Relationship of Sexual Activity to Cervical Cancer: Cancer of the Cervix in a Prison Population. *Obst. & Gynec.,* 17: 154, 1961.

Pollack, R. S., and Taylor, H. C., Jr.: Carcinoma of the Cervix during the First Two Decades of Life. *Am. J. Obst. & Gynec.,* 53: 135, 1947.

Rao, P. S., Reddy, R. S., and Reddy, D. J.: Study of Aetiological Factors in Carcinoma of the Cervix Uteri in Guntur. *J. Indian M.A.,* 32: 463, 1959.

Rotkin, I. D.: Studies on the Inheritance of Cancer of the Human Uterine Cervix. *Cancer,* 14: 179, 1961.

Stern, E., and Dixon, W. J.: Cancer of the Cervix: A Biometric Approach to Etiology. *Cancer,* 14: 153, 1961.

Stocks, P.: Cancer of the Uterine Cervix and Social Conditions. *Brit. J. Cancer,* 9: 487, 1955.

Towne, J. E.: Carcinoma of the Cervix in Nulliparous and Celibate Women. *Am. J. Obst. & Gynec.,* 69: 606, 1955.

Weiner, I. L., Burke, L., and Goldberger, M. A.: Carcinoma of the Cervix in Jewish Women. *Am. J. Obst. & Gynec.,* 61: 418, 1951.

Wynder, E. L., and Licklider, S. D.: The Question of Circumcision. *Cancer,* 13: 442, 1960.

Wynder, E. L., Mantel, N., and Licklider, S. D.: Statistical Considerations on Circumcision and Cervical Cancer. *Am. J. Obst. & Gynec.,* 79: 1026, 1960.

Life History

Brunschwig, A., and Pierce, V.: Necropsy Findings in Patients with Carcinoma of the Cervix. Implications for Treatment. *Am. J. Obst. & Gynec.*, 56: 1134, 1948.

Burns, B. C., Jr., Everett, H. S., and Brack, C. B.: Value of Urologic Study in the Management of Carcinoma of the Cervix. *Am. J. Obst. & Gynec.*, 80: 997, 1960.

De Alvarez, R.: The Causes of Death in Cancer of the Cervix Uteri. *Am. J. Obst. & Gynec.*, 54: 91, 1947.

Diddle, A. W., O'Connor, K. A., and Jenkins, H. H.: Cervical Carcinoma: Growth and Spread and Some Adjunctive Therapeutic Measures. *Am. J. Obst. & Gynec.*, 81: 166, 1961.

Dodds, J. R., and Latour, J. P.: Relationship of Age to Survival Rate in Carcinoma of the Cervix. *Am. J. Obst. & Gynec.*, 82: 33, 1961.

Fluhmann, C. F.: Squamo-Columnar Transitional Zone of Cervix Uteri. *Obst. & Gynec.*, 14: 133, 1959.

Friedell, G. H., and Parsons, L.: The Spread of Cancer of the Uterine Cervix Seen in Giant Histological Sections. *Cancer*, 14: 42, 1961.

Gusberg, S. B., and Corscaden, J. A.: The Pathology and Treatment of Adenocarcinoma of the Cervix. *Cancer*, 4: 1066, 1951.

Gusberg, S. B., Fish, S. A., and Wang, Yin Ying: The Growth Pattern of Cervical Cancer. *Obst. & Gynec.*, 2: 557, 1953.

Hamperl, H., and Kauffman, C.: Cervix Uteri at Different Ages. *Obst. & Gynec.*, 14: 621, 1959.

Henriksen, E.: Distribution of Metastases in Stage I Carcinoma of the Cervix. A Study of 66 Autopsied Cases. *Am. J. Obst. & Gynec.*, 80: 919, 1960.

Hepler, T. K., Dockerty, M. B., and Randall, L. M.: Primary Adenocarcinoma of the Cervix. *Am. J. Obst. & Gynec.*, 63: 800, 1952.

Holzaepfel, J. H., and Ezell, H. E.: Sites of Metastases of Uterine Carcinoma. *Am. J. Obst. & Gynec.*, 69: 1027, 1955.

Isbell, N. P., and Dean, R. E.: Errors in Clinical Staging of Cervical Cancer: The Effect on Prognosis. *Obst. & Gynec.*, 10: 654, 1957.

Javert, C. T.: The Natural History of Cancer of the Cervix. *Am. J. Obst. & Gynec.*, 82: 56, 1961.

Kelly, J. W., Parsons, L., Friedell, G. H., and Sommers, S. C.: A Pathologic Study in 55 Autopsies after Radical Surgery for Cancer of the Cervix. *Surg., Gynec. & Obst.*, 110: 423, 1960.

Kinch, R. A.: Factors Affecting the Prognosis of Cancer of the Cervix in Pregnancy. *Am. J. Obst. & Gynec.*, 82: 45, 1961.

Lawson, J. G.: Cancer of the Uterine Cervix—Some Factors Influencing Survival Rates. *J. Obst. & Gynaec. Brit. Emp.*, 63: 819, 1956.

Lock, F. R., Greiss, F. C., and Blake, D. D.: Stage I Carcinoma of the Uterine Cervix. Comparison of Results with Variations in Treatment. *Am. J. Obst. & Gynec.*, 80: 984, 1960.

Masterson, J. G., and Pomerance, W.: Factors Influencing Mortality Rates in Gynecologic Malignancy. *Am. J. Obst. & Gynec.*, 81: 140, 1961.

Parente, J. T.: Metastases in Cancer of the Cervix. *Am. J. Surg.*, 99: 343, 1960.

Shier, C. B.: Prognosis in Carcinoma of the Cervix as Determined by Vaginal Smear. *Am. J. Obst. & Gynec.*, 82: 37, 1961.

Silva, T. F., Friedell, G. H., and Parsons, L.: Pelvic Exenteration for Carcinoma of the Cervix: Clinicopathological Study of Sixty Operations. *New England J. Med.*, 260: 519, 1959.

Sotto, L. S. J., Graham, J. B., and Pickren, J. W.: Postmortem Findings in Cancer of the Cervix. An Analysis of 108 Autopsies in the Past 5 Years. *Am. J. Obst. & Gynec.*, 80: 791, 1960.

Stone, B. H., and Mansell, H.: Procidentia and Cervical Cancer. *Obst. & Gynec.*, 5: 198, 1955.

Tremblay, P. C., Latour, J. P., and Dodds, J. R.: Adenocarcinoma of the Cervix Uteri. *Obst. & Gynec.*, 15: 299, 1960.

Tweeddale, D. N., and Tanner, F. H.: Malignant Cervical Polyps. *Am. J. Clin. Path.*, 24: 1259, 1954

Pathology of Leukoplakia and Invasive Carcinoma

Antoine, T., and Grunberger, V.: *Atlas der Kolpomikroscopie*. Stuttgart, G. Thieme, 1956.

Bowing, H. H., and Fricke, R. E.: Late Results of Radium Therapy for Carcinoma of the Uterine Cervix. *J.A.M.A.*, 137: 935, 1948.

Broders, A. C.: The Microscopic Grading of Cancer; in G. E. Pack and Livingston: *Treatment of Cancer and Allied Diseases*. New York, Paul B. Hoeber, Inc., 1940, Vol. 1, p. 55.

Ewing, J.: *Neoplastic Diseases*. Philadelphia, W. B. Saunders Company, 1928.

Fluhmann, C. F.: *The Cervix Uteri and Its Diseases*. Philadelphia, W. B. Saunders Company, 1961, Chaps. 18 and 19.

Gates, O., and Warren, S.: The Grading of Epidermoid Carcinoma. *Surg., Gynec. & Obst.*, 58: 962, 1934.

Glucksmann, A., and Cherry, C. P.: Incidence, Histology and Response to Radiation of Mixed Carcinomas (Adenoacanthomas) of the Uterine Cervix. *Cancer*, 9: 971, 1956.

Graham, J. B., Sotto, L. S. J., and Paloucek, F. P.: *Carcinoma of the Cervix*. Philadelphia, W. B. Saunders Company, 1962.

Hinselman, H.: *Colposcopy*. W. Giraudet, Wuppertal-Elberfeld, 1955.

Martzloff, K. H.: Carcinoma of the Cervix Uteri. A Pathological Clinical Study with Particular Reference to the Relative Malignancy of the Neoplastic Process as Indicated by the Predominant Type Cancer Cell. *Bull. Johns Hopkins Hosp.*, 34: 141, 1923.

Meyer, R.: The Histological Diagnosis of Early Cervical Carcinoma. *Surg., Gynec. & Obst.*, 73: 129, 1941.

Novak, E., and Novak, E. R.: *Gynecologic and Obstetric Pathology*. Philadelphia, W. B. Saunders Company, 1958.

Reagan, J. W., Hicks, D. J., and Scott, R. B.: Atypical Hyperplasia of Uterine Cervix. *Cancer*, 8: 42, 1955.

Schiller, W., Daro, A. F., Gollin, H. A., and Primiano, N. P.: Small Pre-ulcerative Invasive Carcinoma of the Cervix—The Spray Carcinoma. *Am. J. Obst. & Gynec.*, 65: 1088, 1953.

Warren, S.: The Grading of Carcinoma of the Cervix Uteri as Checked at Autopsy. *Arch. Path.*, 12: 783, 1931.

Wentz, W. B., and Reagan, J. W.: Survival in Cervical Cancer with Respect to Cell Type. *Cancer*, 12: 384, 1959.

Cancer Stages and Methods of Choosing Therapy

Davis, H. J., Jones, H. W., Jr., and Dickson, R. J.: The Bioassay of Host Radiosensitivity, an Index of Radiocurability Applied to Cervical Carcinoma. *Cancer*, 13: 358, 1960.

Day, E., and Glucksmann, A.: Panel Discussion: Radiation Changes in Carcinoma of the Cervix as Revealed by Cytology and Their Role in Determining Prognosis. *Acta Internat. Cancer*, 14: 355, 1958.

Fricke, R. E., and Dockerty, M. B.: The Prognostic Value of End-of-Treatment Biopsies in Treatment of Cancer of the Cervix. *Am. J. Roentgenol.*, 77: 448, 1957.

Friedell, G. H., and Graham, J. B.: Regional Lymph Node Involvement in Small Carcinoma of the Cervix. *Surg., Gynec. & Obst.*, 108: 513, 1959.

Graham, J. B., and Graham, R. M.: The Sensitization Response in Patients with Cancer of the Uterine Cervix. *Cancer*, 13: 5, 1960.

Gusberg, S. B., Tovell, H. M. M., Emerson, R., and Allina, H.: Radiosensitivity Testing of Cervical Cancer. A Preliminary Report. *Am. J. Obst. & Gynec.*, 68: 1464, 1954.

Hertig, A. T., and Gore, H.: Can Radiosensitivity and Histopathology of Cervical Cancer Be Correlated? *Am. J. Roentgenol.*, 87: 48, 1962.

Kottmeier, H. L.: *Annual Report on the Results of Treatment in Carcinoma of the Uterus*. Stockholm, P. A. Norstedt & Sons, 1958, Vol. 11.

Martzloff, K. H.: Epidermoid Carcinoma of the Cervix Uteri. A Histologic Study to Determine the Resemblance between Biopsy Specimens and the Parent Tumor Obtained by Radical Hysterectomy. *Am. J. Obst. & Gynec.*, 16: 578, 1928.

Meigs, J. V., and Brunschwig, A.: A Proposed Classification for Cases of Cancer of the Cervix Treated by Surgery. *Am. J. Obst. & Gynec.*, 64: 413, 1952.

Radiation Sensitivity

Agnew, A. M., Fidler, H. K., and Boyes, D. A.: Evaluation of Radiation Response. *Am. J. Obst. & Gynec.*, 79: 698, 1960.

Bourne, A. W., and Williams, L. H.: *Recent Advances in Obstetrics and Gynecology*. Cancer of the Cervix. 9th Ed. Boston, Little, Brown & Company, 1958, Chap. 12, p. 289.

Burns, B. C., Jr., and Brack, C. B.: Prognostic Factors in Radio-Resistant Cervical Cancer. *Obst. & Gynec.*, 16: 1, 1960.

Davis, H. J.: A Review—Radiosensitivity and Cervical Cancer. *Obst. & Gynec. Surv.*, 15: 301, 1960.

Glucksmann, A.: Relation of Radiosensitivity and Radiocurability to Histology of Tumour Tissue. *Brit. J. Radiol.*, 21: 559, 1948.

Glucksmann, A., and Spear, F. G.: Qualitative and Quantitative Histologic Examination of Biopsy Material from Patients Treated by Radiation for Cervical Carcinoma. Brit. J. Radiol., 18: 313, 1945.

Glucksmann, A., and Way, S.: On the Choice of Treatment of Individual Carcinomas of the Cervix Based on Analysis of Serial Biopsies. *J. Obst. & Gynaec. Brit. Emp.*, 55: 573, 1948.

Graham, J. B., and Meigs, J. V.: Earlier Detection of Recurrent Cancer of the Uterine Cervix by Vaginal Smear. *Am. J. Obst. & Gynec.*, 64: 908, 1952.

Graham, J. B., Graham, R. M., and Liu, W.: Prognosis in Cancer of the Uterine Cervix Based on the Vaginal Smear before Treatment. SR. The Sensitization Response. *Surg., Gynec. & Obst.*, 99: 555, 1954.

Graham, R. M.: Cytologic Prognosis in Cancer of the Cervix. *Am. J. Obst. & Gynec.*, 79: 700, 1960.

Gusberg, S. B.: A Consideration of the Problems of Radiosensitivity in Cancer of the Cervix. *Am. J. Obst. & Gynec.*, 72: 804, 1956.

Gusberg, S. B., Tovell, H. M. M., Long, M., and Hill, J. C.: Studies on Nucleoprotein Patterns in Radiosensitivity Testing. *Ann. New York Acad. Sc.*, 63: 1447, 1956.

Herman, G. G., Hughes, H. E., and Gusberg, S. B.: The Endocrine Basis for the Sensitization Response. *Surg., Gynec. & Obst.*, 108: 463, 1958.

Jones, H. W., Jr., Goldberg, B., Davis, H. J., and Burns, B. C., Jr.: Cellular Changes in Vaginal and Buccal Smears after Radiation—An Index of the Radiocurability of Carcinoma of the Cervix. *Am. J. Obst. & Gynec.*, 78: 1083, 1959.

Kiekhofer, W., and Peckham, B. M.: The Heterologous Transfer of Cervical Carcinoma, with Certain Histologic Observations. *Am. J. Obst. & Gynec.*, 77: 1228, 1959.

Lanier, R. R., and Wikle, W. T.: The Clinical Significance of "SR" (Sensitization Response to Radiation) in Normal Vaginal Mucosa. *Radiology*, 72: 217, 1959.

Mellors, R. C., Keane, J. F., Jr., and Papanicolaou, G. N.: Nucleic Acid Content of the Squamous Cancer Cell. *Science*, 116: 265, 1952.

Miller, N. F., Ludovici, P. P., Christian, R. T., and Riley, G. M.: Irradiation Sensitivity of Cervix Cancer: Response of Cultured Cervix Cancer Cells to Irradiation. *Am. J. Obst. & Gynec.*, 76: 1071, 1958.

Moore, G. E., and Grace, J. T.: Cancer Immunity. *Surg., Gynec. & Obst.*, 110: 234, 1960.

Puck, T. T., Marcus, P. I., and Cieciura, S. J.: Clonal Growth of Mammalian Cells in Vitro: Growth Characteristics of Colonies from Single HeLa Cells with and without a "Feeder" Layer. *J. Exper. Med.*, 103: 273, 1956.

Smith, C. J., Stepto, R. C., Schack, C. B., and Schmitz, H. E.: The Evaluation of the Basal Cell in the Radiosensitivity Studies of Carcinoma of the Cervix. *Am. J. Obst. & Gynec.*, 73: 598, 1957.

Warren, S., Meigs, J. V., Severance, A. O., and Jaffe, H. L.: The Significance of the Radiation Reaction in Carcinoma of the Cervix Uteri. *Surg., Gynec. & Obst.*, 69: 645, 1939.

Radiation Therapy

Arneson, A. N., and Williams, C. F.: Long Term Follow-up Observations in Cervical Cancer. *Am. J. Obst. & Gynec.*, 80: 775, 1960.

Barnes, A. C.: Use of Cobalt-60 in Radiation Therapy of Gynecologic Malignancies; in J. V. Meigs and S. H. Sturgis, eds.: *Progress in Gynecology.* New York, Grune & Stratton, Inc., 1957, Vol. III, p. 633.

Blakey, P. R.: Optimum Radium Distribution in the Treatment of Cancer of the Cervix. *Obst. & Gynec.*, 16: 679, 1960.

Buschke, F.: Common Misconceptions in Radiation Therapy. *Am. J. Surg.*, 101: 164, 1961.

Cherry, C. P., and Fraser, W. D.: The Influence of Focal Size on Local Radiocurability of Tumors of the Uterine Cervix. *Cancer*, 13: 951, 1960.

Corscaden, J. A.: Cancer of the Cervix; in *Gynecologic Cancer.* Baltimore, Williams & Wilkins Company, 1956, p. 179.

Corscaden, J. A., Gusberg, S. B., and Kosar, W.: Interstitial Radium Treatment of Cancer of the Cervix Uteri: Clinical Appraisal. *Am. J. Roentgenol.*, 72: 278, 1954.

Cosbie, W. G.: The Contribution of Radiotherapy to the Modern Treatment of Female Pelvic Cancer. *J. Obst. & Gynaec. Brit. Emp.*, 66: 843, 1959.

Fletcher, G. H.: The Present Status of Cobalt-60 Teletherapy in the Management of the Cancer Patient. *J.A.M.A.*, 164: 244, 1957.

Fletcher, G. H., Brown, T. C., and Rutledge, F. N.: Clinical Significance of Rectal and Bladder Dose Measurements in Radium Therapy of Cancer of the Uterine Cervix. *Am. J. Roentgenol.*, 79: 421, 1958.

Grande, P.: Calculation and Measurement of Doses from a Radium Applicator for Treatment of Cancer of the Uterine Cervix. *Brit. J. Radiol.*, 31: 336, 1958.

Hahn, G. A.: Comments on the Use of Local Radium in the Treatment of Carcinoma of the Cervix. *Am. J. Obst. & Gynec.*, 75: 882, 1958.

Leucutia, T.: Heuristic Glimpses into the Evolution of Radiation Therapy, Particularly in Reference to Gynecologic Cancers. Caldwell Lecture. *Am. J. Roentgenol.*, 85: 3, 1960.

Merrill, J. A.: Cytohistologic Evaluation of Radiation Response in Carcinoma of the Cervix: Its Present Clinical Significance; in *Progress in Radiation Therapy*. New York, Grune & Stratton, Inc., 1958.

Nolan, J. F.: Postoperative Radiotherapy for Carcinoma of the Cervix. A Study of 38 Cases. *Am. J. Obst. & Gynec.*, 79: 892, 1960.

Schmitz, H. E., and Smith, C. J.: Radiation Treatment of Cervical Cancer; in Symposium on Genital Cancer. *Clin. Obst. & Gynec.*, 1: 1013, 1958.

Silverstone, S. M., and Melame, J. L.: Effective Irradiation with Radium for Cancer of the Cervix. *Radiology*, 69: 360, 1957.

Tanzman, J.: Radiation Therapy for Carcinoma of the Cervix. *Am. J. Obst. & Gynec.*, 82: 42, 1961.

Trump, J. G.: Supervoltage Radiation Therapy in the Next Decade. *S. Clin. N. Amer.*, 40: 839, 1960.

Vasicka, A., Popovich, N. R., and Brausch, C. C.: Postradiation Course of Patients with Cervical Carcinoma. A Clinical Study of Psychic, Sexual and Physical Well-Being of Sixteen Patients. *Obst. & Gynec.*, 11: 403, 1958.

Radioactive Gold Therapy

Allen, W. M., Sherman, A. I., and Camel, H. M.: Radiogold in the Treatment of Cancer of the Cervix. *Radiology*, 70: 523, 1958.

Kottmeier, H. L., and Moberger, G.: Experience with Radioactive Colloidal Gold as an Additional Treatment in the Radiotherapy of Uterine Cancer: Review of Article in Acta Obstet. Scand. *J. Obst. & Gynaec. Brit. Emp.*, 62: 995, 1955.

Taylor, E. S., Isbell, N. P., and Dean, R. E.: An Experiment in the Use of Radioactive Gold for Cervical Cancer. *Am. J. Obst. & Gynec.*, 80: 899, 1960.

Urologic Complications of Therapy

Brack, C. B., Everett, H. S., and Dickson, R.: Irradiation Therapy for Carcinoma of the Cervix: Its Effect upon the Urinary Tract. *Obst. & Gynec.*, 7: 196, 1956.

Carlin, M. R.: Urological Complications Following Use of Radioactive Gold for Carcinoma of Uterine Cervix. *J. Urol.*, 78: 650, 1957.

Collins, C. G., Pent, D., and Jones, F. B.: Results of Early Repair of Vesicovaginal Fistula with Preliminary Cortisone Treatment. *Am. J. Obst. & Gynec.*, 80: 1005, 1960.

Dean, R. E., and Taylor, E. S.: Surgical Treatment of Complications Resulting from Irradiation Therapy of Cervical Cancer. *Am. J. Obst. & Gynec.*, 79: 34, 1960.

Kickham, C. J. E.: Urologic Problems in Carcinoma of the Cervix. *Surg., Gynec. & Obst.*, 112: 27, 1961.

Mallik, M. K. B.: A Study of the Ureters Following Wertheim's Hysterectomy. *J. Obst. & Gynaec. Brit. Emp.*, 67: 556, 1960.

Racker, D. C., and Braithwaite, J. L.: The Blood Supply to the Lower End of the Ureter and Its Relation to Wertheim's Hysterectomy. *J. Obst. & Gynaec. Brit. Emp.*, 58: 608, 1951.

St. Martin, E. C., Pasquier, C. M., Jr., and Campbell, J. H.: Ureteral Complications of Radical Surgery for Carcinoma of the Cervix. *South. M.J.*, 47: 832, 1954.

Other Complications of Therapy

Colock, B. P., and Hume, A.: Radiation Injury to the Sigmoid amd Rectum. *Surg., Gynec. & Obst.*, 108: 306, 1959.

Craig, M. S., Jr., and Buie, L. A.: Factitial (Irradiation) Proctitis—Clinicopathologic Study of 200 Cases. *Surgery*, 25: 472, 1949.

Kottmeier, H. L., and Gray, M. J.: Rectal and Bladder Injuries in Relation to Radiation Dosage in Carcinoma of the Cervix. *Am. J. Obst. & Gynec.*, 82: 74, 1961.

McCormick, N. A.: A Study of Complications Resulting from Treatment of Cancer of the Cervix. *Canad. M.A.J.*, 67: 25, 1952.

Simpson, W. J., and Spaulding, W. B.: Long-Delayed Bowel Complications of Radiotherapy. *Canad. M.A.J.*, 80: 810, 1959.

Smith, F. M.: Fractures of the Femoral Neck as a Complication of Pelvic Irradiation. *Am. J. Surg.*, 87: 339, 1954.

Stander, R. W. Rhamy, R. K., Henderson, W. P., Lansford, K. G., and Pearcy, M.: The Intravenous Pyelogram and Carcinoma of the Cervix. *Obst. & Gynec.*, 17: 26, 1961.

Surgical Treatment

Antoine, T.: Surgical Approach to Cervical Carcinoma and the Problem of Lymphadenectomy. *J. Internat. Coll. Surg.*, 29: 620, 1958.

Braasch, J. W.: The Surgical Treatment of Carcinoma of the Cervix Uteri. *S. Clin. N. Amer.*, 39: 809, 1959.

Brunschwig, A.: Surgical Treatment of Stage I Cancer of the Cervix. *Cancer*, 13: 34, 1960.

Brunschwig, A., and Daniel, W. W.: The Surgical Treatment of Cancer of the Cervix. *Am. J. Obst. & Gynec.*, 82: 60, 1961.

Carter, F. B.: Radical Hysterectomy with Bilateral Dissection of the Pelvic Lymph Nodes; in J. V. Meigs, ed.: *The Surgical Treatment of Cancer of the Cervix*. New York, Grune & Stratton, Inc., 1954.

Kelso, J. W.: Surgical Management of Carcinoma of the Cervix. *South. M.J.*, 52: 681, 1959.

Liu, W., and Meigs, J. V.: Radical Hysterectomy and Pelvic Lymphadenectomy: A Review of 473 Cases, Including 244 for Primary Invasive Carcinoma of the Cervix. *Am. J. Obst. & Gynec.*, 69: 1, 1955.

Meigs, J. V.: Radical Hysterectomy with Bilateral Pelvic Lymph Node Dissections. Report of 100 Cases Operated on Five Years or More. *Am. J. Obst. & Gynec.*, 62: 854, 1951.

Idem: in J. Heyman, ed.: Annual Report on Results of Treatment in Carcinoma of the Uterus, Vol. 10 (collated in 1954), p. 182.

Idem: Radical Hysterectomy with Bilateral Pelvic Lymph Node Dissections for Cancer of the Uterine Cervix. *Clin. Obst. & Gynec.*, 1: 1029, 1958.

Mitra, S.: The Schauta Operation; in J. V. Meigs: *Surgical Treatment of Cancer of the Cervix*. New York, Grune & Stratton, Inc., 1954, p. 267.

Idem: Radical Vaginal Hysterectomy and Extraperitoneal Lymphadenectomy for Cancer of the Cervix. *J. Obst. & Gynaec. Brit. Emp.*, 62: 872, 1955.

Navratel, E.: Radical Vaginal Hysterectomy, the Scharta-Amreich Operation; in J. V. Meigs, Ed.: *Surgical Treatment of Cancer of the Cervix*. New York, Grune and Stratton, Inc., 1954, p. 219.

Parsons, L., Cesare, F., and Friedell, G. H.: Primary Surgical Treatment of Invasive Cancer of the Cervix. *Surg., Gynec. & Obst.*, 109: 279, 1959.

Pratt, J. H.: Surgical Treatment of Carcinoma of the Uterine Cervix. *Proc. Staff Meet., Mayo Clin.*, 35: 523, 1960.

Riva, H. L., Andreson, P. S., Hathaway, C. R., Jr., Des Rosiers, J. L., and Stoehr, N. U.: Surgical Experience in Cancer of the Cervix. *Am. J. Obst. & Gynec.*, 82: 64, 1961.

Pelvic Lymphadenectomy

Black, M. M., and Speer, F. D.: Lymph Node Reactivity in Cancer Patients. *Surg., Gynec. & Obst.* 110: 477, 1960.

Brown, W. E., Meschan, I., Kerekes, E., and Sadler, J. M.: Effect of Radiation on Metastatic Pelvic Lymph Node Involvement in Carcinoma of the Cervix. *Am. J. Obst. & Gynec.*, 62: 871, 1951.

Cherry, C. P., Glucksmann, A., Dearing, R., and Way, S.: Observations on Lymph Node Involvement in Carcinoma of the Cervix. *J. Obst. & Gynaec. Brit. Emp.*, 60: 368, 1953.

Claiborne, H. A., Jr., Thornton, W. N., and Wilson, L. A., Jr.: Pelvic Lymphadenectomy for Carcinoma of the Uterine Cervix. *Am. J. Obst. & Gynec.*, 80: 672, 1960.

Meigs, J. V., Parsons, L., and Nathanson, I. T.: Retroperitoneal Lymph Node Dissection in Cancer of the Cervix. *Am. J. Obst. & Gynec.*, 57: 1087, 1949.

Nathanson, I. T.: Extraperitoneal Iliac Lymphadenectomy in the Treatment of Cancer of Cervix; in

J. V. Meigs and S. H. Sturgis, eds.: *Progress in Gynecology.* New York, Grune & Stratton, Inc., 1946, Vol. I, p. 358.

Parsons, L., Cesare, F., and Friedell, G. H.: The Evaluation of Lymphadenectomy in Therapy of Cervical Cancer. *Ann. Surg.,* 151: 961, 1960.

Rutledge, F. N., and Fletcher, G. H.: Transperitoneal Pelvic Lymphadenectomy Following Super-voltage Irradiation for Squamous-Cell Carcinoma of the Cervix. *Am. J. Obst. & Gynec.,* 76: 321, 1958.

Taussig, F. J.: Iliac Lymphadenectomy for Group II Cancer of the Cervix. *Am. J. Obst. & Gynec.,* 45: 733, 1943.

Idem: Iliac Lymphadenectomy with Irradiation in Treatment of Cancer of the Cervix. *Am. J. Obst. & Gynec.,* 28:650, 1954.

Way, S.: Comparison of Radiosensitivity of Primary Tumours and Their Regional Lymphatic Metastases: Response to Irradiation of Carcinoma of the Cervix at Primary and Secondary Sites. *Brit. J. Radiol.,* 27: 651, 1954.

Welch, J. S., Pratt, J. H., and Cantrell, G.: Involvement of Regional Lymph Nodes in Squamous Cell Epithelioma of the Uterine Cervix. *S. Clin. N. Amer.,* 39: 1067, 1959.

Combined Treatment with Radiation and Surgery

Burch, J. C., Chalfant, R. L., and Lavely, H. T., Jr.: Preoperative Radium Irradiation in Treatment of Cancer of the Cervix; in J. V. Meigs and S. H. Sturgis, eds.: *Progress in Gynecology.* New York, Grune & Stratton, Inc., 1957, Vol. III, p. 555.

Crawford, E. J., Jr., Robinson, L. S., Hornbuckle, L. A., and Godfrey, W. E.: Combined Radiologic-Surgical Therapy of Stage I or II Carcinoma of the Uterine Cervix. A Progress Report. *Am. J. Obst. & Gynec.,* 81: 148, 1961.

Dahle, T.: Combined Radiologic-Surgical Treatment of Carcinoma of the Cervix. *Surg., Gynec. & Obst.,* 108: 600, 1959.

Gray, M. J., Gusberg, S. B., and Guttmann, R.: Pelvic Lymph Node Dissection Following Radiotherapy. *Am. J. Obst. & Gynec.,* 76: 629, 1958.

Liegner, L. M., Olson, M., and Nickson, J. J.: Postoperative Irradiation of 86 Cases of Carcinoma of the Cervix. *Surg., Gynec. & Obst.,* 108: 313, 1959.

Stevenson, C. S.: The Combined Treatment of Carcinoma of the Cervix with Full Irradiation Therapy Followed by Radical Pelvic Operation. Second Report on a Series Now Numbering 95 Cases. *Am. J. Obst. & Gynec.,* 81: 156, 1961.

Carcinoma of the Cervical Stump

Archer, G.: Carcinoma of the Cervical Stump. *Mississippi Doctor,* 31: 6, 1953.

Braund, R. R., and Green, C. R.: Cancer of the Cervical Stump: Plea for Its Early Recognition and Prevention. *Am. Surgeon,* 17: 830, 1951.

Creadick, R. N.: Carcinoma of the Cervical Stump. *Am. J. Obst. & Gynec.,* 75: 565, 1958.

Decker, D. G., Hunt, A. B., Fricke, R. E., and Nelson, G. A.: Carcinoma of the Cervical Stump. *Am. J. Obst. & Gynec.,* 73: 974, 1957.

Dodds, J. R., and Latour, J. P. A.: Carcinoma of the Cervical Stump. *Am. J. Obst. & Gynec.,* 69: 252, 1955.

Dunn, M. R.: Prevalence of Carcinoma Arising in Cervical Stumps. *Am. J. Obst. & Gynec.,* 82: 83, 1961.

Fricke, R. E., and Decker, D. G.: Late Results of Radiation Therapy for Cancer of the Cervical Stump. *Am. J. Roentgenol.,* 79: 32, 1958.

Hahn, G. A.: Carcinoma of the Cervical Stump, with Special Reference to the Causes of Delay in Therapy. Observations from Data of the Philadelphia Committee for the Study of Pelvic Cancer. *Am. J. Obst. & Gynec.,* 71: 413, 1956.

Treatment of Advanced or Recurrent Carcinoma of the Cervix

Bricker, E. M., Butcher, H. R., Jr., Lawler, W. H., Jr., and McAfee, C. A.: Surgical Treatment of Advanced and Recurrent Cancer of the Pelvic Viscera. *Ann. Surg.,* 152: 388, 1960.

Brunschwig, A.: Complete Excision of Palvic Viscera for Advanced Carcinoma. A One-State Abdomino-perineal Operation with End Colostomy and Bilateral Ureteral Implantation into the Colon above the Colostomy. *Cancer*, 1: 177, 1948.

Brunschwig, A., and Daniel, W.: Total and Anterior Pelvic Exenteration. Report Based on 315 Operations. *Surg., Gynec. & Obst.*, 99: 324, 1954.

Idem: Pelvic Exenteration Operations with Summary of 66 Cases Surviving More than 5 Years. *Ann. Surg.*, 151: 571, 1960.

Cromer, J. K.: The Role of Surgery in the Management of Late Vaginal Recurrence Following Irradiation and/or Surgical Treatment of Carcinoma of the Uterine Cervix. *Am. Surgeon*, 23: 920, 1957.

Daniel, W. W., and Brunschwig, A.: Treatment of Carcinoma of the Cervix Recurrent after Surgery. *Cancer*, 9: 1208, 1956.

Friedell, G. H., Cesare, F., and Parsons, L.: Surgical Treatment of Cancer of the Cervix Recurring after Primary Irradiation Therapy. *New England J. Med.*, 264: 781, 1961.

Nathanson, I. T.: In J. V. Meigs: *Surgical Treatment of Cancer of the Cervix.* New York, Grune & Stratton, Inc., 1954.

Nolan, J. F., Vidal, J. A., and Anson, J. H.: Treatment of Recurrent Carcinoma of the Uterine Cervix with Cobalt-60. *West. J. Surg., Obst. & Gynec.*, 65: 358, 1957.

Parsons, L.: Pelvic Exenteration. *Clin. Obst. & Gynec.*, 2: 1151, 1959.

Parsons, L., and Bell, J. W.: An Evaluation of Pelvic Exenteration Operation. *Cancer*, 3: 205, 1950.

Parsons, L., and Leadbetter, W. F.: Urologic Aspects of Radical Pelvic Surgery. *New England J. Med.*, 242: 774, 1950.

Parsons, L., and Taymor, M.: Longevity Following Pelvic Exenteration for Carcinoma of the Cervix. *Am. J. Obst. & Gynec.*, 70: 774, 1955.

Schmitz, R. L., Schmitz, H. E., Smith, C. J., and Molitor, J. J.: Details of Pelvic Exenteration Evolved during an Experience with 75 Cases. *Am. J. Obst. & Gynec.*, 80: 43, 1960.

Schwarz, H., 2nd, and Nolan, J. F.: The Salvage of Treatment Failures in Cancer of the Uterine Cervix. *West. J. Surg., Obst. & Gynec.*, 66: 120, 1958.

Watkins, E., Jr., Hering, A. C., Luna, R., and Adams, H. D.: The Use of Intravascular Balloon Catheters for Isolation of the Pelvic Vascular Bed during Pump-Oxygenator Perfusion for Cancer Chemotherapeutic Agents. *Surg., Gynec. & Obst.*, 111: 464, 1960.

Therapy for Pain

Perese, D. M.: How to Manage Pain in Malignant Disease. *J.A.M.A.*, 175: 75, 1961.

Turnbull, F.: A Basis for Decision about Cordotomy in Cases of Pelvic Carcinoma. *J. Neurosurg.*, 16: 595, 1959.

Idem: The Nature of Pain in the Late Stages of Cancer. *Surg., Gynec. & Obst.*, 110: 665, 1960.

Wetzel, N.: The Surgical Relief of Intractable Pain. *S. Clin. N. Amer.*, 39: 245, 1959.

Chapter 62

Cancer of the Breast

THE BREAST is the most common site for malignant disease to develop in American women. This is responsible for more deaths than cancer appearing anywhere in the genital tract and actually now exceeds the combined figure for cancer of the cervix, endometrium and ovary in some parts of the United States.

Primarily, cancer of the breast is a pathologic entity found in older women, for the peak incidence occurs in the years immediately preceding the menopause. Following a plateau or slight drop in the number of cases seen during the years when the menopause generally occurs, a secondary rise is noted thereafter. It is, therefore, generally fair to say that the older the patient becomes, the greater the chance that malignant disease will appear in her breast.

Because benign forms of dysplastic or neoplastic growth tend to disappear or are not seen as often after the menopause, the physician can be reasonably certain that any tumor which develops after that time is in all probability malignant. Although cancer of the breast is common to the years preceding and beyond the menopause, one should constantly keep in mind that any mass in the breast, however small or large, is potentially a cancer and must be considered so until the true diagnosis is established. Breast cancer has been reported as early as ten years of age, and there are a half-dozen documented cases occurring before the age of twenty. These instances, of course, are exceptions to the concept that cancer of the breast is a disease of older women, but it is true that in actual practice cancer of the breast is rarely encountered before the age of thirty—less than 2 per cent of cancer cases.

What Are Some of the Interesting Factors That Bear on the Etiology of Breast Cancer?

There are a number of common denominators in the patients who suffer cancer of the breast. Among them are (*a*) the role played by the steroid hormones, particularly estrogen, (*b*) the influence of parity and the frequency of nursing, (*c*) the part played by trauma, (*d*) the relation of pre-existing benign lesions in the breast, and finally (*e*) the influence of heredity and the genes.

WHAT ROLE DOES ESTROGEN PLAY IN THE DEVELOPMENT OF BREAST CANCER? There can be little doubt that the etiology is linked to the activity of the steroid hormones, particularly estrogen. In support of the contention that estrogenic stimulation of mammary epithelium is in part responsible for the subsequent development of carcinoma, one may point to the following observations: (*a*) Seemingly, breast carcinoma is less likely to appear in the breasts of women who have had both ovaries

956

removed. (*b*) The menstrual span, during which estrogen may be active, is longer, with earlier menarche and later menopause, in the patient who suffers breast cancer than in the woman who does not. (*c*) Circumstantial evidence suggests that mammary cancer can be induced in some susceptible women by prolonged administration of estrogen. That in all probability the patient must needs be sensitive to the effect of estrogen suggests a genetic influence.

In animal experiments, for example, carcinoma is produced with greater ease and frequency when estrogen is given to mice from a high mammary cancer inbred strain.

WHAT INFLUENCE DOES MAMMARY FUNCTION HAVE ON THE SUBSEQUENT DEVELOPMENT OF BREAST CANCER (PARITY AND NURSING)?   It is interesting that breast cancer tends to appear with greater frequency in women who (*a*) are unmarried, (*b*) have no pregnancies or few children, (*c*) fail to nurse their offspring. There has been a pronounced tendency in modern life in some groups to restrict the family size and to avoid nursing the infant whenever possible. In many instances when there is more than one child in the family the mother will frequently breast-feed the first child, but choose not to do so when the other children come along. Since the incidence of mammary cancer seems to be on the increase, one may well speculate on the importance of these non-nursing factors as etiologic causes. It would appear that the more the lactating breast is used, the less the chance of malignant disease. Statistical studies support this contention. Wherever custom or economic conditions make large families and nursing popular the incidence of carcinoma of the breast diminishes as compared to the United States, for example, where the reverse is true.

It is well known that cancer of the breast is uncommon in certain racial groups widely separated in geographic locations. Racial characteristics and the genes might have nothing to do with it, because these groups tend to marry early, have a lot of children and nurse them. In Puerto Rico economic conditions in the past have predisposed to the neglect of the pregnant woman and made formula feeding in the postpartum period too expensive. There the incidence of cancer of the breast is surprisingly low, while that for cancer of the cervix is abnormally high.

DOES PRE-EXISTING INJURY OR IMMEDIATE TRAUMA LEAD TO THE DEVELOPMENT OF MAMMARY CANCER?   In their exposed positions the breasts likely must be subjected to repeated trauma as the patient goes through life. It is not surprising, then, that in many instances the patient, in recounting her history, will recall a previous blow to the breast and will associate the trauma with the appearance of tumor. There is little evidence that trauma has anything to do with the subsequent development of mammary cancer. Some investigators have noted that malignancy in a right-handed person is found with greater frequency on the left or relatively unprotected side. It is far more likely that the trauma simply calls attention to the damaged area in the breast, and in palpating it a tumor, previously unrecognized, is discovered.

IS THERE SUCH A THING AS A PRECANCEROUS LESION OF THE BREAST?   Since cancer may (*a*) develop in otherwise normal breast tissue, (*b*) appear in a breast that contains predominating cystic disease or sclerosing adenosis, (*c*) arise in the postmenopausal breast which is no longer functional and has undergone atrophy, or (*d*) occur in a breast that is undergoing hyperplasia because of hormonal stimulation during pregnancy, it is difficult to decide whether any of these conditions predispose toward malignant disease. Undoubtedly, unbalanced hormonal stimulation that leads to ductal hyperplasia has something to do with the development of cancer of the breast, but we actually do not know in general whether and which type of hyperplasia inevitably progresses to cancer, if left untreated.

Pathologically, one can see progressive changes in duct hyperplasia and intraductal papillomas that lead to well established cancers, but cancer can also arise in other regions in the breast where no other abnormality in structure can be detected. We have noted that cancer of the breast is found about four times as frequently in the woman who has cystic disease as in her sister who has none. This pathologic entity is perhaps the only pre-existing lesion that one can consider truly precancerous. From a practical point of view the gynecologist will do well to remember that a cancer can develop anywhere in the breast in any woman from puberty onward, regardless of whether she demonstrates any clinical abnormality.

WHAT PART DOES HEREDITY PLAY IN THE ETIOLOGY OF BREAST CANCER? There does appear sometimes to be a strong familial inheritance factor in breast carcinoma. Roughly, the chances of carcinoma developing in a patient born to a mother who has cancer of the breast are about four times as great as for the daughter of a noncancerous woman. There is certainly a notable increase in the frequency with which cancer of the breast appears, not only in mothers and sisters, if they have malignant disease, but also in homologous twins, in whom carcinoma has been found to be increased in occurrence at the same time in the same location in the breast. Extensive epidemiologic studies of family groups carried back through several generations have supported the contention that cancer of the breast is actually partly due to a hereditary predisposition.

Just what the genetic factor is, is not known. The possibility of an extrachromosomal substance, which is believed to be present in milk, has been suggested as the causative agent in the transmission of carcinoma from mother to offspring. Despite exhaustive investigations using the most sensitive modern laboratory equipment such as the electron microscope, no one has been able yet to isolate and identify any human milk factor. About all that can be said at this time is that although there is some evidence that a milk factor, linked to the genes, may be present and responsible for the transmission of carcinoma in mice, there is no proof that the extrachromosomal milk factor is concerned with the etiology of breast cancer in the woman. In fact, several studies have fairly well excluded any milk factor in human cases.

LIFE HISTORY OF CANCER OF THE BREAST

It is important that we have an understanding of the natural history of cancer of the breast in order that our diagnostic acumen be heightened and our therapy be basically sound.

Cancer of the breast, in most instances, appears as a primary tumor with a tendency to develop in the left breast somewhat more often than the right.

How Often Is More than One Cancer Found in the Same Breast?

Occasionally one encounters, usually after pathologic review of the operative specimen, another cancer in the same breast. Rarely is it evident clinically, and the likelihood of another carcinoma being present is probably no greater than 5 per cent.

How Often Are Both Breasts Involved?

In most cases carcinoma appears in only one breast. It is possible, particularly when carcinoma in one breast is in the advanced stage, to have the opposite breast involved, either by lymphatic extension from one side to the other or on occasion by metastasis through the blood stream. The likelihood of the bilateral occurrence of a primary carcinoma, however, is fairly remote. In roughly 3 per cent a primary carcinoma may develop either simultaneously or several years after a radical mastectomy on the contralateral side. It is important to keep this in mind, for some authorities advocate prophylactic removal of the opposite breast when a carcinoma develops in one.

It is true that cancer cannot develop in the breast if it is not there, but such a radical attitude is completely unjustified. It is far more logical to check the opposite breast at regular intervals than to remove it, because the chances of cancer appearing in the other breast are scarcely any greater than one would expect in a woman who has some familial tendency to breast cancer. Nevertheless the old axiom is still true that the most common second cancer in a woman with a malignant tumor of the breast is a cancer of the other breast.

How Does the Malignant Process Develop and Spread within the Breast Itself?

The primary site is most often in the upper outer quadrant of the breast, with the central area the next most common location. Two thirds of all breast carcinomas will be found in these two locations. Tumors in the medial half of the breast in either upper or lower quadrants are seen less often.

The malignant lesion is entirely microscopic at the outset (Fig. 62–1, *A*). It may begin with invasion into the stroma by cords of small isolated epithelial cells, or more often by the plugging of ducts with carcinoma cells. Ninety per cent of breast carcinomas are of duct origin, and the majority appear to begin as purely intraductal carcinomas.

Chronic cystic mastitis, it will be recalled (Chap. 57), may have papillomas or intraductal epithelial hyperplastic changes as accompaniments. When the hyperplastic ductal lining cells lose their regular arrangement and develop variations in the cellular and nuclear staining qualities, this anaplastic appearance is justly regarded with suspicion (Fig. 62–1, *B*).

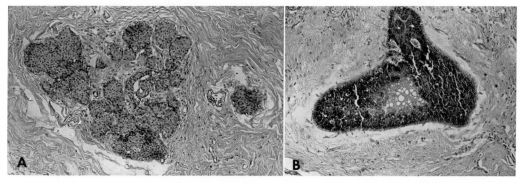

Fig. 62-1.   *A*, Microscopic breast carcinoma with early invasion of stroma that was found incidentally in a specimen removed for cystic disease. It was too small to be visible or palpable grossly. *B*, Atypical intraductal epithelial hyperplasia may have an ominous, hyperchromatic appearance.

Exactly how much anaplasia is required for a pathologic diagnosis of intraductal carcinoma is difficult to define, and criteria differ among individual pathologists. Some cases illustrated by Stewart in his fascicle would likely be called atypical hyperplasia rather than cancer by some other experienced students of breast disease. When the intraductal epithelium forms a solid mass that fills a medium-sized duct, and it contains some giant nuclei, or when the proliferation forms glands within glands, most observers would diagnose this as intraductal carcinoma.

What Is Meant by Carcinoma in Situ of the Breast?

Actually, intraductal carcinoma is a noninvasive form of breast cancer, which appears to grow along the lumens of the ducts. For some reason it is usually not called carcinoma in situ.

Lobular carcinoma in situ is a rarity in that a noninvasive cancer is recognized arising in a breast lobule within the ductules, rather than by the usual type of origin in larger ducts. Some localized lobules are observed that microscopically vaguely resemble sclerosing adenosis. Closer scrutiny reveals cells much too large, with disproportionate enlargement of their nuclei. Nuclear anaplasia is usually rather obvious (Fig. 62–2).

Most often lobular carcinoma in situ, like other noninvasive carcinomas, occurs in an organ that elsewhere manifests invasive cancer. One case has been recorded in which retrospective examination of a biopsy made about five years before breast cancer was recognized showed carcinoma in situ.

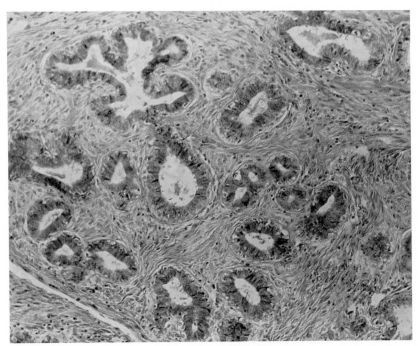

Fig. 62-2.   Lobular carcinoma in situ shows a rounded zone within which the ductular epithelium is variable and anaplastic, but without invasion. The paler, periepithelial cells are myoepithelial and non-neoplastic.

What Happens to Intraductal Breast Carcinoma?

Most often an invasive growth occurs at some break in the duct lining, and the usual spread of carcinoma cells into nearby fibrous stroma and fat develops.

Occasionally the ducts may become grossly distended by carcinoma cells, with little or no stromal invasion. The term *comedocarcinoma* refers to masses of intraductal tumor cells that can be squeezed like toothpaste from sections of a gross tumor. Ordinarily in comedocarcinoma there is some invasion into the stroma as well as along ducts, and the comedo aspect is simply part of an ordinary breast carcinoma (Fig. 62–3, *A*).

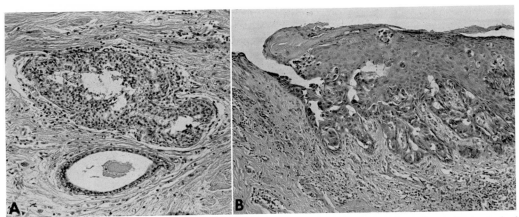

Fig. 62-3. *A*, The upper duct is filled with carcinoma cells growing along the walls, typical of intraductal breast cancer. The lower duct is uninvolved. *B*, The edge of a nipple erosion shows the intact epithelium to be infiltrated at different levels by single or grouped, pale rounded "pagetoid" cells. These carcinoma cells growing intraepidermally are the basic lesion of Paget's disease of the nipple.

Sometimes intraductal carcinoma spreads along ducts until the cells invade the epidermis of the nipple. This produces a grossly eroded red appearance often confused with eczema. Biopsy shows large clear carcinoma cells in the skin of the nipple, and this constitutes *Paget's disease of the nipple* (Fig. 62–3, *B*).

Most cases of Paget's disease of the breast have a palpable tumor deeper in the breast that proves to be an ordinary carcinoma on sectioning. In these women invasion along the large ducts to reach the nipple is simply one route of spread of a versatile cancer that simultaneously is using all other routes of invasion. Consequently the prognosis in these women is poor.

If no mass is found in the breast accompanying pathologically proved Paget's disease of the nipple, and only intraductal carcinoma is observed in the deeper ducts, the prognosis after mastectomy is favorable. This constitutes, in fact, a noninvasive carcinoma with extension to the nipple, and is somewhat analogous to carcinoma in situ of the cervix with endocervical glandular spread.

How Is Breast Carcinoma Most Commonly Recognized?

Usually there is no opportunity to see the mode of origin of a breast cancer, which actually may have begun to change its pattern of growth before it can be detected clinically and confirmed by the microscope. When the differentiation in cell growth, or lack of it, has progressed far enough to produce a mass that can be recognized, the

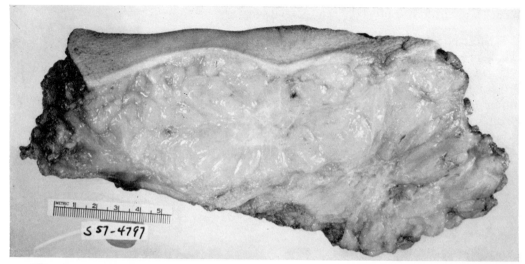

Fig. 62-4.   A typical scirrhous breast carcinoma, about 2 cm. in diameter. It is stellate, pale and granular, and is producing local skin retraction. This is about the average size of breast cancers when first discovered clinically.

characteristic tumor cells can be seen infiltrating and extending both along the ducts and into the fibrous tissue septa until finally the fatty supporting tissue is invaded. In this manner the entire breast segment becomes involved, and as the process progresses other segments are implicated so that finally an entire quadrant of the breast may be infiltrated. As a protective measure designed to confine the invader, fibrous tissue appears. It is the fibrosis that gives substance to the tumor and is the reason why a cancer feels firm and often stony hard. Invasion into the fatty tissue follows no standard pattern, and the outlines of the tumor may tend to be less circumscribed or rounded and more stellate (Fig. 62–4).

What Happens When Cancer Invades the Local Lymphatic Channels within the Breast Tissue?

The lymphatic channels tend to follow along with the nerves and the ducts. Once in the lymphatics, the cells by rapid division and multiplication tend to clog and block the central channels. It is interesting to note that the path followed by the central or main lymphatics tends to be in a vertical direction. The cancer then tends to extend deeply in the direction of the fascia overlying the pectoral muscle beneath the breast before it spreads laterally. The lateral spread occurs because the main channels are plugged with tumor and there is nowhere else for it to go except via the smaller collateral lymphatic system.

Pathologists have noted that at times it is a difficult problem to decide whether the tumor cells are actually within the lymphatics or are simply lying in tissue spaces. The same observations are now being made in studying local spread of cancer in other primary sites such as cervix and prostate. The tumor may, of course, spread by blood vessels as well as lymphatics, for tumor emboli can occasionally be seen within the lumens of both arteries and veins.

As the cancer spreads beyond its point of origin it may also involve the skin overlying the tumor. The first clinical indication of this is the appearance of edema

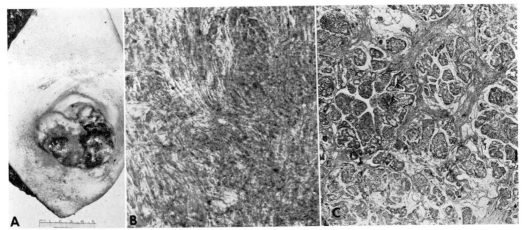

Fig. 62-5. *A,* Neglected, untreated breast carcinomas eventually break through the skin and ulcerate. The clawlike extensions of carcinoma on the chest wall are believed to have given the name "cancer" to the whole group of malignant neoplasms. *B,* Carcinoma simplex growing in cords within a fibrous stroma. This is a frozen section, usually the technique by which breast cancer is first confirmed microscopically. *C,* Papillary adenocarcinoma, an unusual histologic type of breast cancer.

of the skin itself. The edema appears because the lymphatics are completely clogged by tumor cells. Eventually the skin takes on the appearance of the covering of an orange (*peau d'orange*), which is highly characteristic of cancer involving the skin. The skin becomes fixed to the tumor and it to the deeper underlying structures. In neglected cases the skin over the tumor may turn red, break down and either ulcerate or permit papillary excrescences to grow out from the underlying tumor. Foul discharge and frequently bleeding can be so troublesome that amputation of the breast is necessary even though all chance of cure has long gone (Fig. 62–5, *A*).

In rare instances and again in extensive or neglected cases the skin lymphatics are so saturated that satellite skin nodules appear in areas remote from the primary tumor site.

How Fast Does Cancer of the Breast Grow?

The life history of cancer of the breast is a progressive one, since spontaneous cures do not occur. The actual passage of time in an untreated case from the date of the first symptom to death has been calculated, in several large studies, to be in the general range of forty months. This will depend in part on the age of the patient at the time she acquired the neoplasm and the differentiation of the tumor as determined by pathologic grade. Naturally the more highly malignant the tumor, the shorter the duration of life. It can be as short as three months. Although there is no statistical confirmation, there is a general impression that the disease progresses in the direction of death more rapidly in the young than in the old.

As far as the growth of the tumor within the breast is concerned, similar factors are present, because it is obvious that some tumors grow faster than others. The rate of growth is not easy to measure, for we are unable to determine how long the tumor had been there or how rapidly it had grown before it was recognized clinically. Based on observations made by measuring the size of pulmonary metastases, a carcinoma seems to have been present for a long time before it is evident clinically. This may explain the occasionally long latent period between the appearance of a local recurrence and distant metastases.

As far as we can determine, the local cancer growth seems to increase at the rate of about 1 cm. in 3 months. Since the eventual prognosis depends on the size of the primary tumor, it is obvious that early diagnosis and early treatment are of great concern. It is a well documented fact that between 60 and 70 per cent of lesions 1 cm. in size have no metastases.

What Is the Ordinary Gross Appearance of a Breast Cancer?

Usually a breast carcinoma is either firm or stony hard. A knife cuts carcinoma with a gritting sensation, like that of an unripe pear, as the tiny fibrous stromal strands tear one by one. The cut surface typically has a granular tan or pink appearance that resembles moist, unpolished granite.

The outlines of a carcinoma are poorly demarcated. If there are stellate, pointed invasive strands of tumor penetrating the fat, the carcinoma is said to be scirrhous. If the outline is rounded and the tumor not so hard, it may be called a medullary carcinoma. Rarely, cancer arises in the wall of a large cyst, and is called intracystic. These descriptive terms have little prognostic or practical value, and are no longer frequently used.

What Is the Histologic Appearance?

Cords of individual carcinoma cells invading a dense fibrous stroma and fat are most commonly seen (Fig. 62–5, *B*). This growth pattern is called carcinoma simplex (Ewing) or adenocarcinoma grade III or IV (Broders). Less often, ductlike glandular

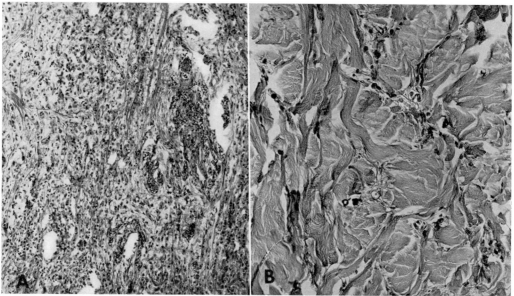

Fig. 62-6. *A,* In medullary breast carcinoma with lymphoid stroma the tumor cells are rather pale and disorderly, and numerous lymphocytes occur around and between them. This is a favorable subtype. *B,* In the rare fibrocarcinoma the stroma is excessive, and the carcinoma cells are visible only as small, darkly stained nuclei. Stains for mucus, however, may indicate their epithelial nature.

spaces are formed, usually in tumors that grossly were medullary. These are called adenocarcinoma (Ewing) or grade II adenocarcinoma (Broders). Rarely tumors occur so well differentiated as to justify the histopathologic diagnosis of papillary adenocarcinoma grade I (Fig. 62–5, *C*).

Since no special significance of histologic pattern in relation to growth activity or prognosis has been established after over forty years of intensive investigation of the usual types of breast carcinoma, some pathologists are satisfied to diagnose simply carcinoma of breast.

A number of uncommon growth patterns exist. One significant variation is the *medullary carcinoma with lymphoid stroma*. Here the individual tumor cells are large and pale and mingled with many lymphocytes. Either the carcinoma cells are defective or the lymphocytes represent a defense reaction, because prognosis in this form of breast cancer is better than usual (Fig. 62–6, *A*). *Parvicellular carcinoma or fibrocarcinoma* has so few carcinoma cells in a fibrous stroma that they are difficult to identify (Fig. 62–6, *B*). This cancer has a long period of creeping growth. Apocrine carcinoma is composed of large, eosinophilic, Schimmelbusch-type cells with invasion. It appears to spread more slowly than most other mammary carcinomas.

Mucinous (or colloid) carcinoma and breast sarcomas will be considered with the older age group (Chap. 67).

How Does Cancer Spread beyond the Confines of the Breast?

It is generally believed that the tumor spreads from primary site to the regional lymph nodal areas either by permeation along lymphatic channels or by emboli. Although in all probability the principal spread is via lymphatic emboli carried to the lymph nodes, blood vessel invasion may be more important than we have hitherto believed.

Of the two possibilities of spread by lymphatic pathways, the majority of pathologists lean to favoring emboli rather than direct permeation. It is an interesting fact that in the breast, just as in the cervix, although tumor may be seen in lymphatic channels adjacent to a primary tumor and again in the periphery of a regional lymph node, one rarely ever sees carcinoma in the intervening lymphatics. It has been postulated that peristaltic movement in the lymphatics pushes the tumor cells along, leaving only a rare residuum that can be recognized, but this seems highly unlikely.

Once the tumor appears in an afferent blood vessel or lymphatic in the capsular sinus of a regional lymph node it tends to block the lumen, and the multiplying cells then invade the substance of the node. How often this occurs is not known, but all too frequently only one pathologic section of a node is made, and this is usually taken from the larger rather than the smaller lymph nodes. Many large lymph nodes will contain cancer, but many more smaller nodes have also microscopic evidence of cancer. When the lymph nodes are cleared by special technique and the smaller nodes are thoroughly examined, the number of metastases recovered increases by 20 per cent.

What Lymph Nodes Are Involved, and What Is the Normal Order of Progression?

Approximately 70 per cent of patients seen today will have regional lymph node metastases. The percentage is higher in patients in the younger age categories and in those who are in the poorer economic strata. Thus the incidence will be appreciably less when patients have the means, intelligence and willpower to consult a private physician early in the course of the disease.

Axillary Lymph Nodes.   The regional nodes in the axillary area are the site of metastases from breast carcinoma nearly twice as often as other areas into which the lymphatics drain. They are the first natural line of defense. The carcinoma may remain confined to this chain of nodes, or it may spread from there to involve nodes in the subclavicular, internal mammary or supraclavicular regions. It is rare to find metastases in other areas without first finding them in the axillary lymph nodes.

Internal Mammary Lymph Nodes.   In recent years there has been a considerable amount of interest in the role of the internal mammary nodes, located along the under side of the sternum in the region of the second, third and fourth intercostal spaces, in the prognosis of breast carcinoma. In the past they received little consideration in therapy. Now there has been a certain amount of enthusiasm for dissection of this nodal chain, after removing the cartilaginous attachments to the sternum of the second, third and fourth ribs. More recently the main lymphatic channels in this area have been isolated surgically and a cobalt wire inserted so that the area can be more selectively irradiated than is possible by the usual x-ray therapy technique. Both methods have the same disadvantage, since the lymph nodes in this area are often small (1 or 2 mm.), a fact which makes adequate local therapy difficult, since cancer may well appear in the peripheral sinuses of a small node.

There can be no doubt that the internal mammary chain does become involved, particularly when the primary carcinoma is situated in the medial half of the breast or in the region of the nipple. Reports in the literature suggest that they will show metastases in approximately 20 per cent of all cases, the incidence rising to 33 per cent when only medial quadrant tumors are considered. Unfortunately, short of surgical exploration, there is no clinical test to indicate whether or not these nodes are involved. In the more advanced case a poorly delineated, fixed parasternal mass can be detected, but there are no clinical signs in the early case as to who is a suitable candidate for radical mastectomy. Haagensen summarizes his experience and that of others as follows:

1. Before metastases to the axillary lymph nodes occur, internal mammary lymph node involvement is so infrequent that it has little therapeutic significance.

2. After metastases to the axillary nodes have occurred, involvement of the internal mammary nodes in the upper 3 interspaces may be expected in between 30 and 50 per cent of cases.

3. Metastases to the internal mammary nodes are more frequent from carcinomas in the inner half and central region of the breast than from those in the outer half.

This is the present trend of thought concerning the importance of the internal mammary node in cancer of the breast. If the observations are accurate, then greater concentration in therapy should be placed on this area, whether it be by surgery or some form of radiation. One might prefer to use radiation, because adequate dissection of these lymph nodes is rather difficult, and the patient may well have passed beyond the point where a reasonable chance of cure can be expected.

Supraclavicular Lymph Nodal Area.   After the involvement by tumor of regional nodes in the upper axillary area, metastases may appear in the supraclavicular space. The tumor extends along the lymphatics, following the subclavicular vein to the point where it joins the external jugular vein at the base of the neck. These lymph nodes are never involved unless the axillary nodes already contain metastases and are less often implicated than the internal mammary chain.

At one time there was some enthusiasm for extensive radical dissection of these nodes in continuity with the axillary group and the primary tumor in the breast. The enthusiasm subsided when it soon became evident that the survival statistics did not improve despite the radical nature of the surgery. External roentgen therapy is now the treatment of choice.

INVOLVEMENT OF LYMPH NODES ON THE CONTRALATERAL SIDE. In far advanced cases the surgeon may be surprised to find a mass in the opposite axilla from the side of the original mastectomy. No suspicious areas are felt in the remaining breast, yet the axillary findings are unmistakable. The spread probably occurs through embolism along the deep lymphatic channels that lie on and perforate the fascia of the muscles in the chest wall.

How Do Distant Metastases Occur, and Where Do They Appear?

Once the carcinoma has left the breast and extended to the regional lymph nodes, distant metastases to bone and other organs may be expected. In most instances the spread to remote regions occurs because the tumor cells get into the general circulation. Occasionally tumor emboli enter the vertebral veins or the azygos system after first invading the intercostal veins.

MANNER OF SPREAD THROUGH THE GENERAL CIRCULATION. Cancer cells get into the right side of the heart by way of the innominate veins. These become involved either by embolic spread through the central lymphatic chains or by direct spread after the tumor has broken into the axillary or internal mammary vessels. After entering the heart tumor cells or thrombi are dispatched to the lung, where they become trapped in the small arteriolar branches or capillaries. Some tumor cells will be strangled by the protective fibrous tissue stromal reaction which is common to all normal structures invaded by neoplastic cells, but others survive and grow. When they break through the restrictive barriers, they tend to multiply and infiltrate the lung structures, particularly the alveoli. Eventually, after lymphatic channels have been plugged the tumor enters the left side of the heart and is pumped into the general circulation.

In most instances unless there is a patent interventricular or atrial septum, metastases to liver, bone, ovary, adrenal and spleen appear only after lung metastases have become firmly established. This may occur early or late, depending on how well the primary metastases are encapsulated by the protective fibrous tissue.

MANNER OF SPREAD THROUGH THE VERTEBRAL VEINS AND AZYGOS SYSTEM. Less frequently metastases occur in brain, bone and ovary because tumor has invaded the intercostal veins that open into the vertebral veins which connect with the azygos system. This manner of spread is common in the development of metastases that appear in the lower vertebrae and pelvis. The tumor cells disseminate widely without ever entering the heart and general circulation. It is therefore possible to have metastases in bone, brain and ovary without lung metastases.

CLINICAL CHARACTERISTICS OF LUNG METASTASES. Metastases to lung from cancer of the breast are more common than those in any other organ or anatomic location. As we have pointed out, cancer gets there because of dissemination of cells via the lymph or blood circulation. We mention this again, because one might expect metastases to occur from lymph nodes situated in the hilar region of the lung. It is true that these nodes may contain tumor, but they are not the source of the metastases within the lung itself.

It is extremely unfortunate that lung metastases produce so few early clinical

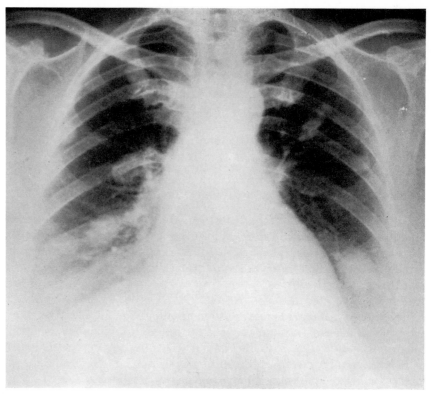

Fig. 62-7.　　Rounded and linear shadows of bilateral breast cancer metastases to the lung are the most common x-ray indications of distant spread.

signs. One might expect pain, cough, dyspnea or cyanosis, but they rarely occur unless the pleura is also involved or the fibrotic response to the carcinoma is excessive. Actually, it is amazing how well the patient with widespread metastases in the lung may appear. The metastases are rarely single, and they come to light only on careful x-ray examination of the lung fields. This is why routine periodic chest plates should be taken after a radical mastectomy.

On x-ray examination the characteristic signs are rounded tumor nodules seen in several areas throughout one or, more often, both lung fields. Occasionally when the fibrotic response to the presence of carcinoma has been extreme, one may see linear streaks extending out into the lung fields from the hilar region (Fig. 62–7).

PLEURAL METASTASES.　　As the disease progresses, tumor cells from the primary metastases within the lung reach the pleura, either by lymphatic extension or by embolic spread through the pulmonary arteries. It is the extension to the pleura that produces the symptoms which call attention to the lung. Involvement of the pleura invariably produces a pain which is typical, as well as cough. Shortness of breath and cyanosis appear particularly when pleural effusion is present. X-ray examination will reveal only the typical opaque picture characteristic of fluid in the pleural cavity. No pleural metastases will be seen unless fluid is aspirated and the same quantity of air is replaced in the chest cavity. The contrast provided by the air will often make it possible to detect pleural extension of the tumor. In some instances, perhaps 10 per cent, the fluid removed from the pleural cavity will be bloody. After centrifuging the fluid, sediment should be (*a*) smeared and stained by the Papanicolaou technique, as well as (*b*) fixed and processed into paraffin blocks or passed through Millipore filters to allow pathologic analyses for tumor cells.

EXTENSION TO LIVER.   Although it is possible to have liver metastases by direct lymphatic extension through channels that lead from the tumor through the rectus fascia and muscle to involve the falciform ligament and finally the liver parenchyma, it is far more common to have blood borne secondary metastases from the primary metastases in the lungs. Next to the lung the liver is the favorite site for metastasis in cancer of the breast. Again, few symptoms appear. The patient will have to have extensive destruction of the liver before any jaundice develops. The first indication may be the palpation of an enlarged liver that feels a little irregular and knobby. Frequently nothing can be felt in the hepatic region.

METASTASES TO BONE.   It is impossible to estimate the number of patients with cancer of the breast who have metastases to bone for the simple reason that they can be detected only by x-ray examinations and autopsy. Pain and tenderness on local bone pressure are the only signs and symptoms, and they may be totally lacking. X-ray films are misleading, because the patient may have suggestive symptoms and physical findings, yet show nothing abnormal when roentgenograms are taken, even when the more refined laminograms are utilized.

The most common alteration in architectural structure produced by metastasis to bone is the osteolytic type of lesion, which gives a characteristic roentgenologic moth-eaten appearance. It may be confused with atrophic bone changes and be misdiagnosed. The other, less common type of change is the osteoplastic type, in which the bone substance actually increases. When the tumor simply occupies the medullary portion of the bone, no recognizable bone changes appear that are suitable for an x-ray interpretation.

Characteristically, the patient has pain in the back, which tends to radiate downward. It is not present all the time, but is apt to be brought out when the patient coughs, sneezes or receives a jolt such as might follow a sudden misstep in walking from a curb to the street or riding in a car. The pain is definitely made worse by motion and accentuated when the moves are sudden and unexpected. Most patients have such symptoms before anything abnormal is discovered by x-ray.

The bones most commonly affected are the vertebrae in the lumbar spine and the pelvis. The upper femur is a common site, but metastases in the thoracic spine, ribs and skull are less frequently seen. Pathologic fractures occur occasionally (perhaps as often as 15 per cent), particularly in the lumbar vertebrae and femurs. Pain in the back, of the type previously described, raises suspicion that the vertebral bodies may have collapsed. It is a common experience to receive a negative report after x-ray examination, only to see complete collapse of the vertebrae when repeat studies are done two months later.

Fractures through a metastatic area in the femur oddly enough heal very well despite presence of the tumor, when the fixation is adequate, but vertebral fractures can be handled only by back braces designed to restrict motion and give support.

Bone destruction is usually accompanied by increased urinary excretion of calcium, which disturbs the calcium-phosphorus relation. Laboratory studies will show this disturbed relation, as well as a rise in the normal blood alkaline phosphatase. As a result of the hypercalciuria the kidney often becomes irreparably damaged, and eventually the patient begins to retain nitrogen as kidney function diminishes. This chain of events may be anticipated when the patient experiences gastrointestinal upsets, such as nausea, vomiting and constipation, while she appears mentally sluggish and apathetic. The physician should be alert for these symptoms when giving a patient hormone therapy such as estrogen or androgen, for these two can precipitate such episodes.

METASTASES TO BRAIN.   We have previously noted that the patient may get metastases to the brain by the passage of tumor cells through the vertebral veins, without any evidence of lung involvement. We recently saw two young women who had cerebellar metastasis two years after radical mastectomy, despite the fact that all the lymph nodes examined were negative and the chest x-rays studies were normal. Brain metastases are less common than those in the lung, liver and bone, but autopsy studies reveal them in approximately one third of breast cancer cases. They are usually multiple and may appear anywhere in the brain substance.

The symptoms are those of intracranial pressure and simulate those produced by primary brain tumor. When the patient complains of headache, vomiting or visual disturbances or has convulsive seizures, one should suspect a primary neoplasm in the brain, but should not overlook the fact that the patient may have an un-recognized primary cancer of the breast or lung.

OVARIAN METASTASES.   Metastasis to the ovary, arising because of dissemination of tumor cells through the general blood circulation or by way of the azygos system, may occur more frequently than we have heretofore supposed. It is probable that spread through the vertebral veins is the most common method, because ovarian metastases are frequently found without any evidence of disease in the lungs. Evidence of ovarian metastases in general is found in the neighborhood of 20 per cent of breast cancer cases, but it approaches 60 per cent when bone metastases are present It is amazing how often cancer secondary to primary breast carcinoma has been found in the ovary when oophorectomy has been done as an adjunct to hormone therapy in young girls. This has been true regardless of whether or not metastases were present elsewhere. There are no symptoms to indicate the presence of ovarian metastases. The fact that they are present so frequently gives added support to the policy of prophylactic oophorectomy when breast carcinoma is first recognized.

What Are Some of the Factors That Bear on the End-Results in Breast Cancer Therapy?

There are several factors that have a direct bearing on the end-results of treatment, notably (1) duration of the lesion, (2) size of the primary neoplasm, (3) the degree of regional lymph node involvement, and (4) the biological nature of the cancer.

DURATION.   In all cancer educational propaganda the need for early diagnosis is constantly stressed, and the breast is no exception. The earlier the lesion is recognized and treated, the better the prognosis. This is true despite the fact that a few carcinomas of the breast remain hidden and manifest themselves only when distant metastases appear. The growth pattern in breast cancer has more variables than malignant disease in practically any other part of the body, so that it is often difficult to determine with any accuracy how long a breast lesion has been present. Nevertheless the duration of the primary cancer and its earliest possible recognition are extremely important. A small carcinoma of short duration will be cured more often than the larger tumor that has been neglected, in the ratio of about 2.5 to 1.

SIZE OF THE PRIMARY CARCINOMA.   Perhaps the most important factor in prognosis is the size of the primary lesion. As the tumor size increases, the five-year cure rate tends to fall. This is true in general whether the lymph nodes are involved or not. Lesions of 1 cm. or less in size have the most favorable prognosis, despite the fact that half these patients will have one or more lymph nodes involved.

In considering the size of the lesion in regard to prognosis it is important to judge the relative rate of growth of the tumor, because the results in therapy may be different in two cases which have tumors of equal size and comparable adenopathy in the axilla. If, for example, one lesion has shown a recent increase in size and the other has remained stationary, the prognosis will favor the latter.

Although the size of the primary carcinoma itself is important in prognosis, it also has a direct relation to the extent of spread to regional lymph nodes. The larger the tumor, the greater the likelihood of nodal involvement and the fewer the five-year survivors. It is an interesting observation, however, that even when the primary tumor is 5 cm. or more in size, approximately 25 per cent of the patients still have negative lymph nodes in the axilla. The histologic nature of the tumor and its growth pattern probably explain this apparent paradox. For example, medullary carcinomas which yield a 75 per cent 5-year survival are usually 4 cm. or more in size, yet have positive nodes in only one third of the cases, in contrast to the infiltrating, scirrhous ductal carcinomas, which, though smaller in size, tend to metastasize to the axillary nodes in nearly 70 per cent and carry a far worse prognosis.

DEGREE OF REGIONAL LYMPH NODE INVOLVEMENT.   There can be little doubt that the spread of cancer beyond the original site in the breast to the regional nodes is a poor prognostic sign. When the metastatic mammary carcinoma appears in recognizable form in the supraclavicular and internal mammary regions, you are no longer dealing with a local but rather a generalized disease, and the cancer is inoperable. There are some authorities, notably McWhirter, who feel that it is useless and perhaps harmful to attempt even to dissect the axillary lymph nodes because of the chance of further disseminating cancer.

Most surgeons feel that radical mastectomy and axillary dissections should be done, provided there is no evidence of distant cancer spread. Clinical staging is of the utmost importance, then, in selecting the mode of therapy as well as in evaluating it in relation to the end-results. Accurate staging is not an easy task. One of the chief difficulties lies in the inability to detect lymph nodes accurately in the axilla. They cannot be felt in the parasternal area. The percentage of error in diagnosis is in the range of 40 per cent.

Approximately 30 per cent of the women seen will have the carcinoma confined to the breast, and another 25 per cent will have discrete axillary lymph nodes as well. These constitute the favorable group. Of the remaining 45 per cent, 30 per cent will have extensive axillary metastases and the other 15 per cent evidence of spread to remote regions of the body.

The importance of clinical staging and lymph nodal involvement in relation to prognosis is clearly evident in the end-result statistics. Seventy-five per cent of patients who have disease confined to the breast and 40 per cent of those who have discrete nodes in the axilla will be alive at 5 years, but only 20 per cent of those with metastatic axillary masses and none with distant metastases survive this period of time.

In evaluating the extent of axillary nodal involvement it is important to compare the location of positive nodes in relation to the pectoralis minor tendon. The prognosis grows progressively worse as lymph nodes are felt higher in the axilla. Involvement of the nodes high in this area has been advanced as a contraindication to surgery, but 16 per cent of patients who have positive nodes at the apex of the axilla still survive 5 years. It is also of interest to note the location of the primary tumor in relation to the site of nodal metastases, although the five-year cures are about the same wherever they are located. Tumors arise in the medial half of the breast about one third as often as they do in the lateral quadrants, but they are theoretically more dangerous because of their tendency to metastasize to the internal mammary lymph node chain, where they are less accessible. There is little difference in the survival rates between the medially and laterally placed cancers, as long as there are metastases in nodes, but the decrease in survival is appreciable with medial carcinomas when there are no regional metastases, roughly 70 versus 82 per cent at 5 years.

BIOLOGICAL NATURE OF THE CARCINOMA.   It is a well known fact that not all tumors of the breast behave alike, even though they have the same histologic appearance. A certain percentage, approximately 20 per cent, have a relatively slow rate of growth and seem little inclined to metastasize. Many of these have a recognizably different pathologic pattern, as described already, while others do not. Roughly 20 per cent of breast cancer patients will be alive 5 years whether you treat them or not.

Because some of the breast lesions are notoriously sluggish in their growth activity, it is unwise to declare a patient inoperable simply on the basis of the size or extent of the primary lesion in the breast. Many patients who have had their tumor a long time are curable despite its extent.

The principal factor that makes some tumors grow rapidly and others in an indolent way is not known, but it is probably linked to the role of the genes in determining the degree of host resistance or the virulence of the growth behavior of the tumor. MacDonald regards this so-called biologic predeterminism as the greatest single factor in evaluating breast cancer prognosis. He feels that in only twenty-five out of a hundred cases are early diagnosis and treatment important to the eventual outcome. In the remaining seventy-five women the pattern of growth is predetermined, and the cure rate depends on this rather than on duration, size of the primary cancer or histologic appearance. Of these seventy-five, twenty can be salvaged, but the remaining fifty-five will succumb to their disease. It is important, then, in evaluating prognosis to correlate the observations on the rate of growth with a clinical evaluation of the extent of disease local, regional or distant.

These views may well support the contention of some authorities that the kind of operation done and the manner in which it is performed have little to do with the end-result. It is true that survival rates from widely dispersed clinics reporting on different types of patients in different geographic areas are similar, with approximately 42 per cent of all breast cancer patients alive at the end of 5 years whether fully treated or not. Any improvement in this figure is traced to the degree of selection in the reported series. Within the same hospital surgeons of widely different training are said to come up with the same five-year survival figure. This is the basis for McWhirter's contention that a simple mastectomy with radiation therapy for the lymph nodes is a more logical approach and gives the same end-results as radical mastectomy and axillary dissection.

No one will deny the variability of the biological nature of different tumors, but this should not be used as an argument for or against the one therapeutic approach that will give the best results with the least trauma to the patient, namely, radical mastectomy. The emotional trauma of mastectomy is considerable, whether it be simple or radical. The addition of intensive radiation therapy to the chest wall and supraclavicular, parasternal and axillary areas after simple mastectomy does nothing to alleviate this mental stress, but does provide a number of complications of its own. Postirradiation necrosis of the chest wall, including both skin and cartilage, radiation pneumonitis with fibrosis of the lung, and lymphedema of the upper extremity so intense that amputation of the arm is required are some of the more serious complications that are noted far too often. The McWhirter approach to the problem of breast cancer in a patient who has disease confined to the breast or involvement of only one or two axillary lymph nodes (clinical stages I and II) has little to offer and should not supplant radical mastectomy and axillary dissection as the procedure of choice. It does have merit when the disease is more extensive. Similarly, one should not condone a sloppy, inadequately performed mastectomy operation simply because some statistics suggest that it does not matter what kind of operation you select or how and when you do it. It has been said that effective treatment will influence the survival statistics by only 10 per cent, but if a relative happened to be the patient, we should want the best informed surgeon with the most accomplished technique in order to take full advantage of the 10 per cent and perhaps add a few per cent more.

Symptoms

The few symptoms of breast carcinoma have been discussed previously in the course of the differential diagnosis of benign lesions. The majority of women discover the breast carcinoma themselves. In less than 10 per cent the physician finds it in the course of a routine physical examination. Usually the woman feels a lump in the breast entirely by accident, and it is amazing how small the lesion may be when the patient becomes aware of the fact that something is grossly wrong. Frequently the lump in the breast is entirely symptom-free, but occasionally the patient notes some local soreness or tenderness. The complaint of nagging or stabbing pain, frequently heard, carries no pathognomonic significance, since it is also one of the main symptoms of benign cystic disease. In many instances the patient notes the lump before she complains of the pain. It seems most probable that fear of the true nature of the lump expresses itself in vague variations of types of pain. Thus the patient may describe pain in terms of twinges, stabbing, burning, throbbing or aching, because she is concerned. In all probability it can be said that the majority of patients who experience pain, together with palpable evidence of a breast disease, do not have breast carcinoma.

In the absence of any erosion of the nipple, a discharge that appears only on manual expression has little significance, unless it comes from a single point within the areola or breast substance. Spontaneous nipple discharge, however, carries much greater significance. The nature of the discharge means little, but there is greater concern when it is bloody. All in all, nipple discharge is an infrequent symptom in breast carcinoma. The chances with discharge are highly in favor of a diagnosis of intraductal papilloma rather than malignant disease. When all factors are considered, approximately 20 per cent of patients who have nipple discharge also have carcinoma.

The signs that suggest breast carcinoma are less readily noted by the patient. Although the physician automatically looks for retraction of the skin, the patient is rarely aware of it. On the other hand, she must have been aware of any redness of the skin overlying the tumor, but rarely thinks anything about it. The size of the lesion and the degree of erythema may be appreciable, but for some reason the patient, although conscious of it, is unwilling to consult her physician. In most instances she suspects the cause, realizes its significance, but does not want to be told what it is.

This is the reason why it is difficult to estimate the length of time the lesion has been present in relation to its size. In general terms the more slowly growing, well

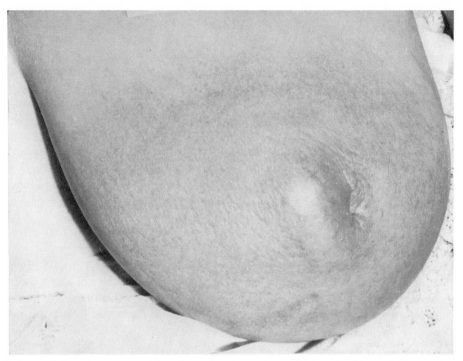

Fig. 62-8.   A large breast cancer has formed a tumor that stretches the skin and distorts the nipple area. It may be slowly growing and curable by adequate surgical therapy.

differentiated cancers have been present for a longer time. Although the emphasis in therapy is on early diagnosis and treatment, many of these patients with unusually large, slowly growing tumors do well clinically and live for a long time after radical surgery (Fig. 62–8). This does not detract from the fundamental concept that the earlier the cancer diagnosis is made and the sooner treatment is undertaken, the better the prognosis, regardless of the cancer's size, microscopic grade or duration of symptoms.

Diagnosis of Malignant Disease in the Breast

We have previously noted that the majority of women who have breast carcinoma discover the lesion themselves. Approximately 5 to 10 per cent of patients are totally ignorant of the fact that the breast contains any abnormality. The discovery is then made in the course of a routine physical examination, depending on whether the physician is alert to the significance of the smallest tumor and how proficient he is in examining the breast.

The most common pitfalls in diagnosis of breast carcinoma spring from the following causes: (*a*) Failure of the physician to attach the proper degree of importance to a tumor pointed out to him by the patient. (*b*) Overconcentration on the symptoms associated with a totally unrelated disease, and failure to do a complete physical examination. (*c*) Failure to attach proper significance to obvious signs of skin retraction overlying a breast cancer. (*d*) A habit of attributing breast signs and symptoms to benign disease or infection without investigating further. (*e*) A tendency to rely on diagnostic methods that are not conclusive and failing to do an incision and biopsy.

As Haagensen points out, the three most difficult types of carcinoma to diagnose are (1) the form of carcinoma that produces neither symptoms nor tumor. The first indication is a mass in the axilla, but nothing can be felt in the breast. Such carcinomas have been called occult or latent primary cancers. Fortunately they are rare. If axillary dissection reveals malignant disease in the lymph nodes, radical mastectomy should be done regardless of the physical findings in the breast. In most reported instances when a policy of delay has been carried out, the patient subsequently had obvious signs of carcinoma in the breast. The chances are so heavily weighted in favor of cancer in the breast, even though no gross tumor is found, that the operation for cancer is justified in these cases, even though the pathologist may fail to find any carcinoma in the surgical specimen.

2. At times women have a prolongation of breast tissue into the axillary fold overlying the pectoral muscle. The confusing factor is the difficulty in deciding whether the irregular nodularity felt is primary in the axillary lymph nodes or in the breast tissue. Such cases are extremely rare.

3. Earlier we discussed the difficulty in deciding what to do about the case that had a spontaneous nipple discharge without any obvious tumor that could be felt or any definite localized point that would produce a discharge when pressure was applied. The fundamental abnormality may be a benign intraductal papilloma, but carcinoma is always a possibility. The nipple area probably should be explored, but this raises the question of where to place the incision. The best policy then is to keep the patient under observation for a short time to await any localizing signs that may appear. If none do, the area should be surgically explored anyhow.

The diagnosis of breast cancer will rarely be missed if the physician's index of suspicion remains high and surgical breast explorations are done when there is any question of the diagnosis. The patient with cystic disease has usually been under observation for some time. The patient who has this form of benign breast condition is statistically more prone to have breast carcinoma. Any change from the pre-existing state that causes her alarm should be investigated and explored. It is also wise to keep in mind that benign disease in the breast is relatively rare in the postmenopausal woman. Any tumor felt is likely to be malignant, and excisional biopsy should be done with a provision for radical mastectomy. Beware of the small carcinoma, for many of the diagnostic criteria such as skin retraction over the tumor are absent. If there is anything odd about the palpation of the small area, it should be explored. It may well prove to be nothing more than cystic disease, adenofibrosis or benign sclerosing adenosis, but it can be carcinoma.

TREATMENT OF CARCINOMA OF THE BREAST

Since the growth pattern of carcinoma of the breast is so variable, no one form of therapy can be designated as the sole definitive method. Selection is made on an individual basis, depending on (1) the age and condition of the patient, (2) the extent of the malignant disease, and (3) the biological nature of the tumor. For example, when the carcinoma is confined to the breast, and no lymph nodes are palpable in the axilla, the patient should have a radical surgical excision of the breast combined with an axillary dissection to remove the regional lymph nodes. For specialized situations the surgeon may elect (*a*) to dissect the internal mammary lymph nodes as part of the radical mastectomy and axillary dissection, (*b*) to use radiation either as definitive therapy or in conjunction with a simple or radical excision of the breast, (*c*) to perform an oophorectomy or administer abdominal radiation as a means of securing "radiation castration," (*d*) to remove the other sources of hormonal stimulation by adrenalectomy or hypophysectomy, or (*e*) to treat the patient with hormones or chemotherapeutic agents.

In order to select properly the right form of treatment for the individual patient the surgeon should have a thorough understanding of what the different forms of therapy have to offer for the different stages of breast carcinoma. A workable clinical classification is therefore an essential part of therapy.

The following clinical classification has been suggested by Haagensen:

Group A: (1) No skin edema, ulceration or solid fixation of tumor to chest wall
(2) Axillary lymph nodes not clinically involved
Group B: (1) No skin edema, ulceration or solid fixation of tumor to chest wall
(2) Clinically involved lymph nodes, but less than 2.5 cm. in transverse diameter and not fixed to overlying skin or deeper tissues of axilla.

Most patients in these two categories should have a radical mastectomy and axillary lymph node dissection. The main object of therapy is to provide a cure, not palliation. When the patients fall into group A, the 5-year survival rate is in excess of 80 per cent. This is an excellent figure, but not entirely surprising, because an all-encompassing operation has been done for a disease that is confined to the breast. This is a clinical classification, and it is possible to have microscopic spread to regional lymph nodes without any commensurate clinical manifestation. This is particularly true of inner-quadrant tumors that have a predilection for the parasternal lymph nodes in the internal mammary chain. They cannot be palpated. The contention that the patient can be cured by radical mastectomy and lymph node dissection so long as the tumor is confined to the breast receives some support when the salvage figures in group B are reviewed.

In group B there is clinical evidence that the cancer has left the breast and spread to the axillary lymph nodes. When the metastatic disease is microscopic there and the enlargement of nodes is due to inflammation or hyperplasia, or only one or two nodes are involved by cancer, the five-year end-result figures approach those of group A. The salvage for the entire group B, however, is about 20 per cent less, for the simple reason that the cancer has spread from its original site. The cure rate, therefore, falls, and the number of patients who have distant metastases increases.

Group C patients either have a more extensive malignant disease or demonstrate clinically obvious signs of a biological pattern of growth that is unfavorable for cure, particularly by surgery. There are five main signs that suggest a poor prognosis:

Group C: Any one of these five grave signs:
(1) Edema of the skin, of limited extent
(2) Skin ulceration
(3) Solid fixation of tumor to chest wall
(4) Massive involvement of axillary lymph nodes (measuring 2.5 cm. or more in transverse diameter)
(5) Fixation of the axillary lymph nodes to overlying skin or deeper structures of axilla.

These patients are on the borderline of operability. The surgeon may elect to perform a radical mastectomy on a patient who has one or two of these signs, but if he does so, he can expect to salvage no more than 33 per cent at the end of 5 years. This is the group that might do better with radiation alone as definitive therapy or perhaps with a simple amputation of the breast followed by radiation therapy for the lymph nodes.

Group D: All other patients are inoperable:
  (1) A combination of any two or more of the five grave signs listed in group C
  (2) Extensive edema of the skin
  (3) Satellite skin nodules
  (4) Edema of the arm
  (5) Supraclavicular metastases
  (6) Distant metastases.

The surgeon must select some form of therapy for this group other than surgery alone. This is the group that will do better with (*a*) radiation therapy, (*b*) hormone therapy, or (*c*) the ablative procedures such as oophorectomy, adrenalectomy or hypophysectomy, (*d*) chemotherapy. The aim in therapy now shifts from hope of cure to palliation.

What Can Be Said about the Contraindications to Surgery?

Radical surgery for cancer of the breast is a mutilating procedure that no patient accepts with equanimity. In electing to perform it, then, the surgeon should have excellent reasons and a reasonable hope for cure. It is possible that he may make a bad situation worse by disseminating cancer, particularly if there is a chance that he may be cutting through malignant disease. The surgeon should be forearmed with full knowledge of the contraindications and why they are so labeled.

1. METASTASES. Obviously there is no point in performing a radical mastectomy if any metastases have already taken place to distant organs or to bone. This is why a so-called metastatic x-ray series is always a prerequisite to surgical intervention. Since the most likely locations for bone metastases are the lumbar spine, pelvis, femurs, dorsal spine and skull, roughly in this order, these are the areas chosen for x-ray study. To these are added x-ray films of the lungs, which also permit study of the ribs. Although x-ray studies are not infallible, they do provide a working guide. If the x-ray films are negative, but the patient complains of pain suggesting the possibility of bone metastases, the surgeon may choose to biopsy the affected bone, particularly when localized tenderness to pressure gives some idea of where to biopsy. If the scout films reveal bone metastases or lung involvement, any plan for radical surgery should be abandoned and either radiation or hormone therapy should be tried instead. The patient now has a generalized, not local, malignant disease.

The only excuse for performing operation other than the ablation procedures might be the presence of a foul fungating or ulcerating mammary mass which, because of the malodorous discharge or tendency to bleed excessively, makes the patient's existence miserable. A simple mastectomy is permissible under these conditions. In most instances irradiation is the preferred therapy.

2. EXTENSION OF CANCER. There is little point in attempting radical surgery when a cancer has escaped from the breast and extended to the supraclavicular lymph nodes or has so blocked the axillary lymphatic channels that the patient has a swollen, edematous arm. The chances of achieving even any lasting palliation diminish appreciably when the nodes are fixed to the axillary vessels or chest wall high in the axilla. The patient simply has too much disease.

Occasionally, particularly when the primary cancer arises in the medial half of the breast, a mass may develop just lateral to the sternal notch along the border of

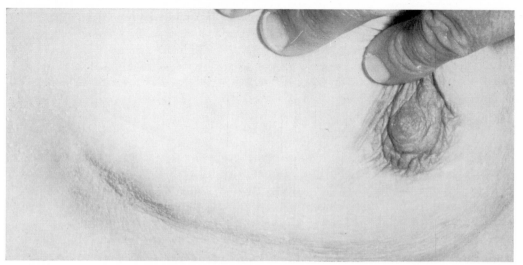

Fig. 62-9.   The area of fixation of the skin to the underlying cancer and chest wall is a poor prognostic sign. This is so-called corset-stay cancer, a localized variant of cancer *en cuirasse*.

the sternum. Some surgeons, notably Urban, have expressed enthusiasm for internal mammary node dissection as a part of the radical operation for breast cancer. The presence of a mass in this area, however, is evidence that the metastases in the internal mammary chain are far beyond the scope of any surgery designed to cure.

3. Fixation of the tumor to the chest wall and underlying pectoral fascia is not a good prognostic sign. There are several degrees of fixation. For example, the patient is a reasonable candidate for radical surgery when the only evidence of fixation is the tendency of the cancer to pull up when the pectoral muscles are contracted. On the other hand, the patient is inoperable when the tumor fails to move on the chest wall. The size of the tumor has little to do with operability. We know, for example, that medullary carcinomas grow to large size, but the 5-year salvage figures are approximately 75 per cent. It is the fixation and other criteria of extensive spread that are the determining factors.

4. Edema of the skin overlying the tumor, however extensive, is a poor prognostic sign, since the five-year cures are about half those achieved by surgery when there is no edema. The more extensive the skin edema, the worse the prognosis. The edema is due to blockage of the skin lymphatics by actively progressing cancer. The same thing may be said about the presence of satellite nodules in the skin overlying the breast. Extensive edema and satellite nodules place the patient in the category of inoperability.

Inflammatory carcinomas are in the same classification. Most of us have had such miserable experiences with this type of cancer that we are almost afraid to confirm our clinical impression by biopsy. The distinction between true inflammatory carcinoma and cancer that has undergone necrosis, but is still a local disease, must be made. When the signs of inflammation are simply those of local tenderness and redness of the overlying skin, the prognosis is no worse than in other forms of carcinoma, provided there are no other signs of extensive disease. If, however, there is widespread edema of the skin as well as erythema and fixation of the tumor to the chest wall or axillary vessels, the prognosis is poor and the patient inoperable (Fig. 62–9).

One or two of the foregoing grave signs in any patient may not be enough to contraindicate radical surgery, but they should make the surgeon stop and think, and when other signs are present as well, the patient is inoperable. For example, fixation of the skin to the tumor does not by itself materially alter the prognosis, but if the other factors mentioned are present, the patient approaches the state of inoperability. Likewise, frank ulceration of the skin need not be a contraindication if other signs of advanced disease are absent.

Principles of Treatment of Cancer of the Breast

It is not enough simply to diagnose a carcinoma of the breast and thereafter to advocate a radical mastectomy and axillary lymph node dissection. The treatment must be individualized. If there is clinical evidence of extensive malignant disease beyond the scope of radical mastectomy and nodal dissection, little good will be forthcoming if attempts are made to widen the operative field. Such patients should be considered inoperable, and some other form of therapy is indicated such as radiation or hormone therapy, the choice depending on the amount of cancerous disease present, its location and pattern of growth.

PALLIATIVE THERAPY

A high percentage of patients—nearly 40 per cent— with cancer of the breast are beyond a reasonable chance of cure at the time they are first seen. The patient has too much malignant disease to hope for permanent salvage from radical mastectomy and axillary node dissection. In recent years attempts have been made to increase the scope of surgery by performing supraradical excisions. After an adequate trial period it has become obvious that en bloc dissections of the supraclavicular nodal areas fail to add appreciably to the salvage, and then only at the price of considerable additional morbidity. If salvage or palliation is to be obtained, we must look to other forms of therapy than surgery. In addition to the patients who have too much carcinoma for primary surgical cure, there are many who have recurrences in the local operative area as well as metastases in distant locations. Consequently there is ample room for the use of therapeutic procedures designed to palliate rather than cure. The media available are (1) radiation therapy delivered by either roentgen rays or radioactive isotopes, (2) hormone therapy, and (3) the ablative procedures such as oophorectomy, adrenalectomy and hypophysectomy.

Radiation as Palliative Treatment of Cancer of the Breast

A variety of problems arise in the treatment of cancer of the breast which are best handled by irradiation, either alone or in conjunction with surgery. The role is a selective one, and the indications for its use should be firmly established. One of the main problems is to decide whether the disease is confined to the breast, and if not, to what extent the regional lymph nodes have become implicated. The mere fact that axillary nodes are involved does not exclude radical mastectomy as the therapeutic choice. If only a few nodes are positive, the 5-year salvage is often surprisingly good, and salvage figures in the range of 75 per cent have been reported. On the other hand, one may well do the patient a disservice by persisting in an operative procedure when the nodes are extensively involved, because of the danger of cutting through carcinoma and disseminating cancer cells. Before selecting any type of therapy, including irradiation, the surgeon should consider the criteria set down to determine operability. These criteria consider both the extent of the disease and biological nature of the tumor.

PRELIMINARY BIOPSY OF REGIONAL LYMPH NODAL AREAS.   To sharpen the accuracy of the clinical estimate of extent of axillary involvement, Haagensen recommends that the lymph nodes at the apex of the axilla, supraclavicular and internal mammary area be biopsied as preliminary steps in the selection of definitive therapy. Unquestionably this biopsy technique can be properly taught if there is a large concentration of breast cancers, such as one finds in a metropolitan treatment center. Since cancer may lie in tissue spaces adjacent to involved nodes and is just as lethal in that position, one may reasonably question from a practical point of view the validity of the information obtained when these biopsies are carried out by surgeons less well trained. The results might well vary, depending on the technical ability of the surgeons and the astuteness of the pathologists.

RADIATION TEST FOR BIOLOGICAL BEHAVIOR.   Not only is there a considerable percentage of error in the clinical estimate of the extent of disease—roughly 30 per cent—but other factors are involved as well, such as the growth pattern. The rate of growth and degree of erythema, edema and fixation of the skin may reflect the biological nature of the malignant tumor. In a certain percentage the surgeon is not quite sure whether the patient is operable or not. The majority of such patients will be subjected to radical operation, which may prove to be inadvisable.

MacDonald attempts to assess the nature of the growth pattern and to make a distinction between those with biological characteristics that favor radiation therapy and those that will do better with surgery. A preliminary trial of radiation, 1500 to 3000 roentgens, is given to the primary tumor. This relatively small dose of radiation is administered slowly over a two- or three-week span. If the tumor is radiosensitive, it should regress at least 50 per cent in size during this period. In his experience such lesions will do well with full irradiation, but relatively badly with surgery. Conversely, a failure to obtain a 50 per cent tumor regression would indicate that it was insensitive to radiation, but will profit by radical surgical excision. This approach is not unlike that currently used by Glucksmann in England or the Grahams in the United States for cancer of the cervix. Both groups feel that they can select the proper cancer patient for either radiation or surgical therapy in this manner.

WHAT IS THE GENERAL ATTITUDE REGARDING POSTOPERATIVE X-RAY TREATMENT?   Throughout the United States most patients with cancer of the breast receive radical mastectomy, combined with axillary lymph node dissection and supplementary x-ray therapy. Not enough attention is paid to the clinical extent of the growth or its biological nature. In many instances both the operation and the radiation therapy are inadequate. Little will be gained from indiscriminate routine use of postoperative x-ray. For example, there is no excuse for using it when the cancer is known to be confined to the breast, and the operation has been adequately performed. It will do no good and can be harmful. On the other hand, it should be used if there is any reason to believe that the operation was less than a complete excision of cancer.

If radiation is to be given, it must be delivered in adequate dosage. The aim is to cure the patient if possible and, if not, to palliate. Irradiation should not be used simply to relieve or placate the minds of the family or the surgeon. There are risks involved in giving the intensive radiation that is required to sterilize the cancer. If the dose is too small, it will be ineffectual; if it is too heavy, the skin may be seriously damaged or the underlying lung so fibrosed that the patient becomes a respiratory cripple.

The main question is whether or not postoperative x-ray treatment should be given to a patient who has only a few lymph nodes positive for cancer among many that are not. Many clinics routinely give such patients radiation therapy, but others do not. It would seem to depend upon how thorough the axillary lymph node dis- section had been. There is little doubt when the nodes are extensively involved. It is well known that routine pathologic examination does not include many small lymph nodes that may contain cancer. For example, a 30 per cent higher yield of positive nodes is obtained when the operative material is subjected to a process that isolates the nodes from the supporting tissue by clearing in oil of wintergreen. This likelihood of hidden nodal metastases would seem to be an argument in favor of postoperative irradiation. There is some evidence also to suggest that if the nodes are not heavily involved, they may be more sensitive to radiation than the primary tumor. The idea behind radiation would be to destroy any lingering metastatic disease at a post- operative time when the cells were most sensitive or, failing in this, to entrap any remaining cancer cells in the fibrous reaction that x-ray therapy evokes.

On the other hand, radiation therapy has its complications. No doubt the lymph nodes can be sterilized if enough radiation is given. It has been estimated that 6000 roentgens are needed to destroy malignant cells in inoperable carcinoma of the breast. When this amount of irradiation is given, however, there is an excellent chance that skin necrosis as well as subcutaneous and pulmonary radiation fibrosis will result. For this reason many clinics have given up supervoltage therapy for metastatic malignant disease in the axillary or supraclavicular regions. In general, amounts in the range of 2000 to 4000 roentgens are administered over a 3- or 4-week period, in the hope that this will destroy the tumor, but avoid the complications. There is considerable doubt that irradiation in these doses will completely sterilize the axillary lymph nodes. The 5 to 10 per cent improvement generally reported in survival statistics can probably be attributed to a small percentage of patients who have radiosensitive tumors.

If the degree of extension of carcinoma to the axillary nodes is minimal and the operative procedures are all-encompassing, it may be a better policy to withhold radiation therapy until there is a clearer indication for its use.

How and in What Situation May Radiation Therapy Be Used?   Radi- ation therapy for advanced or recurrent cancer of the breast may be given in a number of different situations and for a variety of reasons when clinical evaluation of the extent of the disease suggests that surgery will not completely encompass it. Irradiation may be used with profit in the following situations: (1) As a supplement to definitive surgery, when pathologic review of the operative specimen reveals many axillary metastases. (2) When large axillary lymph nodes are felt in the apex of the axilla. They may be matted or fixed to the skin. Radiation may be used as the sole method of therapy or be combined with simple amputation of the breast. (3) When physical examination presents evidence that the biological factors are unfavorable for surgical excision or patient survival. (4) As treatment for local recurrences on the chest wall after radical mastectomy and lymph node dissection. (5) As therapy for metastases in the supraclavicular or internal mammary regions. (6) To provide relief from the pain of bone metastases. (7) As a means of suppressing ovarian activity when castration seems advisable. (8) When carcinoma appears in the pregnant pa- tient and the disease is too extensive to hope for a surgical cure.

What Does Radiation Offer the Patient with Large Fixed Lymph Nodes

IN THE AXILLA? There are two courses open to the physician in treating patients who have large axillary metastases and no other evidence of distant spread: (1) radiation therapy with simple amputation of the breast or (2) radiation therapy alone. In any large series the proportion of patients in this category ranges from 33 to 40 per cent. These cases are too far advanced to expect a reasonable percentage of cure from the standard radical mastectomy and lymph node dissection. One may expect a 70 per cent 5-year survival after surgery when the cancer is confined to the breast or only one or two lymph nodes are involved, but only 40 per cent at the most if the spread is more extensive.

Radiation Therapy Combined with Simple Amputation of the Breast. In recent years there has been considerable controversy about the merits of a simple mastectomy with irradiation therapy for the regional nodal areas, as compared to radical mastectomy and lymph node dissection. The most eager proponent of this program of therapy has been McWhirter in Edinburgh, Scotland. He has expressed great concern that cancer cells may be disseminated by dissection of the axillary lymphatic chain, which might harbor cancer. He reports survival statistics which appear to indicate that not only is a simple breast amputation with radiation therapy to the lymph nodes indicated when the axillary node metastases are clinically evident, but also that it is the equal of radical mastectomy and axillary node dissection when the cancer is confined to the breast. The majority of surgeons agree with the first premise, but are totally out of sympathy with the latter. Ackerman, in a review of McWhirter's material, suggests that there is too high a rate of persistence of cancer in the local area in his reported series and that no histologic proof was offered that radiation affected the lymph nodes, much less sterilized them. Furthermore, one third of the cases reported had other procedures such as oophorectomy or hormone therapy performed concomitantly, which might influence the end-result. It would seem that there is far greater reason to expect dissemination of cancer after cutting through it during a simple amputation than during radical mastectomy and a node dissection which, if performed properly, should remove the axillary nodes, intervening lymphatics and primary tumor en bloc. Although the five-year survival figures presented by McWhirter are excellent and compare favorably, from a statistical point of view, with those reported by surgeons performing radical mastectomy, there appear to be other factors that influence the results.

There is a place for simple amputation of the breast and radiation therapy of nodal areas that are extensively involved by cancer spread. Fletcher, for example, advocates simple mastectomy as a preliminary to irradiation therapy applied to the axillary, supraclavicular and internal mammary regions when a large tumor is present in a pendulous breast. Obviously such cases set up technical difficulties that make irradiation of the primary tumor extremely difficult. This is called a "toilette" mastectomy. He recognizes that there is danger involved in cutting through lymphatics that may contain tumor, and does not do so if the axillary tail of the breast appears to be involved, but the known risks are assumed in the interest of better local radiation therapy when this portion of the breast is clinically free of tumor.

The results obtained from the combination of simple amputation of the breast and irradiation of the nodal areas are in the range of 33 per cent 5-year survivals. This is the equal of or may be superior to results obtained from radical surgery for the same amount of disease. Apparently both simple mastectomy and irradiation contribute to the result, for even the most enthusiastic exponents of radiation therapy prefer to have the primary tumor removed, if at all feasible.

Radiation as the Sole Definitive Therapy for Axillary Node Involvement. When the primary tumor is small, but there is a clinical suggestion that the axillary, supraclavicular or internal mammary nodal regions are involved in cancerous disease, radiation therapy is used alone. McWhirter likewise relies on radiation as the sole method of therapy when the tumor is fixed to the underlying structures, when numerous satellite nodules are present or when the primary cancer in the breast seems to involve the axillary lymph nodes in continuity. In addition it may be wise to use irradiation alone in elderly women who for various reasons may be unsuitable candidates for surgery.

How Should the Radiation Therapy Be Given? In order that irradiation may destroy cancer cells or entrap them sufficiently in fibrous tissue so that they can neither grow nor disseminate, adequate doses must be given. There are also additional factors that bear on successful radiation therapy: (*a*) the source of the radiation and (*b*) the length of time over which the treatments are spread.

Conventional x-ray therapy, as administered to the majority of patients in radiologists' offices and in hospitals throughout this country, is given by the 250-KV machine. Much of it is inadequate, not because of the voltage of the machine, but because insufficient doses are given or the treatments are concentrated in too short a time.

Despite the fact that we now have available in many areas supervoltage x-ray betatrons as therapeutic units, which use isotopic radioactive cobalt, there appears to be no additional salvage so far attributable to their use above that obtained by the 250-KV units.

Serious complications, in the form of radiation osteitis, skin ulceration and pneumonitis, are far more common because of the greater depth dose delivered by the more powerful units. For these reasons there is a tendency to return to the use of the 250-KV machines, giving larger doses, but spreading them out over a longer time.

It has been suggested that a 6000-roentgen tumor dose is needed to destroy malignant cells in an inoperable cancer of the breast. When depth penetration is needed, as in the supraclavicular, internal mammary and mediastinal regions, it is possible to deliver tumor doses of this magnitude, provided they are spread out over ten to twelve weeks. This means that the patient will have to be treated five days a week for approximately three months. In this manner there is less likelihood of skin breakdown and far less radiation pneumonitis. The chest wall and axillary areas are more superficial, and less of a depth dose is required. The radiologist tries to deliver 4500 to 5500 roentgens to these areas. When the therapy is carried out over a four-week period, the complications, particularly radiation skin necrosis, are apt to be both frequent and severe. Distributed over a three-month period in the manner suggested by Bouchard and Baclesse, the adverse effects can be minimized.

What Other Radiation Sources Are Available? To meet specific situations, two other radiation sources are available: (*a*) radium needles and (*b*) radioactive isotopes. When local conditions call for it, radium needles may be implanted in local tumor growths that persist on the chest wall or in the axilla, despite satisfactory radiation response in other areas within the treatment field. Although the needles are usually implanted in the tumor fairly close to the skin and doses up to 3000 to 4000 roentgens are given, erythematous skin reaction is rarely a problem. There has been some temporary enthusiasm for the use of radioactive phosphorus given intravenously at the time of mastectomy in patients with advanced cancer of the breast. When given in conjunction with testosterone, improvement has been noted in a few patients, but there has been no general acceptance of this form of therapy.

WHAT DOES RADIATION OFFER IN INFLAMMATORY CARCINOMA OF THE BREAST OR OTHER FORMS OF BIOLOGICALLY UNFAVORABLE CANCER?   Although the chances of long-time survival are practically nonexistent, radiation therapy does have something to offer in patients who have inflammatory carcinoma. Surgery is contraindicated, because even a biopsy may further activate the growth of the cancer. Many such tumors are sensitive to radiation, and palliation in the form of temporary regression of tumor may be possible when irradiation in doses up to 5000 roentgens is given.

In addition to inflammatory carcinoma of the breast, radiation seems to be the most effective form of treatment when (a) the breast ulcerates because of the size and extent of the malignant tumor within it, (b) there are numerous satellite tumor nodules, (c) the tumor is fixed to the underlying tissues and metastases to other areas outside the breast may be expected.

HOW DO YOU TREAT A SUPRACLAVICULAR AND INTERNAL MAMMARY METASTASIS?   There are two methods of treating supraclavicular and internal mammary node metastases: (a) surgery, (b) radiation. Since spread to these regions is a fair indication that cancer of the breast is now a generalized rather than a localized disease, therapy will naturally tend to fall in the field of radiation. Supraclavicular metastases usually appear only after the axillary chain has become heavily involved. Surgical procedures designed to remove these lymph nodes, along with those in the axillary region in continuity with the primary lesion in the breast, have largely been abandoned. The results were not improved, and the operation is a formidable one.

Internal Mammary Nodes.   Proper management of the internal mammary lymph nodal chain has not been completely established. Although these nodes are rarely involved when the tumor is confined to the breast, they do tend to be implicated to a far greater extent than we formerly believed when the cancer has indeed left the confines of the breast. This is particularly true of tumors located in the inner part of the medial half of the breast, but even when the tumor is laterally placed, extension may occur to these lymph nodes, after first involving the axillary chain. A few patients will demonstrate positive nodes without axillary involvement. When the axillary lymph nodes are the site of metastases, the internal mammary nodes will be positive in 30 to 50 per cent. Figures as high as 60 per cent have been reported.

The internal mammary lymph nodes tend to concentrate in the parasternal area in the first four interspaces. A few surgeons have incorporated dissection of the internal mammary chain as a part of their radical mastectomy and axillary node dissection, with a mortality rate of less than 1 per cent. Statistically, one third of the patients with positive lymph nodes treated in this manner apparently are free of disease at five years.

This procedure, in expert hands, apparently offers a 10 per cent higher cure rate than the standard radical mastectomy and axillary dissection. There are no comparable statistics for radiation therapy of this area, simply because it is a difficult area to biopsy. The majority of surgeons assume that malignant disease has spread to these nodes when the tumor in the breast is medially placed and the axillary lymph nodes are involved. Haagensen has made it a practice to biopsy the subclavicular nodes high in the axillary chain, as well as the internal mammary chain in the first three intercostal spaces as a preliminary procedure. The subsequent plan of therapy is based on the pathologic review of the material obtained. This method is cumbersome and has the disadvantage that the biopsy is done directly in a tumor-bearing area. The cancer may be in the supporting tissue as well as in the lymph nodes, and for this reason tumor cells may be disseminated. A positive biopsy, however, will prevent a useless radical mastectomy.

If the lymph nodes in this area are involved, as they frequently are, and their presence is such a bad prognostic sign, it might be advisable to recommend intensive radiation to these regions in lieu of a biopsy or an extensive operative procedure.

WHAT CAN RADIATION THERAPY DO TO THE INTERNAL MAMMARY CHAIN? Although there is no statistical evidence to support the contention that x-ray treatment will destroy tumor within the lymph nodes of this area, it is reasonable to suppose that some salvage can be obtained. The nodes along the sternum are small, and some of the tumor actually lies in tissue spaces. If the metastasis is a relatively early one, radiation therapy may well destroy it. This is less likely to be the case if the metastases are of long standing. Patients who have died of their disease after irradiation to this area have residual disease present about as often as they are free of tumor. Since many of the patients who have supraclavicular and internal mammary spread have generalized rather than localized malignant disease, it would appear logical to irradiate patients with inner quadrant tumors or axillary metastases, regardless of the location of the primary tumor, rather than to operate on them.

WHAT CAN RADIATION DO FOR THE LOCAL CANCER RECURRENCE ON THE CHEST WALL AFTER SURGERY? Between 5 and 10 per cent of adequately treated cases of carcinoma of the breast will recur on the chest wall after surgery. This is why a wide surgical excision with meticulous dissection of the skin flaps is recommended. Many surgeons make no attempt to cover the defect with skin, but rely entirely on grafting procedures at the time of definitive surgery.

Radiation therapy to the chest wall should not be used as a prophylactic measure. It does not prevent cancer recurrences, simply damages the skin and complicates further therapy if metastases should subsequently appear in this area. X-ray treatment has been useful in controlling both soft part and bony recurrences on the chest wall when they appear in a region previously untouched by x-ray. If the recurrent tumor appears after the chest wall has previously been irradiated, the physician should not reirradiate, but should place his faith on hormone therapy. Occasionally recurrences or metastases will appear on the chest wall while the patient is receiving hormone therapy for distant metastases. If the chest wall has not previously been irradiated, the hormone therapy should be continued while the chest wall recurrence is being irradiated, because one form of therapy often complements the other.

WHAT DOES RADIATION HAVE TO OFFER THE PATIENT WHO HAS PAIN FROM BONE METASTASES? One of the chief problems in the management of a breast carcinoma that has passed beyond the chance of cure is the necessity of trying to make the patient's life more comfortable. Too frequently we, as physicians, lose interest in a patient we cannot cure. These cancer patients should be given suitable relief from their symptoms, whether it be pain or mental anguish.

The most common source of pain is metastatic malignant disease in bone, with pleuritic pain a close second. Pleural pains, along with those from lung and other visceral metastases, are best treated by hormones. X-ray treatment, on the other hand, will relieve pain due to bone metastases in nearly 70 per cent of the cases, despite the fact that less than half of the patients will present any clinical or x-ray evidence of postirradiation recalcification. The lumbar spine is a favorite place for osseous metastases to appear in. In many instances these are the only bones involved, and the situation may remain so for considerable periods of time before widespread cancer dissemination occurs. The usual radiation dosage is in the range of 2400 to 3000 roentgens, given over a period of 2 weeks. The total dosage will vary, depending on the region to be treated. For example, if metastases appear in the cranial bones, the dose would be about half as much. In many instances the addition of steroid therapy will improve the results over those obtained by irradiation alone.

What about Radiation as a Means of Suppressing Ovarian Activity?   It is far better to use surgery than radiation therapy when ovarian castration is indicated. This is particularly true of young women. If for any reason a surgical procedure is contraindicated and suppression of ovarian function is essential, irradiation will be effective, provided enough x-radiation is given and large enough fields are covered. The amount given will depend on the age of the patient. Radiologists use a rule of thumb in estimating the dosage required to castrate the patient. The younger the patient, the more radiation she will require. In most instances ovarian function can be suppressed in a woman who is practically menopausal with 600 to 800 roentgens, but for every decade younger the dose must be doubled and should be given through 20 by 20 cm. fields.

What Does Radiation Offer the Patient Who Has Carcinoma during Pregnancy?   When one speaks of carcinoma of the breast and pregnancy, it is important to distinguish between those patients that have a pregnancy at the same time that they have a carcinoma discovered and those who become pregnant later. The prognosis is generally poor for the former group, but there is little difference between the survival figures for the patient who becomes pregnant after the completion of therapy and for the woman who has carcinoma of the breast without pregnancy.

Since the neoplastic growth characteristics of cancer of the breast are definitely unfavorable when a pregnancy occurs simultaneously, most patients when they are first seen will be inoperable, according to the criteria set forth above for operability. There is little else that can be done except offer the patient radiation therapy. Few patients survive five years, and the average length of prolongation of life is only thirty months. This seems like a relatively short time, but actually the survival time for the patient who is inoperable and not pregnant is only slightly higher, thirty-four months.

Fortunately carcinoma of the breast during pregnancy and lactation is relatively uncommon. Since nearly two thirds of such cases fall into the inoperable category, there is ample reason to rely on irradiation as the definitive therapy, with supplementary help from castration performed at the time of cesarean section.

Oophorectomy as Palliative Therapy for Advanced Cancer of the Breast

It is a well known fact that breast cancer varies appreciably in its rate of growth and manner of spread, not only in different patients, but also in the same subject from time to time. Since the cancer's growth pattern is often only indirectly related to the histologic picture, other factors must be considered to explain the variations that are noted. The difference may be traced to alterations in the internal environment of the host. Long before it became evident that the rate of growth of mammary carcinoma could be influenced by the steroid hormones of either ovary or adrenal, reports appeared suggesting that oophorectomy would result in (a) atrophy of the breast (Shinzinger in 1889) and (b) remission in the growth of advanced cancer of the breast (Beatson, 1896). It is now well established that certain breast carcinomas are estrogen-dependent. The palliative effect of castration, which alters the internal endocrine environment, is clearly evident in 30 to 40 per cent of the patients treated.

WHAT IS THE MECHANISM INVOLVED? It is reasonable to assume that the beneficial effect of castration is due to the fact that the natural source of estrogen has been removed. By laboratory analysis of 24-hour urine specimens it can be shown that the excretion of estrone, estradiol and estriol is reduced. Clinical remissions often follow. If there has been an initial response to oophorectomy, any subsequent re-exacerbation of tumor growth can be further inhibited by bilateral adrenalectomy, removing the remaining major source of estrogen. Unfortunately, the explanation for tumor regression is not quite as simple as this. For example, despite the fact that the combination of oophorectomy and adrenalectomy reduces estrogen secretion to levels so low that they cannot be accurately recorded by present laboratory techniques, cancer often continues to grow. It is also something of a paradox that the administration of large doses of estrogen will cause a breast cancer to regress. Supposedly the growth-inhibiting effect is mediated through the pituitary and the resulting suppression of its gonadotropic function. Actually, we do not know the true mechanism by which the steroid hormones operate. Investigators have now turned to study of the enzyme systems for a more complete explanation of hormonal action. Since the interaction of enzymes and coenzymes chiefly takes place at the cellular level, it is interesting that some of the best results after oophorectomy have come when thyroid extract was given at the same time. Thyroid conditions the metabolism of cells in the hormonal target areas.

WHAT IS THE VALUE OF CASTRATION IN BREAST CANCER? Castration by either surgical or radiologic means is most effective in the patient who is having regular menstruation, and in the woman who is either menopausal or has had the menopause within a five-year period. Cures are not obtained in this manner, but objective improvement is noted more often, and longevity may be extended for months or years. The recurrent carcinoma or distant metastases may be in soft tissue, viscera, bone or in all three. Oophorectomy is particularly effective with soft-tissue and visceral lesions, but it may provide rapid and dramatic relief in patients who have bone pain from osseous metastases. Within twenty-four hours after surgical castration pain diminishes appreciably, to disappear entirely when the urinary calcium levels drop to subnormal levels.

From our experience derived from oophorectomy to date, it would seem that the objective response provides working evidence that many breast cancers are hormone-dependent. If an objective response is not forthcoming within six weeks, the patient's carcinoma is not likely to be hormone-dependent, and there is no point in attempting hormone therapy or other ablative procedures. Since palliative therapy for advanced or recurrent carcinoma of the breast should be used in a definite sequence, any supplementary hormone therapy should be withheld until the remission from oophorectomy shows signs of abating.

HOW SHOULD CASTRATION BE DONE? The majority of physicians prefer oophorectomy to irradiation for purposes of castration, although the proponents of irradiation find no essential difference in patient response. For the younger pre-menopausal woman with breast cancer, when castration is most effective, oophorectomy is both quicker and more reliable. It is well known that the ovaries of young women are more resistant to x-ray therapy than those of the older woman. Surgery removes all the ovarian tissue, leaving nothing behind that could stimulate the growth of the cancer in the breast. Stromal hyperplasia of the ovarian tissue may produce such a stimulating effect. Oophorectomy, then, gives a response which is more predictable.

HOW DO YOU MEASURE THE RESPONSE TO CASTRATION? The measure of the response should be objective evidence of breast tumor regression, not laboratory data based on urinary excretion of the estrogens. The vaginal smear does reflect the suppression of ovarian activity, as shown by the atrophic epithelium that remains, but the observations are sometimes equivocal. One wonders then whether the source of the estrogen is exogenous or whether the adrenal cortex is responsible. Recently we have been interested in the effect that oophorectomy has upon the electro-abdomino-vaginal potential readings. Recordings are in the electro-positive range in castrates, and remissions persist as long as the readings continue at this level. These observations show excellent correlation with the urinary estrogen values, when they are analyzed by the Brown method. By and large, however, the response to castration should be judged by cancer regression in *all, not just one*, of the metastases.

WHAT RESULTS CAN BE EXPECTED FROM OVARIAN ABLATION? The reported palliative results from castration vary, depending on the criteria used to measure improvement, as well as the selection of patients. To evaluate truly the benefits that come from suppression of ovarian activity, there should be clinical evidence that the cancer was actually previously in a phase of progression. In many reports hormone therapy has been given in addition to oophorectomy. The effect of one may supplement that of the other, and it is often hard to evaluate the real cause of any improvement noted. The recorded results usually refer to subjective rather than objective improvement. It is possible, however, to obtain gratifying relief of the pain from osseous metastases without any accompanying measurable changes in tumor size. The results reported from many sources are in the range of 20 to 50 per cent objective remissions. These are palliative results and have little to do with longevity. The average prolongation of life will be measured in months, not years.

IS THERE ANY PLACE FOR PROPHYLACTIC OOPHORECTOMY OR RADIATION CASTRATION? There is no complete agreement among competent observers about the value of prophylactic castration in breast carcinoma. Those who advocate it do so for two reasons: (1) the evidence that longevity is increased, and (2) future pregnancies and lactation are prevented, thus reducing the chances of carcinoma appearing in the remaining breast. Those who oppose it feel that adequate proof of its value has not been established and prefer to wait to perform oophorectomy until actual metastases appear.

Other arguments advanced to discredit prophylactic castration are (1) that early operation eliminates the only yardstick for estimating estrogen dependence of tumor, upon which hormone therapy and ablative procedures depend. (2) Altering the environment at the time of radical mastectomy may promote rather than discourage tumor growth. (3) If the patient is to be cured, this will be accomplished by mastectomy, and castration can produce only palliation, which should be reserved for a time of need. (4) Psychologically, the patient is already traumatized by mastectomy and certainly does not want to become castrate unless there is definite proof that she will benefit thereby. To the emotional stress, castration will add the problems of the menopause in both the fields of physiology and psychosomatics.

The over-all survival figures, however, do suggest that the life of the breast cancer patient who has a prophylactic castration is prolonged when the axillary lymph nodes were negative at the time of radical mastectomy. Benefit is more apparent when the lymph nodes were positive for cancer. Approximately 30 per cent more patients are alive at 5 and 10 years than expected when castration is done at the time of a radical mastectomy in patients who have axillary metastases. Improvement in survival statistics for the patients who have negative lymph nodes is approximately half that of the patients with positive nodes. It must be kept in mind, however, that there is some degree of selection in both the patient and the control groups, and some of the patients had received hormone therapy as well. A clear-cut picture of the true value of castration alone is therefore lacking.

So far as the value of castration and the prevention of pregnancy are concerned as beneficial influences upon the possible development of carcinoma in the remaining breast, the evidence also is not clear-cut. If the original therapy for cancer of the breast has been adequate, when the disease has been relatively confined or the axillary lymph nodes are involved only to a minor degree, the prognosis following surgery for operable cancer in the opposite breast would appear to be no different than if castration were not done.

The majority of surgeons prefer to withhold castration until there is definite proof of cancer recurrence and evidence of progression in the tumor growth process. The best results will be forthcoming in the patient who has generalized rather than localized disease.

What Is the Proper Place for Adrenalectomy or Hypophysectomy?

In the previous discussion, oophorectomy has been shown to be effective in producing long-time remissions in patients who have a hormone-dependent tumor. This is a relatively simple procedure for the patient to undergo, and it can readily be done by the average surgeon with complete assurance that all the ovarian tissue has been removed.

This cannot be said about either adrenalectomy or hypophysectomy. A complete hypophysectomy, which leaves no doubt that all functioning tissue has been removed, is a difficult task for even the most knowledgeable and technically excellent neurosurgeon. Adrenalectomy, though it presents less of a problem, is still a formidable operation for most surgeons, and here, too, one cannot be sure that all adrenocortical function is abolished, since adrenocortical rests are not uncommon.

The endocrine problems that follow these ablative procedures may be formidable. For example, there may be profound disturbances in electrolyte and water metabolism. Sudden strains may precipitate a crisis due to either adrenal or pituitary insufficiency. In addition to the morbidity factors, one must also consider that adrenalectomy or hypophysectomy operations carry a significant mortality, while oophorectomy does not. Both the patient and the surgeon should think twice before accepting or offering the suggestion that such surgery should be undertaken. Knowing that there is a variability in the rate of tumor growth even in the presence of demonstrable breast cancer metastases, it is important to establish the fact that there is an actual progression of tumor growth before considering either.

Adrenalectomy and hypophysectomy in their rightful place can be useful therapeutic tools in the management of the patient with advanced or recurrent cancer of the breast. Certainly adrenalectomy constitutes a surer method of suppressing adrenal function and inducing tumor regression than the use of corticosteroids. The latter have been shown to offer subjective improvement without influencing tumor growth.

The place for hypophysectomy and adrenalectomy is a highly selected one. For example, the most enthusiastic advocates do not recommend either operation when the patient has liver or intracranial metastases. Uniformly these patients have done badly. There is a preponderance of opinion also that adrenalectomy or hypophysectomy has little to offer if the patient has not had a favorable response to castration.

In keeping with the fundamental concept that the various methods of therapy should be used in sequence, the ablative procedures should be tried only after hormone therapy has exhausted its possibilities and the patient has a reactivated tumor. The order in which the therapy is carried out is particularly important, since the patient may gain a remission when adrenalectomy and hypophysectomy follow hormone therapy, but hormone therapy has nothing to offer after surgical excision of the adrenal or pituitary has failed.

In evaluating the reported results of adrenalectomy or hypophysectomy one should remember that the following types of patient are never offered the operation: (*a*) poor-risk patients, (*b*) patients who have failed to respond to castration, (*c*) patients who have liver or brain metastases. If the reported series is otherwise unselected, the objective improvement will be in the range of 20 per cent, which is about what can be expected in breast cancer patients who have been castrated or given androgen or estrogen therapy. If careful selection is made, approximately 40 per cent will register tumor regressions.

Hormone Therapy for Breast Cancer

Since a relatively high percentage (40 per cent) of patients with cancer of the breast are beyond a reasonable chance for cure at the time they are first seen, and others have recurrences after surgical therapy, there is ample scope for the use of palliative procedures. Hormone therapy has much to offer the patient, not in the realm of cure, but in relief of symptoms and rehabilitation. It must be kept in mind (*a*) that steroid therapy does not produce a cure, though life may be prolonged for a span of months or years; (*h*) that there is no real evidence that hormones will either prevent or postpone the subsequent development of cancer recurrence or metastases when given for prophylactic reasons. Hormones do help when there is clinical or x-ray evidence that the malignant disease is no longer local.

The main reason why hormones are effective stems from the observation that certain tumors occurring in different anatomic locations such as breast, thyroid and endometrium are hormone-dependent. It is thus possible to influence their rate of growth by altering the hormonal environment. This may be done in two ways: (1) by eliminating endogenous hormone secretion through removal of its source by oophorectomy, adrenalectomy or hypophysectomy, as discussed already, or (2) by supplying exogenous hormones that upset the endocrine balance and make a less favorable soil for the propagation of tumor cells that are dependent on hormones for their proliferative activities.

Before embarking on a course of hormone therapy it is important to have some estimate of (*a*) the rate of growth of the breast tumor, and (*b*) the extent of the patient's own hormone production. Unfortunately, it is not an easy matter to evaluate the degree of ovarian activity in a menopausal woman, because the output is bound to be variable, and the present analytical methods do not accurately measure small amounts. It is possible, however, to form some idea of the tumor growth rate from information obtained in the patient's history. Some tumors grow relatively rapidly, but others appear to remain static and exhibit little tendency to progress for relatively long periods of time. It is reasonable to assume in the last instance that the patient is living in symbiotic harmony with her tumor or that the tumor is not hormone-dependent. Any substitution therapy will then be useless or actually harmful if the balance is upset.

SHOULD PALLIATIVE THERAPY FOLLOW A DEFINITE PLAN?   It is axiomatic in any palliative therapy of cancer of the breast that the plan of treatment follow an orderly pattern (Table 12). The appearance of cancer recurrence or metastasis is so upsetting emotionally that there is a strong tendency to combine all the therapeutic maneuvers at the same time, but this is an error. It is far better to try one thing at a time and save something for a rainy day ahead. Since cancer of the breast occurs in both premenopausal and postmenopausal women, the program of therapy evolved must take into consideration the patient's age in relation to her own hormone production. The program of Baker and Kelley given below has these virtues.

Table 12.   Sequence of Palliative Treatment for Advanced Cancer of the Breast

REMISSION	NO REMISSION
Premenopausal	
1. Surgical castration 2. Corticosteroids 3. Androgens 4. Hypophysectomy	Androgens Chemotherapy
Menopausal and up to 5 Years Postmenopausal	

1. Establish level of pituitary FSH
2. Review vaginal smears for cornification
  a. If FSH is low and the smear cornified (over 50% of cells), treat as premenopausal patient
  b. If FSH is high and less than 50% of cells in vaginal smear are cornified, treat as postmenopausal patient
3. Corticosteroids
4. Androgens
5. Hypophysectomy
6. Chemotherapy
	Oophorectomy
	Androgens
	Chemotherapy

Postmenopausal	
1. Estrogens 2. Androgens 3. Corticosteroids 4. Hypophysectomy	Androgens Corticosteroids Chemotherapy

WHAT IS THE PLAN FOR THE PREMENOPAUSAL WOMAN?   Since the patient is still having menstrual cycles, it is obvious that hormonal activity is within the range of reasonably normal levels. The best means of upsetting the environment is to use castration.

After oophorectomy one may expect to find in approximately one third to two fifths of the cases that the local tumor, if she has one, will regress or the bone metastases will recalcify. The patient may have a remission of several months or a few years after this procedure alone. If she then has a cancer recurrence, she will probably receive further benefit from adrenalectomy, hypophysectomy or hormone therapy, preferably the last. There is little point in ablative therapy if no initial improvement follows oophorectomy. One may elect to give hormone therapy, but there is little chance that it will do any good.

HOW IS THE MENOPAUSAL WOMAN MANAGED?   The management of the patient who suffers carcinoma of the breast after the cessation of her menstrual periods introduces a different problem. This revolves around the question of how much ovarian activity the patient has, despite the fact that she is no longer having menstrual periods. There is increasing evidence, both on the biochemical and clinical sides, that the ovaries do continue to function. If the patient has a carcinoma of the breast at the same time the menopause occurs, or in the five-year period following it, the extent of ovarian function must be assessed.

The means available to measure such activity are time-consuming, cumbersome and not overhelpful in providing a yardstick by which selection of the proper candidate for the proper mode of therapy can be made. The methods now used are (1) urinary assays for total estrogen, (2) metabolism of the tumor studied with radioactive isotopes, (3) electro-abdomino-vaginal potentials which reflect ovarian activity, (4) uptake of components of nucleic acids. The simplest method is to do pituitary FSH assays on urine and compare them with the extent of cornification seen in the vaginal smears. If, for example, the urinary FSH is low and the vaginal cornification is high, then the patient's ovaries are still functioning, and oophorectomy should be performed. In other words, she should be treated like the premenopausal woman. If the reverse is true, the treatment should follow the program outlined for the postmenopausal woman (Table 12).

WHAT IS THE PROGRAM FOR THE POSTMENOPAUSAL WOMAN? In the postmenopausal woman who has no ovarian activity the physician should attempt to alter the hormonal environment by the use of steroid hormones. Estrogen is the hormone of choice, and improvement may be expected in approximately 40 to 50 per cent of breast cancer patients, provided large enough doses are used. The primary aim is to inhibit the anterior pituitary and its output of gonadotropins. Small doses will not succeed. The usual doses recommended are (*a*) diethylstilbestrol, 5 mg., 3 times daily; (*b*) Premarin, 10 mg., 3 times daily; or (*c*) Ethinyl estradiol, 1 mg., 3 times daily. There is no point in using larger doses than these, because the salvage rate will not be increased.

Many authorities feel that androgen rather than estrogen should be used in the postmenopausal woman. In support of the contention that estrogens are better is the observation that estrogen, administered to a group of women who had cancer of the breast ten years after they had had a natural menopause, produced a 25 to 30 per cent objective regression, as against 12 per cent when androgen was used. The greatest improvement, which averages about one year in duration, will be noted when the patient presents soft part metastatic lesions, although approximately 20 per cent will also recalcify breast cancer metastases in bone.

Estrogen therapy is not without its disadvantages. Some of the undesirable effects observed are (*a*) breakthrough hormone-induced vaginal bleeding, (*b*) pigmentation of the nipples, (*c*) stress incontinence. This last is a distressing complaint that is seen relatively frequently. Why the patient has urinary incontinence is not clear, because estrogen therapy usually helps women in the menopause who have problems with urination. (*d*) Estrogen in this dosage tends to upset the electrolyte balance, and the patient may store excessive intercellular fluid because of sodium retention. With recognition that this contingency is a possibility, the estrogen regimen can usually be continued if the patient is made to follow a low-salt diet with added help from one of the diuretics, such as Diuril. Occasionally digitalis may be needed. (*e*) The most dangerous side effect is the chance that the patient may have hypercalcemia. This can lead to kidney damage and uremia. Approximately 10 per cent of patients on this estrogen regimen will mobilize calcium into the blood. The only thing to do then is stop the estrogen, replace the fluids and give cortisone.

When cancer recurrences appear, and estrogen therapy can no longer control the tumor growth, all is not lost. There is a general observation that if the tumor has once demonstrated that it can be influenced by altering the hormonal environment, it will in all probability respond again either to ablation therapy such as oophorectomy, adrenalectomy or hypophysectomy or perhaps to another hormone such as androgen or prednisone. It is thus possible to obtain another remission which may last one or two years. One should constantly keep in mind that this regimen is palliative, not curative. As a further adjunct to palliation, remissions of breast cancer have been achieved by simply discontinuing all types of supportive therapy.

WHAT ABOUT ANDROGEN THERAPY?   Symptomatic relief can be obtained in patients who have metastatic spread from cancer of the breast by giving testosterone propionate intramuscularly 3 times weekly in dosage of 50 to 100 mg. The intramuscular injection route is stressed because it far surpasses the effects obtained from oral medication. Testosterone is best used when metastatic bone lesions are present, for in addition to improvement in the general sense of well-being, as measured by gain in both appetite and weight, the metastasis in bone will show x-ray evidence of recalcification in about 20 per cent. But nearly 90 per cent will be relieved of bone pain.

It must be firmly kept in mind that, although the patient does get relief of pain and generally feels better, in many instances metastatic tumor growth is not necessarily inhibited. Survival is not greatly influenced by whether androgen or estrogen is given (Table 13).

Table 13.   Influence of Dominant Breast Cancer Metastasis on Survival, from Onset of Therapy

DOMINANT METASTATIC LESION AND THERAPY	CASES	NUMBER OF SURVIVORS	12-MONTH SURVIVAL, %
Androgen, 285 cases			
Bone..........................	122	70	57
Skin, breast, lymph node...................	27	15	55
Visceral (liver, lung, brain)................	36	23	17
Estrogen, 158 cases			
Bone..........................	41	26	63
Skin, breast, lymph node...................	35	30	86
Visceral (liver, lung, brain)................	82	16	19

Many of the undesirable side effects noted in estrogen therapy appear also during the use of androgen. Thus we have the possibility of excessive fluid retention and hypercalcemia to contend with. Hypercalcemia is seen more frequently when testosterone is used in (14 per cent of cases with testosterone, versus 8 per cent with estrogen). At times the patient may have an increase in bone pain after one or two injections of testosterone propionate. In many instances pain disappears as therapy continues, but the physician should remember that the pain may be an indication that tumor growth has been speeded up because of the medication.

The most distressing, though not the most serious, complication of androgen therapy is the virilization that manifests itself by hoarseness and deepening of the voice, hirsutism, loss of temporal hair, clitoral enlargement and increased libido. At present there are a number of androgen-related experimental drugs being used to suppress tumor growth which inhibit the masculinizing effects. They have not been in use long enough for a true evaluation.

WHAT ARE THE SYMPTOMS OF DEVELOPING HYPERCALCEMIA?   Since hypercalcemia may develop during the course of either estrogen or androgen therapy and is so serious that the treatment must be discontinued, it is important to recognize some of the symptoms that herald its onset. When the patient begins to note the following symptoms, her blood calcium level should be checked at regular intervals: (*a*) dry mouth, (*b*) polydipsia, (*c*) polyuria, (*d*) nausea and vomiting, (*e*) sluggish mentality as indicated by apathy, drowsiness or stupor. The serum calcium increases, because the kidney cannot wholly eliminate the excess being produced by osteolytic breakdown. Hypercalcemia develops, and renal failure may follow. Effective treatment, in addition to discontinuance of the steroid medication, involves hospitalization and the administration of large amounts of fluid by the intravenous route, as well as cortisone therapy. The dosage schedule for the corticosteroids must be high to be effective and is in the range of 100 to 300 mg. of cortisone daily. One may choose to use one of the derivatives of cortisone, such as prednisone or prednisolone, in equivalent dosages, 30 to 60 mg. daily.

WHAT CAN YOU EXPECT FROM CORTICOSTEROID THERAPY, AND WHEN DO YOU ELECT TO USE IT?   In recent years adrenalectomy has been performed for patients who had breast cancers that regressed after a successful remission induced by either estrogen or androgen therapy. The results have not been impressive, and corticosteroids have been used instead in an effort to find substances that would (1) suppress the activity of the adrenal cortex, and (2) depress the pituitary gonadotropic hormones without the need of resorting to surgical ablative procedures. Subjective improvement following the use of such corticosteroids as cortisone, prednisone and prednisolone has been dramatic, but authorities differ in their observations about the amount of objective metastatic breast tumor regression that can be obtained from this type of therapy.

For example, the corticosteroids have been used with success in inflammatory carcinoma of the breast. The patient feels better, the erythema disappears. The breast becomes more pliable as the edema disappears and the tumor feels smaller. It is possible, however, that the change in size is more apparent than real, because the actual tumor size may have been masked by the lymphedematous induration that has been dispelled by the hormone. New malignant lesions have been known to appear, and older lesions have been reactivated while the patient is experiencing a subjective improvement.

WHAT ARE THE FAVORABLE EFFECTS NOTED AFTER USE OF CORTICOSTEROIDS? The principal benefits derived from the administration of corticosteroids to a patient with advanced or recurrent carcinoma of the breast are (*a*) An improvement in the general sense of well-being, as measured by an increase in appetite, weight, strength, and the ability to return to the former occupation. (*b*) Fluid accumulations in the pleural, pericardial or peritoneal cavities are materially reduced. This may prove to be lifesaving in a patient with pulmonary metastases. (*c*) Metastatic lesions to the brain improve, and headache, paralysis, papilledema and loss of vision disappear rapidly. (*d*) Edema disappears from the tissues in dramatic fashion, and thus a lymphedematous arm becomes more mobile and less painful. Similarly, hepatomegaly, which is often tender and accompanied by pain, becomes less prominent as the pain lessens. (*e*) Hypercalcemia, which may be lethal, sometimes arises in the course of either androgen or estrogen therapy. The use of cortisone or other corticosteroids may be a lifesaving procedure. (*f*) Any pre-existing anemia tends to improve as therapy continues. Despite the improvement in the aspects noted, there is little evidence that the metastatic breast tumors regress, and they may even enlarge, particularly when the patient has brain metastases.

WHAT IS THE MECHANISM OF ACTION IF SYMPTOMS IMPROVE BUT METASTASES REGRESS TO ONLY A MINOR DEGREE? One can only speculate on the mechanism involved, but in some manner it appears to be linked to the factors that inhibit the production of edema. The most dramatic improvements are observed when edema is present, especially in the brain, lung and abdominal contents. Some part of this may be due to a pituitary suppression, but more likely the effect is a peripheral one that acts to alter the tissue environment in the area of the metastases. In so altering it the edema tends to disappear, but some part of the local tissue resistance to cancer is lost, and the tumor expands. Investigators are aware of this specialized effect of cortisone, and use it, for example, to condition the hamster cheek pouch before attempting human tumor transplants.

The mechanics of corticosteroid action may possibly also be involved in calcium metabolism, for the improvement in patients who have hypercalcemia is dramatic when cortisone is given, even when they have previously had adrenalectomy or hypophysectomy.

Finally it should be made clear that the action of the corticosteroids is not specific for cancer of the breast. Cerebral lesions, secondary to carcinoma of the gastrointestinal tract, for example, also do well on corticosteroid therapy.

WHAT ARE SOME OF THE UNFAVORABLE EFFECTS? Although the patient obtains much subjective improvement from cortisone, prednisone or prednisolone, she often has to pay a price for it in unpleasant sequelae. Chief among these are (*a*) weight gain, (*b*) abnormal fatty deposits, such as one sees in Cushing's syndrome, (*c*) hirsutism, (*d*) moon face, and (*e*) acne. Patients who are on corticosteroid therapy are particularly prone to have bleeding gastric or duodenal ulcers. The likelihood of this complication can be minimized by placing the patient on an ulcer regimen while she is taking the suppressive drugs. In certain patients diabetes mellitus may appear, or if previously existent, it may become severe.

Some patients complain of insomnia and nervousness to such an extent that therapy has to be discontinued. Psychiatric problems may develop. Occasionally a patient will have increasing difficulty in locomotion due to quadriceps weakness. These are distressing symptoms, but they are outweighed by the improvement noted in the cancer patient's sense of well-being.

WHAT IS THE USUAL DOSAGE SCHEDULE? Although it is possible to obtain subjective improvement from the use of 50 to 75 mg. of cortisone daily, and some temporary tumor regression as well when the dose is increased to 200 mg. daily, the majority of physicians conversant with the problems involved in the use of corticosteroids prefer to use prednisone or prednisolone. Fewer electrolyte imbalance problems arise in the course of the therapy, and the steroid potency, measured by the ability to suppress secretions from the adrenal cortex, is three or four times greater than that of cortisone.

There is little point in giving small doses. Symptomatic improvement is much more obvious when larger doses are given. At the outset a patient with known metastases should be given oral medication, 20 mg. twice daily, until the symptoms are under control, after which she continues on a maintenance dose of 50 mg. daily. With dosage of this range pituitary ACTH production should be adequately suppressed. The prednisone dosage is determined by dividing the usual cortisone medication by a factor of five.

What Does Chemotherapy Have to Offer for Patients with Metastatic Breast Cancer?

In recent years there has been a great deal of interest but a decreasing amount of enthusiasm for the use of nonhormonal chemotherapeutic agents in the treatment of patients who show evidence of widespread cancer of the breast. The basis for giving these drugs rests on the well recognized observation that cancer cells circulate in the blood stream in increased concentration after the handling of the tumor at the time of operation. Showers of tumor cells could conceivably provide the explanation for metastases that appear in such remote sites as lung, liver, ovary and bone. It would seem entirely logical to introduce into the blood stream a cancericidal agent that would destroy these free cells while they were still circulating and before they had time to establish themselves and develop a mass in which they could survive and propagate.

It has actually been demonstrated in animal experiments that the growth of cancer cells injected into the blood stream can be materially reduced when a variety of chemotherapeutic agents are injected at the same time or shortly thereafter. There appeared to be more effect on the circulating tumor cells than on those already established in metastases.

The antitumor agents used and their mode of action have been previously described in connection with the use of therapeutic drugs for widely disseminated ovarian cancer. A wide variety of these therapeutic agents has been tried in patients who have breast carcinoma. A few drugs appear to have diminished the recurrence rate, reduced the size of the metastatic or recurrent lesions, diminished the amount of pleural and peritoneal effusions, increased the general sense of well-being and may perhaps have improved the survival rate to a minimal degree.

The most effective agents for use in patients with breast carcinoma are the alkylating compound triethylene thiophosphoramide (Thio-Tepa) and the antimetabolite drugs, Methotrexate and 5-Fluorouracil. Nitrogen mustard seems to have some effect in the patients with lung metastases so far as further lymphatic spread is concerned. Pleural and peritoneal effusions have been improved, and fewer tappings of these cavities have been required. The patients derived subjective benefit even when the actual size of the metastatic deposits has shown little change. Methotrexate, which can be given orally as well as systemically, appears to have some influence on the growth of soft-part tumors. Recently 5-Fluorouracil has been shown to have a similar effect.

The alkylating agent, Thio-Tepa, has had the most extensive trial under controlled conditions. Twenty-four institutions in this country, comprising the Surgical Adjuvant Chemotherapy Breast group, have recently reported their experience with use of Thio-Tepa in over 700 patients. Insufficient time has elapsed to evaluate the true efficacy of the drug in terms of survival, but an encouraging note appeared in the report, when it was shown that the recurrence rate diminished appreciably when compared to the control group treated by radical mastectomy alone. Unfortunately, over one third of the patients had complications of varying severity, depending on individual sensitivity to the drug.

It is well known that all the cancer chemotherapeutic agents are toxic in one way or another. The manifestations are evident chiefly in the hematopoietic and gastrointestinal systems. The antitumor effect is closely linked to the degree of toxicity. The experience with Thio-Tepa is no exception, for the most favorable responses were noted in patients who received the more concentrated doses. In this group the number of complications was significantly higher than in the patients who received a reduced amount of drug. The toxic effects most commonly observed are (1) a depression in both platelets and polymorphonuclear leukocytes; (2) gastrointestinal symptoms, such as anorexia, nausea, vomiting, stomatitis, intestinal cramps and diarrhea; (3) generalized nonspecific symptoms such as malaise, dermatitis, alopecia and hypotension. The severe complications thus are many and varied.

The drugs are dangerous and should not be used indiscriminately without close supervision and thorough knowledge of what complications these agents may produce. It is unfortunate that, with any anticancer drug now available, it seems necessary to produce a toxic effect to secure a significant remission.

How Is Chemotherapy Used?

THIO-TEPA. The dosage schedule recommended by the breast study group called for administration intravenously of a total of 0.6 mg. per kilogram of body weight as follows: (*a*) 0.2 mg. per kilogram at the time of operation; (*b*) 0.2 mg. per kilogram on first postoperative day; and, (*c*) the same dose on the second day. Bateman has had success by injecting the agent directly into the tumor.

In this program no mention is made of a maintenance dose or of repeating the course at a later date if obvious need arose. This could be an important consideration. It is certainly true that the cells within a given tumor have different time cycles in various stages of cell division. If chemotherapeutic drugs exert their effect on the cell nucleus, it might be well to use them over a longer period of time, in order that more cells could be exposed at the time when they were most vulnerable. It is also possible that the agent as given in this fashion might have a tumor effect without severe toxicity. So far as we know at the moment it seems to be a basic point of anti-cancer therapy that drugs be given to the point of toxic side effects.

5-FLUOROURACIL. It has been customary to give 5-Fluorouracil intravenously over a short period of time, in doses of 15 mg. per kilogram of body weight for a period of 5 days, or until signs of toxicity appear. The individual response varies, but the drug is highly toxic to many patients. If control blood studies show no alarming diminution in white blood cells or platelets, the course of therapy may be repeated in 3 to 5 weeks. Recently we have found that a dose of 15 mg. per kilogram given intravenously slowly over an 8-hour period does not produce toxicity, while the same degree of tumor effect is still preserved.

METHOTREXATE. This has been used in breast cancer because of its demonstrated ability to influence some metastatic soft tissue recurrences. It is very toxic when given either systemically or by mouth. To combat the toxic effect citrovorum factor, 3 mg., is usually given intramuscularly 4 times daily.

Because of variations in the individual patient response to Methotrexate, the dose varies widely. Orally, 2.5-mg. tablets of Methotrexate are usually given 2 to 6 times daily, to the point of toxicity. The usual dosage, when given intravenously, is 0.75 to 3.0 mg. with citrovorum factor as a safeguard.

The Rational Place for the Use of Chemotherapeutic Agents

With all these compounds it is important to observe the tumor response. If none is seen, there is little point in continuing the drug. On the other hand, if the initial response is favorable, the physician is fully justified in repeating the course of chemotherapy. None of the agents used for breast carcinoma have any predictable effect on the tumor. All will produce an occasional response. The effect on patient survival is not yet known, but the effectiveness of present-day drugs is questionable.

It should also be kept fully in mind that the remission rate and increased survival possibilities obtained with present-day chemotherapeutic agents are nowhere near comparable to those obtained from adjuvant hormone therapy. Drugs therefore should not be used as the primary form of treatment in lieu of hormone therapy. When hormones have failed to produce the desired result, these agents can be given a try. Hormones obtain their effects by altering the tumor environment over several weeks or months. The physician meanwhile may be justified in giving chemotherapy, while awaiting the effects of hormone therapy. There is some evidence that use of combinations may be effective.

To date chemotherapeutic anticancer drugs have had little influence on the survival rate for carcinoma of the breast, although clinical studies designed to test their efficacy have not yet gone on long enough to document this observation completely. This has been confirmed, however, for carcinoma in other body areas, such as lung, colon and stomach. It may be that the concomitant use of chemotherapy and surgery will destroy cancer cells circulating in the blood and thereby reduce the incidence of metastases, but we still await the development of a drug that will destroy metastatic deposits without creating dangerous toxic complications.

REFERENCES

General References

Cheatle, G. L., and Cutler, M.: *Tumours of the Breast; Their Pathology, Symptoms and Treatment*. Philadelphia, J. B. Lippincott Company, 1931.
Ewing, J.: *Neoplastic Diseases*. 4th ed. Philadelphia, W. B. Saunders Company, 1940.
Geschickter, C. F., and Copeland, M. M.: *Diseases of the Breast*. Philadelphia, J. B. Lippincott Company, 1945.
Haagensen, C. D.: *Diseases of the Breast*. Philadelphia, W. B. Saunders Company, 1956.
Lewison, E. F.: *Breast Cancer and Its Diagnosis and Treatment*. Baltimore, Williams & Wilkins Company, 1955.
Segaloff, A.: *Breast Cancer*. The Second Biennial Louisiana Cancer Conference. St. Louis, C. V. Mosby Company, 1958.
Stewart, F. W.: Tumors of the Breast; in *Atlas of Tumor Pathology*. Washington, D. C., Armed Forces Institute of Pathology, 1950.

Etiology

Andervont, H. B., and Dunn, T. B.: Influences of Heredity and the Mammary Tumor Agent on the Occurrence of Mammary Tumors in Hybrid Mice. *J. Nat. Cancer Inst.*, 14: 317, 1953.
Bittner, J. J.: Relation of Nursing to the Extrachromosomal Theory of Breast Cancer in Mice. *Am. J. Cancer*, 35: 90, 1959.
Clagett, O. T., Plimpton, N. C., and Root, G. T.: Lesions of the Breast. The Relationship of Benign Lesions to Carcinoma. *Surgery*, 15: 413, 1944.
Corbett, D. G., and Abrams, E. W.: Bilateral Carcinoma of Male Breasts Associated with Prolonged Stilbestrol Therapy for Carcinoma of the Prostate. *J. Urol.*, 64: 379, 1950.

Damon, A.: Host Factors in Cancer of the Breast and Uterine Cervix and Corpus. *J. Nat. Cancer Inst.*, 24: 483, 1960.

Dargent, M.: Carcinoma of the Breast in Castrated Women. *Brit. M. J.*, 2: 54, 1949.

Dorn, H. F.: Cancer and Marital Status. *Human Biol.*, 15: 73, 1943.

Foote, F. W., and Stewart, F. W.: Comparative Studies of Cancerous versus Noncancerous Breasts. *Ann. Surg.*, 121: 6, 197, 1945.

Foote, F. W., Jr., and Stewart, F. W.: A Histologic Classification of Carcinoma of the Breast. *Surgery*, 19: 74, 1946.

Frantz, V. K., Pickren, J. W., Melcher, G. W., and Auchincloss, H., Jr.: Incidence of Chronic Cystic Disease in So-Called Normal Breasts. A Study Based on 225 Postmortem Examinations. *Cancer*, 4: 762, 1951.

Hirayama, T., and Wynder, E. L.: A Study of the Epidemiology of Cancer of the Breast. The Influence of Hysterectomy. *Cancer*, 15: 28, 1962.

Horne, H. W., Jr.: The "Milk Factor" in Carcinoma of the Human Breast. An Analysis of 88 Cases. *New England J. Med.*, 243: 373, 1950.

Kilgore, A. R.: Can Injury Cause Breast Cancer? *Am. Surgeon*, 20: 1015, 1954.

Lane-Claypon, J. E.: A Further Report on Cancer of the Breast, with Special Reference to Its Associated Antecedent Conditions. Great Britain, Ministry of Health, Reports on Public Health and Medical Subjects, No. 32. London, His Majesty's Stationery Office, 1926.

Lewison, E. F., and Allen, L. W.: Antecedent Factors in Cancer of the Breast. *Ann. Surg.*, 138: 39, 1953.

Lombard, H. L., and Potter, E. A.: Environmental Factors in the Etiology of Cancer. *Acta Union Internat. contre Cancer*, 6: 1325, 1950.

Macklin, M. T.: Relative Status of Parity and Genetic Background in Producing Human Breast Cancer. *J. Nat. Cancer Inst.*, 23: 1179, 1959.

MacMahon, B., and Feinlieb, M.: Breast Cancer in Relation to Nursing and Menopausal History. *J. Nat. Cancer Inst.*, 24: 733, 1960.

McManus, R. G., and Sommers, S. C.: Breast Cancer Prognosis and Ovarian Cortical Stromal Hyperplasia. *New England J. Med.*, 246: 890, 1952.

Olch, I. Y.: Menopausal Age in Women with Cancer of the Breast. *Am. J. Cancer*, 30: 563, 1937.

Smithers, D. W.: Family Histories of 459 Patients with Cancer of the Breast. *Brit. J. Cancer*, 2: 163, 1948.

Sommers, S. C.: Endocrine Abnormalities in Women with Breast Cancer. *Lab. Invest.*, 4: 160, 1955.

Sommers, S. C., and Teloh, H. A.: Ovarian Stromal Hyperplasia in Breast Cancer. *Arch. Path.*, 53: 160, 1952.

Womack, N. A.: Endocrine Relationships between Chronic Cystic Mastitis and Cancer of the Breast. *Am. Surgeon*, 24: 618, 1958.

Anatomic Features

Busk, T., and Clemmesen, J.: The Frequencies of Left and Right Sided Breast Cancer. *Brit. J. Cancer*, 1: 345, 1947.

Carroll, W. W., and Shields, T. W.: Bilateral Simultaneous Breast Cancer. A.M.A. *Arch. Surg.*, 70: 672, 1955.

Dickinson, A. M.: Carcinoma of the Axillary Tail of the Breast. *Am. J. Surg.*, 49: 515, 1940.

Garfinkel, L., Craig, L., and Seidman, H.: An Appraisal of Left and Right Breast Cancer. *J. Nat. Cancer Inst.*, 23: 617, 1959.

Hubbard, T. B., Jr.: Non-simultaneous Bilateral Carcinoma of the Breast. *Surgery*, 34: 706, 1953.

Moertel, C. G., and Soule, E. H.: The Problem of the Second Breast. A Study of 118 Patients with Bilateral Carcinoma of the Breast. *Ann. Surg.*, 146: 764, 1957.

Owen, H. W., Dockerty, M. B., and Gray, H. K.: Occult Carcinoma of the Breast. *Surg., Gynec. & Obst.*, 98: 302, 1954.

Pierce, E. H., Kirklin, J. W., McDonald, J. R., and Gage, R. P.: Carcinoma in the Medial and Lateral Halves of the Breast. *Surg., Gynec. & Obst.*, 103: 759, 1956.

Factors Bearing on Prognosis

Ackerman, L. V.: The Examination of Regional Lymph Nodes in Carcinoma of the Breast. *Proc. Second Nat. Cancer Conf.*, New York, 1: 194, 1952.

Alrich, E. M., Liddle, H. V., and Morton, C. B.: Carcinoma of the Breast: Results of Surgical Treatment. Some Anatomic and Endocrine Considerations. *Ann. Surg.*, 145: 799, 1957.

Andreassen, M., Dahl-Iversen, E., and Sorensen, B.: Glandular Metastases in Carcinoma of the Breast: Results of a More Radical Operation. *Lancet*, 1: 176, 1954.

Barber, K. W., Jr., Dockerty, M. B., and Clagett, O. T.: Inflammatory Carcinoma of the Breast. *Surg.. Gynec. & Obst.*, 112: 406, 1961.

Batson, O. V.: Vertebral Vein System. Caldwell Lecture. *Am. J. Roentgenol.*, 78: 195, 1957.

Berg, J. W.: The Significance of Axillary Node Levels in the Study of Breast Carcinoma. *Cancer*, 8: 776, 1955.

Black, M. M., Opler, S. R., and Spear, F. D.: Survival in Breast Cancer Cases in Relation to the Structure of the Primary Tumor and Regional Lymph Nodes. *Surg., Gynec. & Obst.*, 100: 543, 1955.

Chris, S. M.: Inflammatory Carcinoma of the Breast. *Brit. J. Surg.*, 38: 163, 1950.

Daland, E. M.: Untreated Cancer of the Breast. *Surg., Gynec. & Obst.*, 44: 264, 1927.

Danckers, V. F., Hamann, A., and Savage, J. L.: Postoperative Recurrence of Breast Cancer after 32 Years. *Surgery*, 47: 656, 1960.

Dao, T., and Moore, G. E.: Clinical Observations of Conditions Which Apparently Enhance Malignant Cell Survival. *Surg, Gynec. & Obst.*, 112: 191, 1961.

Gray, S. W., Skandalakis, J. W., Mitchell, W. E., Nicholson, W. P., Jr., and McRae, F. W.: Tumor Size, Duration of Symptoms and Prognosis in Carcinoma of the Breast. *Surgery*, 49: 143, 1961.

Handley, R. S., and Thackray, A. C.: Invasion of Internal Mammary Lymph Nodes in Carcinoma of the Breast. *Brit. M.J.*, 1: 61, 1954.

Hickey, R. C.: Cancer of Breast: 1661 Patients. Considerations in the Failure to Cure after Radical Mastectomy. *Am. J. Roentgenol.*, 77: 421, 1957.

Kreyberg, L., and Christiansen, T.: Prognostic Significance of Small Size in Breast Cancer. *Brit. J. Cancer*, 7: 37, 1953.

Lumb, G., and Mackenzie, D. H.: The Incidence of Metastases in Adrenal Glands and Ovaries Removed for Carcinoma of the Breast. *Cancer*, 12: 521, 1959.

MacDonald, I.: Clinical Evidence of Biologic Variability in Mammary Carcinoma; in A. Segaloff, ed.: *Breast Cancer*. The Second Biennial Louisiana Cancer Conference, 1958. St. Louis, C. V. Mosby Company, 1958, p. 37.

McDonald, J. J., Haagensen, C. D., and Stout, A. P.: Metastases from Mammary Carcinoma to the Supraclavicular and Internal Mammary Lymph Nodes. *Surgery*, 34: 521, 1953.

Meyer, A. C., Dockerty, M. B., and Harrington, S. W.: Inflammatory Carcinoma of the Breast. *Surg.. Gynec. & Obst.*, 87: 417, 1948.

Moore, C., and Shaw, H. W.: Carcinoma of Breast. Extent of Original Disease Related to End-Results. *A.M.A. Arch. Surg.*, 75: 598, 1957.

Moore, G. E., Sandberg, A., and Schubarg, J. R.: Clinical and Experimental Observations of the Occurrence and Fate of Tumor Cells in the Blood Stream. *Ann. Surg.*, 146: 580, 1957.

Moore, O. S., Jr., and Foote, F. W., Jr.: The Relatively Favorable Prognosis of Medullary Carcinoma of the Breast. *Cancer*, 2: 635, 1949.

Pawlias, K. T., Dockerty, M. B., and Ellis, F. H., Jr.: Late Local Recurrent Carcinoma of the Breast. *Ann. Surg.*, 148: 192, 1958.

Robbins, G. F., and Bross, I.: The Significance of Delay in Relation to Prognosis of Patients with Primary Operable Breast Cancer. *Cancer*, 10: 338, 1957.

Rosahn, P. D.: Results of Treatment of Carcinoma of Breast: Comparison of 5 Year Survival Rates Obtained by Two Different Groups of Surgeons in a Community Hospital. *Ann. Surg.*, 146: 912, 1957.

Smithers, D. W.: Cancer of Breast. A Study of Short Survival in Early Cases and of Long Survival in Advanced Cases. *Am. J. Roentgenol.*, 80: 740, 1958.

Stapley, L. A., Dockerty, M. B., and Harrington, S. W.: Comedocarcinoma of the Breast. *Surg., Gynec. & Obst.*, 100: 707, 1955.

Treves, N.: The Inoperability of Inflammatory Carcinoma of the Breast. *Surg., Gynec. & Obst.*, 109: 240, 1959.

Treves, N., and Holleb, A. I.: Report of 549 Cases of Breast Cancer in Women 35 Years of Age or Younger. *Surg., Gynec. & Obst.*, 107: 271, 1958.

General Aspects of Therapy

Barnett, C. P.: Survival Rate of Patients with Breast Cancer in a Small Community. *J.A.M.A.*, 171: 1180, 1959.

Carroll, W. W., and Shields, T. W.: Judgment in Breast Cancer. *S. Clin. N. Amer.*, 38: 1393, 1959.
Collins, V. P.: Breast Cancer. The Influence of Treatment That Fails to Cure. *Cancer*, 9: 1177, 1956.
Copeland, M. M.: Precancerous Lesions of the Breast: How to Treat Them. *Postgrad. Med.*, 27: 332, 1960.
Idem: Clinical Staging System for Cancer and End Result Reporting. *Ca*, 11: 42, 1961.
Crooke, A. C.: Treatment of Advanced Carcinoma of the Breast. *Brit. M.J.*, 2: 1425, 1958.
Firor, W. M.: A Critical Review of the Treatment of Mammary Carcinoma. *Surgery*, 46: 996, 1959.
Harrison, R. C.: The Management of Breast Problems in Practice. *Canad. M.A.J.*, 83: 849, 1960.
Jessiman, A. G., and Moore, F. D.: *Carcinoma of the Breast. The Study and Treatment of the Patient*. Boston, Little, Brown & Company, 1956.
Montgomery, T. L., Bowers, P. A., and Kittleberger, W. C.: The Diagnosis and Management of Breast Cancer. *Obst. & Gynec.*, 17: 19, 1961.
Powell, R. W., and Rooney, D. R.: A Study of Fatal Breast Cancer. *Am. Surgeon*, 25: 692, 1959.
Segaloff, A.: Investigations in Breast Carcinoma. *J. Nat. Cancer Inst.*, Monograph #3, 1959, p. 257.

Adrenalectomy

Block, G. E., Vial, A. B., McCarthy, J. D., Porter, C. W., and Coller, F. A.: Adrenalectomy in Advanced Mammary Cancer. *Surg., Gynec. & Obst.*, 108: 651, 1959.
Cade, S.: Adrenalectomy for Breast Cancer. *Brit. M.J.*, 1: 1, 1955.
Dao, T. L.-Y., and Huggins, C.: Bilateral Adrenalectomy in the Treatment of Cancer of the Breast. *Arch. Surg.*, 71: 645, 1955.
Huggins, C.: The Adrenal Component in Mammary Cancer. *Acta Internat. Union against Cancer*, 10: 6, 1954.
Krieger, D. T., Gabrilove, J. L., and Soffer, L. J.: Adrenal Function in a Pregnant Bilaterally Adrenalectomized Woman. *J. Clin. Endocrinol. & Metab.*, 20: 1493, 1960.
Lipsett, M. B., and others: Bilateral Adrenalectomy in Palliation of Metastatic Breast Cancer. *Cancer*, 10: 111, 1957.
Nelson, T. S., and Dragstedt, L. R.: Adrenalectomy and Oophorectomy for Breast Cancer. *J.A.M.A.*, 175: 379, 1961.
Perlia, C. P., Kofman, S., Nagamani, D., and Taylor, S. G.: A Critical Analysis of the Palliation Produced by Adrenalectomy in Metastatic Cancer of the Female Breast. *Ann. Int. Med.*, 45: 989, 1956.

Hypophysectomy

Jessiman, A. G., Matson, D. D., and Moore, F. D.: Hypophysectomy in the Treatment of Breast Cancer. *New England J. Med.*, 261: 1199, 1959.
Kennedy, B. J., French, L. A., and Peyton, W. T.: Hypophysectomy in Advanced Breast Cancer. *New England J. Med.*, 255: 1165, 1956.
Pearson, O. H., and Ray, B. S.: Results of Hypophysectomy in the Treatment of Metastatic Mammary Carcinoma. *Cancer*, 12: 85, 1959.
Idem: Hypophysectomy in the Treatment of Metastatic Mammary Cancer. *Am. J. Surg.*, 99: 544, 1960.
Van Wyk, J. J., Dugger, G. S., Newsome, J. F., and Thomas, P. Z.: The Effect of Pituitary Stalk Section on the Adrenal Function of Women with Cancer of the Breast. *J. Clin. Endocrinol.*, 20: 157, 1960.

Endocrine Therapy

A Preliminary Statement by the Joint Committee on Endocrine Ablative Procedures in Disseminated Mammary Carcinoma. Adrenalectomy and Hypophysectomy in Disseminated Mammary Carcinoma. *J.A.M.A.*, 175: 787, 1961.
Baker, W. H., Kelley, R. M. and Sohier, W. D.: Hormonal Treatment of Metastatic Carcinoma of the Breast. *Am. J. Surg.*, 99: 538, 1960.
Block, G. E., McCarthy, J. D., and Vial, A. B.: Adrenal-Corticoid Depression of Adrenal Estrogens in Cases of Mammary Cancer. *A.M.A. Arch. Surg.*, 78: 732, 1959.
Brennan, M. J., Beckett, V. L., Kelly, J. E., and Betanzos, G.: Treatment of Advanced Mammary Cancer with 3-Beta, 17-Beta-Androstranediol. *Cancer*, 13: 1195, 1960.
Council on Drugs: Report to the Council. Androgens and Estrogens in Treatment of Disseminated Mammary Carcinoma. Retrospective Study of Nine Hundred Forty-Four Patients. *J.A.M.A.*, 172: 1271, 1960.

Emerson, K., Jr.: The Endocrine Management of Breast Cancer. *M. Clin. N. Amer.*, 44: 1393, 1960.

Emerson, W. J., Kennedy, B. J., and Taft, E. B.: Correlation of Histological Alterations in Breast Cancer with Response to Hormone Therapy. *Cancer*, 13: 1047, 1960.

Herrmann, J. B., Kirsten, E., and Krakauer, J. S.: Hypercalcemic Syndrome Associated with Androgenic and Estrogenic Therapy. *J. Clin. Endocrinol.*, 9: 1, 1949.

Lemon, H. M.: Cortisone-Thyroid Therapy of Metastatic Mammary Cancer. *Ann. Int. Med.*, 46: 457, 1957.

Idem: Prednisone Therapy of Advanced Mammary Cancer. *Cancer*, 12: 93, 1959.

Lewison, E. F., Grow, J. L., and Trimble, F. H.: The Hormone Treatment of Advanced Breast Cancer. Comparative Therapy with Testosterone and Two Experimental Androgens. *Am. Surgeon*, 26: 278, 1960.

MacDonald, I.: Sex Steroids for Palliation of Disseminated Mammary Carcinoma. *J.A.M.A.*, 172: 1288, 1960.

Nathanson, I. T., and Kelley, R. M.: Medical Progress: Hormonal Treatment of Cancer. *New England J. Med.*, 246: 135, 1952.

Oberhelman, H. A., Jr., Hormonal Treatment of Mammary Cancer. *S. Clin. N. Amer.*, 39: 3, 1959.

Segaloff, A., Weeth, J. B., Rongone, E. L., and Bowers, C. Y.: Hormonal Therapy in Cancer of the Breast. XVII. The Effect of Androsterone on Clinical Course and Hormonal Excretion. *Cancer*, 14: 195, 1961.

Chemotherapy

Ansfield, F. J., and Curreri, A. R.: Further Clinical Studies with 5-Fluorouracil. *J. Nat. Cancer Inst.*, 22: 497, 1959.

Bateman, J. C., and Carlton, H. N.: The Role of Chemotherapy in the Treatment of Breast Cancer. *Surgery*, 47: 895, 1960.

Conference on Experimental Clinical Cancer Chemotherapy. National Cancer Institute Monograph #3. Washington, D.C., U.S. Department of Health, Education, and Welfare, Public Health Service, 1960.

Editorial: Malignancy, Metabolism and Mustard. *J.A.M.A.*, 174: 1728, 1960.

Hurley, J. D., Ellison, E. H., Riesch, J., and Schulte, W.: Chemotherapy of Solid Carcinoma. Indications, Agents and Results. *J.A.M.A.*, 174: 1696, 1960.

Staley, C. J., Kerth, J. D., Cortes, N., and Preston, F. W.: Treatment of Advanced Cancer with 5-Fluorouracil. *Surg., Gynec. & Obst.*, 112: 185, 1961.

Vaitkevicius, V. K., Brennan, M. J., Beckett, V. L., Kelly, J. E., and Talley, R. W.: Clinical Evaluation of Cancer Chemotherapy with 5-Fluorouracil. *Cancer*, 14: 131, 1961.

Wright, J. C., and others: Chemotherapy of Disseminated Carcinoma of the Breast. *Ann. Surg.*, 150: 221, 1959.

Surgical Therapy

Adair, F. E.: Cancer of the Breast. *S. Clin. N. Amer.*, 33: 313, 1953.

Ariel, I. M.: A Conservative Method of Resecting the Internal Mammary Lymph Nodes en Bloc with Radical Mastectomy. *Surg., Gynec. & Obst.*, 100: 623, 1955.

Benninghoff, D., and Tsien, K. C.: Treatment and Survival in Breast Cancer. A Review of Results. *Brit. J. Radiol.*, 32: 450, 1959.

Berkson, J., and others: Mortality and Survival in Surgically Treated Cancer of the Breast. A Statistical Summary of Some Experience of the Mayo Clinic. (1) Relation of Survival to Various Biometric Factors. (2) Comparison of Radical Mastectomy (Mayo Clinic) with Simple Mastectomy (McWhirter). *Proc. Staff Meet., Mayo Clin.*, 32: 645, 1957.

Crile, G., Jr.: Cancer of the Breast. A Surgeon's Dilemma. *Cleveland Clin. Quart.*, 23: 179, 1956.

Fanger, H.: Long Term Survival in Cancer of Breast, Stomach, and in Malignant Melanomas. *Rhode Island M.J.*, 38: 551, 1955.

Gray, E. B., Jr., and Anglem, T. J.: Radical Mastectomy for Carcinoma of the Breast. *New England J. Med.*, 261: 1310, 1959.

Haagensen, C. D., and Stout, A. P.: Carcinoma of Breast. III. Results of Treatment, 1935–1942. *Ann. Surg.*, 134: 151, 1951.

Halsted, W. S.: Results of Operation for Cure of Cancer of Breast Performed at Johns Hopkins Hospital from June 1889 to January 1894. *Ann. Surg.*, 20: 497, 1894.

Harrington, S. W.: Three-Year to Forty-Year Survival Rates Following Radical Mastectomy for Carcinoma of Breast. *West. J. Surg.*, 63: 272, 1955.

Jessiman, A. G., and Moore, F. D.: Medical Progress: Carcinoma of the Breast. The Study and Treatment of the Patient. *New England J. Med.*, 254: 846, 1956.

Lewison, E. F.: Practical Aspects of Surgical Treatment of Breast Cancer. A.M.A. *Arch. Surg.*, 74: 251, 1957.

Miller, E. B., and Kennedy, C. S.: Some Factors in the Choice of Treatment of Carcinoma of the Breast. *Ann. Surg.*, 150: 993, 1959.

Richards, T. A., Palmer, J. D., and Martin, S. J.: Results of Treatment of Cancer of Breast at Montreal General Hospital. *Surg., Gynec. & Obst.*, 104: 451, 1957.

Robbins, G. F., Brothers, J. H., III, Eberhart, W. F., and Quan, S.: Is Aspiration Biopsy of Breast Cancer Dangerous to the Patient? *Cancer*, 7: 774, 1954.

Taylor, G. W.: Clinical Management of Breast Tumors. *New England J. Med.*, 223: 538, 1940.

Urban, J. A.: Early Diagnosis of Breast Cancer. Salvage Data with Lesions Considered Clinically Benign or Doubtful Prior to Operation. *Cancer*, 9: 1173, 1956.

Urban, J. A., and Baker, H. W.: Radical Mastectomy in Continuity with en Bloc Resection of Internal Mammary Lymph-Node Chain. A New Procedure for Primary Operable Cancer of the Breast. *Cancer*, 5: 992, 1952.

Wangensteen, O. H.: Another Look at the Super-radical Operation for Breast Carcinoma. *Surgery*, 41: 857, 1957.

Watson, T. A.: Results of Treatment of Cancer of the Breast. *Surg., Gynec. & Obst.*, 104: 106, 1957.

Simple Mastectomy

Abramson, P. D., Clifton, R. B., and Slagle, G. W.: Cancer of the Breast. Comparison of Two Methods of Treatment. *Surgery*, 42: 689, 1957.

Ackerman, L. V.: An Evaluation of Treatment of Cancer of the Breast at University of Edinburgh (Scotland), under Direction of Dr. Robert McWhirter. *Cancer*, 8: 883, 1955.

Byrd, B. F., Jr., and Stephenson, S. E., Jr.: Simple Mastectomy for Cancer of Breast. *Ann. Surg.*, 145: 807, 1957.

Deaton, W. R., Jr.: Simple Mastectomy for Carcinoma of the Breast. Reported Results. *Surgery*, 37: 720, 1955.

Fletcher, G. H.: Quoted by R. L. Clark. *Ann. Surg.*, 145: 811, 1957.

McWhirter, R.: Simple Mastectomy and Radiotherapy in Treatment of Breast Cancer. *Brit. J. Radiol.*, 28: 128, 1955.

Radical Mastectomy and Radiation Therapy

Garland, L. H., Hill, H. A., Mottram, M. E., and Sisson, M. A.: Cancer of the Breast. Results of Radical Mastectomy and Radiotherapy in Two Hospitals. *Surg., Gynec. & Obst.*, 98: 700, 1954.

Marshall, S. F., and Hare, H. F.: Carcinoma of the Breast: Results of Combined Treatment with Surgery and Roentgen Rays. *Ann. Surg.*, 125: 688, 1947.

O'Brien, F. W., and O'Brien, F. W., Jr.: Surgery and Radiation in Cancer of the Female Breast. *Radiology*, 63: 192, 1954.

Smith, G. V., and Smith, O. W.: Carcinoma of the Breast. Results, Evaluation of X-radiation, and Relation of Age and Surgical Castration to Length of Survival. *Surg., Gynec. & Obst.*, 97: 508, 1953.

Trout, H. H., Jr.: Five-Year Followup of Carcinoma of the Breast Treated with Radical Mastectomy and Postoperative Irradiation. *Tr. South. Surg. A.*, 62: 231, 1950.

Williams, I. G., Murley R. S., and Curwen, M. P.: Carcinoma of the Female Breast: Conservative and Radical Surgery. *Brit. M.J.*, 2: 787, 1953.

Radiation Therapy

Ash, C. L., Peters, V., and Delarue, N. C.: The Argument for Preoperative Radiation in the Treatment of Breast Cancer. *Surg., Gynec. & Obst.*, 96: 509, 1953.

Baclesse, F.: Roentgen Therapy as the Sole Method of Treatment of Cancer of the Breast. *Am. J. Roentgenol.*, 62: 311, 1949.

Brasfield, R. D., and Henschke, U. K.: Treatment of the Internal Mammary Lymph Nodes by Implantation of Radioisotopes into the Internal Mammary Artery. *Radiology*, 70: 259, 1958.

Fletcher, G. H.: Radiotherapeutic Management of Advanced Breast Cancer; in A. Segaloff, ed.: *Breast Cancer*. St. Louis, C. V. Mosby Company, 1958, p. 109.

Hochman, A., and Robinson, E.: Eighty-Two Cases of Mammary Cancer Treated Exclusively with Roentgen Therapy. *Cancer*, 13: 670, 1960.

Keynes, G.: The Place of Radium in the Treatment of Cancer of the Breast. *Ann. Surg.*, 106: 619, 1937.

Lenz, M.: Radiocurability of Cancer. *Am. J. Roentgenol.*, 67: 428, 1952.

Lumb, G.: Changes in Carcinoma of the Breast Following Irradiation. *Brit. J. Surg.*, 38: 82, 1950.

Williams, I. G., and Cunningham, G. J.: Histological Changes in Irradiated Carcinoma of the Breast. *Brit. J. Radiol.*, 24: 123, 1951.

Radiation Therapy of Metastases

Bouchard, J.: Skeletal Metastases in Cancer of the Breast: Study of Character, Incidence and Response to Roentgen Therapy. *Am. J. Roentgenol.*, 54: 156, 1945.

Burch, H. A.: Osseous Metastases from Graded Cancers of the Breast, with Particular Reference to Roentgen Treatment. *Am. J. Roentgenol.*, 52: 1, 1944.

Mueller, H. P., and Sniffen, R. C.: Roentgenologic Appearance and Pathology of Intrapulmonary Lymphatic Spread of Metastatic Cancer. *Am. J. Roentgenol.*, 53: 109, 1945.

Turner, J. W., and Jaffe, H. L.: Metastatic Neoplasms. A Clinical and Roentgenological Study of Involvement of Skeleton and Lungs. *Am. J. Roentgenol.*, 43: 479, 1940.

Warren, S., and Witham, E. M.: Studies on Tumor Metastasis. The Distribution of Metastases in Cancer of the Breast. *Surg., Gynec. & Obst.*, 57: 81, 1933.

Oophorectomy

Atkins, H.: A Comparison of Adrenalectomy and Oophorectomy with Hypophysectomy in the Treatment of Advanced Cancer of the Breast. *Proc. Roy. Soc. Med.*, 53: 638, 1960.

Beatson, G. T.: On the Treatment of Inoperable Cases of Carcinoma of the Mamma. Suggestions for a New Method of Treatment with Illustrative Cases. *Lancet*, 2: 104, 162, 1896.

Idem: The Treatment of Inoperable Carcinoma of the Female Mamma. *Glasgow M.J.*, 76: 81, 1911.

Block, G. E., Lampe, I., Vial, A. B., and Coller, F. A.: Therapeutic Castration for Advanced Mammary Cancer. *Surgery*, 47: 877, 1960.

Brinckley, D. M., and Pillers, E. K.: Treatment of Advanced Cancer of the Breast by Bilateral Oophorectomy and Prednisone. *Lancet*, 1: 123, 1960.

Dragstedt, L. R., Humphreys, E. M., and Dragstedt, L. R., II: Prophylactic Bilateral Adrenalectomy and Oophorectomy for Advanced Cancer. *Surgery*, 47: 885, 1960.

Horsley, G. W.: Treatment of Cancer of the Breast in Premenopausal Patients with Radical Amputation and Bilateral Oophorectomy. *Ann. Surg.*, 125: 703, 1947.

Huggins, C., and Dao, T. L.-Y.: Adrenalectomy and Oophorectomy in Treatment of Advanced Carcinoma of the Breast. *J.A.M.A.*, 151: 1388, 1953.

Osborne, M. P., and Pitts, R. M.: Therapeutic Oophorectomy for Advanced Breast Cancer. The Significance of Metastases to the Ovary and of Ovarian Cortical Stromal Hyperplasia. *Cancer*, 14: 126, 1961.

Strong, J. A., and others: Sex Hormone Excretion after Bilateral Adrenalectomy and Oophorectomy in Patients with Mammary Carcinoma. *Lancet*, 2: 955, 1956.

Taylor, G. W.: Evaluation of Ovarian Sterilization for Breast Cancer. *Surg., Gynec. & Obst.*, 68: 452, 1939.

Thomson, A.: Analysis of Cases in Which Oophorectomy Was Performed for Inoperable Carcinoma of the Breast. *Brit. M.J.*, 2: 1538, 1902.

Treves, N., and Finkbeiner, J. A.: An Evaluation of Therapeutic Surgical Castration in Treatment of Metastatic, Recurrent, and Primary Inoperable Mammary Carcinoma in Women. An Analysis of 191 Patients. *Cancer*, 11: 421, 1958.

Chapter 63

Lacerations of the Pelvic Floor

LACERATIONS of the vulva, vagina and perineum may occur from a variety of causes in all age groups as the results of trauma secondary to accidental injury, instrumental delivery of the newborn, rape, or forceful spontaneous delivery of an oversized infant through a relatively small or unprepared vaginal canal. For example, the unruptured hymen may be forcibly torn in an adult virgin as a result of the initial sexual penetration. If force is used, as in rape, the laceration may extend into the vaginal canal or even the perineum. The patient may suffer the same sort of injury by a fall on a sharp object that projects into the vaginal canal. She may then have an extensive hematoma in the vulvar region or an actual tear extending into the vagina. There are many instances in which objects inserted into the vaginal canal, with or without the consent of the patient, have produced lacerations of the vaginal wall. Most vaginal wall lacerations occur in delivery, whether or not instruments are used.

The chief symptom of vulvar and vaginal lacerations is hemorrhage. The tissues themselves may simply be contused, or actual hemorrhage may extravasate into the surrounding tissues, forming a hematoma. The seriousness of the injury depends on the size of the vessels that may be torn and the extent of the hemorrhage. It can be fatal, though in the majority of instances the bleeding produces pain and discomfort, but rarely is of serious moment. The hematoma generally absorbs slowly and seldom becomes infected or produces an abscess.

The treatment consists largely in the application of hot packs or sitz baths. For the most part lacerations of the perineum and vaginal wall heal quickly and do not require suturing. Extensive bleeding must be controlled, however, and the larger lacerations, particularly those that occur during labor, should be repaired. Actually, no permanent damage results from perineal lacerations unless the levator ani muscles and their accompanying fascia are also torn.

What Are the Various Types of Perineal Laceration?

The significance of the laceration depends upon the extent of the tear and the degree to which the levator ani muscles are traumatized. The vaginal introitus has been compared to the mouth, which is also an elliptical structure, but with a transverse slit. Both structures have a movable lower border and a fixed upper segment. Closure of the mouth is accomplished by the masseter muscles, which elevate the mandible, and constriction of the vagina by contraction of the levator ani muscles. In either case, if the muscle is damaged, the orifice cannot close. There are three types

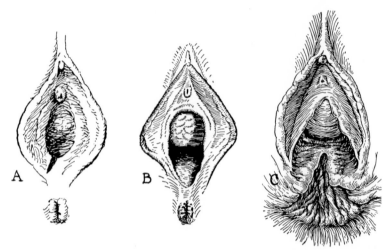

Fig. 63-1.   First- (*A*), second- (*B*) and third-degree (*C*) perineal lacerations. Pelvic relaxation commonly accompanies second-degree lacerations, and in third-degree tears the anal sphincter is involved anteriorly.

of perineal tear that progress in their serious import, depending on the degree of damage to the levator ani muscles.

FIRST-DEGREE TEAR.   The perineal body in its anatomic position lies below the pelvic floor. Lacerations of the perineum that are of the *first degree* may follow delivery when the patient is an elderly primipara, when the delivery has been precipitate or when the tissues are unusually rigid and nonyielding. Overdistention of lower parts of the vaginal wall then produces a tear of the posterior fourchet, some of the overlying skin and the posterior vaginal wall. It is confined to this area and does not extend beyond the anterior half of the perineum. The levator muscles and their fascia are undamaged. On rare occasions the perineal body may be severely damaged without any external evidence of injury. Pressure exerted by a finger on the posterior vaginal wall and a thumb on the fourchet will reveal the loss of substance (Fig. 63–1, *A*).

SECOND-DEGREE TEAR.   In the second-degree tear the injury extends farther beyond the middle portion of the perineum, forming a deep sulcus that runs upward along one or both sides of the posterior vaginal wall. This is secondary to damage to the anterior portion of the levator ani muscles and their supporting rectovaginal fascia. This can be felt by inserting the finger in the vagina and exerting external pressure on the perineal body by the thumb. A line of fibrous scarlike tissue can be felt at the base of the sulcus. When damage has occurred bilaterally and two sulci are present, extensive damage to the levator muscles and their fascia has taken place, and the anterior rectal wall bulges through. Not infrequently the damage to the perineal body is so complete that relaxation of the vaginal outlet occurs, sufficient to admit the introduction of several fingers (Fig. 63–1, *B*).

THIRD-DEGREE TEARS.   The most extensive injuries to the perineum and perineal body usually arise as the result of complicated deliveries which frequently have required the use of instruments. The damage now involves the entire perineum and extends through the spincter ani muscles into the rectum. The anus becomes wholly or partially incompetent, and the reddened rectal mucosa is exposed in the opening. The separated ends of the muscle can be identified by well-marked dimples on either side of the anus (Fig. 63–1, *C*).

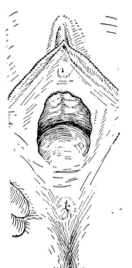

Fig. 63-2. When a perineal laceration is accompanied by weakening of the posterior vaginal wall, the rectum may bulge into the vagina, thereby forming a rectocele.

How Do You Recognize the Presence of Other Injuries Associated with Perineal Tears?

The three types of perineal tear are the most common, and they may appear without other damage to the birth canal. All manner of variations are encountered, however. Inspection of the vagina usually reveals that the perineum has been injured, but often it does not tell the full extent of the damage. For example, the perineum may appear to be intact, but other lacerations in the pelvic floor may have occurred higher up in the vaginal canal.

The extent of damage to the levator ani muscles, which provide the lateral support to the vagina, can best be detected by introducing two fingers into the vaginal canal, and pulling downward and forward while the thumb presses against the perineal body in the midline just above the anus. The loss of muscle support is apparent both in the region of the perineal body and laterally where the levator ani muscles seem to droop along the pubic rami rather than resting in the midline. One must be careful not to confuse scar tissue which is present in quantity from the firm support provided by muscle.

Looking directly at the vulva in a typical case, one sees the gaping vaginal orifice which is retracted backward along with the anus. The failure of the walls of the vagina to appose is evident to an even greater extent when the patient is placed in the Sims position and the vagina is allowed to fill with air. Through the relaxed opening either a cystocele or rectocele, or both, can be seen jutting outward (Fig. 63–2).

In some women relaxation of the pelvic floor follows delivery, yet no sign of pelvic floor injury is evident at the time of birth or later. This is particularly true of women who have been depleted in health or whose muscles have become atonic because of too frequent pregnancies.

How Important Is It to Repair These Tears Early?

The need for early repair depends on the extent of the injury. In general the earlier the repair, the greater the chance of success, because lacerated muscles tend to atrophy, and the fascia becomes more frayed.

The pelvic organs, bladder and rectum tend to prolapse through the weakened pelvic floor. This becomes more apparent the longer the damaged structures are left unrepaired. The ideal time to recognize the injury and treat the laceration is at the time of delivery. If repair is not done at that time, several months should be allowed to elapse before contemplating later repair because of the vascularity of the tissues. The decision for or against reconstructive surgery depends on the extent of the damage and the likelihood of subsequent pregnancies that might undo the repair.

How Does One Recognize Damage to the External Sphincter Ani Muscle?

Incompetence of the anal sphincter is a distressing complication that should be recognized early and corrected. The longer repair is delayed, the more difficult it becomes. It is important, therefore, to know when the external sphincter ani muscle has been seriously damaged. It is obvious when the tear is complete, but damage may occur without any external sign of injury.

Under normal conditions one immediately notes shallow folds of skin that radiate outward from the anal opening in all directions. When the sphincter muscle is damaged, the radiating folds can no longer be seen in the area intervening between the anterior margin of the anus and the posterior wall of the vagina, though they are still present posteriorly and laterally. The muscle has been replaced by scar tissue, which can be felt as a fibrotic band. The retracted ends of the divided muscle can also be felt in a lateral position where they tend to dimple the skin.

What Lesions Are Commonly Associated with Perineal Lacerations?

Herniation of the pelvic viscera often accompanies lacerations of the pelvic floor. The levator ani muscles, combined with the condensation of the pelvic fascia to form ligaments, act to support the pelvic viscera in their normal position. The muscles provide the greater portion of the supporting element. The pelvic fascia or ligaments in themselves are not sufficiently strong and will eventually give way. Weakness of the muscles or fascial supports allows pelvic structures such as bladder, urethra, rectum, uterus and vaginal vault to descend into the vaginal canal.

In most instances damage to the levator ani muscles occurs because of the actual birth trauma, although stretching or incomplete involution of the supporting structures at the time of a later delivery also plays a role. Certainly prolapses of the pelvic viscera are more common in women who have had children than in those who have not. Occasionally, however, one sees a virginal or congenital prolapse. This suggests that there may also be a factor of weakness inherent in some supporting structures from the beginning. Many women who have repeated pregnancies show little disturbance in pelvic floor support. Prolapse of the pelvic organs occurs with increasing frequency with advancing years. It is uncommon before the age of forty despite the fact that the obstetrical trauma occurred some years before the hernia. Various types of prolapse of the pelvic organs are common occurrences after the menopause.

PROLAPSE

There are three well-recognized types of prolapse of the pelvic organs. They vary in degree, depending on the extent of pelvic floor damage, and they occur for the

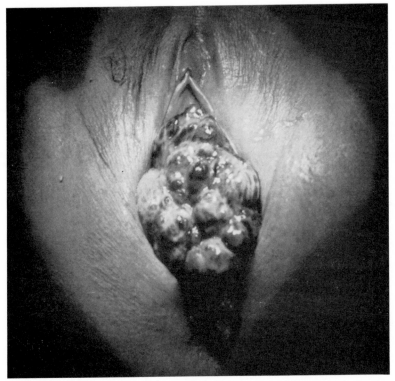

Fig. 63-3.   Prolapse of the uterus, with the protrusion of a large benign cervical polyp through the introitus, is a serious complication of advanced pelvic relaxation.

most part in combinations, although they may appear on rare occasions as single entities.

Clinical evidence of the prolapse is manifest by the presence of (1) A *cystocele*. This is simply a herniation of the bladder through a defect in the anterior vaginal wall at the upper part of the vagina. When the weakness occurs lower down in the vagina, the floor of the urethra descends, and a *urethrocele* is formed.

2. A *rectocele* follows a prolapse of the posterior vaginal wall. A defect in the muscle and fascia allows the anterior wall of the rectum to pout out through it, at the lower end of the vaginal canal. When the supporting structures are weak in their upper portion, an *enterocele* is formed, complete with hernial sac, often containing small intestine.

3. A prolapse of the entire *uterus* or *vaginal vault*. In this instance the damage to the pelvic floor is more serious, since both the muscle and fascial supports are weakened (Fig. 63–3). It is rare to have a cystocele without some element of rectocele or uterine prolapse. The most common association finds a uterine prolapse combined with a cystocele, because of the intimate anatomic attachments of bladder and uterus.

Cystocele and Urethrocele

What Are the Symptoms of Cystocele and Urethrocele?

Primarily the patient with a cystocele complains of a fullness or bulging in the vagina and a sense of bearing-down discomfort as though her pelvic organs were dropping out. The severity of the complaints varies widely with the patient and the degree of prolapse. In general, the cystocele develops slowly and progresses to a certain point. During this period the patient may have discomfort or pain which ceases when the herniation reaches its height. Small cystoceles rarely produce more than minor symptoms, but larger ones are invariably troublesome. The bearing-down discomfort is usually aggravated by physical exercise or fatigue caused by jobs that keep the patient on her feet for long hours. If descent of the bladder is extreme, the patient may be uncomfortable when she sits down, or she may have difficulty in walking. Because of the exposed position and thin overlying vaginal epithelium, the cystocele may ulcerate and cause bleeding or discharge.

Urinary symptoms are common in women who have a cystocele, largely because of their difficulty in completely emptying the bladder. Bladder descent drops the anterior portion below the level of the bladder neck, which makes for a mechanical problem in evacuation. This leads to irritability of the bladder and urinary frequency. Since the retained urine easily becomes infected, *cystitis* is common. Stress incontinence does not occur in the patients who have a cystocele unless there is an accompanying urethrocele.

Stress incontinence is the chief symptom in patients who have a urethrocele. It is usually partial and often diurnal. The symptom is aggravated by any strain, such as laughing, coughing, sneezing or other exertion that increases the intra-abdominal pressure. The patient may experience some difficulty in walking, because of bearing-down pressure and feeling the presence of a mass in the vagina. The symptoms are due to a disturbance in the sphincter mechanism at the base of the bladder. The same symptoms may sometimes occur in the absence of a urethrocele.

How Does One Identify a Cystocele or Urethrocele?

CYSTOCELE.   In the majority of cases one has no difficulty in deciding whether or not the patient has a cystocele. The correct diagnosis is evident when a bulging anterior vaginal wall can be seen and palpated. The bulge is usually spherical and frequently fills the vaginal orifice. The mass is soft in its consistency and has a rather elastic feel on palpation (Fig. 63–4). The herniation increases in size on coughing or straining, particularly if the patient is in a standing position. The urethra is displaced forward and upward and occupies a more prominent position than it does under normal conditions. The urethra runs a straight course into the bladder when a catheter or cystoscope is inserted. In the same manner, one can demonstrate that the bladder is prolapsed and lies beneath the bulging anterior vaginal wall. When the cystocele is large and protrudes beyond the vaginal outlet, the vaginal epithelium becomes thickened and loses its transverse folds, at least in the upper portion. Under normal conditions these folds are prominent.

The cystocele may be so small as not to be obvious with the patient in the supine position. It may be demonstrated by having the physician depress the perineum with the examining fingers and asking the patient to strain downward. The cystocele will become most apparent if this maneuver is carried out with the patient in an upright position. The cystocele may on rare occasions appear only when a patient is relaxed under anesthesia.

There are few pathologic entities except the rather rare vaginal cysts to confuse the examiner in making this diagnosis. We recently encountered a Gaertner's duct cyst that had dissected beneath the anterior vaginal wall epithelium and assumed the position of a cystocele.

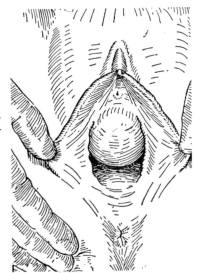

Fig. 63-4. A cystocele bulges into the vagina anteriorly. The urinary bladder becomes displaced posteriorly and downward, owing to a weakened anterior vaginal wall.

URETHROCELE.   Normally the urethra and bladder neck are attached beneath the pubic bone. When the muscle and fascial supports are stretched and damaged, the urethra and bladder neck become detached from their usual position, the relation of the bladder neck to the bladder itself becomes distorted, and the patient has stress incontinence.

In most instances the presence of a urethrocele is readily demonstrated. When the patient is asked to strain down, the urethra can be seen to bulge outward beneath the sagging anterior vaginal wall. The greater the amount of straining, the larger the bulge. When this happens, the urethral meatus curls outward around the symphysis, and she can no longer control the flow of urine, which then gushes out. At times this can be shown best with the patient in the upright position. Because of its exposed position the urethral meatus becomes thick and papillomatous and may bleed easily.

How Do You Treat a Cystocele?

SURGERY.   Unless the patient is having repeated bouts of cystitis or other kinds of urinary infection, there is no urgency about advising the patient with a small or moderately large cystocele to have it repaired. This is particularly true of the younger patient, who may have more children, which would destroy the surgical repair. On the other hand, the repair of even a small cystocele may be advisable if (*a*) the patient is having distressing symptoms, (*b*) the cystocele is becoming larger, or (*c*) there are recurrent bouts of cystitis.

The recurrent nature as well as the actual cause of the symptoms usually lies in the residual urine, which the patient is unable to evacuate completely. The best method of testing this is to catheterize the patient after she has voided as much as she normally can. If more than 2 or 3 ounces are left in the bladder, or the bacteriologic cultures and microscopic studies of the sediment show any infection, the cystocele should be repaired. Large lesions should be repaired unless the patient plans to have more children or there is some contraindication to surgery, such as intercurrent disease or advanced age.

The patient with pelvic abnormalities that require abdominal intervention may

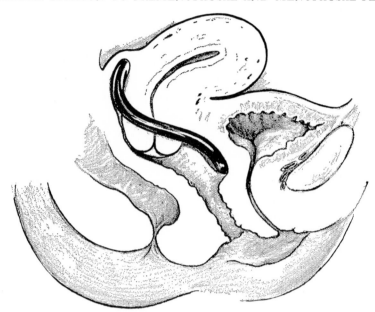

Fig. 63-5.   A pessary properly placed holds the uterus up in the normal position. It should be comfortable. Constant use of pessaries is undesirable because of local irritation and possible urethral compression.

also have a large cystocele. The surgeon will have to rely on his judgment as to when in the course of the operation he repairs the cystocele, if at all. The abdominal procedure is more important. If it is to be a prolonged operation, or the diagnosis is uncertain, the repair of the cystocele had best be postponed to a later date at another separate operation.

There is no problem about when to repair a cystocele when vaginal surgery is to be done for other reasons. This is a regular step in performing vaginal hysterectomy or pelvic floor repair.

Nonsurgical Therapy in Young Women.   If the patient is young and desires to have more children and the symptoms are not too persistent or disabling, surgery should be postponed until the family is completed or the symptoms become more severe. Much can be accomplished in the younger patient after delivery by outlining a course of postnatal exercises designed to strengthen the levator ani muscles. A Hodge pessary may be useful immediately after delivery, particularly if the uterus is retroverted and produces a strain on the supporting ligaments (Fig. 63–5). The elevation of the uterus and its replacement in normal position allow the muscles to regain their normal tone. The measure is entirely temporary, and it should not be relied upon for any protracted time. The pessary cannot hope to cure a long-standing prolapse. At best it can only prevent it from becoming worse. If the younger woman's pelvic relaxation is sufficient to require the constant use of a pessary, she had better be operated upon, unless there is some contraindication to surgery.

Nonsurgical Therapy in Older Patients.   The various types of supporting pessary have their chief usefulness in the patient who has symptomatic pelvic relaxation, but is an unsuitable candidate for surgical repair. Pessaries are effective when the uterus prolapses with the cystocele, but are useless if there is so much relaxation of the outlet that they are promptly expelled with any particular muscular effort, such as during coughing or the act of defecation. Contraindications to surgery should

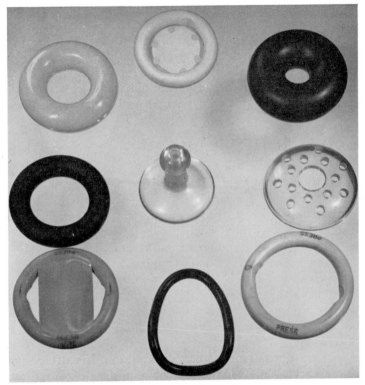

Fig. 63-6. A collection of various types of pessary. Clockwise, beginning with the 12 o'clock position, they are (1) round solid ring, plastic, (2) rubber doughnut, (3) plastic disk with perforation, (4) collapsible ring, (5) Smith Hodge pessary, (6) Gellhorn pessary (center), (7) collapsible ring with a central support, (8) solid rubber ring, (9) rubber doughnut, inflatable.

be based on medical grounds rather than age alone. Many older women withstand vaginal surgery and the minor complications that may go with it far better than the discomfort that follows use of an ineffective pessary.

The choice of pessary is of some importance. The ring pessary, which is effective for uterine prolapse, is of little use when the patient has a cystocele. The rubber doughnut or plastic types of pessary with a collapsible ring and a perforated transverse base are useful, provided the cystocele is not too large (Fig. 63–6).

RECTOCELE

The rectocele is actually a rectovaginal hernia that results from trauma to the levator muscles, stretching or tearing of the supporting fascia and perhaps an associated congenital or inherent weakness in those structures. It usually follows delivery and develops slowly over the years. The rectocele cannot occur without a definite fascial defect which is a part of the extensive perineal injury that occurs with a traumatic birth. Rarely does this type of hernia appear in a nulliparous woman. When it does, there is obviously a congenital or constitutional weakness in the muscle and fascial supports. Of all the types of prolapse, the pure rectocele is the least common. It is usually associated with a cystocele, some degree of uterine descent and laceration of the perineum. This is a measure of the total injury to the structures that make up the pelvic floor.

It is interesting, however, to note that when uterine prolapse is extreme, as in a procidentia, a rectocele is not a part of it. The reason is that in a procidentia the damage has been so great that the rectum has been separated from its attachment to the posterior vaginal wall. When the uterus descends completely, the vaginal canal actually becomes inverted without implicating the rectum. A rectocele can occur only when the anterior rectal and the posterior vaginal walls are adherent. The rectum then simply protrudes into the posterior vaginal wall through the fascial defect.

What Are the Symptoms of a Rectocele?

The symptoms arising from the presence of a rectocele are actually few and far less than one finds when a cystocele is present. The patient may have some minimal bearing-down discomfort or be aware of a bulge in the vagina, but the symptoms are rarely severe enough either to require a pessary or to demand surgical intervention. It is usually the associated elements in the prolapse such as the cystocele and uterine descent that produce the discomfort and disability. The rectocele develops slowly, as the result of repeated straining at stool. The weakened fascial supports gradually give way. This is particularly prone to occur after the menopause.

When the rectocele becomes large, the patient has a difficult time in fully evacuating the lower rectum on defecation. This is due to the saclike bulge above the anal sphincter that allows fecal matter to accumulate. The damage to the levator ani muscles, which have been pushed to the side and no longer attach to the perineal body, interferes with the normal mechanism of expulsion. In extreme cases the patient may actually have to press with a finger along the posterior vaginal wall in order to flatten out the bulge so that defecation can be complete.

How Does One Identify a Rectocele?

The diagnosis is readily made on direct inspection and palpation. When the vaginal orifice is first inspected, it is difficult to distinguish between a cystocele and a rectocele. When a finger is placed in the anal canal, and pressure is exerted toward the upper part of the vagina, the defect in the posterior vaginal wall becomes obvious. When the patient is asked to strain as though she were in the act of defecation, the protrusion of the posterior vaginal wall increases in size. Usually the defect is noted just above the anal sphincter, which is also apt to be damaged.

When the upper part of the posterior wall rolls out over the perineal body, as it sometimes does, one should be suspicious of the presence of an *enterocele*. A "high" rectocele is far more likely to be an enterocele.

ENTEROCELE

What Is an Enterocele?

In contrast to the rectocele, in which the posterior vaginal and anterior rectal walls are adherent, but simply protrude through a defect in the fascial support, an enterocele is a true hernia. It may be either *congenital* or *acquired*. In the congenital type the opening of the sac, which is lined with peritoneum, is found between the attachments of the uterosacral ligaments posterior to the cervix. In its descent it passes between the anterior rectal and posterior vaginal walls. In the *acquired* type

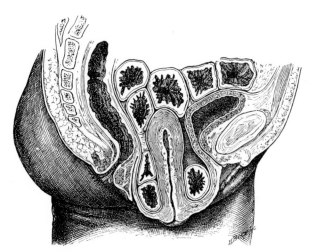

Fig. 63-7. Enteroceles may develop both anterior and posterior to the uterus, with uterine prolapse and eversion of the vaginal walls. The bladder is detached from the uterus and vagina, and the hernia sac containing intestine becomes interposed. (From Kelly: *Operative Gynecology*, New York, Appleton & Co., 1900.)

the cul-de-sac or pouch of Douglas elongates, after delivery, as part of the prolapse of the uterus. One occasionally finds both types of enterocele in the same patient. Both types tend to increase in size, owing to the constant intra-abdominal pressure. As they enlarge they fill with small intestine and occasionally omentum (Fig. 63–7).

How Does One Recognize the Presence of an Enterocele?

It is important to distinguish between a rectocele and an enterocele, since the latter is a true hernia complete with peritoneal sac and small bowel contents. If it is not recognized at the time a rectocele is repaired, the patient is very likely to have the same complaints and a protrusion of the posterior vaginal wall similar to the one she had before the repair was done.

When the patient is examined in the horizontal position, only the rectocele may be in evidence, although it may seem to extend from farther up the vaginal canal than usual. If one keeps in mind that a high rectocele is probably an enterocele, he will search for certain physical findings that may betray its presence. If there is any doubt, the patient should be examined in the standing position.

In a well established enterocele a bulge can be seen in the posterior vaginal wall immediately behind the cervix. The protrusion may expand and contract as the patient breathes, suggesting that there is some communication with the abdominal cavity. From within the abdominal cavity at operation one can often see a definite defect lined with peritoneum, which extends downward anterior to the rectum in the area between the attachments of the uterosacral ligaments and the posterior boundary of the cervix. This is the finger-like projection that one feels at the upper part of the vagina when the patient is examined from below. Frequently it contains small bowel, which can be displaced. One often finds a rectocele and an enterocele in the same patient. With a finger in the rectum and the thumb along the posterior vaginal wall one notes an increase in the thickness of the rectovaginal wall above the thinned-out rectocele. The examining finger enters the sacculation formed by the rectocele, but it cannot enter the upper protrusion which is the enterocele.

The differentiation between an enterocele and a prolapse of the vaginal vault after operation will be discussed in the next chapter.

How Are Posterior Vaginal Wall Herniations Treated?

Since a small rectocele gives the patient little trouble, it may well be disregarded unless a surgical repair is being done for prolapse of other pelvic viscera. The larger rectoceles, particularly those that cause faulty fecal elimination, should be repaired surgically. It is also a good idea to correct a large rectocele, even though it be relatively asymptomatic, when an abdominal hysterectomy is being done. Some women who were previously unaware of the rectocele complain of it after the uterus has been removed. If the rectocele extends high in the vagina, the physician should be on the lookout for an enterocele. A high repair will not correct such a defect.

The *enterocele*, like the rectocele, causes little discomfort unless it is so large that it protrudes outside the vaginal outlet. It should be repaired, however, whenever it is found in the course of a rectocele repair or other reconstruction of the pelvic floor. This can usually be accomplished as a vaginal procedure. The sac is dissected free, as in any hernia operation. It is then excised, and the neck of the sac is fixed to the cervix before the uterosacral ligaments are approximated behind it. At times it is necessary to perform a combined abdominovaginal operation to ensure obliteration of the posterior cul-de-sac, particularly when the enterocele is of the acquired type associated with a broad, deep pouch of Douglas.

REFERENCES

Pelvic Lacerations and Prolapse

Copenhaver, E. H.: Surgical Management of Complete Prolapse of the Uterus and Vagina. *S. Cïin. N. Amer.*, 40: 743, 1960.

Davidson, S.: Prolapse and Its Management. *Practitioner*, 185: 271, 1960.

Fothergill, W. E.: Supports of Pelvic Viscera: A Review of Some Recent Contributions to Pelvic Anatomy, with a Clinical Introduction. *J. Obst. & Gynaec. Brit. Emp.*, 13: 18, 1908.

Gibson, G. B.: The Repair of Genital Prolapse. *Am. J. Obst. & Gynec.*, 78: 1275, 1959.

Goff, B. H.: The Surgical Anatomy of Cystocele and Urethrocele, with Special Reference to the Pubocervical Fascia. *Surg., Gynec. & Obst.*, 87: 725, 1948.

Gordon, R. E.: The Manchester Operation for the Treatment of Uterine Prolapse. *Clin. Obst. & Gynec.*. 4: 179, 1961.

Halban, J., and Tandler, J.: The Anatomy and Etiology of Genital Prolapse in Women: The Supporting Apparatus of the Uterus. *Obst. & Gynec.*, 15: 790, 1960.

Krantz, K. E.: The Gross and Microscopic Anatomy of the Human Vagina. *Ann. New York Acad. Sc.*, 83: 89, 1959.

Malpas, P.: *Genital Prolapse and Allied Conditions.* New York, Grune & Stratton, Inc., 1955.

Mengert, W. F.: Complete Perineal Tear and Perineorrhaphy. *Clin. Obst. & Gynec.*, 4: 168, 1961.

Percy, N. M., and Perl, J. I.: Total Colpectomy. *Surg., Gynec. & Obst.*, 113: 175, 1961.

Phaneuf, L. E.: The Management of Prolapse of the Uterus and Vagina; in J. V. Meigs and S. H. Sturgis, eds.: *Progress in Gynecology.* New York, Grune & Stratton, Inc., 1950, Vol. II, p. 654.

Porges, R. F., Porges, J. C., and Blinick, G.: Mechanisms of Uterine Support and the Pathogenesis of Uterine Prolapse. *Obst. & Gynec.*, 15: 711, 1960.

Ricci, J. V.: Gleanings and Technical Details from 500 Vaginal Hysterectomies for Prolapse. *Am. J. Surg.*, 79: 377, 1950.

Symmonds, R. E., and Pratt, J. H.: Vaginal Prolapse Following Hysterectomy. *Am. J. Obst. & Gynec.*, 79: 899, 1960.

Tanner, J. M.: The Development of the Female Reproductive System during Adolescence. *Clin. Obst. & Gynec.*, 3: 135, 1960.

Uhlenhuth, E., Wolfe, W. M., Smith, E. M., and Middleton, E. B.: The Rectogenital Septum. *Surg., Gynec. & Obst.*, 86: 148, 1948.

Ulfelder, H.: The Normal Mechanism of Uterine Support and Its Clinical Implications. *West. J. Surg., Obst. & Gynec.*, 68: 81, 1959.

Watson, B. P.: Complete Tear of Perineum; in J. V. Meigs and S. H. Sturgis, eds.: *Progress in Gynecology.* New York, Grune & Stratton, Inc., 1950, Vol. II, p. 684.

Enterocele

Austin, R. C., and Damstra, E. F.: New Fascia Plastic Repair of Enterocele. *Surg., Gynec. & Obst.*, 101: 297, 1955.

Hiller, R. I.: Repair of Enterocele with Preservation of Vagina. *Am. J. Obst. & Gynec.*, 64: 409, 1952.

Kinzel, G. E.: Enterocele: A Study of 265 Cases. *Am. J. Obst. & Gynec.*, 81: 1166, 1961.

McCall, M. L.: Posterior Culdeplasty. Surgical Correction of Enterocele during a Vaginal Hysterectomy. A Preliminary Report. *Obst. & Gynec.*, 10: 595, 1957.

Meigs, J. V.: Enterocele; in J. V. Meigs and S. H. Sturgis, eds.: *Progress in Gynecology.* New York, Grune & Stratton, Inc., 1950, Vol. II, p. 698.

Read, C. D.: Enterocele. *Am. J. Obst. & Gynec.*, 62: 743, 1951.

Waters, E. G.: Culdoplastic Technique for Prevention and Correction of Vaginal Vault Prolapse and Enterocele. *Am. J. Obst. & Gynec.*, 81: 291, 1961.

Chapter 64

Abnormal Positions of the Uterus

By the very nature of the fact that the uterus must adapt itself in position to the changing demands of pregnancy, which produce a progressive enlargement, the uterus cannot be a fixed organ. Normally the adult uterus occupies a position midway between the bladder, which lies anteriorly and slightly below it, and the rectum, located posteriorly. With the patient in the upright position the uterus lies in a horizontal plane at right angles to the long axis of the vagina. The anterior surface of the uterus then rests lightly on the fundus of the bladder. The pressure exerted by the overlying intestine tends to keep it in that position. Since the uterus is not fixed, however, it is subject in the nonpregnant state to variable pressures exerted by distention of either the bladder or the rectum, particularly the former. A bladder full of urine will tend to force the uterus backward, and an accumulation of fecal matter in the rectum pushes the uterus upward. It is thus evident that the uterus may alter its position, depending upon forces exerted in a variety of ways. Mobility is also necessary to combat the sudden changes in intra-abdominal pressure associated with trauma, lifting, straining at stool, breathing, walking or running, coughing, or in fact any act that will increase the tension within the abdomen. The range of motion is not inconsiderable in both the anterior and posterior directions where it may move as much as 180 degrees, or laterally where the displacements are restricted, but can be in the range of 45 degrees of motion.

It is a well documented observation, however, that once the forces of displacement are withdrawn, the uterus will resume its natural position, provided the normal structures that support it have not been damaged through trauma caused by accident, pregnancy or the simple processes of aging.

What Are the Supporting Elements That Maintain the Uterus in Position?

In addition to the role played by the pressure of the overlying intestine, the uterus is well suspended and in part supported by a number of so-called ligaments. Some of the ligaments are little more than peritoneal folds or reflexions, and practically speaking they are not very effective in supporting the uterus. In this category one might place familiar structures such as the broad ligaments, vesicouterine fold and to a certain extent the uterosacral ligaments. The last have a part in holding the uterus back in the hollow of the sacrum. Their very laxness, which is apparent when they are seen at the time of an abdominal exploration, allows them to respond to the

1018

demands of pregnancy through their ability to stretch, but their main function is not that of maintaining the uterus in position.

The round ligaments appear to provide a sling type of suspension, since they attach to the uterus and to the inguinal canals. In the nonpregnant state, however, they are often loose and redundant and may be attenuated. They do little to support the uterus. During pregnancy they tend to undergo hypertrophy. Their function then is to prevent the pregnant uterus from rotating as it enlarges.

The cardinal ligaments provide the chief elements in the support of the uterus. They are made up of thick, fibrous, condensed areolar tissue and are found on either side of the cervix. Within their substance they contain important blood vessels, lymphatics and nerves. This condensed mass of areolar tissue blends with the fascial envelopes that surround the bladder and vagina, as well as the muscle bundles of the pelvic floor. In this location they serve to maintain the uterus in a midline position at a fairly constant level in the pelvis (Fig. 64–1).

One becomes aware of their key function in the positioning of the uterus when

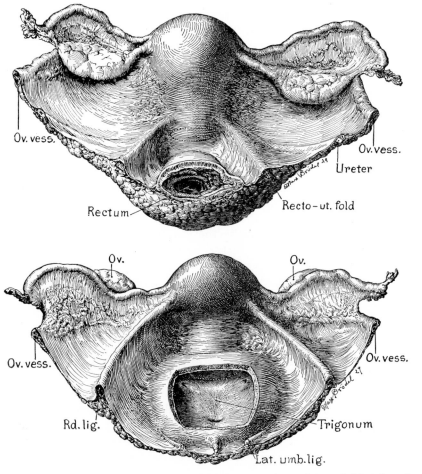

Fig. 64-1.   The uterus, adnexa and their ligaments are pictured from behind (*above*) and from in front (*below*). The broad ligaments contain the tubes and ovarian vessels; the round ligaments pass from the uterus to the canals of Nuck. The cardinal ligaments are at the level of the dotted ellipses. (From Wislocki.)

doing pelvic surgery to remove the uterus. Little mobility is obtained by sectioning the other ligamentous attachments. The uterus moves only after the cardinal ligaments have been divided.

How Does the Position of the Uterus Vary with Age?

Although the normal adult uterus tends to occupy a position horizontal to the long axis of the vagina, this is not true in infancy or after the menopause. In the infant the uterus is customarily retrocessed, paralleling the axis of the bony pelvis, with a tendency to bend backward on itself, i.e., retroversion. Under the influence of the sex hormones and the gradual rotation of the pelvic girdle, the symphysis is forced downward and the sacrum and coccyx upward, so that the uterus finally comes to assume what we regard as the normal or anterior position, with forward flexion. The change in position of the uterus takes place slowly over a period of time and may not be complete before the eighteenth or twentieth year.

The important fact is that many malplacements are congenital or developmental in origin. This could come about through failure of the bony pelvis to go through the normal rotation or through congenital weakness in the supporting musculofascial bundles. As a result the uterus may never achieve the normal anteverted position.

In the menopause, as the supporting structures become more relaxed, the uterus tends to take a position in the long axis of the vagina with a mild degree of retroversion, either through inherent weakness in or damage to the musculofascial ligamentous attachments. The intra-abdominal pressure acting on the anterior surface of the uterus aggravates the malposition and even encourages prolapse.

What Are the Common Types of Uterine Malposition?

Malposition of the uterus may take place in a number of different directions and in a variety of ways. The deviation from the normal may be forward, backward or downward.

The terminology used to describe the various positions of the uterus is often confusing. This is particularly true of the terms "version" and "flexion." Actually, one rarely finds the uterus in a position of flexion without some degree of version, whether the uterus be forward or backward. It is largely a question of the degree of angulation that the fundus makes with the cervix. The more extreme form should be designated as a flexion.

ANTERIOR DISPLACEMENT OF THE UTERUS

The normal position of the uterus is forward with a slight angulation of the fundus on the cervix, i.e. anteversion. Occasionally this position may be accentuated by the pressure of a posteriorly placed tumor which forces the uterus anteriorly against the symphysis pubis. The relation of the fundus to the cervix is not altered, but the uterus now is displaced in relation to the axis of the vagina.

ANTEFLEXION

In some women, particularly in the younger age group, the uterus is bent so sharply forward that an acute angle is made between the fundus and the cervix.

Young women with an infertility problem frequently have such severe anteflexion. The condition carries with it some of the stigmata of maldevelopment, for not infrequently the uterus is infantile in type with a typical cervix elongated in proportion to the size of a relatively small fundus. Though the majority of cases of acute anteflexion are congenital in origin, one occasionally sees a normally developed uterus with acute anteflexion. It is possible to acquire this type of pathologic anterior displacement as an aftermath of puerperal infection and pelvic cellulitis.

How Do You Distinguish between Congenital and Acquired Anteflexion of the Uterus?

The diagnosis of anteflexion is made by bimanual vaginal and abdominal examination. In evaluating the position of the uterus, it should be firmly kept in mind that some angulation of the fundus on the cervix is normal.

There are two points which help in deciding whether the degree of flexion is pathological: (*a*) the size of the fundus in relation to the cervix, and (*b*) the mobility of the uterus. A small uterus with an elongated cervix in a girl in her late teens suggests a congenital maldevelopment. A probe gently introduced through the cervix to the top of the fundus may be helpful in determining the relative proportions of cervix to fundus. The degree of angulation is detected by placing the index finger of the examining hand in the anterior fornix. The differentiation between the congenital and acquired type of pathologic anterior displacement can be made by evaluating the degree of uterine motility. If there appears to be some diminution in the ease with which the uterus can be moved on examination, one may suspect that chronic inflammatory changes in the broad ligaments are responsible.

What Symptoms Are Produced by Acute Anteflexion?

The two chief complaints are dysmenorrhea and sterility. Some women with severe anteflexion, however, are asymptomatic. In all probability the two main symptoms are interrelated, particularly when the uterus is underdeveloped. The underlying defect is a hormonal imbalance. With a normally developed uterus the loss of uterine motility in association with the acute angulation is probably responsible. Many women with acute anteflexion complain of severe, incapacitating dysmenorrhea. One can easily postulate that the cause of the uterine cramps is the inability of the uterus to get rid of the menstrual debris, owing to the obstruction caused by the acute angulation of the fundus on the cervix. Cervical edema can be expected to exaggerate the obstruction during the time of menstruation.

How Do You Treat Acute Anteflexion of the Uterus?

The patient with a normally developed uterus in acute flexion needs no treatment if the condition is asymptomatic. If the uterus is normal in size, sharply flexed forward and restricted in motion, the treatment is the same as that given for chronic pelvic inflammatory disease.

The treatment of the undeveloped uterus in acute flexion should be directed along the lines of hormonal replacement. Uterine enlargement, with a restoration of a more normal balance between the size of the fundus and the cervix, can be achieved by placing the patient on estrin therapy for six months to one year. Premarin, 1.25 mg.; estinyl, 0.5 mg.; diethylstilbestrol, 1 mg., may be used as oral medications, given daily for 25 days out of the month. Thyroid in 1-grain doses daily is often given along with the estrin, depending on the degree of obesity and the indications provided by such tests of thyroid function as the blood protein-bound iodine, blood cholesterol, basal metabolism or the uptake of radioactive iodine. In many instances thyroid extract in small doses has proved to have clinical value when given in the absence of any laboratory indication of hypofunction of the gland.

Occasionally a dilatation and curettage may be helpful in adjusting the angulation of the fundus on the cervix. Its chief value will be the disruption of nerve endings in the cervix and the relief of dysmenorrhea. If a patient can become pregnant after this simple maneuver, and some have, the consequent physiologic enlargement of the uterus will correct the displacement permanently. If pregnancy does not follow, dilatation of the cervix rarely has any lasting benefit.

The angulation of the cervix with the fundus can be corrected and permanent enlargement of the uterus can be obtained by inserting a stem pessary in the uterus and fixing it there so that it cannot be extruded for three to six months. Advocates of this procedure feel that the disadvantages are more theoretical than real. The menstrual flow is not obstructed, infection is said not to occur, and sexual activities are not restricted. Some have advocated the combined use of stem pessaries and estrin. Uterine enlargement has not been augmented by this method. In general, therapy involving the use of hormones alone will accomplish the same thing as well without risks.

POSTERIOR DISPLACEMENTS OF THE UTERUS

The two most common forms of posterior uterine displacement are (*a*) retrocession and (*b*) retroversion or retroflexion (Fig. 64–2).

RETROCESSION

This condition, in which the entire uterus drops back into the hollow of the sacrum, frequently accompanies acute anteflexion of the congenital type. Unlike retroversion, the fundus retains its anteversion in relation to the axis of the cervix. The symptoms are those of the acute anteflexion that accompanies it. When the patient is symptomatic, the primary treatment is hormonal substitution with estrin. If the patient is without symptoms, no treatment is required.

RETROVERSION AND RETROFLEXION

When the fundus of the uterus turns backward while the cervix points in the direction of the vaginal canal or toward the anterior vaginal wall, the patient is said to have a retroversion. It becomes a retroflexion only when the posterior angulation of the fundus on the cervix is extreme. Since the pathologic significance and the symptoms produced are the same, the terms may be used interchangeably.

What Are the Probable Causes of Retroversion?

The retroverted position can, but need not, be due to a pathologic cause. It is possible for a uterus in this position to function normally and to be completely

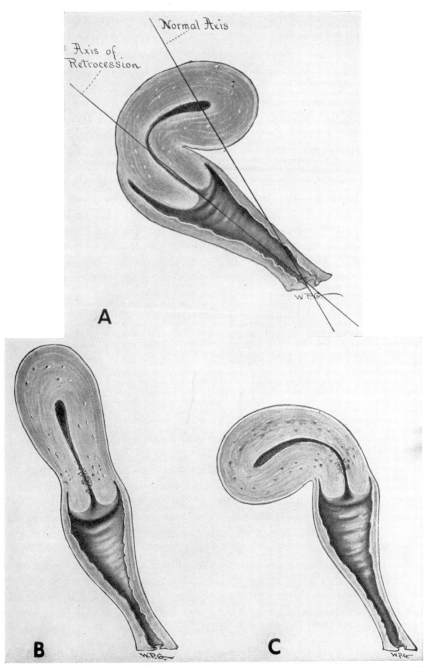

Fig. 64-2. Drawings to illustrate (*A*) retrocession, (*B*) moderate retroversion and (*C*) severe retroversion. The anterior abdominal wall in each case would be to the right. (Drawn by the author from W. P. Graves: *Gynecology*.)

compatible with normal health. In many instances retroversion is asymptomatic, and the position no deterrent to gestation. Patients with a retroverted uterus must be evaluated individually when the problem of treatment arises. The final decision will depend on a careful review of the associated symptoms. If there are no symptoms and no infertility problem, the uterus had best be left in its backward position.

Approximately 20 per cent of all women will have their uterus in the retroverted position. This may in part be due to a congenital cause, since it is frequently found in nulliparous women. The defect then would appear to be in inherent weakness in the musculofascial support of the uterus. Retroversion is common in *women who have had repeated or severe strains in the course of childbirth.* The cause then lies in the relaxation of the supporting structures of the uterus. The size and weight of the uterus frequently contribute to the retroverted position. It is a common finding in the weeks immediately post partum. As further involution in the size of the fundus takes place, the uterus gradually resumes its normal position. In the majority of instances the uterus is held in retroversion by some form of associated disease. The size and weight of the uterus may be increased by a tumor within the uterus or the immediately adjacent adnexa. The most common explanation, however, is some form of pelvic abnormality that binds the uterus in the cul-de-sac. Old pelvic peritonitis from a ruptured appendix, pelvic inflammatory disease or endometriosis frequently produces pelvic adhesions that fix the uterus posteriorly in the hollow of the sacrum.

What Symptoms May Be Attributed to Retroversion?

UNCOMPLICATED RETROVERSION.   When the retroverted uterus is present without evidence of other pelvic disease, the patient rarely has symptoms. She may have some difficulty in becoming pregnant. Before attributing the cause of the infertility to the altered position of the uterus, every other known source of obstruction to conception should be investigated. Most women with retroverted uteri have no trouble getting pregnant—many of them repeatedly. If investigations have proved negative, and the patient with a retroverted uterus is still not able to become pregnant, one might reasonably consider restoring the uterus to the normal position. There is always the possibility that the cervix, which points toward the anterior vaginal wall when retroverted, does not have a chance to bathe in the seminal pool left in the posterior vaginal fornix after intercourse in the supine position. Rarely, one may attribute habitual abortion or miscarriage to the retroverted position of the uterus, but there are many other more fundamental causes that are better explanations of repeated abortion.

BACKACHE.   It is a common habit for women to place the blame for all pelvic pain on the uterus. In most instances the retroverted uterus, when not associated with other pelvic disease, is rarely the cause of backache. Low back pain is far more likely to be due to a faulty posture while sitting or standing. If the patient is overworked or in poor general health, pain in the back may be aggravated by retroversion, but the underlying difficulty is not the position of the uterus. In most instances the activating cause is commonly found in the bony skeleton or its muscular supports. Scoliosis, lordosis, abnormalities of the bony spine, protruding intervertebral disks, myositis or nerve root pressures all are better explanations of backache than a backward displacement of the uterus, and these must be ruled out before treating the retroversion per se. To this end a board under the mattress or a supporting corset may give symptomatic relief. One is justified in treating the patient for backache, but not in attributing its cause to uterine retroversion.

THE CHRONIC PELVIC PASSIVE CONGESTION SYNDROME.   It is not uncommon to find at operation that the pelvic veins are enlarged, tortuous and engorged in the presence of a congested uterus in the retroverted position. Along with these findings the ovaries are frequently prolapsed and enlarged and appear to contain many small follicular cysts. It has been said that this condition, if allowed to continue uncorrected, may lead to permanent uterine and adnexal fibrosis.

This syndrome is frequently accompanied by a low bearing-down backache secondary to pelvic congestion and traction on the nerve trunks, which have been compressed by the fibrosis within the broad ligaments. Along with this, one finds an abnormal menstrual bleeding pattern and other evidences of hormonal imbalance. Headache, increased irritability, abdominal distention, breast engorgement and disturbance in bowel habit—in fact all the symptoms that are classified under the general term of premenstrual tension—appear in the patient who has had a long-standing uterine retroversion associated with congestion.

SYMPTOMS THAT ACCOMPANY A UTERUS FIXED IN RETROVERSION.   Most symptoms commonly attributed to retroversion are actually due to the associated condition that maintains the uterus in this position. The common symptoms are low pelvic pain and backache, dyspareunia, dysmenorrhea, and abnormalities in the menstrual bleeding pattern.

For example, the patient may have a sense of dull, dragging pain in the lower part of the abdomen and back. Usually the patient relieves this sort of pain by resting and getting off her feet. The pain may be worse during menstruation because of the pelvic congestion or perhaps the obstruction to the passage of the menstrual debris due to the retroverted uterine position. Rarely does she wake up in the morning with the pain if the uterus is simply retroverted and not fixed there by other disease.

If the uterus is fixed, however, the backache may be severe throughout the month and worse at the time of the menstrual period. Rest and the prone position do not provide the same measure of relief that is obtained when the uterus is simply retroverted.

Abnormalities in the bleeding pattern and pain accompanying the menstrual flow are usually due to pelvic congestion or incomplete involution of the uterus secondary to childbirth. They are not part of the picture of uncomplicated uterine retroversion.

The dyspareunia that is attributed to the abnormal uterine position is frequently actually due to endometriotic implants on the pelvic floor or the stretching of pelvic adhesions that bind the uterus in a backward position.

How Is the Diagnosis Made and the Extent of Fixation Determined?

The diagnosis is made by bimanual vaginal or rectal examination. By vagina one is immediately impressed with the finding that the cervix is pushed upward toward the bladder. No uterine fundus can be felt anteriorly, and the entire uterus seems to descend into the vaginal canal farther than one would expect. Posteriorly, the fundus of the uterus can be felt in the cul-de-sac. The actual outline and contour of the uterus can best be felt on rectal examination.

Usually there is no question that the smooth, rounded mass felt posteriorly is the actual uterine fundus, but occasionally the differential diagnosis between a retroversion, fibroid or ovarian tumor must be made. It is important to try to delineate the connection of this posterior mass with the uterine cervix. If the cervix is long, and it frequently is when any degree of associated prolapse is present, the fundus of a sharply retroflexed uterus may be thought to be a fibroid. This error in evaluation is common.

In order to estimate the degree of fixation an attempt should be made to replace the uterus in normal position. This is best done with the examining finger in the rectum. If the uterus can be displaced easily, one may assume that it is not fixed in retroversion by adhesions, although on rare occasions uterine mobility is possible despite the adhesions. If the uterus cannot be displaced, it is reasonable to suspect that it is being held backward by some form of other pelvic abnormality. When nodules are felt on the pelvic floor, endometriosis is usually the cause of a fixed retroversion. Sometimes the patient's pelvis is so tender, and she has so much pain when attempts are made to replace the uterus, that a true evaluation of the extent of fixation can be made only under anesthesia.

Treatment of Posterior Uterine Displacements

When the patient is either young or past the climacteric, a retroverted uterus that produces no symptoms and has no complicating disease should be left alone. In the older woman one must also, however, evaluate the degree of uterine prolapse, because the two conditions do go together in this age group.

In the absence of other disease there are two indications for the correction of a persistent uterine retroversion. Both have a relation to pregnancy: (1) After pregnancy and for a few postpartum weeks or months the uterus tends to remain in retroversion. One then may choose to restore the uterus to its normal position until involution is fully completed and the uterus spontaneously assumes the anterior position. (2) The patient has been thoroughly investigated for sterility, and no other cause in either wife or husband has been found except the retroversion. The correction of retroversion may be made as noted above, or one of the suspension operations may be indicated.

Before deciding whether a pessary insertion or operation is indicated, one should clearly understand the advantages and limitations of the supporting pessary. At best a pessary is a temporary expedient and will never cure the nonpregnant patient. Furthermore, to be effective it must accomplish the aim of maintaining the uterus in its normal position. If it is unsuccessful in accomplishing this, use of a pessary should be discontinued. For the same reason a pessary should not be used in acute retroflexion of the uterus, because it cannot hope to restore the uterus to a normal position or to keep it there.

The chief value of the pessary will appear in the following conditions: (1) Older women may have a uterine prolapse as well as a retroversion and are unsuitable candidates for surgical correction. In such cases the patient should return at regular intervals to have the pessary changed and the vagina inspected. If there is any indication of vaginal irritation, the use of the pessary should be discontinued for a few weeks. (2) The patient does have an uncomplicated retroversion with symptoms which may or may not be due to the malposition of the uterus. In this instance the gynecologist may try to replace and hold the uterus with a pessary to see whether the change in position has any effect upon the symptoms. (3) The postpartum patient has an incompletely involuted uterus that tends to persist in the retroverted position.

Replacement of the uterus and its maintenance in the anteverted position for three to four months may result in a permanent cure of the retroversion.

When used in its proper place, a pessary adequately fitted to maintain the uterus in normal position should cause the patient no discomfort and in no way interfere with her activities, including sexual intercourse.

WHAT IS THE TECHNIQUE FOR REPLACING THE UTERUS IN POSITION? In most instances the retroverted uterus uncomplicated by other pelvic lesions can be replaced in a normal position without recourse to anesthesia. Bimanual examination with the patient in the lithotomy position is usually satisfactory, though some gynecologists prefer the Sims and others the knee-chest position. In a simple case pressure is applied in an upward direction by the index and middle fingers of the left hand against the posterior vaginal vault. Once the uterus has been dislodged from its posterior position and raised in the direction of the pelvic brim, the right hand of the operator placed just above the symphysis can gently manipulate the posterior wall of the uterus and direct it forward toward the symphysis. The fingers of the left hand aid in this maneuver by pushing the cervix upward and backward. If difficulty is encountered, the procedure is made easier when a tenaculum is applied to the cervix and it is pushed upward and backward, while the abdominal hand directs the fundus forward.

When the patient is obese, the manipulations with the abdominal hand may be less than satisfactory. If the cervix and vagina harbor no obvious infection, a probe or sound may be introduced into the uterine cavity, after first painting the cervix with iodine and swabbing the endocervical canal. By the combined use of the tenaculum on the cervix and the probe in the uterine cavity, which acts as a lever, it is frequently possible to elevate the uterus gently into a normal position.

PROLAPSE OF THE UTERUS

Although the less serious forms of prolapse, such as the cystocele and rectocele, may on rare occasion occur as individual entities, they are most commonly associated with some degree of uterine descent. The underlying cause is similar to that which permits the formation of a cystocele and rectocele. Obstetrical trauma is the main etiologic factor, with resultant damage to the levator ani muscles and stretching of the accompanying fascial ligaments that go to make up the pelvic floor. Since many women have many babies or traumatic deliveries without exhibiting any signs of prolapse, one must assume that there is some weakness inherent in the supporting connective tissue structures of those that do. As further evidence of this, extreme degrees of prolapse are sometimes seen in nulliparous women. Furthermore, the signs and symptoms usually develop slowly with age as both muscles and fascia tend to atrophy.

There are three types of uterine prolapse: (1) Prolapse of the first degree is said to be present when the uterus descends into the vaginal canal from its normal position high at the apex. It has not yet descended or protruded through the introitus. It is not uncommon for the patient to have an element of uterine retroversion as well. This tends to prevent the uterus from descending further. (2) In second-degree prolapse the cervix appears outside the vaginal orifice, either in part or in total. The cervix elongates at the expense of the fundus, but both descend. The fundus is displaced backward into the axis of the canal in a position to encourage further descent. (3) Prolapse of the third degree calls for a complete descent of the entire uterus with

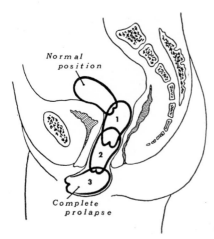

Fig. 64-3.   Diagrammatic representation of first- and second-degree prolapses and procidentia of the uterus.

inversion of the entire vaginal canal. Both have now dropped out of the vagina entirely. This condition has been called a "complete prolapse" or procidentia. These are synonymous with prolapse of the third degree (Fig. 64–3).

In the first degree of prolapse there is minimal prolapse of the vagina. This increases in the second-degree prolapse as the fundus falls back into the axis of the vagina. It is intensified when the uterine prolapse is complete. Yet it is not the downward traction exerted by the descending uterus that brings about the inversion of the vaginal canal. Actually, it is the descent or inversion of the anterior vaginal wall that pulls the uterus down out of the vagina. To test this observation one should replace the procidentia and ask the patient to strain. The first thing that appears is the lower part of the vaginal wall, followed by the upper portion along with the cervix. As a final stage the posterior vaginal wall, which is not attached to the anterior rectal wall—as is true in a rectocele—descends, beginning from above downward.

The covering of the hernia is made up of the anterior and posterior vaginal walls. Within the abdomen the pouches formed by the anterior and posterior reflections of the uterus are drawn into the sac and disappear from the abdomen. The base, or at times all, of the bladder is included in the contents of the hernial sac. The rectum on the other hand, does not appear, since the posterior vaginal wall is completely separated from it. Since there is no longer any cul-de-sac, either anterior or posterior, small intestine and omentum may also be present in the sac.

What Symptoms Are Produced by a Prolapse of the Uterus?

The symptoms that arise from relaxation of the supporting structures of the uterus are slow in developing, and in most instances the patient does not seek medical help until she is well past forty. With lessening in sex hormonal activity and increasing age the vitality of the pelvic tissues deteriorates to a greater or less degree. Disability begins to appear years after obstetrical trauma. The patient becomes increasingly aware of the bearing-down discomfort and the size of the vaginal mass. Less often the patient notes a sudden appearance of the uterus outside the vagina upon exertion.

The patient usually consults the physician because she feels a *lack of pelvic support* and senses that the womb is *dropping out*. When the prolapse is extreme, she knows it is, because she may have to push the uterus back in order to void. The patient with procidentia often complains of discomfort on walking or sitting. It is not surprising that the patient has urinary difficulty. There are two main reasons for this: (1) The abnormal position of the bladder makes complete urine elimination difficult. Residual urine stagnates and easily becomes infected. The patient is therefore prone to have cystitis.

It is interesting that patients with uterine prolapse, even of third degree, do not have urinary incontinence. When the patient has a prolapse of any magnitude, the bladder descends and the urethra runs upward from the bladder to the meatus. A sharp degree of angulation occurs at the point where the urethra enters the bladder. This increases when the patient strains in the act of micturition, and a mechanical obstruction is produced that cuts off the urinary flow. (2) Because of the descent of the bladder the ureters are also pulled downward. This tends to produce ureteral kinking and partial obstruction. The combination of infection within the bladder and ureteral obstruction predisposes the patient to recurring bouts of upper urinary tract infection.

What Are the Characteristic Physical Findings in Uterine Prolapse?

Occasionally the patient with a first-degree prolapse will complain of bearing-down discomfort and a sense of loss in pelvic support. When she is examined in the lithotomy position, the uterus resumes its normal position, and the prolapse may not be apparent. The patient should be asked to strain down while the examiner's finger is in the vagina. This may recreate the prolapse. If it does not, traction should be applied to the cervix with a tenaculum. Should this fail to demonstrate any prolapse, the patient must be examined while standing up.

When procidentia has been present for any length of time, extensive changes take place in the vaginal epithelium, because of its exposed position. The epithelial

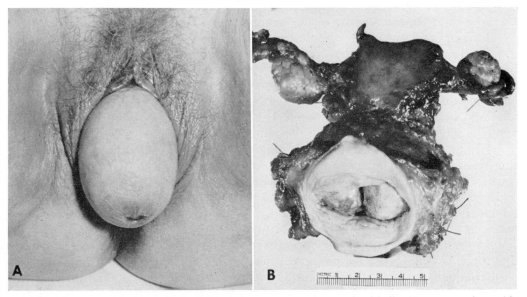

Fig. 64-4. *A,* In procidentia a large amount of everted vaginal epithelium may protrude outside the body. The cervical os is visible in the most dependent portion, where it is subject to frictional trauma and ulceration. *B,* Cervical hypertrophy may imitate uterine prolapse. In this specimen the cervical enlargement was due to a primary carcinoma.

surface is dry and smooth. The usual transverse folds are lacking (Fig. 64–4, *A*). The anterior vaginal wall thickens and frequently becomes edematous. With the cervix outside the vagina chronic ulcerations are common because of pressure, necrosis and constant irritation. Occasionally these ulcerations bleed. It is interesting that, despite the fact that the cervix is constantly subject to frictional trauma when a patient has procidentia, cancer of the cervix is rarely found. A chronic cervical ulcer can produce pelvic cellulitis. Before a vaginal hysterectomy is performed every attempt should be made, through local treatment and chemotherapy, to sterilize the ulcer and to minimize the chance of pelvic infection in the postoperative period.

So far as possible the examiner should try to evaluate the contents of the perineal hernia. This can be done by grasping the procidentia in the hand with the thumb on the anterior vaginal wall. One can then outline the entire uterus and determine whether or not there are any enlargements of the adnexa. This is an important part of the examination for two reasons: (1) Sometimes an elongated cervix may simulate the physical finding of uterine procidentia. In this case the fundus has not actually descended from its normal position, but the cervix has simply hypertrophied (Fig. 64–4, *B*). (2) With too much concentration on the obvious procidentia, the associated lesions may well be missed. Failure to recognize them may cause complications when the vaginal repair is performed.

What Forms of Treatment Are Available for the Various Degrees of Uterine Prolapse?

The symptoms of procidentia, like those of cystocele, are often due to urinary tract complications. It is important, therefore, to catheterize the patient after she has voided, to determine the amount of residual urine and whether or not it is infected. Since there may be an element of ureteral obstruction in the presence of a true procidentia, intravenous pyelograms should be taken.

The choice of therapy will depend on the *age* of the patient, parity or the desire for more children, the severity of the symptoms and the extent of the prolapse.

EXPECTANT THERAPY.   Unless she has severe symptoms or there is associated disease, the patient with a first- or moderate second-degree uterine prolapse should be left alone. Since there is a tendency for the prolapse to become more pronounced, the patient should be examined thereafter at yearly intervals. There is little point in operating on a girl who has only a moderate degree of prolapse with minimal symptoms and wants to have more children. It is better to try and tide her over until the family is complete or the symptoms become more disabling.

USE OF PESSARY.   This can be done by inserting a supporting pessary of the ring type. It does not interfere with the performance of normal function, and intercourse can be carried out satisfactorily. The pessary must be removed, cleansed and replaced at monthly intervals. Though a regimen of this sort is a nuisance, it is preferable to repairing the prolapse, only to have it torn down by a subsequent pregnancy.

In prescribing a pessary for vaginal support the gynecologist should remember that it will not cure a uterine prolapse, since the damage to the supporting structures has been done, but it will, at least for a time, prevent it from becoming worse. It will not improve the situation if the perineal body is damaged so badly that the vagina has lost its power to retain the pessary. Any strain such as coughing or the act of defecation will then expel the pessary.

When the prolapse is well established, the pessary is used chiefly for (*a*) the combination of circumstances mentioned above; (*b*) patients who, because of advanced age or constitutional disease, cannot withstand the rigors of surgery.

When one considers age to be the only contraindication to surgical repair, the decision should be made with care. The patient may be able to withstand surgery better than she or her family think. There is a tendency to avoid operations in older women and to rely on the use of a pessary. The older patient with more relaxed tissues and a greater degree of herniation requires a pessary of the doughnut or Gellhorn type. This, too, must be cleansed and replaced at regular intervals. If cleanliness is not observed, vaginal irritation, or even ulceration, will occur. When this happens, the patient cannot tolerate the further use of a pessary.

Unfortunately, the initial success in the use of a pessary is not always maintained. There is always a group of women in every gynecologist's practice who come to surgery when, after years of wearing it, the pessary no longer provides sufficient support. If the older patient has no medical contraindications, she should be offered surgery, provided the degree of uterine prolapse and the severity of the symptoms warrant.

SURGERY.   The choice of the surgical procedure to correct a prolapse likewise depends on the age, the severity of the symptoms and the extent of the pelvic relaxation. The young woman in the childbearing age who wants more children should not be treated with the same operation that one would use in a menopausal woman with the same degree of prolapse.

When the young woman has so much prolapse that she is miserable and cannot be relieved by a supporting pessary, she should be operated upon, but if at all possible the menstrual and childbearing functions should be preserved. This can be accomplished by one of two operative procedures: (1) If the uterine prolapse is not extensive, but is enough to require surgical treatment, the cystocele and rectocele should be repaired and the uterus suspended by the Olshausen method, in which the round ligaments are simply approximated to the anterior abdominal wall. This combination permits a subsequent delivery without reproducing the pelvic relaxation. A cesarean section will not be required. (2) With a more extensive prolapse the Manchester operation of Donald and Fothergill will also correct the prolapse and still allow a pregnancy to occur. In this operation the bladder is freed from the cervix, the cervix amputated at the level of the internal os, the cardinal ligaments are approximated in front of the amputated cervix, and the cystocele and rectocele are repaired. Enthusiasts who champion this operation claim that a normal delivery can be carried out without incident. Since the cervix has been amputated, there will be less risk of obstetrical complications and disruption of the previous repair if the patient with any subsequent pregnancy is delivered by cesarean section.

The operation of choice in the patient who has completed her family or is in the menopause should be a vaginal hysterectomy combined with repair of the pelvic floor, cystocele and rectocele. It should be done whether she has symptoms or not, since if she has considerable uterine prolapse now, it can only get worse as the pelvic tissues lose more of their vitality. This operation will suffice for even the most extreme degree of prolapse, such as a procidentia. On rare occasions there may be reason to question the strength of the tissues used in the pelvic repair. In this case some form of vaginal obliteration, such as the LeFort or Williams vaginal occlusion procedures, should be done.

PROLAPSE OF THE VAGINAL VAULT

What Does One Do about Prolapse of the Vaginal Vault after Hysterectomy?

The vaginal vault or apex may prolapse after either a total vaginal or a supra-cervical hysterectomy. Fortunately it is rather a rare complication, for it makes for many problems in the correction. The explanation of the mechanisms involved in its development is not altogether clear. Inadequacy of the tissues used in the repair, or perhaps actual sloughing of the tissue, is the probable cause.

There are varying degrees of prolapse. It may be so slight that the patient is scarcely aware of it at all. The apex may descend into the vaginal canal and lie there as a bulging mass. The patient then complains of fullness in the vagina and bearing-down discomfort. If the vagina becomes totally inverted, the protruding mass can interfere with the patient's ability to walk or sit comfortably.

Before deciding on the best method for correcting the prolapse, the surgeon should be sure that he is dealing with a vaginal vault prolapse and not an enterocele. This is especially true if the prolapse follows a previous vaginal hysterectomy. Too frequently the enterocele is not recognized at the time of the first operation.

The problem is not particularly difficult if a cervical stump is present. If the presenting mass is an enterocele, it will be found in the usual position, and the mass protruding into the posterior vaginal wall is seen behind it. If there is any doubt about the position of the cervix, it should be checked by exerting traction on it with a tenaculum.

The differential diagnosis becomes more complicated when the uterus has been totally removed, by either the abdominal or vaginal route. The landmark that will help most in distinguishing between an enterocele and a vaginal vault prolapse is the location of the scar that should be present high up in the vagina. If the scar is in the expected position, the bulging mass is an enterocele. There is no question that the vaginal vault has descended if the operative scar is found well down the canal or outside the vaginal orifice.

What Are the Problems in Repair of a Vaginal Prolapse?

The main problem in the correction of vaginal vault prolapse is the preservation of an unobstructed vaginal canal. Total hysterectomy or supracervical hysterectomy may be done for a wide spectrum of pathologic entities early in the patient's reproductive life. It is important that any operative procedure should not occlude or fore-shorten the vagina. There may be a cystocele or rectocele present which was not obvious at the time of the original operation. Vaginal hysterectomy may have been done for a fibroid tumor as well as for pelvic floor relaxation. A cystocele or rectocele is less likely to be found, but an enterocele may well have been missed.

When vaginal vault prolapse occurs in a woman past the menopause, the problem is less acute, but still important. In most instances it can be corrected satisfactorily by vaginal plastic procedures, although some foreshortening of the canal may be expected. If both enterocele and prolapse are present, they can be corrected at the same time. If the prolapse is complete and the patient no longer has any interest in sexual activity, the vagina should be obliterated. For the patient who is a poor operative risk, or if the older patient refuses operation, a pessary may suffice, provided there is a good perineal body.

The surgeon has a problem in the younger woman who has a vaginal prolapse. If the prolapse is not extensive and not too troublesome, it may be wise to do nothing. When the prolapse is complete or the symptoms are severe, some form of operative procedure is indicated. The choice of the proper operation should be made with great care. A combined abdominal and vaginal operation may be indicated if there is also a cystocele or rectocele present, after a total hysterectomy for pelvic disease unassociated with damage to the levator ani muscles or their fascia. If the prolapse follows a vaginal hysterectomy, another procedure performed from below is not indicated unless the patient has an associated enterocele. In this case a direct abdominal surgical approach should be tried.

Some means of supporting the sagging vaginal canal must be found. It may be possible to use the round ligaments, suturing them to the back wall and sides of the vagina, provided they appear to have enough resilience to rely upon them for support. The uterosacral ligaments should be shortened, so that their backward pull will keep the upper part of the vagina open. If the round ligaments appear to be inadequate, strips of rectus abdominus fascia may be freed up and led retroperitoneally through the same path taken by the broad ligaments to reach the top of the vagina. There they are attached to the lateral and posterior walls of the vagina.

If an enterocele is present, it may be cured by obliterating the posterior cul-de-sac with a series of puckering purse-string sutures.

REFERENCES

Bailey, K. V.: A Clinical Investigation into Uterine Prolapse with Stress Incontinence. Treatment by Modified Manchester Colporrhaphy. *J. Obst. & Gynaec. Brit. Emp.*, 63: 663, 1956.

Ball, T. L.: Discussion of E. G. Waters: Culdoplastic Techniques for Prevention and Correction of Vaginal Vault Prolapse and Enterocele. *Am. J. Obst. & Gynec.*, 81: 296, 1961.

Bayan, F. B.: Increased Incidence of Prolapse of the Uterus as a Probable Effect of War. *Philippine J. Surg.*, 2: 201, 1947.

Bickel, D. A.: Prolapse of the Vagina Following Abdominal Hysterectomy. *Am. J. Obst. & Gynec.*, 56: 152, 1948.

Burch, J. C.: Urethrovaginal Fixation to Cooper's Ligament for Correction of Stress Incontinence, Cystocele, and Prolapse. *Am. J. Obst. & Gynec.*, 81: 281, 1961.

Colmer, W. M., Jr.: Use of the Pessary. *Am. J. Obst. & Gynec.*, 65: 170, 1953.

Curtis, A. H., Anson, B. J., and McVay, C. B.: The Anatomy of the Pelvic and Urogenital Diaphragms, in Relation to Urethrocele and Cystocele. *Surg., Gynec. & Obst.*, 68: 161, 1939.

Falk, H. C., and Bunkin, I. A.: A Study of 500 Vaginal Hysterectomies. *Am. J. Obst. & Gynec.*, 52: 623, 1946.

Goff, B. H.: The Surgical Anatomy of Cystocele and Urethrocele, with Special Reference to the Pubocervical Fascia. *Surg., Gynec. & Obst.*, 87: 725, 1948.

McElin, T. W., and Paalman, R. J.: Pessary Complications in the Management of Uterine Prolapse. *Am. J. Obst. & Gynec.*, 78: 643, 1959.

Symmonds, R. E., and Pratt, J. H.: Vaginal Prolapse Following Hysterectomy. *Am. J. Obst. & Gynec.*, 79: 899, 1960.

Williams, J. T.: Vaginal Hysterectomy and Colpectomy for Prolapse of the Uterus and Bladder. *Am. J. Obst. & Gynec.*, 59: 365, 1950.

Chapter 65

Incontinence of Urine

THE INABILITY of a patient to prevent the escape of urine has been called urinary incontinence. There are a number of different types and degrees of urinary leakage, as well as a wide variety of causes.

What Are the Types and Degrees of Urinary Incontinence?

Whatever the cause, incontinence of urine is an unpleasant situation for the patient who has it. It may be *very slight* and occur intermittently, but if the patient cannot count on her ability to control her bladder function voluntarily, she may experience an unexpected loss that can be embarrassing. The incontinence may be considered *moderate* when it is not enough to require wearing a protective pad, but enough to soil the patient's underclothing constantly and to keep her moist or wet most of every day. It becomes *severe* when multiple pads or rubber pants are required at all times. The patient who has such extensive uncontrollable urinary loss gradually gets to be so unnerved by her condition that she becomes asocial and retires into herself.

If the urinary loss is *complete* and the leakage constant, there is usually a major defect in bladder, urethra or ureters, which generally takes the form of a fistula. Partial or intermittent loss of urinary control is in most instances due to stress incontinence. For a variety of reasons the shut-off mechanism is defective, and urine escapes as the intravesical pressure rises. The patient at times may simply be unable to avoid urinating when she has a sudden urge to empty a full bladder. This is called "urgency incontinence." Obviously, many of the factors that are concerned with stress incontinence are also present in urgency incontinence. Thus a sudden increase in intravesical pressure, such as laughing or sneezing in a patient with a full bladder, may result in urinary leakage. The difference between stress and urgency incontinence would seem to have academic interest only, but the differential diagnosis is really of great practical importance. Correction of stress incontinence may prove to be difficult, as demonstrated by the wide variety of operations designed to correct the deficiency. The implications of urgency incontinence are far less severe. Some women void infrequently from force of habit. A full bladder may then be entirely normal for them. If incontinence subsequently develops, cure may be achieved simply by correcting a life-long habit.

A variety of nerve lesions increases the tone of the bladder musculature, thereby

1034

increasing the intravesical pressure, so that the patient simply dribbles urine. This has been called "overflow incontinence."

What Factors Contribute to Urinary Incontinence?

By and large, urinary incontinence is a problem encountered in the older woman who has experienced obstetrical trauma with damage to the muscular support of the bladder base. Symptoms are accentuated as estrin production by the ovary declines upon the onset of the menopause. The two factors combine to set up a problem and concentrate numbers of patients in this age group. Far less often incontinence is encountered in the nulliparous woman. It may then be due to spinal cord defects, some of them anatomical such as spina bifida or cord injury, others due to neurologic diseases such as diabetic neuropathy, multiple sclerosis, tabes dorsalis, or brain or spinal cord tumors.

A number of other causes contribute to incontinence. We have noted that a complete loss of urinary control is usually due to fistula formation. It may arise as a result of operative or obstetrical trauma or be secondary to extensive pelvic infection, cancer spread or radiation therapy. In the young child complete urinary incontinence is usually due to such congenital defects as absence of the urethra or ectopically placed ureters that open not into the bladder, but into the uterus or vagina.

Anything that will (*a*) increase intra-abdominal pressure generally, such as laughing, coughing, sneezing or lifting, or (*b*) produce local pressure on the bladder such as pregnancy, large cervical or broad ligament fibroids, ovarian tumors or inflammatory masses can be a causative agent in defeating the patient's attempts to control retention of the urine. Atrophy of the bladder, urethral or vaginal epithelium also may contribute to the spontaneous leakage of urine from a full bladder. This is a common complaint in women of menopausal age, when estrin lack becomes increasingly apparent.

Low-grade infections of the urethra and bladder frequently accompany the epithelial changes. Thus we have *trigonitis* and *urethritis*, both of which provide a constant irritation and make it difficult to control the flow of urine completely. Severe endocervicitis produces the same train of events. It is not surprising that many older women are plagued intermittently by minimal degrees of urine leakage that do no more than soil her underclothes. Older women are also prone to evacuate the bladder incompletely and to carry a residual urine constantly. Any sudden increase in bladder filling then may cause the patient to dribble in small quantities. This may be the explanation for the overflow type of incontinence, but one should always be suspicious of the presence of a neurologic lesion, particularly tabes dorsalis.

Functional urinary disturbances without anatomic or neurologic cause may at times be the explanation of incontinence. Hyperactivity of the bladder with incontinence can occur in disturbed mental or emotional states. This is particularly true in conditions that induce anxiety or anger. The mechanism is probably that of increasing the intravesical pressure. The same factors have been noted in patients with schizophrenia.

The Physiology of Micturition

The various types of incontinence could be explained more adequately if the physiology of micturition were more clearly understood. We know that the bladder acts automatically to discharge its urine content, but at the same time it is under voluntary nervous control. Under normal conditions the bladder distends as it fills with urine. This may or may not be associated with an increase in the intravesical pressure. If the bladder capacity is limited by some disease such as interstitial fibrosis, the intravesical pressure may rise abruptly. The capacity and frequency of urination are also influenced by a variety of factors, some of them infectious or otherwise pathological, others in the realm of the psychosomatic.

The initial response to urine distention manifests itself by wavelike contractions of the bladder musculature, of varying degrees of frequency and intensity. This is interpreted by the patient as a desire to void and usually begins when the volume of urine fills but half the total capacity of the bladder.

It is generally believed that contraction of the bladder musculature, along with a simultaneous shortening of the muscles in the trigone where the ureters open into the bladder, brings about a depression of the base of the bladder and forces the orifice of the internal sphincter (the so-called involuntary sphincter) to open. The external sphincter (compressor urethrae muscle) relaxes only when the internal sphincter has already opened. The actual expulsion of urine is the result of the combined action of bladder, abdominal wall and levator ani muscles (pubococcygeus and ileococcygeus muscles). The conscious act of micturition depends then on proper function of the muscles that go to make up the pelvic floor. If the patient desires not to void, the external sphincter, which can be closed, but not opened, at will, and the perineal muscles contract. The action raises the bladder neck, closes the internal sphincter and thus prevents the escape of urine.

It is obvious that in a dysfunction of the bladder, such as incontinence, there must be some disruption of the anatomic arrangement of the muscles of the bladder base or urethra, or some alteration in the reciprocal action of the sphincter mechanism. The problem may be entirely mechanical or the result of faulty innervation of the sphincter, acting through the parasympathetic and sympathetic nerve chains. Unfortunately, the actual function of the sphincter mechanisms has not been worked out completely.

STRESS INCONTINENCE

The most common type of involuntary loss of urinary control appears in so-called stress incontinence. This usually occurs after a rise in the intravesical pressure brought on by the act of laughing, coughing or sneezing. Anything that will increase intra-abdominal pressure, such as heavy lifting, will also result in stress incontinence. In most instances there has been a past history of obstetrical trauma to the supporting structures of the bladder neck and urethra. Incontinence may appear directly after delivery and correct itself for a period of years, only to prove troublesome again in the years approaching the menopause and beyond. The amount of urine lost and the degree of disability are in direct relation to the amount of damage done in the region of the bladder neck and proximal urethra. The incapacity becomes progressively more severe as the patient grows older.

As a direct result of the old injury the pelvic support to the bladder neck is diminished. The urethra moves downward and backward away from its usual position under the pubis. Because of the damage to the tissues that normally support the urethra, the walls relax and permit the internal sphincter to open. The upper portion of the urethra then simply becomes an extension of the bladder itself. Thus one might expect to find the observations that appear characteristically in x-ray studies of the urethrovesical area in patients who have incontinence: namely, (*a*) descent of the bladder, funneling of the bladder neck and a loss of the normal posterior urethrovesical angle when the patient is in the upright position. Along with the alteration in anatomic arrangement there also appears to be (*b*) an element of damage to the delicate sphincter mechanism (Fig. 65–1).

It has been suggested that distortion of the upper urethra occurs as a result of scar tissue that fixes the urethra to the pubic rami. For this reason the urethral sphincter muscles, which normally assume a circular pattern, lose this because of scar tissue fixation to the pubic rami. The sphincter becomes elliptical as it contracts. This kind of closure is inadequate to control the escape of urine. Whatever the cause, the internal bladder sphincter is almost invariably relaxed and incompetent. Since the proximal urethra now becomes the lower portion of the bladder cavity, the urethral canal shortens from a normal length of 4 cm. to approximately 2 cm. There appears to be some disagreement as to the part played by the external sphincter in the voluntary control of urination. Many investigators feel that the pubococcygeus, bulbocavernosus and deep transverse perineal muscles have an entirely secondary role, but others are equally certain that they are a part of the external sphincter mechanism involved in controlling urinary loss.

All who have had experience with the radical removal of the vulva for carcinoma are aware of the fact that the extent of the tumor is occasionally widespread enough to demand the removal of all but 1 to 1.5 cm. of the distal urethra. With careful suturing of the bladder neck these patients are continent of urine. It is difficult to see how urinary control can be ascribed to the external sphincter alone.

It is interesting to contrast the obstetrical trauma which results in the formation of a cystocele with that involved in stress incontinence. The location of the traumatic

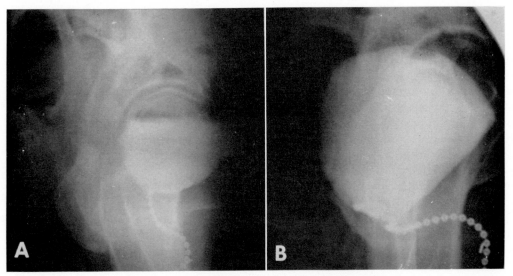

Fig. 65-1. With radiopaque beads in a urethral catheter and contrast medium in the bladder, it is possible to analyze the causes of incontinence by an x-ray urethrocystogram. *A*, In the standing position the urethra is in an abnormally straight and vertical position. This predisposes to stress incontinence. *B*, The urethrovesical angle is preserved, and any incontinence would more likely involve sphincter dysfunction. (Courtesy of Dr. T. H. Green, Jr.)

effect in stress incontinence is anterior, in the region of the supporting structures of the bladder neck and urethra, while that of the simple cystocele is much more posterior along the bladder base. *The posterior urethrovesical angle, therefore, may not be disturbed in the presence of a cystocele.*

A well known clinical observation is that, although some degree of bladder descent is present in patients who have stress incontinence, symptoms to indicate its presence are rarely noted when the bladder prolapses outside the introitus (procidentia). This is also true of patients who have a large cystocele. By virtue of its position in procidentia, a sharp angulation occurs posteriorly between the base of the bladder and the urethra that prevents the unexpected loss of urine. Replacement of the uterus in a proper position will bring out the fact that sometimes symptoms of stress incontinence are being masked by extreme descent of the uterus, because with the uterus in the new position the patient becomes incontinent. This becomes a practical matter when a vaginal hysterectomy is contemplated. Symptoms of stress incontinence may appear in the postoperative period if the true condition is not recognized and corrected at the time of the hysterectomy.

How Is the Differential Diagnosis of Stress Incontinence Established?

Since there is a wide variety of causes, such as anatomic alterations in the support of the bladder neck and urethra, relaxation and fibrous fixation of the internal sphincter, prolapse of the uterus and bladder, funneling of the bladder neck, loss of the posterior urethrovesical angle and perhaps some deficiency in the external sphincter, it is important (*a*) to pinpoint the most likely cause in a given patient and (*b*) to establish the fact that she has stress incontinence.

As noted in the general discussion of incontinence there are many causes of stress incontinence. Stress incontinence secondary to loss of muscle support of the bladder neck and urethra must be separated from (*a*) "urgency" or a false incontinence caused by urethritis, trigonitis or cystitis. One should look for the common types of infection that produce these pathologic changes, such as senile vaginitis, moniliasis, *Trichomonas vaginalis* infection and endocervicitis. (*b*) Diseases of the nervous system, such as multiple sclerosis, diabetic neuropathy, tabes dorsalis and central nervous system tumor; (*c*) fistula formation, due to congenital causes such as absence of the urethra, ectopic ureter, fistulas acquired because of surgical complications, or as the aftermath of pelvic infections or malignant diseases; (*d*) lesions of the bladder or urethra itself, such as calculi, urethral diverticula, infection or tumors; (*e*) pelvic tumors, such as pregnancy, ovarian cysts, inflammatory masses or fibroids (Fig. 65–2). The diagnostic workup must be complete to exclude the various uninvolved possibilities that could provide the etiology. The effort to pinpoint the exact cause will be worth while, because a poorly chosen operation is sure to fail.

A *careful history* will be extremely helpful in suggesting a possible diagnosis of diabetes, tabes dorsalis, multiple sclerosis, ectopic or acquired fistulas, previous pelvic infection, trauma of pregnancy, menopausal change—to name a few of the many possible causes. From the history one finds that at some time, perhaps years after a traumatic delivery, the patient becomes unable to control the urine. The loss is small at first and is considered to be of no great consequence, since many of the older age group have this complaint. Gradually, however, the symptoms become more severe, until finally the patient is constantly wet and miserable because of it. Also evident from the history is that the urinary loss occurs only while the patient is in the upright position, and incontinence is aggravated by such acts as coughing, sneezing, laughing, or lifting heavy objects. For the most part patients who have stress incontinence are dry at night.

PHYSICAL EXAMINATION.   From the examination one can promptly rule out pregnancy, genital tract tumors, or inflammatory masses as causes of stress incontinence. A thorough neurologic examination, combined with suitable x-ray films of the head and pelvis, will exclude most of the nerve lesions, including spina bifida and brain tumor. Any cervicitis, vaginal infection or atrophic epithelial change should be evident on inspection.

There are a few anatomic changes in stress incontinence that are fairly characteristic. Almost invariably there is some element of prolapse of both the bladder and uterus, owing to the lack of muscle support. Varying degrees of cystocele, urethrocele and generalized pelvic floor relaxation are usually present. It should be noted, however, that (a) older multiparae may have a large cystocele without incontinence, and (b) stress incontinence is frequently found in the absence of any urethrocele or cystocele. This is particularly true of older nulliparous patients. Since there is no element of obstetrical trauma, one can only postulate that stress incontinence here is due to malfunction of the pubococcygeus and other muscles of the pelvic diaphragm. It can be due to an inadequate sphincter mechanism. One should always be alert to the possibility that stress incontinence in the nulliparous can have a neurologic basis.

One of the most distinctive findings in patients with stress incontinence is the anatomic position of the urethra. In the normal woman who has had no children the urethral opening beneath the symphysis points straight out, when the patient is in the lithotomy position. In contrast, the urethral meatus of the multiparous woman who has stress incontinence flattens out and tends to be directed toward the ceiling. With it one may find a bulging area either in the posterior wall of the proximal urethra (urethrocele) or in the anterior vaginal wall itself (cystocele).

TEST FOR STRESS INCONTINENCE.   The best method of proving whether the patient has a true urinary incontinence in the presence of a cystocele is to have her strain as she would in the act of voiding. The anterior vaginal wall, particularly in the region of the bladder base, can be seen to bulge outward. If much stress incontinence is present, there will be some evidence of urinary leakage. There is less chance of urinary loss if the patient is in the supine position. The same straining effort should

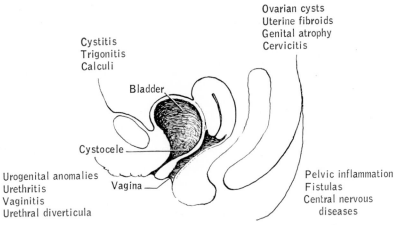

Cystitis
Trigonitis
Calculi

Ovarian cysts
Uterine fibroids
Genital atrophy
Cervicitis

Bladder

Cystocele

Urogenital anomalies
Urethritis
Vaginitis
Urethral diverticula

Vagina

Pelvic inflammation
Fistulas
Central nervous
diseases

Fig. 65-2.   Some pathologic states associated with incontinence.

therefore be made with the patient standing up. Not infrequently the urine can be seen to spurt out from the urethra when the patient exerts voluntary muscle pressure on the bladder. The flow of urine can be stopped abruptly by placing two fingers in the vagina, one on either side of the urethra with the tips at the bladder base. Upward pressure on the bladder neck is applied as the patient forcefully strains. If she has stress incontinence, she is promptly made continent.

Another method of testing for the presence or absence of stress incontinence is to apply Allis clamps on the bladder neck at the site of the bulge in the anterior wall that is produced as the patient strains. When traction is applied to the clamps as the patient bears down, urinary loss occurs, which is immediately stopped when the clamps are pushed upward. This is the so-called vesical neck elevation test.

LABORATORY PROCEDURES. Urinalysis and bacteriologic culture to determine the presence or absence of infection are primary requirements in the diagnostic work-up. It also is important to know whether the patient normally carries a residual urine. She should therefore be catheterized after voiding. Cystoscopy should be done, together with inspection of the urethral canal, to rule out fistula, calculus, tumor formation, trigonitis, cystitis and urethritis. Cystometrograms should be done to determine the extent of bladder capacity and the degree of intravesical pressure required to bring out the urge to evacuate the bladder contents. The most important diagnostic laboratory procedure is the urethrocystogram.

What Do We Learn from the Urethrocystogram? Patients with stress incontinence exhibit permanent changes in urethrovesical relations which closely resemble the temporary alterations that occur in the first stages of voiding in the normally continent woman: (1) loss of the posterior urethrovesical angle; (2) descent and funneling of the bladder neck; (3) a variable degree of backward and downward rotation of the course of the urethra.

Technique of Performing the Test. After the patient has emptied her bladder, exactly 150 cc. of 12 per cent sodium iodide solution, warmed to body temperature, is instilled slowly into the bladder via a glass catheter. The next step calls for the fitting of a metallic beaded chain, 25 cm. in length, into the lumen of a no. 18 rubber urethral catheter that has previously been bisected. The first or most proximal bead extends over the catheter tip. The lubricated catheter, with its chain, is then introduced into the bladder. The chain is disengaged from the catheter by gently pulling down on the chain while the catheter is advanced upward. Lipiodol, 15 cc., is then injected into the bladder through the catheter before removing it entirely, leaving the chain in place. This increases the sharpness of the outline of the vesical neck. Anatomic landmarks are established by (1) placing a metal Michel clip on the external urethral meatus, and (2) laying a thin strip of gauze saturated with Lipiodol from the apex of the vagina to the introitus. This enables an interpretation of the x-ray films, which are now taken, to determine the direction of the vaginal canal (Fig.65–1).

Anterior, posterior and lateral x-ray pictures are then taken in the standing and horizontal positions while (*a*) straining to void and (*b*) resting. The most important and informative view is the lateral view, with the patient straining while in the upright position. This view, combined with the others, will demonstrate (*a*) the loss of the posterior urethrovesical angle, (*b*) the rotational descent of the bladder neck, and (*c*) the change in the inclination of the course of the urethra.

Green finds it helpful to subdivide the patients with stress incontinence into two categories. Type I: In this instance the defect seems to involve only the loss of the posterior urethrovesical angle. Type II: The damage in this case is more pronounced, since in addition to the loss of the posterior angle there is also a downward and backward rotational descent of the urethra and bladder neck, combined with a change in the inclination of the urethra.

Treatment of Stress Incontinence

It would seem to be a simple matter to correct the anatomic derangement of the bladder neck, restore the damaged internal sphincter to its normal circular shape and correct the involuntary loss of urine. One has only to examine the literature and see the number of operations which have been designed to accomplish this simple aim to realize that the problem is much more complex. The reason for this is the simple fact that the results of surgical treatment have, until recently, been far from satisfactory. Medical and nonsurgical methods have a place in therapy for this condition, but only for minor degrees of urinary loss.

SURGICAL REPAIR.   This may be accomplished in a number of different ways. In type I incontinence, in which there is only a loss of the posterior urethrovesical angle, a satisfactory restoration can be accomplished by an extensive dissection that (*a*) mobilizes both the bladder and urethra from their lateral attachments to the pubic rami, and (*b*) advances the bladder upward and away from the uterus. Restorative sutures then approximate the relaxed wall of the bladder in the midline below the bladder neck. If one chooses, one can, in addition, reduce the caliber of the relaxed urethra by a row of infolding sutures. This operation, originally described by Kelly and perfected by Kennedy, will cure a high percentage of patients who have loss of the posterior angle of the bladder alone.

Since there is usually some element of uterine descent as well, the repair is frequently done in association with a vaginal hysterectomy or Fothergill type of operation. Even in type I stress incontinence, one should seriously consider one of the urethral and bladder neck suspension operations, such as the Marshall-Marchetti-Krantz operation, as the sole definitive procedure when there is other pelvic disease present that would call for abdominal surgical intervention.

In type II, in which the urethra is displaced as well, the vaginal procedures are less successful. When faced with this problem or with a recurrence of incontinence after a vaginal repair, one of the urethral-bladder-neck suspension operations should be chosen. A number of such operations are being used at present. The Marshall-Marchetti procedure suspends the tissue in the paraurethral and bladder base area to the under surface of the pubic symphysis. The fascial sling operations, using fascia taken from the abdominal wall or lateral surface of the thigh, elevate the proximal urethra and bladder neck by passing the fascial strip beneath them and attaching it to the fascia of the rectus abdominus muscles on the anterior abdominal wall.

A number of other operations have been devised, but all have attempted to restore the anatomic relation of the bladder neck to the urethra in different ways.

MEDICAL MANAGEMENT.   Medical therapy for stress incontinence is based on the known observations that it is often associated with (*a*) atrophy or dysfunction of the pubococcygeus muscle, (*b*) atrophic vaginitis and cystic urethritis, (*c*) hypotonic muscular action due to a number of neuropathies, (*d*) bladder infections, (*e*) pulmonary disease and obesity. Thus specific therapy can be directed toward specific observations.

Estrin Therapy.   For example, the woman at the menopause or beyond is apt to show evidence of the lack of estrin stimulation. As a result the atrophy in the vaginal, urethral and bladder epithelium is accompanied by low-grade chronic infection that appears in the subepithelial layers. This can be corrected by giving oral estrogen in the dosage normally provided for the postmenopausal woman who has hot flashes. As a result of continued use of estrin, epithelial proliferation is reactivated, and the infection disappears.

Drug Therapy. When cystometrographic studies indicate hypotonic pressures, much can be accomplished by giving Urecholine in dosage ranging from 10 to 40 mg., 4 times daily. This drug is particularly useful for patients who have the overflow type of incontinence.

When the patient has urgency incontinence secondary to bladder irritability, Banthine, 25 to 50 mg., 4 times daily, will often be effective in cutting down on the cause of urgency.

General Medical Therapy. The patient who has weakness of the bladder floor or poor function of the internal vesical sphincter will benefit from a weight reduction diet if she is obese, or from a variety of drugs that are commonly given to suppress a chronic cough, if she has one. In some instances the disability calls for surgery, but the patient is not a sufficiently good operative risk to permit it. In this instance the patient may obtain some relief from the use of supporting pessaries.

Muscle-Setting Exercises. The muscle-setting exercises suggested by Kegel train the pubococcygeus muscles to function more effectively and are useful in overcoming stress incontinence of a slight or moderate degree. The exercises are based on the observation that patients with stress incontinence present evidence of loss of function and occasionally atrophy in the voluntary muscles found about the vesical neck. The weakness manifests itself most often in the pubococcygeus muscles. The exercises are designed to re-educate and strengthen these muscles.

The weakness can be demonstrated when an examining finger is introduced into the vaginal canal and the lateral walls in the upper third are palpated, while the patient attempts to contract the vaginal muscles. The ability to contract the muscles varies in different women. The majority of normal women can do it, but have never thought to try. Muscular atrophy is apparent as shown by the excessive vaginal space noted throughout the circumference, particularly in the upper part of the vagina. The lateral walls are thin, and the vaginal muscles seem to drop away from their attachments to the rami of the pubis. Poor muscle tone is noted on one or both sides.

Since many women have never attempted to contract the vaginal muscles, it is frequently necessary to tell them how to do it. The simplest method of doing this is to tell the patient, while she is lying in the lithotomy position, to tighten the buttock muscles as though she were preventing the involuntary escape of feces from the anal opening. She should then be asked whether she can feel the anus or the urethral opening pull up. The patient who has an extensive degree of stress incontinence usually experiences no such sensation. Any response, however, is a good prognostic sign, since with continuing exercise the magnitude of the contracting ability will increase. A fair estimate of the ability to control these muscles can be obtained by asking the patient to compress the examiner's finger in the vagina. If one cares to measure the degree of contractility, it can be done with a so-called perineometer, which is inserted in the vaginal canal. This is simply a pneumatic resistance chamber with a manometer attached.

When the patient has learned to contract the proper group of muscles, particularly the pubococcygeus, she must carry out the exercises innumerable times a day over a long period of time. All too frequently the patient discontinues the exercises at the first sign of improvement. In simple stress incontinence improvement may be noted as early as six to eight weeks, but in the more severe forms it may take a year or more before any satisfactory degree of control is obtained. There should also be some indication of improving muscular action or hypertrophy. This evidence can be obtained either by palpation or observations made from the manometer of the perineometer.

To obtain the best results the patient should learn to contract the vaginal muscles against the resistance of the perineometer, which completely fills the vaginal canal. This will permit the patient to see whether she is actually accomplishing what she is trying to do and to what degree she is successful.

The muscle-setting exercises provide a practical and effective method of helping the patient to control the involuntary loss of urine. They are most useful in the milder degrees of incontinence and have been particularly helpful in the group of women who have distressing stress incontinence after radical surgery for cervical cancer.

REFERENCES

Aldridge, A. H.: Transplantation of Fascia for Relief of Urinary Stress Incontinence. *Am. J. Obst. & Gynec.*, 44: 398, 1942.

Ball, T. L.: Topographic Urethrography. *Am. J. Obst. & Gynec.*, 59: 1243, 1950.

Bors, E.: Neurogenic Bladder. *Urol. Survey*, 7: 177, 1957.

Brewer, J. I.: *Textbook of Gynecology*. Baltimore, Williams & Wilkins Company, 1953.

Counseller, V. S., and Symmonds, R. E.: Vesicourethral Suspension for Urinary Stress Incontinence. A Study of the Results Obtained in 82 Patients. *Am. J. Obst. & Gynec.*, 75: 525, 1956.

Cullen, P. K., Jr., and Welch, J. S.: Ten Year Results of the Kelly and Kennedy Types of Procedure in Urinary Stress Incontinence. *Surg., Gynec. & Obst.*, 113: 85, 1961.

Davies, J. W.: Urinary Stress Incontinence—Its Relation to Cystocele and Lacerations of the Pelvic Floor. *J. Urol.*, 48: 536, 1942.

Durfee, R. B.: The Anterior Vaginal Suspension Operation. A Report of 110 Cases. *Am. J. Obst. & Gynec.*, 78: 628, 1959.

Dutton, W. A. W.: The Urethrovesical Angle and Stress Incontinence. *Canad. M.A.J.*, 83: 1242, 1960.

Francis, W. J.: The Onset of Stress Incontinence. *J. Obst. & Gynaec. Brit. Emp.*, 67: 899, 1960.

Frost, I. F.: *The Vaginal Approach in the Surgical Treatment of Stress Incontinence, with Special Reference to Certain Factors Necessary to the Cure of This Condition*. Monographs of Surgery. Baltimore, Williams & Wilkins Company, 1952, p. 82.

Gleadell, L. W., and Zacharin, R. F.: Urethral Suspension; A Preliminary Report on a New Approach to the Problem of Stress Incontinence in the Female. *Australian & New Zealand J. Surg.*, 26: 226, 1957.

Green, T. H., Jr.: *Surgery: A Concise Guide to Clinical Practice;* edited by G. L. Nardi and G. D. Zuidema. Boston, Little, Brown & Company, 1961.

Idem: Development of Plan for the Diagnosis and Management of Urinary Stress Incontinence in the Female. *Am. J. Obst. & Gynec.*, 83: 632, 1962.

Hodgkinson, C. P., and Cobert, N.: Direct Urethrocystometry. *Am. J. Obst. & Gynec.*, 79: 648, 1960.

Ingelman-Sundberg, A.: *The Use of the Pubo-coccygeal Muscle in the Repair of Stress Incontinence*. Monographs of Surgery. Baltimore, Williams & Wilkins Company, 1952, p. 108.

Janssens, J.: Results of Urethrocystographically Differentiating Operative Treatment for Stress Incontinence. Obst. & Gynec. Surv., 15: 611, 1960.

Jeffcoate, T. N. A., and Roberts, H.: Observations on Stress Incontinence of Urine. *Am. J. Obst. & Gynec.*, 64: 721, 1952.

Jones, E. G., and Kegel, A. H.: Treatment of Urinary Stress Incontinence with Results in 117 Patients Treated by Active Exercise of Pubococcygei. *Surg., Gynec. & Obst.*, 94: 179, 1952.

Kegel, A. H.: Physiologic Therapy for Urinary Stress Incontinence. A Survey of 34 Cases Treated by the Millin I Sling Operation. *J.A.M.A.*, 146: 915, 1951.

Kelley, H. A.: Incontinence of Urine in Women. *Urol. & Cutan. Rev.*, 17: 291, 1913.

Kennedy, C.: Stress Incontinence of Urine. *Brit. M.J.*, 2: 263, 1960.

Kennedy, W. T.: The Muscle of Micturition. Its Role in the Sphincter Mechanism with Reference to Incontinence in the Female. *Am. J. Obst. & Gynec.*, 52: 206, 1946.

Idem: *Operative Technique for Stress Incontinence of Urine in the Female.* Monographs of Surgery. Baltimore, Williams & Wilkins Company, 1952, p. 74.

Lapides, J., Ajemian, E. P., Stewart, B. H., Lichtwardt, J. R. and Breakey, B. A.: Physiopathology of Stress Incontinence. *Surg., Gynec. & Obst.*, 111: 224, 1960.

Lund, C. J., Fullerton, R. E., and Tristan, T. A.: Cinefluorographic Studies of the Bladder and Urethra in Women. II. Stress Incontinence. *Am. J. Obst. & Gynec.*, 78: 706, 1959.

McCrea, L. E. and Kimmel, D. L.: New Concept of Vesical Innervation. Relationship of Vesical Innervation to Bladder Management Following Abdominal Perineal Proctosigmoidectomy. *Arch. Surg.*, 66: 84, 1954.

Marchetti, A. A.: Female Bladder and Urethra before and after Correction for Stress Incontinence. *Am. J. Obst. & Gynec.*, 58: 1145, 1949.

Marshall, V. F., Marchetti, A. A., and Krantz, K. E.: The Correction of Stress Incontinence by Simple Vesicourethral Suspension. *Surg., Gynec. & Obst.*, 88: 509, 1949.

Marshall, V. F., Pollack, R. S., and Miller, C.: Observations on Urinary Dysfunction after Excision of the Rectum. *J. Urol.*, 55: 409, 1946.

Meigs, J. V.: Fascial Sling Operation for Incontinence of Urine. *J. Mt. Sinai Hosp.*, 14: 504, 1947.

Muellner, S. R.: The Physiologic Components of the Urinary Bladder. Their Clinical Significance. *New England J. Med.*, 241: 769, 1949.

Idem: *The Etiology of Stress Incontinence.* Monographs of Surgery. Baltimore, Williams & Wilkins Company, 1952, p. 54.

Idem: The Anatomies of the Female Urethra—A Critical Review. *Obst. & Gynec.*, 14: 429, 1959.

Rashbaum, M., and Mandelbaum, C. C.: Nonoperative Treatment of Urinary Incontinence in Women. *Am. J. Obst. & Gynec.*, 56: 777, 1948.

Read, C. D.: Stress Incontinence of Urine, with Special Reference to Failure of Cure Following Vaginal Operative Procedure. *Am. J. Obst. & Gynec.*, 59: 1260, 1950.

Roberts, H.: Observations on Micturition in the Female. *J. Obst. & Gynaec. Brit. Emp.*, 60: 621, 1953.

Salmon, U. J., Walter, R. I., and Geist, S. H.: The Use of Estrogens in the Treatment of Dysuria and Incontinence in Postmenopausal Women. *Am. J. Obst. & Gynec.*, 42: 845, 1941.

Studdiford, W. E.: The Problems of Stress Incontinence and Its Surgical Relief. *Surg., Gynec. & Obst.*, 83: 742, 1946.

Symmonds, R. E.: Present Concepts and Management of Urinary Stress Incontinence. *S. Clin. N. Amer.*, 39: 933, 1959.

Talbot, H. S.: Medical Progress: Functional Disorders of the Urinary Bladder. *New England J. Med.* 258: 643, 1958.

Thompson, I. M.: The Surgical Relief of Urinary Incontinence. *Surg., Gynec. & Obst.*, 108: 493, 1959.

Ullery, J. C.: *Stress Incontinence in the Female.* New York, Grune & Stratton, Inc., 1953.

Wharton, L. R., Jr., and TeLinde, R. W.: An Evaluation of Fascial Sling Operation for Urinary Incontinence in Female Patients. *J. Urol.*, 82: 76, 1959.

Chapter 66

The Climacteric and the Menopause

THE FINAL phases of the reproductive capacity of the female patient come to an end when all menstrual periods cease. This has been called the *menopause*, and in approximately one-half of women it is complete between the ages of forty-five and fifty years. This period in a woman's life has also been called the "change of life." Such a term tends to create in the patient's mind the thought that steady downhill deterioration, physically, mentally and sexually, can be expected from then on. This is unfortunate. A gradual slowdown in ovarian function precedes the cessation of periods over a span of several years and continues after menstruation has permanently ceased. The gradually diminishing ovarian function causes its own train of symptoms. These are distressing in their own right, but they are magnified and often overpowered by the psychic unrest that follows a woman's thought that she is no longer useful except to manage the household affairs and may no longer be able to attract her husband either physically or sexually.

This period in a woman's life is one of adjustment to the waning potential of the ovary which takes place over a period of years. It has rightfully been called the climacteric, a term derived from the Greek, meaning "rung of the ladder." The climacteric, then, is a transition period which gradually evolves and continues for varying stretches of time after the menstrual periods have ceased. We have noted that anovulatory menstruation is common in the years preceding the menopause. This is the direct result of deficiency on the part of the ovarian hormones. Ovarian activity, on the other hand, does not cease when menstruation disappears, since there is ample clinical, and recently laboratory, evidence that the ovary continues to secrete estrin in variable quantities for many years thereafter. Though the terms "menopause" and "climacteric" are used interchangeably, the use of climacteric best describes the period of physiologic adjustment and is to be preferred. The menopause then is simply one incident among the many that occur over the longer interval which is the climacteric.

At What Age Do Menstrual Periods Normally Cease?

The average age at the menopause is approximately fifty years. This is later than the age reported in the older writings (forty-seven years) and suggests that with better nutrition, planned parenthood, less hard work and better health the modern American woman can expect to experience the menopause later in life than her grandmother did.

1045

On the other hand, there is a tendency for the daughter to follow the menstrual pattern of the mother. This is particularly noticeable in the group who tend to have the menopause before the age of forty. Hereditary, racial, constitutional and social factors are all implicated in the woman who has a premature cessation of her menstrual flow.

There appears to be little relation between the date of onset of the menarche and the age at which menstruation ceases. Many investigators insist that the earlier the menarche, the later the menopause. This is an interesting observation, particularly as it bears on the findings of polycystic ovaries in the girl who does not menstruate until she is eighteen. Such observations need further confirmation, but such data as are now available show that it makes little difference when the periods begin in relation to when they cease. This statement is not changed when one considers the childbearing factor or the age when the patient married.

What Are the Characteristic Symptoms of the Climacteric?

It is important to remember in this discussion of symptomatology that the climacteric covers a span of years during which the ovarian activity is on the wane. The menopause is simply a dramatic incident that takes place during this phase of menstrual activity. The symptoms, then, precede and follow the menopause in greater or lesser degree.

Approximately 20 per cent of women enter and complete the climacteric period without any other symptoms than a changing pattern of menstrual flow and final amenorrhea. The remainder have varying degrees of discomfort from symptoms based on vasomotor instability, psychosomatic unrest or constitutional changes. The cessation of the menstrual periods, either real or anticipated, for many women is a disheartening and alarming experience. The severity of the symptoms will depend in large part on the patient's general and mental health, as well as her adjustment to the pressures of her life and circumstances. If she is sick, bored or unhappy, the symptoms will be worse.

The symptoms of the climacteric tend to fall into four main categories, recorded roughly in order of their appearance: (*a*) disturbance in the menstrual pattern, (*b*) vasomotor manifestations, (*c*) psychosomatic response, and (*d*) factors of aging, as they apply to other endocrine glands.

What Are the Changes in the Menstrual Pattern?

The principal change in ovarian function that occurs during the climacteric and is reflected in the menstrual period is the disappearance of the luteal phase. Estrin production, unbalanced by progestin, continues in varying amounts for several years after the periods have ceased.

The first indication of the oncoming climacteric is the appearance of anovulatory cycles. Sampling of the endometrium shows a persistence of the proliferative phase at a time when secretory endometrium should be evident. Lessening amounts of estrin produced without wide fluctuations in amount set the irregular menstrual pattern. This also determines the nature of the menstrual flow and bears on its duration. The detailed description and therapy for bleeding in this age group appear in Chapter 58.

In brief, an irregular menstrual bleeding pattern is to be expected. The change in the type of menstrual bleeding begins with foreshortened anovulatory cycles. The transition is gradual. Rarely do the periods suddenly cease without some preliminary alteration in the type of flow. As the ovarian function declines, one commonly encounters periods that are spread farther apart with diminished flow of shorter duration. Amenorrhea may persist for two or three months followed by excessive and prolonged flow. This is the *metropathia hemorrhagica* pattern of bleeding and comes about through continuous estrogenic stimulation of the endometrium, but no actual sloughing occurs because there is insufficient fluctuation in the blood levels of circulating estrogen. When breakthrough bleeding does appear, the endometrium is shed only in patches rather than in its entirety, and the periods are both prolonged and heavy.

The important thing to keep in mind is the possibility of bleeding from organic causes, of which cancer is the most important. In general, if the menstrual periods have progressively diminished in amount of flow and appear at increasingly long intervals, uterine bleeding is probably functional. The regular foreshortened cycle likewise is less dangerous. When, however, the bleeding is excessive in quantity, duration and frequency, then bleeding from a pathologic source should be suspected and ruled out.

What Are the Other Clinical Signs of Ovarian Failure?

LOCAL EFFECTS ON GENITAL TRACT. The primary evidence of ovarian failure is amenorrhea. The ovaries, as part of the aging process, tend to atrophy, and the graafian follicles and ova disappear. With the gradual decline in estrin production atrophy occurs in all target organs that were formerly stimulated. This takes place over a period of time, which is longer for some patients than for others. The gross effect involves varying degrees of avascularity, as seen in the entire genital tract.

When firmly established, atrophy is evidenced by the reduction in size of the labia majora of the external genitalia. The subcutaneous fat vanishes and the labia shrink. The clitoris becomes smaller, and the skin of the vulvar area loses its elasticity and thins out so much that it looks like parchment. The changes in the vaginal epithelium are variable and depend on the amount of estrin being produced. Apparently less estrin is needed to maintain the vaginal epithelium than the endometrium. When estrin deprivation is at its worst, the epithelium no longer has its moist, bluish-red appearance, but looks pale and pink. The vaginal canal is dry, because there is less secretion produced. The cells of the vaginal epithelium are inactive and contain no glycogen (Fig. 66–1).

Adhesive vaginitis is prone to develop. Constricting fibrosis may close off the upper part of the vagina. The entire uterus becomes fibrotic and diminishes in size. The cervix shrinks, retracts and becomes flush with the wall of the vagina. Not infrequently the cervical canal becomes stenotic, and on rare occasions the patient may have a pyometra or hematometra. The fundal portion of the uterus takes part in the regressive process and comes to contain more connective tissue than muscle. Contrary to a general impression, a pre-existing fibroid becomes smaller, but it does not disappear. The endometrium atrophies, although focal areas of hyperplasia are occasionally seen. It retains its power to respond to estrin stimulation, however, and bleeding may follow the use of exogenous estrin.

GENERAL MANIFESTATIONS OF ESTRIN LACK. The effects of estrin deprivation are noted throughout the body, as well as locally in the genital tract. For example,

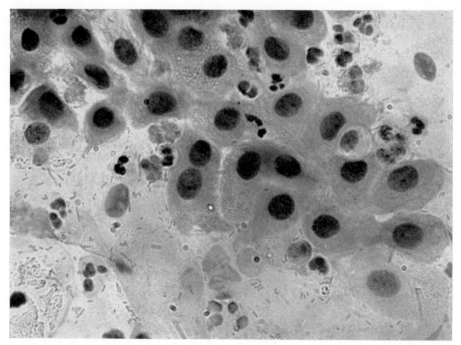

Fig. 66-1. Atrophic vaginal epithelial cells are of smaller size and more rounded than those that show estrogen effects. The nuclei appear comparatively larger and darker-stained in vaginal smears.

not only is there a loss of pubic hair, but hair on the head also becomes sparse. At the same time the patient may have a slight growth of hair on the upper lip and chin. The breast tissue atrophies and becomes replaced by areolar tissue. Since elasticity is lost, the breasts droop and become pendulous.

The body habitus also changes to become less rounded and less feminine. The skin generally loses its elasticity and tends to wrinkle. Osteoporotic changes appear in the bones, particularly of the spine and pelvis. It is interesting that the primary failure is in the bone matrix and not in the process of calcification. For this reason, calcium replacement therapy accomplishes little, while estrin therapy may induce calcium deposit and pain relief. Obesity and hypothyroidism are common in this age group. Obesity may be secondary to reduced thyroid activity.

What Are the Vasomotor Manifestations?

Hot flashes are the chief source of distress at the time of the climacteric. In a few instances the hot flashes appear before the menopause is definitely established, during the period when the estrin level is known to fluctuate, but the majority of women have them concomitantly with the cessation of the periods.

Hot flashes are hard to describe and mean many things to many people. A sensation of warmth begins over the upper part of the chest and characteristically spreads up over the neck and face.

The response may be generalized over the entire body and be accompanied by a prickling sensation in the skin, particularly of the scalp. The patient is acutely aware of the blushing sensation, which is visible at times. The flashes may appear as often as fifteen or twenty times a day and last as long as two minutes. They are apt to be more troublesome at night, because they produce such profuse sweating that the patient spends the night alternately throwing off the bed clothes and trying to recover them, as she experiences first hot spells and then chills. The severity of the flashes provides an accurate index of the degree of endocrine imbalance, since there is little doubt that they reflect alterations in hormonal output.

Some 65 per cent of women will have hot flashes. Of these, approximately 20 per cent have them badly enough to require medical help for relief, though a much higher percentage are treated.

Other vasomotor symptoms accompany the hot flashes and perspiration. Numbness and tingling, cold hands and feet, palpitations, headache, vertigo and fainting all bring their own measure of distress.

WHAT IS THE PROBABLE CAUSE OF THE VASOMOTOR INSTABILITY AND THE HOT FLASH?   The explanation for the vasomotor symptoms is not completely established. The apparent cause is the loss of the ovarian response to stimulation by pituitary gonadotropins. As a result (1) the ovarian follicle develops improperly or not at all, and no progesterone is secreted. (2) There is also a sharp reduction in the amount of estrin produced. (3) The pituitary hormones (FSH) are produced in excess in an attempt to stimulate the aged ovary to secrete more estrin. Twenty times the normal amount of FSH may be recovered in the urine. The titer may rise because of increased production on the part of the pituitary or more likely under-consumption on the part of the ovary.

It is not clear just how the increase in the FSH or the drop in estrin produces the flushing. Supposedly the decrease in the output of the steroids changes the neurovascular mechanism and lowers the threshold for external stimuli. It is interesting, however, that both the decrease in estrin levels and the increase in FSH persist throughout the remainder of the patient's life, yet the hot flashes have a self-limited course. That course may be over one or two years or it may last for ten.

Not all authorities accept the explanation that the increase in FSH titer is responsible for the flashes. It is true that, although all women have an increased amount of FSH in the face of ovarian failure, not all such patients have symptoms. Furthermore, a high gonadotropic titer may be recorded both before and after symptoms develop. There appears to be little correlation between the amount of circulating FSH and their severity. As added evidence it is well known that small doses of estrin relieve the symptoms without changing the amount of circulating FSH. The inference to be drawn from these observations is that the symptoms are due to ovarian failure rather than to an excess production of pituitary FSH. Other investigators are not convinced that the diminished supply of estrin is the entire explanation since (*a*) after oophorectomy estrogen disappears long before the hot flashes appear; (*b*) the estrin level is raised by treatment some time before the symptoms disappear; (*c*) low estrin determinations are commonly found in pituitary disease, but they are not associated with hot flashes. In the minds of some observers the high levels of FSH are the responsible factor.

Actually, it is of little practical importance, because relief from medication may result either from depression of pituitary function or from replacement of the diminishing supply of estrin.

What Other Bodily Symptoms Appear in the Climacteric?

In addition to disturbances in the menstrual pattern and the presence of hot flashes, a train of seemingly unrelated symptoms appears. Among them are insomnia, headache, fatigue, joint pains, tendency to gain weight and loss of libido.

During the climacteric period the woman complains of being tired all the time, regardless of how much sleep she gets. She tires easily with a minimal expenditure of effort. In part, the explanation may be traced to metabolic disturbances that are common in this age group. It is well known that thyroid function is impaired at this time. Patients are apt to have dry skin and brittle fingernails and to note a tendency for the hair to fall out, not only in the pubic region but on the scalp as well. The basal metabolic rate is usually low and blood cholesterol elevated.

The definite trend toward weight gain during the climacteric can be traced in part to decreased thyroid function, but perhaps more to decreased physical activity and increased food intake. Regardless of whether the patient gains weight or not, a change in the distribution of the fat takes place. The areas of concentration seem to be on the lower abdominal wall, buttocks and hips, with less fat deposited elsewhere.

Headaches are common, frequent and severe and have many of the characteristics of migraine. There is a variety of explanations for the headaches, which often appear at the time of the menopause. Before attributing the discomfort to a functional cause, hypertension, sinus infections and allergies should be ruled out. In some women the headaches occur only at the time of menstrual bleeding, but other patients have them almost continuously.

Insomnia is not confined to this period of life, but it seems to be aggravated by the other problems that arise at this time. In many instances the patient had insomnia before, but the climacteric-related nervous tension, anxiety state and instability make the insomnia worse.

Diminished estrin secretion produces changes in bone as well as skin. In addition the patient frequently has pain in all the joints. Osteoporosis is prone to develop, particularly in the lower lumbar vertebrae and pelvis. Estrin apparently relieves the pain by increasing the rapidity of osteoid formation and calcium deposit, as well as by reducing the extent of bone resorption in osteoporosis. Increasing the bone vascularity, a known property of estrin, probably explains the favorable effect of estrin therapy.

The *libido* is a variable thing in patients in this age group. The normal expectancy in the intensity of the sex drive is one of gradual tapering off with age. In some instances, however, the woman in the climacteric experiences a notable and frequently exaggerated need for sexual gratification.

What about the Psychosomatic Symptoms?

The principal problems of the menopause which have some physiologic or endocrinologic basis are often complicated by a large group of symptoms that have a tinge of the psychosomatic. In too many instances medical treatment has been directed toward their relief without sufficient evidence that the patient is approaching, or is actually in, the climacteric period.

Chief among the symptoms of this type are increasing nervousness, apprehension, lack of concentration, uncertainty in the face of unexpected situations, irritability, depressions and melancholia. Many of these symptoms may be traced to folklore.

Through the medium of old wives' tales the menopause has been transformed from a natural process into a bleak abyss that women must traverse whether they want to or not.

The majority of women who are sound in health and mind and well adjusted to their surroundings will pass through the menopause with the minimum of distress. Not more than 20 per cent require any intensive medical therapy. The explanation of many psychosomatic symptoms is obvious, and they can be managed by simple sedation and reassurance without the services of a psychiatrist.

The emotional instability experienced by women during the climacteric is well documented. The patient is frequently nervous and apprehensive without apparent cause. She is disturbed because she cannot think consecutively and complains that she cannot remember anything. Combined with depression and some tendency toward melancholia, this is enough to make her think that she is losing her mind. She cries with or without the slightest provocation and is subject to sudden changes in mood during which she may flare up at the children and family or become extremely irritable with her oldest friend. Insomnia is a frequent complaint. She has probably had this to a minor degree before, but it becomes exaggerated during the menopause. She is therefore tired all the time.

There is a perfectly reasonable explanation for such symptoms. They have little to do with the menopause, except that they do provide an indication that the patient is no longer young. This disturbs the patient as much as the obvious manifestations. The children have usually grown up, have their own problems and no longer need mother's help. For years this has been her chief role in life. Without the children the job of simply keeping house does not seem to be enough to justify her existence. She feels that she is no longer useful.

The aging process she is sure has detracted from her physical appeal, and her security becomes threatened. The husband does not help her much, because he may be preoccupied with his own interests outside the family and may not be as tolerant or sympathetic as he might. It is also true that he may be noting the physiologic changes inherent in the aging process. It may well be a time of adjustment for both wife and husband to a changing physiologic state, but it need not be catastrophic and will not be if the woman is healthy and thinks objectively about it. Actually, some women anticipate the menopause with enthusiasm, since they no longer have to worry about the minor degrees of physical discomfort they have long associated with the menstrual flow, and pregnancy is no longer possible.

How Does One Evaluate the Symptoms of the Menopause?

Primarily the physician must decide whether the patient's symptoms are actually due to the menopause. Many women, particularly if they are unhappy or bored with their existence, display diverse symptoms that they are apt to attribute to the menopause, since it provides a convenient excuse for their inadequacies. The situation frequently constitutes a plea for the attention, sympathy and understanding of the husband. In too many instances the physician aids and abets the woman's explanation of her troubles by treating her for menopausal symptoms when none exist. This is particularly true of women in the thirties or early forties.

It is rare to have symptoms of vasomotor instability when the menstrual pattern is normal. When the periods become irregular and the progestin element disappears, the patient will have vaginal bleeding and breast symptoms commonly attributable to estrogenic stimulation in varying degrees, depending on the level of the hormones in the blood. The symptoms conversely should be most pronounced in the climacteric when there is an established estrogen insufficiency. One may determine the degree of estrogen lack by laboratory studies such as (1) the cornification index of the vaginal smear, (2) the endometrial biopsy, (3) the progesterone withdrawal test, and (4) urinary assays for FSH.

The symptoms in all probability are not due to any great degree of estrogen deficiency if (*a*) the vaginal epithelial cytoplasm with Papanicolaou stain is orange-pink or acidophilic and more than 10 per cent of the cells in the smear are fully cornified; (*b*) the endometrial biopsy shows proliferative activity, and certainly no estrogen lack exists if a secretory phase is found; (*c*) the patient has withdrawal bleeding 3 to 4 days after Proluton, 50 mg., has been administered daily for 3 days; (*d*) the urinary FSH shows no elevation above normal values.

WHAT IS THE BEST METHOD OF TREATMENT FOR THE MAJORITY OF PATIENTS WITH TRUE MENOPAUSAL SYMPTOMS?

ABNORMAL BLEEDING

We have established that the patient is truly in the climacteric period. During this phase it is important to rule out any possible organic cause for an abnormal vaginal bleeding pattern. This may be done by an endometrial biopsy, though a curettage is preferable and more informative. If the bleeding is truly functional, the patient may be treated by intramuscular injection of progesterone. This is available in a number of different forms, which have different dosage schedules. Proluton, 20 mg. given intramuscularly every day for 5 days, beginning on about the eighteenth day of a 28-day cycle, produces a medical curettage approximately 5 days after the last dose.

The newer progestational compounds, norethindrone (Norlutin), norethynodrel (Enovid), ethisterone or anhydrohydroxy-progesterone (Pranone, Lutocylol) may be taken by mouth and have much the same progestational action as the other compounds given intramuscularly. For anovulatory bleeding Norlutin, 10 to 15 mg. daily for 3 days; Enovid, 10 mg. daily for 3 weeks; Delalutin, a longer-acting progesterone, 2 cc. given by injection on the sixteenth day, will produce withdrawal bleeding and simulate the action of natural progesterone by producing a "medical curettage." Except for the obvious advantage of being oral medications the new progesterone relatives do nothing that cannot be achieved with intramuscular progesterone, and they have the distinct disadvantage of not being as predictable.

If the patient resumes an abnormal vaginal bleeding pattern or fails to respond to progesterone therapy, curettage and possibly hysterectomy are indicated. In most instances an organic explanation will be found.

GENERALIZED SYMPTOMS

We have noted that (*a*) the climacteric period is one of adjustment to physiologic processes of aging and carries its own train of symptoms; (*b*) although all women go through some physiologic change, only a few have symptoms severe enough to require concentrated treatment; (*c*) not all the symptoms that appear at this time are due to the climacteric, but some are simply manifestations of organic disease; (*d*) the symptoms that do accompany the climacteric, in the absence of organic disease, are made worse if the patient is in a poor state of physical and mental health.

All these factors have a bearing on the therapy, which may then take the form of (*a*) simple reassurance and education, (*b*) general measures to improve the physical condition, (*c*) special therapy designed to relieve specific complaints such as the hot flashes.

What Form Should Reassurance Take?

Much can be accomplished by explaining to the patient that the climacteric period and the cessation of menstruation are natural processes which cannot be avoided, but they need not be a nightmare. All women know of some friend or member of the family who has had an unpleasant emotional experience and may even have been admitted to a sanitarium because of extreme nervous symptoms. It will help the patient to know that women do not become mentally unbalanced simply because of the menopause. Women who do so have almost always had psychiatric manifestations of a similar pattern in the past. The physiologic changes of the menopausal period simply provide another aggravation.

There is no reason for most women to feel that they too "are going out of their minds" simply because they have anxieties, cannot remember things or concentrate for any length of time. The physician should make it clear to the patient that her present situation is but temporary, for the climacteric period is a self-limiting one. She need not, therefore, expect to carry her anxieties, fears and lack of concentration to the end of her days. The patient should be encouraged to take a greater interest in outside activities, provided they are not too diffuse and can be carried on within the limits of her strength.

If she is concerned about losing her sexual drive or her husband's affection, she should be told that her interest in sex or her husband's interest in her is not altered by the menopause. The impulse and response to the sexual act in human beings are not dependent on ovarian function. This observation is supported by the experience of many women who have had a Wertheim hysterectomy, which removes the uterus, ovaries and a large part of the vagina, yet they retain their sexual urge and obtain satisfaction from intercourse. The probable explanation lies in the fact that the clitoris, like the nipple, responds to stimulation through a reflex arc involving the spinal cord and brain.

What Measures Should Be Taken to Improve the General Health?

We have noted that the patient's reaction to the symptoms common to this age group varies with her physical and mental condition. Overwork, undue fatigue and unpleasant home surroundings exaggerate the symptoms. The patient should be encouraged to take an objective view of life, realizing that she will not feel as she does now forever. She should be encouraged to do more and not to retire into her misery. Senseless overactivity, on the other hand, can only increase her fatigue and augment her complaints. The patient should be encouraged to take plenty of exercise, coupled with adequate rest and sleep.

She should also avoid putting on weight and should embark on a sensible diet to keep it under control. She should be told that she may be expected to gain weight more easily now than she has done in the past and that more attention should be directed toward avoiding the obvious reasons for any increase in weight. Chiefly these are decreased activity and overeating. If the patient has placed herself on a weight reduction diet of her own choosing, it should be closely examined. Many bizarre diets are in vogue which change with passing fashions, contain scant life-sustaining elements and are usually woefully lacking in vitamins and minerals.

What Specific Medications May Be Given to Relieve Symptoms?

In many instances the patient's response to the physician's program of education and reassurance is good, but she is still unduly jumpy, nervous and apprehensive. Supportive measures designed to alleviate specific complaints are then indicated. Estrin will not control the nervousness, alter the libido or counteract depression. Such patients need sedatives, not estrin.

SEDATION.   Small doses of phenobarbital are enormously helpful to the patient who understands the menopause, but still needs additional support. Phenobarbital may be given with impunity in ¼- or ½-grain dosage several times daily. One is perhaps less justified in giving tranquilizing drugs, though they can be useful if the physician retains control of the dosage schedule. It should certainly be kept in mind that (*a*) patients who have a tendency to be depressed may be more so when taking tranquilizers, (*b*) withdrawal symptoms are often acute when the drug is omitted. Physician-control is essential, for too many patients take medications on the theory that if a little will help, more benefit will be obtained by larger and more continuous dosages.

THERAPY OTHER THAN ESTRIN.   It is well known that the thyroid functions less well at this time of life. The lowered basal metabolism reflects the accuracy of this observation. The fact that patients tire easily with little expenditure of effort and regardless of the amount of sleep they obtain suggests that thyroid hormone might be helpful in combating fatigue. Thyroid extract in ½- to 1-grain doses daily has been used effectively in helping to overcome the sense of exhaustion and perhaps to help alleviate the general endocrine imbalance.

Many patients are distressed that hair tends to fall out both in the pubic region and on the scalp. The nails also get brittle and chip off. The physician may choose to give iron and calcium along with the small doses of thyroid extract. Vitamins C and E in large doses have been used in combination with thyroid hormone. Theoretically, the threshold to aggravating stimuli may be raised by the action of vitamin E on the nerve receptors. The effect, however, actually may be in the realm of psychosomatic medicine.

FOR WHAT SYMPTOMS IS ESTRIN EFFECTIVE?   Estrogen lack produces varying symptoms, depending on the extent of deprivation. The primary reason for giving estrin is to relieve hot flashes. Many of these patients are utterly miserable and need estrin replacement badly. The dosage need not be large and should not be continuous.

Other vasomotor symptoms such as tingling of the hands and feet and painful finger joints will be materially improved when estrin is given. Through its power to increase vascularity estrin is helpful in improving joint function and may justifiably be given in the absence of hot flashes.

Vaginal spotting, burning and itching may be so intense that enough estrin should be given to relieve the discomfort.

Frequency of urination, dysuria and cystitis may well improve with the use of estrin.

As ovarian activity diminishes, the epithelium of the urethral canal atrophies, and chronic infection appears. Urethritis can be most uncomfortable. Estrin therapy causes a re-epithelialization, and the chronic infection disappears.

Osteoporosis, which manifests itself as pain in the lower back and pelvis, requires estrin for relief. The underlying defect is a failure to deposit bone connective tissue matrix as well as calcium, and the addition of calcium to the diet does not alone produce recalcification. Estrin is necessary in order that bone connective-tissue osteoid be produced and thereafter calcium be properly deposited to form bone trabeculae.

Estrin is specific in its action on the target organs and should be given only when there is evidence of real estrogen deficiency.

WHEN, HOW AND ON WHAT DOSAGE SCHEDULE SHOULD ESTRIN BE GIVEN? *When?*   Nearly 70 per cent of women will respond to a regimen of explanation, reassurance, revision of living habits, exercise and re-evaluation of their point of view on life, supplemented when needed by mild sedative and tranquilizing drugs. Approximately 15 per cent, however, need specific estrin substitution therapy.

The wide spectrum of menopausal symptoms will not be relieved by estrin medication alone, despite the fact that the whole period is ushered in by a decline in ovarian activity in general and decreased estrin production in particular. It will not relieve anxiety or calm depressive states, for example, but estrin replacement therapy is rewarding when the patient has real symptoms that are primarily due to lack of estrin stimulation.

How Much?   Primarily the hormone should be given to relieve symptoms and not to restore the full physiologic effect on the target organs. If, for example, the patient has atrophic vaginitis, estrin is given in small doses adequate to relieve the burning discomfort and pinkish discharge, but not with the idea of achieving complete cornification of the vaginal epithelium.

There are disadvantages in overstimulation by estrin. The chief indication that too much is being given over too long a period is the appearance of vaginal bleeding. Small doses are as effective as large ones in relieving hot flashes and other symptoms when they are taken on a schedule that calls for periodic interruptions in the continuity of estrin administration. Another indication of overenthusiastic estrin ingestion is tenderness and soreness of the breasts and pigmentation of the nipples.

By What Route Should Estrin Be Given?   Despite the insistence of many patients that oral estrin medication is completely ineffective and that only intramuscular injections will suffice, the facts are in contradiction. Insistence on the intramuscular route of estrin administration is a reflection of the psychic and mental unrest that goes with this period of life. Oral medications with estrin will do everything equally well. Too often estrin therapy is given by injection. It is more costly, calls for more dependence on the physician and is no more helpful than in pill form given by mouth.

The majority of patients receive benefit from synthetic diethylstilbestrol in nightly 0.5-mg. doses. Others prefer the more costly estrin derived from natural sources. Whatever the type of the estrin preparation, it should be given as an oral medication, whenever possible. A few patients will complain of nausea when taking the estrin pills by mouth, particularly if they have become dependent on the injection method. In many instances phenobarbital in small doses should then be taken with the nightly dose of synthetic estrin. For the 15 per cent who either cannot or will not take estrin by mouth, estradiol dipropionate, 1.25 mg. intramuscularly once a week, may be given.

What Estrin Dosage Schedules Are Recommended?   Estrogen therapy should follow a definite plan. As noted before the main idea is (a) the relief of symptoms, not the restoration of the full effects of estrin on the target organs; (b) too intensive therapy frequently results in a reappearance of vaginal bleeding. One then is concerned with the possible cause and wonders whether the bleeding is due to the hormones or whether it has a more important organic cause. To these two factors one may add the fear that estrin, a known epithelial stimulant, might produce cancer in the target end-organs it acts upon, such as the breasts and genital tract.

The best method of avoiding (a) breakthrough bleeding, and (b) possible carcinogenic effects of estrin is to plan the therapy so that it is not continuous. For this reason the estrin, in whatever form the physician elects to use it, should be given daily for a period of three weeks, followed by a week of rest. To help the patient's possibly faulty memory it is a good practical point to have the patient start the medication on the first day of the month and stop it on the twenty-fifth day. It has been well demonstrated that estrogenic stimulation sufficient to induce malignant changes depends more on the continuity than the size of the dose administered.

It is also possible to avoid the disadvantages of estrin therapy mentioned above by combining estrin and androgen in the same medication. A variety of proprietary preparations is available for this purpose. The ratio of methyltestosterone to estrin should be between 1:15 and 1:20 if bleeding is to be avoided and masculinization prevented. The addition of androgen has other advantages. Testosterone is a potent anabolic stimulant, as well as having a protein-sparing effect. The patient therefore feels better. Androgen also tends to increase the libido. The combination of estrin and androgen appears to be synergistic in its effects on the vaginal epithelium. The favorable action of both is probably partly mediated through the effect on the pituitary. Symptoms based on physical, mental and emotional depletion tend to improve under the combined estrogen and androgen therapy.

Some women are afraid to take hormone treatment, because they have been told that it increases the chance of cancer and may prolong the period of physiologic adjustment. No one wishes to interfere with a normal and natural process. If the patient can live satisfactorily with her symptoms, aided only by mild sedation, this approach should be encouraged. There is no reason, however, for her to be miserable and deny herself the relief that hormone therapy can bring because of her fear of cancer or concern about prolongation of the climacteric. These theoretical disadvantages can be safely overcome by (a) interrupting the dosage schedule, and (b) giving estrogen and androgen together in the same cyclic manner.

REFERENCES

Banner, E. A.: The Menopause. Its Symptoms and Care. *S. Clin. N. Amer.*, 39: 1113, 1959.

Barnes, A. C.: The Menopause. *Clin. Obst. & Gynec.*, 1: 203, 1958.

Black, E. F.: Treatment of the Climacteric Woman. *J. Obst. & Gynaec. Brit. Emp.*, 66: 784, 1959.

Brewer, J. I., and McCune, W. W.: Management of Abnormal Uterine Bleeding during the Climacteric. *Clin. Obst. & Gynec.*, 1: 796, 1958.

Danforth, D. N.: The Climacteric. *M. Clin. N. Amer.*, 45: 47, 1961.

Evans, T. N.: Post-menopausal Bleeding. *Clin. Obst. & Gynec.*, 1: 809, 1958.

Faber, J. E.: Dyspareunia in Older Women. *S. Clin. N. Amer.*, 39: 1105, 1959.

Greenblatt, R. B.: Newer Concepts in Management of the Menopause. *Geriatrics*, 7: 263, 1952.

Jeffcoate, T.N.A.: Drugs for Menopausal Symptoms. *Brit. M.J.*, 1: 340, 1960.

Kupperman, H. S., Wetchler, B. B., and Blatt, M. H. G.: Contemporary Therapy of the Menopausal Syndrome. *J.A.M.A.*, 171: 1627, 1959.

Masukawa, T.: Vaginal Smears in Women Past 40 Years of Age, with Emphasis on Their Remaining Hormonal Activity. *Obst. & Gynec.*, 16: 407, 1960.

Moldawer, M.: Senile Osteoporosis. The Physiological Basis for Treatment. A.M.A. *Arch. Int. Med.*, 96: 202, 1955.

Novak, E. R.: The Menopause. *J.A.M.A.*, 156: 575, 1954.

Randall, C. L.: Ovarian Function and Woman after the Menopause. *Am. J. Obst. & Gynec.*, 73: 1000, 1957.

Rogers, J.: Medical Progress: The Menopause. *New England J. Med.*, 254: 697, 750, 1956.

Shelton, E. K.: The Use of Estrogen after Menopause. *J. Am. Geriatrics Soc.*, 2: 627, 1954.

Soule, S. D., and Burstein, R.: Prophylaxis of the Postsurgical Menopause. Estradiol Pellet Implantation. *Am. J. Obst. & Gynec.*, 77: 1254, 1959.

Struthers, R. A.: Post-menopausal Oestrogen Production. *Brit. M.J.*, 1: 1331, 1956.

PART VI

Gynecologic Problems in the Postmenopausal Era (Age 50 to 65)

Chapter 67

Breast Problems in Older Women

CANCER of the breast may appear in all age groups from adolescence on, the incidence generally increasing in proportion to age. The diagnostic problem decreases appreciably after the menopause, however, for the simple reason that cystic disease and adenosis tend to subside and do not enter into the differential diagnosis when a lump appears in the breast. In this situation the tumor felt by the patient is likely to be a carcinoma.

MAMMARY DUCT ECTASIA

There is one other pathologic entity common to the menopause which does introduce an element of confusion into the diagnosis, namely, *mammary duct ectasia*. This is a benign process associated with atrophy of the duct epithelium. As a sequel to the thinning of the epithelial lining of the ducts, exudation often appears. The inflammatory process spreads from the duct system and involves the periductal tissue and the surrounding extrinsic stroma.

Any inflammation in the supporting tissue of the breast is always accompanied by a fibrous tissue response designed to limit the spread of infection. Thus a mass develops in the breast which is firm or hard and may simulate carcinoma. The lesion may or may not be tender, indicating its inflammatory nature, but even then the surgeon cannot without a biopsy differentiate mammary duct ectasia from a carcinoma that is undergoing central necrosis.

What Is the Clinical Picture of Mammary Duct Ectasia?

The breast lesions that appear as the result of epithelial proliferation of either the ducts, the ductules or the acinar system are concentrated in the age groups in which mammary stimulation is likely to occur because of the action of various hormones. On the other hand, mammary duct ectasia is a pathologic entity associated with the aging breast and is atrophic rather than proliferative.

Because it does produce (*a*) nipple discharge, (*b*) nipple retraction, (*c*) tumors

1061

of varying size, (*d*) evidence of inflammation, accompanied at times by localized erythema, pain and tenderness, duct ectasia is often mistaken for carcinoma.

What Is the Natural Process of Evolution of Mammary Duct Ectasia?

Mammary duct ectasia is first noted in the collecting ducts that lie directly beneath the nipple and the areola. The dilated ducts are often in evidence during the course of surgical exploration of the breast for other causes, undoubtedly because the first clinical suggestion of their presence is the spontaneous appearance of a nipple discharge. They show up as bluish or green discolorations, varying in size from 3 to 5 mm., in the tissue at the base of the nipple and areola. Unlike the intraductal papilloma, which often develops from proliferation of the epithelium of a single duct, mammary duct ectasia arises as a degenerative process not in one but in many ducts, varying in number from four to twenty. Atrophy of the lining epithelium is present rather than proliferation. The duct itself is tortuous, thick and fibrosed, owing to the irritation by the material contained within and leaking from the dilated lumens. Since locally there is no adequate epithelial protective lining, the walls themselves become infiltrated with lymphocytes and macrophages that appear in response to the chemical properties of the stagnant duct contents. The true nature of the thick amorphous material within the ducts is not known, but much of it is debris, and in all probability it includes decomposition products of fatty nature. Microscopically, the debris is evident, and characteristic crystalline bodies of cholesterol can at times be identified.

As the process progresses—and it may take place over several years—the inflammatory changes in the duct wall extend from the areolar area deeper into the substance of the breast. So long as the inflammation is confined to the lumens and walls of the ducts only thickening and fibrosis of the duct itself may be found. Retraction of the nipple begins to appear, since the more thickened they become, the greater the foreshortening of the ducts. It is the contraction in duct length that produces the nipple retraction. As yet no tumor has appeared, because the inflammation is mainly confined to the ducts.

Eventually some portion of the duct wall weakens, and the irritating contents spread into the periductal tissues and extrinsic fibrofatty stroma of the breast. Fibrosis results, owing to damage to the supporting fatty tissue stroma, and a process begins to appear not unlike that of fat necrosis, such as one sees after trauma to the breast. This is evident because a tumor develops beneath the areola, gradually extends down into the substance of the normal breast and increases in size as it progresses.

The mass feels stony hard, is fixed to the skin and underlying breast tissue and is practically indistinguishable from either fat necrosis or carcinoma. The involved breast lumps have a tendency to break down and become red, hot and tender. In a sense these areas resemble a carbuncle. The architecture of the breast does not lend itself to free drainage, and abscess formation that recurs at varying intervals of time is not uncommon.

How Do You Differentiate Mammary Duct Ectasia from True Breast Carcinoma?

Since the process does have many of the characteristics of carcinoma, including skin retraction, fixation of the underlying breast tissue and even enlarged axillary lymph nodes, it is important to establish the true diagnosis, because in one instance only adequate drainage is indicated, but in the other a radical mastectomy is imperative. It is also important to decide whether you are dealing with a benign inflammatory process or an inflammatory carcinoma that does not lend itself readily to radical surgery.

For all practical purposes the only way by which *an accurate* differentiation can be made is by biopsy. It is true that many of the cases of mammary duct ectasia that go on to tumor formation do tend to become painful and tender to touch. In general this is not true of carcinoma. This is not a safe guide, however, for occasionally a malignant tumor will necrose and present ample evidence of inflammation. Although it may be practically impossible to tell on gross inspection of the excised specimen whether you are dealing with a carcinoma or duct ectasia, it is usually possible to differentiate the two accurately by frozen section and microscopic examination.

What Are the Pathologic Characteristics of Mammary Duct Ectasia?

Once the specimen is sectioned, many duct ectasias become obvious grossly. Tortuous, cylindrical, wormlike ducts about 5 mm. in diameter are seen to bulge from the white flat surface of the breast stroma. When cut, these enlarged ducts exude on pressure a thick green or yellow putty-like material vaguely resembling toothpaste (Fig. 67–1, *A*).

Microscopically, there is usually a periductal accumulation of leukocytes, chiefly lymphocytes and macrophages. As mentioned above, the duct epithelium either is atrophic or has completely disappeared in places. There may be foci of fat necrosis and fibrosis between ducts. Sometimes pockets of necrosis develop that are surrounded by lymphocytes, giant cells and fibroblasts, and they may form granulomas vaguely resembling tuberculosis (Fig. 67–1, *B*). Caseation necrosis and acid-fast bacilli are lacking, however.

The uninvolved breast usually is atrophic, without many ductules or lobules. Mammary duct ectasia is usually localized to the largest breast ducts close beneath the nipple.

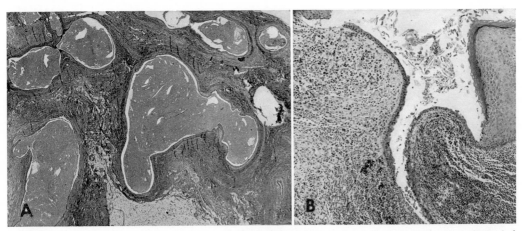

Fig. 67-1.   *A,* In mammary duct ectasia the large ducts beneath the nipple become distended with thick, inspissated secretion. *B,* Inflammation, shown here at the duct outlet onto the nipple, may be severe. It is attributed to leakage of the stagnant secretion through the ectatic duct walls rather than to infection.

How Do You Treat Mammary Duct Ectasia?

Once the diagnosis is established, the principles of treatment follow those established for a carbuncle. If there is no extension into the breast substance, one need only excise the tissue that contains the dilated ducts. When the breast tissue itself is involved, the entire area should be excised with margins well into the normal tissue to ensure a complete removal. Whether it is necessary to establish drainage after excision is a matter of personal preference and custom.

CYSTOSARCOMA PHYLLOIDES

Older women who have neglected a slowly growing rounded tumor of the breast sometimes present with an impressively enlarged mammary gland. On occasion the skin has become so stretched over the tumor that it has ulcerated. At first glance such a patient appears to have an inoperable carcinoma in the last stages of its growth. This may prove to be the case.

Not infrequently, however, such a large tumor proves to be a cystosarcoma phylloides. The term is ominous and misleading, since the mass is neither cystic, sarcomatous nor phylloid—meaning leaflike. Actually, pathologic examination will show an overgrown fibroadenoma, and some writers would prefer to rename this condition giant intracanalicular fibroadenoma—a much more accurate if less picturesque term.

What Is the Clinical Picture of Cystosarcoma Phylloides?

The presence of a slowly enlarging spherical solid breast tumor over a prolonged period of time is perhaps most characteristic. The breast is movable on the chest wall,

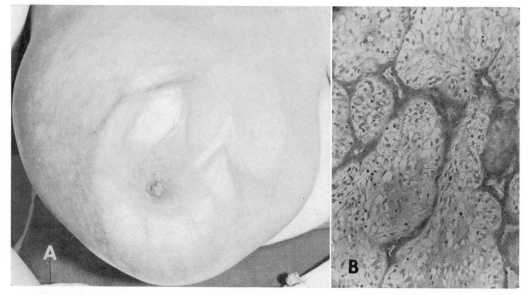

Fig. 67-2. *A,* An extremely bulky breast tumor with stretching and atropy of the overlying skin proved pathologically to be a giant fibroadenoma (cystosarcoma phylloides). *B,* Microscopically, the edematous and cellular intrinsic stroma of the breast has proliferated and crowded the adenomatous ductular epithelium. This is the usual appearance of a benign cystosarcoma phylloides.

and unless the overlying skin is extremely stretched, it is movable over the tumor. In view of the impressive size of the tumor and the likelihood of local skin damage and ulceration over it, axillary lymph nodes are enlarged slightly or not at all (Fig. 67–2, *A*).

Although, with a carcinoma of this size, a loss of appetite and weight would be expected, with a cystosarcoma the patient's general health remains good and in fact robust. One marvels that such a healthy woman could be so obtuse as to allow a breast mass to develop to the size of a baseball or a volleyball before doing anything about it.

What Does Cystosarcoma Phylloides Look Like Pathologically?

On section of the tumor it is clear that there has been a complete restricting fibrous capsule surrounding it, because the cut tumor bulges, and soft finger-like masses of pale fibrous tissue unfold and project from the cut surface. These were likened to leaves by the pathologists who named the tumor "phylloides." In the literature some spell it without the "i," but several Greek physicians have assured us that the proper spelling is "phylloides."

Any hardness of an intact cystosarcoma is lost on sectioning, and the consistency becomes that of a fibroadenoma or adenofibrosis. There is no fluid content in this solid tumor.

Microscopically, cystosarcoma phylloides differs from an ordinary benign fibroadenoma mainly in having a more abundant, edematous-appearing stroma. The loosely arranged, overgrown intrinsic breast stroma produces lumps and nodules covered by ductal epithelium and myoepithelial cells (Fig. 67–2, *B*). The architectural pattern formed is the same as that which characterizes the benign fibroadenoma with an irregular arborization of ducts compressed by intracanalicular and pericanalicular overgrowths of breast stroma. No anaplasia or invasion is found. Pressure necrosis or ischemic degenerative changes may occur locally in a cystosarcoma, sometimes with hemorrhage, hyaline degeneration, microcysts or calcification that develop secondarily.

A small percentage, 1 or 2 per cent of cystosarcomas, are actually malignant. Usually it is the stromal element that is invasive and grows with the appearance of a myxosarcoma or fibrosarcoma. Anaplasia of the malignant stromal cells is obvious, and there may be blood vessel invasion. This cancer may be called malignant cystosarcoma phylloides, but this can be confusing. Perhaps the term "adenosarcoma of breast" arising in cystosarcoma phylloides is to be preferred.

What Is the Treatment of Cystosarcoma Phylloides?

Once the diagnosis has been made by biopsy and frozen section, simple excision of a cystosarcoma phylloides is the treatment of choice. Since the tumor may involve practically the whole breast, a simple mastectomy may be required.

Because of its rarity, a cystosarcoma may catch both the surgeon and the pathologist unaware. On frozen section the benign, proliferating, edematous stroma may look suspicious, and the pathologist would not be certain whether the cystosarcoma was benign or malignant. Because of the tumor size, possible skin ulceration, and the uncertainty of diagnosis on frozen section, the surgeon may decide that it is wiser to proceed with a radical mastectomy and axillary dissection. Actually, even the malignant cystosarcoma, or adenosarcoma, rarely metastasizes to lymph nodes.

One would hope that, with a wider appreciation that cystosarcoma phylloides usually is only a giant benign fibroadenoma, less radical surgical breast excisions for this rare condition might be practiced. The cure rate is practically 100 per cent if the cystosarcoma is completely excised, and axillary lymphadenectomy generally is not necessary.

OTHER BENIGN SOFT TISSUE TUMORS OF THE BREAST

Soft tissue tumors of the breast are relatively rare and may occur at any age. Older women occasionally have one of these uncommon neoplasms.

Since fat is the principal component of breast tissue, it is not surprising that *lipomas* may occasionally be found. They tend to appear as solitary tumors and are completely symptom-free. Their size depends on the length of time they have been present. When they become sufficiently large, the patient becomes concerned and finally consults her physician. There should be little confusion in diagnosis, since on gross palpation these tumors tend to be encapsulated and are freely movable within the breast tissue. They are firm rather than hard and never produce skin retraction. At times the actual outline of the tumor may not be distinct, because they tend to blend into the surrounding fatty tissue of the breast; nevertheless a definite capsule is immediately apparent when the breast is surgically explored. The only problem in differential diagnosis at the time operation is performed is the possibility that the patient has one of the rarer forms of sarcoma such as adenosarcoma. If there is any doubt about the gross appearance of the tumor, frozen section will provide the correct diagnosis. If it is simply a benign lipoma, the tumor may be enucleated, but if it is a sarcoma, at least a wider section of normal breast tissue should accompany the local excision.

On rare occasions some of the epithelial glandular elements may be found within a predominantly fatty tumor. These benign neoplasms are called *adenolipomas*. Since smooth muscle is normally present in the erectile tissue of the nipple, an occasional *leiomyoma* may appear in the areolar area. Equally rare are the *myoblastoma*, *rhabdomyoma* and the *smooth-muscle tumors* that appear deep in the breast substance. Here leiomyomas probably take origin from blood vessels.

PAGET'S CARCINOMA OF THE BREAST

Paget's disease of the breast, as already briefly discussed, is a rather unusual and specialized form of intraductal carcinoma, characterized by an inflammatory response in the nipple and surrounding areola that closely simulates chronic eczema. For this reason it can be a dangerous form of carcinoma, since there is a large delay factor, to which both the patient and the physician contribute. Unless there is a high index of suspicion, its true carcinomatous nature may be long overlooked. Nearly 50 per cent will have positive lymph nodes by the time of radical mastectomy and axillary node dissection. The over-all prognosis is somewhat less favorable than for other forms of intraductal carcinoma.

What Does a Typical Lesion of Paget's Disease of the Nipple Look Like?

Paget's disease of the nipple has many of the characteristics of a chronic eczema.

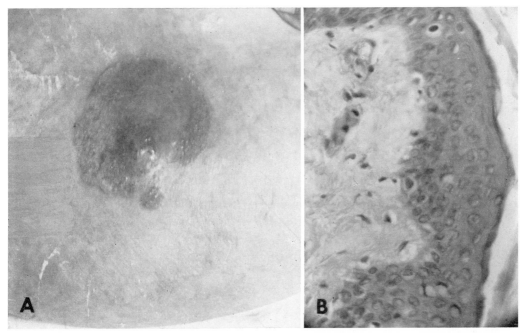

Fig. 67-3. *A,* Paget's disease of the nipple is a superficial, spreading duct carcinoma within the skin of the nipple and areola that masquerades as a dermatitis. *B,* Individual clear cells in the epidermis are the pagetoid cells of intraepithelial carcinoma. Special stains show that they contain PAS-positive mucoprotein, indicative of their ductal origin.

The entire process appears raw, strawberry-red with a granular base where the superficial epithelium has been denuded. The maceration and profuse serous discharge that accompany it keep the area moist, soft and covered with crusts and scabs. The entire lesion seems to be limited to the nipple and surrounding areola, with only rare instances of spread to the adjacent skin (Fig. 67–3, *A*). At times bacterial infection is superimposed on the underlying lesion and produces tissue necrosis. As a result the true nature may be masked by fissures and ulcerations.

There is nothing, then, about the appearance of the lesion that should ordinarily arouse suspicion that the underlying cause is not a localized dermatitis, but carcinoma. The physician should keep in mind that dermatitis of the nipple, without manifestation elsewhere on the body, is extremely rare and far less common than Paget's type of carcinoma.

Why Is the Diagnosis of Paget's Carcinoma Missed So Frequently?

Paget's disease of the nipple, which is fundamentally another form of intraductal carcinoma, should be the easiest of all carcinomas to diagnose and treat. It produces symptoms, such as burning and itching, distressing enough that the patient is bound to be aware of the fact that something is wrong with the nipple. She is simply not cognizant of its sinister significance. There is a strong resemblance between Paget's carcinoma of the nipple and carcinoma of the vulva in the patient's and physician's attitudes. Neither carcinoma is silent, and both produce lesions that can be seen and felt, yet both are about as badly diagnosed and treated as any carcinoma anywhere. The average delay in diagnosis of fifteen months is approximately twice as long as for several other forms of carcinoma, and the number of missed diagnoses is twice as great as for other cancer sites.

The patient is not alert to the possibility of carcinoma, but the physician should be, yet he continues to treat the lesion with salves, ointments and frequently even cauterization without ever resorting to a biopsy. Not only is the general practitioner guilty of this form of procrastination, but also the dermatologist and the surgeon frequently make the same mistake. The true diagnosis is suspected only when the lesion fails to heal. Paget's disease is notoriously resistant to local treatment. If epithelialization ever occurs, it does not persist.

What Is the Differential Diagnosis?

There are three main objectives in considering the differential diagnosis between Paget's disease of the nipple and the other entities that may imitate it. We must (1) establish whether the erosion is a benign dermatologic lesion, (2) distinguish between benign intraductal papilloma and intraductal carcinoma, and (3) decide whether the carcinoma is primarily intraductal or whether the nipple has become involved because of skin extension of carcinoma from a mass in the breast, rather than solely via the duct system.

Erosion Due to Dermatologic Lesions.   There are several clinical observations which will help in distinguishing between a simple erosion of dermatologic nature and Paget's type of carcinoma.

1. A benign dermatitis tends to spread rapidly to involve the whole areola and often the surrounding skin, in contrast to Paget's carcinoma, which is a chronic process that tends to limit itself to the area of the nipple and areola. Months may go by before an erosion of the Paget's type involves much of the nipple.

2. The location and extent of the lesion help in distinguishing between the two. If the erosion involves only the nipple epithelium, the lesion is *carcinoma*. Conversely, when the erosion is present in the areola and surrounding skin, but not in the nipple, you are generally dealing with a dermatologic entity, not carcinoma.

3. Benign dermatologic processes do not destroy the nipple, but carcinoma, if it is extensive enough, will produce nipple destruction. In the early phases of its development carcinoma does not disturb the nipple, which continues to be of a normal contour and mobility. It is only in the later stages that this point of distinction is of value. The surgeon must also be careful to distinguish between a chronically inverted nipple with maceration or discharge and Paget's carcinoma. The former will clear up rapidly when everted and cleaned, the latter will not.

4. An erosion based on dermatologic cause will respond readily to treatment, but Paget's carcinoma will resist all forms of treatment.

Benign Intraductal Papilloma.   At times a benign intraductal papilloma may take origin in the terminal ducts within the nipple and extrude itself out onto the surface of the nipple as a red, fragile, weeping lesion that bleeds easily on trauma. The appearance of such a lesion may closely simulate the nipple erosion seen in Paget's carcinoma. There is one point of difference. In most patients who have a benign intraductal papilloma a firm nodule can be seen and felt in the nipple itself. This is not true of early Paget's disease. Later in its development the Paget's erosion may be accompanied by tumor formation.

Secondary Invasion of Nipple by a Carcinoma Elsewhere in the Breast. In most the nipple in Paget's carcinoma does not change in its physical characteristics or mobility. It continues to be erect and mobile. When the nipple retracts and its base broadens, then an ordinary invasive carcinoma arising in other parts of the breast likely has extended to the subareolar area and involved the nipple.

How Is the Final Diagnosis Established?

The final, unequivocal diagnosis of Paget's type of carcinoma of the breast is made by biopsy. As already mentioned, large pale cells containing prominent, irregular nuclei with occasional mitoses, lying in the epidermis either singly or in clumps, are typical and pathognomonic of Paget's carcinoma.

The more experienced you are clinically with oncologic problems, the more you biopsy and the less you rely on your clinical astuteness. Since benign erosions of the nipple area are uncommon in the absence of dermatologic disease elsewhere, every such lesion, however small or unpretentious it may seem, should be biopsied under local anesthesia when the patient is first seen in the office or clinic. In this manner a definite working diagnosis is established. This is important for two reasons: (1) If it is Paget's carcinoma, a radical mastectomy with lymph node dissection is usually indicated. (2) If it is a benign erosion, a radical surgical procedure is avoided.

Pathologic Criteria of Paget's Disease of the Nipple

As we have discussed, Paget's carcinoma is diagnosed histologically by finding so-called Paget cells in the epidermis of the nipple. They occur singly or in groups of two or three cells within the epithelium of the skin. Since the Paget's carcinoma cells are larger, rounder and paler than normal epidermal epithelium, they look definitely out of place. By their anaplastic variations in nuclear size, shape and chromatin content Paget cells can be identified as carcinomatous. When stains for mucus or glycogen are used, Paget cells often are found to contain these substances, as evidence of their glandular origin. This glycoprotein content explains why the cytoplasm ordinarily has a clear, pale appearance with routine stains (Fig. 67–3, *B*).

Usually the large ducts beneath the nipple will show either an intraductal carcinoma in continuity with the nipple lesion, or discontinuous foci of Paget cells within uninvolved duct-lining epithelium. At times an invasive breast carcinoma of the usual appearance is found deeper in the breast.

Sometimes Paget's carcinoma of the nipple has a sluggish course. A few patients were apparently cured years ago by excision of the nipple and areola. In one case Paget's cells persisted in the skin around the scar of such a local operation for at least eight years without any clinical or pathologic evidence of further growth. Unfortunately, more often Paget's disease of the breast involves a carcinoma of greater than average malignancy.

What Are the Origin and Nature of Paget's Carcinoma?

Paget's disease is fundamentally an intraductal carcinoma. The surgeon should not make the mistake of assuming that the carcinoma is confined to the terminal portion of the duct system alone, for in most instances this tumor has multicentric points of origin. It is frequently found in the ducts deep in the substance of the breast and appears not in one but in many ducts. If one of these areas happens to be close to the nipple, the epidermis of the nipple becomes involved, and an erosion appears.

On the other hand, one of the intraductal lesions deep in the breast tissue may break through into the supporting stroma and behave like any other infiltrating carcinoma of the breast. The latter occurrences are far more common and much more malignant. In the early phase of its development, before the cancer has extended into the main portion of the breast and produced gross tumor formation, the existence of any deep lesion may be entirely unsuspected in a large breast. The surgeon may then be trapped into performing a local excision of the tumor or simple amputation of the breast when a radical mastectomy with axillary lymph node dissection is really called for. Surprisingly enough, axillary metastases are found in nearly half of these patients.

There are two types of Paget's carcinoma that are recognizable clinically: (1) Intraductal carcinoma is present, confined to the ducts of the nipple with extension only to the epidermis of the nipple and the areola. The clinical symptoms are simply burning, itching, and nipple discharge, and the presenting sign an erosion.

2. Carcinoma is present in the ducts of the nipple, but a gross tumor is also present, indicating that the deeper ducts and stroma are involved as well. This group is ten to fifteen times more common than an intraductal carcinoma appearing clinically only in the nipple.

There has been some pathologic controversy about the direction of spread taken by intraductal carcinomas of the Paget type. Paget originally made the observation that nipple erosion generally precedes the appearance of an obvious tumor. The assumption was then made that the deeper lesions appeared because the tumor extended down into the duct system. In all probability this is incorrect, and multicentric ductal carcinomatous foci that spread upward provide the true explanation.

What Is the Proper Treatment of Paget's Carcinoma?

It is obvious from the preceding discussion that radical mastectomy with axillary lymph node dissection is ordinarily the only logical treatment for Paget's carcinoma. Multiple malignant foci occur too frequently to justify a local excision. Simple mastectomy is not enough, because 60 per cent of patients with more than one intraductal carcinoma in the breast will have axillary metastases. Radiation should not be used, for it may mask the growth of the deep-seated lesion while it is controlling the superficial cancer.

The prognosis is excellent if the patient has an erosion of the nipple without a palpable tumor. When gross tumor is present and the axillary lymph nodes are positive, the clinical cure rate varies from 30 to 45 per cent. Without the usual element of delay the prognosis for the majority of cases should approach the respectable salvage figure of 67 per cent that Haagensen has obtained when Paget's carcinoma is confined to the nipple.

MUCINOUS CARCINOMA OF THE BREAST

Because of its sluggish behavior in older women, usually in their sixties and seventies, mucinous carcinoma of the breast constitutes a separate clinical and pathologic entity. Many otherwise ordinary breast carcinomas will contain foci of mucin-secreting epithelium, evident either grossly or microscopically, or both. These tumors behave clinically like other breast cancers, and it is not this subtype of breast carcinoma to which we refer.

What Is the Clinical Appearance of Pure Mucinous Carcinoma?

When an older woman, probably over sixty years of age, has a mass in the breast that grows slowly and progressively, mucinous carcinoma is a possibility. Usually the tumor is not well demarcated, and it may be attached to the skin or pectoral muscle, or to both. Axillary lymph nodes typically are not enlarged.

To the extent that the history and physical examination help to make a diagnosis, the problem involved is one of a mass in the breast, probably malignant.

How Does the Pathologic Picture Differ from That of Other Breast Carcinomas?

When it is biopsied, the mucinous carcinoma has a sticky, wet, mucoid or colloid appearance. This may or may not be obvious grossly, but microscopically the bulk of the tumor is seen to consist of lakes and pools of mucus secreted by carcinoma cells. The malignant epithelium may form some glands filled with mucus, but more often nests of dark-stained small carcinoma cells lie surrounded by extensive collections of mucinous secretion (Fig. 67-4).

The entire tumor may have a rounded, medullary appearance or be rather dense and fibrous grossly. It is important to remember that the pure mucinous carcinoma produces mucus through its entire mass, not just focally, if any accurate clinicopathologic distinction is to be made.

Characteristically, a genuine mucinous carcinoma of the breast involves the axillary lymph nodes either late in its course or not at all. Its growth activity appears deficient.

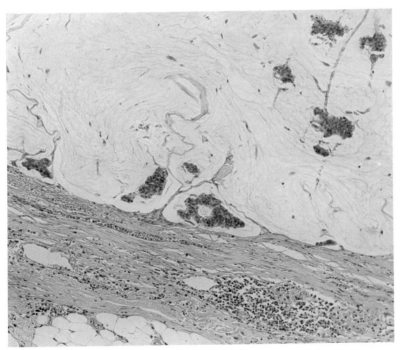

Fig. 67-4.   Cancer cells in a mucinous carcinoma of the breast lie in small groups, surrounded by masses of faintly basophilic mucoid secretion. Invasive activity may be sluggish, both clinically and pathologically.

What Is the Therapy of Mucinous Carcinoma?

If the surgeon and the pathologist are in agreement that a true mucinous carcinoma, or what was once called a "colloid carcinoma," is present, it is justifiable to consider leaving the axillary contents and proceeding with a sufficiently wide local excision of the cancer in an aged patient of dubious physical condition to undergo more radical surgery. This is practically the only breast cancer for which a simple mastectomy in the hope of a cure could ever be justified.

On the other hand, if (*a*) the patient is younger and (*b*) can withstand a radical mastectomy with axillary dissection, or (*c*) there is any doubt as to whether the mucinous secretion is localized or generalized throughout the tumor, the usual therapy for any breast carcinoma had probably better be carried out. Simple mastectomy for a genuine mucinous carcinoma is best reserved for the aged and infirm woman who does not have a long natural life expectancy.

SARCOMAS OF THE BREAST

Although they are not common, a number of different forms of sarcoma appear in the breast. They do not have the same malignant potential as carcinomas, and the treatment often need not be as radical. At most a simple amputation of the breast with removal of the fascia overlying the pectoral and intercostal muscles may be all that is required. The majority will be cured by a wide local excision, leaving the rest of the breast intact.

Fibrosarcoma is the most common malignant tumor of soft tissue origin found in the breast. It may take origin from the skin itself or from the deeper structures in the breast. The latter type of fibrosarcoma appears less well differentiated and has a greater lethal potential. In either case, however, wide local excision is adequate therapy, since the more malignant types metastasize, not through lymphatic channels, but by blood stream invasion. There is no reason to do a radical mastectomy and axillary dissection.

Grossly the fibrosarcoma has a moist, smooth, "fish-flesh" appearance closely resembling a leiomyosarcoma. It is unencapsulated and nonspherical and often has invasive processes that penetrate the nearby fat. Microscopically, the cells are spindly with enlarged, darkly stained nuclei. Giant nuclei and mitoses are common. There is an irregular tumor growth pattern as bands of cells cut across each other in a haphazard manner (Fig. 67–5). Blood vessel invasion may be found.

In the *adenosarcoma* variant of fibrosarcoma, some ducts or cysts are found that suggest that the tumor began as a benign cystosarcoma. Actually, the epithelial component does not appear malignant, and the tumor usually looks and behaves more like a fibrosarcoma.

Liposarcomas appear in other parts of the body and may appear in the breast, where they form sizable tumors. Their true nature is recognized only when they are removed and examined microscopically. Their malignant potential is high, because they tend to be undifferentiated in type and very invasive.

Invasive hemangioendothelial sarcoma, or angiosarcoma, is a rare tumor of vascular origin which can appear in the breast at any age, but usually in younger women in their teens or early twenties. The outward manifestation may simply be a bluish-red discoloration that reflects the vascularity of the tumor felt beneath. It grows rapidly

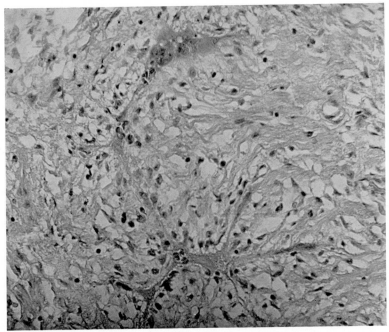

Fig. 67-5. Mammary fibrosarcoma is commonly composed of rather immature myxomatous and collagen-producing spindle cells arranged loosely and irregularly. Nuclear hyperchromatism and cellular anaplasia are usually relatively prominent.

and metastasizes by both blood stream and lymphatic pathways, with the former the more common method of spread. Although this form of sarcoma is usually fatal, a few patients with more highly differentiated lesions have survived for long periods of time.

Usually the tumor invades deeply and disseminates widely without any suggestion of demarcation. An angiosarcoma is usually bulky without limiting factors and appears as a mass of soft pale gray or red tissue, not unlike brain in its appearance. Because of its size it usually undergoes central degeneration as the tumor outruns its blood supply.

Microscopically atypical, large anaplastic endothelial cells are easily recognized. The tumor cells line vessels filled with blood. At times there may be some difficulty in distinguishing between a hemangioendothelial sarcoma and a fibrosarcoma or leiomyosarcoma. When masses of anaplastic endothelial cells appear within and line the lumens of blood vessels, there is no question of the diagnosis.

The treatment, whether it be by surgery or irradiation, is not very effective, because the tumor spreads too widely and too fast. Simple mastectomy offers as much chance of cure as a radical mastectomy with node dissection.

Postmastectomy Lymphangiosarcoma

After a radical mastectomy for breast carcinoma, women who suffer from persistent lymphedema of the arm as a complication occasionally develop years later reddish-blue tumor masses in and beneath the skin of the edematous extremity. The nodules resemble benign capillary hemangiomas at first, but they progress, enlarge, coalesce and become larger and more necrotic. This is a form of sarcoma not unlike Kaposi's sarcoma of the skin. Eventually the patient succumbs to lung metastases.

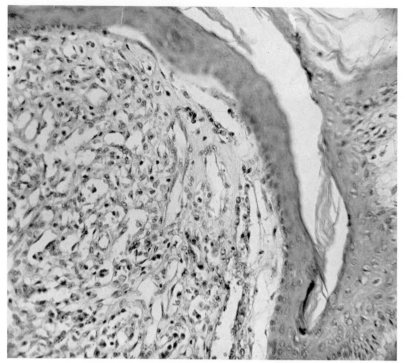

Fig. 67-6.   A lymphangiosarcoma that developed years after a radical mastectomy for carcinoma, in the dermis of the chronically edematous arm.

Microscopically, the lesions are primarily spindle cell in type, very cellular, and show most of the characteristics of a fibrous endotheliosarcoma (Fig. 67–6). Tumor cells are seen lining lymphatic spaces, instead of blood vessels as in Kaposi's sarcoma and hemangiosarcoma.

Any treatment offered must be radical. Nothing short of an interscapular-thoracic amputation of the arm is likely to do any good surgically. A few cases have been noted to respond to radiation therapy. There is something of a paradox here, because some of the patients who have postmastectomy lymphangiosarcoma have already had irradiation of the axilla and operative areas after their original operation. In all probability lymphangiosarcoma arises because of the long-standing edema of the arm. Of course, radiation reaction may be followed by the development of skin carcinomas and sarcomas, as well as by osteogenic sarcomas, but it does not seem to be the cause of postmastectomy lymphangiosarcoma.

REFERENCES

Mammary Duct Ectasia

Adair, F. E.: Plasma Cell Mastitis—A Lesion Simulating Mammary Carcinoma. A Clinical and Pathologic Study with a Report of Ten Cases. *Arch. Surg.*, 26: 735, 1933.

Bloodgood, J. C.: The Clinical Picture of Dilated Ducts beneath the Nipple Frequently to Be Palpated as a Doughy Wormlike Mass—Varicocele Tumor of the Breast. *Surg., Gynec. & Obst.*, 36: 486, 1923.

Manoil, L.: Plasma Cell Mastitis. Am. J. Surg., 83: 711, 1952.

Tice, G. I., Dockerty, M. B., and Harrington, S. W.: Comedomastitis. A Clinical and Pathologic Study of Data in 172 Cases. *Surg., Gynec. & Obst.*, 87: 525, 1948.

Cystosarcoma

Cooper, W. G., Jr., and Ackerman, L. V.: Cystosarcoma Phylloides, with a Consideration of Its More Malignant Variant. *Surg., Gynec. & Obst.*, 77: 279, 1943.
Lester, J., and Stout, A. P.: Cystosarcoma Phyllodes. *Cancer*, 7: 335, 1954.
Nelson, H. M.: Case Report of Cystosarcoma Phyllodes. *Ca*, 9: 98, 1959.
Rogers, J. C. T.: Benign Tumors of the Breast. *Illinois M.J.*, 114: 166, 1958.
Ross, D. E.: Cystosarcoma Phyllodes (Giant Intracanalicular Myxoma). *Am. J. Surg.*, 84: 728, 1952.
Treves, N., and Sunderland, D. A.: Cystosarcoma Phyllodes of the Breast: A Malignant and Benign Tumor. A Clinicopathological Study of Seventy-Seven Cases. *Cancer*, 4: 1286, 1951.

Benign Soft Tissue Tumors

Craig, J. M.: Leiomyoma of the Female Breast. *Arch. Path.*, 44: 314, 1947.
Haagensen, C. D., and Stout, A. P.: Granular Cell Myoblastoma of the Mammary Gland. *Ann. Surg.*, 124: 218, 1946.
Tedeschi, C. G.: Mammary Lipoma. *Arch. Path.*, 46: 386, 1948.

Paget's Disease of Breast

Cheatle, G. L., and Cutler, M.: Paget's Disease of the Nipple. Review of Literature, Clinical and Microscopic Study of Seventeen Breasts by Means of Whole Serial Sections. *Arch. Path.*, 12: 435, 1931.
Colcock, B. P., and Sommers, S. C.: Prognosis in Paget's Disease of the Breast. *S. Clin. N. Amer.*, 34: 773, 1954.
Congdon, G. H., and Dockerty, M. B.: Malignant Lesions of the Nipple Exclusive of Paget's Disease. *Surg., Gynec. & Obst.*, 103: 185, 1956.
Culberson, J. D., and Horn, R. C., Jr.: Paget's Disease of the Nipple. Review of 25 Cases, with Special Reference to Melanin Pigmentation of "Paget's" Cells. *Arch. Surg.*, 72: 224, 1956.
Dockerty, M. B., and Harrington, S. W.: Preclinical Paget's Disease of the Nipple. *Surg., Gynec. & Obst.*, 93: 317, 1951.
Haagensen, C. D.: *Diseases of the Breast.* Philadelphia, W. B. Saunders Company, 1956.
Inglis, K.: Paget's Disease of the Nipple, with Special Reference to the Changes in the Ducts. *Am. J. Path.*, 22: 1, 1946.
Jones, D. B.: Florid Papillomatosis of the Nipple Ducts. *Cancer*, 8: 315, 1955.
McGregor, J. K., and McGregor, D. D.: Paget's Disease of the Breast; 20 Year Survey of Cases Presenting at a Large General Hospital. *Surgery*, 45: 562, 1959.
Nichols, F. C., Dockerty, M. B., and Judd, E. S.: Florid Papillomatosis of the Nipple. *Surg., Gynec. & Obst.*, 107: 474, 1958.
Quero, R., and Maso, C.: A Rapid Method, Useful in the Differential Diagnosis of Paget's Disease of the Nipple. (Cytological Procedure.) *J. Invest. Dermat.*, 31: 307, 1958.

Mucinous Carcinoma

Foote, F. W., Jr., and Stewart, F. W.: Histologic Classification of Carcinoma of the Breast. *Surgery*, 19: 74, 1946.
Frantz, V. K.: Prognostic Significance of Intracellular Mucicarminophilic Material in Carcinoma of Female Breast. *Am. J. Cancer*, 33: 167, 1938.
Saphir, O.: Mucinous Carcinoma of the Breast. *Surg., Gynec. & Obst.*, 72: 908, 1941.

Sarcomas of Breast

Adair, F. E., and Herrmann, J. B.: Sarcoma of the Breast. *Surgery*, 19: 55, 1946.
Barber, K. W., Jr., Harrison, E. G., Clagett, O. T., and Pratt, J. H.: Angiosarcoma of the Breast. *Surgery*, 48: 869, 1960.

Botham, R. J., MacDonald, J. R., and Clagett, O. T.: Sarcoma of the Mammary Gland. *Surg., Gynec. & Obst.*, 107: 55, 1958.

Cahn, M. M., Aaronson, L., and Beerman, H.: Differential Diagnosis of Tumors Involving the Skin of the Breast. *GP*, 20: 154, 1959.

Kay, S.: Lymphosarcoma of the Female Mammary Gland. A.M.A. *Arch. Path.*, 60: 575, 1955.

McClanahan, B. J., and Hogg, L., Jr.: Angiosarcoma of the Breast. *Cancer*, 7: 586, 1954.

Stephenson, S. E., Jr., and Byrd, B. F., Jr.: Malignant Melanoma of the Breast. *Am. J. Surg.*, 97: 232, 1959.

Lymphangiosarcoma

Hall-Smith, S. P., and Haber, H.: Lymphangiosarcoma in Postmastectomy Lymphoedema. (Stewart-Treves Syndrome.) *Proc. Roy. Soc. Med.*, 47: 174, 1954.

Stewart, F. W., and Treves, N.: Lymphangiosarcoma in Postmastectomy Lymphedema. A Report of Six Cases in Elephantiasis Chirurgica. *Cancer*, 1: 64, 1948.

Chapter 68

Carcinoma of the Endometrium

THE PROBLEMS pertaining to the etiology, diagnosis and treatment of carcinoma and other malignant neoplasms of the endometrium differ materially from those of carcinoma of the cervix, despite the fact that the two cancers arise in the same organ, although in different locations. Although many physicians have, in recent years, been very much interested in the early detection of and therapy for cervical cancer, the same cannot be said of endometrial cancer. For some reason gynecologists have been complacent in their attitude toward carcinoma of the endometrium, for it is felt that we handle the problem rather well. This is probably because we have come to believe that (a) cancer of the uterine fundus is encountered less often than cervical cancer, (b) it has a less lethal potential, and (c) treatment can be carried out by surgeons who have had no special training in the surgery of malignant disease with a far higher chance of cure than in cervical cancer.

All these factors are in part true, but a close scrutiny of the over-all cure rate for all types of endometrial cancer, in both the favorable and unfavorable categories, should make us less confident of our ability to cure. Since the incidence of endometrial cancer appears to be on the increase, it is extremely important that we appraise the management of endometrial cancer with a critical eye.

It is true that cancer of the endometrium has a different growth pattern, which progresses less rapidly and is less lethal than cervical cancer. This is partly because the endometrial cavity is surrounded by thick myometrial walls that tend to restrict cancer spread. The favorable factors, however, are more than balanced by the facts that (a) cancer of the endometrium grows in a location where it can be neither seen nor felt, (b) the symptoms are not pathognomonic, and (c) diagnostic aids such as the vaginal smear are of much less help. An early diagnosis can be made only when there is a high index of suspicion which encourages the surgeon to sample the endometrium, by either endometrial biopsy or curettage.

Owing partly to the apparent increase in incidence, but more to expanding interest in the role of hormones in the etiology of endometrial carcinoma, the clinician and the pathologist are becoming more actively concerned with the many fascinating problems that it presents. The surgeon has begun to question the standard methods of therapy previously outlined for carcinoma of the endometrium. Gradually we gynecologists are becoming aware that we should not remain satisfied with our management of this type of uterine cancer.

What Is the Present Incidence of Endometrial Carcinoma?

In the past, the ratio of cancer of the cervix to cancer of the endometrium was usually placed at eight to one. Today this disparity in incidence has practically disappeared. There has been a gradual but steady change in the United States over the last twenty years. In the mid 1940's the ratio was about 5 to 1, dropping approximately to 3 to 1 in most clinics in the early 1950's. At present the relative incidence is slightly less than two to one. Randall, in a recent report, states that in upper New York state, where accurate statistics are kept, at the present time 23 women per 1000 are now suffering cervical cancer as opposed to 17 per 1000 women who have endometrial cancer. Thus 4 out of every 100 women will at some time during their life have carcinoma of either the fundus or cervix. This experience is a general one.

In the future we may look to a steady increase, rather than a decline, in the number of patients who will be found to have cancer in the uterine fundus, since more women now survive to the age when it commonly occurs. Corscaden has noted that though the population of New York City doubled between 1900 and 1940, the number of persons over the age of 65 quadrupled. We must therefore heighten our index of suspicion in this group of women, who have minimal symptoms and negligible physical findings, if we are to make the diagnosis early enough in the disease to offer the best possible chance of cure.

At What Age Is Cancer of the Endometrium Apt to Be Found?

Seventy-five per cent of all cases of carcinoma of the endometrium will appear in the years past the menopause. The significance of any sort of bleeding at this time is thereby emphasized. A variety of causes of postmenopausal bleeding exist, but practically four out of every ten women who consult their physician because of the reappearance of vaginal bleeding after one or two years of amenorrhea will have endometrial carcinoma.

The other 25 per cent appear in the reproductive age group. Although adenocarcinoma of the cervix appears in infancy, carcinoma of the endometrium, though reported, is extremely rare in the teen-age adolescent girl. Approximately 2 per cent occur between 20 and 30 years of age, and roughly 5 to 8 per cent appear between the ages of 30 and 40 years. The youngest woman we have seen with cancer of the endometrium was nineteen.

The remainder occur in the forty- to fifty-year age group, in which abnormal bleeding is a more common occurrence. The symptoms are all too frequently explained on a functional basis. In view of (a) the frequency with which carcinoma of the endometrium is noted at this time, and (b) the fact that the peak incidence of carcinoma of the cervix is approximately at forty-five years of age, the first consideration in evaluating any abnormal uterine bleeding in a woman of this age should be the possibility that a cancer may be present.

What Is the Etiology of Endometrial Carcinoma?

One of the things that have prompted a returning and increasing interest in endometrial cancer has been the debatable role that the ovarian hormones, notably estrin, play in its histogenesis.

In the past chronic irritation was believed to be a precursor of the subsequent development of carcinoma within the endometrial cavity. Older writers like Graves were particularly impressed by the fact that many of the patients who had endometrial cancer also had cervical obstruction and particularly pyometra (Fig. 68–1). There seems to be little evidence that such violent intrauterine infections as postabortional or postpuerperal sepsis predispose to endometrial cancer. It is possible that the chronic irritation theory was based on a misinterpretation of the pathologic differences between metaplastic endometrial responses secondary to infection and hyperplastic endometrial reactions to hormonal stimuli.

For the most part the chronic irritation theory has given way to the theory of the role played by overproduction of ovarian hormones, especially estrogen unbalanced by progesterone, in relation to the development of both endometrial hyperplasia and carcinoma.

THE ESTRIN THEORY.   The basis for considering estrin as an etiologic factor partly lies in the observation that hyperplasia of the endometrium is frequently associated with carcinoma. The relation is clearer in the postmenopausal age group, in which 75 per cent of cancer of the endometrium is found. It is in this group that estrin stimulates the endometrium and is usually unopposed by the action of progestin. Preceding the menopause corpora lutea may be present in the ovary of a patient who demonstrates not only an endometrial carcinoma, but also a normal secretory response to hormonal stimulation in the remaining uninvolved portion of the endometrium.

In all probability hyperplasias, excluding adenomatous hyperplasia, in the reproductive period have no particularly intimate relation to carcinoma, but the same entity encountered in the postmenopausal age is more suspect. In view of the relative frequency with which a uterus is stimulated by estrogen, either naturally or synthetically through the use of hormone therapy, and the relative rarity of carcinoma

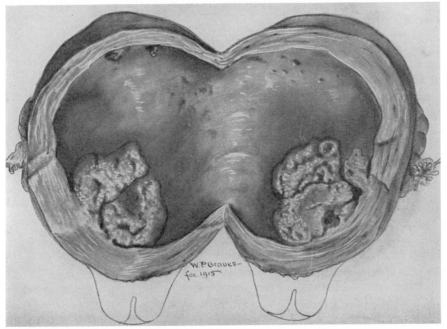

Fig. 68-1.   Drawing of a case of pyometra with distention of the uterine cavity and endometrial carcinoma growing as a papillary mass in the lower segment. (From W. P. Graves: *Gynecology.*)

of the endometrium, it is obvious that the evidence for hyperestrinism as the sole etiologic explanation is unsatisfactory. We must also assume the presence of a properly sensitive substrate that is sensitized and overreacts to estrogenic stimulation.

Clinical Support for the Estrin Theory.   There appears to be considerable evidence on the clinical side that estrin does play an etiologic role. The frequent association of endometrial carcinoma with uterine fibroids and endometrial polyps is well known. Ovarian functioning tumors such as the granulosa cell and theca cell types are thought to secrete estrin and accompany both fibroids and carcinoma of the endometrium with increased frequency. The other typical finding in the endometrium of these patients is hyperplasia. Well documented cases are found in which continued synthetic estrin stimulation was succeeded by a hyperplasia of the endometrium and later carcinoma.

Coexistence of Uterine Fibroids and Endometrial Carcinoma.   There can be little doubt that the two often coexist. Any large series of cases with fibroids will have cancer of the fundus in only 2 to 4 per cent, but approximately 35 per cent of cases with cancer of the endometrium will have associated fibroids in the uterus. The coexistence may be entirely coincidental, for 20 per cent of all women over 30 years old will have fibroids. Where leiomyomas are so commonly found it would be surprising that carcinoma and fibroids did not often coexist.

It may be that the association of fibroid and carcinoma is merely an indication of the uterine growth potential. Given the proper stimulation, both benign and malignant tumors may appear in a susceptible uterus. The source of the stimulation in both instances may be hormonal, and in all probability estrin is implicated. Since only 11 per cent of cases with uterine fibroids have an endometrial hyperplasia, a poor endometrial substrate must be present, relatively speaking. The stimulation, however, may really be more selective for the endometrium than for the cervix in the same uterus, because fibroids occur eight times more frequently with cancer of the endometrium than with neoplasms of the cervix. The importance of the tissue substrate is again apparent when one considers the Negress, in whom carcinoma of the cervix and uterine fibroids are common, though endometrial carcinoma is rare.

Regardless of the etiologic relation, it is well to remember that uterine fibroids and carcinoma do coexist. Abnormal bleeding at the time of the menopause should be considered due to carcinoma and not to a fibroid, lest valuable time be lost in instituting the proper treatment.

Association of Endometrial Cancer with Endometrial Polyps.   The occasional finding of carcinoma with benign endometrial polyps suggests that malignancy may have arisen on the basis of a pre-existing hyperplasia of the endometrium in a uterus subjected to continuous unbalanced estrogenic activity. It is this coexistence, coupled with a history of repeated removal of polyps in a uterus that subsequently develops carcinoma, that has given support to the contention that carcinoma of the endometrium may arise from a pre-existing polyp. Polyps found within the uterus do not have the same malignant potential as those found elsewhere, e.g., in the large intestine, because rarely does a carcinoma arise from a pre-existing polyp. In most instances the base of the polyp is invaded from a carcinoma growing in the adjacent epithelium. Primary carcinoma in a polyp is a rarity mostly found in rather old women.

The coexistence, however, is more than a coincidence, since polyps occur eight times more often with carcinoma than in uteri without malignant disease. Hertig and Sommers reported a case of adenocarcinoma of the endometrium developing in a woman at the age of thirty-nine years, who (*a*) at the age of twenty-nine had a polyp removed that showed cystic hyperplasia, (*b*) at thirty years of age had another polyp excised that showed adenomatous hyperplasia, (*c*) at the time of curettage at age thirty-one showed all transitions from normal glands to adenomatous hyperplasia to frank endometrial carcinoma in situ, and finally (*d*) at the time of hysterectomy had a frankly invasive adenocarcinoma. Other authors have reported repeated instances of the removal of an intrauterine polyp from a patient who subsequently had carcinoma of the endometrium.

The finding of adenomatous hyperplasia at the time of a curettage years before the final diagnosis of invasive cancer has been documented repeatedly. Prior endometrial biopsies have adenomatous hyperplasia in approximately one third of the cases. TeLinde noted that in those cases in which the distinction could not be made histologically with any assurance of accuracy, endometrial carcinoma was later found practically universally and that all who had suspicious pathologic interpretations, but were not operated on thereafter, had full-blown cancers, anywhere from one to twenty-three years later. Hertig and Sommers found that the prior specimens taken within about twelve years from patients who subsequently had carcinoma had some degree of endometrial hyperplasia. The majority of the specimens reviewed that showed adenomatous hyperplasia were taken within five years of the final cancer diagnosis, but some went back as far as twelve years.

Both endometrial polyps and adenomatous hyperplasia should, therefore, be regarded with suspicion—the latter because it may change through gradual stages to become a true adenocarcinoma. Polyps are important because the symptoms of abnormal bleeding may be interpreted as being due to the polyp, while an unrecognized carcinoma exists in the same uterus.

Endometrial Carcinoma and Feminizing Tumors of the Ovary. Increasing numbers of reports are found establishing a relation between functioning tumors of the ovary such as granulosa and theca cell tumors and the appearance of hyperplasia of the endometrium. Since such tumors not only secrete estrogen, but also actually contain it in measurable quantities, as shown by biochemical analysis, it is reasonable to infer that there is a direct relation between estrogenic stimulation, the development of endometrial hyperplasia and probably the later appearance of carcinoma of the fundus. Not all granulosa cell tumors are hormonally active. Many, however, have some theca cell component. The more theca cells there are, the more active the tumors are endocrinologically and the greater the chance of malignancy in the endometrium.

Some authors believe that the association of feminizing tumors and endometrial carcinoma is no more than casual. Most, however, feel that the coexistence is more than one would expect from mere chance. It is generally believed that four fifths of the endocrinologically active granulosa and theca cell tumors will be accompanied by cystic and adenomatous endometrial hyperplasia, and 20 per cent will also have endometrial cancer.

Since the estrogen source in these hormonally active tumors is unopposed by progestin, there appears to be good circumstantial evidence here in support of the estrin theory of causation of some endometrial hyperplasias and carcinomas.

Carcinoma of the Endometrium and Estrin Therapy. Today untold numbers of women are taking estrogenic hormones as replacement therapy for the failing ovary. These women, despite the fact that they have extreme degrees of endometrial hyperplasia to the point that they are sometimes distinguishable with difficulty from microscopic cancer, rarely have true adenocarcinoma of the uterus. Nearly all gynecologists interested in malignant disease can produce, however, one or more cases in which carcinoma has followed the prolonged ingestion of estrin.

The total amount ingested need not be great, for there is experimental evidence that it is the continuity of the dosage rather than its size that is the important consideration. For this reason common clinical practice interrupts estrin therapy for one week out of each month. Small doses over too long a period may produce endometrial carcinoma, based on documentary evidence. But when one considers the myriads of women in the menopausal age group who are regularly exposed to the stimulating effects of this known carcinogen, it is indeed surprising that more cases of carcinoma do not make themselves evident. Thus to make the estrin to hyperplasia to carcinoma theory tenable we must presuppose that a genetic substrate is present which makes these patients more than normally susceptible to the development of endometrial carcinoma.

Experimental Evidence for Estrin as Stimulating Factor.   Support for the estrin theory as the principal etiologic factor in the development of carcinoma of the endometrium is derived chiefly from clinical observations, and until recently obtained little support from the laboratory. A prolonged estrin stimulation will produce both fibroids and a polypoid proliferative hyperplastic endometrium in animals, but carcinoma does not appear in the rat, mouse, guinea pig or monkey uterus after prolonged administration of large amounts of estrin.

Endometrial carcinoma occurs naturally in old rabbits. The tumor arises in the epithelium, spreads by local extension and metastasis and is associated with estrin effects in the cervix, breast and pituitary. By injecting long-acting "depot" estrogen in oil into young rabbits, Meissner and co-workers succeeded in producing several endometrial carcinomas. Not all rabbits treated in this way had cancer; some had only pyometra.

Study of the endocrine glands of these two groups of rabbits showed that the animals in which carcinoma developed had more enlargement of their adrenal glands, ovaries and pituitaries. These animals apparently had overreacted to the injected estrogen to an extent not usually seen. In this respect they showed evidence of the abnormally susceptible tissue substrate also postulated to exist in some women. Both in susceptible rabbits and in women with endometrial carcinomas there were indications of excessive hormonal secretion by the anterior pituitary lobe, adrenal cortex and ovarian stroma, which may have stimulated the development and growth of the carcinomas.

The Relation of Endometrial Hyperplasia to Carcinoma.   The same suggestive but inconclusive evidence is present when one regards hyperplasia as an inevitable and essential precursor of endometrial cancer. Not all pathologists agree as to what constitutes hyperplasia. Some will admit that the uninvolved endometrium with carcinoma of the fundus is stimulated, but will deny that it represents true hyperplasia. The two conditions do coexist and occur naturally together in the presence of functioning ovarian tumors.

Part of the considerable difference of opinion as to the role played by hyperplasia in the development of carcinoma of the endometrium depends upon whether inferences are drawn from data acquired from cases in the reproductive period or in the postmenopausal age group. Carcinoma in younger women may be found in an endometrium that elsewhere has responded normally both to estrogenic and progestational stimulation. The majority of patients with endometrial hyperplasia in the reproductive period manifest changes that have no close resemblance to carcinoma, e.g., the ordinary "swiss cheese" type of *cystic* hyperplasia.

In this same age group there is a small number of women whose endometrium is so abnormal that even the most experienced pathologist is concerned about the malignant possibilities. When hormones have been administered, the diagnostic problems of the pathologist may be magnified. In certain instances the suggestion of malignancy is so strong that practical considerations may call for a hysterectomy. In general, endometrial hyperplasia before the menopause has little obvious significance in relation to cancer development.

After the menopause the finding of endometrial hyperplasia is important. The incidence of endometrial hyperplasia in women with cancer of the endometrium is approximately four times as great as in normal women. It is here that the two conditions coexist, with evidence at times of a gradual transition from one to the other. The difference may be one of degree only. The unopposed action of estrin upon the endometrium may be observed in all stages from a minimal effect in the thin, atrophic endometrium with fibrotic-appearing stroma and moderately dilated cystic atrophic glands to thick, succulent, piled-up glandular epithelium that forms adenomatous glands within an active-appearing stroma. It is in this latter group that borderline cases difficult to classify are found and errors of interpretation may be made. The differences depend on what is interpreted as hyperplasia and as neoplasia.

In general, the finding of hyperplasia of the endometrium in a woman past the menopause should be regarded with grave suspicion.

What Is the Source of the Estrin Stimulation?   Circumstantial evidence exists that hyperplasia of the endometrium is the result of the unopposed action of estrin. In the postmenopausal period, in which the association of hyperplasia and carcinoma is the strongest, ovarian function normally is at its lowest ebb. Actually, carcinoma may be found in the uterus of a patient previously castrated some years before by surgery or irradiation. Once the endometrium has become hyperplastic, primed so to speak by ovarian estrogenic stimulation, other processes can carry the hyperplasia on to carcinoma without further need of ovarian participation. The suggestion has therefore been made that extragenital sources of estrin or other hormonal stimulants may exist, such as the adrenal cortex and pituitary. It is doubtful whether extragenital sources, such as the adrenal cortex, can secrete enough estrin to produce an endometrial hyperplasia, although they may exaggerate a hyperplasia that has already developed.

It is a common clinical observation that most women with endometrial hyperplasia or carcinoma, perhaps as many as 80 per cent, have abnormally active ovaries for their age. In this group there is usually evidence of hyperplasia of the ovarian cortical stroma, with abundant lipoid content, so-called thecomatosis, and occasionally the finding of small granulomas in the cortex that represent a local inflammatory reaction to excess lipoid. Ovarian stroma synthesizes estrogens experimentally in vitro. Stromal hyperplasia is a common finding in patients with endometrial carcinoma in a ratio of better than two to one compared to the noncancerous controls.

Hyperplastic ovarian stroma, when the follicles in the ovary have been exhausted, is the principal source of estrogen secreted postmenopausally (Fig. 68–2). There is some recent evidence that estrin is responsible for endometrial hyperplasia, but that the anterior pituitary and adrenal hormones are essential if endometrial carcinoma is to develop from hyperplasia in a susceptible uterus.

Clinical Evidence to Support the Estrin-Hyperplasia-Carcinoma Concept.   Although the relation between hyperplasia and carcinoma of the endometrium is often not

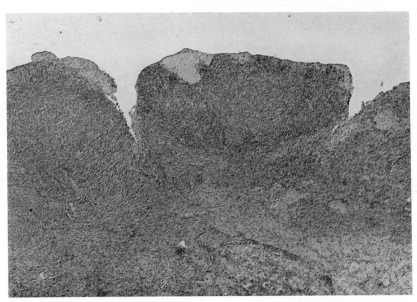

Fig. 68-2.   Nodular cellular masses of hyperplastic ovarian cortical stroma are found in the ovaries of more than 80 per cent of women with endometrial carcinoma. Biochemical, cytologic and pathologic studies indicate this tissue to be a source of postmenopausal estrogen secretion.

obvious clinically, there is ample circumstantial evidence from the clinical side to permit judicious speculation on the role played by estrin. For example, carcinoma of the endometrium does not develop while a woman is having hot flashes, particularly if the vaginal epithelium indicates by its atrophy that estrin deprivation exists. Conversely, vaginal bleeding in a patient who presents symptoms of estrin activity that persist into the menopause is three times more likely to be due to endometrial carcinoma than in her contemporary with an atrophic vaginal epithelium.

LIKELY CANDIDATES FOR ENDOMETRIAL CANCER.   From a consideration of clinical histories and physical findings there appears to be a definite type of woman who may have carcinoma of the body of the uterus. It is not essential that she have all the factors, but when they exist, the chances of endometrial cancer are enhanced.

1.   *Late or Delayed Menopause.*   In all probability the menopause has been prolonged for several years and the periods have been excessive in the woman who has carcinoma of the endometrium. Such a history increases the likelihood of endometrial cancer fourfold. The normal expectancy of continuing the menstrual cycle beyond the age of 50 is approximately 15 per cent, in contrast to the 60 per cent noted for patients with endometrial cancer. Along with the delayed menopause, which on the average occurs about six years later than at the normal age reported in these studies as forty-eight, the patient continues to show some evidence of estrin activity. Approximately one third of these patients will show endometrial hyperplasia on curettage. Hot flashes are absent, and the vaginal epithelium is succulent rather than atrophic.

2.   *Irregular Menstrual Pattern.*   Many patients who have endometrial cancer give a history of an abnormal vaginal bleeding pattern in the past. This is true regardless of the age period at which cancer of the endometrium is discovered. Before the menopause nearly one half will give a past history of excessive menstrual bleeding. In many instances this begins at the menarche when prolonged and profuse bleeding takes place from an anovulatory condition.

Some of these patients show stigmata of the polycystic ovary syndrome. There is a suggestion, though no actual proof, that the polycystic ovary in youth may later become the ovary that shows cortical stromal hyperplasia, which, as already discussed, is frequently associated with endometrial cancer.

The same abnormal menstrual pattern is observed in a review of the past histories of women who demonstrate endometrial carcinoma in the postmenopausal era. In most instances the history will show that one or more diagnostic curettages have been performed for the control of excessive menstrual bleeding. The patient who bleeds heavily at the time of the menopause is far more likely to have an endometrial carcinoma than the patient who either abruptly stopped having monthly menstrual cycles or gradually ceased over a period of months.

In many histories it is revealed that the patient has received intrauterine radium for control of the excessive menstrual bleeding. Usually the carcinoma appears some ten to fifteen years later. One may choose to implicate radiation as the cause of the neoplasia within the uterine cavity, feeling that either it served as the stimulating carcinogenic agent or that cancer developed on a previously irradiated site. It is true that the number of women who have cancer of the endometrium after irradiation is higher than the normal expectancy, but it seems far more likely that the substrate in these patients was wrong from the beginning. The abnormal vaginal bleeding pattern would be an indication of this, and the radiation was not the activating source, but simply a therapeutic agent given to control the hemorrhage in a woman who was probably destined to have uterine adenocarcinoma in any case.

Heredity. The problem of heredity always appears in any discussion of malignant disease, and endometrial carcinoma is no exception. Just as there seems to be a body type present in the patient who has cancer of the fundus, so there also appears to be some familial tendency. We recognize that the menstrual pattern of the daughter tends to repeat that of the mother. If the substrate is wrong in one, it may be passed to the other. Roughly 20 per cent of patients with endometrial carcinoma will have a family background of a similar cancer. Hauser and Weller reported a "cancer family" in which many of the women had endometrial carcinoma and many of the men gastrointestinal cancer.

Obesity. A further suggestion that patients with endometrial cancer may have a particular type of body configuration is the well known observation that these patients tend to be obese. On an average, patients with carcinoma of the endometrium are about 10 per cent overweight, and nearly half of the patients with endometrial cancer will be clearly obese. It is true that women tend to put on weight after the menstrual periods have ceased, but the same tendency is noted earlier in the woman who has endometrial cancer. Not only do these patients seem to be obese, but also they actually look bigger than they are, for they are prone to have small hands and feet with large rounded hips. A woman does not have to be fat to have cancer of the endometrium, but if the physician confronts a woman with a body configuration of this type who is having an abnormal bleeding history, either before or after the menopause, he should be alert to the possibility that she may have endometrial cancer. Corscaden calls these "burgeoning women."

The obesity does not appear by accident, but is rather an indication of a fundamental endocrine imbalance. The heavy, broad-chested, broad-hipped woman who has carcinoma of the endometrium is also apt to have hypertension, diabetes mellitus and arthritis. Between 10 and 20 per cent of patients with endometrial cancer will have clinical diabetes, and over 50 per cent will have a diabetic type of glucose tolerance test. Nearly half will have hypertension, called "endocrine hypertension" by Schroeder. In all probability there is no direct association between hypertension and diabetes, but they do tend to appear together in the patient with cancer of the endometrium, probably because the body types are so similar. Way has written that these medical abnormalities suggest pituitary hyperactivity.

5   *Marital Status and Diminished Fertility.*   In general, patients with endometrial carcinoma marry about as frequently as women in the general population, although some reports find a proportion of unmarried women that runs as high as 25 per cent. This is in contrast to cervical cancer, where over 90 per cent are married.

The percentage of nulliparous married women with carcinoma of the uterine fundus, on the other hand, is in striking contrast to carcinoma of the cervix. Approximately one third of the endometrial cancer patients have never borne a child, and only 40 per cent have more than one. These observations hold true regardless of the age at marriage or when the endometrial carcinoma is discovered. The younger woman who gets endometrial cancer has frequently either had difficulty in getting pregnant or has had problems in bearing a live baby if she does. Few have more than one child. Nulliparous women make up only 10 per cent of patients who have cervical cancer, and the average size of the family approaches three.

The fact that parity does not contribute to the etiology of endometrial cancer as it does in cancer of the cervix, and the infertility factor known to be present, lend support to the contention that the uterine substrate is wrong from the start.

Summary.   Both the delayed menopause and the previous history of an irregular menstrual pattern suggest that estrogenic stimulation is an important, but not the only, factor in the etiology of endometrial cancer. It may be that estrogen sometimes is a carcinogenic agent, but whether opposed by progestin or not it becomes effective only when it acts upon the proper soil. Estrogen may prime the endometrium so that other stimuli result in cancer development. Some such qualifying interpretation is necessary to explain the many incongruities in what is otherwise an acceptable theory. There are, for example, many instances of endometrial hyperplasia, but relatively few women have carcinoma. The obesity, diabetes, hypertension, abnormal vaginal bleeding pattern and the infertility suggest that there is an endocrine imbalance, but they also seem to indicate that the genital substrate is faulty. The kind of woman who acquires a cancer of the endometrium appears to have something in her genes that makes her cancer-susceptible.

What Evidence Is There That Endometrial Cancer Can Develop Independently of Any Estrogenic Stimulation?

There is some clinical evidence that carcinoma can develop from an endometrium that responds cyclically to the rhythmic action of the two principal types of ovarian hormones. In other words, one does not need to have evidence of an endocrine imbalance to explain the appearance of every endometrial cancer. Certainly cancer of the endometrium can be present without any contemporary evidence of stimulation by estrogenic source. Not all the patients who have endometrial cancer have coexistent endometrial hyperplasia, and only a minority of the patients who have endometrial hyperplasia have carcinoma of the endometrium.

A few cases of endometrial carcinoma have occurred in women only recently successfully pregnant, and we have seen one such patient, in whom the uninvolved endometrium appeared to function normally. Also patients with bicornuate uteri have been reported in whom endometrial carcinoma was found in one uterine horn, and a normal pregnancy or cyclic endometrial changes in the other horn. It is clear that some endometrial carcinomas arise from purely localized abnormalities.

THE NATURAL HISTORY OF ENDOMETRIAL CARCINOMA

Carcinoma may arise anywhere in the uterine cavity and in a number of different ways. Commonly it appears where the endometrial lining is the thickest, namely, at the top of the fundus, usually in one cornu. There may be multicentric points of origin, or it may arise in a single isolated area.

How Does Carcinoma Develop within the Endometrium?

The growth pattern of endometrial carcinoma varies widely, both in the nature and the rapidity of its spread. By and large the rate of growth is far less rapid and the carcinoma much less lethal than a cervical cancer. There is a general feeling that as long as the cancer is confined to the endometrium it is relatively less dangerous and is amenable to therapy with a high expectancy of cure. As soon as the myometrial muscle wall becomes involved, it has the same lethal potential attributed to cervical cancer, and when it has spread beyond the confines of the uterus, it is more deadly than carcinoma of the cervix.

Unfortunately we have no way of knowing the site of origin, the nature and mode

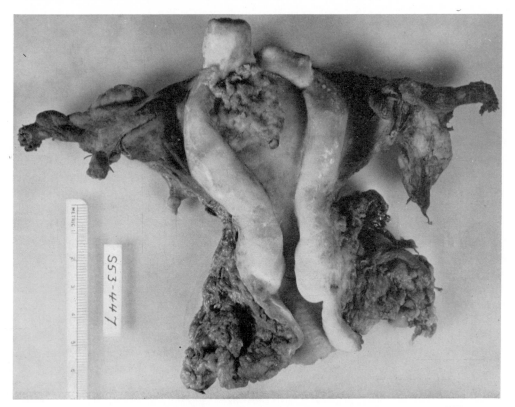

Fig. 68-3. A localized polypoid endometrial carcinoma of the fundus is invading the myometrium at its base.

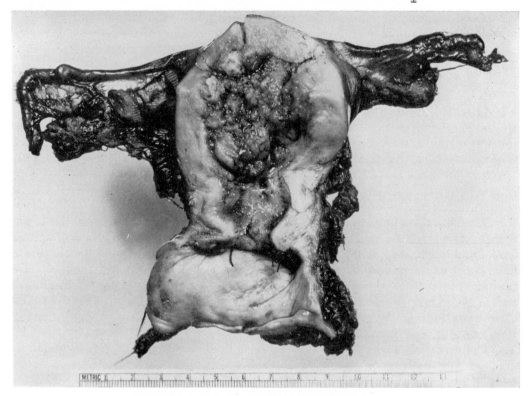

Fig. 68-4.   Diffuse endometrial carcinoma, with polypoid foci and areas of necrosis and hemorrhage, is the most common gross type of uterine adenocarcinoma.

of spread or the degree of invasion until after the uterus has been removed. There are two main growth patterns.

THE CIRCUMSCRIBED TYPE.   This represents the earliest phase of a frank invasive carcinoma within the uterine cavity. A slight thickening of the mucosa grows slowly, forming papillary or polypoid projections sharply demarcated from the rest of the uterine mucosa. Grossly, the lesions appear as flat, velvety, polypoid masses which have a tendency to be pedunculated (Fig. 68–3). Curettage may remove such areas, and the uterus may show no other evidence of carcinoma when it later is removed. Hysterectomy is essential, for curettage, regardless of the size of the lesion, can never be adequate therapy. From the primary site the cancer may do one of two things: (1) It may invade and diffusely infiltrate the myometrium at its point of origin, but with little involvement of the surrounding epithelium. (2) The growth may extend from the primary source as a superficial growth and implicate the rest of the mucosa.

THE DIFFUSE TYPE.   About 50 per cent of all endometrial cancers will involve at least half of the entire mucosa. There seems to be a protective barrier at the internal cervical os, so that the endocervical epithelium is rarely involved unless (a) the cancer has spread by lymphatic channels from a source higher in the uterine cavity, or (b) the cancer takes origin from the lower uterine segment or upper portion of the endocervical canal. Cancers that arise in this area are regarded as a separate entity by some observers. They are called "carcinoma of the corpus and cervix" or adenocarcinoma of lower uterine segment and are given an individual classification, because they are far more lethal than the ordinary fundal carcinoma. Actually, they behave more like a cervical carcinoma. Because of their anatomic location they tend to follow the same pattern of spread beyond the uterus as that taken by cervical cancers.

The diffuse type of endometrial cancer spreads widely through the lining of the uterine cavity, but shows little tendency to invade muscle. In a few instances areas are present that show varying depths of penetration, depending on how long the carcinoma has been present and the growth rate of the tumor. By and large the endometrium is thickened and shaggy in appearance, exhibiting irregularly placed polypoid areas of varying size (Fig. 68–4). Occasionally, superficial ulceration is present, and frank necrosis may occur as the tumor outruns its blood supply. It is amazing how much superficial growth of carcinoma may be present in the endometrial cavity without any myometrial muscle invasion.

Direct invasion of the muscle wall is the earliest serious manifestation of spread of endometrial cancer. This invasion may come from a small focus or be widespread throughout the uterus. Within the uterine wall the lymphatics run horizontally from the endometrium to communicate with a longitudinal network that extends from the fundus to the cervix. These lymphatics drain into collecting channels which form along the lateral sides of the uterus beneath the serosa. Cancer of the endometrium is therefore potentially a disease of the entire uterus. Extension along lymphatic pathways is slow compared with cervical carcinoma.

It is important to remember that the surgeon can obtain little idea of the extent of the carcinoma within the uterus by trying to estimate its size. In many instances fibroids are present within the same uterus, and whether they are present or not the uterus that contains an endometrial carcinoma rarely gets to be as large as a three-month pregnancy.

How Does Cancer of the Endometrium Spread beyond the Uterus?

Extension of the carcinoma beyond the confines of the uterus takes place rather late in its course, along the following channels: (1) lymphatics, (2) fallopian tubes, (3) blood stream, (4) transperitoneal spread.

LYMPHATIC SPREAD.   The route chosen for extension via lymphatic channels depends for the most part on the site and extent of the carcinoma within the uterus. If it arises at the top of the fundus, as it most often does, the lymphatic drainage will disseminate the cancer *along the upper portions of the broad ligaments*. A free anastomosis takes place in the lymphatic channels between the fallopian tube and the hilus of the ovary before proceeding to the lateral aortic lymph nodes on the left and the lateral vena caval lymph nodes on the right, and thence to the kidney regions. Approximately 12 per cent of endometrial cancers will metastasize to the ovary.

From the same primary source the disease may follow *the lymphatics of the round ligaments* to involve the superficial inguinal lymph nodes. This is far less common. When the carcinoma arises in the central portion of the body of the uterus, the lymphatic spread occurs *laterally along the courses of the ureters and uterine vessels* to involve the ureteral, iliac, obturator and hypogastric lymph nodes. The expectancy of such nodal involvement has been placed as high as 25 per cent. Growth in the lower portion of the uterus may be expected to follow the same pathway in its lymphatic spread as cervical carcinoma, but less readily.

Carcinoma arising on the posterior uterine wall may extend into the posterior plexus coursing *along the uterosacral ligaments to communicate with the rectal lymphatics* and thence to the promontory of the sacrum. The possibility of *retrograde lymphatic spread to the cervix and vaginal region* cannot be overlooked. The fact that solitary nodules found along the course of the urethra and multiple areas appearing in the lower part of the vagina are located beneath the vaginal epithelium, usually on the anterior vaginal wall, suggests that these areas represent lymphatic extensions rather than implant metastases. The frequency of their appearance ranges from 6 to 12 per cent.

SPREAD BY FALLOPIAN TUBE.   Cancer cells have been observed in the lumens of the fallopian tubes when muscle invasion has been minimal and lymphatic permeation absent. Implants of endometrial cancer upon the ovary are thus possible. To prevent the possibility of spread of cancer in this manner it is common practice to clamp the tubes as the initial step in abdominal hysterectomy. There is no evidence, however, that tumor cells, displaced into the tubal lumens, implant as cancer. Since many tubal metastases are interstitial or submucosal, it is more logical to assume that cancer of the endometrium reaches the tube and ovary by extension along the lymphatics in the majority of instances.

SPREAD BY BLOOD STREAM.   It is possible that distant metastases to lungs, liver and bones occur by tumor invasion of blood vessels. Extension to the brain has been observed without primary involvement of the lung, perhaps through the azygos vein system and the vertebral veins. It is also possible that tumor cells are dislodged from their primary source and enter the blood stream either at the time of curettage or in handling of the uterus during the course of its surgical removal. The fact that tumor cells are in the general venous system has been documented. It is still debatable whether these groups of cells can implant and form the nucleus of metastases in viscera or in bones.

Experimentally, the chances seem to be greater when showers of cancer cells are discharged. Isolated metastases have been found in lungs and liver years after a total hysterectomy with removal of the adnexa had been performed. Severe back pain has been traced to vertebral body metastases in the absence of local uterine symptoms. Distant metastases from endometrial cancer do not invariably mean an early demise. One of our patients had stationary lung metastases for fourteen years and died of heart disease. This is in keeping with the experience with malignant disease in general and is more understandable in view of the known slow rate of tumor growth in cancer of the uterine cavity.

TRANSPERITONEAL METASTASES.   It is a common clinical observation that once endometrial carcinoma has reached the peritoneum, progression of the course of the malignant disease is accelerated. Subserosal extension of the carcinoma is clinically obvious when multiple, firm white nodules are seen and felt. Rupture of these foci may take place with dissemination of cancer cells throughout the pelvic peritoneum. In this manner the disease tends to involve adjacent structures such as the bladder and rectum. Discrete peritoneal implants are found in more than half of the terminal cases.

What Are the Symptoms of Endometrial Carcinoma?

VAGINAL BLEEDING.   The most important single symptom of endometrial cancer is abnormal uterine bleeding. The nature of the bleeding depends upon the age of the patient at the time the carcinoma develops. Bleeding in some form is present in nearly 100 per cent and appears as the first symptom in approximately 80 per cent of affected women.

The nature of the bleeding varies. It may manifest itself as (1) *irregular vaginal bleeding with a tendency to increasing quantity of flow*. This kind of bleeding is characteristic of the group that develops carcinoma before the menopause. (2) *Irregular vaginal spotting*, usually of no great quantity. It may appear after straining on defecation or voiding. Rarely is it aggravated by coitus or douches. (3) *Minimal vaginal spotting or staining in the postmenopausal period*. This is often intermittent in frequency. (4) *Sudden gushing of blood*, which is not uncommon in the premenopausal age, but is of greater significance after the menopause.

These types of uterine bleeding are well known to the medical profession, yet their significance seems to be sadly overlooked. There is a tendency to explain away the symptoms rather than to investigate the cause. Cancer of the endometrium can be diagnosed only by the symptoms it produces, with confirmation and proof by endometrial sampling. Carcinoma of the fundus is relatively slow growing, but early diagnosis and treatment are reflected in better survival rates just as positively as in cancer anywhere else in the body.

PREMENOPAUSAL BLEEDING. Irregular uterine bleeding, with a tendency to increase steadily in the amount of flow, is common in the years before the menopause. The majority of patients will be found to be bleeding from functional causes. This is the same sort of vaginal bleeding that we encounter at puberty. Bleeding occurs from a proliferative endometrium in the absence of any progestrin influence. Only one in ten will show carcinoma on curettage. Nevertheless 25 per cent of all endometrial cancers appear before the menopause. The common error is to ascribe the uterine bleeding to the presence of a fibroid or an endocrine imbalance. The most important cause is carcinoma. It must be ruled out by curettage before instituting any therapy.

POSTMENOPAUSAL BLEEDING. Vaginal spotting in the postmenopausal age is by far the most common symptom. This may be continuous or intermittent. Because it is small in amount and infrequent in appearance, the patient is lulled into a sense of security by the inconstancy of the symptom and may fail to consult her physician. When this symptom arises one or more years after the menopause, two thirds of the patients will prove to have carcinoma.

Occasionally the patient may experience a sudden severe hemorrhage from the uterine cavity years after the cessation of the menstrual periods. This is sometimes due to other lesions, but carcinoma is the most credible explanation.

Other Causes of Postmenopausal Bleeding. There are other explanations of postmenopausal bleeding than endometrial carcinoma, but it occurs sufficiently often to cling to the old axiom that such bleeding is considered due to carcinoma of the uterus until proved otherwise. *Cancer of the cervix* is the most important condition to rule out, since the treatment designed to cure endometrial cancer is inadequate for cervical neoplasms. Too often the bleeding is explained on the basis of the presence of a *cervical polyp*, *senile vaginitis* or *urethral caruncle*. *Hypertension* is known to produce uterine bleeding. *Functioning tumors of the ovary*, such as the granulosa and theca cell tumors, tend to produce a recurrence of cyclic bleeding after the menopause. Excessive bleeding from a *heavy polypoid endometrium* is occasionally seen in the late menopause. We have seen this at age eighty-three.

The most troublesome type of postmenopausal bleeding follows the use of *hormone therapy*. Estrogenic hormones are widely used for hot flashes or simply to make women "feel better" at the time of the menopause. Bleeding occurs either as a result of prolonged administration or from withdrawal of the estrogenic hormone. The physician falls into the trap of blaming the vaginal bleeding on the use of the drug, without considering that the bleeding may either mask the presence of a carcinoma or perhaps cause it.

Too much estrin therapy is being prescribed for a variety of disorders of the menopause, including vaginal bleeding, without first ruling out the possibility of a pre-existing carcinoma.

A curettage is indicated. Great care must be exercised in the interpretation of endometrium in a patient who has been under estrin therapy. It is in this group that the pathologist is most likely to be confused or to err. The greatest error, however, is neglecting to do the curettage.

VAGINAL DISCHARGE.   Vaginal discharge may precede the onset of bleeding. Its diagnostic significance cannot be stressed particularly, for there are many other entities that may explain it. A clear, watery discharge, however, is important. It frequently comes in bursts after heavy exertion, defecation or micturition. The discharge may be preceded by indefinite cramps as the uterus tries to expel its contents through a stenosed cervical canal. This is particularly true if a *pyometra* is present. A gradual progression to a brownish or blood-tinged vaginal discharge is commonly noted. The secretion becomes malodorous only as tumor within the uterus breaks down and becomes necrotic.

PAIN.   This symptom is difficult to evaluate. Many women will have a sense of pressure and lower abdominal discomfort, particularly if a pyometra or hematometra is present. It is unwise to be guided in the choice of treatment by the symptom of pain. Severe pain does not necessarily indicate that we are dealing with a hopeless or inoperable cancer case. Such pain may be due to carcinoma invading the parametrium, but it is more likely to be secondary to other pelvic lesions that are commonly found with an endometrial cancer. A high percentage of patients who demonstrate extrauterine cancer extension at the time of surgery have no pain at all.

WEIGHT LOSS.   Since carcinoma of the endometrium appears to be relatively slow in its development, the general appearance of the patient does not reflect the extent of the disease. Weight loss is not significant.

ANEMIA.   Though the primary symptom is bleeding, neither blood loss nor the necrosis of the tumor is sufficient to influence the blood picture. Anemia is not a common finding.

What Are the Physical Findings?

The diagnosis of carcinoma of the endometrium is made by histologic confirmation of endometrial samplings, after suspicion has been aroused by the history. Little further information is gained by physical examination. To treat successfully, one should have some idea of how much carcinoma is actually present. This is impossible with cancer of the endometrium. It cannot be seen or palpated. Carcinoma of the endometrium arises within thick myometrial muscle walls in the uterine cavity. Neither the primary site, the nature of the spread nor the degree of invasion can be determined until the entire uterus has been removed.

UTERINE SIZE AND PROGNOSIS.   Attempts have been made to forecast the prognosis of endometrial cancer on the basis of the size of the uterus. Any such correlation is pure chance. A small carcinoma may arise within a uterine cavity that is expanded by the presence of submucous fibroids, which appear in approximately 35 per cent of all uteri containing endometrial carcinoma. The cancer may fill the entire cavity of a small uterus. Rarely does the uterus that contains a fundal cancer increase in size beyond that of a two-month pregnancy.

The fact that these patients are often obese makes an accurate appraisal of uterine size inaccurate if not impossible. The uterus may be fixed by invasion of the parametrial tissues once the tumor has traversed through the uterine wall, but fixation may be secondary to endometriosis or pelvic inflammation in a uterus that also contains an endometrial cancer. Fixation is not indisputable evidence of advanced cancerous disease. When, however, the size of the uterus is correlated with the histology of the carcinoma, there appears to be a somewhat better relation of uterine size to the eventual prognosis.

The general examination is important in outlining therapy. Since endometrial cancer is hormone-dependent, it is not surprising that approximately 4 per cent will have *concomitant cancers primary in the breast or ovary.* Diabetes mellitus and hypertension are handmaids of the obesity. Choice of therapy is influenced by their presence.

Evaluation of the cardiac status is important in the older age group in which endometrial cancer appears, since standard therapy calls for an abdominal hysterectomy. Since blood vessel invasion occurs, evidence of distant metastases should be sought in lungs, bones and liver.

The local examination gives useful information.

VAGINAL INSPECTION.   A suspicious history may gain further support by the finding of a bluish, moist vaginal epithelium that suggests estrin activity in a postmenopausal patient. Retrograde lymphatic extension may take place, and multicentric cancer foci may appear as nodules beneath an intact vaginal epithelium, particularly along the anterior vaginal wall. At times these nodules may ulcerate or produce fungating tumors.

CERVICAL EXAMINATION.   Normally endometrial cancer is confined to the uterine cavity, and it rarely extends below the level of the internal os. Papillary tumor may prolapse through the endocervical canal to present at the external os. If myometrial invasion has occurred, the longitudinal lymphatics may carry the malignant disease to the cervical musculature.

EXAMINATION OF THE UTERUS.   Pliability of the pelvic floor is of particular interest, together with determining the presence or absence of nodular thickenings. The uterine size and mobility should be determined. This can best be done by rectal examination. These observations have greater value in evaluating the operability than in determining the extent of the cancerous disease.

General Observations on Cancer Spread

There is a striking tendency for carcinoma of the endometrium to remain local even in the face of an extensive local malignant process. Postmortem examinations of fatal cases show no involvement of the regional lymph nodes in two thirds of the cases. Necrosis of the carcinoma may produce an inflammatory reaction within the lymphatics and nodes of the parametrium that serves as a check upon the further spread of the cancer. When the main lymphatic channels are involved, however, metastases may be expected in regional lymph nodes and more distally in liver, lungs and bones.

How Is a Diagnosis Made of Endometrial Carcinoma?

Early recognition of cancer of the endometrium is much more difficult than that of cancer of the cervix, for the obvious reason that the lesion can be neither seen nor felt. The symptoms are varied and are not pathognomonic for cancer of the endometrium alone. Physical examination is helpful in determining the presence of associated diseases and remote spread, but it offers little in determining whether a carcinoma is present, or if so how much. The problem is accentuated if the clinical evaluation is carried out before the menopause, largely because abnormal menstrual bleeding from benign causes is common to the younger age group, in which cancer of the uterus also has a significant incidence. The final diagnosis is made only after samples of the endometrial lining have been obtained.

Abnormal vaginal bleeding at any age should arouse suspicion of the possible presence of a carcinoma. We recently confirmed the diagnosis of endometrial cancer in a girl of twenty-two. It has been reported in the teens. As the menopause approaches, the likelihood of cancer as the cause of bleeding increases sharply. It is further accentuated in the years past the menopause. Fifty per cent of patients with postmenopausal bleeding will have carcinoma. The presence of uterine fibroids, polyps, ovarian cysts or endometriosis should not distract the physician from considering cancer the most important, if not the most frequent, source of the uterine bleeding. Too many hysterectomies are done and too much hormone therapy given without first performing a diagnostic curettage. If the surgeon will make a definite rule, without exception, to perform a curettage and a thorough cervical biopsy in every operative case, tragedies incident to a mistaken diagnosis will be materially reduced.

Beware of the bleeding fibroid. A patient may bleed from a uterus that contains a fibroid, but the bleeding is generally due either to cancer within the uterus or to functional causes, not to the fibroid itself. The lone exception is the submucous fibroid, but this likewise can be neither seen nor felt. Bleeding may come from the endometrium, but the cervix is still suspect. It is of the utmost importance that the source of the uterine bleeding be determined.

The one diagnostic aid of much importance in making the diagnosis is a curettage. It is amazing, despite the fact that this is well known, that 70 per cent of a large series reported never had a curettage. There is a tendency to explain away the cause of abnormal uterine bleeding or discharge rather than investigate it.

ENDOMETRIAL SAMPLING. In the postmenopausal age group there can be no question that curettage is indicated when vaginal spotting, staining or sudden gushing appears after a period of amenorrhea. In the age immediately preceding the menopause the abnormal uterine bleeding is usually functional, but the most important cause is carcinoma. Before instituting hormone therapy an endometrial sample must be obtained. Every effort should be made to encourage the patient to have a curettage, but some patients will be uncooperative. An *endometrial biopsy* taken in the office without anesthesia gives some evidence of the state of the endometrium. A positive finding of carcinoma allows the physician to plan therapy. A negative biopsy, though it is only a sample, gives a sounder basis for hormone therapy. If the bleeding persists, curettage is imperative. The *endometrial biopsy should not be regarded as a substitute for a diagnostic curettage.*

VAGINAL SMEAR. The same observations may be made from the vaginal or Papanicolaou smear. A positive smear for cancer should be regarded as significant; a negative smear means nothing. The reports in endometrial carcinoma have less accuracy than in carcinoma of the cervix. A diagnostic error of about 25 per cent false-negatives is reported for cancer of the endometrium. These figures are based on material aspirated from the vaginal pool.

Direct aspirations from the endometrial cavity will be more accurate, but this is a much more difficult procedure than simple aspiration of the vaginal secretions. It is sounder practice to insist on a curettage, which must be done in any case before definitive treatment can be carried out.

CURETTAGE. This is the most important procedure in establishing the diagnosis of endometrial cancer. *Gentleness* is essential for there is (1) danger of perforating the uterus with either the dilator or curet; (2) forcing malignant cells through the fallopian tube into the abdominal cavity by the forceful plunger effect of the dilator; (3) causing tumor cells to escape into the general circulation.

The curettage should be *fractional*. The abnormal uterine bleeding may be coming from a cancer of the cervix rather than endometrium. The treatment given for endometrial cancer is totally inadequate for cancer of the cervix. Thus the source of bleeding must be accurately identified. After the endocervical canal has been thoroughly curetted and the samples separately labeled, the surgeon proceeds to the curettement of the endometrial cavity. This must be *methodical*. Every surgeon has had the experience of missing a carcinoma lurking in the cornu of the uterus. A flat polypoid growth may also be overlooked when it occurs at the top of the fundus. It is excellent practice to follow the curettage by exploration of the uterine cavity with a common-duct forceps, in order to pick up an occasional polypoid growth which has rolled away from the curet.

Further useful information may be obtained from the curettage which will aid in both diagnosis and treatment. The *Clark test* for carcinoma of the fundus has stood the test of time and may be a helpful adjunct to curettage. Carcinoma is suspected when profuse bleeding is noted from the canal as the uterine probe is withdrawn. Evaluation of the uterine cavity is of the greatest importance. Not infrequently the uterine cavity is found to be distorted by the presence of a totally unsuspected submucous fibroid which militates against the proper application of radium. Since we have no idea where the disease arises, a uniform dose of radiation has to be given to the entire cavity. The size and depth of the cavity are important observations if we are to give radium effectively.

Collection and Gross Examination of the Curettings. The curettings should be collected on moist fine-meshed gauze, lest the material become entangled in the coarse gauze interspaces. Rubber dam or a spoon may be used. *All curetted material, however small, should be saved* for histologic examination.

The curettings should be carefully examined in a good light and by running the fingers over them gently. The diagnosis of carcinoma can often be made on the gross appearance of the curetted material, which is usually yellowish-white, crumbling, granular and firm or hard. It may at times even be possible to differentiate an adenocarcinoma from adenoacanthoma by gross palpation. There is greater sense of resistance to the adenoacanthoma tissue with less tendency to disintegrate than one encounters with adenocarcinoma. This is a helpful maneuver, for differentiation may be difficult on frozen section. It is significant, because adenoacanthoma does less well with radiation therapy.

The most important distinction to make is that between endometrial hyperplasia and cancer. In hyperplasia the curettings are usually abundant and come away in long strips which are smooth, moist, firm and pink, not easily confused with carcinoma. Polyps have a shiny surface. When the curettings are polypoid, the strips may break up when the finger runs over them and dissolve much as one finds in carcinoma. In this instance only the microscope can make the diagnosis.

Frozen Section Diagnosis.   In most cases there are no particular problems in histologic identification of the specimens. If enough material is given the pathologist, curettings of the postmenopausal uterus usually present no great difficulty. If hormones have been given or the material is obtained from a patient before the menopause, the diagnosis may be more difficult or remain in doubt. When doubt exists, it is best not to rely on the frozen section diagnosis to make a therapeutic decision, but to wait for the permanent paraffin sections.

In certain types of endometrial disease the differential diagnosis is so highly controversial that multiple serial sections and consultations may be required before a definite diagnosis can be made. If the diagnosis is still in doubt after further review, it is possibly better to err on the side of the suspicion of cancer and to remove the uterus and adnexa.

Accuracy of Curettage.   It is important to keep in mind that a negative report from the curettings means only that no cancer has been found in the material examined. Human error in collection of the curettings or their interpretation is always possible. Carcinoma may hide in the cornua of the uterus and be missed entirely at curettage. Any resumption of uterine bleeding after a negative curettage should alert the physician, and the possibility of cancer within the uterus should be reconsidered.

What Is the Histopathology of Endometrial Carcinoma?

Since the diagnosis of endometrial cancer is made by curettage in an age group when abnormal bleeding patterns are common, it is well to point out the pitfalls in microscopic interpretation of the endometrium that may lead to confusion in diagnosis.

PATHOLOGIC ENTITIES SIMULATING CARCINOMA.   *Atypical Hyperplasia.*   The differentiation between glandular hyperplasia and endometrial cancer becomes increasingly difficult as the menopause approaches and passes. Mild degrees of hyperplasia and the "swiss cheese" cystic type of proliferation, when they occur before the menopause, rarely set up a diagnostic problem.

As growth stimulation becomes more pronounced, heaping up of the glandular epithelium becomes increasingly evident. Cysts and adenomatous glands of varying shapes and sizes form; some of the abnormal glands are small and round, and others are irregularly elongated, flattened and distorted by finger-like outgrowths. The nuclei are often eccentrically placed within cells that show varying degrees of immaturity. Dark-staining, irregular nuclear chromatin is noted, and at times a prominent nucleolus may be found. There is a disparity in the size and shape of the glands, which tend to demonstrate locally increased thickenings of the epithelium and papillary infoldings as the epithelial layers become crowded. Whenever there is abnormal growth stimulation, the stroma also usually becomes abundant and of active appearance (Fig. 68–5, *A*).

Such atypical hyperplasias may be found in localized foci in a field of otherwise benign hypertrophy, or may be uniformly distributed throughout the endometrial lining. It is these abnormal areas of proliferation that cause confusion in the differential diagnosis from carcinoma. These findings are commonly observed in patients when hormonal therapy has been given interruptedly. Adenomatous hyperplasia is frequently noted when the pathologic material taken from curettings obtained months or years preceding the final diagnosis of cancer is reviewed.

Carcinoma in Situ.   Though less common and well known, there are histologically recognizable changes in the endometrium that may be called carcinoma in situ. They present the same noninvasive characteristics as are noted in carcinoma in situ of the cervix, but authentic cases are recorded of the progression to invasive endometrial carcinoma. The average latent period is placed at three to five years.

The earliest changes are noted focally in the glandular cells. The endometrial glands are found to be composed of large cells heaped irregularly and frequently varying in size and shape. Palisading occurs, and there is sometimes an increased thickness to the glandular epithelial lining. The glands themselves become crowded, but they are not placed back to back. Carcinoma in situ is frequently encountered in a localized area amid an otherwise ordinary background of endometrial hyperplasia.

The nuclei typically are round, pale and swollen and often have folded or wrinkled nuclear membranes. Mitoses are infrequent and much less common than in invasive endometrial cancer. The eosinophilic nature of cytoplasm of the cells and the finely granular chromatin in the nuclei are notable (Fig. 68–5, B).

The homogenous pink stain they take in itself is not evidence of cancer, for eosinophilia has been noted in normal premenstrual glands, endometritis and squamous metaplasia. If the nearby cellular elements show degeneration, and the stroma contains numerous leukocytes, the eosinophilic reaction alone is likely of no consequence. In carcinoma in situ the cells in question are sharply outlined and clean-looking, and evidently do not respond to either estrin or progestin stimulation.

The final diagnosis between carcinoma in situ and frankly invasive carcinoma must rest on the presence of an intact basal membrane and the absence of stromal invasion by carcinoma in situ.

Chronic Endometritis. Inflammatory infiltration of the endometrial stroma by plasma cells, lymphocytes and macrophages is less common during and after the menopause, but it does occur. The endometrial glands that are trapped in or lie adjacent to inflammatory exudate may become distorted, with irregular degeneration and regeneration, apparent anaplasia and at times a really sinister appearance (Fig. 68–6, A).

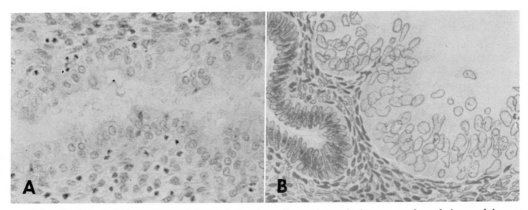

Fig. 68-5. *A,* In endometrial anaplasia the cells are irregularly arranged, and the nuclei vary abnormally in size and staining. Frequently they stain irregularly with poorly defined cell walls and leukocytic infiltration of the stroma. *B,* Carcinoma in situ of endometrium. In contrast to the hyperplastic gland at the left, the nuclei are pale, swollen and folded. The cytoplasm is clear and acidophilic. No degeneration or leukocytes are present. (*B* from T. S. Cullen: *Cancer of the Uterus.* New York, Appleton & Co., 1900.)

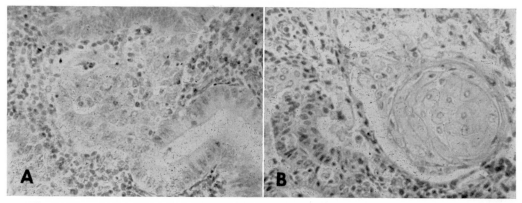

Fig. 68-6.   *A*, In chronic endometritis plasma cells and other leukocytes are found in the stroma, and the glands often show bizarre shapes and staining qualities, of no neoplastic significance. *B*, A nest of squamous-like cells in endometrial hyperplasia. Squamous endometrial metaplasia is a histologic curiosity that should not be confused with carcinoma.

Once plasma cells in reasonable numbers are identified, and the diagnosis of chronic endometritis is consequently made histopathologically, the anaplasia in general can be discounted as having any precancerous significance. The changes are considered a reaction to inflammation, and it is uncommon to find a carcinoma developing later. Neither pyometra nor chronic endometritis nowadays is regarded as a precancerous condition.

Squamous Metaplasia.   In endometrial hyperplasia or chronic endometritis nests of squamous-like cells may be found lining parts of some glands (Fig. 68–6, *B*). They lack the prickle-cell margins of true squamous cells and do not form pearls, but do resemble keratinized epithelial foci. By themselves such cells have no precancerous significance, nor should they be confused with carcinoma cells.

What Are the Main Pathologic Types of Endometrial Adenocarcinoma Encountered?

There are two main types of carcinoma that arise in the endometrium. The *papillary adenocarcinoma* arises from the proliferation of the more superficial cells of the surface epithelium and gland necks. The carcinoma cells are generally columnar. The adenomatous adenocarcinoma pattern forms glands within glands and is more solid. It differs more dramatically in architecture from the normal endometrial glands (Fig. 68–7, *A*). The line of demarcation of carcinoma from the surrounding uninvolved glands is often indefinite, and the exact boundary between the hyperplastic and malignant glands is hard to determine. In addition to the two main types of adenocarcinoma, another cancer growth type occurs that contains islands of squamous epithelium scattered through the malignant gland pattern. This pathologic picture is usually called adenoacanthoma (Fig. 68–7, *B*).

PATHOLOGIC GRADING OF ENDOMETRIAL ADENOCARCINOMA.   The degree of clinical malignancy generally is correlated directly with the maturity of the cancer cell and inversely with the extent of its undifferentiation. The fully differentiated adenocarcinoma grade I and the highly anaplastic grade IV are more easily recognized. The intervening grades are harder to classify with certainty, for the simple reason that varying degrees of differentiation are frequently encountered in different sections or even within the same section of a single carcinoma.

Grade I (Malignant Adenoma, or Adenoma Malignum). This tumor usually rises from the surface epithelium. It may be limited to a small portion of the cavity and forms a villous or lumpy polypoid mass. The gland pattern is not uniformly disturbed. The glands tend to be increased in number, and have much the same general appearance as normal glands, but they are abnormally closely pressed together as the intervening stroma becomes less abundant. The cells are usually columnar and are arranged in palisades. The nuclei show mild hyperchromatism. The cytoplasm is eosinophilic. Large gland spaces may be found containing a few large cells with an occasional mitosis. Mitoses are not common. It takes experience to distinguish a malignant adenoma from a polypoid atypical hyperplasia.

Grade II (Adenocarcinoma). The picture is an exaggeration of the neoplasm in grade I. The entire tumor is filled with enlarged, dilated and elongated, poorly oriented glands. Multiple papillary convolutions may be present. The cells are so closely packed, one on the other, that they appear to be in layers which locally tend to push into and occlude the gland lumens. Abundant mitoses and hyperchromatic nuclei may be present. The glands are so numerous that they encroach on the stroma to the point that in places it is practically nonexistent. The adjacent glands are "back to back." Glands are formed within the lumens of other glands. Because there is so little supporting stroma the tumor tends to necrose, and hemorrhage may be present. The tumor breakdown produces vaginal bleeding early in its life cycle.

Secretory Adenocarcinoma. A few carcinomas of grades I and II are so well differentiated that the glands actually demonstrate subnuclear and supranuclear vacuoles like a functioning postovulatory secretory endometrium. Most such cases occur before the menopause, and evidently are responding to normal ovarian hormonal stimuli.

In the postmenopausal age group secretory endometrial adenocarcinoma should arouse a suspicion of the presence of a functioning ovarian tumor, such as a thecoma or granulosa cell tumor. Perhaps half the endometrial carcinomas found with estrogenic ovarian tumors show secretory activity.

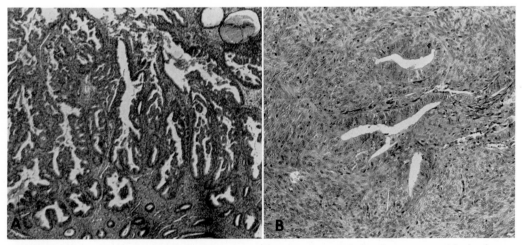

Fig. 68-7. *A,* Endometrial adenocarcinoma has a rather solid glanular pattern with the formation of secondary glands within other glands, small papillary foci and epithelium of 2 adjacent glands growing back to back. It merges in places with atypical hyperplastic glands. *B,* In adenoacanthoma solid nests of squamous-like acidophilic cells are present in reasonable abundance mixed with adenocarcinomatous glands.

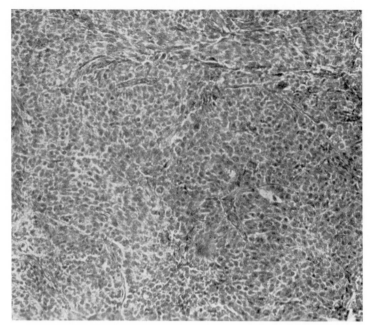

Fig. 68-8.   Endometrial carcinoma simplex is a solid, sheetlike epithelial growth containing only occasional glands to indicate the tissue of origin. It is usually highly invasive.

There is a traditional gynecologic belief that a secretory endometrial adenocarcinoma is easier to cure than the average adenocarcinoma.

Grade III (Carcinoma Simplex).   There may be elements of tumor growth resembling grades I and II, but in general there is a definite loss in polarity, the tumor growing in solid masses, cell cords and columns throughout (Fig. 68–8). These masses usually extend into the musculature. In some portions there may be a thwarted effort to reproduce the gland pattern. The cells are more close-packed and atypical, though some may show evidence of maturity. Signs of anaplasia are more evident, with dedifferentiation noted in at least 50 to 75 per cent of the tumor constituents.

Grade IV (Undifferentiated Carcinoma).   Here the loss of cellular polarity is complete. Masses of atypical cells, both round and polyhedral, grow in sheets and cords replacing entirely what remains of the gland structure. For the most part uninvolved endometrium has disappeared. It would be hard to classify this neoplasm as a carcinoma unless the source is known. The nuclei are small and hyperchromatic, there is scanty cytoplasm, and abundant mitoses occur. Sheets of cells can be found deeply invading muscle. In undifferentiated carcinomas, metastases appear early, and the entire pathologic picture may be reproduced in the regional lymph nodes.

Prognosis on the Basis of the Grade of Endometrial Adenocarcinoma.   Approximately 60 per cent of the patients with fundus cancer will have low (grade I) to medium (grade II) grades of malignancy. It is in this group that the best therapeutic results are noted. These patients have symptoms over a relatively short period. The less differentiated carcinomas (grades III and IV) appear in a somewhat older age group, and more of them are inoperable. Too much difficulty is experienced in the accurate grading of adenocarcinoma, owing to the local variables in the rate of growth within the tumor, to attempt to use the tumor grade as a guide to the kind of treatment that should be given. This is especially true if the information is gathered from frozen sections of the endometrium.

Adenoacanthoma of Endometrium. Islands of proliferating squamous-type cells appear not infrequently in cases of adenocarcinoma. There appears to be a combination of intermingled malignant glandular and epidermoid-like epithelium, varying in quantity and extent. In most instances the glandular element greatly predominates. The diagnosis is best based on a reasonably balanced mixture of the glandular elements with squamous cells. The incidence of adenoacanthoma will be low if abundant material is not studied. Conversely, if any focus of malignant squamous cells in any part of an otherwise glandular tumor results in a diagnosis of adenoacanthoma, the incidence will be high.

Sheets of keratinized malignant cells may occur in some areas separate from the adenocarcinomatous element, or more often they may be intermingled. When the metaplasia is extensive, broad solid fields of eosinophilic cancer cells may obliterate the glandular epithelium. Invasion of the myometrial wall is often noted.

There is an impression that adenoacanthoma is a more vicious form of tumor than adenocarcinoma in the endometrium. The response to radiation is not as favorable, metastases are noted more often, and more extensive surgery is necessary to achieve a comparable salvage. It is doubtful whether any statistically significant differences exist between adenoacanthoma and adenocarcinoma of the endometrium, in their five-year survivals or over-all malignant behavior, however.

TREATMENT OF ENDOMETRIAL CARCINOMA

Until recent years the medical profession has been complacent about the results of therapy in carcinoma of the endometrium. A close scrutiny of the survival statistics in relation to the amount, nature and spread of fundal cancer will show that the results are satisfactory only in the group in which the growth pattern is superficial. Since the majority spread in this fashion, the over-all survival figures reflect the excellent results obtained in this group.

When attention is focused on the type of endometrial carcinoma that invades the myometrium, the end-results of therapy are not outstanding. In our own experience the 5-year survival figures were close to 90 per cent when the growth was superficial, but dropped to approximately 65 per cent when any degree of invasion of the myometrium was noted, despite the fact that a radical Wertheim hysterectomy and node dissection were done.

Excellent survival statistics are found, but when an extensive compilation is reviewed, such as one finds in the "Annual Report of Results of Treatment in Carcinoma of the Uterus," Volume XI, it is evident that general experience fails to keep pace with the individual series reported (Table 14). The 5-year end-results in a total of over 11,000 cases is 56.5 per cent survival. This is a commendable salvage rate, not quite as high as the figure we often regard as the normal expectancy for endometrial cancer cases, but better than that obtained in cancer of the cervix. It is possible, however, that these favorable results are due to the fact that more early cases showing superficial growth formed the bulk of the material on which the report was made. Breaking down the statistics in this report, we note that over 6000 cases or more than half the total number, were in the operable group, with localized tumors. In this classification the 5-year favorable results are 71 per cent, as opposed to the 45 per cent salvage in the one third of the cases in which the cancer was oper-

Table 14.   **Survival Data in Carcinoma of the Endometrium**

TOTAL NUMBER OF PATIENTS		
Alive with no evidence of disease	6,376	56.5%
Alive with carcinoma present	247	2.2%
Died of carcinoma	3,720	32.9%
Lost to follow-up	196	1.7%
Died from intercurrent disease	752	6.7%
Total	11,291	100.0%

DISTRIBUTION BY STAGES		
Stage I (growth confined to the uterus):		
Group I (operation advisable)	6,157	54.5%
Group II (bad operative risks)	3,532	31.3%
Stage II (growth spread outside of uterus)	1,602	14.2%
Total	11,291	100.0%

RESULTS OF TREATMENT		
Number of patients treated:		
Stage I, group I	6,157	
Stage I, group II	3,532	
Stage II	1,602	
Total	11,291	
Patients alive with no evidence of disease:		
Stage I, group I	4,417	
Stage I, group II	1,609	
Stage II	350	
Total	6,376	
Relative recovery rate:		
Stage I, group I	71.7%	
Stage I, group II	45.6%	
Stage II	21.8%	
Total	56.5%	

Experience in 29 world institutions, 1947–1951.

able, but the disease more extensive. In the remainder, stage II, the unfavorable classification, the 5-year survival rate is only 22 per cent. These same factors are present in most series reported today.

We become complacent about what we can accomplish in the treatment of endometrial cancer because we falsely assume, for some reason or another, probably because the majority of cases seen are in the favorable group, that the 70 or higher per cent 5-year salvage rate that we obtain from the favorable cases applies to all cancer of this type in this location. Since more and more cases of endometrial cancer will be seen, as more women reach the age in which it may appear, it is important that we take a close look at what we are trying to accomplish in endometrial cancer from the points of view of both early diagnosis and individualization in therapy.

Attempts are made to classify material on the basis of a clinicopathologic study of the uterus after removal. The most recent classification is that proposed by Blaikley, Kottmeier, Martius and Meigs:

Stage I: Carcinoma confined to the corpus
    II: Carcinoma has involved the corpus and cervix
    III: Carcinoma has extended outside the uterus, but not outside the pelvis
    IV: Carcinoma has involved the bladder or the rectum, or has extended outside the pelvis.

Such a classification is helpful in evaluating the results of therapy, but it is of little help in selecting therapy for the individual patient. The information is obtained only after the uterus has been removed. Since cancer of the endometrium can be neither seen nor felt, the true nature of the disease and its mode of spread cannot be determined with accuracy before the uterus has been removed.

Gusberg has attempted to correlate uterine size with the degree of differentiation of the carcinoma and has used it as a guide to therapy. If this observation can be widely confirmed, it will be a distinct aid in the selection of therapy on an individual basis. It is our impression, however, that the size of the uterus has little to do with the prognosis.

Another reason why the results are poor in the patients regarded as unsuitable candidates for the therapeutic procedures commonly used is the fact that so many of these patients are obese and have a variety of medical complications, such as hypertension and diabetes. Many die of intercurrent disease and are considered dead of their carcinoma, unless an autopsy has been obtained. When selection of therapy is based on the spread of the disease, the survival figures reflect the life history of the cancer.

How Can We Select Therapy for the Individual Case?

It is obvious from the previous discussion that we are handicapped in selecting the ideal form of therapy for the individual case. At the moment we have no satisfactory method of evaluating the clinical stage of the disease. Our best chance, then, to improve the results of therapy is a high index of suspicion when an abnormal bleeding pattern is noted. Obviously, better results are obtained when the endometrial cancer is discovered early in its course before much invasion has taken place. The best means of investigating the cause of vaginal bleeding is curettage, which provides an opportunity to look at all the uterine epithelium. Unfortunately, many women who have been told that a curettage is essential have refused to have it done. We are inclined to use the term "diagnostic curettage," which promptly raises a doubt in the patient's mind of the actual need. It might be better if we stressed the curative effects of curettage. If the uterine bleeding has a functional or hormonal background, which is possible, a curettement will frequently prove curative. If the curettings show frank carcinoma, the patient has no doubts about the necessity of subsequent therapy.

In the past few years we have made it a practice to do an endometrial biopsy on any patient past the age of forty years who has a history of abnormal vaginal bleeding. The material obtained is only a sample and is obtained from one or, at best, two locations within the endometrial cavity. It is possible, then, to miss a small area of cancer located in the cornu, just as it is on curettage, but we have been impressed with how rarely this happens. Our experience would support the contention of Randall that endometrial biopsy will be accurate better than 90 per cent of the time. If the findings are negative for cancer, there is a working basis for hormone therapy. If the vaginal bleeding is not controlled by the use of hormones, then curettage is a must. A curettage is a more accurate procedure, but at least the endometrial biopsy gives a measure of evidence if the patient refuses to accept your advice and have the curettement. It is far better than prescribing hormone therapy without the benefit of any histologic examination.

What Are the Common Methods of Treatment?

The accepted forms of therapy for cancer of the endometrium may be surgery, x-radiation or a combination of both. The pathologic nature of the tumor, associated local lesions, coexistent systemic disease, age and the size of the patient all have a direct bearing on the proper choice of treatment for the individual patient.

Optimum Treatment for the Good-Risk Patient

There is general acceptance among modern gynecologists that the ideal type of treatment for the good-risk patient is preoperative irradiation followed by a total hysterectomy, with bilateral removal of the adnexa at a later date. The radiation may be either intracavitary or external. Routine postoperative x-ray treatment following surgery has some advocates, while others irradiate the vaginal vault with radium plaques after removing the uterus. The hysterectomy and bilateral salpingo-oophorectomy were formerly done after a six-week interval of time. There is a tendency in recent years to shorten the interval to three weeks or, in some clinics, to ten days.

RATIONALE OF PREOPERATIVE RADIATION.   The reasons advanced for preoperative radiation therapy turn on the frequent appearance of vaginal and parametrial metastases following surgery when radiation was not used. These may appear because of implantation of tumor tissue at the time of operation, or as the result of lymphatic extension. Radiation is given in the attempt to (1) render the tumor cells nonviable, (2) reduce the bulk of the tumor, (3) block the adjacent lymphatics.

THE PROBLEM OF PREOPERATIVE INTRACAVITARY RADIATION.   It is not easy to apply radium properly to endometrial cancer. A cancericidal dose of radiation must be delivered in a blind cavity of varying size and contour to an invisible tumor that may be obscured by submucous fibroids or polyps. There may be a small carcinoma in a large uterine cavity. A wide variety of applicators and methods is available to provide a uniform lethal dose to the entire uterine cavity, since we are usually totally unable to determine where the carcinoma is located or the extent of its penetration of the uterine wall. The multiple capsule method advocated by Heyman achieves this end most effectively.

With the best of applicators and the most careful technique residual tumor is a frequent finding when hysterectomy is later performed. The incidence has been placed as high as 55 per cent in cases studied routinely. When serial sections are done, the percentage is much higher. It is impossible to tell whether these cells are viable. Certain sensitive tumors will have vanished, independent of the amount of irradiation. Regardless of how well the tumor has responded to radiation, hysterectomy must be performed. Neither mortality nor morbidity has been appreciable from surgery following irradiation.

PROBLEMS INVOLVED IN THE PREOPERATIVE USE OF EXTERNAL RADIATION. X-ray may be used as a preoperative preparation for surgery in lieu of irradiation with radium. The two main advantages are that (1) the ease of application involves no manipulation of the uterus other than that necessary to make a diagnosis and tends to reduce the danger of manipulative spread at the time of a later operation. (2) The chief advantage would appear to be the effect on the outlying cancer cells and the partial obliteration of the lymphatic network. Just what the effect on the primary carcinoma within the uterus may be is problematical. Some observers find less residual tumors following preoperative x-ray therapy than radium. The effect is therefore twofold, since the lymphatics as well as the intrauterine tumor are treated.

The disadvantage lies in the fact that many of the patients are obese. It is possible with the new supervoltage x-ray machines that an adequate tumor dose of cancericidal x-ray may be given without an overdestructive action upon the skin of the portals of entry or the adjacent viscera. The obesity of the patient remains as a definitive objection to the use of x-ray. The second disadvantage is the time that must elapse between the initial diagnosis and the final definitive cancer treatment by surgery. Nearly a month is needed to introduce sufficient lethal x-radiation to the tumor site.

RATIONALE OF TOTAL HYSTERECTOMY WITH BILATERAL SALPINGO-OOPHO-RECTOMY. The standard operation for cancer of the endometrium following preoperative irradiation calls for a total abdominal hysterectomy with removal of a wide vaginal cuff and both tubes and ovaries. The abdominal approach provides an ample opportunity to explore the liver and the remainder of the abdominal cavity, and it gives wider latitude to the surgeon if more cancer is encountered than was expected in the preoperative evaluation. The vaginal hysterectomy, which a few surgeons prefer, should be reserved for the decidedly obese patient who is also a poor surgical risk.

The reasons why a total hysterectomy with removal of the vagina and the adnexa is considered essential spring from (1) knowledge of the natural spread of the disease, (2) the known fact that residual malignant tumor may be present in uteri subjected to radiation therapy alone.

Within the uterus the cancer may arise over a wide area and spread superficially, with little tendency to invade, or it may spring up in one or more isolated spots with superficial growth but early invasion of the myometrial wall. The extent of the disease, the degree of penetration of the muscle wall and the effectiveness of the radiation therapy cannot be determined until the uterus is removed. An appreciable number will show no evidence of residual tumor on the surface, but nests of active cells in the myometrium.

The cervix and adnexa become involved by direct extension of the carcinoma or permeation along the lymphatic channels. Thus cancer of the endometrium is a disease of the entire uterus. There is no place for a supravaginal hysterectomy in the treatment of endometrial cancer.

THE RESULTS OF PREOPERATIVE RADIATION AND SURGERY. The results after the combined method of treatment show some improvement over those after surgery alone. Compiled statistics indicate about a 60 per cent survival for surgery as compared with 70 per cent from radium and surgery. The best results, 86 per cent, have been obtained when preoperative x-ray treatment has been given. Because these patients are prone to have diabetes mellitus, obesity and hypertension, deaths from intercurrent diseases tend to reduce the salvage figures. They also reduce the operability rate, which is approximately 70 per cent. The operative mortality rate at 4 per cent is higher than after hysterectomy for benign cause. This increase is largely due to the associated abnormalities.

RADIATION THERAPY AS THE DEFINITIVE TREATMENT. Ionizing radiation is used as the only form of treatment in cancer of the endometrium for two reasons: (1) the firm conviction that radium will cure as many patients, without the morbidity and mortality associated with surgery used either alone or in combination with radium; (2) the case is inoperable. The patient may be considered inoperable for a variety of reasons: (a) she may be too old or too obese; (b) she may have too much hypertension or diabetes; or (c) the carcinoma may be too extensive. Any one or all of these reasons would make her a poor candidate for surgery.

THE USE OF RADIUM INSTEAD OF SURGERY.   Advocates of radiation therapy claim that they obtain results from radiologic treatment comparable to those achieved by surgery either alone or in combination with radium. To them surgery should be reserved for radiation failures.

Kottmeier at the Radiumhemmet in Stockholm, using the method devised by Heyman, which fills the uterus with multiple capsules each containing a radium source, reports a 5-year survival rate of 63 per cent for all stages of endometrial cancer. For stage I (the favorable classification) a 79 per cent salvage rate was achieved. These figures challenge the best offered by surgery. Perhaps the criticism of radiation should be directed toward our deficiencies in its use. It is questionable, however, whether all clinics will have the wide variety of equipment and the detailed knowledge required for its proper use to duplicate the experience quoted.

The average salvage rate is approximately 50 per cent. In criticism of the use of radium instead of surgery, it should be noted that (1) all the problems inherent in the application of lethal ionizing radiation to a cancer hidden in a uterine cavity of variable contour are magnified when radium is to be the only form of treatment the patient receives. Since the amount of radiation therapy to be given is increased, there is the added danger of overirradiation. The amount usually given is in the neighborhood of 6000 mg.-hrs. (2) There are many contraindications to the use of radium. Pelvic inflammation, pyometra, submucous fibroids and multiple polyps increase the hazards of intracavitary radiation. One or all may be present in a uterus that harbors an endometrial cancer. (3) Increasing the dosage within the uterine cavity will not destroy a cancer that has permeated the lymphatics beyond the confines of the uterus.

When there is a choice of therapy, surgery should be used in combination with ionizing radiation.

Radium in the Poor-Risk Patient

The favorable results observed from the radium treatment of operable cases is encouraging, since an effective instrument is available for use in the patient who cannot withstand the rigors of abdominal surgery. Approximately 30 per cent of all patients with endometrial cancer will be in the inoperable group.

The patient who is inoperable because of systemic disease, or who is too old and too obese, may expect a 40 per cent chance of being alive after 5 years. It may be necessary to divide the total radiation into several applications two or more weeks apart to avoid the dangers of overirradiation in the group least able to withstand any complications.

Equally satisfactory results cannot be expected when the patient is inoperable because of extensive malignant disease. At best a 15 to 20 per cent cure rate should be anticipated. The surgeon should carefully consider what he hopes to achieve by irradiation in this group of patients. In relatively few the full course of radiation therapy may be given with profit, but with some danger. Others may be irradiated with palliation alone in mind. In this instance radium is given largely to control excessive uterine bleeding.

External Ionizing Radiation as Supplemental Therapy

X-ray treatment has proved value in the treatment of cancer of the endometrium when it is used as a supplement to surgical or radium treatment. It is less useful when the patient is obese. Used preoperatively instead of radium, it has the disadvantage of requiring time to secure the desired effect.

There would appear to be a real place for external radiation following surgery both in the control of implant metastases and of unrecognized lymphatic spread. Five-year end-results have improved in the clinics where it is used routinely.

When external irradiation is used with radium in the absence of surgical removal of the uterus, great care must be exercised to avoid a too concentrated radiation effect at any one point. The *primary mortality* rate rises sharply from 2 to 8 per cent when full doses of x-ray follow complete intrauterine irradiation. It is well to have a planned attack designed to give proper balance to each factor, in order that uniform radiation may be given to the primary cancer as well as to the field of its potential spread. It may be necessary to reduce the dosage of the intracavitary radiation if full tolerance doses of x-ray are to be administered.

Local Application of Radium as Added Therapy

It is common practice in many areas today to perform total hysterectomy, bilateral salpingo-oophorectomy and removal of an upper vaginal cuff as the primary treatment for endometrial cancer with addition of a radium bomb to the apex of the vagina. The radium is designed to minimize the chance of recurrence or persistence of the cancer in this region. The radium application is made approximately two weeks after the hysterectomy when the vaginal apex is reasonably well healed. Small 10-mg. radium sources are enclosed in a round bomb usually totalling 50 mg. The duration of the application is in the neighborhood of 3000 mg.-hr., which provides a dose of 4500 roentgens to the tumor site at 0.5 cm. depth.

This method of handling the potential spread of endometrial cancer beyond the primary site carries less risk than the extended surgical procedures which remove the intervening paravaginal and paracervical lymphatics, particularly in the obese patient who is a borderline surgical risk.

If radium is given routinely without regard to the spread of the cancer within the endometrial cavity, it may take care of any implant metastases that theoretically occur, but otherwise this method would seem to have little rationale. If the cancer has invaded the myometrium, it likely is in the lymphatic channels, and one may expect multiple foci located subepithelially, rather than a single neoplastic mass. It would seem logical to remove these channels at the time of the original surgical attack. Nevertheless many patients with endometrial cancer are not good candidates for extended surgical excisions. A postoperative application of radium to the upper vaginal canal is therefore a useful adjunct to therapy, as we attempt to adjust our treatment program to the individual needs of the patient.

Treatment of the Recurrence of Endometrial Carcinoma

Cancer of the endometrium, as we noted in the discussion of its life history, is a relatively sluggish form of malignant disease so long as the cancer is confined to the endometrial cavity. A limited amount of myometrial invasion, however, adversely influences the recovery rate appreciably. As soon as this takes place, cancer dissemination by lymphatic channels and blood stream is prone to occur. Furthermore, we have noted that cancer cells appear in the peripheral blood stream after a curettage for endometrial cancer. Thus we may expect to find remote as well as local metastases. These may take place fairly promptly and be clinically evident within a space of four to six months, or they may not manifest themselves for years.

We have seen local recurrences in the vaginal canal, always on the anterior vaginal wall, appear three, seven and eleven years after irradiation and surgery in the same patient. Lung metastases may develop or become evident by x-ray years after a local cure has been obtained. These may take the form of large "snowballs," the commonest variety, or as scattered nodules throughout the lung fields, giving an appearance not unlike bronchopneumonia.

In the past we had little to offer patients who had extensive local recurrence or metastatic disease in the lung fields. Recently some, though limited, salvage can be obtained by (*a*) more extensive surgical excision and (*b*) the use of the newer progestational agents.

What Do We Have to Offer the Patient with a Localized Cancer Recurrence at the Vaginal Apex?

Recurrences of carcinoma following preliminary radiation therapy and surgery in the vaginal wall, either along its course or at the apex of the foreshortened canal, may be treated by (1) direct application of radium plaques, or the implantation of radium needles into the area of cancer recurrence; (2) surgical removal of the remaining portion of the vagina. The choice depends on the findings in the individual case.

If the local recurrence occurs in a limited area and there is no clinical evidence of cancer elsewhere in the vagina, radiation therapy may be effectively used. With little infiltration of the surrounding tissue the introduction of a surface applicator containing a radium source will often suffice. When the local recurrence has depth, radium needles at 1-cm. intervals should be implanted in the tumor, giving a total dose of about 1000 mg.-hr.

When the patient is a good surgical risk, and there is a clinical suggestion that multiple cancer foci are present, a total vaginectomy with transperitoneal lymph node dissection should be done. In the less favorable risk the vaginectomy may be done through the perineal approach, without a node dissection. In the poor-risk patient therapeutic recourse must rest with (*a*) radium treatment to the entire vaginal canal, using a large radium bomb; (*b*) external radiation therapy, using the perineal port; or (*c*) progestational therapy.

What Treatment Can Be Offered the Patient with a Sizable Parametrial Carcinoma Recurrence?

When the carcinomatous recurrence in the vaginal vault is large, a surface application of radium will not suffice. If radiation therapy is to be given, it must be in the form of (1) introduction of radium needles into the mass, or (2) external irradiation by x-ray or cobalt units. When the lesion is centrally placed, however, enough radiation to cure the recurrence may severely damage the bladder or rectum, however carefully it is given or whatever the modality. If the patient is a poor operative risk, this chance must be taken.

Pelvic Exenteration

With a patient in good general condition and no evidence of remote endometrial cancer metastases the surgeon may, if he has had sufficient experience, elect to use one of the ultraradical exenteration procedures. The results are not as rewarding as they have been in cancer of the cervix, since fewer patients with cancer of the endometrium localize their metastases to a manageable area. A few patients, including two who had positive lymph nodes for carcinoma, continue to survive without malignant disease, five or more years after the extirpation of the pelvic contents, in our experience.

What Do the New Progestational Agents Have to Offer?

In the past few years encouraging results have been obtained by parenteral injection of the new progestational agents in patients who have lung metastases of endometrial adenocarcinoma or local recurrences in the vaginal vault not amenable to surgical extirpation because of their size or the condition of the patient. Recognizing that endometrial cancer does appear to be influenced by hormonal activity, chiefly estrin, one may reasonably contemplate the possibility of altering the internal milieu by using such an estrin antagonist as progestin.

Accordingly, Kelley and Baker gave biweekly intramuscular injections of Delalutin (17-alpha-hydroxyprogesterone caproate) in 250-mg. doses to patients who had either lung, bone or local vaginal vault metastases of endometrial carcinoma. Objective improvement was shown by (*a*) the disappearance of x-ray shadows considered to be metastases by the radiologists, (*b*) the reduction in the size of malignant tumor masses that occurred in areas where they could be measured, (*c*) the recalcification of bony metastases, which occurred in one third of the patients treated. No adverse side effects such as drug toxicity, androgenic stimulation or abnormal weight gain appeared. As an additional dividend, subjective improvement such as gain in strength and appetite was noted in many patients, including some who showed no objective changes. The durations of remissions have run from two to five years.

The mode of action of the progestational agents is not known. The effect may be mediated through the pituitary, since there is some evidence that the LH production is diminished, or the drug may act directly on the tumor itself. Bioassays for LH have the disadvantage of being so variable, depending on the method used, that the final answer on pituitary action must be reserved.

There is also evidence that the progestational drug may exert its effect locally. This is based on the now well documented observation that the newer progestational agents can convert a hyperplastic to a resting or atrophic endometrium.

Regardless of its mode of action, we now have an additional adjunct to therapy to offer the patient with endometrial cancer who either did not respond to the standard methods of therapy or had too much neoplastic disease to hope that she would. As yet no prediction can be made as to which patient will do well with this hormone therapy. In general, better results can be expected when the endometrial adenocarcinoma is well differentiated, and the interval between the original treatment and the development of the cancer recurrence is prolonged.

Criticism of the Present Attitude toward Treatment of Endometrial Cancer

Although radiation techniques have improved and more powerful and flexible instruments are available for delivery, a wave of skepticism has appeared as to the value of ionizing radiation in the treatment of endometrial cancer. There is a tendency to go back to the simple total hysterectomy with removal of the adnexa and a section of the upper part of the vagina. This is little more than the operation customarily performed for benign disease such as a fibroid uterus. Undoubtedly it will be adequate for patients—and they do form the majority of the cases—who have the type of carcinoma that spreads superficially and fills the endometrial cavity, but does not invade the muscle wall.

To our mind this is a step backward toward standardization in cancer therapy. It stems from our complacent attitude toward the treatment of endometrial cancer and gives no consideration to the patient who is unfortunate enough to have myometrial invasion.

If preoperative radiation therapy is to be abandoned, it would seem far more logical to extend the operation and do a more extensive dissection of the paravaginal and paracervical lymphatics. The vaginal apex along its anterior wall is a common place for local metastases to occur in. The incidence reported in the literature is in the range of 10 per cent. There is a common conception that such recurrences appear because carcinoma is implanted on the cut edges of the vagina at the time of operation. Attempts are made at the start of the operation to suture the cervix to prevent spillage of cancer cells.

There is increasing evidence to indicate that the cancer actually arrives at these locations through lymphatic spread rather than by implants. The question is therefore raised as to whether a more vigorous surgical attack should not be made upon the block of tissue that contains these lymphatic channels. Spread of carcinoma to the regional lymph nodes in the external iliac and obturator regions has been noted with increasing frequency in recent years. The incidence, based on autopsy findings, runs as high as 25 per cent, but in the kind of case usually encountered at the time of operation positive nodes will be found in not much more than 12 per cent. The regional lymph nodes then should also be dissected, and a few patients who have nodes positive for cancer will be saved. The important aspect of the extended surgical procedure, however, will be the more complete dissection of the lymphatic channels adjacent to the uterus and vagina.

If one is prepared to perform this type of cancer surgery, the advisability of abandoning preoperative radiation might well be considered. Such an operation obviously should not be offered as a standard therapy for endometrial cancer. It is possible that the morbidity and mortality from such a procedure in the older age group might increase to the point at which the five-year salvage would not improve significantly. In the interests of individualization in therapy it may offer the best chance for cure in the properly selected endometrial carcinoma case, especially since we have as yet no way of knowing in advance of hysterectomy which cases will have myometrial invasion. This surgical approach is now receiving attention in a number of clinics.

If our results are to improve in the management of endometrial cancer, it is obvious that more advances will come from early recognition of the malignant tumor and a better understanding of the factors that cause it, rather than from improved methods of therapy. We should continue efforts to improve our therapy, but should give the same concentrated thought to achieving an early diagnosis as we have given to the cervical cancer problem, with hope that such attention will provide the same rewards.

MIXED MESODERMAL TUMORS OF THE UTERUS

Sarcomas of the uterus that arise from the endometrium or its stroma are extremely rare, but when they do occur they present fascinating problems to both clinician and pathologist. Usually there is a bleak outlook for the patient. It is estimated that barely 250 cases have been reported. Since no one physician or clinic is apt to encounter this bizarre pathologic entity with any frequency, cases that do appear are unlikely to be reported. The incidence, therefore, is actually higher than that commonly reported.

Unlike the genuine teratoma, mixed uterine tumors of a sarcomatous nature arise from a single germ layer; hence the name "mesodermal." They are called mixed tumors, because they have components of both epithelial and stromatogenous cells. In general there are two main types: (a) The simple homologous type, in which varied amounts of carcinoma and sarcomas are present in the same tumor. Such neoplasms are called *carcinosarcomas*. (b) The heterologous type of tumor that may arise either from endometrium or myometrium and which has a highly bizarre histologic composition. These sarcomas contain cells that would not normally be found in the uterus at all. Thus we find mixed tumors of sarcomatous type that contain bone, cartilage, fat and striated muscle. The neoplasm usually derives its name from the type of tissue that is predominant. Thus we encounter such terms as rhabdomyosarcoma, osteosarcoma, chondrosarcoma, myxosarcoma, fibrosarcoma, liposarcoma and angiosarcoma. In general this heterologous group of tumors is classified under the heading of mixed mesodermal tumors, while the homologous type tends to retain the name of carcinosarcoma.

When and Where Do They Occur?

The majority of these unusual tumors are discovered in the fundus of the uterus when the patient has passed the menopause. The greatest concentration appears in the age span between fifty-five and sixty-five years. Occasionally, however, mixed mesodermal tumors are encountered in infancy, as well as during the years of active sex life. A dramatic form, *sarcoma botryoides*, for example, was discussed with problems of infancy (Chap. 9), and it occurs also after the menopause. In general such tumors arise in the upper part of the vagina during infancy, in the cervix during the reproductive years, and in the fundus after menstruation has ceased. The genital tract is a common site of origin for the mixed tumors of mesenchymal type, but they have also been found in kidney, ureter, bladder, breast, neck, pharynx, gastrointestinal tract and bone. The histogenesis of these bizarre forms of malignant disease provides a constant challenge to pathologists.

CARCINOSARCOMA

The term is widely used to describe neoplasms of the endometrium that are composed both of epithelial elements that form adenocarcinoma and stromal or myometrial components that provide the sarcoma. Not all pathologists are agreed on whether carcinosarcoma is a true pathologic entity. Some eminent authorities, for example, feel that this type of tumor is simply an anaplastic form of carcinoma that manifests bizarre reactive alterations in its stroma which may simulate a sarcomatous change. To support this contention they point to the fact that many of the metastases appear in the form of pure adenocarcinoma, despite the mixed histologic appearance of the primary tumor. Others, equally prominent, feel that a carcinogenic stimulus is present that may either bring about a sarcomatous change in the stroma of an adenocarcinoma or a carcinomatous alteration of glands that are caught in a sarcoma. Whatever concept of their histogenesis one prefers, these tumors tend to follow a similar pattern of progressive growth which is clinically recognizable and almost invariably lethal.

What Is the Commonly Used Pathologic Classification of Carcinosarcoma?

Meyer felt that changes took place in the stroma of an antecedent carcinoma when a carcinogenic stimulus as yet unknown was present. He set up a classification consisting of four main types:

1. The "collision" type of carcinosarcoma, in which the two types of cancer have separate points of origin, but tend to grow together, intermingle and coalesce. One may find adenocarcinoma growing as an independent neoplasm around the base of a polyp or into a pedunculated type of submucosal sarcoma. At times the sarcoma seems to spread from an involved polyp across into an obvious area of adenocarcinoma. In some other instances the adenocarcinoma appears conversely to invade a sarcoma.

There will be less doubt about the histologic classification if the sites of origin of the two separate tumors can be identified, despite their tendency to coalesce. If not, the question will arise as to whether this might be simply an anaplastic tumor whose stroma has taken on the spindle-like characteristics of a sarcoma. Willis, for example, considers that endometrium and its stroma, being basically of the same mesenchymal origin, can respond to carcinogenic stimulation by proliferating in a variety of different ways.

2. Malignant transformation may take place in both tissue components of a benign lesion of mixed nature, such as a fibroadenomatous polyp or an area of adenomyosis. To support this concept the pathologist must find an uninvolved benign remnant of the original lesion.

3. In some mixed tumors, one or the other element would seem to have undergone malignant change before the other. The stroma may be stimulated to undergo sarcomatous morphologic alterations as a secondary result of the growth of the adenocarcinoma. On the other hand, the sarcoma may have had priority, and it apparently provided the impetus for neoplasia of the endometrium. Suggestive evidence would be present if, for example, a superficial growth of adenocarcinoma could be seen invading a sizable sarcomatous polyp.

4. The so-called müllerian or composite type is probably closest to being a true carcinosarcoma. Here the two cellular elements seem to arise from a common matrix. It is a well known embryologic fact that the primitive mesenchymal cells not only line the celomic cavity, but also contribute to the development of the underlying urogenital ridges. The endometrial lining of the uterine cavity is derived from the celomically originating epithelium that also covers the urogenital ridge. Hence the epithelium and the stroma of the endometrium have the same embryologic background, and they can readily develop in various directions. Both the epithelium and stroma of the endometrium inherently have less limited possibilities for aberrant differentiation than tissues of ectodermal or entodermal origin.

What Provides the Stimulus for the Combined Type of Neoplasia?

The actual reason why the endometrium and its stroma both undergo neoplasia and develop in this unusual fashion is unknown. Attempts have been made to implicate the use of intrauterine radium to control previous benign menstrual bleeding. It is true that study of most series of cases of carcinosarcoma will uncover a number of patients who present such a history.

Since one can find reviews of large numbers of irradiated cases without a single instance of the subsequent development of a carcinosarcoma, one wonders whether the uterine substrate in these patients was not at fault. The abnormal uterine bleeding for which the radium was given may simply have been an indication of this, and irradiation had nothing to do with the subsequent development of carcinosarcoma. There is also a suggestion that the stimulus is hormonal, but convincing proof is lacking.

What Do These Tumors Look Like Grossly?

For the most part carcinosarcoma grows as a polypoid mass of moderate size. It usually arises in the upper part of the endometrial cavity and seems to prefer the posterior wall. It may progress to such size that it protrudes from the cervical os. In most instances, however, it is found only at the time of curettage. It is fibrous in appearance, but is friable and bleeds easily.

On cut section the surface appears shiny and gelatinous, with none of the granular element common to adenocarcinoma. Around the base of the polypoid mass the endometrium is thick, rough and friable (Fig. 68–9).

The carcinosarcoma may be discrete, but more often invasion of the uterine wall has taken place, with occasional evidence of spread into the broad ligaments and adnexa. Once in the uterine wall, spread may take place through the blood stream, since these tumors are vascular and microscopically reveal tumor cells in their sinus-

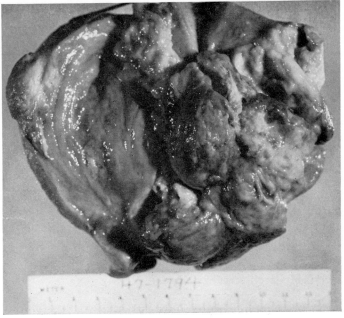

Fig. 68-9.   A friable, hemorrhagic endometrial carcinosarcoma with extensive myometrial invasion.

oids. It may also spread by lymphatic channels and present vaginal metastases in the same areas as when the basic lesion is an adenocarcinoma of the endometrium. Metastases may occur in remote as well as local areas. Interestingly enough, the remote metastatic deposits are usually either a pure adenocarcinoma or a sarcoma. Rarely are they found coexisting. With extensive local invasion the patient may have severe pain as the function of intra-abdominal organs is compromised. Lymph nodal metastases, however, are infrequent.

What Do Carcinosarcomas Look Like Microscopically?

With low magnification it is obvious, because of the cellular nature of the process, that a neoplasm is present, and higher magnification shows a wild tangle of bizarre, crowded cells of undoubted malignancy. The problem is how to classify this undifferentiated cancer.

Careful scrutiny shows some cuboidal or columnar cells lined up in rows and perhaps forming a rare incomplete gland. This growth pattern would indicate carcinoma simplex. Other intermingled spindly cells, mostly composed of large, darkly stained anaplastic nuclei, are evidently not epithelial, but do caricature the specialized endometrial stroma. This is the sarcomatous element (Fig. 68–10).

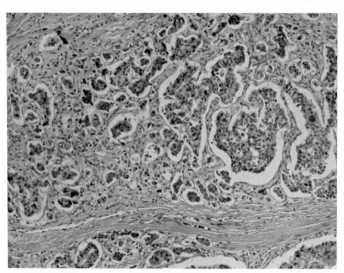

Fig. 68-10.   Mixed with the poorly differentiated endometrial carcinoma is a stroma of malignant appearance, partly undifferentiated and resembling endometrial stromal cells elsewhere. The combined pattern is that of carcinosarcoma.

The intimate admixture of both cell lines and two growth patterns, with apparent histologic transitions between them in places, is best satisfied by the pathologic diagnosis of endometrial carcinosarcoma.

Possibilities of collision tumors and the invasive proclivities of carcinosarcomas have already been considered.

How Is the Diagnosis of Carcinosarcoma Made?

Since the carcinosarcoma grows as a polypoid mass and is highly vascular, it is prone to have its blood supply jeopardized. Foul discharge and uterine bleeding in varying amounts are the predominant symptoms. The uterus tends to be large, but may be mobile unless invasion of the adnexa, broad ligaments or peritoneum has taken place. If the polypoid growth protrudes through the external os and presents in the vagina as a friable sloughing mass, the diagnosis is fairly obvious. In the majority of instances a fibroadenomatous polyp, with which it may be confused, does not grow to a size that will permit it to pass through the cervix. This is not invariable, however. Without the appearance of a mass protruding from the uterine os the diagnosis is made on suspicion when a foul discharge and bleeding appear in a postmenopausal woman. The final diagnosis awaits tissue confirmation after biopsy of the mass or curettage.

What Is the Most Effective Method of Treatment?

The prognosis is uniformly bad, regardless of the method of therapy. The majority of patients are dead within a year. Total hysterectomy with removal of the adnexa and upper part of the vagina offers as good a chance as any for a cure. Radiation therapy is effective only in the treatment of the metastatic deposits. This may reflect the histologic nature of the metastasis, which differs from the primary tumor in that it tends to grow as a pure tumor rather than in the mixed form found in the primary site. Although the carcinosarcoma spreads by vascular channels and infrequently involves lymph nodes, a wide dissection of the paravaginal and paracervical lymphatics, combined with pelvic lymphadenectomy and a Wertheim type of hysterectomy, may have a place. In our own experience one such patient is alive and free of disease after seven years.

Mixed Mesodermal Uterine Sarcomas of Heterologous Nature

These bizarre and unusual forms of endometrial and myometrial sarcoma differ from the homologous type such as the carcinosarcoma because of their strange histologic patterns and the finding of mesodermal derivatives that would not be present in the uterus under normal conditions. Thus we may find bone, cartilage and skeletal muscle as well as an undifferentiated sarcomatous component. Such peculiar mixed mesodermal tumors are reported infrequently, but there are undoubtedly many that are encountered and never recorded. The histogenesis is both fascinating and controversial, but regardless of this they are a distinct pathologic entity with a recognizable and unfavorable clinical course.

One reason why they are not reported more often is the uncertainty that exists in assigning the tumor to its proper histologic category. Some pathologists, for example, refuse to call such tumors mixed mesodermal growths unless they find embryonal myoblasts to go along with other heterotopic elements, such as myxomatous tissue, cartilage or glands. In recent years restrictive criteria have been relaxed so that the diagnosis can now be made when two or more heterologous connective tissue elements are present, regardless of the presence or absence of striated muscle cells.

Histogenesis of Mixed Mesodermal Sarcomas

Complete agreement is lacking as to why these strange tumors appear in the uterus. In general, pathologists accept the Wilms theory that mesodermal cells from the myotome and urogenital ridge are carried down as the wolffian duct develops and are deposited along its course where they lie dormant until the proper stimulus is applied. Why they should remain quiescent all through the active childbearing period only to burst into activity after the menopause is mysterious. It could be that the endometrial cells undergo dedifferentiation to a more primitive state, while the stromal cells enter a proliferative neoplastic phase. The endometrial stroma is known to be unstable and to have the power to develop into a wide variety of aberrant tissues. Years ago it was suggested that the neoplastic cells derived from undifferentiated connective tissue thereafter undergo metaplasia. It is possible to explain the cartilage and bone on this theory, but metaplasia does not ordinarily occur into striated muscle, which is often present in these tumors. Ober has provided a scholarly classification and discussion of the origin of these neoplasms.

Some pathologists subscribe to the theory of primitive cell rests, derived from the müllerian duct system, being incorporated within the mature myometrium. Thus one may see a carcinosarcoma or one of the more complex tumors develop, depending on the strength of the stimulus and the degree of alteration in the intrauterine environment. The causative factors then may be either (a) accidents of development, (b) metaplasia or (c) the rejuvenation of rests. The activating carcinogenic stimulus is unknown. Hormonal stimulation may be important, but parity seems to have little to do with it. Three times as many parous women have these tumors as nulliparous.

What Is the Life History of Mixed Mesodermal Sarcomas?

The growth rate of these mixed mesodermal tumors is rapid, and the clinical course is one of progressive deterioration. In the menopausal years, when most of these tumors occur, the primary growth appears in the fundus as a solitary, soft, bulky polypoid growth, usually on the posterior wall (Fig. 68–11, A). At times solid, hard portions are felt within the primary tumor. This is usually an indication that

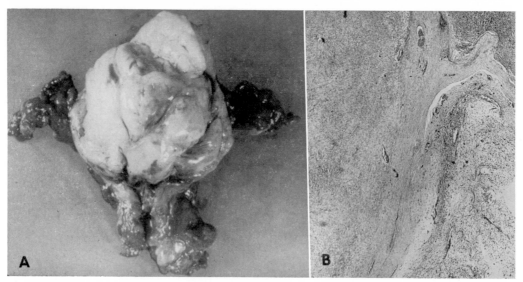

Fig. 68-11.   *A*, Mixed mesodermal uterine sarcoma grossly is indistinguishable from other sarcomas, with which it shares the characteristic smooth, moist, shining cut surface. *B*, The central fibrous stromal septum separates undifferentiated sarcoma at the top right from chondrosarcomatous foci at the lower right and fibrosarcoma along the left side of the field.

cartilage or bone is present. The prognosis, which is poor whether the tumor is encapsulated or not, seems to be much worse when cartilage is present.

The tumors are vascular, and sarcomatous tumor cells invade the vessels, often clogging their lumens. Thromboses therefore are common. As a result of the obstruction to the blood supply the tumor is purplish-red and is prone to undergo necrosis and liquefaction.

Fundamentally, in an intracavitary lesion, spread occurs rapidly in two directions: (a) the growth may protrude out through an uneffaced but dilated cervical os, or (b) it may grow directly through the wall of the uterus to involve the adjacent pelvic peritoneum and organs. The uterus is invariably larger, therefore, than one would expect from an uncomplicated adenocarcinoma of the endometrium. It tends to be symmetrical unless the invasion has localized or fibroids are present. Though the uterus is mobile in the early phases of growth, it rapidly becomes fixed when the tumor has grown through the uterus and invaded adjacent structures. Distant and local metastases are common. Metastases to lung are almost universal, and liver deposits are common. When a polypoid mass appears in the vagina, immediate suspicion is aroused. If it is confined to the uterus, the final diagnosis must await curettage and tissue confirmation.

What Are the Symptoms?

There are no pathognomonic symptoms. Bleeding and vaginal discharge are present, but the pattern is not very different from that of a pure adenocarcinoma of the endometrium. The bleeding is usually persistent or irregular and is rarely profuse. The nature of the discharge may alert the physician, for unlike in carcinoma of the endometrium, it is apt to be watery and to have a foul odor because of the necrosis of the primary tumor. Pain becomes part of the symptomatology rather earlier than in carcinoma of the endometrium, probably owing to more rapid invasion of the uterine wall and spread beyond it. Although extensive blood loss is rarely a part of the clinical picture, these patients lose weight, have a fever and become cachectic very rapidly. In all probability this is due to the tendency on the part of all sarcomas to necrose and become infected. This contributes to the rapid downhill course of patients who have mixed mesodermal sarcomas.

What Is the Microscopic Picture of Mixed Mesodermal Sarcoma?

The true nature of the tumor may be suspected grossly, but is confirmed by histologic review of the specimen. As with carcinosarcoma, it is easy to identify the malignant neoplastic nature of the growth, which has no capsule and is poorly delimited.

Much of a mixed mesodermal sarcoma is usually made up of loosely arranged, primitive stellate or elongated cells with abnormally large nuclei and nucleoli. These undifferentiated sarcomatous cells lie in an edematous myxoid stroma, or may be crowded together, but they demonstrate no collagenous or myomatous fibrils. Intermingled are usually some straplike or cigar-shaped cells that contain longitudinal cytoplasmic myofibrils. Careful search with high magnification may be rewarded by finding a sarcoma cell, or several, with cross-striated cytoplasm, indicating that the tumor contains foci of rhabdomyosarcoma.

Traditionally, the pathologist searches diligently for striated muscle cells in an undifferentiated sarcoma as a clue to its heterologous nature. Occasionally the entire sarcoma may be a mixture of myosarcoma, with its longitudinal cytoplasmic striations, and rhabdomyosarcoma, with its cross-striations.

More often, additional types of sarcomatous differentiation are identifiable (Fig. 68–11, *B*). Chondrosarcomatous foci are characterized by prominent chondroblastic nuclei spaced irregularly through a glassy, slightly bluish, chondromucoid matrix. Osteogenic foci are forming along the edges of irregular bands of bright eosinophilic osteoid, and malignant osteocytes are found trapped within the primitive osteoid trabeculae. Liposarcomatous cells have small or large cytoplasmic lipoid vacuoles. Vascular invasion is common.

Typically, no adenocarcinoma or benign glandular neoplastic component occurs in mixed mesodermal sarcomas, but only connective tissues. If adenocarcinoma were found, the tumor would then be classified as an *adenosarcoma, or Wilms's tumor* of the uterus. These actually occur, as Wilms reported.

What Are the Treatment and Prognosis of Mixed Mesodermal Sarcomas?

The only form of treatment that offers any hope for the patient is total removal of the uterus and adnexa. Although the components that go to make up the tumor are embryonal, these tumors are not radiosensitive, as one might suppose. One may choose to irradiate, particularly postoperatively when the surgeon is uncertain as to whether he has removed all neoplastic tissue, but there is little chance that any improvement will follow. The prognosis is poor, at best, since the patients rarely survive for any appreciable time, and 90 per cent are dead within one year of the diagnosis.

In young children and sometimes in the menopausal age group, when grapelike polypoid masses characteristic of sarcoma botryoides can be seen arising in the cervix, from the upper part of the vagina or beneath the mucous membrane of the bladder, there may be a place for the exenteration operations that are designed to remove the entire contents of the pelvis. Meigs reported a child alive and well eight years after an exenteration for a moderate-sized tumor of this sort (see Chap. 9).

In the exercise of good surgical judgment the operator may, on rare occasions, be justified in performing a total hysterectomy and removal of the adnexa when the uterine bleeding is uncontrollable by any other means, even in the presence of known metastases in remote regions. Removal of the primary tumor will have little effect on the metastatic growths, but the hysterectomy is performed to control hemorrhage when all other methods, including irradiation, have failed.

REFERENCES

Incidence and Etiology of Endometrial Carcinoma

Andrews, W. C.: Estrogens and Endometrial Carcinoma. *Obst. & Gynec. Surv.*, 16: 747, 1961.

Andrews, W. C., and Andrews, M. C.: Stein-Leventhal Syndrome with Associated Adenocarcinoma of the Endometrium. Report of a Case in a 22 Year Old Woman. *Am. J. Obst. & Gynec.*, 80: 632, 1960.

Benjamin, F.: Glucose Tolerance in Dysfunctional Uterine Bleeding and in Carcinoma of the Endometrium: A Preliminary Report. *Brit. J. Med.*, 1: 1243, 1960.

Chun, L., Gong, G., and Roddick, J. W., Jr.: The Epithelium of the Uterine Tube and Cervix in Patients with Endometrial Carcinoma: A Search for Estrogenic Effect. *Am. J. Obst. & Gynec.*, 78: 174, 1959.

Copenhaver, E. H.: Atypical Endometrial Hyperplasia. *Obst. & Gynec.*, 13: 264, 1959.

Corscaden, J. A., Fertig, J. W., and Gusberg, S. B.: Carcinoma Subsequent to the Radiotherapeutic Menopause. *Am. J. Obst. & Gynec.*, 51: 1, 1946.

Dockerty, M. B., and Mussey, E.: Malignant Lesions of the Uterus Associated with Estrogen-Producing Ovarian Tumors. *Am. J. Obst. & Gynec.*, 61: 147, 1951.

Ehrmann, R. L., McKelvey, H. A., and Hertig, A. T.: Secretory Behavior of Endometrium in Tissue Culture. *Obst. & Gynec.*, 17: 416, 1961.

Garnet, J. D.: Constitutional Stigmas Associated with Endometrial Carcinoma. *Am. J. Obst. & Gynec.*, 76: 11, 1958.

Graves, W. P.: *Gynecology*. Philadelphia, W. B. Saunders Company, 1928.

Greene, J. W., Jr.: Feminizing Mesenchymomas (Granulosa-Cell and Theca-Cell Tumors) with Associated Endometrial Carcinoma. Review of the Literature and Study of the Ovarian Tumor Registry. *Am. J. Obst. & Gynec.*, 74: 31, 1957.

Gusberg, S. B.: Precursors of Corpus Carcinoma: Estrogens and Adenomatous Hyperplasia. *Am. J. Obst. & Gynec.*, 54: 905, 1947.

Gusberg, S. B., and Hall, R. E.: Precursors of Corpus Cancer. III. The Appearance of Cancer of the Endometrium in Estrogenically Conditioned Patients. *Obst. & Gynec.*, 17: 397, 1961.

Gusberg, S. B., Moore, D. B., and Martin, F.: Precursors of Corpus Cancer. II. Clinical and Pathological Study of Adenomatous Hyperplasia. *Am. J. Obst. & Gynec.*, 68: 1472, 1954.

Hauser, I. J., and Weller, C. V.: A Further Report on the Cancer Family of Warthin. *Am. J. Cancer*, 27: 434, 1936.

Hecht, E. L.: The Cytology of Endometrial Cancer; in J. V. Meigs and S. H. Sturgis, eds.: *Progress in Gynecology*. New York, Grune & Stratton, Inc., 1957, Vol. III, p. 119.

Hertig, A. T., and Sommers, S. C.: Genesis of Endometrial Carcinoma. I. Study of Prior Biopsies. *Cancer*, 2: 946, 1949.

Hertig, A. T., Sommers, S. C., and Bengloff, H.: Genesis of Endometrial Carcinoma. III. Carcinoma in Situ. *Cancer*, 2: 964, 1949.

Jackson, R. L., and Dockerty, M. B.: The Stein-Leventhal Syndrome: Analysis of 43 Cases with Special Reference to Association with Endometrial Carcinoma. *Am. J. Obst. & Gynec.*, 73: 161, 1957.

Jensen, E. I., and Ostergaard, E.: Clinical Studies Concerning the Relationship of Estrogens to the Development of Cancer of the Corpus Uteri. *Am. J. Obst. & Gynec.*, 67: 1094, 1954.

McKay, D. G.: Ovarian Cortical Stromal Hyperplasia; in J. V. Meigs and S. H. Sturgis, eds.: *Progress in Gynecology*. New York, Grune & Stratton, Inc., 1957, Vol. III, p. 1.

Meissner, W. A., Sommers, S. C., and Sherman, G.: Endometrial Hyperplasia, Endometrial Carcinoma and Endometriosis Produced Experimentally by Estrogen. *Cancer*, 10: 500, 1957.

Merriam, J. C., Jr., Easterday, C. L., McKay, D. G., and Hertig, A. T.: Experimental Production of Endometrial Carcinoma in the Rabbit. *Obst. & Gynec.*, 16: 253, 1960.

Miller, N. F.: Carcinoma of the Endometrium: Some Facts, Figures and Fancies. *Obst. & Gynec.*, 15: 579, 1960.

Nash, A. B.: Symposium: Incidence of Endometrial Carcinoma. *Am. J. Obst. & Gynec.*, 81: 1100, 1961.

Novak, E. R.: Uterine Adenocarcinoma in a Patient Receiving Estrogens. *Am. J. Obst. & Gynec.*, 62: 688, 1951.

Novak, E. R., and Mohler, D. I.: Ovarian Stromal Changes in Endometrial Cancer. *Am. J. Obst. & Gynec.*, 65: 1099, 1953.

Novak, E. R., and Santa, U. V.: Factors Influencing the Ratio of Uterine Cancer in a Community. *J.A.M.A.*, 174: 1395, 1960.

Papanicolaou, G. N., and Maddi, F. V.: Diagnostic Value of Cells of Endometrial and Ovarian Origin in Human Tissue Cultures. *Acta Cytologica*, 5: 1, 1961.

Peel, J. H.: Observations upon the Etiology and Treatment of Carcinoma of the Corpus Uteri. *Am. J. Obst. & Gynec.*, 71: 718, 1956.

Randall, C. L.: Ovarian Conservation. *Clin. Obst. & Gynec.*, 4: 857, 1961.

Randall, J. H., and Goddard, W. B.: A Study of 531 Cases of Endometrial Carcinoma. *Surg., Gynec. & Obst.*, 103: 221, 1956.

Roddick, J. W., Jr., and Greene, R. R.: Relation of Ovarian Stromal Hyperplasia to Endometrial Carcinoma. *Am. J. Obst. & Gynec.*, 73: 843, 1957.

Idem: Relation of Ovarian Stromal Hyperplasia to Endometrial Carcinoma. II. A Comparison of Autopsy and Surgical Controls. *Am. J. Obst. & Gynec.*, 75: 1015, 1958.

Scheffey, L. C.: Malignancy Subsequent to Irradiation of the Uterus for Benign Conditions. *Am. J. Obst. & Gynec.*, 44: 925, 1942.

Schroeder, H. A.: *Mechanisms of Hypertension*. Springfield, Ill., Charles C Thomas, 1957, pp. 133–40.

Sommers, S. C., Hertig, A. T., and Bengloff, H.: Genesis of Endometrial Carcinoma. II. Cases 19 to 35 Years Old. *Cancer*, 2: 957, 1949.

Taw, R. L.: Histology in Relation to Carcinogenesis in Endometrial Carcinoma. *Am. J. Obst. & Gynec.*, 81: 1103, 1961.

TeLinde, R. W., Jones, H. W., and Galvin, G. A.: What Are the Earliest Endometrial Changes to Justify a Diagnosis of Endometrial Cancer? *Am. J. Obst. & Gynec.*, 66: 953, 1953.

Traut, H. F.: Problems in Diagnosis of Cancer of the Endometrium. *Am. J. Obst. & Gynec.*, 81: 1102, 1961.

Vander, J. B.: The Association of Diabetes Mellitus and Carcinoma of the Endometrium. *Am. J. Obst. & Gynec.*, 77: 243, 1959.

Way, S.: Aetiology of Carcinoma of Body of Uterus. *J. Obst. & Gynaec. Brit. Emp.*, 61: 46, 1954.

West, C. D., and Rawson, R. W.: The Role of Hormones in the Growth and Control of Tumors Arising in the Female Reproductive System; in J. V. Meigs and S. H. Sturgis, eds.: *Progress in Gynecology*. New York, Grune & Stratton, Inc., 1957, Vol. III, p. 277.

Woll, E., Hertig, A. T., Smith, G. V. S., and Johnson, L. C.: The Ovary in Endometrial Carcinoma, with Notes on Morphological History of the Aging Ovary. *Am. J. Obst. & Gynec.*, 56: 617, 1948.

Diagnosis and Course

Benson, R. C., and Miller, J. N.: Surgical Curettage; Its Value in Abnormal Uterine Bleeding. *Obst. & Gynec.*, 8: 523, 1956.

Blaikley, J. B., Kottmeier, H. L., Martius, H., and Meigs, J. V.: Classification and Clinical Staging of Carcinoma of the Uterus. A Proposal for Modification of the Existing International Definitions. *Am. J. Obst. & Gynec.*, 75: 1286, 1958.

Bunker, M. L.: The Terminal Findings in Endometrial Carcinoma. *Am. J. Obst. & Gynec.*, 77: 530, 1959.

Finn, W. F.: A Clinicopathological Classification of Endometrial Carcinoma Based upon Physical Findings, Anatomical Extent, and Histological Grade. *Am. J. Obst. & Gynec.*, 62: 1, 1951.

Henriksen, E., and Murrieta, J.: Adenocarcinoma of the Corpus Uteri. A Clinicopathological Study. *West. J. Surg., Obst. & Gynec.*, 58: 331, 1959.

Javert, C. T.: Prognosis of Endometrial Cancer. *Obst. & Gynec.*, 12: 556, 1958.

Jordan, M. J., Bader, G. M., and Nemazie, A. S.: Comparative Accuracy of Preoperative Cytologic and Histologic Diagnosis in Endometrial Lesions. *Obst. & Gynec.*, 7: 646, 1956.

McCartney, C. P.: Adenocarcinoma of the Uterine Corpus. *S. Clin. N. Amer.*, 33: 241, 1953.

McGuire, T. H.: Efficacy of Endometrial Biopsy in the Diagnosis of Endometrial Carcinoma. *Obst. & Gynec.*, 19: 105, 1962.

McKelvey, J. L., and Prem, K. A.: Adenocarcinoma of the Endometrium; in J. V. Meigs and S. H. Sturgis, eds.: *Progress in Gynecology*. New York, Grune & Stratton, Inc., 1957, Vol. III, p. 465.

Roberts, S., and others: The Isolation of Cancer Cells from the Blood Stream during Uterine Curettage. *Surg., Gynec. & Obst.*, 111: 3, 1960.

Schlink, H.: Cancer of the Female Pelvis. *J. Obst. & Gynaec. Brit. Emp.*, 67: 402, 1960.

Stander, R. W.: Vaginal Metastases Following Treatment of Endometrial Carcinoma. *Am. J. Obst. & Gynec.*, 71: 776, 1956.

Varangot, J., and others: Detection and Diagnosis of Carcinoma of the Endometrium by Vaginal and Endometrial Smears. *Am. J. Obst. & Gynec.*, 68: 474, 1954.

Wall, J. A., and Mastrovito, R.: Malignant Neoplasia in the Endometrium. A Ten Year Experience in Private Practice. *Am. J. Obst. & Gynec.*, 74: 866, 1957.

Way, S.: Vaginal Metastases of Carcinoma of the Body of the Uterus. *J. Obst. & Gynaec. Brit. Emp.*, 58: 558, 1951.

Therapy

Arneson, A. N.: Symposium: Continuing Evaluation of Endometrial Carcinoma. *Am. J. Obst. & Gynec.*, 81: 1106, 1961.

Bateman, J. C., Carlton, H. N., and Thibeault, J. P.: Chemotherapy for Carcinoma of the Uterus. *Obst. & Gynec.*, 15: 35, 1960.

Braasch, J. W.: Carcinoma of the Endometrium; Follow-up and Future. *S. Clin. N. Amer.*, 39: 821, 1959.

Brunschwig, A., and Murphy, A. I.: The Rationale for Radical Panhysterectomy and Pelvic Node Excision in Carcinoma of the Corpus Uteri. Clinical and Pathological Data on the Mode of Spread of Endometrial Carcinoma. *Am. J. Obst. & Gynec.*, 68: 1482, 1954.

Corscaden, J. A., and Tovell, H. M. M.: The Management of Carcinoma of the Corpus. *Am. J. Obst. & Gynec.*, 68: 737, 1954.

Costolow, W. E., Nolan, J. F., Budenz, G. C., and De Sault, L.: Radiation Treatment of Carcinoma of the Corpus Uteri. *Am. J. Roentgenol.*, 71: 669, 1954.

Dobbie, B. M. W.: Vaginal Recurrences in Carcinoma of the Body of the Uterus and Their Prevention by Radium Therapy. *J. Obst. & Gynaec. Brit. Emp.*, 60: 702, 1953.

Finn, W. F.: Time, Site and Treatment of Recurrences of Endometrial Carcinoma. *Am. J. Obst. & Gynec.*, 60: 773, 1950.

Gusberg, S. B.: Standard Practices at Sloane Hospital. The Management of Carcinoma of the Corpus. *Bull. Sloane Hosp. for Women*, 5: 53, 1959.

Gusberg, S. B., Jones, H. C., Jr., and Tovell, H. M. M.: Selection of Treatment for Corpus Cancer. *Am. J. Obst. & Gynec.*, 80: 374, 1960.

Hendricks, C. H., Callendine, G. W., and Morton, J. L.: A Bead Packing Technique for the Application of Uniform Doses of Irradiation to the Endometrial Cavity. An Experimental Approach. *Am. J. Obst. & Gynec.*, 69: 1039, 1955.

Heyman, J.: Improvement of Results in Treatment; with Special Reference to Radium Therapy and Applicators for Its Use. *J.A.M.A.*, 135: 412, 1947.

Idem: The Radiotherapeutic Treatment of Cancer of Corpus Uteri. *Brit. J. Radiol.*, 20: 85, 1947.

Hubbard, T. B., Jr.: The Effect of Adrenalectomy on Adenocarcinoma of the Uterus. A Case Report. *Cancer*, 13: 1032. 1960.

Javert, C.: The Spread of Benign and Malignant Endometrium in the Lymphatic System, with a Note on Coexisting Vascular Involvement. *Am. J. Obst. & Gynec.*, 64: 780, 1952.

Javert, C., and Hofammann, K.: Observations on Surgical Pathology, Selective Lymphadenectomy and Classification of Endometrial Adenocarcinoma. *Cancer*, 5: 485, 1952.

Kelley, R. M., and Baker, W. H.: Progestational Agents in the Treatment of Carcinoma of the Endometrium. *New England J. Med.*, 264: 216, 1961.

Kistner, R. W.: Histological Effects of Progestins on Hyperplasia and Carcinoma in Situ of the Endometrium. *Cancer*, 12: 1106, 1959.

Kottmeier, H.-L.: Carcinoma of the Corpus Uteri: Diagnosis and Therapy. *Am. J. Obst. & Gynec.*, 78: 1127, 1959.

McCartney, C. P., and Hayden, G. E.: Adequacy of Surgical Treatment for Endometrial Cancer. *Obst. & Gynec.*, 9: 293, 1957.

McLennan, C. E.: The Argument against Preoperative Radium for Endometrial Cancer. *Tr. Pacific Coast Obst. Gyn. Soc.*, 25: 122, 1957.

Meigs, J. V.: Adenocarcinoma of Fundus of Uterus; Report Concerning Vaginal Metastases of This Tumor. *New England J. Med.*, 201: 155, 1929.

Montgomery, J. B., Lang, W. R., Farell, D. M., and Hahn, G. A.: End Results in Adenocarcinoma of the Endometrium Managed by Preoperative Irradiation. *Am. J. Obst. & Gynec.*, 80: 972, 1960.

Nolan, J. F., and Harrison, L. A., Jr.: Carcinoma of the Endometrium. An Evaluation of Preoperative Radiation Therapy. *Obst. & Gynec.*, 17: 601, 1961.

Parsons, L.: *Carcinoma of the Endometrium*. Monographs of Surgery, edited by B. N. Carter. New York, Thomas Nelson Co., 1950, p. 203.

Parsons, L., and Cesare, F.: Wertheim Hysterectomy in the Treatment of Endometrial Carcinoma. *Surg., Gynec. & Obst.*, 108: 582, 1959.

Scheffey, L. C., Thudium, W. J., Farell, D. M., and Hahn, G. A.: Controversial Factors in the Management of Fundal Carcinoma. *Am. J. Obst. & Gynec.*, 52: 529, 1946.

Schmitz, H. E., Smith, C. J., and Fetherson, W. C.: Effects of Preoperative Irradiation on Adenocarcinoma of the Uterus. *Am. J. Obst. & Gynec.*, 78: 1048, 1959.

Schwartz, A. E., and Brunschwig, A.: Radical Panhysterectomy and Pelvic Node Excision for Carcinoma of the Corpus Uteri. *Surg., Gynec. & Obst.*, 105: 675, 1957.

Stroup, P. E.: Surgical Treatment of Endometrial Carcinoma: Analysis of 97 Cases. *Obst. & Gynec.*, 13: 608, 1959.

Endometrial Adenoacanthoma

Chanen, W.: A Clinical and Pathological Study of Adenoacanthoma of the Uterine Body. *J. Obst. & Gynaec. Brit. Emp.*, 67: 287, 1960.

Jones, E. G., Drake, T., Fox, J. B., and Taw, R.: Adenoacanthoma of the Uterus. *Tr. Pacific Coast Obst. & Gynec. Soc.*, 27: 25, 1959.

Liggins, G. C., and Way, S.: A Comparison of the Prognosis of Adenoacanthoma and Adenocarcinoma of the Corpus Uteri. A Report of 24 Cases and a Review of Squamous Metaplasia. *J. Obst. & Gynaec. Brit. Emp.*, 67: 294, 1960.

Marcus, S. L.: Adenoacanthoma of the Endometrium. *Am. J. Obst. & Gynec.*, 81: 259, 1961.

Novak, E. R., and Nalley, W. B.: Uterine Adenoacanthoma. *Obst. & Gynec.*, 9: 396, 1957.

Mixed Mesodermal Tumors and Carcinosarcoma

Carter, E. R., and McDonald, J. R.: Uterine Mesodermal Mixed Tumors. *Am. J. Obst. & Gynec.*, 80: 368, 1960.

Charache, H.: Carcinosarcoma of the Uterus: A Review of the Literature and Report of 4 New Cases. *Am. J. Surg.*, 100: 522, 1960.

Corscaden, J. A., and Singh, B. P.: Leiomyosarcoma of the Uterus. *Am. J. Obst. & Gynec.*, 75: 149, 1958.

Glass, M., and Goldsmith, J. W., Jr.: A Review of Ninety-Four Mixed Mesodermal Tumors of the Uterus, with Report of an Additional Case. *Am. J. Obst. & Gynec.*, 41: 309, 1941.

Gruenwald, P.: Developmental Basis of Regenerative and Pathologic Growth in the Uterus. *Arch. Path.*, 35: 53, 1943.

Hardy, J. A., Jr., and Moragues, V.: Mesodermal Mixed Tumors of the Body of the Uterus, with Report of Two Cases. *Am. J. Obst. & Gynec.*, 63: 307, 1952.

Herbut, P. A.: *Gynecological and Obstetrical Pathology.* Philadelphia, Lea & Febiger, 1953, p. 323.

Hill, R. P., and Miller, F. N., Jr.: Combined Mesenchymal Sarcoma and Carcinoma (Carcinosarcoma) of the Uterus. *Cancer*, 4: 803, 1951.

Horn, R. C., Jr., and Enterline, H. T.: Rhabdomyosarcoma: A Clinicopathological Study and Classification of 39 Cases. *Cancer*, 11: 181, 1958.

Laufe, L. E., and Meyers, L. L.: Mixed Mesodermal Tumors of the Uterus. *Obst. & Gynec.*, 4: 548, 1954.

Laurain, A. R., and Monroe, T. C.: Mixed Mesodermal Sarcoma of the Corpus Uteri Associated with Bilateral Thecoma. *Am. J. Obst. & Gynec.*, 78: 613, 1959.

McElin, T. W., and Davis, H., Jr.: Mesodermal Mixed Tumor of the Corpus Uteri. *Am. J. Obst. & Gynec.*, 63: 605, 1952.

MacFarlane, K. T., and Pritchard, J. E.: Two Cases of Müllerian Carcinosarcoma. *Am. J. Obst. & Gynec.*, 68: 652, 1954.

Marcella, L. C., and Cromer, J. K.: Mixed Mesodermal Tumors. Report of 11 Cases. *Am. J. Obst. & Gynec.*, 77: 275, 1959.

Meyer, R.: Beitrag zur Verstandigung über die Namengebung in der Geschwulstlehre. *Centralbl. allg. Path. u. path. Anat.*, 30: 291, 1919–1920.

Nicholson, G. W. de P.: *Studies of Tumour Formation.* London, Butterworth & Co., Ltd., 1950, pp. 147, 279.

Novak, E.: *Gynecologic and Obstetric Pathology, with Clinical and Endocrine Relations.* 3rd Ed. Philadelphia, W. B. Saunders Company, 1952, p. 236.

Ober, W. B.: Uterine Sarcomas: Histogenesis and Taxonomy. *Ann. New York Acad. Sc.*, 75: 568, 1959.

Ober, W. B., and Tovell, H. M. M.: Mesenchymal Sarcomas of the Uterus. *Am. J. Obst. & Gynec.* 77: 246, 1959.

Radman, H. M., and Korman, W.: Mixed Mesodermal Tumors of the Uterus. *Am. J. Obst. & Gynec.*, 80: 1115, 1960.

Scheffey, L. C., Levinson, J., Herbut, P. A., Hepler, T. K., and Gilmore, G. H.: Osteosarcoma of the Uterus: Report of a Case. *Obst. & Gynec.*, 8: 444, 1956.

Schmidt, E. C. H., and Schutz, R. B.: Mesodermal Mixed Tumors of the Uterus. *Am. J. Obst. & Gynec.*, 56: 966, 1948.

Sternberg, W. H., Clark, W. H., and Smith, R. C.: Malignant Mixed Müllerian Tumor (Mixed Mesodermal Tumor of the Uterus); Study of 21 Cases. *Cancer*, 7: 704, 1954.

Symmonds, R. E., and Dockerty, M. B.: Sarcoma and Sarcoma-Like Proliferations of the Endometrial Stroma: A Clinicopathologic Study of 19 Mesodermal Mixed Tumors. *Surg., Gynec. & Obst.*, 100: 232, 1955.

Tammes, A. R.: Carcinosarcoma of the Uterus. *A.M.A. Arch. Path.*, 70: 343, 1960.

Willis, R. A.: *Pathology of Tumours.* London, Butterworth & Co., 1948, p. 739.

Wilms, M.: *Die Mischgeschwulste der Vagina und der Cervix Uteri.* Leipzig, Geirgi, 1900.

Wolfe, S. A., and Pedowitz, P.: Carcinosarcoma of the Uterus. Report of Sixteen Cases. *Obst. & Gynec.*, 12: 54, 1958.

Chapter 69

Carcinoma of the Fallopian Tube

CARCINOMA of the fallopian tube is regarded as a rare form of genital cancer. When hospital statistics from large metropolitan centers are considered, the frequency of occurrence of malignant disease of the fallopian tube, among all tumors of the genital tract, is somewhere in the range of 0.5 per cent. Undoubtedly there are more cases never reported, for no one surgeon will likely encounter a sufficient number to make a report worth while. Owing to the awakened consciousness of the medical profession toward the cancer problem generally, there is some suggestion that the incidence may be on the increase.

The important point in the consideration of tubal carcinoma lies not in its rarity, but in the fact that it is one of the most malignant forms, not only of genital cancer, but of carcinoma anywhere in the body. The 5-year survival rate, despite improvements in surgical and roentgen therapy, is somewhere in the range of 5 per cent at best. Despite many reports, diagnostic errors made preoperatively are about as frequent as they were twenty years ago. Since the chance of cure varies inversely with the progression of the disease, it is obvious that there can be no improvement in prognosis until earlier diagnoses can be made.

Why Is the Clinical Diagnosis Made So Infrequently?

There are a number of different reasons which contribute to the likelihood of error in diagnosis. The most obvious of these, of course, is that owing to its rarity tubal carcinoma is almost never considered in the differential diagnosis. Furthermore, because of its location, it cannot be seen or felt with any accuracy. Many of these patients are obese. An atrophic, inelastic vagina, combined with a thick layer of abdominal wall fat, is not conducive to an accurate evaluation of adnexal disease.

Cancer of the fallopian tube is primarily a disease of menopausal or older women, though there are reported occurrences in girls as young as eighteen years. Unfortunately in the earlier phases of its development the symptoms are vague. Lower abdominal soreness and pain may be associated with a variety of pelvic diseases. In many instances they are regarded as functional disturbances common to the menopause. It is small wonder, then, that the correct diagnosis is not made more often; yet there are a few pathognomonic signs and symptoms that should arouse suspicion of the possible existence of carcinoma of the fallopian tube.

What Are the Symptoms and Physical Findings That Suggest a Correct Diagnosis?

BLEEDING.   In all reported series a sudden onset of vaginal bleeding, after several years in the menopausal state, appears as the most consistent observation. In nearly every instance the bleeding is continuous, although often of no great quantity. In our own experience, however, we have seen a patient who had bled for three days one year before admission and not thereafter. Recognition of the true cause came only when exploration was done for an enlarging abdominal tumor. Better than 50 per cent of patients, however, will have menorrhagia as their most prominent symptom, regardless of the age in which it occurs.

One of the pitfalls in the interpretation of the causes of postmenopausal bleeding stems from our teaching that it is due usually to carcinoma of either the cervix or endometrium. Hence, with the attention of the surgeon directed primarily toward the endometrial cavity and the cervical canal, the finding of an atrophic uterus with a negative endometrium practically excludes thereafter the thought of a cancer from the mind of the operator. Carcinoma of the tube, however, frequently presents just such a picture. In all probability an adnexal mass is also present. With a history of vaginal bleeding, carcinoma of the ovary is rarely present unless the endometrium is either involved by extension of the cancer or stimulated by estrin elaborated by a functioning ovarian tumor. Thus a curettage can become diagnostic. In the presence of postmenopausal bleeding and a palpable adnexal tumor we should suspect the ovary if the endometrial curettings reveal cancer or hyperplasia, and the tube if a negative or atrophic endometrium is encountered.

Any older patient who (1) has an adnexal mass and vaginal bleeding and (2) has a curettage with negative results, but not surgical exploration, should be carefully watched. We have seen carcinoma of the tube develop and become apparent several years after such a curettage. Other authors have reported the same observation. It may be said and taken as a warning that if no adequate cause has been found to explain vaginal bleeding after a curettage, a carcinoma of the adnexa, and possibly the tube, should be suspected. Any reappearance of bleeding calls for further investigation.

PAIN AND VAGINAL DISCHARGE.   In most reported cases an indefinite sense of lower abdominal pain or soreness is consistently noted. Because of its variable nature and location not much attention is paid to it until it is accompanied by enlargement of the abdomen or the sudden appearance of bleeding. Nearly all authors are in agreement that pain appears early in the disease, in contrast to carcinoma of the uterus or ovary, in which the progress is more insidious. The disturbing fact is that no attention is given to the pain, or it is dismissed as unimportant.

In many cases of carcinoma of the tube the patient notes a more or less continuous serosanguineous vaginal discharge in minimal quantity. In any postmenopausal woman this sort of symptom is important. In many reported instances the vaginal smear has shown tumor cells. When smear diagnosis is positive, the source must be discovered. The percentage of error in a negative report is undoubtedly higher than in endometrial cancer. Vaginal smears should be taken, however.

One of the fascinating features in the symptomatology of carcinoma of the tube is the association of an intermittent, colicky pain with a sudden, profuse watery discharge of variable nature, after which the pain subsides and the adnexal mass disappears. In most instances such a course of events is regarded as a manifestation of pelvic inflammatory disease. Actually, when the discharge is serosanguineous, isht combination of symptoms should be regarded as pathognomonic of carcinoma of the tube. Approximately 25 per cent will exhibit such a train of symptoms.

This has been called *hydrops tubae profluens*. The explanation for the phenomenon is an interesting one. By and large, carcinoma of the fallopian tube develops in the outer two thirds. According to Robinson, the outer or fimbriated ends of the tube close late in the course of the disease. This is in contrast to gonorrhea, which also produces a hydrosalpinx. Thus the early symptoms are vague, and pain appears only as the tubal lumen distends and the serosa is stretched. When the fimbriae finally close, the tube may reach enormous dimensions as the lumen becomes distended with secretions and products of tumor necrosis. The tube now attempts to discharge the contents by peristaltic action, thereby accounting for the intermittent, colicky nature of the pain. The sudden discharge of tubal contents into the uterus takes place as the obstruction at the uterine end that was produced by kinking of the tube or peritubal adhesions is released.

If no discharge takes place, the patient has the same intermittent colicky pain without relief, along with abdominal tenderness and a backache that radiates down the leg. Because there is no accompanying sudden vaginal discharge and disappearance of the adnexal mass, the symptoms are usually ascribed to an acute flareup of an antecedent pelvic inflammation.

PHYSICAL FINDINGS.   Since the correct diagnosis is unsuspected, because of the vague symptoms, the patient frequently presents herself to the physician with little else than a story of an enlarging abdomen and some abdominal pain, which may have increased in severity in recent weeks.

Unfortunately there is nothing very characteristic about the physical findings with carcinoma of the tube. The tender mass found may be due to fibroids, a twisted ovarian cyst or pelvic inflammation in an acute recurring phase. In most instances carcinoma of the tube presents itself in the form of a unilateral hydrosalpinx. The diagnostic problem, however, is made no easier by the fact that the patient may also have a simple ovarian cyst on the same side.

Early diagnosis of carcinoma of the tube can be made only when the index of suspicion is high, and proper consideration is given to the symptomatology. This further emphasizes the feeling we have about adnexal or eccentrically placed lesions. Certainly in the postmenopausal woman at least, the palpation of such a mass should call for surgical abdominal exploration, particularly when the patient also has pain and vaginal bleeding, however minimal they may be.

What Is the Gross Appearance of Tubal Carcinoma?

The most important single fact about the spread of tubal carcinoma, as reported by many authors, is that the tubal muscular wall becomes involved in the disease. Microscopically, then, it is important to decide whether the carcinoma actually arises within the tubal epithelium or appears as the result of secondary invasion from a carcinoma elsewhere, the endometrium or ovary, for example. Late involvement of the tubal wall would speak for a primary carcinoma of the fallopian tube, in contrast to a metastatic carcinoma, implants of which might be found in the muscular wall with normal mucosal epithelium in the lumen.

Before further extension has occurred through metastasis, continuity or contiguity, a primary carcinoma of the tube may grossly resemble a benign, thin-walled, hugely dilated, retort-shaped, simple hydrosalpinx. It is reddish-purple, with a smooth

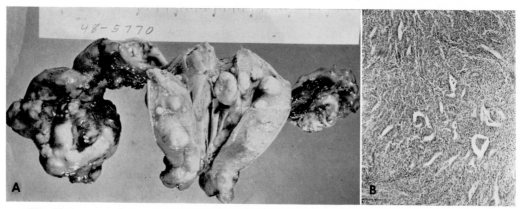

Fig. 69-1.　　*A,* Carcinoma of the fallopian tubes is characterized by a fleshy tumor in the tubal wall, both undemarcated and unencapsulated. Both tubes are often involved, as here, although one carcinoma is much more advanced than the other. *B,* An adenocarcinoma that is rather undifferentiated, but contains some glandular structures, is the most common histologic type of tubal carcinoma.

serosal surface. The true nature is not suspected until the tube is sectioned (Fig. 69–1, *A*). There is a double danger in suspecting that a single large hydrosalpinx is evidence of a benign condition. Not only may tubal carcinoma actually be involved, but the apparently normal-looking tube on the opposite side may also be the site of malignancy. Primary carcinoma of the tube is frequently bilateral.

Approximately 30 per cent of tubal carcinomas show metastases. Their extension is largely by lymphatic channels to the lumbar, iliac and sacral lymph nodes. We have seen one case of inguinal node metastasis in the groin that appeared before the tubal wall became involved. Metastases are usually limited to the lower part of the abdomen, and the liver rarely becomes involved. Ascites and large abdominal masses are late manifestations of the disease.

Microscopically, adenocarcinomas have been classified in a variety of ways, but by and large they fall into one of three patterns: (*a*) adenomatous, (*b*) medullary, or (*c*) papillary. The tubal carcinomas most often form atypical glands within glands, and a solid tumor of adenomatous architecture is seen with obvious anaplasia and invasive capacity (Fig. 69–1, *B*). The less common medullary carcinoma is a solid, sheetlike growth of cells not easily identified as of tubal origin. Ordinarily one first thinks of a solid ovarian carcinoma, and later, on finding that the ovaries are completely negative, one realizes that the primary site was in the fallopian tube. The papillary tubal carcinomatous pattern resembles a serous cystadenocarcinoma of the ovary and is the rarest and least malignant subtype.

Actually, little is gained by attempting to divide the tubal cancers into different types of carcinoma. The earliest forms are papillary, but since they merge into one another, an attempt to divide them may be more confusing than helpful.

What Is the Differential Diagnosis Pathologically?

Grossly and microscopically, one should consider other tubal diseases that might prove confusing.

Salpingitis rarely causes difficulty because there is insufficient epithelial hyperplasia to produce a solid tissue mass or to arouse suspicion of cancer microscopically. Tuberculous salpingitis, however, typically is accompanied by an epithelial hyperplasia of sinister appearance, but without precancerous significance. No invasion or obvious anaplasia is found. The presence of granulomatous inflammation with tubal epithelial hyperplasia favors tuberculosis and is against a carcinoma.

SALPINGITIS ISTHMICA NODOSA.   This curious nodular thickening of parts of both fallopian tubes, most characteristically their isthmic portions, is seen in multiparous women both before and after the menopause. Alone, it has little clinical importance, and is usually an incidental finding after uterine surgery for fibroids or adenomyosis.

Grossly, the tubes are lumpy, tortuous and locally firm. On section the muscular walls are thickened, but the appearance is not similar to carcinoma.

Microscopically, instead of a single central tubal lumen, one sees multiple tubal epithelial outpouchings irregularly mingled with the fibromuscular wall, so that there seem to be multiple, separate small lumens and blind pouches. Muscular hypertrophy is present, but there is no epithelial anaplasia or invasion (Fig. 69-2, A).

The process is believed to have an identical pathogenesis with that of adenomyosis of the uterus. Neither the uterus nor tube has a submucosal buffer zone, and epithelium can herniate outward directly via weak spots in the smooth muscle. A similar condition occurs also in the gallbladder. None of these lesions are neoplastic.

ADENOMATOID TUMOR OF TUBE.   In common with the male spermatic cord, sometimes one fallopian tube is distorted by a firm, spherical, sharply demarcated fleshy nodule, averaging about 1 or 2 cm. in diameter. Microscopically, in both sites the tumor is composed of well formed ductlike spaces lined by irregularly flattened or bulging watery cells. The epithelial-like linings are practically identical with those of the uterine mesonephroma (Fig. 69-2, B).

The term "adenomatoid tumor" is now preferred for these benign lesions, which once were called lymphangioma, mesothelioma or angioma and were even confused with cancer. The mesonephric origin of these tumors from wolffian duct remnants in the tubal region and spermatic cord appears reasonable.

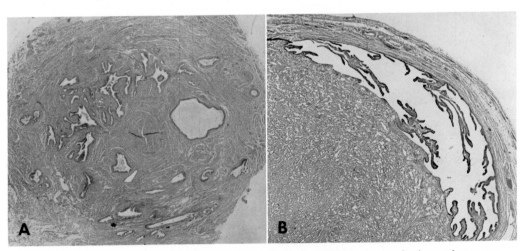

Fig. 69-2.   A, In salpingitis isthmica nodosa the main tubal lumen remains intact, but numerous diverticular outpouchings develop that mingle with locally hypertrophied smooth muscle. Together these form irregular nodules, most characteristically of the tubal isthmus, that give the condition its name. B, Distortion of the tube lining by a rounded mass composed of small, closely packed spaces is found in the adenomatoid tumor. The glandlike spaces are lined by benign-appearing, watery mesonephric-type cells. (B, Courtesy of Dr. Cesar Tedeschi, Framingham Union Hospital.)

What Is the Proper Treatment?

It is obvious, when survival statistics are considered, that either the therapy used in the past was inadequate, or, owing to their insidious growth pattern, tubal carcinomas have been too far advanced when treatment is undertaken. The greatest mistake, of course, is assuming that the existing disease is benign, unilateral pelvic inflammation. If the surgeon will make it a routine practice to section the excised specimen at the operating table, there will be less chance of making this mistake. The next mistake is assuming that the opposite tube is benign because of its innocuous appearance.

The operation of choice is a total hysterectomy with removal of both adnexa. This should be followed by external roentgen therapy. We have personal knowledge of one patient who survived seventeen years and died at the age of seventy-five without any suggestion of recurrence after this program of therapy.

To improve the prognosis in the future one might speculate on the wisdom of doing a Wertheim type of hysterectomy with a bilateral pelvic lymphadenectomy, when the diagnosis is confirmed at surgical exploration.

The life history of carcinoma of the tube is similar to that of carcinoma of the endometrium and cervix. Meigs has noted that vaginal metastases are present in 60 per cent of the cases. This is a common finding when inadequate surgery is done for cancer of the cervix. The fact that carcinoma of the tube tends to remain local, but with metastases to the regional iliac and obturator lymph nodes, is another point of similarity. Exceptions to this pattern occur, for metastases have appeared in the inguinal region before the tubal wall became involved, and other metastases have been reported in the supraclavicular lymph nodes as well as nearly every organ in the body. In all probability spread in these instances was by blood stream rather than by lymphatic channels.

As yet there is no precedent for a more radical surgical approach, which has been suggested in the hope that the results in the future may prove to be more rewarding.

REFERENCES

Carcinoma of Fallopian Tube

Anderson, H. J., Bantin, C. F., Giffen, H. K., Olson, L. J., and Shack, C. B.: Primary Carcinoma of the Fallopian Tube. *Obst. & Gynec.*, 3: 89, 1954.

Anspach, B. M.: Early Diagnosis of Adnexal Cancer. *Am. J. Obst. & Gynec.*, 20: 571, 1930.

Bose, K.: A Case of Bilateral Primary Carcinoma of the Fallopian Tubes. *Brit. J. Clin. Pract.*, 16: 19, 1962.

Brewer, J. I., and Guderian, A. M.: Diagnosis of Uterine Tube Carcinoma by Vaginal Cytology. *Obst. & Gynec.*, 8: 664, 1956.

Corscaden, J. A.: *Gynecologic Cancer*, 2nd ed. Baltimore, Williams & Wilkins Company, 1956, p. 442.

Cron, R. S., and Claude, J. L.: Primary Papillary Carcinoma of the Uterine Tube and Report of a Case. *Obst. & Gynec.*, 13: 734, 1958.

Edwards, E. A., and Beebe, R. A.: Primary Carcinoma of the Fallopian Tube. *Am. J. Obst. & Gynec.*, 53: 1049, 1947.

Fidler, H. K., and Lock, D. R.: Carcinoma of the Fallopian Tube Detected by Cervical Smear. *Am. J. Obst. & Gynec.*, 67: 1103, 1954.

Finn, W. F., and Javert, C. T.: Primary and Metastatic Cancer of the Fallopian Tube. *Cancer*, 2: 803, 1949.

Frankel, A. N.: Primary Carcinoma of the Fallopian Tube. *Am. J. Obst. & Gynec.*, 72: 131, 1956.

Hayden, G. E., and Potter, E. L.: Primary Carcinoma of the Fallopian Tube with Report of 12 New Cases. *Am. J. Obst. & Gynec.*, 79: 24, 1960.

Helo, A.: Carcinoma of the Fallopian Tube, with Special Reference to the Yellow Discharge Which Appears with It. *Acta obst. et gynec. Scandinav.*, 39: 259, 1960.

Hu, C. Y., Taymor, M. L., and Hertig, A. T.: Primary Carcinoma of the Fallopian Tube. *Am. J. Obst. & Gynec.*, 59: 58, 1950.

Israel, S. L., Crisp, W. E., and Adrian, D. C.: Preoperative Diagnosis of Primary Carcinoma of the Fallopian Tube. *Am. J. Obst. & Gynec.*, 68: 1589, 1954.

Krugman, P. I., and Fisher, J. E.: Primary Carcinoma of the Fallopian Tube. *Am. J. Obst. & Gynec.*, 80: 722, 1960.

Lombardo, F. A., and Wood, H. T.: Primary Adenocarcinoma of the Uterine Tube. Report of 6 Cases. *Obst. & Gynec.*, 17: 611, 1961.

Meigs, J. V.: *Tumors of the Female Pelvic Organs.* New York, Macmillan Company, 1934.

Mitchell, R. M., and Mohler, R. W.: Primary Carcinoma of the Fallopian Tube. *Am. J. Obst. & Gynec.*, 50: 283, 1945.

Parsons, L.: Carcinoma of the Fallopian Tube. *New England J. Med.*, 221: 367, 1939.

Robinson, M. R.: Report of Three Cases of Primary Cancer of the Fallopian Tubes, with Summary of Cases Omitted from Nürnberger's Report (1931) and Those Recorded to 1935. *Am. J. Obst. & Gynec.*, 32: 84, 1936.

Roddick, J. W., Jr., and Danforth, D. N.: Primary Carcinoma of the Uterine Tube. Report of an Unusual Case. *Am. J. Obst. & Gynec.*, 80: 67, 1960.

Sedlis, A.: Primary Carcinoma of the Fallopian Tube. *Obst. & Gynec. Surv.*, 16: 209, 1961.

Tatum, H. J., and Golden, A.: Carcinoma of the Fallopian Tube. *Clin. Obst. & Gynec.*, 1: 1113, 1958.

Salpingitis Isthmica Nodosa and Adenomatoid Tumor

Benjamin, C. L., and Beaver, D. C.: Pathogenesis of Salpingitis Isthmica Nodosa. *Am. J. Clin. Path.*, 21: 212, 1954.

Jackson, J. R.: The Histogenesis of the Adenomatoid Tumor of the Genital Tract. *Cancer*, 11: 337, 1958.

Leach, W. B.: Adenomatoid Tumor of Fallopian Tube Associated with Chronic Salpingitis; Report of Case. *Am. J. Clin. Path.*, 20: 970, 1950.

Ragins, A. B., and Crane, R. D.: Adenomatoid Tumors of the Fallopian Tube. *Am. J. Path.*, 24: 933, 1948.

Chapter 70

Dermatologic Lesions of
the Vulva and Perineal Region

Owing to its exposed position, which subjects it to constant trauma, and its anatomic configuration to which the upper thighs are in apposition, a wide variety of dermatologic infections and dermatoses tends to appear in the vulvar area. The problems are accentuated in the postmenopausal woman, who may have put on weight as her physical activities decline and hormonal activity lessens. Since the skin of the vulvar area is under hormonal control, atrophic conditions are apt to manifest themselves at this time. Likewise the skin of the vulvar area is prone to develop neoplastic changes. Malignant melanomas, for instance, occur not infrequently in the vulvar area. Approximately 3 per cent of all malignant genital processes appear as carcinoma of the vulva.

It is manifestly impossible to describe all the dermatologic lesions or infections that may appear in the vulvar area. A few will be described in brief fashion. The manifestations of dermatoses in the vulvar area are often so unusual, even for the more commonplace lesions, that the most experienced of dermatologists may need to rely on darkfield examinations and biopsy rather than their clinical acumen.

VULVAR FOLLICULITIS, FURUNCULOSIS AND CARBUNCLES

Pyogenic organisms are prone to infect hair follicles in the anogenital region because of the difficulty in keeping this area dry. This is particularly true if the patient is obese, if the weather is hot or she lives in a damp climate. The trauma produced by scratching or friction is enough to provide a break in the skin through which superficially located bacteria may enter the deeper skin layers. Depending on the depth of their penetration, she may have either a superficial folliculitis or a deep one (furunculosis). In the majority of instances the infecting organism is a coagulase-positive staphylococcus.

When the infection is superficial, small pustules are seen with the shaft of hair piercing the centers. The pustules tend to break and crust over. Simple soap and water cleansing and the application of antibiotic ointments are all that is needed to clear up the infection. With deeper penetration of the bacterial infection the hair follicles themselves become involved, and inflammation spreads to the perifollicular tissues

1130

around them. As long as the infection is confined to a single hair follicle there is no particular problem in therapy.

With more extensive spread of the infection we may find a widespread furunculosis or actual carbuncle formation. When there are only a few isolated, firm, tender furuncles (boils), hot saline applications should be used to encourage tissue breakdown so that drainage can be established simply by puncturing the fluctuating top coverings. One should carefully avoid squeezing the area, because infection can be spread beyond the normally protective barriers by so doing. Again, the entire area should be kept clean with soap and water, and antibiotic ointments should be used to protect the adjacent uninvolved hair follicles.

With even deeper infection in the lower corium and subcutaneous layers of the skin, such as one sees in a carbuncle, there is no longer any reason to use topical antibiotics. If they are to be effective, they now should be given systemically, usually in the form of adequate amounts of penicillin. When the infection has localized sufficiently, it should be drained extensively with cruciate incisions after the manner advocated for the treatment of a carbuncle wherever it is found. Once the infection is cured, a strict regimen of cleanliness must be instituted to avoid subsequent recurrence of the folliculitis and furunculosis.

TINEA CRURIS

This type of fungus disease which takes the form of what was once called eczema marginatum, now usually termed tinea cruris, occurs largely on the upper inner

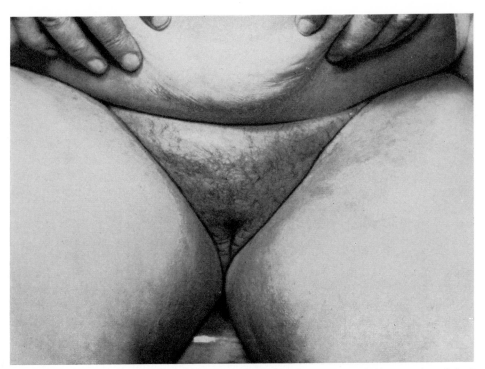

Fig. 70-1.   Tinea cruris is associated with a reddish, slightly elevated skin eruption of the intertriginous areas adjacent to the vulva. Obese women are more often affected. (Courtesy of Dr. H. Mescon, Massachusetts Memorial Hospitals.)

portions of the thighs as well as on the pelvic and gluteal areas. It is far more common in men, but is occasionally seen in women, particularly in the inguinal regions. It begins as a sharply demarcated, red circular patch with tiny vesicles and papules around the periphery. The advancing margins of the lesion tend to be elevated above the surface of the surrounding skin (Fig. 70–1). The lesion is likely to expand along the margins while it heals in the central portion, although this is not invariably true. It is known to be contagious and has been reported in epidemics within a boarding school. The fungus, *Epidermophyton floccosum*, or sometimes Trichophyton, receives its impetus for propagation in the moist, warm medium established by the anatomic arrangement of the vulva, thighs, buttocks and groins.

Itching is the most prominent symptom. Though it is not intense, it does lead to scratching. In this manner small lesions coalesce to become larger. Although it does occur around the anus, tinea cruris is rarely the cause of pruritus ani.

The *treatment* of tinea cruris is relatively simple. One should be cautioned about overtreatment, which may do more harm than good. Hot water baths and mild dusting powder may be all that is needed. The area must be thoroughly dried and all the soap removed before the powder is applied, or caking will result. If the infection is more extensive, topical hydrocortisone ointment or emulsion may be used.

Prophylactically, emphasis should be placed on dryness and aeration. Loose cotton underwear, rather than nylon panties, should be worn, since the latter may generate both heat and moisture. Tight-fitting underclothing may produce irritation by friction and allow secondary infection to enter through skin abrasions. The process has a tendency to recur, but it need not if simple precautionary hygiene measures are observed.

DERMATITIS MEDICAMENTOSA

It is possible for a wide variety of dermatitides to appear on the vulvar area, as the result of systemic ingestion or local application of drugs. There seems to be no particular specific variety of skin eruption that can be attributed to any given drug, nor does the dosage or duration of its use have much relationship. A patient may have taken some particular drug for a long time without adverse effect, only to become sensitive later. An individual sensitization factor is obviously present, since some patients can tolerate continued use of a drug in high concentrations without any skin manifestations, but others will react violently to infinitesimal amounts. Frequently the patient is unaware of any particular sensitivity. It is an interesting observation that local eruptions in the genital areas, traceable to drug therapy, may occur without any accompanying systemic manifestation of hypersensitivity such as fever, malaise or joint pains.

Drug allergy and individual sensitivity are far too complex problems to be discussed in a gynecologic treatise. Nevertheless any kind of drug can produce a dermatitis in the genital area. In the presence of such a dermatitis the possibility of an underlying cause traceable to drug therapy should be kept in mind and the patient interrogated along that line.

Some drugs that produce the vulvar and genital dermatitis are in common use. A rash may be acquired from preparations given for ordinary headache or migraine, which contain antipyrine. Phenolphthalein is a common ingredient in many laxative prescriptions (e.g. Ex-Lax, Agoral, Feen-a-mint). Vesicular and urticarial eruptions may appear on the genital as well as the oral mucous membranes in a person who is sensitive to phenolphthalein. The same thing may be said about pyramidon, phenacetin or the salicylates, which are frequently used either alone or in combination with other drugs for pain relief. It is also well known that erythematous and vesicular eruptions, some of them bullous, may follow the use of even minimal doses of the barbiturates.

Perhaps two of the most common of drugs now in general use that may, in a given individual, produce drug reactions in the skin of the vulva and genital area are the sulfonamides and antibiotics. Penicillin in a sensitized person may produce swelling of the vulva, as well as of other mucous membrane areas. The reaction may appear in a matter of hours or after a lapse of a week or ten days. The reactions are more likely to occur in the vulva after the topical use of penicillin ointments than when the drug is given systemically (Fig. 70–2). One should therefore be cautious about using preparations that contain penicillin for genital dermatitis, particularly if there are other forms of treatment available that will serve as well. The same observations may be made for other antibiotic drugs, such as Aureomycin, streptomycin, Chloromycetin, tetracycline and Terramycin. We have previously mentioned, for example, the mycotic dermatitis that may follow the use of Aureomycin.

Unfortunately, there does not appear to be any test to determine drug sensitivity in an individual patient, short of trial and error. Before prescribing any of the antibiotic preparations it will be well to question the patient about any past reaction to their use. Furthermore, if other preparations will be effective, they should be tried first, rather than running the risk of creating hypersensitivity to a drug which may have lifesaving value in the face of a more severe disease than vulvar dermatitis. When

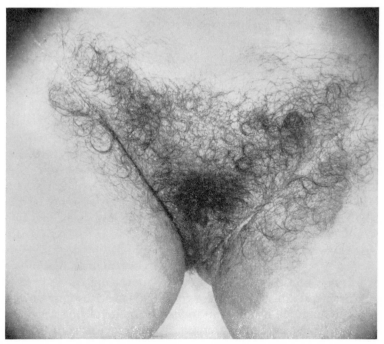

Fig. 70-2.   Hypersensitivity reaction with vulvar dermatitis following the use of penicillin. (Courtesy of Dr. F. Ronchese, Providence, R.I.)

a dermatitis is already present, the patient should be thoroughly questioned about the previous use of drugs in any form.

Antihistaminic drugs to relieve the itching caused by a drug reaction are a well known form of treatment. When the drug-induced dermatitis is accompanied by a severe rash, erythema and swelling of the skin in the vulvar and inguinal areas, dramatic relief can be obtained by giving 100 mg. of cortisone, twice daily, for 48 hours.

SEBORRHEIC DERMATITIS

Seborrheic dermatitis is common in the hairy portion of the vulva as well as in the inguinal folds and intergluteal cleft. It usually occurs in combination with involvement of other regions such as the scalp, ears, umbilicus, axillae and presternal region. It is particularly apt to occur in obese patients and may be difficult to assess if there is an associated intertrigo. In most instances the diagnosis is not difficult, because the typical greasy, yellow scales are usually present in other areas as well as the vulva.

In the acute phases moist compresses and shake lotions are preferred to the use of ointments, because ointments may turn the seborrheic dermatitis into an eczema. When the acute phase has subsided, preparations containing sulfur, salicylic acid and tar or 6 per cent precipitated sulfur in a zinc paste will be effective in most instances when applied every night for two or three occasions. In the obese patient, who has intertrigo as well, one may either give hydrocortisone lotion or apply 2 to 5 per cent silver nitrate to the fissured lesions in the groins.

PRURITUS VULVAE

Pruritus vulvae is a common gynecologic complaint that affects women of all ages, but it is particularly apt to appear in the postmenopausal woman. It is important to stress that pruritus is just a symptom and not a disease entity. Pruritus vulvae is simply a localized form of neurodermatitis for which there are multiple explanations. Before any therapy can begin the underlying cause for the itching (pruritus) and the actual site of the irritation should be determined. It is impossible within the scope of this text to discuss all the possibilities, but a few generalizations may be made.

The anogenital area is constantly being contaminated by secretions and excretions from the vagina, urethra and rectum. Furthermore, the area is hard to keep perfectly clean. Under normal conditions the vaginal secretions are nonirritating. They are usually acid, and the skin of the vulva is partially protected by the secretion of the sebaceous glands. This is less likely to be true in the years that follow the menopause, when sweat-gland activity diminishes and the normal vaginal secretions become neutral or alkaline in reaction. With accompanying pathologic conditions, such as cervicitis or vaginitis, the secretions are more copious and tend to macerate the vulvar and perineal skin. Under these conditions pruritus may develop. Any local treatment of the itching will usually fail unless the contributing cervicitis or vaginitis is controlled. There is less agreement among dermatologists as to the roles played by monilial and trichomonad vaginal infections in the causation of pruritus, since the symptoms often persist after the primary infections have been cleared up.

The accumulation of minute amounts of fecal matter in crypts and crevices of the vulvar area can frequently account for the itching. In some instances, because of external hemorrhoids, anal fissures or previous surgery, there may be some involuntary leakage from the anus. This excretion, like pathologic or menopausal vaginal discharges, is apt to be on the alkaline side, which the vulvar and perianal skin tolerates less well. Constant or periodic irritation from this source may produce pruritus. Leakage from the bladder when the patient has urgency or stress incontinence may contribute to the etiology of pruritus by setting up an irritation and keeping the area moist and macerated.

In addition to the change in the vulvar skin produced by secretions and excretions, one should keep in mind the possibility of a local skin sensitivity that may be produced by douches, contraceptive devices, both of male and female, hygienic pads or inserts, underclothing and soap.

Any factor that will irritate the vulva or perineal area will be enough to cause pruritus. Friction of tight undergarments or the rubbing of a girdle may trigger a pruritus vulvae. Edema and congestion are also contributing factors. Thus we find that itching is more severe on or about the time of menstruation. Not all of this is due to the friction of the hygienic pads, but can be traced in part at least to edema, congestion and nervous tension (Fig. 70–3).

Excluding all other causes, there remains a psychosomatic component in the problem of pruritus vulvae. Some dermatologists feel that a high percentage of all pruritus vulvae is due to sexual frustration, inhibitions or maladjustments. Others feel that, though there may be basic fears such as a fear of cancer or venereal infection,

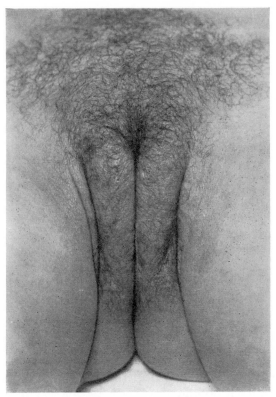

Fig. 70-3.   Pruritus vulvae is associated with reddening and edematous swelling of the labia and adjacent vulvar soft tissues in some cases. (Courtesy of Dr. F. Ronchese, Providence, R.I.)

psychogenic cause is less likely to be present in pruritus vulvae than in pruritus ani. One cannot deny that pruritus vulvae tends to be worse at night, when the day's activities are over, or that the symptoms invariably become more pronounced during periods of anxiety or emotional stress. Frequently the physical findings such as vaginal discharge are minimal, indeed. One must conclude that psychogenic causes are prominent in the etiology of pruritus vulvae.

Treatment

It is practically impossible to outline any standard form of therapy for pruritus vulvae, because of the many possible explanations as to cause. In general, however, one should (1) prescribe hot baths or douches followed by thorough drying; (2) keep the area cool, dry and well aerated; (3) apply cold applications as compresses to the vulvar area; (4) use lotions rather than ointments, which are poorly tolerated; (5) give antihistaminic preparations to relieve the itching, such as Benadryl, 50 mg., or Pyribenzamine, 3 times a day and at bedtime; (6) give the patient sedatives at night to minimize the insomnia produced by the itching.

Specifically, one may give hydrocortisone lotions, although the corticosteroids have proved less effective for pruritus vulvae than for pruritus ani. In rare instances, and probably more for the psychogenic effect than for any specific reason, x-ray treatment might be given in very mild doses to the vulvar area. Surgical procedures, such as undermining of the entire skin of the area, vulvectomy or alcohol injection, have all been tried with varying degrees of success.

PRURITUS ANI

One of the other more common manifestations of neurodermatitis is *pruritus ani*. The itching may be intense and the impulse to scratch almost uncontrollable. The social implications are therefore formidable. There is a wide variety of possible explanations for pruritus in this area, such as pediculosis pubis, intestinal parasites like pinworms, lichen planus, psoriasis, seborrheic dermatitis and other infections, allergic responses and irritations produced by contact (Fig. 70–4). The problems are compounded by the fact that it is difficult to keep the area dry and clean, since it is intermittently contaminated by fecal and vaginal discharges. Despite all these possible etiologic explanations, the most likely cause of true anal pruritus can be traced to psychic imbalance. The anxiety, frustration, grief, depression and hostility states all contribute to explain it. In addition, psychiatrists point out that anal fixations are common and that erotic and homosexual tendencies may contribute to the anal itching.

In the patient who has true neurodermatitis of the anal area no eruption is seen, but the skin itself is edematous, excoriated and grayish-white. In some instances it may simulate leukoplakia. On rarer occasions the skin may be covered with dry, scaly, papular lesions arranged in circular fashion about the anus, but tending to extend in the direction of the vulva or onto the buttock (Fig. 70–5).

The initial phase of *treatment* concerns itself with the establishment of an accurate diagnosis. Thus both the vaginal and the rectal canals must be thoroughly investigated to rule out possible etiologic conditions. A proctoscopic examination is as important as a vaginal examination in this regard. The possibility of psychiatric maladjustments must be considered and evaluated. In addition, a number of generalized disease entities common in general medical practice are capable of producing anal pruritus.

The primary aim of course is to relieve the itching. To this end all possible irritating sources must be eliminated. It may therefore be advisable to be concerned with the proper regulation of bowel habit. Chemical changes in the stool of a patient who has diarrhea, for example, may be responsible for the local skin sensitivity. Avoidance of any food that seems to cause anal itching should be axiomatic.

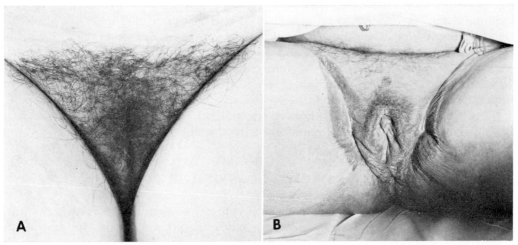

Fig. 70-4.   *A,* Pediculosis pubis is commonly associated with pruritis. A sharp and experienced eye will discern the *Phthirus pubis,* crab lice, on the skin and their nits attached to the pubic hairs. *B,* Psoriasis of the vulva may be a cause of pruritus vulvae et ani. (Courtesy of Dr. F. Ronchese, Providence, R.I.)

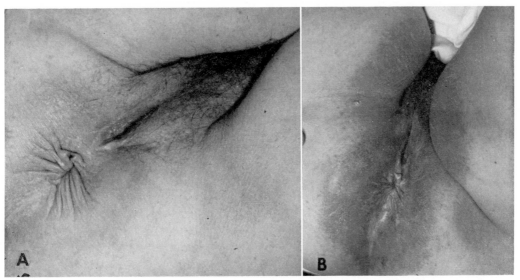

Fig. 70-5.   *A,* Pruritus ani may be associated with a perianal ring of lichenified dermatitis with fine wrinkling and scaling. (Courtesy of Dr. H. Mescon, Massachusetts Memorial Hospitals.) *B,* Severe excoriated dermatitis with pruritis ani may result partially from scratching or overtreatment. (Courtesy of Dr. F. Ronchese, Providence, R.I.)

Anal hygiene is therefore of fundamental importance. Since anatomic considerations make this difficult, it is often wise to have the patient use moistened cotton or facial tissue rather than coarse toilet paper. At times an anal fissure, external hemorrhoid or infected anal crypt makes adequate toilet of the anal area difficult, since minute collections of fecal matter tend to hide in small skin crevices. Gentle use of soap for cleansing after a bowel movement should be encouraged, but the patient must be instructed to remove the soap thoroughly.

Hot sitz-baths are comforting, although cold applications such as ice and witch hazel are frequently more effective. Cortisone, applied locally as a lotion if there is an inflammatory reaction or as an ointment if there is none, is highly successful in relieving the itching when used in small amounts three or four times daily. Even the most resistant case usually resolves and disappears after one week of such treatment. Many surgical procedures, such as undermining of the skin or alcohol injections, were advocated and used in the past. Like x-ray treatment, there appear to be fewer indications today for their use.

As an obvious adjunct to therapy the patient should be given sedatives and barbiturates to ensure peace of mind and a good night's rest.

DEGENERATIVE LESIONS OF THE VULVA

Older women past the menopause, or younger women who for one reason or another no longer have ovarian function, may undergo changes in the skin of the vulvar area that produce painful fissuring, intense pruritus, burning sensations or an uncomfortable sense of dryness. The four most common entities that produce this train of events are (1) senile atrophy, (2) kraurosis, (3) leukoplakia, and (4) lichen sclerosus et atrophicus.

SENILE ATROPHY

This condition is common after diminution in the output of the ovarian hormones. The skin becomes thin and shiny as well as dry and smooth. At times areas of telangiectasia appear, and occasionally the skin thickens to a leathery consistency and takes on a splotchy, brownish discoloration. Signs of atrophy are apparent in the loss of subcutaneous fat and elasticity of the skin, which results in a shrinkage of the labia majora and minora, and at times the clitoris, to the point at which they are hardly recognizable as anatomic structures. There may be some associated leukoplakia.

Since the atrophied skin is easily traumatized, minute breaks occur in its integumentary covering that permit the introduction of low-grade pathogenic bacteria. The patient then suffers from an intense itching which induces her to scratch for relief. A vicious circle then develops because the scratching produces more minute excoriations and further infection.

Treatment

The simplest forms of therapy are the best. The area should be kept cool, dry and clean. Cold applications will tend to relieve the itching. Benadryl, 50 mg., in the middle of the afternoon and at bedtime is a useful remedy. Since the condition may be exasperating enough to keep the patient awake, a barbiturate such as Nembutal or Seconal should be given to prevent insomnia. If the itching is intense and cannot be relieved by squeezing the tissue rather than scratching it, and cold applications fail, relief may be obtained by 1 per cent liquid cortisone, applied and rubbed in with the little finger.

Leukoplakia and Kraurosis Vulvae

The two most serious degenerative diseases of the vulva are kraurosis and leukoplakia. Although both have atrophy as their end-stage, often occur in the same patient and may, at times, have the same external appearance, actually the two entities are dissimilar in their etiology, microscopic appearance and malignant potentialities.

Leukoplakia at inception actually represents a hyperplasia rather than atrophy. The epithelium thickens and forms a superficial scale that reflects light, giving the plaque the white color responsible for the name of the process. In kraurosis, conversely, the epithelium becomes abnormally thin and shiny so that the vascularized tissue beneath shows through and gives the area a pinkish-red hue. Despite the dissimilarity the two lesions do tend to coexist to such an extent that many authors feel that they are actually one and the same condition, but in different stages. It is of the utmost importance to differentiate between the two, however, for leukoplakia is a precancerous lesion, while kraurosis is not.

Kraurosis Vulvae

The term "kraurosis" means dry or brittle. One may expect to find a shrunken atrophic vulva covered by an abnormally smooth, thin, parchment-like skin layer. The subcutaneous fat disappears, and the labial folds flatten and fade away. The clitoris vanishes behind the preputial cover. The pubic hair becomes brittle and sparse. The vaginal orifice contracts.

Because the parchment-like epithelial covering is easily traumatized, small breaks and fissures appear. Low-grade infection is prone to develop in these shallow crevices, and itching may become so intense that scratching for relief produces further trauma and recurring exacerbations of inflammation.

What Are the Histologic Characteristics of Kraurosis?

The differentiation between kraurosis and leukoplakia is made by a histologic review of the biopsy specimen. Pathologically, kraurosis reveals a thinning of the vulvar epithelium to perhaps three or four cells in depth over a wide or, less typically, a limited area.

The atrophic epithelium is smoothly and precariously attached to a connective tissue that is abnormally hyaline, afibrillar, acellular and generally degenerated in appearance, particularly in the superficial strata. Blood vessels present may appear both dilated and stiffened. Beneath the glassy, hyaline superficial layer of stromal tissue are leukocytes, chiefly lymphocytes, massed in abundance around and between the blood vessels in a fairly well demarcated layer (Fig. 70–6, *A*). In many ways the appearance resembles lichen sclerosus et atrophicus (see p. 1142).

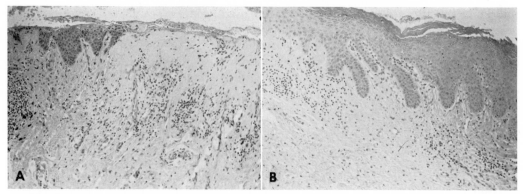

Fig. 70-6.   *A*, In kraurosis vulvae the epithelium is thin and often eroded. The stroma beneath is hyalinized, and at a deeper level there are leukocytes around the thickened small blood vessels. *B*, Leukoplakia is characterized by epithelial hyperplasia, dyskeratosis, and a superficial scale of hyperkeratotic and parakeratotic type. Stromal inflammation is usually rather prominent.

Treatment

This is described with that of leukoplakia later. So far as hormonal deficiency may be responsible, estrin replacement is desirable.

LEUKOPLAKIA

In contradistinction to kraurosis, which is an atrophic process from the outset, leukoplakia begins as a chronic inflammatory and hyperplastic process. The first manifestations may appear on the labial folds around the vaginal outlet. The vulvar skin hypertrophies and becomes dry, thick, red and swollen. As the disease progresses the labial folds tend to flatten out, since chronic inflammation in the deeper tissues destroys the elastic fibers. Narrowing of the introitus follows. The normal vulvar pigment tends to disappear, and the red color changes to opaque white, with a bilaterally symmetrical butterfly-type of distribution that covers the entire vulvar area from clitoris to perianal region. Less frequently the distribution is unilateral.

Eventually, white raised patches made up of thickened hyperkeratotic squamous epithelium develop (1) in isolated areas on an atrophic background or (2) diffusely cover the entire vulva. As the later atrophy progresses, the surface epithelium thins out. Such tissue breaks easily under any trauma. Cracks and fissures appear. Superficial infection enters, intensifying the intense pruritus. In these cracks carcinoma may develop. The final or resting stage of leukoplakia is not unlike that of kraurosis. One may find a complete atrophy of all anatomic landmarks with loss of hair, underlying fat, sebaceous glands and pigment. A thin, smooth, shining white layer of epithelium covers the degenerated inelastic tissue beneath.

What Is the Histologic Appearance of Leukoplakia?

As already discussed in considering the cervix, the essence of the histopathology of leukoplakia is a laggardly maturation and irregular keratin formation of the epithelial cells. It is the same process wherever leukoplakia is found. The basal cells of the vulvar epithelium may form from two to several layers instead of the normal single stratum. Hyperplastic epithelial pegs bulge downward into the underlying connective tissue. Here a lymphocytic and plasma cell infiltration can be seen beneath and surrounding the proliferating epithelial projections. The formation of keratin is confined to the upper half of the epithelium, where it is irregular and incomplete to a variable extent. Further toward the surface the superficial layers of fully keratinized cells retain their nuclei and are abnormally interadherent. This produces a firmly attached, superficial keratinized scale in which pyknotic nuclei remain visible. This last condition is called *parakeratosis* by dermatologists (Fig. 70–6, *B*).

What Are the Histologic Differences between Kraurosis and Leukoplakia?

Microscopically, leukoplakia has a more definite pattern than that encountered in kraurosis. The chief point of difference lies in the appearance of the basal layers of the vulvar epithelium. In leukoplakia a proliferation of the basal layers is noted with finger-like or branching epithelial projections extending downward into the supporting connective tissue. Sometimes this is called pseudoepitheliomatous hyperplasia. In kraurosis basal cell activity is missing.

The chronic inflammatory aspect of leukoplakia is emphasized by the presence of many plasma cells and lymphocytes surrounding the hyperplastic epithelial projections. In these areas hyaline degeneration takes place later, and most of the normal elastic tissue fibers disintegrate and disappear. This explains the contraction of the vulvar tissue that is seen in advanced leukoplakia. In kraurosis the elastic tissue fibers usually remain everywhere except in local areas of intense inflammation.

The malignant potentiality of leukoplakia stems from the cellular activity that is often noted within the epithelium that extends into the surrounding stroma. This may have anaplastic features like those seen in carcinoma in situ The increased cellular growth activity, together with the proliferation of the interpapillary downgrowths, is perhaps increased by the loss of the restricting elastic tissue fibers.

The appearance of the superficial layers in leukoplakia varies with its stage of development. In early phases the keratinization may be slightly more than normal, and hyperkeratosis may progress to the point that more than half the epithelial thickness is a keratinized scale. In the final stages the overlying keratinized layer is cast off, the inflamed connective tissue stroma is replaced by acellular fibrous tissue, and the vulva finally comes to be covered by a thin layer of epithelium devoid of all papillary proliferations. This is the end or resting stage of leukoplakia. It is a dangerous condition as regards cancer development only in the proliferating phase.

Treatment

Once the diagnosis of leukoplakia is established, some surgeons believe that there is no reason to postpone a surgical excision of the entire vulva. Authors have reported an association of leukoplakia with squamous carcinoma in as high as 80 per cent of cases, though others record an incidence no higher than 12 per cent. The majority of surgeons believe that 50 per cent of all carcinomas of the vulva develop on a background of leukoplakia. With the incidence of malignancy so high, there is much to be said for a prophylactic excision. Pathologists, conversely, feel that a vulvectomy for leukoplakia alone is unjustified, just as a glossectomy would not be used to treat leukoplakia of the tongue. We badly need some kind of group study to resolve these wide differences of opinion. In a single hospital controversy about how to treat leukoplakia often generates more heat than light.

Since the microscopic changes in leukoplakia are often widespread, there is little merit in mere local excision of an obvious area. At least 1.5 or 2 cm. of apparently normal skin margin should be included in performance of a total surgical removal of the vulva. Not to do so is to invite recurrence, the incidence of which has been placed as high as 25 per cent. Particular attention should be directed toward the involved areas around the anus. Despite the fact that carcinoma rarely develops in the leuko-plakic area posterior to the anus, it may be wise also to include an excision of a triangle of skin in this area.

If the biopsy fails to show evidence of leukoplakia, one is justified in using a variety of forms of therapy for the intolerable itching that plagues the patient.

Since the process is one of atrophy probably associated with ovarian hormonal deficiency, one may elect to give estrin ointment as a topical application, supplemented by oral stilbestrol therapy. Temporary improvement may be noted as the affected area epithelializes, and the fissures and minor breaks in the skin heal. The long-range results from this sort of therapy are disappointing.

Certain patients with leukoplakia appear to have allergies, and approximately one fourth will have an established abnormal neuropsychiatric background.

The most satisfactory form of conservative treatment follows the use of vitamin A, supplemented by an oral intake of dilute hydrochloric acid. A regimen of daily oral doses of 250,000 to 500,000 units of vitamin A is recommended, supplemented by biweekly intramuscular injections of 50,000 units. Fifteen minims of dilute USP hydrochloric acid are given with a glass of water three times daily after each meal. Reports of the efficacy of this combination vary widely. It has been successful sufficiently often to advise a trial course. If no improvement is noted, a total surgical removal of the vulva may be indicated to relieve the intense itching and to prevent any possibility of malignant change.

LICHEN SCLEROSUS ET ATROPHICUS

The chief gynecologic interest in lichen sclerosus et atrophicus lies in its similarity to kraurosis vulvae. It tends to appear in an older age group, but like leukoplakia and kraurosis it may occur in much younger women. Primary lesions are often confined to the vulvar and perineal areas, although the axillae, neck, shoulders and forearms are also favored locations.

What Does Lichen Sclerosus et Atrophicus Look Like?

The lesions have a fairly characteristic appearance. At the outset one usually encounters an isolated group of polygonal macules or papules. The papules have an ivory white or yellowish flat top and may either be raised slightly above the surface of the skin or appear as depressed lesions. The most characteristic finding is the central depression or black spot that occurs on the surface of the papule. The depression is due to the tendency for the lesion to set up follicular plugging. The surface itself may be either smooth or horny and rough. The smooth-surfaced papules are customarily like yellow parchment in color, and the rough patches are ivory white. Frequently both types are found in adjoining areas. At the outset the macules or papules appear in discrete areas, but as the process develops they tend to coalesce. In the vulva one may observe rows of papules, but in many instances they coalesce to form nodules. Occasionally a collection of rough white papules with depressed black centers simulates the appearance of warty growths that spread from the outer surface of the labia majora to the skin around the perineum, anus, genitocrural folds and buttocks.

How Does It Progress?

The chronic process usually goes on for years, although it may clear spontaneously in a matter of weeks. In the course of its resolution the appearance of the vulva is appreciably altered. This is particularly true in the region of the labia minora and clitoris. The skin in these areas is much more delicate than that of the rest of the vulva. There are no sweat glands or hair follicles, and the subcutaneous tissue is less abundant. The dermatitis largely destroys the elastic tissue component in the dermal layers, so that when the connective tissue beneath becomes fibrosed, the clitoris and labia minora tend to shrink and disappear. Thus one frequently finds a smooth, shiny, thin skin cover that is freely movable over the underlying tissue and is completely devoid of all pigment. There is little scarring, and the white parchment-like skin is only slightly depressed below the level of the uninvolved skin (Fig. 70–7). The loss of connective and elastic tissue, however, does tend to contract the outlet of the vaginal canal.

There are many characteristics of this clinical picture that are common to both kraurosis and lichen sclerosus et atrophicus. In the former, however, there does appear to be some connection with a deficiency in the sex hormones that is not true of the latter.

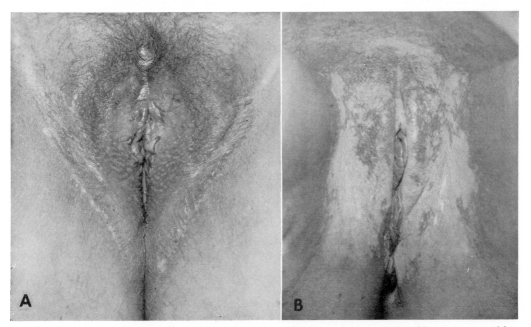

Fig. 70-7. *A,* Coalescent white papular lesions of lichen sclerosus et atrophicus are seen with a linear pattern on both sides of the vulva. *B,* By use of the Wood's ultraviolet light the extent of atrophy in vulvar lichen sclerosus et atrophicus may be shown to be more widespread than is apparent in ordinary light. (Courtesy of Dr. F. Ronchese, Providence, R.I.)

What Are the Symptoms?

The symptoms are variable and depend upon the stage of the process, the manner in which it develops and the location. Thus one finds less irritation and discomfort when the patches are smooth than when they are rough and horny. The latter need not be symptomatic, but when irritation is present, one usually finds the coarser type of lesions. In the earlier phases, when coalescing papules cover the inner surface of the vulva, the entire vulva may be swollen, red, hot and tender, as one might expect in any inflammatory process. Oddly enough, pruritus is not a severe or even a common symptom. It is minimal, and 50 per cent of the patients do not have any. In the more chronic phases any irritation is usually due to some other cause, such as an infection incident to trauma, rather than to the eruption itself.

If the lesions develop around the urethral meatus, the patient usually suffers considerable irritation during and after the act of voiding. Because of the sclerotic nature of the dermatitis, vulvar and anal contractions may make problems. Dyspareunia, for example, is a common complaint. If fissures develop between the labia or between the clitoris and the mons veneris as the result of scratching, secondary infections may contribute to the discomfort and irritation. Rarely do the lesions of lichen sclerosus et atrophicus ulcerate, however.

What Is the Differential Diagnosis?

Lichen sclerosus et atrophicus does not occur as often as kraurosis or leukoplakia, but it so closely resembles both entities that the differential diagnosis must be established before instituting therapy. Vulvectomy has been performed for lichen sclerosus et atrophicus under the mistaken impression that the local condition was leukoplakia. There are indications for surgery in the latter, but not in the former.

LEUKOPLAKIA.   As we have noted previously, leukoplakic vulvitis is commonly associated with intense itching, but this is minimal or absent in lichen sclerosus et atrophicus. Leukoplakia is typically confined to the inner surfaces of both labia, the perineum and the clitoris. It rarely extends laterally to involve the labia majora or posteriorly to include the anal region. Although lichen sclerosus et atrophicus is particularly prone to occur in the vulvar area, it can be found also in the perianal region, groins and upper thighs as well as on the skin of the breast, neck, axillae and forearms. Rarely is it confined to the vulva alone.

Although leukoplakia begins as a hyperplasia, unlike lichen sclerosus et atrophicus, which is an atrophic process from the beginning, it eventually progresses to a state of atrophy as chronic inflammation within the dermis destroys the elastic fibers. In the end the patient with leukoplakia is apt to suffer atresia and stenosis of the vaginal outlet. This rarely occurs in lichen sclerosus et atrophicus.

The most important point in the differential diagnosis between the two entities is the frequent association of leukoplakia with cancer. Lichen sclerosus et atrophicus is a benign process. One justifiably could advocate vulvectomy for the former, but never for the latter. A biopsy will readily establish the diagnosis.

KRAUROSIS.   The only similarity between kraurosis and lichen sclerosus et atrophicus is that they are both basically benign atrophic processes. Since it is often impossible clinically to differentiate kraurosis from leukoplakia, everything said about distinguishing leukoplakia from lichen sclerosus et atrophicus applies to kraurosis.

What Is the Histologic Picture of Lichen Sclerosus et Atrophicus?

The final differential diagnosis is established by the histologic sections obtained at biopsy. Characteristically, in lichen sclerosus et atrophicus one finds a uniform atrophy of the epidermis as well as liquefaction and degeneration in the basal cell layers. In the immediately underlying supporting connective tissue there is a distinct superficial zone of homogenized hyaline collagen. Beneath this zone are leukocytes (Fig. 70–8).

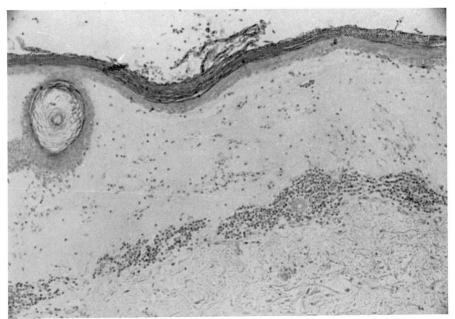

Fig. 70-8.   Lichen sclerosus et atrophicus has keratotic plugs both in and separate from the hair follicles and sebaceous ducts, as shown at the left. The epidermis is thin and hyperkeratotic. The subepithelial zone of collagen degeneration and the underlying stratum of lymphocytic infiltration are the most distinctive lesions in this condition.

Both keratotic plugging and collagen homogenization are absent in leukoplakia. Instead of atrophy of the epithelial layers, leukoplakia tends to show hyperplasia together with a loss of elastic connective tissue fibers. In kraurosis the keratotic plugging seen in lichen sclerosus is absent, and one may find hyperkeratosis in the dermis. Leukocytes come right up to the epithelium in kraurosis, without any zone of hyalinized collagen devoid of cells being evident.

Treatment

The treatment likewise depends on the extent of the process, its duration and the location. There is no specific therapy. In the acute inflammatory phase the simplest form of therapy should be used. Hot baths are helpful, but they should not be prolonged. The area must be thoroughly dried with soft cotton cloth rather than rough toweling. The treatment of a vulvar dermatitis in the stage of acute inflammation has been outlined already. The great danger is in overtreatment. A simple inflammatory process may be converted into an eczematous one by injudicious use of strong keratolytic ointment, for example. To superimpose a dermatitis medicamentosa will not help the patient.

When itching is present and the lesions are excessively keratotic, local applications of a 2.5 per cent lotion of hydrocortisone acetate may be helpful. The patient should also be given some mild sedative at night to secure adequate rest.

Some dermatologists feel that corticosteroid therapy has actually reversed the course of the disease. If so, it is worth trying, although the final assessment of its effectiveness must take into consideration the well known observation that spontaneous regressions do occur and the dermatitis may tend to be self-limited.

REFERENCES

Vulvar Dermatitis and Dermatosis

Allen, A. C.: *The Skin*. St. Louis, C. V. Mosby Company, 1954, Chaps. 13, 14.

de Sousa, H. M., and van Uden, N.: The Mode of Infection and Reinfection in Yeast Vulvovaginitis. *Am. J. Obst. & Gynec.*, 80: 1096, 1960.

Hunt, E.: *Diseases Affecting the Vulva*. 4th Ed. St. Louis, C. V. Mosby Company, 1954.

Parks, J., and Martin, S.: Reactions of the Vulva to Systemic Diseases. *Am. J. Obst. & Gynec.*, 55: 117, 1948.

Schoch, E. P., Jr., and McCuistion, C. H.: Diagnostic and Therapeutic Errors in Certain Dermatoses of the Vulva. *J.A.M.A.*, 157: 1102, 1955.

Sulzberger, M. B., Baer, R. L., and Hecht, R.: Common Fungous Infections of the Feet and Groin. Negligible Role of Exposure in Causing Attacks. *Arch. Dermat. & Syph.*, 45: 670, 1942.

Taussig, F. J.: *Diseases of the Vulva*. New York, D. Appleton & Co., 1926.

Woodruff, J. D.: Lesions of the Vulva. *Postgrad. Med.*, 18: 340, 1955.

Pruritus Vulvae and Pruritus Ani

Cornell, E. L.: Vaginal and Rectal Pruritus—Etiology and Treatment. *Am. J. Obst. & Gynec.*, 55: 691, 1948.

Hailey, H., and Hailey, H.: Pruritus Ani et Vulvae. *Arch. Dermat. & Syph.*, 40: 726, 1939.

Kevorkian, A. Y.: The Treatment of Chronic Pruritus Vulvae with Local Applications of Estrogen. *New England J. Med.*, 220: 661, 1939.

Parker, R. T., Jones, C. P., and Carter, F. B.: Pruritus Vulvae in the Postclimacteric Woman. *Geriatrics*, 11: 235, 1956.

Parks, J.: Pruritus, Kraurosis and Leucoplakia of the Vulva; in J. V. Meigs and S. H. Sturgis, eds.: *Progress in Gynecology*. New York, Grune & Stratton, Inc., 1957, p. 451.

Spinka, H. M.: Pruritus Ani—Diagnosis and Treatment. *Am. J. Proctol.*, 12: 309, 1961.

Swinton, N. W.: Pruritus Ani. *New England J. Med.*, 236: 169, 1947.

Degenerative Diseases

Brewer, J. I.: Kraurosis and Leucoplakia of the Vulva. *Illinois M.J.*, 77: 26, 1940.

Graves, W. P., and Smith, G. V. S.: Kraurosis Vulvae. *J.A.M.A.*, 92: 1244, 1929.

Hyman, A. B., and Falk, H. C.: White Lesions of the Vulfa. Discussion of Lichenification (Lichen Chronicus Simplex), Leucoplakia, Bowen's Disease, "Kraurosis Vulvae," Lichen Sclerosus et Atrophicus and Senile Essential Atrophies of the Vulva. *Obst. & Gynec.*, 12: 40, 1958.

McKay, D. G., Street, R. B., Jr., Benirschke, K., and Duncan, C. J.: Eosinophilic Granuloma of the Vulva. *Surg., Gynec. & Obst.*, 96: 437, 1953.

Montgomery, H., and Hill, W. R.: Lichen Sclerosus et Atrophicus. *Arch. Dermat. & Syph.*, 42: 755, 1940.

Montgomery, H., Counseller, V. S., and Craig, W. McK.: Kraurosis, Leukoplakia and Pruritus Vulvae. Correlation of Clinical and Pathologic Observations with Further Studies Regarding the Resection of the Sensory Nerves of the Perineum. *Arch. Dermat. & Syph.*, 30: 80, 1934.

Seibel, D. I.: Glycogen Content of the Epidermis of the Vulva in the Presence of Leukoplakia and of Squamous-Cell Carcinoma. Histochemical Study of 98 Specimens. *Am. J. Obst. & Gynec.*, 77: 298, 1959.

Wallace, E. G., and Nomland, R.: Lichen Sclerosus et Atrophicus of the Vulva. *Arch. Dermat. & Syph.*, 57: 240, 1948.

Chapter 71

Malignant Diseases of the Vulva

MALIGNANT diseases of the vulva are uncommon, but occur sufficiently often to account for approximately 3 per cent of all the cancerous processes that occur in the genital tract. When vulvar cancer is compared with carcinoma of the uterus, the ratio varies between 1:20 and 1:30, according to reported world statistics. The neoplasms may be either primary or secondary, carcinoma or sarcoma.

What Is the Background for the Subsequent Development of Vulvar Cancer?

Atrophy of the vulvar tissue secondary to ovarian failure, castration or menopause seems to be a predisposing factor in the etiology of malignant disease in this area. The epithelium appears to be extremely sensitive to the action of the ovarian hormones, as noted experimentally in the monkey during estrus and in the woman during pregnancy. Cessation of hormonal activity results in profound atrophic changes. The entire area from the clitoris to the coccyx is under hormonal control, yet it is interesting to note that cancer develops only in the anterior two thirds. The areas posterior to the fourchet and anal opening become involved only secondarily as the neoplastic process spreads.

There can be little doubt that leukoplakic vulvitis can serve as a precursor of later development of carcinoma of the vulva. Reports vary as to the actual incidence, as already mentioned, from 12 to 50 per cent association. Most patients who exhibit leukoplakic changes will be in the menopause, but 10 per cent of cases appear among patients in whom ovarian function has ceased prematurely, either because of surgery, irradiation or natural causes. The relation between leukoplakia and estrin deprivation seems definite, despite the fact that leukoplakia has been reported in pregnancy, when the level of circulating estrin should be high. A few instances occur in infancy.

Leukoplakia has a strong epidemiologic relation to venereal disease, particularly syphilis. Lymphogranuloma venereum and chancroid have also been implicated. The relation may sometimes be coincidental, since some British authors could not establish an association. A reported series of cases with carcinoma of the vulva among Negroes, in whom the incidence of venereal disease was high, showed a relatively minor tendency of leukoplakia. Though there is little doubt that carcinoma may develop on a background of leukoplakic vulvitis, the connection between it and venereal infections has not been generally established.

There is some evidence that leukoplakia can be a nutritional disease related to vitamin A deficiency. Although normal blood levels of vitamin A have been reported

1147

in patients with leukoplakia, the association could still hold, since the leukoplakic tissue response may be due to nonutilization of vitamin A. Also there is an observation that patients with leukoplakia have inadequate free hydrochloric acid on gastric analysis.

It seems clear that carcinoma of the vulva develops on a background of epithelial atrophy and subsequent hyperplasia in an area normally under hormonal control and in an age group in which ovarian activity has ceased. It is surprising, however, that no more patients have cancer of the vulva. There must be other, unknown factors.

PRIMARY CARCINOMA OF THE VULVA

Rare cases have been reported in infancy and an occasional instance has been noted in a pregnant woman. The majority, however, appear in the postmenopausal age group. Atrophy of vulvar tissues secondary to ovarian failure, castration or the menopause seems to be a predisposing factor. The mean age incidence lies somewhere between fifty-eight and sixty-eight years.

Carcinoma of the vulva has a tendency to develop on a background of leukoplakic vulvitis, as discussed previously. This is by no means a constant finding, but several authors have noted the coincidence of the two conditions.

What Is the Growth Pattern of Vulvar Carcinoma?

Carcinoma of the vulva is typically epidermoid in type, well differentiated and in its growth pattern similar to carcinomas of the lip or skin. Most often it is an epidermoid carcinoma grade I that tends to remain localized to the primary site and immediately adjacent lymph nodes for a considerable time. True carcinomas of the vulva arise in the labia majora, usually on the lateral margins and commonly in the lower half. The clitoris and fourchet are less frequent primary sites, but they frequently become involved by extensions of the lateral growth. The vaginal epithelium and urethra are rarely involved, except in the most advanced stages.

The earliest forms of malignant disease in the vulvar region are forms of carcinoma in situ called Bowen's disease or erythroplasia of Queyrat. The lesion may present as red raised plaques with a finely granular surface or appear as superficial, shallow ulcerations. They represent the earliest change toward invasive cancer. Though these lesions tend to appear on one side, examination of the seemingly normal tissues of the opposite side may show similar pathologic changes that are less pronounced. For the most part the malignant alterations are confined to intraepithelial changes, but there is a tendency with time for invasion of the basement membrane in some portion of the growth.

The initial invasive lesion is often inconspicuous and may present as a simple fissure or shallow ulceration that fails to heal. Frequently the patient complains only of a small lump which persists. The earlier phases of the disease appear to bother the patient very little, and early clinical diagnosis is not common. When ulceration appears, infection produces pain.

A fully developed carcinoma grows either as (1) a papillary fungoid growth with overhanging edges and a strawberry-like surface, or (2) in the form of an indurated ulcer that may be either superficial or deep (Fig. 71–1). Not infrequently a papillary exophytic growth may outrun its blood supply and necrose to become a large ulcerating area. Nonulcerating forms of carcinoma are not common. Usually they are firm and hard with an intact skin covering. When they are lateral to the introitus deep in the adjacent tissues, they may simulate an indurated Bartholin's gland. They may reach a fair size before they break down and ulcerate.

Gradually the malignant ulceration spreads, either superficially or as a deep induration that involves all of one side of the labium. The opposite side is included by direct extension of the growth across the midline, both at the site of the clitoris and

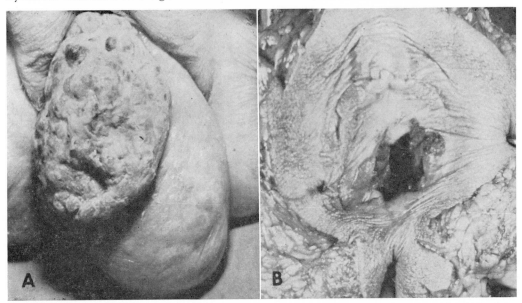

Fig. 71-1.   *A,* A large exophytic carcinoma of the vulva associated with a procidentia is of the usual well differentiated epidermoid type. *B,* Ulcerative carcinoma of the vulva, with atrophic changes of the uninvolved skin and mucous membranes, from an operative specimen.

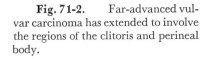

Fig. 71-2.   Far-advanced vulvar carcinoma has extended to involve the regions of the clitoris and perineal body.

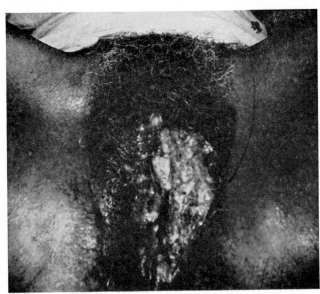

at the fourchet. In the advanced stages both the external portion of the urethra and the perineal body may be extensively ulcerated (Fig. 71–2).

Vulvar carcinoma may arise in the region of the clitoris. This is less frequently seen than similar epidermoid carcinomas that arise on the lateral sides of the labia minora and majora. The danger is greater, for though the primary ulcerations are usually small, there is less of a tendency for the lesion to remain local. Lymphatic extension seems to occur bilaterally and to the deep lymph nodes.

The predominant cell types of the primary vulvar neoplasms are epidermoid. Rarely are they adenocarcinomas. When adenocarcinoma is encountered in an advanced lesion, one may suspect that the cancer took origin from Gaertner's duct, Bartholin's gland or an accessory vaginal gland.

How Does the Cancer Spread beyond the Primary Site?

Because of the free lymphatic anastomoses around the vulva, carcinoma of the vulva metastasizes freely to the adjacent regional lymph nodes. The spread is by embolus rather than permeation. Lymphatic permeation occurs only in the immediate vicinity of the tumor. When recurrences appear, they localize either at the primary site or in the regional nodes. Rarely is it possible to demonstrate cancer cells in the intervening lymphatics.

It appears to make little difference whether the pathologic picture is that of a well differentiated form of epidermoid carcinoma or whether the tumor is more anaplastic; lymph nodal metastases are equally common in either. In the same histologic groups there are evident differences in the trend toward metastasis. The size of the primary growth has but a slight bearing on the likelihood of regional lymph node involvement. The carcinoma may be either extensive and remain localized or may be minimal in size and metastasize.

The most common extension occurs to the superficial inguinal and femoral regions. Groups of lymph nodes are found both lateral and medial to the inguinal ligament, the medial collection lying below the external ring. Those in the femoral group collect around the saphenous opening. Free lymph communication exists, and efferent lymphatics are given off to the chain of nodes that lie not only lateral, but also underneath the external iliac veins above Poupart's ligaments. Rosenmuller's or Cloquet's node lies just above the ligament on the medial side of the external iliac vein (Fig. 71–3).

The deep lymph nodes could be involved directly without passing through the superficial inguinal group if the carcinoma is in the midline near the clitoris. In the majority of instances, however, the superficial nodal chain will also have metastases when the deep nodes are implicated. Here the pathway is direct. Occasionally, further extension takes place to the lymph nodes located in the triangle between the external and internal iliac arteries and from there to the lateral side of the common iliac artery. Postmortem examinations suggest that cancer extension rarely occurs in the lymph nodes as high up as the chain around the aorta.

Contralateral cancer extension to the opposite side occurs frequently, owing to the rich intercommunicating lymphatic drainage. The location of the primary tumor is important. If the disease arises near the clitoris or fourchet, or encroaches upon the midline from a primary growth on the lower labia, the likelihood of bilateral metastases is materially increased. The opposite side is always suspect, and not

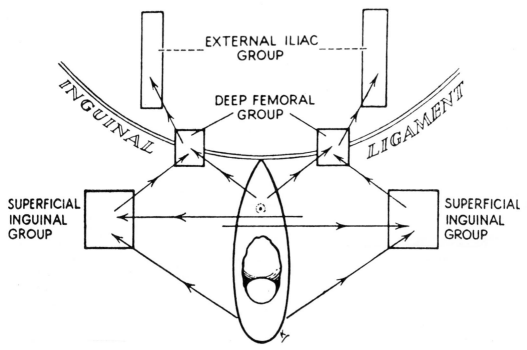

Fig. 71-3.   The pattern of lymphatic drainage from the vulva is primarily to the superficial inguinal lymph nodes, and from there secondarily to the deep femoral nodes and thereafter to the external iliac nodes. From the clitoral region the drainage is to the deep femoral lymph nodes.

infrequently positive nodes are found on the uninvolved side where they were not palpable.

There appears to be a fairly rapid spread from the primary carcinoma site to the regional lymph nodal areas. In lymph nodes the rate of cancer growth appears to slow down. Not infrequently the nodes in the superficial inguinal and femoral areas enlarge and ulcerate, yet dissection of the lymph nodes above fails to produce any evidence of further extension. The patient may die a miserable death from invasion of local structures before metastasis has occurred to distant organs.

What Are the Usual Symptoms?

The fact that the history of carcinoma of the vulva is characterized by procrastination and delay both in diagnosis and in treatment seems to emphasize the fact that symptoms are minimal. The prevailing symptom is intense itching. In general the patient has tried innumerable ointments in search for relief before consulting her physician. The next most common patient complaint is the discovery of a lump that does not disappear. When the lump ulcerates or the process begins as an ulcerated area or fissure, the patient complains of burning after urination, together with local tenderness in the involved area. When ulceration is established, the patient has pain. Cancer of the vulva is one of the few malignant tumors which are tender and painful. This is due either to exposed nerve endings or to sepsis. Rarely does bleeding appear in sufficient quantity to alarm the patient. If the ulceration is extensive, the patient may be concerned with a discharge.

If the malignant process has arisen in an area of leukoplakic vulvitis, all these symptoms except those related to the ulceration may have been present for some time. This in part may explain the prolonged delay before medical consultation. It is difficult to understand the procrastination.

The patient's reluctance may stem from the increasing modesty that comes with advancing years. This seems far to transcend the shyness of virginity. The itching vulva is far too personal a matter about which to consult a physician. The ulceration or lump is too insignificant to bother him with. She prefers to try her own salves and ointments. In an area that can be both seen and felt the average size of the primary cancer lesion is greater than 4 cm. when the patient first presents herself for definitive treatment.

How Do You Make the Diagnosis of Vulvar Carcinoma?

There are a few lesions that can be confused with cancer of the vulva. Infectious lesions are extremely common, and the various types of tissue reaction are so protean in the vulvar area that they may defy even the trained dermatologist to make an accurate diagnosis. He is cognizant of the difficulties and rarely tries to make a diagnosis without first doing a darkfield examination and biopsy of the involved area. Therapeutically caused or factitious ulcerations in the senile or feebleminded may be confusing. Condylomata may resemble nonulcerating carcinomas even to the point of presenting enlarged lymph nodes in the groin, but like lupus vulgaris, another widespread vulvar lesion, they tend to arise around the perianal area where carcinoma is rarely found. Gummas and tuberculosis can be ruled out by biopsy.

Failure to biopsy is the principal error of the physician in the diagnosis of cancer of the vulva. Why are more biopsies not performed? The medical profession may have been taught that malignant ulcerations are not tender. This is a good axiom, except that it does not apply to lesions of the lip, mouth and vulva. These cancerous lesions are tender, and a small injection of Novocain is all that is necessary to obtain a biopsy without pain. Tenderness seems to establish a mental block, particularly if the physician is habitually reluctant to suspect malignant disease. Any ulceration or tumor should be biopsied, regardless of the age of the patient or size of the lesion.

Once a biopsy is obtained, the pathologist does not find it difficult to diagnose

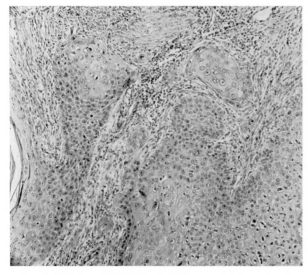

Fig. 71-4.   Epidermoid carcinoma of the vulva typically has abundant keratinized cells, forms numerous prickle cells and shows relatively few mitoses. It is most often considered of grade I malignancy, but has a considerable propensity for metastasis.

the usual vulvar carcinoma. Nests and cords of well differentiated cells have broken loose from the surface and are found within the connective tissue. The invasive epithelial cells most often are well keratinized, not particularly anaplastic, with many intercellular bridges and fairly abundant keratin pearls. Ordinarily a diagnosis of epidermoid carcinoma grade I is made (Fig. 71–4).

Sometimes there is deeper invasion, and the cells show more anaplasia, mitoses and less keratinization, so that the cancer represents an epidermoid carcinoma grade II or III, as described to occur in the cervix also. Invasion of perineural lymphatics may be present.

Treatment of Carcinoma of the Vulva

The same procrastination and uncertainty already noted in the diagnosis of carcinoma of the vulva carry over into the field of therapy. Because these women are in an older age group, the physician is reluctant to subject them to an extensive surgical procedure, which is the only form of treatment that offers any hope of cure. The accepted form of therapy for cancer of the vulva is a radical surgical removal of the local lesion with an en-bloc dissection of the regional lymphatics.

It is important to keep in mind in the treatment of cancer of the vulva that the entire substrate of the block of tissue that goes to make up the vulva is pathologically unsound. Furthermore, carcinoma of the vulva often has multicentric points of origin. It is for this reason that excision of what is grossly a unilateral lesion is to be strongly condemned.

Carcinoma of the vulva is an external form of malignancy with a life history that indicates a tendency for the cancer to remain confined to the local site and adjacent regional lymphatics. It can be cured, provided the physician attacks the problem promptly and carries out an adequate surgical procedure. It will not be cured by underestimating the growth potential or by temporizing in the choice of therapy. Review of the histories of patients with cancer of the vulva serves to emphasize the following points of controversy in therapy:

1. Can radiation therapy cure vulvar malignancy?
2. Is there any place for local excision or hemivulvectomy?
3. Does a wide vulvectomy suffice?
4. Should the dissection be unilateral or bilateral?
5. Should the dissection be en bloc?
6. Should the dissection be extended to include the glands above Poupart's ligament?

RADIATION TREATMENT. Radium therapy, whether by local application, infiltration of platinum needles, or irradiation by x-ray treatment centered over the vulva, has no place in the treatment of carcinoma of the vulva, except for the patient who is totally unsuitable for a surgical excision. Experimental use of x-ray therapy in inoperable cases has produced a minimal salvage.

The vulva does not tolerate irradiation very well. This may have been due in part at least to the fact that low-voltage therapy has been used, on the theory that the superficial cancer location makes a deeper dose unnecessary. If radiation is the only treatment possible, it had best be given by the medium of high-voltage x-ray machines, not for reasons of depth penetration, but because of the quality of the roentgen beam. Prolonged postirradiation ulceration, however, may be anticipated with widespread necrosis of uninvolved tissue, great suffering and actual reduction in the anticipated life span. Radiation therapy appeals to the physician, since it causes no initial mortality. This advantage is more than offset by its complete ineffectiveness and the profound discomfort that follows its use.

Some surgeons have removed the vulva by either surgery or electrocoagulation, combined with a supplementary treatment of the regional lymphatics in the groin by either x-ray therapy or teleradium. Five-year survival end-results approaching 40 per cent are reported from electrocoagulation and teleradium. Few clinics have the equipment or the experience necessary to use them and can hardly be expected to duplicate the results. X-ray therapy has the disadvantage of producing discomfort through excessive destruction of tissue. Furthermore, the metastatic lymph nodal areas appear to be more resistant to irradiation than the local lesion. The radiation response varies, not only in the adjacent lymph nodes, but also in different areas in the same node. There appears to be general agreement that the treatment of choice for carcinoma of the vulva is radical surgery, not irradiation.

WHAT PARTS DO LOCAL EXCISION AND HEMIVULVECTOMY HAVE IN THERAPY? It may be categorically stated that there is no place for partial excision or hemivulvectomy in the treatment of carcinoma of the vulva. More disaster has accompanied local excision of carcinoma of the vulva than any other procedure tried. Regardless of the fact that cancer appears to be unilateral, radical surgical removal of the complete vulva is indicated. Carcinoma of the vulva is a disease of the entire vulva. The substrate has gone wrong. There is a tendency toward the development of contralateral lesions and local recurrence.

The treatment of choice is a wide complete vulvectomy. The only possible exceptions might be a small basal cell carcinoma or a small warty growth low on the lateral side of the vulva, or a hopelessly inoperable patient.

DOES A WIDE VULVECTOMY SUFFICE?   There appears to be a good deal of uncertainty as to how far the surgeon must go in order to do an adequate surgical removal of vulvar cancer. Because these patients are older, the surgeon all too frequently performs a radical removal of the vulva, but procrastinates in the treatment of lymph nodes until they can actually be felt.

HOW ACCURATE IS OUR CLINICAL APPRAISAL OF REGIONAL LYMPH NODES BY PALPATION?   The error approaches 30 per cent. Little can be told from the size of the nodes. When lymph nodes are larger than 1 cm., approximately 65 per cent will be positive, but the remainder are free of disease. About 20 per cent are positive for cancer when the nodes are less than 1 cm. in size. Moreover, 30 per cent have metastatic disease locally when no lymph nodes are palpable in the groins.

Any surgeon who pursues a policy of watchful waiting, under the misguided impression that he is following a conservative course, is doing so at considerable peril. Biopsy of doubtful lymph nodes in the groin should be condemned. Tumor tissue may be transplanted and the subsequent dissection made more difficult. Furthermore, the tumor may bypass one or more nodes in the group. A negative biopsy therefore means nothing, and a positive biopsy is dangerous.

The network of lymphatics in the vulva is so extensive that a bilateral dissection of the lymph nodes is a necessary requirement, if adequate surgery is to be performed. Vulvectomy alone cannot be considered adequate treatment for anything but carcinoma in situ.

The five-year end-result figures from vulvectomy alone are about 28 per cent survival. This figure increases to 40 per cent when the superficial regional lymphatics in the inguinal area are included and to 60 to 80 per cent when the lymph nodes above Poupart's ligaments are dissected.

SHOULD THE DISSECTION BE UNILATERAL OR BILATERAL? Bilateral spread from a unilateral lesion occurs in about 20 per cent of the cases, increasing to 40 per cent when the tumor encroaches on the midline. Contralateral extension is a common finding. Since 50 per cent of the cases seen may be expected to have regional lymph node metastasis, it is important that the nodes on both sides should be dissected out.

SHOULD THE DISSECTION BE EN BLOC? In the past it was common practice to wait for complete healing of the vulvectomy wound before beginning the attack on the superficial lymph nodes. This was a mistake. Some patients disappeared after the vulvectomy. Others refused further surgery, and, most important, there were too many local cancer recurrences. The latter were probably due to the fact that the lymphatics intervening between the regional lymph nodes and the primary vulvectomy excision were not removed.

Present-day therapy calls for an en-bloc removal of both the superficial inguinal and femoral lymph nodes, together with a complete removal of the vulva and the communicating lymphatics.

The older patient tolerates a dissection of this magnitude far better than either the physician or her family anticipate. An en-bloc dissection has been successfully carried out under Novocain anesthesia in several patients over 80 years old with a mortality rate of but 10 per cent. Age is a factor, but with proper attention to detail the operability should be better than 80 per cent. Age should not dissuade the physician from advising surgical intervention. To do less than the amount of surgery necessary to control the disease, on the mistaken impression that this is the conservative approach, is a grave mistake that fails to consider the destructive life history of vulvar cancer.

SHOULD THE LYMPH NODES ABOVE POUPART'S LIGAMENTS BE DISSECTED? This is a highly controversial point. Statistics vary as to the likelihood of cancer involvement of the lymph nodes along the external iliac vessels and obturator spaces. Theoretically, lesions arising in or encroaching on the midline could metastasize directly to these areas. Actually, the deep lymph nodes are rarely involved unless metastasis has already taken place to the superficial nodes. Clouqet's or Rosenmuller's node, lying medial to the external iliac vein just above Poupart's ligament, often harbors metastatic cancer, but the obturator lymph nodes are less frequently involved. Advanced cases with ulcerating lymph nodes in the groins are not uncommonly encountered with the iliac nodes free of disease. The cancer appears to be arrested in the region of the inguinal lymph nodes for long periods of time.

Nevertheless the survival figures indicate an increased salvage rate when the deep lymph nodes are dissected. A recent report from England shows an 83 per cent survival rate in a limited group of cases. This contrasts sharply with the 40 per cent figure when the superficial lymph nodes alone are dissected.

It is doubtful whether the entire operation, involving the deep and superficial dissection together with the primary tumor, can be done in one stage in many instances. This is a formidable procedure in a patient who is obviously a poor risk. With routine performance the operative mortality rate mounts and has been reported at 14 per cent. In a selected case the operation is far less dangerous. For other than the ideal case it would be more logical to do the operation in stages. An en-bloc removal of the superficial inguinal and femoral lymph nodes, combined with radical vulvectomy, is first performed. Dissection of the deep nodes could then be done three months later.

OTHER TUMORS OF THE VULVA THAT MAY SIMULATE CARCINOMA

Hidradenoma of the Vulva

This lesion is mentioned at this point simply because it is frequently confused with cancer. It has an odd gross appearance, but is strictly a benign lesion. Hidradenomas take origin from the sweat glands in the vulvar skin and may appear elsewhere, particularly along the embryonic milk lines. The tumor is often called a sweat gland adenoma. It is usually small, raised, papillary, and reddish-gray in appearance. It tends to be sharply circumscribed.

The confusion may come less from the gross than the microscopic picture. Typically, the hidradenoma is formed of close-packed papillary glands. The number of glands both dilated and small, together with the numerous large dilated intervening ducts, produce the general picture of cellularity, but without any anaplasia. There is no atypicality to the cells lining the ducts and glands, though occasional palisading is noted. Finally, the lesion is entirely encapsulated by fibrous tissue (Fig. 71–5, *A*).

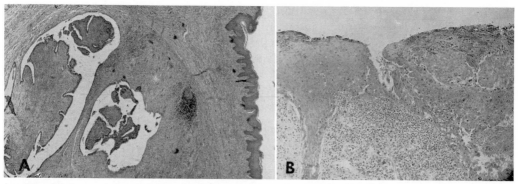

Fig. 71-5.   *A,* Portion of a papillary hidradenoma of the vulva. The vascular stroma accounts for the redness of the lesion grossly. The papillary processes are covered by sweat-duct type of epithelium. *B,* Low-power view of a vulvar apocrine carcinoma invading upward into the epidermis, where it is spreading intraepithelially as so-called extramammary Paget's disease.

Paget's Disease of the Vulva

In contrast to hidradenoma, Paget's disease arises from the apocrine glands, and it is malignant. It is a rare lesion of the vulva. The malignant change seems to be confined to the epithelial layers. The typical, large, clear Paget cells are found in the basal portions of the epidermis, after invasive upward extension from an intraductal sweat gland carcinoma in the connective tissue beneath (Fig. 71–5, *B*). Pathologically, it is identical with the same process that occurs in the nipple, except that there is less tendency for it to be associated with an underlying invasive carcinoma. To judge from the scanty information available, surgical treatment for both Paget's disease and the underlying apocrine carcinoma should include a total vulvectomy, with or without lymph node dissection, depending upon the extent of deep invasion.

BOWEN'S DISEASE

This is the one of the two earliest forms of malignant disease found in the vulvar area. The lesion may present as red raised plaques with a finely granular surface or as superficial ulcerations. Though these areas tend to appear on one side only, pathologic examination of the seemingly normal tissue of the opposite side may show a similar intraepithelial carcinoma or precancerous hyperplasia. The malignant alteration by definition is confined to intraepithelial changes, with giant nuclei and anaplastic multinucleated epithelial cells in some portion of the growth (Fig. 71–6). The bowenoid change is more dramatic than is usually seen in carcinoma in situ of the cervix. Bowen's disease occurs preceding invasive epidermoid carcinoma of the skin, as well as in the vulva.

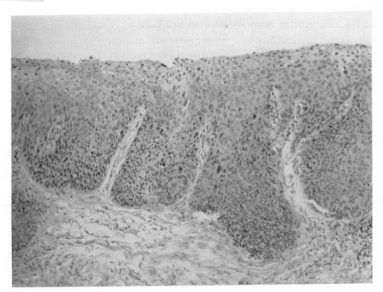

Fig. 71-6.   Bowen's disease of the vulva shows anaplastic changes through most layers of the epidermis, with giant nuclei and multinucleated, so-called bowenoid cells. This is regarded as a special variety of epidermoid carcinoma in situ.

ERYTHROPLASIA OF QUEYRAT

This is the exotic name of a rare precancerous lesion more common on the penis, but sometimes seen in the vulva and vagina. It appears as a red velvety patch of mucous membrane and is often painful. Microscopically, the epithelium is without any surface scale and is either thinned or of normal thickness. All the individual epithelial cells are so abnormal, with close-packed darkly stained irregular nuclei, that they appear either already cancerous or about to become malignant. The cellular pattern is monotonous but anaplastic (Fig. 71–7). The picture closely resembles carcinoma in situ of the cervix. Queyrat's erythroplasia is clinically a precancerous situation, and epidermoid carcinomas develop from it.

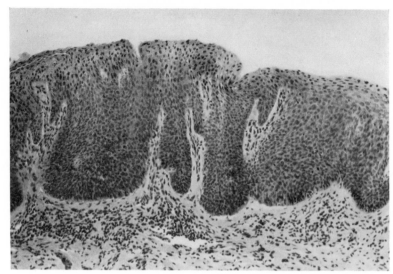

Fig. 71-7.   Closely packed hyperchromatic cells with abnormally large, dark nuclei are found histologically in the erythroplasia of Queyrat. Whether this is to be regarded as precancerous hyperplasia or carcinoma in situ is a moot point.

SARCOMA OF THE VULVA

This is a rare lesion. It may arise spontaneously from the underlying connective tissue or occur secondarily from malignant change within a pre-existing fibroma. When sarcoma does occur, it usually takes the form of either a fibrosarcoma or myxosarcoma. These are highly malignant, and metastasize readily to lungs and bone. Despite the fact that metastases may be established by both lymphatic and blood stream emboli, the treatment recommended is the same as that for a primary carcinoma of the vulva. The final results are not as satisfactory.

MALIGNANT MELANOMA OF THE VULVA

Although nevi appear in the skin in all areas of the body and may undergo malignant change wherever they are encountered, malignant melanomas have a distinct tendency to appear in the genital area fairly frequently. It is estimated that approximately 5 per cent of all melanomas occur on or around the vulva, and that roughly 10 per cent of all malignant lesions that occur in this location are classified as malignant melanomas.

What Is the Prognosis in Malignant Melanoma?

Melanomas are potentially extremely dangerous and should never be regarded lightly. The small lesions carry the same lethal possibilities as the larger melanomas. The growth pattern is so completely unpredictable that metastases either develop with astonishing rapidity, and in the absence of any striking change in the patient's clinical appearance, or they may either never appear or do so years later. Once metastases have developed, the results from surgical excision, however radical, are extremely poor.

What Does Prophylactic Excision of Nevi Have to Offer?

Since the size of the nevus has little to do with the possibility of a malignant change and the histologic growth pattern is so unpredictable by clinical appraisal, the best method of dealing with any pigmented lesions in the vulvar area is to excise them all, regardless of size, giving wide margins to the growth.

In the majority of instances pigmented nevi or moles do not suddenly develop; many have been present since birth. It is manifestly impossible to remove all moles in all locations for fear that they will undergo malignant change, but if a nevus occurs in an area that is subject to repeated trauma, such as on the vulva, it should be excised. In the vulvar area plastic surgical considerations are not present, as they are, for example, on the sole of the foot. Emphasis is placed on surgical excision rather than dissection with an electric scalpel, largely because the desiccation that follows makes the problem of the pathologist extremely complicated as he tries to decide whether or not there is any malignant change present. There is no place for a biopsy by electrocoagulation. Radium application has been used as definitive therapy, but it has the disadvantage of failing to provide pathologic material for evaluation, and many observers feel that true melanomas have a measure of radioresistance. If radium is to be used, it should be reserved for the case that either recurs locally after surgical excision, or when the surgeon entertains doubts that his removal has been adequate. Both factors can be avoided simply by excising the lesion at the original operation with extensive margins of adjacent skin.

It is true that we have encouraged the practice of taking a biopsy of lesions of the vulva, simply because grossly similar lesions in this area have a variety of etiologic agents, and a single factor may produce various types of lesions. This, however, does not apply to malignant melanomas. The only acceptable biopsy is a wide surgical excision of the entire lesion. Review of the previous histories of patients who succumb to malignant disease arising in the vulva almost invariably suggests that either no attention has been paid to the lesion or that meddlesome temporizing procedures have been used.

Whenever possible, pigmented nevi of the vulva should be excised. This is mandatory when the nonhairy mole is seen to thicken and increase in size, extend beyond its usual perimeter into the adjacent skin, alter in color to become darker, or undergo either inflammatory changes or frank ulceration. Even in the absence of these changes, pigmented moles of the vulva should be excised whenever the patient has to have anesthesia for either surgical or obstetrical cause. It is well to remember that some nevi are nonpigmented, and papillomatous flesh-colored lesions might better also be excised.

If the excision has been adequate and was performed at the earliest manifestation of malignancy, the end-results at 5 years will approach a 40 to 50 per cent salvage rate, as against approximately 15 per cent when the surgeon has delayed therapy. Unfortunately, survival at five years does not carry a guarantee that the patient may not subsequently have metastases of malignant melanoma and die at a later date. Instances of lymph nodal involvement as late as twenty years after excision of the primary lesion have been reported.

What Are the Pathologic Criteria of Malignancy?

Grossly, the melanotic lesion need not be large to harbor malignant disease. Two

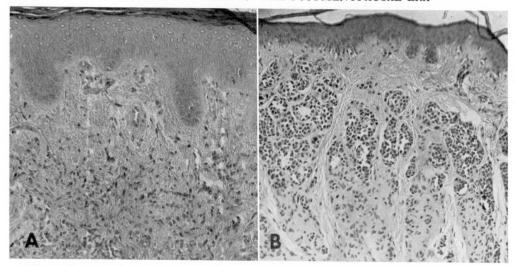

Fig. 71-8.   *A*, In vulvar malignant melanoma the invading pigment-forming or amelanotic cells may be either rounded or spindly, as in this case. Lymphatic invasion is common in the dermis. *B*, A benign nevus has the melanocytic cells growing in clusters, sometimes with transitions that resemble nerve end-organs, as shown at the bottom of the field.

of the melanoma cases recently reported by Symmonds and Pratt from the Mayo Clinic were less than 7 mm. in diameter. Nearly all will show either a local or diffuse deposit of melanin in large tumor cells, polygonal or spindly in shape, usually arranged in an alveolar fashion (Fig. 71–8, *A*). These changes are particularly apparent at the junction where the melanoma is invading normal skin. Although we commonly consider trauma and chronic irritation to be the activating stimuli for malignant change, cancer may be present without any ulceration, and in Symmonds's series when an inflammatory reaction was seen, there was little evidence that it contributed to the growth rate of the tumor. Spreading from the tumor border one may frequently find fine finger-like melanotic cell processes extending laterally in a starlike pattern out into the normal dermis and invading its lymphatics.

Pathologic interpretation of the excised specimen is of the utmost importance in outlining further therapy. If the nevus gives no indication of malignant change (Fig. 71–8, *B*), and the excised margins are sufficiently wide, nothing more need be done, although the patient should be rechecked at regular intervals. If the melanotic tumor is malignant, then consideration should be given to the surgical removal of the regional nodes.

What about Regional Lymph Node Dissection?

Surgical opinion varies widely as to the need for and the timing of regional node dissection with the presence of a primary malignant melanoma. The basis for the controversy lies in the known potential of melanomas to spread by blood stream as well as via lymphatics. It is a difficult matter to find statistical confirmation that long-time survival follows surgical extirpation of positive lymph nodes. Statistically, it does seem to be true, however, that more patients survive when primary excision of the tumor is combined with lymph nodal dissection. Some malignant melanomas will spread chiefly by blood stream, so that one may reasonably question the advisability of removal of lymph nodes. It does seem, nevertheless, that hematogenous spread tends to occur late, and it is possible that it may stem from metastatic disease within the lymph nodes. The same suggestion has been made about the spread of cervical carcinoma. If this is true, it might explain why the survival figures are better when lymph nodes are resected.

For other areas of the body the surgeon also has to consider spread along the superficial as well as the deep lymphatics. If the lesion is eccentrically placed, he may have to consider which lymph nodes drain the area. In the vulvar area the lymphatic drainage pattern is well established, and the standard operation will include the superficial as well as the deep pathways. In addition the surgeon need not be particularly concerned with either the cosmetic or functional result.

WHEN SHOULD THE LYMPH NODES BE DISSECTED? With the diagnosis of malignant disease established, a melanoma of the vulva should be treated without delay by subsequent regional lymph node dissection, together with a complete vulvectomy. Some surgeons prefer to wait for an indefinite time before doing the node dissection, on the theory that with the passage of time any malignant cells will find their way to the lymph nodes and be trapped there. Others wait until the lymph nodes can be palpated. There seems to be little logic in the former and no excuse for the latter point of view. In all probability the nodes will be involved in the early stages of melanomas, or not at all, if all channels are choked with tumor. As regards the palpation of lymph nodes, the clinical error in the evaluation of node involvement is notoriously great. As in carcinoma of the vulva, the statistical reports reflect procrastination in the surgical excision of lymph nodes. Pack and his associates improve their salvage from 17 to 39 per cent when the lymph nodes are dissected immediately after the establishment of a diagnosis of malignant melanoma.

MIXED TUMORS AND TERATOMAS

The gross appearance of these rare vulvar tumors is generally that of a fibroma. Muscle, fat and glandular structures may be found mixed with a fibroma, thus producing a mixed tumor. Embryonal sarcomas of mixed mesodermal type that contain striated as well as unstriated muscle, together with nerve tissue, have been reported. A small percentage of these are actually teratomas and highly malignant.

SECONDARY CARCINOMAS OF THE VULVA

Metastatic deposits from cancers in other organs are occasionally noted in the vulva. Two recent cases, one presenting a solid tumor in the labium and another a shallow superficial ulceration near the urethral opening, were metastases from a hypernephroma or primary renal cell carcinoma. Chorionepithelioma may metastasize to either the vulva or vagina and thus perhaps give the first indication of the primary process within the uterus. Carcinomas of the cervix or endometrium may develop implants on the vulva or within Bartholin's glands.

The appearance of such secondary extensions from a remote carcinoma is an indication of a rather wide dissemination of the original tumor. Biopsy of the vulvar tumor must be done to avoid over-enthusiastic treatment of the secondary manifestations of hopeless cancer.

REFERENCES

Carcinoma of Vulva

Berven, E. G. E.: Carcinoma of the Vulva; Treatment of Cancer of Vulva: Symposium. *Brit. J. Radiol.*, 22: 498, 1949.

Brunschwig, A., and Daniel, W.: Pelvic Exenterations for Advanced Carcinoma of the Vulva. *Am. J. Obst. & Gynec.*, 72: 489, 1956.

Cassidy, R. E., Braden, F. R., and Cerha, H. T.: Factors That Might Influence Prognosis in Malignancies of the Vulva. *Am. J. Obst. & Gynec.*, 74: 361, 1957.

Collins, J. H., and Nolan, J. F.: Symposium on Management of Carcinoma of the Vulva. *Am. J. Obst. & Gynec.*, 79: 1207, 1960.

Cosbie, W. G.: The Treatment of Cancer of the Vulva. *Am. J. Obst. & Gynec.*, 63: 251, 1952.

Eichner, E.: In Vivo Studies on the Pelvic Lymphatics in Women; in J. V. Meigs and S. H. Sturgis, eds.: *Progress in Gynecology.* New York, Grune & Stratton, Inc., 1957, Vol. III, p. 604.

Ellis, F., III: Cancer of the Vulva Treated by Radiation; Analysis of 127 Cases. A Symposium. *Brit. J. Radiol.*, 22: 513, 1949.

Gemmell, A. A., and Haines, M.: Pregnancy Following Radical Vulvectomy for Carcinoma of the Vulva. *J. Obst. & Gynaec. Brit. Emp.*, 67: 199, 1960.

Green, T. H., Jr.: Carcinoma of the Vulva; in J. V. Meigs and S. H. Sturgis, eds.: *Progress in Gynecology.* New York, Grune & Stratton, Inc., 1957, Vol. III, p. 507.

Green, T. H., Jr., Ulfelder, H., and Meigs, J. V.: Epidermoid Carcinoma of the Vulva; An Analysis of 238 Cases. *Am. J. Obst. & Gynec.*, 75: 834, 848, 1958.

Hahn, G. A.: Variables in the Diagnosis and Management of Vulvar Carcinoma as Observed by the Philadelphia Committee for the Study of Pelvic Cancer. *Am. J. Obst. & Gynec.*, 72: 756, 1956.

Langley, I. I., Hertig, A. T., and Smith, G. V. S.: Relation of Leucoplakic Vulvitis to Squamous Carcinoma of the Vulva. *Am. J. Obst. & Gynec.*, 62: 167, 1951.

McKelvey, J. L.: Carcinoma of the Vulva: Treatment and Prognosis. *Obst. & Gynec.*, 5: 452, 1955.

Idem: Carcinoma of the Vulva; in Symposium on Genital Cancer. *Clin. Obst. & Gynec.*, 1: 1101, 1958.

Merrill, J. A., and Ross, N. L.: Cancer of the Vulva. *Cancer*, 14: 13, 1961.

Nolan, J. F.: Carcinoma of the Vulva. *Am. J. Obst. & Gynec.*, 78: 833, 1959.

Palmer, J. P., Sadugor, M. G., and Reinhard, M. C.: Carcinoma of the Vulva. Report of 313 Cases. *Surg., Gynec. & Obst.*, 88: 435, 1949.

Parry-Jones, E.: Lymphatics of the Vulva. *J. Obst. & Gynaec. Brit. Emp.*, 67: 919, 1960.

Parsons, L.: Carcinoma of the Vulva; in J. V. Meigs and S. H. Sturgis, eds.: *Progress in Gynecology.* New York, Grune & Stratton, Inc., 1946, Vol. I, p. 395.

Parsons, L., and Meigs, J. V.: Medical Progress in Gynecology: Carcinoma of the Vulva. *New England J. Med.*, 234: 860, 1946.

Taussig, F. J.: Cancer of the Vulva: An Analysis of 155 Cases (1911–1940). *Am. J. Obst. & Gynec.*, 40: 764, 1940.

Tod, M. C.: Carcinoma of the Vulva: Radium Implantation Treatment of Carcinoma of the Vulva. *Brit. J. Radiol.*, 22: 508, 1949.

Ulfelder, H.: Radical Vulvectomy with Bilateral Inguinal, Femoral and Iliac Node Resection. *Am. J. Obst. & Gynec.*, 78: 1074, 1959.

Way, S.: Carcinoma of the Vulva. *Am. J. Obst. & Gynec.*, 79: 692, 1960.

Other Neoplasms

Ackerman, L. V.: Malignant Melanoma of the Skin. Clinical and Pathologic Analysis of 75 Cases. *Am. J. Clin. Path.*, 18: 602, 1948.

Ariel, I. M.: Malignant Melanoma of the Vagina. Report of a Successfully Treated Case. *Obst. & Gynec.*, 17: 222, 1961.

Buckingham, J. C., and McClure, J. H.: Reticulum Cell Sarcoma of the Vulva: Report of a Case. *Obst. & Gynec.*, 6: 138, 1955.

Folsome, C. E.: Benign and Malignant Tumors of the Vulva. *J.A.M.A.*, 114: 1499, 1940.

Foraker, A. G., and Miller, C. J.: Extramammary Paget's Disease of Perianal Skin. *Cancer*, 2: 144, 1949.

Hertig, A. T.: Seminar on Tumors of the Gynecologic System. *Proc. 18th Seminar, Am. Soc. Clin. Path.*, 1953, p. 6.

Jeffcoate, T. N. A., Davie, T. B., and Harrison, C. V.: Intraepidermal Carcinoma (Bowen's Disease) of the Vulva. Report on 2 Cases. *J. Obst. & Gynaec. Brit. Emp.*, 51: 377, 1944.

Kaufman, R. H., Boice, E. H., and Knight, W. R., III: Paget's Disease of the Vulva. *Am. J. Obst. & Gynec.*, 79: 451, 1960.

Marcus, S. L.: Basal Cell and Basal-Squamous Cell Carcinomas of the Vulva. *Am. J. Obst. & Gynec.*, 79: 461, 1960.

Meyer, H. W.: Malignant Melanoma; The Importance of Early Aggressive Treatment. *Surgery*, 41: 335, 1957.

Mitchell, J. A., and Kaplan, D.: Granular-Cell Myoblastoma of the Labium Majus. *Am. J. Obst. & Gynec.*, 71: 901, 1956.

Newman, W., and Cromer, J. K.: The Multicentric Origin of Carcinoma of the Female Anogenital Tract. *Surg., Gynec. & Obst.*, 108: 273, 1959.

Novak, E., and Stevenson, R. R.: Sweat Gland Tumors of the Vulva, Benign (Hidradenoma) and Malignant (Adenocarcinoma). *Am. J. Obst. & Gynec.*, 50: 641, 1945.

Pack, G. T.: Problem of Malignant Melanoma. *Proc. Second Nat. Cancer Conf.*, New York, American Cancer Society, 1952, p. 54.

Simmons, R. J.: Melanoma of the Vagina and Cervix Treated by Radical Surgery. *Am. J. Obst. & Gynec.*, 71: 1137, 1956.

Symmonds, R. E., Pratt, J. H., and Dockerty, M. B.: Melanoma of the Vulva. *Obst. & Gynec.*, 15: 543, 1960.

Woodruff, J. D.: Paget's Disease of the Vulva. Review—Report of a Case. *Obst. & Gynec.*, 5: 175, 1955.

Chapter 72

Carcinoma of the Vagina and Urethra

THE VAGINAL canal may be the site of a malignant process as the result of (1) a primary growth, (2) direct invasion from a cancer in adjacent organs, or (3) metastases of a primary tumor from a distant site. It is often difficult to distinguish between primary and secondary carcinomas, largely because the tumor is usually well advanced when first seen. The anticipated primary lesion is an epidermoid carcinoma. When adenocarcinoma is found, search should be made for a primary source other than in the vagina such as in the uterine fundus, ovary, kidney or gastrointestinal tract.

PRIMARY SQUAMOUS CELL CANCER OF THE VAGINA

This is one of the rarer forms of malignant disease that appears in the genital tract, with an incidence of perhaps 0.5 per cent of all cancer. It is usually a disease of older women. Chronic irritation from the prolonged use of a pessary to correct a prolapse seems to play some role in the etiology. Cancer of the vagina also has been reported in infancy, as well as the twenty- to thirty-year age group.

How Does It Grow and Spread?

Though cancer may arise anywhere in the vaginal canal, it is most often found in the upper vaginal fornices on the posterior wall near the cervix. One is more inclined to suspect a secondary carcinoma when the tumor arises on the anterolateral aspect near the urethra. Multicentric points of origin and diffuse spread through the entire vagina are not uncommon. The tumor may appear either as a papillary, everting mushroom-like growth or as a circumscribed area of induration, nodule or plaque (Fig. 72–1). Rarely, the growth is subepithelial with a fixed induration noted throughout the length of the vaginal canal. Occasionally an annular constriction may develop at the midportion of the canal, as the growth spreads in all directions. Superficial widespread ulceration is the rule.

Extension of epidermoid carcinoma through the lymphatics occurs relatively early. The direction of the spread depends in large part upon the site of the primary tumor. When the point of origin is in the upper part of the vagina, invasion or permeation of the lymphatic pathways will produce metastases in the iliac, hypogastric and

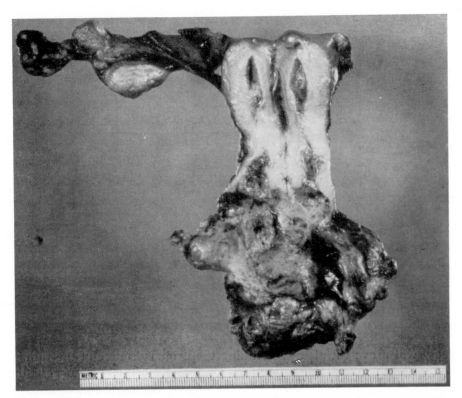

Fig. 72-1.   Extensive primary epidermoid carcinoma of the vagina is shown growing laterally as well as upward into the vaginal fornices.

obturator lymph nodes. The lower vaginal sites metastasize to the superficial inguinal regions. Direct extension of the growth may result in an invasion of the bladder, rectum and, if the disease has attained considerable dimension, ulcerations and fistula formation. Since posterior vaginal wall origin is the most common, rectovaginal fistulas appear more often. The parametrium may also become fixed by malignant disease, either as the result of lymphatic permeation or by direct extension of the growth. Distant metastasis to lungs, liver and bone, as well as to tube and ovary, have been reported.

Symptoms

When ulceration has occurred, the symptoms may be a thin vaginal discharge, often bloody, which may or may not follow intercourse. The ulcerating lesions are tender, owing to secondary sepsis. The nodular form of primary carcinoma, if not ulcerated, may be the only positive finding on physical examination, and may cause no symptoms. The symptoms present are indistinguishable from those produced by cancer of the cervix. The diagnosis is made by vaginal smear, palpation and biopsy.

Treatment

The treatment to date has been unsatisfactory and the prognosis uniformly poor. Until recently radiation was the sole therapy. This took the form of (1) topical applications of radium plaques molded to fit the vagina, or (2) interstitial applications of platinum-screened radium needles. X-ray treatment through vaginal ports proved more effective for tumors located in the upper part of the vagina than for those located lower in the vaginal tract.

With the increased enthusiasm for radical surgery, new avenues have opened with a promise of greater ultimate success. Depending on the location of the growth, its size and the general condition of the patient, the surgeon who is properly trained may elect to do a total vaginectomy with bilateral pelvic or inguinal lymphadenectomy. In the more advanced cases when the bladder or rectum or both are invaded, a complete or posterior exenteration may be performed.

SECONDARY CANCER OF THE VAGINA

The vagina may be involved in a malignant process in one of two ways: (1) direct extension from a carcinoma primary in the bladder, urethra or rectum, as well as cervix; (2) metastases may occur from adenocarcinoma of the endometrium, ovary, tube, kidney or gastrointestinal tract.

Direct Extension

Biopsy will prove useful in establishing the primary source of the tumor. In a biopsy from the upper part of the vagina, epidermoid carcinoma suggests that the disease was primary in either the cervix or vagina. Taken from the anterolateral aspect in the lower vagina, a squamous cell carcinoma points to either urethra or vagina. Adenocarcinoma, on the other hand, implicates either the base of the bladder, the rectum or rare primary carcinomas arising in embryologic anlage (Fig. 72–2).

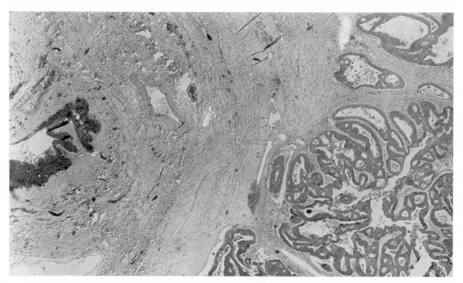

Fig. 72-2. Primary adenocarcinoma of the vagina may arise from accessory vaginal glands or from Gaertner's duct rests, or in the rectovaginal septum it may be thought to be of cloacogenic origin. If the adenocarcinoma is of average grade malignancy, as in this case, the gland of origin is difficult to identify.

Metastatic Cancer

Adenocarcinoma appearing in a biopsy also calls attention to the fact that the vagina may be involved secondary to cancer originating elsewhere. Malignant disease in the fundal portion of the uterus frequently involves the vagina not through implants, but by lymphatic permeation. This is true of both chorionepithelioma and adenocarcinoma of the endometrium. The metastatic areas are usually subepithelial and in many instances are widespread. It is interesting to observe how frequently such metastatic lesions are located in the anterior vaginal wall. This is particularly true when the site of the primary tumor is in such a remote area as intestine, kidney, ovary or tube.

OTHER PRIMARY TUMORS OF THE VAGINA

SARCOMA

In adults, sarcoma usually appears in the form of a diffuse subepithelial growth completely surrounding the vaginal canal and distorting its lumen, but often without destroying the epithelium. The induration is most irregular to direct palpation. The prognosis is usually poor, though external irradiation therapy has produced gratifying results in one patient treated seven years ago.

Another form of sarcoma in children produces diffuse infiltration as well as degeneration of the epithelial lining. It usually begins as a small area of induration on the posterior vaginal wall. This breaks down, and ulceration is followed by a diffuse sarcomatous infiltration involving the entire circumference of the vagina.

SARCOMA BOTRYOIDES

This form of vaginal sarcoma is most frequently encountered in infancy, though it may be seen also at puberty or in old age. The gross appearance of grapelike vesicular masses of tumor is most striking. It begins probably as a polyp on the anterior vaginal wall, but when first seen, it is usually a large mass that distends the vagina and appears externally at the introitus.

The *treatment* of sarcoma botryoides is most discouraging, because nothing short of massive extirpative surgery will cure. Total exenteration of the pelvic contents in a baby of eighteen months has produced at least one five-year cure.

CARCINOMA ARISING IN EMBRYOLOGIC ANLAGE

A few isolated cases of adenocarcinoma arising in Gaertner's duct have been reported. One large tumor with the histologic appearance of thyroid tissue has been removed from the rectovaginal space. No suspicion of tumor was found in the thyroid gland. Such tumors are rare (Fig. 72–2).

ADENOMA AND CARCINOMA OF BARTHOLIN'S GLAND

Carcinoma of Bartholin's gland is a rare form of malignant disease. Approximately 2 to 3 per cent of all vulvar cancers will take origin in a Bartholin's gland.

Among all the disease processes that implicated the gland in the records of the Mayo Clinic, 1 per cent were carcinomas. The true incidence is probably higher than the one carcinoma of Bartholin's gland among 1000 genital malignancies as suggested by Crossen. The lesion is encountered largely by general practitioners who performed operations for what they thought was a benign condition, and few of the actual number are ever reported. Masterson in 1955 could find only 117 cases in the medical literature.

Because the cancer arises in a secretory gland it is generally taken to be an adeno-carcinoma, but actually in collected series from the literature, there are nearly as many epidermoid carcinomas as adenocarcinomas. A few primary sarcomas have occurred.

One reason why more carcinomas of Bartholin's gland are not recorded can be attributed to the growth pattern. When the disease has left the confines of the gland and spread to the deeper structures in the vagina and labia, it can hardly be distinguished from a carcinoma of the vulva. The point of origin is thus completely obscured, and the difficulties are further compounded when the structure is that of an epidermoid carcinoma.

How is the Diagnosis Made?

In the early phases there is little to differentiate cancer from a chronic infection in Bartholin's gland or from adenofibroma. All that the patient notes or the physician discovers is a small, firm or hard, painless nodule in the lower third of the vulvar area where Bartholin's gland is normally found. The tumor moves in the underlying tissue, and the skin is intact.

As the cancer continues its slow growth the restraining capsule ruptures, and the tumor begins to invade the deeper structures. The tumor fixes to the underlying tissue, and the skin over it ulcerates. Partial necrosis ensues, and infection appears, so that the area now becomes semifluctuant and tender. For this reason many are missed and drained surgically under the mistaken impression that the pathologic process is a simple Bartholin's abscess. The patient rarely consults a physician in the early stages of growth, since she has no pain and suffers no inconvenience. The delay from probable date of onset to final definitive treatment ranges from eight to fifteen months.

In the early stages when the tumor is encapsulated there is little likelihood of spread to the regional nodes in the superficial inguinal and femoral areas or to the nodes above Poupart's ligament. When the tumor has spread beyond the confines of the gland, enlarged lymph nodes are frequently palpated in the groin. The enlargement may be due to carcinoma or perhaps to infection secondary to tumor necrosis.

In the later stages a possible diagnosis of cancer should be considered, and a biopsy taken to confirm or exclude it. In the earlier phases when the tumor simply appears to be a nontender, movable lump the index of suspicion is low. Taussig has stressed that any such lesion in a woman over the age of forty should be regarded as potentially dangerous and should be removed. Although cases have been reported as early as eighteen and as late as ninety-one years, the majority of carcinomas of Bartholin's gland appear in the forty- to sixty-year age group.

Little help can be obtained by considering the symptomatology. In the earlier stages the patient has no symptoms and may or may not be aware of a tumor. In the later stages there is nothing about such symptoms as pruritus, pain, bleeding or discharge that will distinguish carcinoma from any other lesion of the vulva or from an inflammatory process in Bartholin's gland. The important point is that the lesion may be carcinoma, and its true nature must be established before any surgical procedure is carried out.

What Is the Pathologic Appearance?

Bartholin's gland neoplasms are either adenomas or carcinomas. The adenoma has a solid, spherical, encapsulated appearance. Closely crowded small nests of mucinous glands and nests of transitional-type ductal epithelium are present in a rather prominent fibrous stroma, all with a peripheral fibrous capsule (Fig. 72–3, *A*).

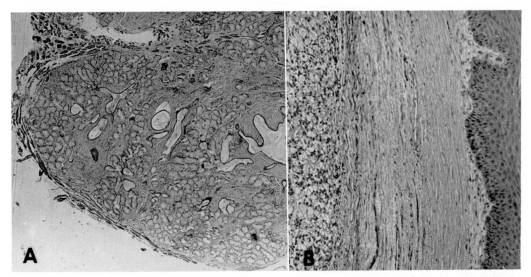

Fig. 72-3. *A*, The rare benign Bartholin's gland adenoma is encapsulated and reproduces the architecture of the acini and ducts in the form of a compact fibroadenomatous tumor. *B*, Bartholin's gland carcinoma has a variety of histologic types, in this case a mucinous carcinoma simplex, growing deep beneath the labial vestibular epithelium.

Carcinomas grossly have a poorly demarcated outline and are either granular and friable or sticky and mucinous on sectioning. Microscopically, as mentioned, either an epidermoid carcinoma of duct origin or a solid type of mucinous adenocarcinoma may be found, depending on whether the ducts or the acini have undergone neoplastic change. Sometimes the tumor has a transitional appearance reminiscent of a bladder carcinoma (Fig. 72–3, *B*). Local invasion is evident.

What Is the Best Form of Treatment?

According to the literature, the prognosis after therapy would seem to be poor. This is rather hard to understand, because in its early stages the neoplasm would seem to be confined to the gland itself. The prognosis appears to depend more on the size of the primary lesion than on the extent of metastases to lymph nodes.

The therapy that has proved effective for cancer of the vulva should be utilized for cancer of Bartholin's gland; namely, a radical vulvectomy and bilateral superficial inguinal node dissection. It is true that (*a*) cancer of Bartholin's gland is a unilateral lesion and that (*b*) the lymph drainage from Bartholin's gland has not been established. Nevertheless, particularly when the lesion is no longer confined, the principle of a large operation for a small lesion applies. The lymph nodes should therefore be removed.

Unlike carcinoma of the vulva, malignant disease of Bartholin's gland is unicentric in origin. If the operation is radical enough, we should be able to cure more patients with cancer of Bartholin's gland than with carcinoma of the vulva. If the lesion proves to be a sarcoma, the radical approach still applies. It would appear that the poor prognosis after therapy for cancer in this gland is due, for the most part, to failure to recognize the true nature of the growth and to inadequate attempts to deal with it. The primary approach to therapy is radical surgical extirpation. There have been a few advocates for the supplementary use of local radium applicators.

CARCINOMA OF THE URETHRA

The female urethra may be involved in malignant disease because it is either (1) the primary source of the cancer or (2) the site of secondary extension from an initial cancer source in bladder, bowel, uterus, vulva or vagina. It is a relatively rare form of malignant disease in women. The etiologic factors are not well established, but circumstantial evidence suggests that chronic irritation plays a role.

Natural Course of the Disease

There are two types of carcinoma of the urethra, depending on the point of origin. The tumor may arise, (1) either in and around the urethral meatus or (2) at the bladder neck.

CANCER AT THE URETHRAL MEATUS.   This tumor is usually an epidermoid carcinoma. It arises in one of three ways: (*a*) It may appear as a friable papillary type of tumor that closely resembles a urethral caruncle or prolapse of the epithelial lining of the urethra. It bleeds easily to the slightest trauma. (*b*) More often it appears as a frank ulceration, with overhanging undermined edges, located just beneath the urethral outlet. (*c*) It may appear as a heavy induration around the meatus.

CANCER OF THE BLADDER NECK.   This tumor usually arises from the paraurethral glands at the bladder neck and is an adenocarcinoma histologically. In its growth it tends to extend down along the urethral wall as a drawn-out elongated ulcer, or it spreads into the paraurethral tissues along the course of the urethra. There seems to be little tendency to invade the bladder wall in the early phases.

When the carcinoma has taken origin from the urethral meatus, lymphatic extension may occur to the regional lymphatics in the inguinal regions. When carcinoma arises from the bladder neck, the deep regional lymph nodes along the iliac and obturator vessels are implicated.

Symptoms

The growth is insidious, and the patient may not be aware of trouble until ulceration of the tumor appears. Then follows bloody and painful micturition. A tumor nodule may make its appearance and produce a sense of discomfort in the region of the external urethral orifice. This usually brings the patient to the physician.

If the tumor arises in the paraurethral glands, the first symptom may be an increasing difficulty in initiating a urinary stream. Encroachment of the tumor upon the lumen produces obstruction.

How to Make a Diagnosis of Urethral Carcinoma

When an ulceration or friable growth is present, the diagnosis may be made by palpation, inspection and biopsy. Papilloma, urethral prolapse and caruncle produce many of the symptoms of carcinoma, but rarely the palpable impression of malignancy. If any question exists, the suspicious lesion should be biopsied. Early diagnosis is important, for the prognosis reflects the size of the primary tumor.

The greatest difficulty comes in trying to put the proper interpretation on the induration that is sometimes felt along the whole course of the urethra. The thickening noted may be due to neoplasia or the inflammatory response to a chronic urethritis, periurethritis or possibly infected urethral cysts. Normally a shallow sulcus can be felt on either side of the urethra between it and the bony rami of the pubis. When this can no longer be felt, the induration in all probability is a tumor that has spread beyond the borders of the urethra. The diagnosis may be confirmed either by biopsy under local anesthesia through the anterior vaginal wall, or occasionally by biopsy of the urethral epithelium through a urethroscope.

Treatment

Because of the location of the primary carcinoma, rather than differences in its pathologic classification, the plan of treatment varies with the individual case.

1. When the initial lesion is located near the urinary meatus and seems to be localized to the adjacent paraurethral tissue, radiation therapy is given. Long low-intensity 2- or 3-mg. platinum-screened radium needles are placed in the tumor at 1-cm. intervals in the long axis of the urethra. A total dosage of 2500 mg.-hr. frequently controls the growth without producing irreparable damage to urinary control through destruction of the urethra. The total amount given varies with the amount of tumor tissue to be irradiated. Since carcinoma in this area spreads to the regional lymph nodes in the inguinal regions approximately 20 per cent of the time, node dissection must be considered. It is debatable whether node dissection should be postponed until lymph nodes are palpable in the groin.

2. When the tumor has its primary site of origin in the paraurethral glands at the neck of the bladder, radiation can no longer be considered an adequate therapeutic agent. With this form of tumor the symptoms are minor, the diagnosis is delayed, and the malignant tumor usually extensive when the case is first presented for treatment. Radical surgery that permits bilateral lymphadenectomy, cystectomy and vaginectomy is alone adequate for the control of the cancerous disease. The urinary stream is diverted to the bowel by ureterointestinal anastomoses.

REFERENCES

Carcinoma of Vagina

Arronet, G. H., Latour, J. P. A., and Tremblay, P. C.: Primary Carcinoma of the Vagina. *Am. J. Obst. & Gynec.*, 79: 455, 1960.

Bivens, M. D.: Primary Carcinoma of Vagina: A Report of 46 Cases. *Am. J. Obst. & Gynec.*, 65: 390, 1953.
Brack, C. B., Merritt, R. I., and Dickson, R. J.: Primary Carcinoma of the Vagina. *Obst. & Gynec.*, 12: 104, 1958.
Douglas, G. W.: Observations on the Pathology of Primary Carcinoma of the Vagina and Its Relation to Therapy. *Surg., Gynec. & Obst.*, 98: 456, 1954.
Kaiser, I. H.: Primary Carcinoma of the Vagina. *Cancer*, 5: 1146, 1952.
Lang, W. E., Menduke, H., and Golub, L. J.: The Delayed Period in Carcinoma of the Vagina, with Observations in Age Incidence and Survival Rate. *Am. J. Obst. & Gynec.*, 80: 341, 1960.
Livingstone, R. G.: *Primary Carcinoma of the Vagina.* Springfield, Ill., Charles C Thomas, 1950.
Marcus, S. L.: Primary Carcinoma of the Vagina. *Obst. & Gynec.*, 15: 673, 1960.
Merrill, J. A., and Bender, W. T.: Primary Carcinoma of the Vagina. *Obst. & Gynec.*, 11: 3, 1958.
Murphy, W. T.: Primary Vaginal Cancer: Irradiation Management and End-Results. *Radiology*, 68: 157, 1957.
Palmer, J. P., and Biback, S. M.: Primary Cancer of the Vagina. *Am. J. Obst. & Gynec.*, 67: 377, 1954.
Singh, B. P.: Primary Carcinoma of the Vagina. *Cancer*, 4: 1073, 1951.
Smith, F. R.: Primary Carcinoma of the Vagina. *Am. J. Obst. & Gynec.*, 69: 525, 1955.
TeLinde, R. W., and Brack, C. B.: Carcinoma of the Vagina. *Clin. Obst. & Gynec.*, 1: 1108, 1958.

Sarcoma of Vagina

Johnson, C. E., and Soule, E. H.: Malignant Lymphoma as a Gynecologic Problem. Report of 5 Cases, Including One Primary Lymphosarcoma of Cervix Uteri. *Obst. & Gynec.*, 9: 149, 1957.
Salm, R.: Botryoid Sarcoma of the Vagina. *Brit. J. Cancer*, 15: 220, 1961.
Weseley, A. C., and Berrigan, M. V.: Reticulum-Cell Sarcoma of the Vagina: Report of a Case. *Obst. & Gynec.*, 11: 192, 1958.

Carcinoma of Bartholin's Gland

Boughton, T. G.: Carcinoma of Bartholin's Gland. *Am. J. Surg.*, 59: 585, 1943.
Bowing, H. H., Fricke, R. E., and Kennedy, T. J.: Radium Therapy for Carcinoma of Bartholin's Glands. *Am. J. Roentgenol.*, 61: 517, 1949.
Crossen, R. J.: Primary Carcinoma of Bartholin's Gland. *Am. J. Surg.*, 75: 597, 1948.
Masterson, J. R., and Goss, A. S.: Carcinoma of Bartholin's Gland. Review of the Literature and Report of a New Case in an Elderly Patient Treated by Radical Operation. *Am. J. Obst. & Gynec.*, 69: 1323, 1955.
Newman, B., and Gray, D. B.: Primary Carcinoma of Bartholin's Gland. *Am. J. Surg.*, 92: 490, 1956.
Pattison, D. S., and Shute, D.: Carcinoma of Bartholin's Gland. *Canad. M.A.J.*, 64: 249, 1951.

Carcinoma of Urethra

Buschke, F., and Cantril, S. T.: Roentgen Therapy of Carcinoma of the Female Urethra and Vulva. *Radiology*, 51: 155, 1948.
DeHaan, Q. C., and Johnson, C. G.: Adenocarcinoma of the Paraurethral Glands. *Am. J. Obst. & Gynec.*, 80: 1108, 1960.
Graves, R. C.: Carcinoma of the Female Urethra; in J. V. Meigs and S. H. Sturgis, eds.: *Progress in Gynecology.* New York, Grune & Stratton, Inc., 1946, Vol. I, p. 401.
Knoblich, R.: Primary Adenocarcinoma of the Female Urethra. A Review and Report of 3 Cases. *Am. J. Obst. & Gynec.*, 80: 353, 1960.
Marshall, F. C., Uson, A. C., and Melicow, M. M.: Neoplasms and Caruncles of the Female Urethra. *Surg., Gynec. & Obst.*, 110: 723, 1960.
Monaco, A. P., Murphy, G. B., and Dowling, W.: Primary Cancer of the Female Urethra. *Cancer*, 11: 1215, 1958.
Teoh, T. B.: Papillary Adenocarcinoma of the Female Urethra. A Case Report. *Brit. J. Surg.*, 48: 151, 1960.

PART VII

Gynecologic

Problems in Old Age

Chapter 73

Geriatric Gynecology

Since we have elected to relate symptoms and diseases peculiar to women according to the most likely causes within each age group, it is important that we carry out the plan and discuss gynecologic problems in the aged. This section is called "Geriatric Gynecology" simply because the terms are in general usage. As Adair points out, however, geriatrics is derived from the Greek roots "geron," meaning old men, and "iatrikos," signifying medical treatment. In all probability the problems of the aged have received this designation because much of the older literature dealt with the male rather than the female. Adair suggests that elderly women may be more "appealing to their relatives and descendants," but perhaps no one wishes to assume responsibility for a poor old man. Thus his problems have become the focal point of much discussion. It is obvious, however, that many disease processes in the elderly are common to both sexes.

It is a difficult matter to assess the aging process or to determine exactly when it begins. Technically, it starts when the spermatozoon impregnates the ovum. All too frequently the usefulness of woman is judged by her ability to produce children. As metabolic processes slow down and the menopause appears, the woman tends to resign herself to a life of diminishing activity and responsibility. Until recent years it has been customary to link productivity to chronologic age in both men and women. Unfortunately, productivity seems to have an essentially sexual connotation. The sexual powers certainly get no stronger with advancing years, but the ability to function physically and mentally otherwise does not necessarily follow a parallel course.

Too many men and women are forced into retirement at an age when they are most useful. This is an error, for the process of aging is a relative one with manifestations peculiar to each person. Some women, for example, are in amazingly good health in both mind and body in their seventies, despite the fact that their path through life may not have been easy, but others deteriorate rapidly before their time without experiencing stressful situations.

Heredity, for example, plays an obviously important role both in determining longevity and in the rate at which senescence occurs. The retrogressive process in function as well as structure of organs varies from person to person and in different organs within the same person. In evaluating problems of the aged it is far more important to consider the physiologic rather than the chronologic age. It has a bearing, in the first place, on whether an elderly woman has any gynecologic problems, and it is also intimately concerned with what you can achieve and to what extent you can correct her difficulties.

1175

How Much of a Problem Does Geriatric Gynecology Present?

It is a well known fact reflected in statistical reports from state Health Departments and actuarial figures of Life Insurance Companies that more of the population is reaching the older age groups in which degenerative disease processes may be expected. A woman in good health at fifty years, for example, can expect to live at least twenty years more. Lash suggests that for each year a woman lives after the age of fifty years one can project a six-month period of life beyond the age of seventy years. A woman of sixty years can then be expected to live to be seventy-five years old, and one at eighty can anticipate five more years.

Not only are more women living longer, but also they are presenting themselves in increasing numbers for correction of many of their difficulties. If the expectancy of life is short, a patient may be reluctant to have elective surgery performed, but if there is a reasonable chance of survival for a respectable period of time, the patient may request it. The basic point in offering surgical correction to a patient of advanced years is not simply to permit her to live longer, but to make her more comfortable, useful and happy as long as life continues. We now know, through increasing experience, that age alone is not a contraindication to surgery that may be needed, nor need the surgeon perform a palliative operation on this basis when a more extensive procedure might have a chance to cure the patient. The aging public is becoming aware of these facts, and more and more elderly women are becoming interested in early gynecologic diagnosis and treatment.

There can be no question that in this age group the physician will uncover more cardiovascular, renal and pulmonary abnormalities, but they need not contraindicate any needful surgery, provided reasonable surgical judgment is exercised and the modern principles of preoperative and postoperative care are followed. The chances of success improve, however, when the condition is attacked early in the course of its development. Unfortunately, in too many instances there is a factor of neglect before the aged patient applies for definitive correction of her problem. This emphasizes the value of the modern concept of practicing medicine through prevention by periodic examinations at any age.

What Are the Most Common Gynecologic Problems in the Aged?

The same primary symptoms of bleeding, pain and discharge prevail in this age group as in the earlier years of woman's life, but their significance changes. No longer is the physician mainly concerned with the activity of the sex hormones as they bear on the symptoms, but rather considers that the symptoms may appear because of hormonal deficiency. Many symptoms and physical findings actually relate to damage experienced during labor many years before.

High among the list of complaints that plague women beyond the age of sixty-five years are those referable to the bladder and the urinary tract. Their causation is in part attributable to the inadequacy of hormonal secretion, and in part to the ravages of obstetrical delivery. Parturition has so weakened the pelvic floor support that symptoms may appear and become most troublesome decades later when the supporting structures are weaker because of age.

In this age group the appearance of a mass anywhere in the breast, abdomen or genital tract carries with it a high index of suspicion that a malignant disease may be present, particularly when accompanied by vaginal bleeding.

A general statement may be made that fully 80 per cent of all gynecologic problems in patients over 60 years old are traceable to (*a*) postmenopausal bleeding, (*b*) genital prolapse, (*c*) infections or (*d*) alterations in normal bladder function.

What Manifestations of Age Appear in the Vulvar Area, and How Do They Contribute to Gynecologic Disease?

Recognizable changes appear in the skin throughout the body in the process of aging, and the vulva is no exception. In fact, since the area was one of the main target organs for the hormones in the past, the deficiency is sometimes most evident in this area. The anatomic changes that are immediately apparent are as follows:

(a) Atrophy is noted in the thin, flabby skin of the vulva.

(b) The skin itself is now only a few cell layers thick, and much of the vascularity and nearly all the elastic fibers are lost.

(c) The hair becomes noticeably less abundant, and there is a disappearance of subcutaneous fat.

(d) As a result the labial folds are much less prominent and tend to fade into the surrounding skin.

We noted in the infant that the exposed position of the vulva predisposed it to the development of a wide variety of skin infections because of the increased likelihood of trauma. As the estrogenic hormones came into play, physiologic alterations took place which resulted in an increased deposition of perineal subcutaneous fat and epithelial changes in the vagina. With the chance of trauma thus minimized and

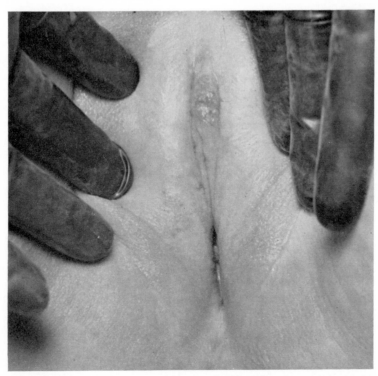

Fig. 73-1.   Atrophic vulvitis, with thin, shiny mucous membranes and skin. There is also a carcinoma of the clitoris present.

resistance to infection increased through hormonal action the problem of vulvar infection diminished. The situation is reversed in the older woman. As the hormone output falls off, she reverts to the susceptible condition of infancy. The fact that the older woman frequently pays less attention to her nutritional needs and is often more careless about the hygienic requirements in this area tends to contribute to dermatologic infections. Through neglect the vulvar and perineal skin frequently macerates and may even progress to the fissuring stage, particularly if the patient is obese. In part, this situation is made worse by the intense itching that results from a superficial infection which enters the skin through the abrasions. The patient compounds her problem by scratching, which simply produces more trauma and introduces more infection.

The end-result of all this is the common condition known as *atrophic* and *hypertrophic vulvitis*. It acquires this name because of the tendency to show atrophy and shrinkage in some areas, while hypertrophy, induration and even lichenification appear in others. Areas of fissuring and ulceration are common (Fig. 73–1). The perineal as well as the vulvar area may be involved. Since lichenification, in many instances, may resemble leukoplakia, which has some relation to cancer, it is important to biopsy such areas, particularly if they do not respond to estrogen or vitamin A therapy. In many instances atrophic and hypertrophic vulvitis will revert to something like the normal state after such therapy, but in all probability leukoplakia is irreversible.

Treatment of Vulvar Lesions

Most vulvar infection is troublesome to the older patient, not because of the ulceration, but because of intense itching and burning. Treatment therefore is frequently directed toward the pruritus rather than the underlying cause. It should be kept constantly in mind that pruritus is a symptom, not a disease. If you want to cure it, you must do two things: (*a*) eliminate the underlying cause, and (*b*) break the scratch reflex. Too frequently overenthusiastic efforts are made to eradicate the underlying defect. The primary aim in therapy should be to make the patient more comfortable. If the patient is overtreated, the vulvar dermatitis can be made worse rather than better.

By and large more cures and relief are obtained by a regimen of cleanliness, nutritional and vitamin replacement, particularly vitamins A and B complex, reassurance and the application of bland soothing lotions than can be had from too intense application of ointments or the use of x-ray therapy or alcohol injections.

Many pitfalls in therapy can be avoided if a few simple rules are followed. (1) It is always a wise move to try to establish a diagnosis before outlining a program of therapy. Thus you may need a urine specimen or blood sugar determination to rule out diabetes mellitus. Other generalized systemic diseases can produce vulvar lesions with itching, and they must be considered possible explanations. Chief among these are pernicious anemia, leukemia and hepatitis. If the lesion is ulcerating or a lump is present and epithelialization does not occur promptly under therapy, a biopsy is indicated. A macerated vulva may harbor pathogenic bacteria mixed with mycotic organisms which can be identified by culture.

2. Some of the dermatologic lesions in the vulvar area arise in response to chemical irritation or food and drug hypersensitivity. As high as 10 per cent of vulvar pruritus has been traced to this source. Some women are sensitive to soaps or dis-

infectants. Others are allergic to nylon or rayon underclothing. A careful history will help in detecting the underlying cause.

3. General experience emphasizes two important factors in the use of topical applications in the region of the vulva: (a) There is a tendency to apply oily-base ointments, many of which are too strong and tend to superimpose a medical dermatitis on the original infection. Oily-base ointments should not be used. It is far better to use simple soothing antiseptic lotions rather than ointments. (b) It is also well known that any topical application, whether it be an antihistaminic, an antibiotic or a simple anesthetic agent, can produce skin sensitivity if it is given over too long a period.

4. In evaluating the response to therapy the physician should remember that itching, which may be paroxysmal or continuous, accompanying any dermatologic lesion in the vulvar and perineal areas will be more severe at night and during periods of stress, either physical or mental. For the most part the skin lesion itself is not a neurodermatitis, as it frequently is in the reproductive age group, but certainly there is a large psychic component associated with pruritus. If the physician is aware of this, he can accomplish a great deal through patience and a sympathetic interest in the problem. A little reassurance combined with mild sedation may accomplish as much as the specific topical therapy prescribed.

The treatment of vulvar infection in the elderly patient should stress the importance of keeping the area cool, clean and dry. Since some part of the problem is commonly associated with malnutrition and avitaminosis, measures should be taken to provide an adequate diet with a vitamin supplement.

We have discussed in the previous section the more important dermatologic lesions commonly found in the vulvar area in the postmenopausal patient (see Chap. 70). Because of neglect in both nutrition and hygiene, the problems are magnified in the older age group. Furthermore, an attitude of indifference may be the patient's chief reaction to any ulceration or lump that may appear in this area. Old patients often prefer to ignore it and will continue to unless the itching and burning become so intense that they have to consult a physician for relief. It is important to stress the fact that malignant disease of the vulva may mimic vulvar infection. Any ulceration that does not heal, a leukoplakic area or tumor of the vulva, however small, should be biopsied.

Parker and his associates have outlined a useful table that may be of help in treating local vulvar infections associated with pruritus.

Local Symptomatic Therapy
1. Starch water sitz baths to alleviate itching and burning
2. Plain water douches
3. Simple lotions

For Secondary Infection
1. Potassium permanganate soaks, 1:5000 dilution
2. Saline compresses
3. One-half per cent acetic acid compresses in the presence of Pseudomonas infection

Drying Regimen (after Toilet and Bath)
1. Avoid the use of a rough towel. Pat with soft tissue
2. Lie exposed with legs akimbo after the bath. A hair dryer or perineal heat lamp may be used to facilitate drying
3. Wear loose-fitting, clean, dry underclothing. Cotton panties are better than silk, rayon or nylon

Improvement in General Health
Any malnutrition, vitamin deficiency or anemia should be corrected

Sedation
1. This is important, particularly at night and during the early phase of treatment
2. Antihistaminic preparations should be used as a mild sedative and antipruritic

Psychogenic Therapy
  1. The patient should be reassured that she does not have a cancer or venereal disease
  2. Frequent visits should be encouraged during the early phase of treatment
  3. An all-out effort should be made to break the scratch habit.

In the majority of instances simple therapeutic measures should be tried. There is a tendency to overtreat this troublesome problem. X-ray therapy should not be used, and alcohol injections are both temporary in their effect and dangerous in their application.

VAGINAL LESIONS

Estrogen lack and the accompanying atrophy of the vulvar and vaginal tissues provide the background for a majority of problems that have the vagina as their focal point. Vaginal discharge, with or without bleeding, and abdominal discharge, with or without pruritus, are the main reasons why patients in this age group consult the physician. The evidence pointing to estrogen lack is found in the morphologic changes that appear in the vaginal epithelium and the alteration in the vaginal flora seen on smear and culture.

The same changes go on within the vaginal canal that we noted in the vulva. The epithelium thins out, and loses much of its blood supply and nearly all the elastic tissue fibers. Connective tissue tends to replace elastica. As a result the vaginal epithelium no longer looks moist, edematous and succulent. Now the rugae disappear, and the epithelial covering of the vaginal canal appears smooth, shiny and dry and has a pinkish-red tinge to its glazed surface. Actually, both the canal and its opening, the introitus, become smaller. If the woman has borne children, the lacerated walls of the outlet tend to gape open and roll outward. Because the epithelium is thinned out, it is much more susceptible to trauma and subsequent infection, both specific and nonspecific.

As a part of the altered physiologic state, vaginal secretions are scanty, and when examined a notable lack of the Döderlein bacillus is apparent. Again, the flora reverts to the condition previously noted in early childhood before the hormones become active. Carter, in studying the bacteria found in the senile vagina, noted a mixed flora made up of nonsporulating anaerobic organisms, diphtheroids, nonhemolytic streptococci and *Staphylococcus albus*. As the Döderlein bacilli disappear, the pH rises to 6.7, instead of the 4.5 reading that is normal for women in their reproductive years. All the factors mentioned contribute to the increased sensitivity of the vaginal epithelium to trauma, which allows breaks to occur and permits the introduction of low-grade infection.

ATROPHIC VAGINITIS

What Are the Common Types of Atrophic Vaginitis?

Two of the most common gynecologic conditions with this background are senile vulvovaginitis and senile vaginitis per se.

In *senile vulvovaginitis* the patient complains of intense itching in and around the vagina, often with burning. There may be little to see except the changes we have noted. Occasionally subepithelial hemorrhages are noted in localized areas within the vagina or at its outlet. They often have a muddy brown appearance. The striking thing is the almost complete lack of secretion. The symptoms are out of proportion to the gross appearance. About the only thing that can be seen is evidence of tissue atrophy.

In *senile vaginitis* superficial erosions may be apparent, with varying amounts of filmy adhesions that are often so extensive that the entire vaginal lumen is occluded. The adhesions can be broken up readily enough, but the maneuver is usually associated with a moderate amount of bleeding. Sometimes the adhesive vaginitis is so extensive that an actual stenosis exists.

Treatment

Both senile vulvovaginitis and senile vaginitis have estrogen deficiency in their background. Lack of cleanliness and inadequate nutritional and vitamin requirements provide additional causes.

The primary treatment should be to provide estrogen locally in the form of estrin cream or suppositories in order to obtain a better vaginal epithelialization. This regimen should be carried out nightly for at least two or three weeks. Local topical treatment is better than estrogenic substances given orally, because the latter may produce uterine bleeding through their power to activate even a senile endometrium. Bleeding will not occur if the estrogen is applied locally.

In addition the diet should be placed in proper balance, and vitamins, particularly A and B complex, should be added. Perineal and vulvar hygiene should be stressed. In some instances vinegar douches (2 tablespoonfuls to a quart of water) are helpful, since they themselves promote epithelialization, tend to make the vaginal pH more acid and form a soil unfavorable for many pathogenic organisms.

Trichomonas Vaginalis and Monilial Infections

Without diabetes or antibiotic therapy, monilial infection in the elderly patient is a rather rare finding. *Trichomonas vaginalis*, on the other hand, is not uncommon, though it is found much less often than in the reproductive years. Not only is it less often encountered, but also the symptoms are appreciably less severe when it is. It can produce a considerable amount of trouble and discomfort in the obese old lady who is not particularly careful about her perineal hygiene. *Trichomonas vaginalis* then complicates the intertrigo that spreads from the vulvar area to involve the groins and inner surfaces of the upper thighs. It is perpetuated by the moisture that collects, as the skin on the obese thighs becomes apposed. Without the element of intertrigo the itching in older women is limited to the labia, vestibule and clitoris. In gross appearance the discharge from *Trichomonas* has the same bubbly green-yellow appearance that we see in other age groups. The vaginal canal is edematous and appears hyperemic. The typical granular, strawberry-like areas are spotted throughout the epithelium.

The diagnosis is made by finding the typical motile protozoa in the wet vaginal smear.

The *treatment* is the same as that outlined for *Trichomonas* in the twenty-to-thirty age section. It is particularly important to incorporate vaginal douches of vinegar or lactic acid in the therapeutic program, for fungicides will destroy the protozoa, but do nothing to restore the normal acidity of the vagina.

CERVICAL LESIONS

What Gynecologic Conditions Appear in the Senile Cervix?

The same physiologic changes noted in the vulva and vagina take place in the aging cervix. As part of the general atrophy that goes on in the cervix, the muscle fibers tend to disappear, to be replaced by connective tissue. As in the vaginal epithelium, the vascular supply is restricted by an obliteration of many of the small vessels. Many may show hyaline degeneration in the walls. They are less prominent both in number and in caliber of lumen.

In addition, the epithelium of the endocervix shows the same atrophic change. The epithelium thins and flattens out, and the occasional cilia are no longer present in the cells of the glands within the lower uterine segment. As a result normal secretions, though less in quantity, become trapped in the glands as their ducts seal over. It is not uncommon then to find many so-called nabothian cysts. If the process goes far enough, an actual stenosis of the endocervical canal takes place. Since secretory

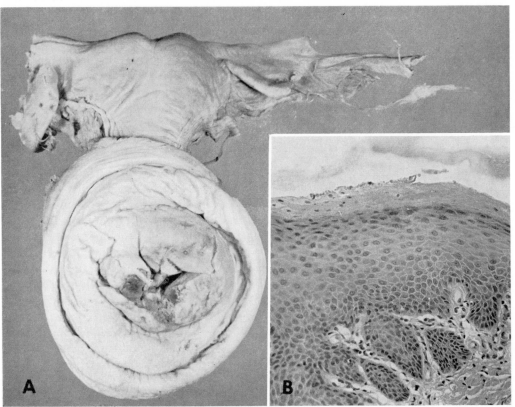

Fig. 73-2.   *A*, Exceedingly hypertrophied and eroded cervix and atrophic uterine fundus, from an aged woman. The hypertrophy is not exaggerated particularly by the perspective. *B*, The cervix in procidentia develops hyperkeratosis and epithelial hyperplasia due to frictional trauma, as well as erosions and ulcerations.

activity is at a minimum, this can happen without setting up any particular problem. It can, however, lead to the development of a pyometra when secretions are trapped in the endometrial cavity.

One of the most dangerous symptoms in older women is irregular vaginal bleeding or spotting, mixed with varying amounts of discharge or occurring without it. It can be due to senile vaginitis or to *Trichomonas vaginalis*, but the physician should keep constantly in mind that cancer of the cervix can occur in both the portio and endocervix of older women. Vaginal smears, a Schiller test involving Lugol's solution to stain the cervix, and biopsy of both the external portions and endocervical canal are indicated. It is also important to remember that such spotting may be due to a cancer of the endometrium. If results of the cervical smears and biopsies are negative, a curettage is indicated. A *pyometra* may have a benign cause and be due to simple atresia of the cervical canal, but all too frequently pyometra and endometrial cancer are found together.

The cervix occasionally contains benign polyps in this age group, which may or may not produce bleeding. Occasionally the cervix becomes hypertrophied and inflamed (Fig. 73–2, *A*). A hypertrophied cervix may be badly eroded and often ulcerated when it is the presenting portion of a complete procidentia (Fig. 73–2, *B*). Actually, this will not clear up until the prolapse is corrected, through a pelvic floor repair, pessary support or hysterectomy. The important factor to remember is that such an ulcerated cervix can occasionally be cancerous. For some reason it is far less likely than one might think to be carcinoma, but nevertheless Diaz Bazan and others have collected a number of cases in which cervical cancer has been found with a procidentia (see Chap. 61).

UTERINE LESIONS

What Geriatric Problems Arise in an Aging Uterus?

In the section on problems that arise directly after the menopause we have discussed the symptoms and physical findings of carcinoma of the endometrium and the mixed mesodermal tumors of the uterus. Any unexplained bleeding vaginally, however small in amount or infrequent in appearance, can be due to either uterine carcinoma or sarcoma. The bleeding in this age group can come from a benign endometrial polyp or senile endometritis or at times be without a pathologic explanation, but the most obvious as well as the most probable cause is cancer. Among the gynecologic problems of older patients there is always a high incidence of neoplasms, both benign and malignant.

It is also well to keep in mind that a benign fibroid tumor can cause problems in the older woman. The statement is often made that one need not worry about fibroids in the postmenopausal period, because they will atrophy once ovarian hormonal function ceases. To be sure, some retrogressive changes go on in the uterus just as they do in the rest of the genital tract. The uterine musculature thins out as smooth muscle atrophies and is replaced by fibrous tissue. The vascularity diminishes. The epithelium of the endometrial cavity loses many of its glands, and much of the stromal component disappears (Fig. 73–3). It is interesting, however, that endometrium never really loses its capacity to respond to estrogenic stimulation. One must keep this in mind when giving estrogenic substances, orally or parenterally, for what-

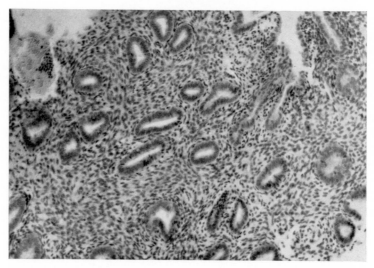

Fig. 73-3.   In endometrial atrophy the glands and stroma shrink, and no mitotic activity is found.

ever cause. A fibroid therefore may well regress to a certain extent, but it is also a well documented fact that fibroids in old ladies are prone to undergo degenerative changes, probably because of their diminished blood supply. It is unwise to assume that the vaginal bleeding of an elderly woman is due to the presence of a fibroid. Far more likely, the fibroid masks the presence of a coexistent carcinoma in the endometrium. A curettage is indicated, because a negative vaginal smear means little.

GENITAL PROLAPSE

What about Genital Prolapse in the Geriatric Patient?

The most common cause for a gynecologic complaint in the elderly woman is pelvic floor prolapse. In most instances the bladder, uterus and rectum have all descended, but occasionally a cystocele or rectocele appears separately. Less frequently the entire cul-de-sac descends, and an enterocele is noted.

The cause for the failure of pelvic-floor support can be traced back to the time of childbirth, for the original damage was done at that time. There may be no obvious evidence of it at the time of delivery, or in subsequent years, so long as the hormonal function continues to be active. As the patient enters the menopause and grows older, the muscular and ligamentous supports weaken, and the uterus begins to sag, carrying the bladder and rectum downward with it. The vaginal hernia may give little in the way of symptoms during reproductive years, but later on the patient begins to complain of a dragging sensation, pulling or a sense that everything is dropping out. She is apt to have a low chronic backache and a feeling of heaviness in her pelvis. Subsequently the bladder or bowel may fail to function properly, since both are implicated when the prolapse is at all extensive. The patient has recurring bouts of cystitis and increasing constipation.

It is amazing how patiently some women will put up with complaints of this sort. No man would permit himself to have these symptoms for long, but apparently some women expect to feel poorly and regard this as part of woman's lot in this world.

Once established, however, the symptoms get worse, because the condition is both irreversible and progressive. Eventually the elderly woman presents herself for relief simply because she cannot stand a prolapse any longer. Some women continue through life with a complete procidentia, perhaps through fear of hospitalization or surgery, or perhaps because they have learned to live with the problem.

What about Prolapse and the Urinary Problem?

In almost every instance any real descent of the uterus is accompanied by a cystocele as well. As a result of the bladder prolapse the patient has great difficulty in completely evacuating the bladder contents. Thus she carries a residual urine which is apt to become infected. Contributing factors are the atrophic changes that occur in the bladder musculature, just as they do in all organs at different phases of the aging process. Despite frequent attempts at voiding, based on the sense of urgency due to the reduced bladder capacity, the patient is still unable to eliminate all the urine the bladder holds, because of the altered anatomic state that exists when a genital prolapse is present. A chronic cystitis develops when the stagnant urine in the bladder becomes infected, and it is difficult to cure until the anatomic landmarks are restored.

There are variable degrees of prolapse, as we have noted in more detailed discussions in the previous section (Chap. 63). If the patient has a simple urethrocele or prolapse of the bladder neck, she may have stress incontinence and no residual urine. True stress incontinence is rare in the presence of a cystocele or procidentia. Thus, when the patient has an obvious prolapse of the uterus and bladder, and has symptoms which suggest stress incontinence, the differentiation should be made between simple *overflow* or *urgency incontinence* and true stress incontinence. This is important, for the corrective measures used are different.

What Can Be Done for Uterine, Bladder and Rectal Prolapses?

The best way to avoid these troublesome gynecologic complaints in the older woman is to perform better and less traumatic obstetrics in the reproductive years. Since obstetrical techniques have improved in the last thirty years, the problem of dealing with genital and bladder prolapse may be a diminishing one. It is here for those of us who are practicing medicine now.

Since the elderly patient has tolerated her disordered anatomic state for a considerable time before she consults the physician, it is obvious that she is now seriously troubled. Some part of the reason for delaying her visit may come from fears as to what may be necessary to provide correction. If she can avoid surgery, she will do everything in her power to do so. For this reason the too sympathetic surgeon may elect to use mechanical supporting devices of various sorts, including the old-fashioned rubber doughnut pessary, in lieu of surgery. This form of therapy will please the old lady, but it does not always provide the answer to her problem.

In the first place, uterine prolapse accompanied by relaxation of the muscular support to the bladder is a progressive, not a static, condition. A prolapse may be held in place by a pessary with relief of symptoms for a few years, but if the patient lives on, there will usually come a time when the mechanical contrivance fails to provide adequate support. The patient, now several years older and no better able to stand an operation, may still have to undergo surgery to obtain relief. In addition, since the pessary exerts continued pressure against the thin vaginal epithelium, ulcerated areas may develop and become infected, despite the fact that the patient is instructed to return for cleansing and replacement of the device at six-week intervals. With their symptoms relieved, many older women will either neglect themselves or not take the trouble to douche regularly to keep the vagina clean. They also frequently fail to return on schedule. Furthermore, some of the pessaries made today are of plastic construction. Not only are certain women allergic to any foreign body in the vagina, but also they are particularly sensitive to a plastic type of pessary.

The pessary does have a place in therapy, but only in the patient who has such severe medical complications that surgery of any sort is contraindicated.

At the end of this section we shall discuss the changing concept toward surgery in the aged, with special reference to the geriatric problems. Unless the medical contraindications are valid, as well as pronounced, or unless the patient is totally unwilling to undergo surgery, there is no place for the pessary as a permanent form of treatment for genital prolapse in the medicine of today.

OTHER UROLOGIC COMPLAINTS

Although women in all age groups are frequently harassed by complaints referable to their urinary bladder, even the mildest form of urethritis is apt to produce an exaggerated train of symptoms in the elderly woman. In many instances little in the way of disease can be demonstrated. The annoyance and degree of disability far exceed the magnitude of the physical findings.

History

The patient may complain of frequency, burning, urgency, pressure, hematuria, inability to eliminate completely and finally urinary incontinence. Before any attempt can be made to track down the cause of the complaint, the physician must have the time and above all the patience to obtain a detailed history.

It will do no good to accept the older patient's casual recounting of her symptoms, for she will frequently hide her true feelings because of fear of the consequences. The elderly patient is prone to minimize her symptoms before operation and to exaggerate them afterward. To this end the family should be questioned, for the urologic pattern of the elderly female is apt to be well known to the rest of the family.

Flint has outlined a few points that should be sought in the history and physical examination of an elderly woman with urologic complaints:

1. How much urine does the patient eliminate with each voiding? A true polyuria accompanied by polydipsia may suggest the presence of unsuspected diabetes mellitus. On the other hand, a nocturnal type of polyuria may well be due to the fact that the arteriosclerotic kidney does not know the difference between day and night. This is not true of the normal kidney, which seemingly automatically makes the necessary adjustments.

2. As far as possible, the true source of any bleeding should be checked. It is important to know whether it is coming from the urethra or bladder, or whether it has origin in the vagina. It will be unwise to assume, for example, that the bleeding is due to a urethral caruncle when the true source is in the endometrium.

3. If the patient has urinary incontinence, what is its nature?

(a) If it is a continuous dribble, overflow incontinence should be suspected.

(b) Urgency incontinence suggests bladder infection.

(c) A true stress incontinence points to loss of sphincter control.

(d) An intermittent involuntary loss often has a neurogenic background, either central or local.

(e) On physical examination the physician should pay attention to the patient's gait, because it may indicate the presence of a neurologic lesion.

(f) Before outlining any therapy, whatever the abnormality, it is important to evaluate the patient's mental competence. Will she tolerate any appliance that may be needed, even though she is mentally alert and intelligent enough to wear it?

(g) What is the patient's general condition, as judged by the state of her nutrition, her pulmonary capacity and her cardiac status? The tone of the skin and the color of her mucous membranes will give some indication of her nutritional state, and her breathing and the appearance of her extremities aid in estimating the pulmonary and cardiovascular situations.

(h) A palpable bladder in the absence of symptoms points to the possibility that the cause may be neurogenic, or possibly such systemic diseases as diabetes or pernicious anemia.

Chronic Urethritis and Vesical Neck Obstruction

These two entities, which frequently go hand-in-hand, account for many of the urologic complaints in elderly women. They are often seen in patients who have senile vaginitis as well. It is therefore fair to assume that the underlying defect can be traced to a hormonal deficiency.

It is surprising that the normal woman can hold as much urine for as long as she does. Despite the relatively short female urethra, women can hold as much as 500 cc. in the upright position. The urethra, surrounded as it is by numerous glands, can be rather easily infected with low-grade pathogenic organisms. Even a minor degree of low-grade infection will often give rise to severe symptoms and at times to a loss of control of micturition. The catheter specimen of urine may be microscopically negative.

Mild forms of urethritis are common in postmenopausal women and more elderly females, for the simple reason that estrogen lack has allowed changes in the urethral epithelium and that of the bladder trigone, just as it has in the vagina, vulva and the rest of the genital tract.

Because of connective tissue and epithelial atrophy in the vaginal epithelium, the vaginal canal becomes not only narrow, but also short. Foreshortening carries the external meatus of the urethra back along the roof of the vagina. Sometimes it is even hard to find. If attempts are made to catheterize the urethra with the patient in the usual position, the catheter has to be pushed almost vertically up toward the symphysis before it can finally pass along the rest of the urethra into the bladder.

Fortunately, even the elderly woman tolerates cystoscopy fairly readily. It should be kept in mind that, though the normal urethra can be distended to a size no. 28 French dilator with ease, the atrophied old-age urethra will not tolerate a size much greater than a no. 14 French, particularly if there is even a mild degree of urethritis present. The atrophic, often inflamed trigone of the bladder can be readily seen by cystoscopy, and the extent of residual urine determined. The degree of trabeculation should be recorded, and the urologist may wish to do a cystometrogram at the same

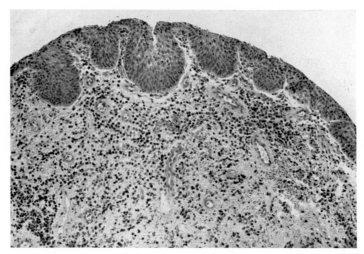

Fig. 73-4.   Chronic urethritis with caruncle formation is characteristically associated with a thin epithelial layer beneath which is vascular granulation tissue containing abundant leukocytes, including lymphocytes and plasma cells. True caruncles are painful; ectropions are not.

time to determine the tone of the bladder musculature. On withdrawing the cystoscope the extent of atrophy of the urethral mucous membrane should be noted. The urine should be cultured and its specific gravity determined. If it is below 1.010, for example, this may point to a diminished renal reserve.

That the urethra in its atrophic state is actually often chronically infected can be proved by biopsy. Microscopic sections will show a thin epithelium with infiltration of lymphocytes in the supporting stroma, which also shows evidence of atrophy (Fig. 73-4). This condition can be reversed by administering estrogen orally or by the insertion of estrogen suppositories in the urethra. After a month of therapy the urethral mucous membrane resembles that of a woman in her reproductive years, and all evidence of chronic infection has gone. *Urethral caruncles* are also said to vanish.

What Is the Treatment of Chronic Urethritis and Vesical Neck Obstruction?

With the diagnosis established, this distressing problem in elderly women can be met simply by (*a*) giving estrogen in the form of urethral suppositories, or orally if desired, for several months and periodically thereafter. There will be less chance of activating the endometrium if hormone is given locally. (*b*) Gently dilating the urethral canal and bladder neck at weekly intervals. This should not be carried higher than a no. 25 French. The effect can be increased at times by irrigating the bladder with a mild silver proteinate solution (or 1:5000 silver nitrate). (*c*) If there is an element of stress incontinence, it will be well to encourage the patient to practice starting and stopping the urinary stream. The muscle-setting exercises of Kegel (Chap. 63) should also be used.

MASSES IN THE EXTERNAL GENITALIA, ABDOMEN AND BREAST

One of the most common complaints that bring the older woman to the physician is the discovery of a mass in the vulva, vagina, abdomen or breast. In many instances the mass has no pathologic significance, but in others it is extremely important. In no case can it be dismissed without adequate investigation, simply because the patient is elderly. If the lesion proves to be benign, the older patient will need a great deal of reassurance, since most have a mortal fear of cancer.

VULVA AND VAGINA

In previous discussions we stressed the need for particular attention when any lump or ulceration appears in the area of the vulva and vagina. Cancer of the vulva can have a poor prognosis, not because of its life history or difficulties in carrying out adequate definitive treatment, but mainly because there has been such a delay between the time of cancer initiation and when the patient first presents herself for care. Unfortunately, elderly patients become more alarmed by the finding of a bulging mass in the vagina, which is in all probability simply a cystocele, than by any ulcerating lesion or small lump in the vulva.

If our educational propaganda about cancer can finally penetrate far enough to reach the older female members of the family and convince them that they should seek advice from a physician when they note vaginal bleeding of any sort, whatever the amount, much will be accomplished. The older a patient gets, the greater the chance of malignant disease. Since more people are living until an age when they may become candidates to acquire cancer, the best chances we have of reducing the continually increasing death rate from malignant disease are (a) prevention and (b) early recognition and treatment. The problem centers sharply on the reproductive tract of women, since the greatest number of cancer deaths in women come from cancer of the breast and female genitalia.

ABDOMINAL TUMOR

Benign as well as malignant tumors occur in the elderly woman. It is unwise to assume that an abdominal tumor mass is malignant simply because it occurs in an older woman, but it is equally wrong to proceed as though it were benign. The final diagnosis cannot be made until abdominal exploration is performed and the tumor and its contents are inspected and biopsied.

We pointed out in the section on Ovarian Tumors that there is no aspect of the neoplasm's life history, tumor pattern of growth, patient's history or physical findings that will permit accurate preoperative differentiation of a benign from a malignant tumor in its early stages, when surgical treatment is most rewarding. It was noted that the more solid the tumor, the greater the chance of cancer. There is a double reason, then, for operating on an elderly woman who has an eccentrically placed adnexal tumor, whether the site of its apparent origin be uterus, tube or ovary, because neither the point of tumor origin nor its true pathologic nature can be determined without abdominal surgical exploration.

Carcinoma of the ovary is on the increase, and since it commonly is discovered in postmenopausal patients, we may expect to run into the problem more often in the future. The end-results in the more advanced stages of the disease are extremely poor. Our sole chance of having the patient survive for a long time in peace and comfort is to achieve early complete operative removal. We should not deny the patient a chance to live simply because (a) there is a chance that the tumor may be benign, and (*b*) the patient may not survive the operation. Age in itself is no contraindication.

An operation was performed recently on a patient with known cancer metastases in the chest because life was unbearable, owing to the pressure of a huge ovarian tumor against the stomach, intestines, liver and diaphragm. The aim was not to prolong life, but to make the patient more comfortable.

A considerable amount of surgical judgment is needed in making a decision for or against operation. The physician may elect to use other means of cancer therapy such as x-ray or the newer alkylating or antimetabolic agents. By and large, however, surgery offers the greatest chance in the older patient. With proper preoperative preparation and postoperative care, surgery—even intra-abdominal procedures—can be done far more often than we ever believed in the past. This problem will be further discussed subsequently.

Other sites than ovary, uterus or tube may give rise to abdominal tumors. Some may be benign, and not all are neoplastic. For example, a centrally placed mass in the midline that rises above the pubic symphysis and can be palpated without pain may simply be a large, distended bladder in an older patient who has a vesical neck obstruction. A fixed cystic mass in the adnexal area may be the residuum of a long-standing pelvic infection. If a mass occupies a flank position, the point of origin may be the kidney rather than uterus or adnexa. The most likely urologic causes of a mass are hydronephrosis, due to a staghorn calculus; an abscess of the kidney, usually with obstruction and nephrolithiasis; a renal cyst; and finally a neoplasm. Renal cysts and cancers account for about 15 per cent of all masses that arise in the flank of a woman over the age of 70 years.

The mass could have a retroperitoneal origin or arise from a müllerian duct rest. Such a mass can encroach on bladder or rectum, causing alterations in the function of both. A huge carcinoma can sometimes arise in a Gaertner's duct remnant. Several such tumors have been operated on in elderly women, with both long-time survival and relief of symptoms.

Brunschwig has repeatedly stressed that age itself is not as important as the cardiovascular-renal component in the individual patient. Major surgical procedures are well tolerated by elderly patients when no serious degenerative factor is present. Generally, the patient who has survived to the age of seventy years and beyond is made of sterner stuff than her sisters who died earlier. The important thing to remember is that, once the patient has been thoroughly evaluated as to her general condition, the surgeon should perform whatever operation is necessary and not do a lesser procedure simply because the patient is in the older age group.

Statistically, the mortality figures from extensive surgical procedures are approximately the same for patients in the sixty- to seventy-year group as they are in the fifty- to sixty-year-old patients. The decision must be made on an individual basis, and if it favors operation, the surgeon should go all out or not operate at all.

BREAST PROBLEMS

Breasts, like all other organs in the reproductive tract, tend to undergo atrophy when the stimulus of the various hormones is either entirely withdrawn or goes into decline. Directly after the menopause there seems to be an increased deposit of subcutaneous fat, but as the patient progresses into more advanced age this resorbs, and the breast becomes loose and flabby, with wrinkled skin and a pronounced tendency to droop. If the breasts were large to begin with, the patient may have intertrigo or superficial dermatitis in the submammary fold where skin is apposed to skin, should she not be careful enough about keeping the skin cool, dry and clean. If any eczematous eruption appears in the nipple area, Paget's disease should be immediately considered, particularly if the superficial epithelial ulcerations do not heal under simple therapy or break out again after they have epithelialized. Too frequently such lesions are disregarded as benign dermatologic entities.

Carcinoma of the breast is common in women past the age of sixty years and not uncommon after the age of seventy years. In some statistical reports 40 per cent occurred after the age of 60 years and 18 per cent beyond the age of 70 years. One patient was ninety-one years of age, with an estrogen effect in her vaginal smear and a large carcinoma of the breast. Her reaction to radical mastectomy did not differ from that of women many years younger.

Despite the suggestion of hormone dependence in this particular case, by and large patients beyond the age of sixty-five years do not have much indication of ovarian activity. There is considerable evidence that, even though the patient is postmenopausal, ovarian activity may continue in some, but not all, older women until they are well into their sixties. In the age group under discussion we must assume that a carcinoma of the breast is not being activated by hormonal action. It is rather difficult to prove, but the impression is general that cancer of the breast in older women grows at a more leisurely pace than is true of the younger women.

Since cancer incidence is high in the elderly patient and confusing elements such as mammary cystic disease and adenofibrosis are less often found, any mass in the breast should be regarded with grave suspicion. The means of establishing a diagnosis are no different in this age group, and the various procedures have been previously outlined (Chap. 57).

To repeat, age should not be the sole factor in deciding for or against a breast operation or in dictating the kind of operation to be performed. If the patient is in good condition, so far as her pulmonary and cardiovascular status is concerned, she should have the usual radical mastectomy and axillary lymph node dissection. On the other hand, if the condition is doubtful or borderline, the surgeon may elect to do a simple amputation and irradiate the axilla after the manner of McWhirter. When the cancer is more advanced, as it may be in the older woman because she has chosen not to recognize that a mass is present, there may sometimes be a place for a simple breast amputation, particularly if the tumor is necrotic, ulcerated and bleeding.

Chemotherapy and x-ray treatment have their place in the treatment of recurrent or advanced breast cancer. Although there is only a slight chance that the tumor may be hormone-dependent, individual variations are such that treatment of this sort is justifiable. We have seen a mass appear on the chest wall twenty-five years after a radical mastectomy. Despite the fact that this patient was 83 years old at the time of the cancer recurrence, she was given 15 mg. of stilbestrol daily by mouth for several months. The tumor completely disappeared and remained healed until she died three years later.

Thus we have radical mastectomy with axillary lymph node dissection to offer the elderly patient who has cancer confined to her breast and axilla. If she is less than a good surgical risk, she can have either a simple mastectomy plus irradiation, or solely chemotherapy or irradiation. When cancer recurrences appear or distant metastases are present, chemotherapy or x-radiation is a helpful adjunct in palliation.

THE CHANGING ATTITUDE TOWARD SURGERY
IN THE GERIATRIC PATIENT

Since more of the population are surviving to the age of sixty-five years and over, we speak nowadays in terms of an increased life expectancy. This does not provide a true picture, because the improvement has chiefly been noted in infant mortality. Nevertheless modern medicine, through the use of such drugs as digitalis, insulin, antibiotics, hormones and antihypertensive medications, now assists the aging patient to live not only longer, but also more comfortably. If simple survival were the only factor, little would be gained. The primary aim in treating elderly patients should be to try to prolong a useful functional life and to avoid the pitfall of being overenthusiastic in attempts to delay the natural processes of deterioration.

We cannot restore youth, but we can teach the patient how to live by adjusting her physical and emotional strains to the capacity of the organs she has. There is no reason why the aging patient cannot live a useful, happy and productive life. In too many instances the patient is encouraged to think that she is no longer needed and is therefore a burden. No woman, whatever her age, wants to think she is old, but she is apt to have the feeling thrust upon her. In recent years there have been more concentrated efforts at all levels from the government to the family to see that the older members lead more productive and happy existences.

What Is the Attitude toward Surgery?

One has only to tour the wards of any general hospital to realize that an increasingly high percentage of the patients there are in the old-age group. It has been estimated that at least 5 per cent of all hospitalized persons are in the geriatric phase of life. This is not due entirely to the fact that more patients are alive in the old-age groups, in which the processes of deterioration require correction of functional and anatomic defects. In the past older women patients had the same problems, but either they refused to be hospitalized or they were never offered a curative procedure, because it was believed to be poor medical judgment to attempt to treat the patient other than symptomatically when the expected duration of life was limited. Patients are now beginning to realize that a hospital entry is not tantamount to a death sentence and that they need not put up with an ailment that could be corrected, for example, by surgical measures. It seems much more reasonable to submit to an operation if the expectancy of life at the age of seventy is ten years; at eighty, five to eight years; or at ninety, three years. The older woman may not wish to put up with a deformity that can be corrected, if this is going to persist for so long.

It is, therefore, completely justifiable to offer surgery or other definitive types of therapy to patients in the old age group, provided there are no serious defects in the cardiovascular, pulmonary or renal systems. Furthermore, when proper attention has been given to the preoperative evaluation and the decision for surgery has been made, the surgeon need not settle for a palliative procedure when a more extensive operation will cure. In the past surgeons had a tendency to compromise on the magnitude of the operation because, often without adequate cause, they felt that older patients could not possibly stand a rigorous surgical attack on the problem. As Lash points out, in the present day older patients who have had adequate preoperative care can be cured by a type of surgery that is tailored to the disease and not the age of the patient. With good postoperative care such patients can resume their normal position in society and be happy in so doing.

What Is the Nature of the Preoperative Workup?

The preoperative surgical evaluation in the older patient does not differ from that of a patient in any other age group. It is, however, more important.

There is no question that in this age group there is a higher concentration of such degenerative diseases as diabetes, hypertension, arteriosclerosis, myocardial damage, emphysema, asthma, bronchiectasis and particularly renal disease. In all probability, renal function is the most important single factor that must be thoroughly evaluated before any operation is undertaken, whatever is planned. The necessary laboratory tests are well known and will not be elaborated upon. Perhaps the simplest of all is a close scrutiny of the urine specific gravity. If it is consistently below 1.010, the surgeon should strongly suspect a serious impairment of kidney function.

The mere fact that a patient has hypertension, however, need not deter the surgeon from performing needful surgery. Approximately 80 per cent of patients in this age group will have a systolic pressure over 140 mm. of mercury, and in 40 per cent it will exceed 170. Obviously the choice of anesthesia will be an important factor in a patient who has hypertension, just as it is when the patient has emphysema or bronchiectasis. An estimate of the cardiac reserve is also naturally a primary requisite. The patient with but minimal cardiac damage can weather the necessary surgery without too much risk. Approximately 4 per cent with severe coronary disease may fail to survive an operation or may succumb in the postoperative period. The surgeon must then balance the seriousness and the degree of incapacity produced by the condition for which he is doing the surgery against the probable risk.

There is an additional factor, which is often either not considered at all or is minimized, that has an important bearing on successful surgery in the aged, namely, the nutritional state. Surgeons have always been wary of operating on the pale, fat, flabby patient, because experience has taught them that such patients do not do very well; however, too frequently the underlying condition is suspected, but not treated. In all probability such a patient is in a serious state of malnutrition. As we noted earlier, the elderly patient is often indifferent to food. If she is depressed, feels that no one cares what happens to her, has little purpose in life, or even any great desire to live, she may well neglect the essential food and vitamin intake requirements to such an extent that she is a poor candidate for any stressful situation, especially surgery.

In a normal nutritional state the older patient has more resistance to infection than her younger sisters, but all this is lost if the dietary requirements are inadequate. The malnourished older patient heals less well, can less readily cope with infection and is less resilient in her response to shock. Before any operation is undertaken in an elective situation, drastic steps should be made to eliminate all septic foci so far as possible and to restore excessive nitrogen loss through adequate protein and vitamin replacements. Undoubtedly the impaired nutritional state has been of long standing, and the physician cannot be expected to restore the balance in a hurry.

Because the liver in malnutrition loses some of its power to synthesize proteins, it will take approximately 750 gm. of protein in the diet to increase the serum albumin by 1 gm. per 100 ml. One of the best and quickest methods of raising the total serum protein is to give blood by transfusions, to the extent of 40 ml. for each pound of weight lost. When surgery is not of an emergency nature, the surgeon will be well advised to postpone it while he attempts in a more leisurely way to establish a normal state of nutrition, such as by giving the essential amino acids with a high-protein diet at the level of 2 gm. of protein daily for each kilogram of body weight.

Finally, before performing actual operations the surgeon should make an all-out effort to comfort the patient that the anticipation of an operation is actually worse than the ordeal of going through it. Much can be accomplished by reassurance. Many patients are frightened by the prospect of surgery and are inclined to be suspicious of the surgeon. They are also apt to be a bit stubborn. The surgeon can do much to restore their confidence by talking over their problem frankly and convincing them that not only can they cope with the surgery, but also that everyone concerned is depending on them and wants them to get well.

What Are the Criteria for Advising Surgery?

The conditions for which surgery is being considered tend to fall into these groups: (1) Surgery is definitely indicated; (2) operations are justifiable, if the medical complications are either manageable or correctable; and (3) surgical procedures are obviously ill advised.

Before suggesting an operation to the patient or her family, the surgeon will do well to consider the following points:

1. Taking into full consideration the patient's physical condition, does she have a chance of equaling or exceeding the life expectancy for her age?

2. If the condition for which surgery is being considered does not jeopardize her chance of survival, does it produce a train of symptoms that make life an intolerable burden?

3. If the situation is for the moment devoid of symptoms, is it progressive and will it necessitate surgery later?

4. If the patient has two problems, such as hypertension and procidentia, is she so uncomfortable and miserable from the procidentia, which certainly is not life-endangering, that the hypertension—which is serious—is made worse?

5. If the functional, pathologic or anatomic condition is apt to continue and to become worse, are the economic or home conditions such that the family can cope with the unresolved problem if surgery is not done?

6. Has the patient the necessary mental alertness and adaptability to contend with any altered physiologic state that may result from the surgery, such as a colostomy or ileal bladder?

Summary

A gynecologic problem in a geriatric patient can be corrected by surgery with only moderate risk, provided the preoperative evaluation, preparation and the postoperative care are well considered and administered. The choice of any operation necessary should not be made on the basis of chronologic age, but on an estimate of the physiologic condition of the individual patient. If these factors are properly balanced, the physician and the surgeon can carry the patient safely through an essential definitive operation with far greater anticipation of success than either the physicians, the patient or the family may believe. The important objective is for all three to have equal confidence that this can be accomplished.

REFERENCES

Adair, F. L.: Geriatric Gynecology; in E. J. Stieglitz, ed.: *Geriatric Medicine*. Philadelphia, W. B. Saunders Company, 1943, p. 750.

Blumenstock, D. A., and Mithoefer, J.: Studies of the Aged: Selection of Elderly Patients for Major Surgical Operations. *J. Am. Geriatric Soc.*, 4: 781, 1956.

Brunschwig, A.: Age of Patients in Relation to Radical Cancer Surgery. *Geriatrics*, 11: 367, 1956.

Cauter, F. B., and Jones, C. P.: A Study of the Vaginal Flora in Normal Female. *South. M.J.*, 30: 298, 1937.

Davis, D. M.: Vesical Orifice Obstruction in Women and Its Treatment by Transurethral Resection. *J. Urol.*, 73: 112, 1955.

Diaz Bazan, N.: Cancer del cuello uterino associado con prolapso total en El Salvador. Revision de la literatura y reporte complementario de 25 cases. Extrait du Deuxième Congrès International de Gynecologie et d'Obstetrique de Montrèal en 1958, 1: 226, 1958.

Flint, L. D.: Some Aspects of Geriatric Urology. *S. Clin. N. Amer.*, 31: 697, 1951.

Gilchrist, R. K., and de Peyster, F. A.: Principles and Safeguards in Abdominal Surgery of the Aged. *J.A.M.A.*, 160: 1375, 1956.

Haug, C. A., and Dale, W. A.: Major Surgery in Old People. A.M.A. *Arch. Surg.*, 64: 421, 1952.

Hock, E. F.: Vesical Neck Obstruction in the Female: Etiology and Treatment. *J. Urol.*, 72: 657, 1954.

Hosbein, D. J., and Mithoefer, J.: The Treatment of Elderly Women with Cancer of the Breast. *S. Clin. N. Amer.*, 40: 889, 1960.

Hutchins, S. P. R.: Vesical Neck Obstruction in Women. *J. Urol.*, 69: 102, 1953.

Korenchevsky, V.: Effects of Sex and Thyroid Hormones on Process of Ageing in Female Rats. *Brit. M.J.*, 1: 728, 1948.

Kosmak, G. W.: Gynecologic and Other Implications Which Relate to an Ageing Female Population. *Am. J. Obst. & Gynec.*, 44: 897, 1942.

Lash, A. F.: Surgical Geriatric Gynecology. *Am. J. Obst. & Gynec.*, 53: 766, 1947.

Maycock, P. P., and Burns, C. N.: Vesical Neck Obstruction in Women. *Geriatrics*, 11: 79, 1956.

Mithoefer, J.: The Selection and Preparation of Elderly Patients for Operation. *S. Clin. N. Amer.*, 40: 871, 1960.

Monroe, R. T.: Medical Progress: The Effect of Aging of Population on General Health Problems. *New England J. Med.*, 249: 277, 1953.

Parker, R. T., Jones, C. P., and Carter, F. B.: Pruritus Vulvae in the Postclimacteric Woman. *Geriatrics*, 11: 235, 1956.

Pettit, M. D.: Gynecological Conditions Found in Older Women. *Geriatrics*, 4: 353, 1949.

Powers, J. H.: Geriatric Trends in Surgery. *S. Clin. N. Amer.*, 40: 865, 1960.

Pratt, J. H.: Gynecologic Surgery in the Geriatric Patient. *J. Arkansas M. Soc.*, 52: 173, 1956.

Index

1197